Noninvasive Vascular Diagnosis

Second Edition

Ali F. AbuRahma and John J. Bergan, Eds.

Noninvasive Vascular Diagnosis

A Practical Guide to Therapy

Second Edition

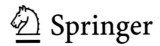 Springer

Ali F. AbuRahma, MD, FACS, FRCS, RVT, RPVI
Professor
Chief, Vascular/Endovascular Surgery
Department of Surgery
Robert C. Byrd Health Sciences Center
West Virginia University
and
Medical Director, Vascular Laboratory
Co-Director, Vascular Center of Excellence
Charleston Area Medical Center
Charleston, WV, USA

John J. Bergan, MD, FACS, Hon FRCS
UCSD School of Medicine
La Jolla, CA
USA

British Library Cataloguing in Publication Data
Noninvasive vascular diagnosis : a practical guide to therapy. – 2nd ed.
  1. Blood-vessels – Diseases – Diagnosis 2. Diagnosis, Noninvasive
  I. AbuRahma, Ali F. II. Bergan, John J., 1927–616.1'3'0754
ISBN-13: 9781846284465
ISBN-10: 1846284465

Library of Congress Control Number: 2006924879

ISBN-10: 1-84628-446-5 2nd edition   e-ISBN 1-84628-450-3 2nd edition   Printed on acid-free paper
ISBN-13: 978-1-84628-446-5 2nd edition
ISBN 1-85233-128-3 1st edition

9 8 7 6 5 4 3 2 1

Springer Science+Business Media
springer.com

To my loving children,
Zachary, Chelsea, and Joseph,
for their patience and support
during the preparation of this book.
Ali F. AbuRahma

I join in that dedication because of my admiration for
Ali and his splendid family.
John Bergan

Foreword to the Second Edition

Rapid development of sophisticated technology, as well as efforts by vascular surgeons to improve vascular care, has resulted in the widespread proliferation of vascular laboratories throughout the United States in the last three decades. Prior to that, only a handful of vascular laboratories were available, and all served as space for an academic surgeon to study peripheral circulation in humans. Early instrumentation included the use of various types of cumbersome plethysmographs. The introduction of ultrasound technology in the 1970s ushered in a new era in noninvasive diagnosis. At present, noninvasive vascular diagnostic techniques have much wider applications, and there is a need for a book on noninvasive vascular diagnosis to guide therapy. After all, effective treatment follows precise diagnosis. *Noninvasive Vascular Diagnosis: A Practical Guide to Therapy*, edited by Ali AbuRahma and John Bergan, is a welcome addition to the field of noninvasive diagnosis.

The continued refinement of duplex ultrasound technology has led to the gradual replacement of indirect tests using plethysmography in the diagnosis of deep vein thrombosis or carotid artery disease. Duplex scan is now the dominant technology in vascular laboratories, and its use has extended to the diagnosis of chronic venous insufficiency, mesenteric ischemia, and disease of the renal artery. In addition to diagnostic use, duplex ultrasound has also found use in surveillance of patency of bypass or hemodialysis grafts and following carotid endarterectomy or stent placement. It also is helpful to map saphenous veins prior to infrainguinal bypass. In addition, use of duplex scan has evolved to therapeutic applications, such as sclerotherapy for varicose veins, newer minimally invasive ablation procedures, injection of thrombin into pseudoaneurysms of the femoral artery after catheterization, and bedside placement of vena cava filter. Meanwhile, ankle systolic pressure recorded by a handheld Doppler probe, first introduced in 1969, has stood the test of time as a simple diagnostic test for arterial occlusive disease of extremities. Doppler ankle pressure is now widely used to grade degree of ischemia objectively and as a screening test for peripheral arterial disease and epidemiology study. Newer ultrasound technologies, such as transcranial Doppler, intravascular ultrasound, and 3-D ultrasound, have found new application in noninvasive vascular diagnosis.

The last three decades also have seen a rapid development of imaging technique, ushering in an era in which diagnosis and early detection of arterial and venous disease can be readily made by a host of noninvasive diagnostic techniques. High-resolution ultrasound, magnetic resonance, and CT technology have completely changed the face of imaging techniques. At present, we have many choices in imaging techniques that can be used alone or in combination to obtain the needed diagnostic information. Arteriography by CT or MR has provided images similar to those obtained by the traditional invasive contrast arteriography, thus significantly decreasing the clinical use of venography or invasive contrast arteriography.

There is no question that advancement of vascular care depends on technology. Noninvasive technology is now an important component in training of future generations of vascular surgeons. However, the widespread use of vascular laboratories calls for quality control and certification of the laboratories as well as the technologists and physicians. Technology, when used wisely, benefits the patient; when used indiscriminately, it results in waste of time, energy, and resources. The reader is advised to follow the excellent guidelines and advice put forth in this volume by the editors and the group of distinguished contributors that they have assembled.

James S.T. Yao, MD, PhD
Emeritus Professor of Surgery
Division of Vascular Surgery
Department of Surgery
Northwestern University, Feinberg School of Medicine
Chicago, Illinois

Foreword to the First Edition

This book is remarkable when compared with books concerning the vascular diagnostic laboratory of a few years ago, one of which Dr AbuRahma co-authored. At the present time, noninvasive diagnosis is dominated by duplex scanning and other imaging modalities. Physiologic studies are being down-played. This is due to the increasing dominance of the field by radiology-based laboratories. Therefore it is a pleasure to see this book which covers both imaging and physiologic studies well, and does so in a problem-oriented format.

This volume does more than that. It addresses the full gamut of vascular laboratory operations including accreditation of laboratories and their personnel; it covers the basic physics of ultrasound instrumentation; and it treats thoroughly each of the four important components of vascular laboratory accreditation: cerebrovascular, peripheral arterial, venous and abdominal studies. The book also deals with a number of special areas which are peripheral to most vascular diagnostic laboratories but are included in their operations by some – three-dimensional imaging, intravascular ultrasound, magnetic resonance angiography and Doppler flow wire to name just a few. This breadth of coverage has not been seen since the mammoth volumes of a decade ago that the late Gene Bernstein published as proceedings of his San Diego meetings. But this book differs from those volumes in that it is not a compendium of focused presentations for a meeting. It is instead a carefully organized comprehensive coverage of everything one would need to know and could expect to encounter in the most complete vascular laboratory operation conceivable. For example, the section on cerebrovascular diagnosis not only includes overviews of clinical considerations and the various techniques, it provides individual chapters on carotid duplex examination, evaluation of the proximal aortic arch vessels, examination of the vertebral arteries and even descibes use of the transcranial Doppler. This then ends up with a clinical correlation chapter that critiques these competitive techniques and discusses their relative value in specific clinical settings. The intraoperative assessment of technical adequacy of carotid endarterectomy or angioplasty is described, for example; then the survey of a patient developing neurological deficits after operation is addressed; the postoperative surveillance after endarterectomy or angioplasty is detailed; the laboratory evaluation of the trauma victim is included; and examination of the patient presenting with vertebrobasilar symptoms is explained. Each major section has a final chapter such as this which brings all the preceding information together in a practical and meaningful summary for the clinician.

As organized, this book is ideal for any physician of any specialty background, whether in training or in practice, who wants current and in-depth coverage of noninvasive vascular diagnosis from operations and administration, to credentialing, to fundamental techniques and their instrumentation or specific clinical applications in every conceivable setting.

The authors are to be commended for putting together such a comprehensive text at this time of need to hold all the components of noninvasive diagnosis together as a traditional vascular diagnostic laboratory. The reader will

benefit from their vision and from efforts of their well-selected contributing
authors.

Robert B. Rutherford, MD
Emeritus Professor of Surgery
University of Colorado

Preface

The purpose of this revision of what has become a very popular textbook is to high-light recent advances in the investigation of vascular disorders. The additions to this volume describe new methods of investigation and how they can be used to the best advantage of the patient by the physician. This volume is designed to instruct physicians on how to make a greater number of correct decisions regarding care and how to save some patients from unnecessary and expensive procedures.

Although it is nearly 200 years since John Hunter transformed vascular surgery from a terrifying craft to a positive scientific success, there have been long stagnant periods during which little progress could be seen. That is not true of the past 10 years. During this time, the noninvasive vascular laboratory has become an essential part of every general hospital. It is now a place where objective measurements can be obtained on which prognosis and treatment can be based. There is a growing sophistication of methods and new terms have emerged that are at first sight unfamiliar. This volume is designed to help guide the reader through these problems.

The rapid expansion of this field in the past several years, in terms of new modalities and new applications, justifies this second edition. A few examples of these are the role of duplex technology in carotid stenting, the diagnosis of temporal arteritis, surveillance after percutaneous transluminal angioplasty/stenting of peripheral arteries, abdominal stent grafts for abdominal aortic aneurysms, and the use of duplex ultrasound for bedside insertion of inferior vena cava filters. Interestingly, noninvasive vascular technology has spread from a very few early pioneers, mostly vascular surgeons influenced by the late Gene Strandness, to a much broader group of physicians, including neurologists, radiologists, cardiologists, and internists. An entire corps of vascular technologists has evolved. There are now vascular sonographers, a number of whom participate in the development of new and important applications of ever changing diagnostic equipment. With this in mind, this textbook is designed to be comprehensive enough to address the needs of all who are involved in vascular diagnostic technology.

A new level of maturity and technological advancement in the field of noninvasive testing has been reached and, as a result, 14 chapters of the current edition are new and 24 chapters have been radically revised. The section on cerebrovascular diagnosis includes several new chapters: Carotid Plaque Echolucency Measured by Grayscale Median (GSM) Identifies Patients at Increased Risk of Stroke during Carotid Stenting: The ICAROS Study, Duplex Ultrasound in the Diagnosis of Temporal Arteritis, Duplex Ultrasound Velocity Criteria for Carotid Stenting Patients, Use of Transcranial Doppler in Monitoring Patients during Carotid Artery Stenting, and the Use of an Angle-Independent Doppler System for Intraoperative Carotid Endarterectomy Surveillance. The section on peripheral arterial disease includes the following new chapters: Rationale and Benefits of Surveillance after Prosthetic Infrainguinal Bypass Grafts, Rationale and Benefits of Surveillance after Percutaneous Transluminal Angioplasty and Stenting of Iliac and Femoral Arteries, Duplex Ultrasound in the Diagnosis and Treatment of Femoral Pseudoaneurysms, Lower Extremity Arterial Mapping: Duplex Ultrasound as an Alternative to Arteriography Prior to Femoral and Popliteal Reconstruction, Noninvasive Diagnosis of Upper Extremity Vascular Disease, and Protocol and Technique for Dialysis Ultrasound Surveillance. The section on venous disorders includes new chapters on

Duplex Ultrasound Use for Bedside Insertion of Inferior Vena Cava Filters and Venous Stenting Using Intravascular Ultrasound (IVUS). In the section on deep abdominal Doppler, a new chapter was added on The Role of Color Duplex Ultrasound in Patients with Abdominal Aortic Aneurysms and Stent Grafts. These reflect the development of better methods and display the changing indications for use of the new technology. The earlier techniques must be placed in a proper perspective.

Several modalities are now described in this edition by new authors who were selected because of their comparative knowledge of alternative and supplementary approaches. These new contributors and their increasingly diverse backgrounds have added immeasurably to the breadth of this volume. To these contributors, the previous authors, and all of their staffs, the editors wish to express their full and most sincere appreciation. We hope that the reader will enjoy dipping into this volume as much as we have enjoyed updating it.

Ali F. AbuRahma
John J. Bergan

Acknowledgments

This book owes much to our colleagues, who have contributed a great deal to the text. Their particular interests and expertise add substance to this book. Without exception, they managed to submit intelligent and up-to-date contributions.

This volume survived thanks to the support of our technical staff, particularly Mona Lett in Charleston for transcribing and revising the various versions of the chapters and for maintaining contact with contributing authors regarding guidelines and deadlines.

Our profound appreciation goes to Maynard Chapman for producing the majority of the illustrations used in this book. We appreciate the efforts of Kimberly S. Jarrett, Chief Vascular Technologist, Vascular Laboratory, Charleston Area Medical Center, Charleston, West Virginia for her assistance in providing some of the illustrations for this book.

The Springer-Verlag publishing team and Grant Weston recognized the worth of this project. Hannah Wilson provided much invaluable support and guidance. Without the support of those named here, and many others, this edition could not have seen the light of day.

Ali F. AbuRahma
John J. Bergan

Contents

SECTION I VASCULAR LABORATORY OPERATIONS

SECTION II BASIC PHYSICS

SECTION III CEREBROVASCULAR DIAGNOSIS

SECTION VI   DEEP ABDOMINAL DOPPLER

SECTION VII   MISCELLANEOUS

Contributors

Ali F. AbuRahma, MD, FACS, FRCS, RVT, RPVI
Professor
Chief, Vascular/Endovascular Surgery
Department of Surgery
Robert C. Byrd Health Sciences Center
West Virginia University
and
Medical Director, Vascular Laboratory
Co-Director, Vascular Center of Excellence
Charleston Area Medical Center
Charleston, WV, USA

Cameron M. Akbari, MD, MBA, RVT
Senior Attending in Vascular Surgery
Director, Vascular Diagnostic Laboratory
Department of Vascular Surgery
Washington Hospital Center
Washington, DC, USA

Andrei V. Alexandrov, MD, RVT
Director
Stroke Research and Neurosonology Program
Barrow Neurological Institute
Phoenix, AZ, USA

Jose I. Almeida, MD, FACS
Medical Director
Miami Vein Center
and
Voluntary Assistant Professor of Surgery
University of Miami Miller School of Medicine
Miami, FL, USA

Clifford T. Araki, PhD, RVT
Associate Professor
Department of Medical Imaging Sciences
University of Medicine and Dentistry of New Jersey
School of Health Related Professions
Newark, NJ, USA

Paul A. Armstrong, DO
Assistant Professor
Division of Vascular and Endovascular Surgery
University of South Florida College of Medicine
Tampa, FL, USA

Enrico Ascher, MD
Vascular Institute of New York
Maimonides Medical Center
Brooklyn, NY, USA

J. Dennis Baker, MD
Chief, Vascular Surgery Section
West Los Angeles VA Medical Center
and
Professor of Surgery
David Geffen School of Medicine–UCLA
Los Angeles, CA, USA

Jeffrey L. Ballard, MD, FACS
Clinical Professor of Surgery
University of California,
Irvine School of Medicine
and
Staff Surgeon
Department of Vascular Surgery
St. Joseph Hospital
Orange, CA, USA

Dennis F. Bandyk, MD
Division of Vascular and Endovascular Surgery
University of South Florida College of Medicine
Tampa, FL, USA

Mark C. Bates, MD
Senior Scientist
Cardiovascular Research CAMC Health Education and
    Research Institute
Clinical Professor of Medicine and Surgery
Robert C. Byrd Health Sciences Center of West Virginia
    University
Charleston, WV, USA

Kirk W. Beach, PhD, MD
Research Professor
Department of Surgery
University of Washington
Seattle, Washington, USA

Phillip J. Bendick, PhD
Director of Surgical Research
Director, Peripheral Vascular Diagnostic Center
Department of Surgery
William Beaumont Hospital
Royal Oak, MI, USA

George L. Berdejo, BA, RVT, FSVU
Director, Vascular Diagnostic Laboratories
Montefiore Medical Center and Jack D. Weiler Hospitals
Vascular Laboratory
Bronx, NY, USA

John J. Bergan, MD, FACS, Hon FRCS
Professor of Surgery
UCSD School of Medicine
La Jolla, CA, USA

G.M. Biasi, MD, FACS, FRCS
Department of Surgical Sciences and Intensive Care
University of Milano-Bicocca
Vascular Surgery Unit
San Gerardo Hospital
Monza (MI), Italy

John Blebea, MD, FACS
Professor
Chief, Section of Vascular Surgery
Temple University Health Sciences Center
Philadelphia, PA, USA

Peter N. Burns
Department of Medical Biophysics and Radiology
Imaging Research
Sunnybrook Health Centre
University of Toronto
Toronto, Ontario, Canada

Ruth L. Bush, MD
Assistant Professor
Division of Vascular Surgery
and
Endovascular Therapy
Michael E. DeBakey Department of Surgery
Baylor College of Medicine
Houston, TX, USA

Keith D. Calligaro, MD
Chief, Section of Vascular Surgery
Pennsylvania Hospital
Philadelphia, PA, USA

V. Camesasca, MD
Department of Surgical Sciences and Intensive Care
University of Milano-Bicocca
Vascular Surgery Unit
San Gerardo Hospital
Monza (MI), Italy

Sandra C. Carr, MD
Department of Surgery
University of Wisconsin
Madison, WI, USA

Kathleen A. Carter, BSN, RN, RVT, FSVU
Technical Director
Vascular Laboratory
Vascular and Transplant Specilists
Virginia Beach, VA, USA

Benjamin B. Chang, MD
Associate Professor
The Vascular Group, PLLC
The Institute for Vascular Health and Disease
Albany Medical College, Albany Medical Center
   Hospital
Albany, NY, USA

R. Clement Darling III, MD
Professor
Chief, The Vascular Group, PLLC
The Institute for Vascular Health and Disease
Albany Medical College
Albany Medical Center Hospital
Albany, NY, USA

G. Deleo, MD
Department of Surgical Sciences and Intensive Care
University of Milano-Bicocca
Vascular Surgery Unit
San Gerardo Hospital
Monza (MI), Italy

Edward B. Diethrich, MD
Medical Director
Arizona Heart Hospital and Foundation
Phoenix, AZ, USA

Kevin J. Doerr, RVT
Section of Vascular Surgery
Pennsylvania Hospital
Philadelphia, PA, USA

Matthew J. Dougherty, MD
Section of Vascular Surgery
Pennsylvania Hospital
Philadelphia, PA, USA

JimBob Faulk, MD
Vascular Surgery Fellow
Department of Vascular Surgery
Vanderbilt University Medical Center
Nashville, TN, USA

William R. Flinn, MD
Department of Surgery
Division of Vascular Surgery
University of Maryland School of Medicine
Baltimore, Maryland, USA

A. Froio, MD
Department of Surgical Sciences and Intensive Care
University of Milano-Bicocca
Vascular Surgery Unit
San Gerardo Hospital
Monza (MI), Italy

Niki Georgiou, RN
Vascular Ultrasonographer/Nurse
Vascular Screening and Diagnostic Centre
Ayios Dhometios, Nicosia, Cyprus

George Geroulakos
Department of Surgery
Charing Cross Hospital
London, UK

Peter Gloviczki, MD
Division of Vascular Surgery
Mayo Clinic College of Medicine
Rochester, MN, USA

Maura Griffin, MSc (Hons), PhD
Chief Clinical Scientist
Vascular Clinic
Vascular Noninvasive Screening
and
Diagnostic Centre
London, UK

Thomas Grist, MD
Department of Radiology
University of Wisconsin
Madison, WI, USA

Esteban Henao, MD
Vascular Fellow
Division of Vascular Surgery and Endovascular Therapy
Michael E. DeBakey Department of Surgery
Baylor College of Medicine
Houston, TX, USA

Anil Hingorani, MD
Vascular Institute of New York
Maimonides Medical Center
Brooklyn, NY, USA

Robert W. Hobson II, MD
Professor
Department of Surgery and Physiology
UMDNJ-New Jersey Medical School
Newark, NJ, USA

Khalid Irshad, FRCS
Consultant Vascular and Endovascular Surgeon
King Edward Medical College
Lahore, Pakistan

Kimberly S. Jarrett, RVT
Technical Director, Vascular Laboratory
Department of Surgery
Charleston Area Medical Center
Robert C. Byrd Health Sciences Center of West Virginia
   University
Charleston, WV, USA

Anne M. Jones, RN, BSN, RVT, RDMS
Instructor in Neurology
Transcranial Doppler Consultant to Clinical Trials
Department of Neurology
Medical College of Georgia-Augusta
Augusta, GA, USA

Stavros K. Kakkos, MD, MSc, PhD
Department of Vascular Surgery
Imperial College
London, UK

Manju Kalra, MBBS
Assistant Professor
Department of Surgery
Division of Vascular Surgery
Mayo Clinic College of Medicine
Rochester, MN, USA

Stephen Kolakowski, Jr.
Section of Vascular Surgery
Pennsylvania Hospital
Philadelphia, PA, USA

Paul B. Kreienberg, MD
Associate Professor
Department of Surgery
The Vascular Group, PLLC
The Institute for Vascular Health and Disease
Albany Medical College
Albany Medical Center Hospital
Albany, NY, USA

Athena Kritharis, BA
Medical Student
New York University School of Medicine
New York, NY, USA

Ann Marie Kupinski, PhD, RVT
Director, Karmody Vascular Laboratory
The Vascular Group, PLLC
The Institute for Vascular Health and Disease
Albany Medical College
Albany Medical Center Hospital
Albany, NY, USA

Efthyvoulos Kyriacou, PhD
Visiting Lecturer
Department of Computer Science
University of Cyprus
Nicosia, Cyprus

Michel Lafortune, MD
University of Montreal
Hôpital Saint-Luc
Montreal, Quebec, Canada

Brajesh K. Lal, MD
Assistant Professor
Division of Vascular Surgery
UMDNJ-New Jersey Medical School
Newark, NJ, USA
and
Assistant Professor
Department of Biomedical Engineering
Stevens Institute of Technology
Hoboken, NJ, USA

M. Lavitrano, PhD
Department of Surgical Sciences and Intensive Care
University of Milano-Bicocca
Vascular Surgery Unit
San Gerardo Hospital
Monza (MI), Italy

A. Liloia, MD
Department of Surgical Sciences and Intensive Care
University of Milano-Bicocca
Vascular Surgery Unit
San Gerardo Hospital
Monza (MI), Italy

Evan C. Lipsitz, MD
Associate Professor
Department of Surgery
Medical Director, Vascular Diagnostic Laboratory
Montefiore Medical Center
and
The Albert Einstein College of Medicine
Vascular Laboratory
Bronx, NY, USA

Alan Lumsden, MB ChB, RVT, FACS
Professor and Chief Baylor College of Medicine
Division of Vascular Surgery
   and Endovascular Therapy
Michael E. DeBakey Department of Surgery
Baylor College of Medicine
Houston, TX, USA

M. Ashraf Mansour, MD
Department of Surgery–Division of Vascular Surgery
Spectrum Health Butterworth Hospital
Grand Rapids, MI, USA
and
Southern Illinois University School of Medicine
Springfield, IL, USA

Natalie Marks, MD, RVT
Vascular Institute of New York
Maimonides Medical Center
Brooklyn, NY, USA

Sandy McAffe-Benett, RVT
Section of Vascular Surgery
Pennsylvania Hospital
Philadelphia, PA, USA

Manish Mehta, MD, MPH
Assistant Professor
Department of Surgery
The Vascular Group, PLLC
The Institute for Vascular Health and Disease
Albany Medical College
Albany Medical Center Hospital
Albany, NY, USA

George H. Meier, MD, RVT, FACS
Chief of Vascular Surgery
Program Director–Fellowship
Department of Vascular Surgery
Eastern Virginia Medical School
and
Vascular and Transplant Specialists
Norfolk, VA, USA

Lisa Mekenas, RVT
Vein Institute of La Jolla
La Jolla, CA, USA

Bruce L. Mintz, DO
Clinical Assistant Professor of Medicine
University of Medicine and Dentistry of New Jersey
   (UNDNJ)
New Jersey Medical School (NJMS)
and
Director, Venous Discase Clinic
UMDNJ-NJMS University Hospital
Nework, NJ, USA

Gregory L. Moneta, MD
Professor and Chief
Division of Vascular Surgery
Oregon Health Science University
Portland, OR, USA

Kathy Mueller, RVT
Section of Vascular Surgery
Pennsylvania Hospital
Philadelphia, PA, USA

Thomas C. Naslund, MD
Associate Professor
Chief, Vascular Surgery
Department of Vascular Surgery
Vanderbilt University Medical Center
Nashville, TN, USA

Peter Neglén, MD, PhD
Vascular Surgeon
River Oaks Hospital
Flowood, MS, USA

Courtney Nelms, BS, RVT, RDMS
Senior Vascular Technologist
Vascular and Transplant Specialists
Virginia Beach, VA, USA

David G. Neschis, MD
Department of Surgery
Division of Vascular Surgery
University of Maryland School of Medicine
Baltimore, MD, USA

Marsha M. Neumyer, BS, RVT, FSVU, FAIUM
International Director
Vascular Diagnostic Educational Services
Vascular Resource Associates
Harrisburg, PA, USA

Andrew N. Nicolaides, MS, FRCS, FRCSE
Emeritus Professor of Vascular Surgery
Imperial College
London, UK
and
Special Scientist
Department of Biological Sciences
University of Cyprus
Nicosia, Cyprus
and
Director
Vascular Screening and Diagnostic Centre
Nicosia, Cyprus

Lyssa N. Ochoa, MD
Surgery Resident
Michael E. DeBakey Department of Surgery
Baylor College of Medicine
Houston, TX, USA

Kathleen J. Ozsvath, MD
Assistant Professor
Department of Surgery
The Vascular Group, PLLC
The Institute for Vascular Health and Disease
Albany Medical College
Albany Medical Center Hospital
Albany, NY, USA

Luigi Pascarella, MD
Department of Bioengineering
UCSD School of Medicine
La Jolla, CA, USA

†Heidi Patriquin, MD
Department of Radiology
University of Montreal
Hôpital Sainte-Justine
Montreal, Quebec, Canada

Philip S.K. Paty, MD
Associate Professor
Department of Surgery
The Vascular Group, PLLC
The Institute for Vascular Health and Disease
Albany Medical College
Albany Medical Center Hospital
Albany, NY, USA

Marla Paun, BS, RDMS, RVT
Research Trauma Sonographer
Department of Surgery
University of Washington
Seattle, WA, USA

C. Piazzoni, MD
Department of Surgical Sciences and Intensive Care
University of Milano-Bicocca
Vascular Surgery Unit
San Gerardo Hospital
Monza (MI), Italy

Jean F. Primozich, BS, RVT
Research Vascular Technologist
Department of Surgery
University of Washington
Seattle, WA, USA

†Deceased

Jeffrey K. Raines, PhD
Director
Vascular Laboratory and Research
Miami Vein Center
and
Professor Emeritus of Surgery
University of Miami Miller School of Medicine
Miami, FL, USA

Todd E. Rasmussen, MD
Wilford Hall USAF Medical Center
Lackland Air Force Base
TX, USA

Donald B. Reid, MD, FRCS
Consultant Vascular and Endovascular Surgeon
Wishaw Hospital
Scotland, UK

Marc Ribo, MD, PhD
Unitat Neurovascular Vall d'Hebron
Barcelona, Spain

Michael A. Ricci, MD, RVT
Professor of Surgery
Division of Vascular Surgery
University of Vermont College of Medicine
Burlington, VT, USA

Sean P. Roddy, MD
Associate Professor
Department of Surgery
The Vascular Group, PLLC
The Institute for Vascular Health and Disease
Albany Medical College
Albany Medical Center Hospital
Albany, NY, USA

Robert B. Rutherford, MD
Emeritus Professor of Surgery
Formerly at University of Colorado Health Science
   Center
Colorado, USA

Sergio X. Salles-Cunha, PhD, RVT, FSVU
Clinical Research Director
Jobst Vascular Center
Toledo, OH, USA

Jocelyn A. Segall, MD
Vascular Fellow
Division of Vascular Surgery
Oregon Health and Science University
Portland, OR, USA

Dhiraj M. Shah, MD
Professor
Department of Surgery
Director
The Vascular Group, PLLC
The Institute for Vascular Health and Disease
Albany Medical College
Albany Medical Center Hospital
Albany, NY, USA

Anton N. Sidawy, MD, MPH, FACS
Chief, Surgical Services
VA Medical Center
and
Professor
Department of Surgery
George Washington and Georgetown Universities
Washington, DC, USA

Niten Singh, MD, MS
Vascular Fellow
Department of Vascular Surgery
Washington Hospital Center/Georgetown University
Washington, DC, USA

Patrick A. Stone, MD
Assistant Professor
Vascular and Endovascular Surgery
Robert C. Byrd Health Sciences Center
Charleston, WV, USA

David S. Sumner, MD
Department of Surgery–Division of Vascular Surgery
Spectrum Health Butterworth Hospital
Grand Rapids, MI, USA
and
Southern Illinois University School of Medicine
Springfield, IL, USA

William D. Turnipseed, MD
Department of Surgery
University of Wisconsin
Madison, WI, USA

Section I
Vascular Laboratory Operations

1
Improving Quality in Noninvasive Testing by Certification and Accreditation

J. Dennis Baker and Anne M. Jones

Noninvasive testing had its roots in early research laboratories more than half a century ago. The first facility in this country was established at the Massachusetts General Hospital in 1946 and others appeared over the following years. The work focused on research efforts with little thought about providing routine clinical testing. By the 1960s arterial reconstructive procedures became increasingly frequent and there was a surge in interest in the clinical investigation of blood flow. The ability of the early measurement methods to provide objective noninvasive determination of vascular parameters attracted the interest of vascular surgeons and by the 1970s there was regular clinical use of a number of tests. What had been quiet (and often esoteric) research laboratories expanded, providing an increasing volume of routine examinations directed toward patient management. By the late 1970s the majority of hospital-based facilities were dedicated to routine clinical service rather than to research. At the same time, physicians took the testing modalities into the office, thus increasing the availability of the tests.

Education and Training

Physician

The testing in the early laboratories was done and supervised by the physicians who worked on developing and validating the techniques. These researchers were committed to critical evaluation of the tests being developed and careful work preceded widespread clinical application. Once the value of vascular testing was promulgated, increasing numbers of physicians became interested in the field. The majority of physicians who established clinical laboratories in the late 1970s and early 1980s lacked the research background and the experience of the original investigators. The newcomers relied on learning what they could from the few published articles and visits to observe the work done in established laboratories. Over time there has been an increase in the quality and availability of courses and teaching materials available. Some specialties require training in vascular testing in the core curriculum. Many programs include didactic presentations, direct participation in examinations, and experience in test interpretation. As the result of these programs many doctors come out of training much better prepared for vascular testing.

Technologist

With the expansion of vascular testing into the clinical arena and the increasing demand for services came a need for additional personnel and the training of these people. The most important change was adding personnel whose job was to perform the different testing protocols. People from a variety of technical backgrounds were recruited, including nurses, radiology technicians, and catheter laboratory specialists. With time this hybrid group evolved into vascular technologists. Adequate training and supervision became an obvious problem. These people were initially taught the basics by the supervising physician, who might or might not have an adequate background. With time there was a growth in meetings and courses dedicated to teach the principles and practice of the different testing methods. In general, most technologists learned by a hit-or-miss approach of "on-the-job" training. Where a knowledgeable physician supervised the experience, a reasonable level of expertise could result, but often trainees were on their own, learning by rote without understanding what was being done. In the past two decades, noninvasive testing has become more complex both in terms of equipment and procedures. Understanding vascular disease and the instrumentation used has become increasingly important. In many settings physicians rely on the technologists to assess patients with vascular disease and ensure appropriate utilization of noninvasive testing, thus the increased need for better and more advanced education.

Dedicated vascular technology educational programs have continued to evolve over the past decade. Their measured development can be attributed partly to inadequate funding and partly to the classification of vascular technology within the allied health specialty of "cardiovascular technology" (CVT). The CVT specialty was formally recognized by the Committee on Allied Health Education and Accreditation of the American Medical Association in 1981. Essentials and Guidelines of an Accredited Educational Program for Cardiovascular Technology were completed in 1983, and adopted by 12 allied health organizations [including the Society of Vascular Ultrasound (SVU)]. While recognition gave credibility to the cardiovascular technology profession, and established *Standards and Guidelines*, it failed to recognize the practical specialty of vascular technology. In theory, CVT includes invasive and noninvasive cardiovascular technology as well as peripheral vascular testing. As a result, educational programs in CVT routinely included very limited didactic or clinical exposure to peripheral vascular testing.

Increased utilization of noninvasive vascular testing combined with local carrier directives requiring certified vascular technologists to perform noninvasive vascular testing has created a high demand for vascular technology programs. Three baccalaureate programs in vascular technology are currently available (Oregon Institute of Technology, Rush University, and Nova Southeastern University). In addition, vascular programs are offered by 10 CVT-CAAHEP accredited associate degree programs and 2 baccalaureate programs. Several accredited Diagnostic Medical Sonography programs also offer "vascular tracks". This educational information can be accessed through the SVU and CAHEP websites.

The emergence of "distance" or "internet" educational programs is also impacting the educational choices of vascular technologists. Currently, registered vascular technologists desiring a bachelor's degree in vascular technology can do so through the Oregon Institute of Technology (OIT). The school began the first vascular technology bachelor degree program in the nation, and currently enrolls 30 to 40 students on-campus and up to 100 students in the off-campus annually. The Degree Completion Program integrates basic medical science and vascular diagnostic courses with a general college education, allowing students to complete a Bachelor of Science Degree in Vascular Technology. The distance program was developed for vascular technologists desiring a degree without leaving their present employment. The program is available to technologists who lack a bachelor's degree, and credits are awarded for achieving certification as a Registered Vascular Technologist (RVT). Details of the program are available at the school's website.

Certification

From the early days of vascular testing there was concern about the level of knowledge, experience, and competence of the individual technologist. In 1979, the national association of vascular technologists, the Society of Noninvasive Vascular Technologists (SNIVT, which later became the SVU) recognized that validation of the specialty required documentation of competence through certification. The American Registry of Diagnostic Medical Sonographers (ARDMS) was selected to provide the vascular technology certification examination. For 30 years, the ARDMS has developed and administered practice-based examinations in six ultrasound specialty areas. Certified by the National Commission of Health Certifying Agencies (NCHCA), ARDMS has consistently maintained "category A" classification with the National Commission for Certifying Agencies (NCCA). ARDMS has certified more than 45,000 individuals and has become a recognized standard for diagnostic medical ultrasound credentialing by many facility accreditation programs. The ARDMS has well-defined educational and clinical prerequisites for candidates preparing to sit for ultrasound certification examinations. These prerequisites are available on the website. Once the prerequisites are met, applicants are required to pass two comprehensive examinations to earn a credential: (1) a physical principles and instrumentation examination, and (2) a specialty examination. After acquiring a credential, continuing competency must be documented by submitting evidence of continuing medical education to the ARDMS. The first vascular technology examination was administered by ARDMS in 1983; since that time, over 14,000 RVT credentials have been awarded. Nearly 600 RVTs are also MDs. An important component of maintaining information on registrants is the ongoing documentation of the profession of vascular technology through periodic task analysis surveys. These surveys, completed by active RVTs, reflect changes occurring within the practice of vascular technology and assist with examination validation by documenting the tasks routinely performed by vascular technologists in the clinical setting. As new ultrasound technology emerges, and older methods are discarded, the task survey documents the changing clinical practice. The information is used to update examination content so that candidates are assured that the examination reflects technological advances within the profession. The surveys are also required to maintain accreditation by the NCCA. The NCCA establishes accreditation standards; ARDMS is the only certifying body for sonography accredited by NCCA.

Survey results are also used to provide historical data about trends within the specialty. For instance, in 1982, over 75% of practicing vascular technologists were nurses; this number decreased to only 18% by 1994. Similarly, in early surveys, most vascular technologists acquired their training in vascular technology on the job; by 1995, 40% of the respondents had graduated from a technical program in vascular technology, while 37% had a bachelor's or master's degree. In 1988, most RVTs worked in the department of vascular surgery (70%) in dedicated vascular laboratories. By 1994, this number had decreased to 51%, with an increasing number of vascular technologists in radiology (18%) and ultrasound departments (17%). Increasingly, the individual seeking the RVT credential may be "cross-trained" in other areas of ultrasound. Data collected between 2000 and 2004 show that 55% of vascular technologists are "RVT-only," 34% are RVT/RDMS (general sonographers), and 11% are RVT/RDCS (cardiac sonographers).

A second pathway to certification is through Cardiovascular Credentialing International (CCI). Established in 1988, CCI is a not-for-profit corporation founded for the purpose of administering credentialing examinations. The CCI Corporation of today is the result of corporate mergers of the testing components of the National Alliance of Cardiovascular Technologists (NACT), the American Cardiology Technologists Association (ACTA), and the National Board of Cardiovascular Testing (NBCVT). CCI registry examinations are offered in three specialty areas: invasive/cardiac catheterization, noninvasive echocardiography, and vascular technology/ultrasound. The Registered Vascular Specialist (RVS) credential is awarded to candidates who successfully complete the two-part examination in vascular technology. Similar to the ARDMS process, the only mechanism for obtaining the CCI credential is through examination. Candidates for the RVS credential may qualify for exemption for the Cardiovascular Science component of the examination if they hold an "active" CCI registry or meet two additional criteria, as noted on the website. There are currently 950 active CCI registrants with the RVS credential; nearly 40% also hold the CCI Registered Cardiac Sonographer (RCS) credential. Recent data indicate that fewer than 5% of the RVSs also hold the RVT (1%) or RDMS (4%) credentials awarded by ARDMS. Only 13 MDs (less than 1%) have acquired the RVS credential. Not surprisingly, Registered Vascular Sonographers are frequently employed by cardiologists, although a growing number are being hired in radiology departments. Ongoing documentation of continuing medical education is required to maintain active status.

In an effort to demonstrate competence in vascular technology, many vascular surgeons have acquired the RVT credential. The majority of MD/RVTs are vascular surgeons. There has been concern expressed that the RVT credential, designed to evaluate the knowledge and competence of the vascular technologist, is not the appropriate vehicle for a physician. To address these concerns,

in 2003, the Society for Vascular Surgery submitted a formal request to the ARDMS to explore the interest in a voluntary credential for physicians in vascular ultrasound interpretation. A market analysis was conducted, and based on the favorable response, a physician interpretation examination was developed. This examination is designed to target physicians in many medical specialties who practice vascular ultrasound. The Physician Vascular Interpretation (PVI) examination is currently under development by a six-member examination development task force. The group is chaired by R. Eugene Zierler, MD and represents all major medical specialties practicing vascular technology, and one registered vascular technologist. A detailed survey of the tasks and expertise relevant to the practice of vascular interpretation was developed and randomly distributed to 6000 physicians in February 2005. The results of the survey will be used to develop a "blueprint" of the practice, and the foundation of the PVI examination. Prerequisite guidelines and examination format have also been developed. The PVI examination will combine physics and nonphysics questions into a single, 4–5 hour examination, with one single passing score. A pilot examination was delivered in the last quarter of 2005, so that the content, scoring, reliability, and validity of the examination could be determined prior to delivering a qualified PVI examination in 2006. Examination prerequisites and applications are available on the ARDMS website.

Accreditation

An important concern in the late 1980s was the lack of any standards or guidelines for establishing and running a vascular laboratory. For the neophyte there were no benchmarks to be met regarding entry level education and experience for physicians and technologists, what constituted a complete examination, extent of ongoing supervision, quality of equipment, reporting practices, or validation studies. The great escalation in vascular testing that came in the early 1980s was accompanied by a wide range of quality of the work being done. The problem with the accuracy of the diagnostic examinations came in part as the result of the common practice of simply buying equipment and following protocols described in articles or recommended by manufacturers. Likewise, diagnostic criteria were accepted as described, presuming that the accuracies of tests by the newly established laboratory would be similar to those reported by the experts. Internal validation of the work of an individual laboratory was rarely obtained. It became clear that high accuracy of testing is dependent on both (1) technical considerations of protocols and procedures and (2) the knowledge and clinical experience of the technologist performing the examinations. In addition, there was a growing concern among the leaders in noninvasive testing about the calls from the medical insurance companies for regulation of all testing and for elimination of payment for vascular tests. Isolated cases of fraudulent operations were well publicized and caught the attention of many payers. Leaders in the field voiced the need for better self-policing but had no way to bring this about. There was also concern that some state or specialty organization might take the initiative to create standards for vascular laboratories. Often when regulation comes from government or from a single specialty group, there is limited or unbalanced input from the other professionals to be regulated. In some cases the regulation is skewed in favor of one or more special interest groups.

Intersocietal Commission for the Accreditation of Vascular Laboratories

Finally in 1989, an informal meeting of leaders in the field of noninvasive testing proposed the possibility of establishing a voluntary accreditation process. This initial group included vascular surgeons, radiologists, and vascular technologists. They concluded that there was no suitable existing accreditation option and that they needed to study the feasibility of creating an accrediting organization. Support and financial sponsorship were sought from a variety of professional societies whose members were involved in noninvasive vascular testing. The initial goals were (1) to have a broad base of support across different specialty lines and (2) to have an independent entity that was not specifically allied with any one specialty or society. From the very beginning the emphasis was on an intersocietal approach. The American Academy of Neurology, American College of Radiology, American Institute of Ultrasound in Medicine, International Society for Cardiovascular Surgery (North American Chapter), Society for Vascular Surgery, Society for Vascular Medicine & Biology, Society of Diagnostic Medical Sonographers, and Society of Vascular Technology committed to sponsor the initial efforts and an initial work group was formed with two representatives from each society.

The initial meetings were dedicated to defining the scope of vascular laboratory accreditation and the minimum guidelines necessary for the assurance of quality. The overall objective was "To ensure high quality patient care by providing a mechanism that recognizes laboratories providing quality vascular diagnostic techniques through a process of voluntary Accreditation." This goal was to be achieved by establishing an accreditation process, issuing certificates of accreditation, and maintaining a registry of accredited laboratories. An important principle that was established early was that the accreditation should be as inclusive as possible, something that could be achieved by even the smallest laboratory that was doing quality work. Another important principle adopted was that accreditation would not require a specific medical specialty training but would evaluate the particular education and experience of the doctors and the technologists in each laboratory. Standards for the overall laboratory organization addressed the qualifications of the medical and technical personnel, the layout of the laboratory, the support personnel, reports, record keeping, patient safety, and equipment maintenance. Additional standards were developed for specific testing areas (cerebrovascular, peripheral arterial, peripheral venous, and abdominal vascular). Attention was also given to indications, testing protocols, diagnostic criteria, and quality assurance. Not all components of the standards carried equal weight; some aspects were mandatory or required while others were recommended. It was decided that the accreditation would be limited to 3 years, requiring an application for renewal after that time. In March 1990 the group adopted the Constitution and Bylaws for the Intersocietal Commission for the Accreditation of Vascular Laboratories (ICAVL) and in November 1990 it was incorporated as a nonprofit corporation in Maryland. The members of the ad hoc work group became the original Board of Directors and Brian Thiele, MD, who had chaired the work group, was elected the first President. In January 1991 Sandra Katanick, RN, RVT, was selected as the Executive Director and charged with creating the administrative structure for the Commission.

The accreditation process starts with submission of a detailed application form, which includes documentation of all aspects of the facility. The sample cases and their reports are the most important part of the application, for the greatest weight in the evaluation process is on the quality of the testing provided. The final part of each testing section is the laboratory's documentation of validation or quality assurance. The Board of Directors reviews applications quarterly and decides on granting accreditation. Some applications have noted deficiencies and in these cases the decision is delayed. Commonly a laboratory is accredited in some areas while having a postponed decision in others. Once the additional material is received completing the application or documenting the correction of a problem, the final decision is made. If a laboratory is not considered to be in substantial compliance with the Essentials and Standards, a site visit is required to permit more extensive evaluation of the problem areas. While the visit may confirm the problems detected in the application, experience through the years has been that more often than not the problem was not with the laboratory itself but with a poorly prepared application. Also noted is that some laboratories with clearly documented problems have identified these and efforts toward correction are being made by the time of the site visit.

Accreditation is granted for 3 years. Reaccreditation requires an abbreviated application. New personnel complete an information and background section but for prior staff only an updated listing of CME is required. As with the original accreditation, the most important aspect of the application is the quality of the studies performed. A new set of case studies is required along with copies of the current protocols and diagnostic criteria. The other critical part of the reaccreditation is the adequate documentation of correction of the deficiencies or weaknesses identified in the previous accreditation. The review process is the same as described above except that special attention is given to evaluating improvement in problem areas.

From its inception the Commission operated on the principle that vascular testing is an advancing field and that the Essentials and Standards needed regular review and consideration for revision. The revisions to the Standards give examples of the Commission's response to changes in vascular testing. In 1994 the Venous Testing Standard was changed to make duplex scanning the only primary modality, so that laboratories performing only physiologic tests would no longer qualify for accreditation in venous testing. Later, additional testing areas were created for Intracranial Cerebrovascular and Visceral Vascular testing. A more recent policy change concerned the minimum volume required for a laboratory to apply for accreditation. The initial philosophy was that some minimum number was required to maintain competence and proficiency in the procedures. The requirement was set at 100 tests per year for each primary test. Ultimately the Board of Directors went back to its primary philosophy: the most important factor in granting accreditation should be the quality of the work being done. In the experience of the members of the Board, low volume laboratories often have trouble producing good quality studies, therefore the solution adopted was to increase the level of scrutiny for these applications. In 1997 the policy was revised so that laboratories with less than 100 studies per year could apply but would be required to submit a higher number of sample cases, some randomly selected by the ICAVL.

Through the years the ICAVL Board has been concerned about the validity of the review process. Site visits were used only when the review identified serious concerns about the data in the application. For several years consideration was given to instituting a process for random site visits to validate applications the quality of which did not trigger additional scrutiny. In 1998 a policy was established for random site visits to be carried out each quarter. The findings and recommendations of the site visit team will be compared with the recommendations resulting from the regular review of the applications.

The Commission was created as an independent, self-funded organization, so it was critical to generate sufficient interest in accreditation to be able to cover the entire cost of the operation. At first there were low numbers of applicants, but there has been a continuing steady growth in the number of accredited laboratories, currently totaling 1150. It was encouraging that most laboratories chose to reapply for accreditation after the first 3 years. An increasing number of laboratories have completed five cycles. One of the leading goals set by ICAVL was to help improve the quality of testing through the education resulting from completing the application process. Probably the most important evidence of impact of accreditation is the fact that most laboratories applying for reaccreditation show improvement over what was found the first time around. Another indicator of success was the fact that ICAVL was used as the basis for the creation of the Intersocietal Commission for the Accreditation of Echocardiography Laboratories (ICAEL) in 1996 and of the Intersocietal Commission for the Accreditation of Nuclear Medicine Laboratories (ICANL) in 1997.

American College of Radiology

Even though the American College of Radiology (ACR) was one of the original sponsors of ICAVL, its leadership decided to create its own ultrasound accreditation. A major reason put forth for this change was the interest by radiologists in having a single accreditation for all the areas of diagnostic ultrasound. This move certainly came in response to the success of ICAVL. In 1997 the new accreditation was offered to radiology-based laboratories. The vascular component directly paralleled that of ICAVL, but the requirements were less stringent and the application therefore easier to complete. A number of radiology laboratories have stopped renewing their ICAVL accreditation in favor of that offered by ACR. Approximately 900 facilities have this vascular accreditation.

Accomplishments and Impact

Over the years since the introduction of certification, and later accreditation, there has been growth in both these areas. The number of RVT certificates issued was low in the early years but has shown a later growth. In general, laboratory directors have found that people who have obtained the RVT are better prepared and ultimately show better potential for improvement of skills. Many institution-based laboratories use the RVT as a lever to place the technologist at a higher pay level than the average hospital technicians. ICAVL has always recommended that all technical personnel be credentialed, but last year a mandate was introduced requiring that all technical directors hold an approved credential. The growing appreciation of technologist credentialing was reflected by the creation by CCI of a parallel process.

When ICAVL was incorporated in 1991 there were no standards or guidelines for the evaluation of noninvasive laboratories. One of the original expectations of the founding members of the Board of Directors was that the accreditation would gain recognition and come to be used as an index of quality of vascular testing. Once the Commission succeeded in becoming established and surviving as an independent organization, there was growing interest in this type of accreditation. The Standards stood the test of time and became the basis for similar efforts by other national groups. In 1996 the American Institute of Ultrasound in Medicine established an accreditation for the areas of general and obstetrical ultrasound and followed the next year by the creation of the ACR ultrasound accreditation. The ICAVL staff participated in the creation of standards for accreditation in echocardiography and nuclear medicine laboratories.

In the early years of noninvasive testing the insurance companies paying for the work had little to no interest in the quality of testing provided to patients. As one company officer stated, "We assume that anyone billing us for a test is providing a quality examination." This attitude is changing and in recent years different insurance programs including Medicare have developed an interest in the quality of work done in vascular laboratories. There has been a growing recognition of technologist certification and laboratory accreditation as predictors of higher quality. An important step occurred in March 1998 when the Medicare carrier for Virginia implemented a regulation requiring ICAVL accreditation as a prerequisite for reimbursement. Additional carriers have addressed the quality issue, with 27 companies requiring either accreditation or that credentialed technologists perform the tests. An additional 11 recommend (do not require) that these standards be met. It is encouraging to see that groups outside the Medicare carriers are beginning to look at similar mandates. The Coalition for Quality in Ultrasound (CQU), a group of professional organizations participating in diagnostic ultrasound studies, is conducting an active campaign to increase the mandates for certification and accreditation across the country. The ideal would be to achieve these regulations on a national basis. This will fulfill the goal of wide reaching improvement in the quality of vascular testing and hopefully the elimination of poor operations, which have been the bane of the specialty throughout the years.

Appendix

Education
www.oit.edu/zimmermg/mithome/vtdcom/vasgate.html
   (Oregon Institute of Technology)
www.CAAHEP.org (education info)
www.svunet.org

Credentialing
www.ARDMS.org
www.CCI-online.org

Accreditation
www.icavl.org
www.acr.org

2
Qualifications of the Physician in the Vascular Diagnostic Laboratory

Michael A. Ricci and Robert B. Rutherford

The vascular diagnostic laboratory (VDL) is of increasing importance in the care of patients with vascular disease[1-3] while coming under greater governmental scrutiny and economic pressures.[4] In view of these challenges, the qualifications and credentials of physicians who interpret noninvasive diagnostic studies have taken on additional importance. The InterSocietal Commission for the Accreditation of Vascular Laboratories (ICAVL) has established overall standards for vascular laboratories, including credentials for interpreting physicians. Several professional societies[5-10] have published guidelines for credentials for physicians interpreting noninvasive vascular studies but, as yet, there is no universally accepted standard. Physicians from different specialty backgrounds and with different training and clinical diagnostic experience may all read and direct vascular laboratories.[7,11,12] Can these diverse backgrounds and training be accommodated in a single set of standards that qualifies physicians for working in the VDL in these capacities? This chapter will examinationine the desired attributes in regard to formal education and necessary skills, as well as special qualifications required for physicians interpreting noninvasive vascular diagnostic studies.

Educational Background

Although the first vascular laboratories were developed by vascular surgeons,[13] today a variety of other physician specialties are involved in the interpretation of noninvasive vascular studies. These include radiology, cardiology, neurology, and neurosurgery, as well as vascular medicine specialists.[7] However, each of these specialties has, stereotypically, certain deficiencies in their usual training experiences when it comes to understanding and interpreting vascular diagnostic laboratory tests. Neurologists and neurosurgeons have clinical knowledge regarding cerebral vascular disease, particularly stroke, but are less fre-

quently provided the opportunity to acquire significant experience in the VDL evaluation of patients with those conditions. In addition, cerebrovascular diagnosis is only a limited segment of the broad scope of today's VDL. Radiologists often are well-grounded in the principles of ultrasound and have experience interpreting and performing duplex ultrasound examinations, but generally lack knowledge of the principles that govern physiologic vascular testing and the clinical aspects of vascular disease. Training in cardiology includes a focus on the pathogenesis of arterial disease, particularly atherosclerosis, and the clinical aspects of some other peripheral vascular diseases, such as venous thromboembolism, but it infrequently includes adequate exposure to noninvasive vascular diagnosis or nonarterial vascular disease, such as chronic venous insufficiency. Vascular surgeons and vascular internists have broad educational exposure to the hemodynamic principles, the pathogenesis, and clinical aspects of a broad spectrum of vascular disease and how they apply to diagnosis. However, they are less often exposed to the principles and instrumentation of ultrasound and often are not given the opportunity to actually perform duplex ultrasound examinations.

While training requirements in each of these fields has evolved considerably in the past several years, no one specialty characteristically provides adequate exposure to all the educational components of vascular diagnosis that have been recommended[7,12,14] to qualify physicians to interpret noninvasive vascular tests. These educational components, listed in Table 2–1, require a multispecialty approach to the education of residents or fellows in the vascular diagnostic laboratory. The table lists all the areas in which knowledge and skills should be acquired. These components provide a framework for noninvasive vascular diagnosis training within standard specialty training so that individuals can work effectively in the VDL.

Although residency and fellowship training may vary between specialties, and between different programs

TABLE 2–1. Educational components of training in vascular laboratories.[7,12,14]

- **Ultrasound and doppler physics**
- **Plethysmographic principles**
- **Hemodynamic principles**
- **Instrumentation**
- **Extremity arterial disease**
  - Continuous wave Doppler
  - Segmental limb pressures and plethysmography
  - Duplex ultrasound scanning
  - Provocative testing (reactive hyperemia, exercise)
- **Cerebrovascular disease**
  - Duplex ultrasound scanning
  - Transcranial Doppler (TCD)
- **Visceral disease**
  - Renal arterial duplex ultrasound
  - Mesenteric artery duplex ultrasound
  - Organ transplant duplex ultrasound
  - Portal venous duplex ultrasound
- **Venous disease (acute and chronic)**
  - Duplex ultrasound scanning
  - Photoplethysmography
  - Air plethysmography
- **Testing for erectile dysfunction**
- **Ophthalmic ultrasound**

within those specialties, individuals interpreting vascular laboratory studies should have acquired a certain set of basic skills (Table 2–2). A thorough understanding of diseases that affect the vascular system is an absolute requirement. This should include an understanding of the epidemiology and pathophysiology of vascular disorders as well as their clinical signs and symptoms, prognosis, and treatment options. This fundamental knowledge is necessary because noninvasive VDL tests are based upon both normal and abnormal vascular physiology. By the same token, since noninvasive testing is an adjunct to caring for patients with vascular disease, physicians interpreting noninvasive vascular tests should have a thorough understanding of appropriate indications for the performance of these tests. It is incumbent upon the

TABLE 2–2. Prerequisite skills for physicians interpreting noninvasive vascular studies.[5]

- **Thorough understanding of vascular disease**
- **Understanding of principles of vascular testing**
  - Hemodynamics
  - Physiology
  - Ultrasound and Doppler physics
- **Understanding of the appropriate tests and indications for testing**
- **Familiarity with instrumentation**
- **Ability to perform vascular noninvasive tests**
- **Understanding of the clinical utility of noninvasive vascular tests**
  - Reliability
  - Accuracy
  - False-positive and false-negative rates
  - Technical limitations

interpreting physician to understand these indications to ensure appropriate clinical conclusions are reached and wasteful or excess testing is avoided. This, of course, includes an understanding of the false-positive and false-negative rates of VDL studies.

It should also be understood that not every laboratory will be able to produce an equivalent experience for every individual in each listed area, nor is it absolutely necessary (i.e., there is little need for residents in neurology to learn venous testing). Areas of expertise and emphasis can and should be designated by each specialty, although individuals who hope to direct a VDL should seek an educational experience that covers all the components listed in Tables 2–1 and 2–2. Additionally, it is desirable that individuals learn how to utilize instruments by actually performing clinical studies, although this may be more difficult to achieve in some specialty areas. As a minimum, in our opinion, a basic knowledge of the instrumentation and testing is desirable—if not essential. Experience actually performing the various examinations is necessary in order to adequately assist technologists with difficult examinations and, for the surgeon, to perform intraoperative duplex scanning.[1]

Qualifications

The qualifications for physicians interpreting vascular noninvasive studies have been outlined previously.[12] They consist of the following: (1) understand instrumentation (and be able to troubleshoot technical problems); (2) be able to perform and instruct others in performing noninvasive tests; (3) have a thorough knowledge of vascular diseases studied in the VDL; (4) understand the meaning, accuracy, and limitations of test results in light of other tests and the clinical setting; (5) either be completely supported by the VDL or have other activities that do not interfere with the ability to be accessible for the VDL; and (6) have no conflicts of interest between acting as both diagnostician and clinician. The individual should have a valid medical license and be in good standing in the medical community. Some professional organizations have suggested minimum numbers of examinations to qualify interpreting physicians in the VDL, but no consensus exists.[5,7–10,15] In many situations, no single individual will meet those criteria and more than one individual (physician, engineer, or technologist) may need to share these qualifications.

Credentialing

ICAVL encourages all technologists to seek certification as Registered Vascular Technologists (RVT) and considers such certification by physicians suitable evidence of appropriate experience and training. However, it should be noted that a credential specifically for physicians has only recently been introduced by the American Registry of Diagnostic Medical Sonographers (ARDMS). Until there is widespread adoption of this credential it remains up to individual departments and hospitals to set credentialing criteria in a responsible rather than self-serving manner. For examinationple, at the University of Vermont, a Department of Surgery ultrasound credentialing committee reviews and sets criteria for physicians using diagnostic ultrasound.[14] The criteria and subsequent credentialing recommendations are then sent to the hospital's credentials committee. However, this oversight obviously falls short for free-standing VDLs, pointing out the need for a national, multispecialty credentialing system. Such an approach to credentialing should be inclusive, not exclusive, to allow for the variety of specialists who have a stake in vascular noninvasive diagnosis. It may be difficult for certain specialists to obtain the adequate hands-on experience that is necessary, particularly after completing formal training. We would suggest spending an extended period of time in the VDL, e.g., 1–2 hours per week for 6–12 months, depending upon the tests to be interpreted, which could serve as a means to gain adequate experience.

The vascular surgical societies have developed hospital privileging guidelines for vascular surgery, including noninvasive vascular diagnosis.[5] Besides a medical license, these suggested requirements basically include the skill sets listed in Tables 2–1 and 2–2, as well as minimum numbers of cases and experience necessary for physicians in established practices, newly trained physicians, and those without formal training in the VDL during residency.[5]

Initial credentialing must be followed by periodic recertification. Such a process should include, as a minimum, evidence of continued effective clinical activity in the VDL and attendance at continuing medical education courses related to the VDL and vascular diagnosis.[5,12,14] Educational activities should include specific ultrasound and vascular diagnostic training but also continuing education in the vascular diseases being referred to the VDL.

Registered Vascular Technologists Examination

Can the RVT examination, administered by the Registered Physician in Vascular Interpretation (RPVI) examination serve as a suitable substitute for credentialing of physicians interpreting noninvasive studies? First, it should be pointed out that no examination

guarantees competence. Thus, as noted above, it falls to hospital and/or departmental credentialing committees to assess initial and continued competence in the awarding of credentials.[5,12,14] However, many of the criteria noted above may be fulfilled in meeting the eligibility for and passing the ARDMS examinations.[16] The RVT examination requires documentation of significant hands-on clinical experience before one can sit for the examination. The RPVI examination does not require hands-on experience, however. The 3-hour RVT examination uses a two-part format to test the candidate on (1) the principles of physics, hemodynamics, and noninvasive testing, and (2) the clinical aspects of vascular disease. The RVT examination is criterion-referenced; the minimum level for passing is set in advance, and will not be adversely affected by highly trained physicians who might skew the examination results.[16] Although it should not be an absolute requirement, it seems desirable for physicians interpreting noninvasive vascular tests to be qualified as RVTs or RPVIs.

The RPVI credential provides an alternate, and perhaps more appropriate credential for physicians interpreting vascular noninvasive studies.

Requirements for Physicians Directing Vascular Laboratories

In addition to the training, skills, and qualifications outlined above, physician-directors of VDLs must have additional capabilities. Minimum training should cover all the aspects discussed above for physician-readers in the VDL. It has also been suggested that a mandatory requirement should be for the director to have obtained the RVT credential,[17] though in the future this may be the RPVI credential. The broadest clinical experience and skills are desirable for someone to serve as a VDL director. Clinical experience will be necessary for credibility when the director is asked to resolve issues or complaints regarding appropriate selection of diagnostic tests or assistance in understanding test results in light of a clinical situation. In addition to diagnostic skills, the director must also have administrative and budgeting skills, particularly in difficult financial times.[11,17] Directors must be responsible for developing and instituting scanning protocols, interpretation criteria, accreditation applications, personnel decisions, and day-to-day operational management. Additionally, good interpersonal skills are important, for the person in this position must lead as well as direct, but these are judgment attributes. Finally, while an academic career is not essential, a good

VDL director should not only be interested in the performance of the laboratory and its staff, but ideally should be interested in examining and, where appropriate, reporting clinically significant correlations with laboratory tests or their diagnostic criteria. Clearly, directors have much greater responsibility and the selection of those individuals should reflect these needs.

References

1. Ricci MA. The changing role of duplex scan in the management of carotid bifurcation disease and endarterectomy. Sem Vasc Surg 1998;11:3–11.
2. Kasper GC, Lohr JM, Welling RE. Clinical benefit of carotid endarterectomy based on duplex ultrasonography. Vasc Endovasc Surg 2003;37:323–7.
3. Jaff MR. Diagnosis of peripheral vascular disease: Utility of the vascular laboratory. Clin Cornerstone 2002;4:16–25.
4. Zwolak RM. Coding and billing issues in the vascular laboratory. Semin Vasc Surg 2001;14:160–8.
5. Moore WS, Clagett GP, Veith FJ, et al. Guidelines for hospital privileges in vascular surgery: An update by an ad hoc committee of the American Association for Vascular Surgery and the Society for Vascular Surgery. J Vasc Surg 2002;36:1276–80.
6. Spittell JA, Jr, Creager MA, Dorros G, et al. Recommendations for training in vascular medicine. J Am Coll Cardiol 1993;22:626–8.
7. Creager MA, Goldstone J, Hirshfeld JW Jr, et al. ACC/ACP/SCAI/SVMB/SVS: Clinical competence statement on vascular medicine and catheter-based peripheral vascular interventions. J Am Coll Cardiol 2004;44:941–57.
8. Gomez C, Kinkel P, Masdeu J, et al. American Academy of Neurology Guidelines for Credentialing in Neuroimaging; Report from the task force on updating guidelines for credentialing in neuroimaging.
9. Grant EG, Barr LL, Borgestede J, et al. ACR standard for performing and interpreting diagnostic ultrasound examinations. 1992; revised 2000, http://www.acr.org/s_acr/bin.asp?TrackID=&SID=1&DID=12267&CID=539&VID=2&DOC=File.PDF, accessed July 27, 2006 Neurology 1997;49:1734–1737.
10. Johnson B, Moneta G, Oliver M. Suggested minimum qualifications for physicians interpreting noninvasive vascular diagnostic studies. http://www.svunet.org/about/positions/standard.physicianquals.htm, accessed July 27, 2006.
11. Rutherford RB. Qualifications of the physician in charge of the vascular diagnostic laboratory. J Vasc Surg 1988;8:732–35.
12. Rutherford RB. Physicians in the vascular diagnostic laboratory: Educational background, prerequisite skills, credentialing, and continuing medical education. Sem Vasc Surg 1994;7:217–22.
13. Kempczinski RF. Challenging times for the vascular laboratory. Sem Vasc Surg 1994;7:212–16.
14. Shackford SR, Ricci MA, Hebert JC. Education and credentialing. Prob Gen Surg 1997;14:126–32.
15. Ricci MA. Qualifications and competence of vascular laboratory personnel. In: Mansour A, Labropoulos N (eds). Vascular Diagnosis. Philadelphia, PA: WB Saunders Co, 2004.
16. Jones AM. Training and certification of the vascular technologist. Sem Vasc Surg 1994;7:228–33.
17. Kempczinski RF. Challenging times for the vascular laboratory. Sem Vasc Surg 1994;7:212–16.

Section II
Basic Physics

3
Principles and Instruments of Diagnostic Ultrasound and Doppler Ultrasound

Kirk W. Beach, Marla Paun, and Jean F. Primozich

This chapter is an April 2005 revision of a chapter written in April 1998. During that period, the basics of ultrasound examination have been surprisingly stable. Electronics have shrunk so that now full function ultrasound duplex scanners can fit in your pocket. The speed of personal computers has advanced so that the new scanners are just software residing in personal computers equipped with an ultrasound receiver on the front end and a printer or DICOM adaptor on the back end.

In spite of shrinking electronics, all of the "modern" triplex-Doppler, color flow, (three-dimensional real-time) "four-dimensional" scanners have converged on a single standard package. Most instruments are still 20 inches (50 cm) wide, 30 inches (75 cm) long, and 50 inches (125 cm) tall, with a power cord that requires 120 V (240 V in Europe), 60 Hz (50 Hz in Europe), delivering a maximum of 15 A (7.5 A in Europe) or 1800 W (volts multiplied by amps) with a printer included. This standard was developed because doorways are 30 inches (760 mm) wide and the eyes of ultrasound examiners are located 60 inches (150 cm) off the ground, and power outlets are ubiquitous. This way, an examiner can roll the ultrasound instrument through a door while the examiner's view over the top of the instrument is unobstructed and connect the instrument to power at the patient's bedside. Thus the systems are "portable," something that will always be out of reach of the computed tomography (CT) and magnetic resonance imaging (MRI) alternative technologies. It is truly surprising that the manufacturers, over the period from 1979 (when commercial duplex scanners became popular) to 2005, while electronics have shrunk to $(1/2)^{18}$ or 1/250,000 size, have elected to keep the instrument package unchanged until this year with the introduction of notebook size systems. What has changed is that the complexity of the systems has exploded. Now ultrasound scanners are over 4000 times as complex as in 1979. But, that era has come to an end. The first companies to introduce palm size scanners have reverted to mounting them on standard size carts, not because

small size is impossible, but because the customers appear to want ultrasound scanners that look large. Now, all the major manufacturers offer palm size ultrasound scanners as an alternative to the large systems.

This chapter was written in the United States in a world where inches and feet, gallons and quarts are the rule, and room temperature is 72°F (22°C) and body temperature is 98.6°F (37°C). "Science" has "advanced" to use a decimal metric system. The decimal system, however, is misaligned with the computer-friendly binary number system. As an example, 0.1 is an irrational number in binary computer math. In the future, I predict, the decimal system will be discarded in favor of a binary (or hexadecimal) system that is more compatible with computers. In the meantime, the relationship between the decimal and binary systems will require constant explanation.

In this chapter, the MKS (meter kilogram second) system will be used when alternatives are not more convenient. To facilitate understanding, all units will be listed every time a number is given. To make things more difficult, the "scientists" have decided to honor their own by naming often used groups of units after the great people in physics, like Hertz for frequency instead of cycles per second, Pascals for pressure instead of Newton per square meter, and Rayls for impedance instead of kilograms per square meter per second. In this chapter, along with the modern names, the more primitive units of measure will be included in order to foster the ability of the reader to correctly perform important computations, which facilitate the understanding of future instruments and methods. The results of many computations are quite astounding.

Introduction

Medical imaging of the body requires the completion of three tasks: (1) locating volumes of tissue in the body (voxels) to be examined, (2) measuring one or more feature(s) of the tissue within each volume, and (3) delivering the data to the brain of the examiner/interpreter. The primary sensory channel used in medical imaging is the retina, a two-dimensional, analog/trichromatic (color), cine-capable (motion) data path. A secondary channel used exclusively in ultrasound Doppler is dual audio channels (two ears). Although used in physical examination, the tactile, taste, and olfactory senses are not currently used in medical imaging. A two-dimensional medical image presentation involves two tasks: (1) arranging areas on a screen (pixels) that correspond to tissue voxels and (2) displaying the measurement from the corresponding tissue voxel in each pixel. If more than one measurement type is made from each voxel (for example, echogenicity and tissue velocity) then both data types can be shown in a single pixel on the screen by differentiating the echogenicity (shown in gray scale) from the velocity (shown in colors) by using the trivariable (red-green-blue) nature of the eye. If the process is done once to form one image, the image is called "static"; if the process is repeated rapidly (10 or more times per second) to show motion, then the process may be called "real time." These steps are required in all sectional imaging modalities such as CT, MRI, positron emission tomography (PET) imaging, and ultrasound. Note that the voxels used in sectional imaging are different from the voxels used in projectional imaging like conventional X-ray and nuclear imaging. In sectional imaging, the voxels are nearly cubic, whereas in projectional imaging the voxels are long rods penetrating the entire body and viewed from the end as pixels (dots).

In the following discussion, ultrasonic imaging consists of three steps: (1) the voxels will be located, (2) measurements on each tissue voxel will be made, and (3) the tissue data from each voxel in the image plane will be displayed as a two-dimensional array of pixels. This discussion will be limited to pulse echo ultrasound; continuous wave ultrasound will not be covered. There are several alternatives to the popular methods that may become useful in the future.

Locating Voxels with Pulse Echo Ultrasound

A transmitting ultrasound transducer is designed to direct a pulse of ultrasound along a needle-like beam pattern from the transducer through the body tissues. Voxels located along that beam pattern provide echoes that return to the receiving transducer along a needle-like beam pattern. Usually the transmitting transducer aperture and the receiving transducer aperture are at the same location, so the transmit beam path and the receive

beam path are the same. The location of each voxel reflecting ultrasound from along the beam can be determined by the time taken for the echo to return. Data from a reflector at a depth of 1 cm returns to the transducer in 13 μs; data from a depth of 3 cm returns in 40 μs; data from 15 cm returns in 200 μs. Except for the details, this is a complete description of pulse-echo ultrasound. To understand the physics and consequences on the image in more detail, we need to separate four coordinate directions in tissue: (1) distance from the ultrasound transducer (depth), (2) lateral direction in the image (ultrasound beam pattern width), (3) thickness direction in the image (ultrasound beam pattern thickness), and (4) time of image acquisition (frame interval/sweep) in the cardiac cycle. The physics of each of these is different. Thus, each of these has an associated resolution. We will consider each of these in sequence.

Distance from the Ultrasound Transducer Depth

Pulse-echo ultrasound involves transmitting a short pulse of ultrasound into tissue and then receiving the echoes that return from the tissues located at each depth along the ultrasound beam pattern. The echo time, the time after transmission for an echo to return from a voxel at a particular depth, can be computed from the speed of ultrasound in tissue. The speed of ultrasound in tissue is called C. In most body tissues C is about 1500 ($\pm$ 80) m/s = 150,000 cm/s = 1.5 mm/μs.

To compute the time [t] required for an echo to return from a voxel at a particular depth [d], the round trip distance of travel must be used [$t = 2d/C$]. For an echo to return from a depth of 3 cm (30 mm), the time required is [$t = 2 * 30\,mm/1.5\,mm/μs = 40\,μs$]. The result of this computation for a series of depths is given in Table 3–1.

In a typical ultrasound machine, the time when echoes are returning is divided into 200 divisions, each division being 1 μs long. Each division takes data from a 0.75-mm voxel along the ultrasound beam pattern to provide data for a pixel along the beam line on the screen. Each beam line on the screen is thin and straight corresponding to the thin straight ultrasound transmit beam pattern and thin straight ultrasound receive beam pattern. Most ultra-

TABLE 3–1. Ultrasound echo time for depth.

Depth	Time	Vessel
0.75 mm	1 μs	
1.5 mm	2 μs	Finger artery
15 mm	20 μs	Superficial vein
3 cm	40 μs	Carotid artery
9 cm	120 μs	Renal artery
15 cm	200 μs	

sound systems assume that the speed of ultrasound is exactly 1.54 mm/μs; unfortunately the speed in some soft tissues is 7% above or below this value.

Speed of Ultrasound in Tissue

The speed of ultrasound in tissue is determined by the character of tissue. From basic physics, the speed can be computed; it is determined by tissue density (ρ) and stiffness (K). $C = \sqrt{(K/\rho)}$. Ultrasound speed is the square root of the ratio of the tissue stiffness and the tissue density. Both stiffness and density are different in different tissues and both vary with temperature. Temperature is not an issue (unless you examine a lizard or snake) because the normal mammalian body temperature is 37°C. If you examined a body part with ultrasound for a really long time, you might increase the temperature by 1°C, which would increase the sound speed by about 0.2%. For diagnostic ultrasound, the ultrasound speed is the same for all ultrasound frequencies and is the same for all ultrasound intensities. Typical ultrasound speeds have been measured in dead meat. They are used as if they are the correct speeds for living tissue. Most commercial ultrasound systems assume that the "average" speed of ultrasound is 1.54 mm/μs. Thus, the dimensions of the image in the depth direction are correct only in liver. Objects in breast [C(fat) = 1.45 mm/μs] appear to be 6% deeper than the actual depth because the echoes take longer to return due to the lower speed. The diameter of blood vessels appears to be 2% smaller than actual because the ultrasound speed in the tissue between the blood vessel walls (blood) is higher than the assumed "average" [C(blood) = 1.57 mm/μs] (Table 3–2).

Depth Resolution

Depth resolution, the ability to see two independent objects located along the same beam pattern, separated in depth by a small distance, is determined by the length of the burst of ultrasound, which is often near the wavelength of ultrasound. The wavelength of ultrasound can

TABLE 3–2. Ultrasound speeds in tissues.

Tissue	Speed	Difference from standard value	
Air	0.33 mm/μs		
Fat	1.45 mm/μs	−6%	
Urine	1.49 mm/μs	−3%	
Liver	1.54 mm/μs	0%	standard value
Blood	1.57 mm/μs	2%	correct Doppler value
Muscle	1.58 mm/μs	3%	
Cartilage	1.65 mm/μs	7%	
Bone	3.5 mm/μs	130%	
Ultrasound transducer PZT[a]	3.8 mm/μs		

[a] PZT (PbZrTi) = lead zirconium titanite.

TABLE 3–3. Typical ultrasound wavelengths in soft tissues.

Frequency[a]	Wavelength	Use
1.5 MHz	1 mm	Transcranial Doppler
3 MHz	0.5 mm	Adult cardiac and abdomen
5 MHz	0.3 mm	Pediatric cardiac and carotid
7.5 MHz	0.2 mm	Superficial imaging
10 MHz	0.15 mm	Vascular wall
20 MHz	0.075 mm	Intraluminal ultrasound

[a] MHz is megaHertz = 1,000,000 cycles/s = cycles/microsecond = cy/μs.

be computed from the ultrasound frequency (F) and the speed of ultrasound in tissue C (Table 3–3).

$$\lambda(\text{cm/cy}) = C/F[(\text{cm/s})/(\text{cy/s})]$$

Ultrasound Reflection

In pulse-echo ultrasound, an ultrasound burst is sent from the transducer into the tissue. Echoes from the tissues return to the transducer. All of the information that we learn from the tissues is contained in the echo. There are three kinds of information in the echo: (1) the strength or amplitude, (2) the phase or relative timing, and (3) the shape or frequency content. The strength is used for gray scale imaging. The phase of the echo is determined by the exact distance of the reflector from the ultrasound transducer; the phase is used for velocity and motion measurement. The shape of the echo is determined by the propagation and attenuating properties of the tissue between the transducer and the reflector plus the nature of the reflector. The shape of the echo is used in harmonic imaging. If the shape of the echo is not "sinusoidal" then the echo contains harmonics or frequency components at 2×, 3×, 4× . . . times the "fundamental" transmitted ultrasound frequency.

Echoes occur only when the ultrasound encounters changes in a tissue property called ultrasound **impedance**, called Z. The ultrasound impedance (Table 3–4) depends on the same factors as ultrasound speed, the stiffness and the density. $Z = \sqrt{(K \times \rho)}$. But in contrast

TABLE 3–4. Ultrasound Impedance in Tissues.[a]

Tissue	Impedance	Impedance	
Air	0.4 Mg/m²/s	400 Rayls	4 atm s/km
Fat	1,380 Mg/m²/s	1.38 MRayls	13.8 atm s/m
Urine	1,490 Mg/m²/s	1.49 MRayls	14.9 atm s/m
Liver	1,640 Mg/m²/s	1.64 MRayls	16.4 atm s/m
Blood	1,620 Mg/m²/s	1.62 MRayls	16.2 atm s/m
Muscle	1,700 Mg/m²/s	1.70 MRayls	17.0 atm s/m
Bone	7,800 Mg/m²/s	7.80 MRayls	78.0 atm s/m
Ultrasound transducer PZT	29,000 Mg/m²/s	29 MRayls	290.0 atm s/m

[a] Mg/m²/s = megagrams/square meter/second = megaRayls = kiloNewton seconds/cubic meter. Atmosphere = 100,000 Newton/square meter = 100,000 Pascal = 1,000,000 dyne/square cm. PZT (PbZrTi), lead zirconium titanite.

TABLE 3–5. Ultrasound energy reflection at different interfaces between materials.

Tissue	Impedance MRayls	Air 0.0004	Fat 1.38	Urine 1.49	Blood 1.62	Liver 1.64	Muscle 1.7	Bone 7.8
Air	**0.0004**							
Fat	**1.38**	99.88%						
Urine	**1.49**	99.89%	0.15%					
Blood	**1.62**	99.90%	0.64%	0.17%				
Liver	**1.64**	99.90%	0.74%	0.23%	0.00%			
Muscle	**1.7**	99.91%	1.08%	0.43%	0.06%	0.03%		
Bone	**7.8**	99.98%	48.91%	46.13%	43.04%	42.58%	41.23%	
PZT[a]	**29**	99.99%	82.66%	81.41%	79.96%	79.74%	79.08%	33.19%

[a]PZT (PbZrTi), lead zirconium titanite.

to ultrasound speed, ultrasound impedance is the square root of the product of the tissue stiffness and the tissue density.

$$\text{Rayl} = \text{kg/m}^2/\text{s}$$

Some authors prefer to express impedance as the product of tissue density and ultrasound speed. With algebra, you can demonstrate that these are the same.

The difference in impedance between the superficial tissue and the deep tissue at an interface determines the strength of the reflector and therefore is proportional to the amplitude of the ultrasound echo. $R = (Z_2 - Z_1)/(Z_2 + Z_1)$. If the difference between the impedances is greater, then the fraction of the incident ultrasound that is reflected is larger. The pulse energy is proportional to the square of the amplitude, so the energy reflected is equal to R^2. Table 3–5 shows that the reflected energy from an ultrasound pulse as it crosses an interface between two soft tissues is usually less than 1%. Reflections at the surface of bone interfaces are near 50%. Reflections at the surface of air interfaces are greater than 99%. The greatest reflections between solids occur at the surface of a PZT (PbZrTi, lead zirconium titanite) ultrasound transducer. Less than 0.12% of the energy in the transducer will pass into tissue in an ultrasound cycle; less than 0.01% will pass from the transducer into air.

As ultrasound passes from fat into muscle, 1% of the ultrasound pulse energy is reflected and 99% is transmitted. The same percentage is reflected as ultrasound passes from muscle into fat. However, as shown in Table 3–6, there is a difference between the two reflections. As ultrasound is passing from muscle to fat, the shape of the reflected pulse is inverted because the distal tissue has a lower impedance than the proximal tissue; the inversion is indicated by the minus sign in Table 3–6.

Ultrasound Attenuation

As an ultrasound pulse travels through tissue, the energy in the pulse decreases. Some of the energy is reflected by interfaces and scatterers where the impedance changes, some of the energy is absorbed by the tissue causing the tissue to heat, and some of the energy is converted into harmonic ultrasound frequencies that are not received by the ultrasound system. For imaging purposes, the importance of attenuation is that the strength of the echoes received from deep tissues is less than the strength of the echoes from similar superficial tissues. This complicates the interpretation of echo strength. The time gain control (TGC) should be set to compensate for the attenuation. This control is also called depth gain compensation (DGC), system time compensation (STC), and other names.

TABLE 3–6. Ultrasound amplitude reflection at different interfaces between materials.

		Material on the superficial side of the interface							
Tissue	Impedance Mrayls	Air 0.0004	Fat 1.38	Urine 1.49	Blood 1.62	Liver 1.64	Muscle 1.7	Bone 7.8	PZT[a] 29
Air	0.0004	0	−0.99942	−0.99946	−0.99951	−0.99951	−0.99953	−0.99990	−0.99997
Fat	1.38	0.99942	0	−0.03833	−0.08000	−0.08609	−0.10390	−0.69935	−0.90915
Urine	1.49	0.99946	0.03833	0	−0.04180	−0.04792	−0.06583	−0.67922	−0.90226
Blood	1.62	0.99951	0.08000	0.04180	0	−0.00613	−0.02410	−0.65605	−0.89419
Liver	1.64	0.99951	0.08609	0.04792	0.00613	0	−0.01796	−0.65254	−0.89295
Muscle	1.7	0.99953	0.10390	0.06583	0.02410	0.01796	0	−0.64211	−0.88925
Bone	7.8	0.99990	0.69935	0.67922	0.65605	0.65254	0.64211	0	−0.57609
PZT	29	0.99997	0.90915	0.90226	0.89419	0.89295	0.88925	0.57609	0

[a]PZT (PbZrTi), lead zirconium titanite.

The effect of attenuation on the strength of the echo received from a voxel can be computed using the attenuation rate and thickness of the tissues between the ultrasound transducer and the voxel. The attenuation rate is expressed in three different kinds of units: Nepers, decibels, and half-thickness.

As a 1-MHz ultrasound pulse passes through a section of typical soft tissue 10 cm thick, approximately 90% of the energy is reflected (scattered), absorbed (converted to heat), or converted to harmonics, so only 10% of the original energy is present in the pulse leaving the section. Attenuation to 0.1 of the original pulse energy is called 1 bel (B) of attenuation. If the ultrasound passes through an additional 10-cm-thick section, only 0.1 of the previous 0.1 or 0.01 of the original energy survives. This is called 2 B of attenuation. If ultrasound passes through 30 cm of soft tissue, only 0.001 (0.1^3) of the original pulse energy survives. This is called 3 B of attenuation. These units are too large for the engineers that use them so they use decibels: 10 dB is equal to 1 B.

As a 1-MHz ultrasound pulse passes through a section of typical soft tissue 3 cm thick, approximately 50% of the energy is reflected (scattered) or absorbed (converted to heat), so 50% of the original energy is present in the pulse leaving the section. Thus, 3 cm is the half value thickness or half value layer. If the ultrasound passes through 3 half value layers or 9 cm, then ($0.5 \times 0.5 \times 0.5$) 0.125 of the energy in the pulse survives. If the ultrasound passes through 30 cm or 10 half value layers, then (0.5^{10}) 0.001 of the original energy is still in the pulse. Fortunately, the answer is the same for 30 cm of tissue whether computed in decibels or in half value layers.

If E_f is the surviving energy and E_o is the incident energy, then

$$E_f/E_o = 0.1^{d/10} = 0.5^H$$

where d is in decibels and H is in half value layers.

If the ultrasound frequency is doubled, the attenuation for each centimeter is doubled. The attenuation per ultrasound cycle is constant over wide ranges. A half value layer of soft tissue is about 20 wavelengths thick. A tissue layer that attenuates ultrasound by 10 dB is 67 wavelengths. The attenuation rate in some soft tissues is greater than in others.

The attenuation refers to energy or power, but not to intensity. Power is energy/time; intensity is power/area. As ultrasound spreads or converges, the area of the beam changes. Changes in intensity are due to a combination of changes in power and changes in area. In turn, pressure amplitude is dependent on intensity. Attenuation in Nepers is defined as $I_f/I_o = \exp(-\eta)$ where η is the attenuation in Nepers. This would be acceptable if the beam did not diverge or converge so that the beam cross-sectional area did not change. In that case $d = 3 \times H = 8.69 \times \eta$.

TABLE 3–7. Ultrasound attenuation in tissues.[a]

Tissue	Cycles/decibel	Cycles/half thickness	Cycles/Neper
Urine	1000	3010	8690
Blood	37	111	321
Fat	11	33	95.6
Liver	7	21	60.8
Muscle	3	9	38.7

[a]For a nonconverging beam.

Attenuation in some tissues is greater than in other tissues (Table 3–7).

Ultrasound Intensity

The meaning of ultrasound impedance is not as obvious as the meaning of ultrasound speed. To understand impedance, imagine what happens as ultrasound passes through tissue. As the ultrasound wave travels through a portion of tissue, the molecules in that portion of the tissue jiggle in the wave propagation direction, in response to pressure changes in the forward and backward direction as the wave passes. Since the molecular motion is in the same direction as the wave travels, this is called a longitudinal wave. Ultrasound impedance is the ratio of the pressure fluctuation (p) to the molecular velocity fluctuation (v) as the wave passes $Z = p/v$. The instantaneous intensity of the wave is the product of the pressure fluctuation and the velocity fluctuation. $i = p \times v$. P, the instantaneous air pressure, includes two parts, the atmospheric pressure A and the fluctuating part p, $P = A + p$. With algebra, you can show that $i = Z \times v^2$ or that $i = p^2/Z$. Typical medical ultrasound values are shown in Table 3–8.

For continuous wave (CW) ultrasound, a continuous sound wave that can be expressed as a sine wave, the average intensity I can be computed.

TABLE 3–8. Ultrasound intensity wave parameters in soft tissue if $Z = 1.5$ MRayls.

Intensity[a]	Pressure fluctuations	Molecular velocity fluctuations
10 mW/cm^2	17 kN/m^2 = 0.17 atm	1.2 cm/s
100 mW/cm$^{2\,b}$	54 kN/m^2 = 0.54 atm	3.6 cm/s
333 mW/cm^2	100 kN/m^2 = 1.00 atm^c	6.6 cm/s
1,000 mW/cm^2	170 kN/m^2 = 1.70 atm	11.5 cm/s
3,000 mW/cm$^{2\,d}$	295 kN/m^2 = 2.95 atm	20 cm/s
10,000 mW/cm$^{2\,e}$	540 kN/m^2 = 5.40 atm	36.4 cm/s
2,000 W/cm$^{2\,f}$	7.6 MN/m^2 = 76 atm	510 cm/s

[a]Intensity refers to spatial peak temporal peak for pulsed ultrasound.
[b]Maximum "continuous wave" intensity for diagnostic ultrasound.
[c]Pressure fluctuaftion equals 1 atmosphere.
[d]Typical continuous wave intensity used for therapeutic ultrasound.
[e]Spatial peak temporal peak intensity typical of diagnostic ultrasound.
[f]High intensity focused ultrasound cautery.

$$I = \text{time average} \left\{ \left[p_m \times \sin(\omega t)^2 \right] \right\} \Big/ Z = \left(\frac{1}{2} p_m^{\ 2} \right) \Big/ Z$$

or

$$p_{\mathrm{m}} = \sqrt{(2 \times I \times Z)}$$

and similarly

$$v_{\mathrm{m}} = \sqrt{(2 \times I / Z)}$$

Note that the relationships between intensity, the pressure fluctuations, and the molecular velocity fluctuations are independent of ultrasound frequency. Each depends on the ultrasound intensity and the tissue impedance.

At instantaneous intensities of $333\,\text{mW/cm}^2$, the highest pressure at the compression half cycle is 2 atmospheres and the lowest pressure at the decompression half cycle is **zero** according to linear theory. When spatial peak temporal peak (SPTP) intensities exceed that, as they often do in diagnostic imaging, the simple (linear) equations no longer apply. The wave changes in shape; the compression half cycle travels faster than the decompression half cycle causing the decompression half cycles to flatten while the compression half cycles become more sharply peaked.

Harmonic Waves

The change in ultrasound waveshape that occurs when SPTP ultrasound intensities exceed $333\,\text{mW/cm}^2$ can be expressed as the introduction of harmonics: frequencies two or three times as high as the transmitted ultrasound frequency. If the harmonic waves are phase aligned properly (Figure 3–1A), the decompression portions of the wave are flattened and the compression peaks are sharpened. This effect is exploited in harmonic imaging. In Figure 3–1, two cycles of the wave can be seen. If the amplitude were low, then only the fundamental frequency would be seen as in Figure 3–2.

The harmonics permit the transmission of the ultrasound without the necessity of "negative" pressures, which are prohibited by the laws of physics. The actual absolute pressure values are not usually measured, because the transducers used to measure pressure are "AC" coupled, which delivers only differences. Changes

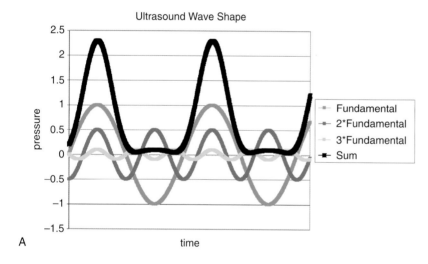

A

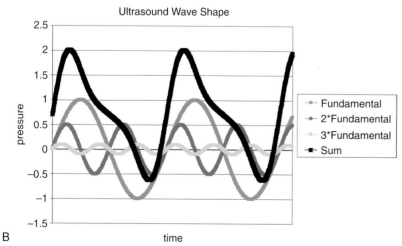

B

FIGURE 3–1. Waveshape of a $1.0\,\text{W/cm}^2$ SPTP intensity ultrasound wave in soft tissue. (A, B) The waveshape seen in tissue is shown as a wide line. Three frequency components of the wave are shown in light lines, the fundamental, the second harmonic, and the third harmonic. The three-component waves are added to form the resulting wave. The phase alignment and amplitude of each harmonic determine the shape of the resulting wave.

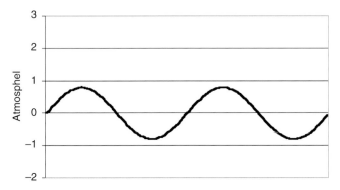

FIGURE 3–2. Waveshape of a $210\,mW/cm^2$ SPTP intensity ultrasound wave in soft tissue. At intensities below $300\,mW/cm^2$ ultrasound behaves as predicted by linear equations and the shape of a sine wave (or any other shape) is preserved.

in wave speed at extreme pressures can alter the waveshape (Figure 3–1B). George Keilman has shown that a focused ultrasound beam that forms peaks like those in Figure 3–1 will revert to a sinusoid like Figure 3–2 if reflected by an inverting reflector in the middle of the path ($Z_2 < Z_1$), but will convert more energy to harmonics if reflected by a noninverting reflector in the middle of the path ($Z_2 > Z_1$).

Harmonics are also formed when ultrasound interacts with bubbles in the ultrasound beam. The history of bubbles and harmonic imaging is interesting. Ultrasound contrast made by agitating saline has been used for years by cardiologists to diagnose patent foramen ovale (PFO). Injected intravenously, the microbubbles are too large to pass through the lung. They are very echogenic in the ventricle. If they appear in the left ventricle, a PFO is diagnosed. Recently ultrasound contrast agents consisting of bubbles smaller than $8\,\mu m$ in size (the size of an erythrocyte) have been manufactured so that they will pass through the capillaries of the lung. When injected intravenously, these will permit ultrasound contrast studies in arteries and organs supplied by the systemic arterial circulation.

Usually, small bubbles are not stable in liquid because the surface tension at the interface between the gas and the liquid squeezes the bubbles and causes the gas to dissolve. The surface tension can be reduced by adding a surfactant that acts like soap. Common surfactants include albumen and sugars. Of course, the chemical properties of the surfactant can be used to cause the bubbles to attach to the endothelial surface of blood vessels. Rather than a bubble filled with air, which has a moderate solubility in water (which shortens the life of the contrast agent in blood), contrast bubbles often contain fluorocarbons that have poor solubility in water and blood plasma. This increases the duration of bubble survival in the tissues. The fluorocarbons do have a high solubility in fat, a factor that has not yet been explored in ultrasound contrast agents.

Unfortunately, ultrasound contrast agent bubbles are not as echogenic as expected. Therefore, new ultrasound imaging systems have been adapted to transmit at one frequency and receive at a harmonic. Contrast agents are conspicuous in harmonic images. Surprisingly, many tissues produce bright harmonic echoes when contrast agents are not present. This is evidence of the harmonic conversion of ultrasound due to the high SPTP intensities common in ultrasound imaging. Thus, there is a new B-mode imaging method called harmonic imaging (Figure 3–3), which changes the appearance of the image, making some structures appear to be more conspicuous and others less conspicuous. There may be some utility in superimposing the colorized images of different received frequencies to form a composite.[1] With current ultrasound systems, that is not possible because they require different software at different frequencies.

Piezoelectric Transducers

An ultrasound transducer is a polarized wafer of crystalline, ceramic, or plastic piezoelectric material that has a conductor applied to each side. Wires connected to the conductors connect to the ultrasound imaging system. If a voltage ranging from 4 to 400 V is applied between the conductors, the thickness of the material will expand or contract depending on the polarity. If a compression or expansion is applied to the transducer from outside, a

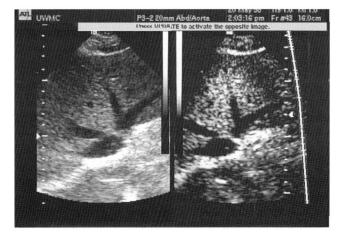

FIGURE 3–3. Fundamental frequency image and harmonic frequency image of liver. The left image was formed with the fundamental frequency echo and the right image was formed with the second harmonic of the transmitted frequency. The echo strengths of the harmonic are much lower than the echo strengths of the fundamental. Of course, attenuation of the echoes from greater depth is more severe at the second harmonic frequency.

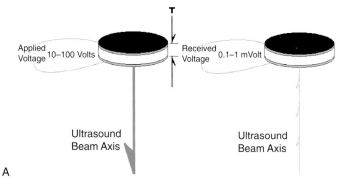

A

B

FIGURE 3–4. (A) Piezoelectric ultrasonic transducer. The transducer is transmitting on the left and receiving echoes on the right. (B) Ultrasound transducer vibrational modes that interact electrically and mechanically. Positive half waves will cancel negative half waves for even harmonics. Only the shaded half cycle interacts effectively with the electric and mechanical fields.

voltage will appear between the conductors. Thus the transducer is able to convert an electrical signal into a mechanical motion for transmitting an ultrasound pulse and is able to convert a mechanical motion into an electrical signal for receiving ultrasound echoes.

Each ultrasound transducer has a natural frequency of oscillation, much like the natural frequency of a bell. As with a bell, the natural frequency of the transducer is determined by a dimension of the transducer; this dimension is the thickness. Thin ultrasound transducers oscillate at high frequencies and thick transducers oscillate at low frequencies. The oscillation occurs because ultrasound is "trapped" in the transducer; the ultrasound energy reflects back toward the center from both surfaces and cannot get out because the impedance difference between the transducer material and the material outside is so great that all of the ultrasound is reflected. A similar trapped wave is a jump rope. The wave traveling down the rope cannot get past the hand holding each end, so the center just vibrates up and down. As with a jump rope, only certain wavelengths are allowed. The allowed wavelengths in a jump rope are $\frac{1}{2}, \frac{2}{2}, \frac{3}{2}, \frac{4}{2}, \frac{5}{2}, \frac{6}{2}, \frac{7}{2} \ldots$ of the total length dimension. In a piezoelectric ultrasound transducer, only the odd values are present. The even values ($\frac{2}{2}, \frac{4}{2} \ldots$) do not interact with the electric or mechanical environment because one-half of the wave exactly counteracts the other (Figure 3–4), so only the odd values are effective ($\frac{1}{2}, \frac{3}{2}, \frac{5}{2}, \frac{7}{2}$). The most common oscillation occurs when the wavelength is half of the transducer thickness (T):

$$\lambda = 2 \times T = C/F$$

So the ultrasound frequency of a transducer is determined by the thickness.

$$F = C/(2 \times T)$$

Other possible oscillation frequencies are shown in Table 3–9. These oscillating crystals are used for many applications, including the clock timing for computers. The "highest quality" (High Q) transducers lose very little energy each cycle and therefore oscillate for a long time at a single frequency. When a short voltage pulse is used to "strike" the transducer, it will ring for a long time at a single frequency.

For ultrasound, three things should be different: (1) transmit a short pulse into tissue to produce good depth resolution, (2) transfer of the mechanical ultrasound pulse energy into the tissue from the transducer, and (3) transfer of the mechanical echo energy coming back into the transducer to create a voltage. When the transducer is in air, 99.99% of the ultrasound energy is reflected back into the transducer, so almost no ultrasound is transmitted. If gel is applied to couple the transducer with skin, only 80% of the energy in the pulse is reflected back into the transducer and 20% is transmitted into the tissue with each cycle of oscillation. CW Doppler transducers are constructed like this. If 20% of the energy leaves the transducer each cycle, then after 5 cycles only 33% of the energy remains in the transducer, and after a total of 10 cycles of oscillation only 11% of the original energy remains. The transducer "rings" for too long to provide good depth resolution for imaging. To "damp" the oscillation more quickly, a backing material is applied to the back of the transducer that removes 50% of the energy

TABLE 3–9. Possible ultrasound transducer frequencies.[a]

Mode	Frequency	Relative amplitude	Relative power
$F = C/(2 \times T)$	3 cy/μs	1	1
$F = 3 \times C/(2 \times T)$	9 cy/μs	1/3	1/9
$F = 5 \times C/(2 \times T)$	15 cy/μs	1/5	1/25
$F = 7 \times C/(2 \times T)$	21 cy/μs	1/7	1/49
$F = 9 \times C/(2 \times T)$	27 cy/μs	1/9	1/81

[a]For a 0.63-mm-thick lead zirconium titanite transducer.

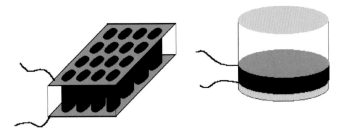

FIGURE 3–5. Advanced transducer damping methods. The left image is a composite transducer and the right image is a backed transducer with matching layer. Black is piezoelectric material. Wires are hooked to electrodes. The damping material between the transducer columns on the left transducer and on the back of the right transducer is shown as clear. Electrodes are dark gray. Light gray is the quarter wavelength matching layer on the bottom face of the right transducer where it comes in contact with the patient. A similar matching layer could be added to the face of the left composite transducer.

each cycle. With 20% leaving through the front and 50% leaving through the back, only 30% remains after 1 cycle, 9% after 2 cycles, and less than 1% after 4 cycles. This is called a low Q transducer because it wastes so much energy, but makes images with good depth resolution because the transmitting pulse is so short and the receiving response is so quick. The wasted energy makes the transducer warm. Such transducers are also inefficient from an energy point of view.

Two new methods are used in modern transducers to lower the Q and improve depth resolution (Figure 3–5). One method is to couple the transducer more effectively to the skin by using a piezoelectric material with lower impedance or using a matching layer of intermediate impedance, one-quarter wavelength thick, between the transducer and the skin. The other method is to combine the damping material with the piezoelectric material in the transducer; piezoelectric columns span from electrode to electrode with damping material between the columns. The first method makes the transducer more efficient as a transmitter and as a receiver. The second method makes transmitting and receiving less efficient.

Broad Band and Narrow Band

Well-damped and well-coupled transducers create short pulses that provide good depth resolution. When tested for the presence of a series of frequencies, positive tests are found over a broad band of frequencies (Figure 3–6).

Lateral Direction in the Image Ultrasound Beam Pattern Width

Ultrasound pulses are sent into tissue along a beam pattern that is established by the location, orientation, widths, and shape of the active ultrasound transducer. The beam pattern is quite complex. It is useful to begin with a simplified view of the ultrasound beam

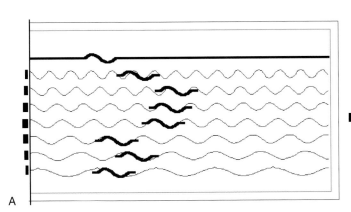

A

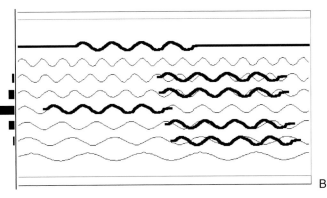

B

FIGURE 3–6. (A) Broad bandwidth pulse. A short pulse has a broad bandwidth because so many frequencies exhibit an equally poor fit with the pulse. The results of each frequency test are shown as a bar graph spectrum on the left. (B) Moderate bandwidth pulse. A long pulse has a moderate bandwidth because several frequencies exhibit a fit with the pulse. Note: the middle frequency is the best fit. The results of each frequency test are shown as a bar graph spectrum on the left. (C) Narrow bandwidth wave. The continuous wave has a narrow bandwidth because only one frequency exhibits a fit with the wave. The results of each frequency test are shown as a bar graph spectrum on the left.

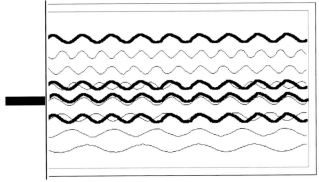

C

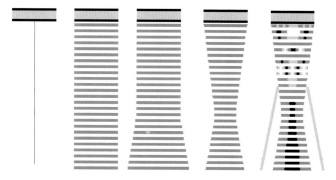

FIGURE 3–7. Concepts of ultrasound beam patterns. Increasingly sophisticated concepts of ultrasound beam patterns. From left to right: thin beam pattern, collimated beam pattern, beam pattern with Fraunhoffer zone, beam pattern with Transition zone natural focus and Fraunhoffer zone, beam pattern with Fresnel zone, Transition zone natural focus, Fraunhoffer zone, and first-order sidelobes.

pattern and then to include aspects of the complexity in steps.

In the simplest view, the ultrasound beam pattern is a straight line that extends into tissue along the axis of the ultrasound transducer. If the ultrasound transducer is a disk, the beam pattern is a line through the center of the disk perpendicular to the surface. In a slightly more complex view (Figure 3–7), the ultrasound beam pattern is a cylinder extending from the face of the transducer. Because ultrasound is a wave, the shape of the ultrasound beam pattern includes diffraction effects that alter the shape of the beam pattern near the transducer (Fresnel zone), far from the transducer (Fraunhoffer zone), and at the boundary between these regions (Transition zone). In

the Fresnel zone, there is a patchwork of regions of high intensity and low intensity. From the Transition zone into the Fraunhoffer zone, the ultrasound beam pattern is smoother. The distance from the transducer face to the Transition zone (L) is determined by half the transducer width ($W/2$) and the wavelength (λ). In a circular transducer ($W/2$) is the radius.

$$L = (W/2)/\lambda$$

Thus, with shorter wavelength or a larger diameter transducer [that is if (W/λ) is larger], the length of the region over which the beam converges increases. The width of the ultrasound beam at the transition zone is half of the transducer width. By increasing the bandwidth of the transducer, unwanted variations in the beam pattern are smoothed out (Figure 3–8).

Focusing and Lateral Resolution

The width of the ultrasound beam pattern may be decreased to improve lateral resolution by focusing. To achieve focusing, a transducer may have a concave face, a lens added to the front, and/or segmentation into an array with delayed action at the center. The beam diameter at the focus is narrow compared to the half transducer width natural focus at the Transition zone (Figure 3–9). Focusing causes the beam to be narrow at one depth. With such a narrow beam, the space between closely positioned reflectors can be identified as the beam passes between them. It is easy to obtain reflections from objects in tissue, but it is difficult to detect and display the space between objects. The minimum separation distance between objects recognized as separate is the resolution. A smaller number is better. The lateral resolution is

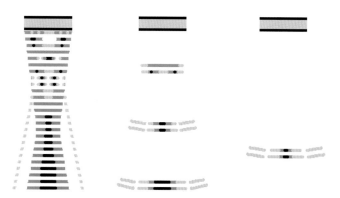

FIGURE 3–8. Beam pattern for damped transducers. The narrow band continuous wave transducer on the left has a complex Fresnel zone and narrow sidelobes. The broad band, high pulse repetition frequency (PRF) transducer in the center and the broad band, low PRF transducer on the right have a smoothed Fresnel zone and broadened sidelobes due to the differences in patterns for each of the frequency components.

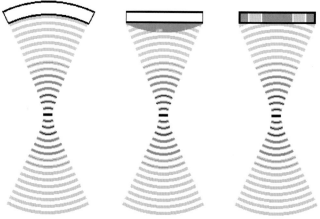

FIGURE 3–9. Focusing of ultrasound beam patterns. Left: transducer with concave face. Middle: transducer with lens. Right: phased focus transducer.

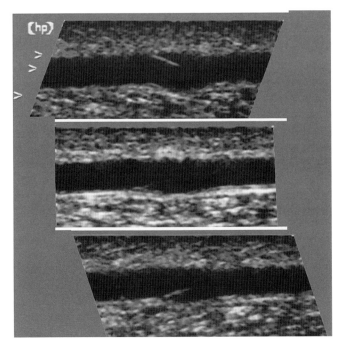

FIGURE 3–10. Venous valve leaflets in a reverse saphenous vein graft seen only when scanlines are perpendicular. In the upper image with the scanlines angled left, the upper venous valve leaflet can be seen because the ultrasound beam patterns are perpendicular to it. In the middle image with the scanlines angled down, the double line of Pignoli (intima-media thickness) can be seen because the ultrasound beam patterns are perpendicular to it. In the lower image with the scanlines angled right, the lower venous valve leaflet can be seen because the ultrasound beam patterns are perpendicular to it.

$A = 2F\lambda/W$. So if the transducer diameter is half of the focal length, then the lateral resolution at the focal depth is four times the wavelength of the ultrasound. The resolution deteriorates in regions shallower and deeper than the focus. Therefore it is very important to adjust the focus of an ultrasound transducer carefully.

It is essential to recognize that depth resolution is always near the wavelength of ultrasound. Lateral resolution is always much larger (poorer). Therefore details can be seen in the depth direction even when features in the lateral direction are obscure. Many examiners see the detail in the depth direction and assume that the resolution is isotropic so that the lateral image detail is also present. This leads to misinterpretation of the image. By steering and angling the transducer, features visible in one view are not visible in another (Figure 3–10). These features become visible when the ultrasound beam is perpendicular to a specular reflector providing superior depth resolution.

Refractive Distortion

As ultrasound travels through and crosses a boundary from one tissue with one ultrasound speed to another tissue with another ultrasound speed, the direction of ultrasound propagation changes due to refraction. The angle of deflection of the beam is determined by Snell's law: $C_2/C_1 = \sin \theta_2 / \sin \theta_1$ where the angle of deflection is equal to $\theta_2 - \theta_1$ (Table 3–10). If ultrasound passes from fat into a prism of muscle at an incident angle of 30°, the deflection angle is 2.7°. If the ultrasound continues through the muscle back into fat leaving the prism at an angle of 30°, the deflection is an additional 3°, which is a total deflection of 5.7°. In the midline of the abdomen, the rectus abdominus muscles and the fat-filled linea alba act as a pair of prisms tilting a left-directed ultrasound beam toward the right and a right-directed ultrasound beam toward the left. These two beams, which are expected to image structures 2.2 cm apart at a depth of 11 cm, cross and provide echoes from the same structure. The ultrasound machine shows two objects when only one is actually present in tissue (Figure 3–11).

Refractive distortion can alter dimensions and numbers of objects in the lateral direction in any ultrasound image. Therefore dimensional measurements in

TABLE 3–10. Ultrasound beam deflection at different interfaces between materials.

Incident angle is 30°		Material on the superficial side of the interface							
Speed in mm/μs		Fat	Urine	Liver	Blood	Muscle	Bone	Cartilage	PZT[a]
	Speed	1.45	1.49	1.54	1.57	1.58	1.65	3.5	3.8
Tissue									
Fat	1.45	0	0.884	1.915	2.498	2.686	3.935	18.05	19
Urine	1.49	−0.92	0	1.068	1.672	1.867	3.159	17.71	18.69
Liver	1.54	−2.08	−1.793	0	0.63	0.834	2.182	17.29	18.31
Blood	1.57	−2.78	−1.793	−0.65	0	0.209	1.591	17.04	18.08
Muscle	1.58	−3.01	−2.019	−0.86	−0.21	0	1.394	16.96	18
Cartilage	1.65	−4.68	−3.621	−2.39	−1.7	−1.48	0	16.37	17.46
Bone	3.5	−120[b]	−120[b]	−120[b]	−120[b]	−120[b]	−120[b]	0	2.579
PZT	3.8	−120[b]	−120[b]	−120[b]	−120[b]	−120[b]	−120[b]	−2.88	0

[a] PZT (PbZrTi), lead zirconium titanite.
[b] Deflection angles greater than 90° means that total internal reflection has occurred.

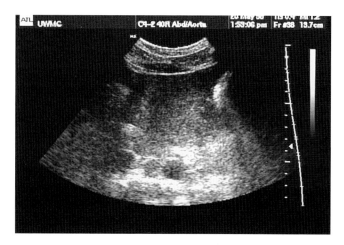

FIGURE 3–11. Duplication of abdominal aorta image due to ultrasound beam refraction. Beginning at a depth of 11 cm at the center of the image, the 1.8-cm-diameter aorta can be seen (pulsating in real time); 2.2 cm to the left of that image is a second image of the aorta (pulsating in real time). A further 2.4 cm to the left is the 2.1-cm-diameter inferior vena cava. The "duplication" of the aorta is due to ultrasound refraction from the linea alba/rectus abdominus muscles.[2]

the lateral direction are hampered by two factors: (1) poor lateral resolution and (2) lateral refractive distortion. This distortion becomes obvious only when duplicated structures are seen. A duplicated aorta is an unbelievable finding. A twin blastocyst in early pregnancy is believable. A duplicated aortic valve due to refraction in the peristernal cartilage is unbelievable.

Reflective duplications also occur such as the duplication of the subclavian artery image due to reflection of ultrasound from the pleura. Refractive duplications show both structures at generally the same depth; reflective duplications usually show the duplicate at a deeper depth. Duplications appear in B-mode images and in color Doppler images. Spectral waveforms can be obtained from both images. Therefore the only defense against misdiagnosis is knowledge of anatomy and of anatomic anomalies.

Sidelobes

Undesired sidelobes are also present in the beam patterns of ultrasound transducers, in addition to the desired central beam patterns. Sidelobes degrade the image. The sidelobes are shown in Figure 3–7 as lines angled out to the left and right of the image. If the transducer is circular, the beam pattern is symmetrical around the axis of the beam pattern. Thus, the sidelobe(s) look like a cone extending from the face of the transducer. The angle at which the sidelobes diverge (μ) can be computed from the ultrasound wavelength and the transducer width (W).

$$\text{Sin } \alpha = [(2n + 1) \times \lambda]/(2 \times W)$$

n is any integer that is equal to 1 or greater. If (W/λ) is large, then n can have many values and therefore many sidelobes form. The position of each sidelobe is determined by the wavelength.

Sidelobes are a problem in imaging because strong reflectors in tissue that are located within a sidelobe at a distance of 3 cm from the transducer will send a weak echo back to the ultrasound transducer that is indistinguishable from an echo from a weak reflector in the strong central beam at the same depth. The ultrasound instrument will show the sidelobe echo in the image as a reflector along the central beam direction. This is one of the causes of poor ultrasound images.

The amplitude of the signal along the sidelobe portion of the beam is about $1/n$ of the central amplitude, diminished further by the divergence of the sidelobe pattern. For $n = 3$, the sidelobe amplitude is 1/3, the power is 1/9, and the receiver sensitivity is 1/9. The overall pulse-echo strength is diminished 1/81 compared to a similar reflector in the central lobe of the beam pattern. The reduction is greater when the effect of divergence is included. So the echo from the sidelobe is suppressed by about 20 dB (about 1/100) compared to echoes from the beam axis. The difference in echogenicity between blood and muscle at 5 MHz is about 30 dB, so a strong reflector in the sidelobe could appear to be along the beam in the image inside a blood vessel where the central lobe echoes are weak.

Other factors and methods can suppress sidelobes. One method is to cut notches in the boundary of the transducer so that the width W is fuzzy. This will smear the sidelobes. A similar method is to reduce the transmit strength and receive sensitivity near the edge of the transducer. This method is called apodization. The sidelobe position depends on wavelength (λ) as well as width (W). Therefore, a broad band transducer with a range of wavelengths will have smeared sidelobes with diminished sensitivity.

Sidelobe effects are more severe in Doppler kinds of imaging because large differences in amplitude are ignored in the signal analysis process, minimizing the difference between sidelobe echoes and beam axis echoes.

Thickness Direction in the Image Ultrasound Beam Pattern Thickness

Most ultrasound instruments use one-dimensional electronic array transducers to sweep the ultrasound beam across a plane in tissue to form an image (Figure 3–12). The fixed focusing in the thickness direction causes the beam pattern to be thick at most depths. Therefore objects in tissue that are outside the tissue "plane" are included in the image (Figure 3–13).

An additional interesting feature of Figure 3–13 is the presence of reflected images. A moderately bright circu-

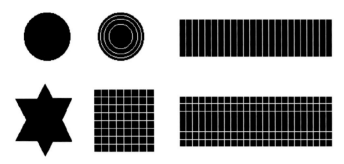

FIGURE 3–12. Different arrangements of ultrasound transducers from the patient view. Upper left: circular single element transducer. Upper center: annular array transducer for electronic focusing. Upper right: linear array transducer for electronic beam pointing in the lateral direction and fixed mechanical focus in the thickness direction. Lower left: single element "star" transducer to suppress sidelobes; a five-point design or seven-point design is preferred because of fewer symmetries. Lower center: two-dimensional array to steer the beam electronically in two directions for three-dimensional imaging. Lower right: 1.5-dimensional array to steer the beam electronically in the lateral direction and electronically focus the beam in the thickness direction.

lar image of the straw appears below the "real" image. This deeper image is formed because of ultrasound that reflects from the lower straw surface, back up to the upper straw surface, then back down to the lower straw

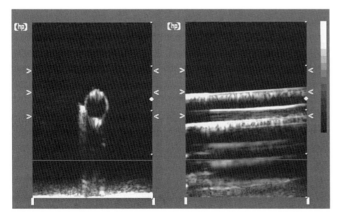

FIGURE 3–13. Five-millimeter-diameter straw in cross section and longitudinal section. To demonstrate the effect of ultrasound image thickness on the image of a 5-mm-diameter vein graft, a 5-mm-diameter drinking straw is imaged in a water tank. A wire was attached to the side, outside the lumen. In cross section (left) the wire can be seen outside the lumen. In longitudinal section on the right, the wire image appears to be within the lumen between the superficial and deep walls. The strong specular (mirror like) reflections from the superficial and deep walls combined with excessive image gain cause a "blooming" of the image that smears the echoes making the superficial and deep walls appear thicker than they are. Reducing the ultrasound transmit power will provide a proper image of the perpendicular wall thickness.

surface and finally back to the transducer. The additional time for that "reverberant" trip forms the moderately bright reflected image. A third deeper image is also barely detectable.

Time of Image Acquisition Frame Interval/Sweep

When ultrasound image data are acquired, data along each line extending from the scanhead into tissue are gathered within one pulse-echo cycle. The conventional two-dimensional image is formed by a series of such lines, each gathered in sequence. Common formats are sector from a phase or curved array or raster from a linear array (Figure 3–14). With modern linear arrays, the location of the aperture can be selected as well as the direction of beam pointing (Figure 3–15).

The time to acquire data from each scan line is determined by two factors: (1) the maximum depth from which data are coming, and (2) the number of pulse-echo cycles required to acquire the data from the scanline (ensemble length). The time for each pulse-echo cycle is $T = 2 \times D/C$ where D is the maximum depth and C is the speed of ultrasound. For a maximum depth of 3 cm, the time required is 40 µs and for a maximum depth of 15 cm, the time required is 200 µs. For B-mode imaging, the ensemble length is 1 and for typical Doppler color flow imaging, the ensemble length is 8 (Table 3–11).

In a typical Doppler color flow image that is 3 cm wide (Figure 3–15), the images are formed from 128 B-mode scanlines and 64 color scanlines. The B-mode scanlines extend to a depth of 6 cm (requiring 80 µs) for each of the 128 scanlines. The B-mode portion of the image requires (80 µs × 128) 10.2 ms for image formation. The color scanlines extend to a depth of 3 cm (requiring 40 µs each cycle) with an ensemble length of 8 requiring (40 µs × 8) 320 µs for each of the 64 scanlines. The color Doppler portion of the image requires (320 µs × 64) 20.5 ms for image formation. The total time to create the image is (10.2 ms + 20.5 ms) 30.7 ms, which nearly matches the 33 ms time for each image in a standard ultrasound

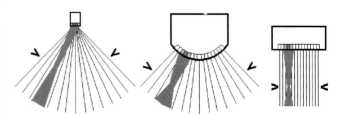

FIGURE 3–14. Image scan formats. Left: sector format from a phase array. Middle: sector format from a curved linear array. Right: raster format from a straight linear array.

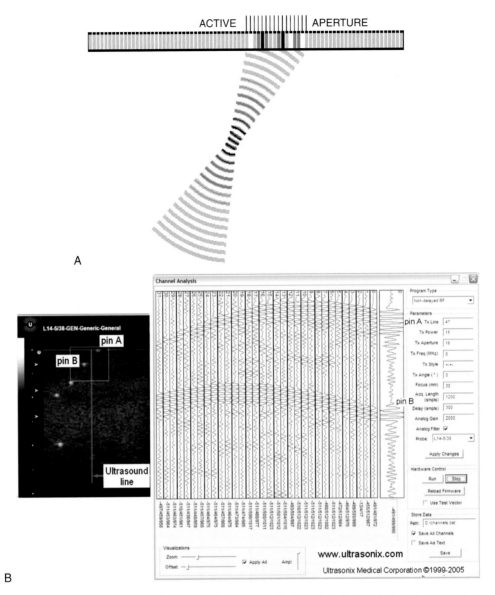

FIGURE 3–15. (A) Modern phased-linear array beam steering. The ability to steer the beam pattern to a variety of angles for B-mode imaging is easier that to steer to a variety of angles for Doppler data. (B) Receiver channel echoes from each transducer. The echoes received by each of 32 transducer elements are displayed. Before adding the transducer data together, "beam forming" time delays are introduced on each channel to align the echoes from a particular depth and location, then the data from the channels are added to produce "beam formed" RF data for demodulation and display.

(National Television Standard Code) at 30 images per second. If greater depths are required, then more time is required for each scanline and either the number of scanlines or the frame rate must be sacrificed.

In "real time" imaging, a frame is not formed instantly, but the data are acquired systematically from left to right. In Doppler color flow imaging, the data for color lines are acquired in sequence across the 3 cm image width in 0.02 s (20 ms); the acquisition proceeds from left to right at a speed of 150 cm/s. This speed should be compared with the speeds in the vascular system: wall motion <1 cm/s, average arterial blood velocity = 30 cm/s, and pulse propagation speed = 1000 cm/s. It takes about five cardiac cycles for blood to travel 150 cm from the heart to the toes; it takes only 0.15 s for the pulse to travel from the heart to the toes. Note that the speed of the Doppler acquisition line moves across the image more slowly than the pulse propagation speed. This causes a time distortion in all color flow images (Figure 3–16).

TABLE 3-11. Ultrasound modes and factors.[a]

Factor	Ultrasound operating modes					
	B-mode	Color power angiography	Color flow imaging	Pulsed Doppler waveform	CW Doppler	Harmonic imaging
Ultrasound frequency	b	c	c	c	c	Depressed Tx Elevated Rcv
Ultrasound bandwidth	Wide	Moderate	Moderate	Moderate	Narrow	Broad split
Demodulation method	Amplitude	Phase	Phase	Phase	Phase	Band filtered/pulse invert
Ensemble length	1	8	8	128	NA	1 or 2
PRF	Max	Low	Max	Max	0	Max or max/2
Filter method	None	Hi pass	Hi pass	Hi pass	Hi pass	Dual band
Analysis method	Square sum	Variance	Lambda	FFT	Heterodyne	Square sum
Display method	Gray	Colorize	Bicolor	Gray/V-t	Audio	Gray
Frame rate	High	Low	Moderate	0	0	High or moderate
Averaging	None	Time and space	Time	None	Time or none	None or difference

[a]CW, continuous wave; PRF, pulse repetition frequency; FFT, fast Fourier transform.

[b]The dynamic range of echogenicity of solid tissues in ultrasound images is about 42 dB (7 bits in a computer) and most instruments are capable of processing a dynamic range of 96 dB (16 bits). Thus, echoes attenuated by 54 dB still have the full dynamic range. A soft tissue layer that attenuates ultrasound by 10 dB is 67 wavelengths (from the attenuation discussion). So the roundtrip path of $(67 \times 54/10)$ 360 wavelengths defines the maximum imaging depth, or 180 wavelengths deep.

[c]The echogenicity of blood is 54 dB (9 bits) lower than the brightest solid tissues in ultrasound images. Thus, for attenuation and Doppler from blood in the presence of solid tissues, 42 dB (7 bits) remains. Blood echogenicity increases with the fourth power of the frequency of ultrasound. Selection of the best ultrasound frequency depends on the balance between increased blood echogenicity and increased attenuation. For blood vessels in liver (0.5 dB/MHz/cm) the best ultrasound frequency is $F = 1.7\,\text{cm MHz}/d$ where d is the depth of the blood vessel in cm.

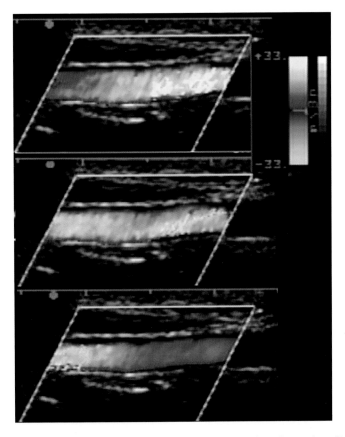

FIGURE 3-16. The effect of image sweep speed on color flow images. These are three images of the same segment of an artery taken in sequence. Although we intend to show distance displayed along the horizontal dimension, because of the slow sweep speed compared to the pulse propagation speed, the horizontal dimension shows time. Peak systole shows as an aliased blue velocity. In the bottom image, the Doppler data were acquired near the left edge of the image during peak systole; in the middle image, the Doppler data were acquired near the right edge of the image during peak systole.

The interaction between the pulse propagation speed and the Doppler acquisition speed suggests that a "systolic velocity bolus" is just 2 cm long, however, high systolic velocities appear at the toes while they are still present at the aortic valve during systole.

Learning about the Tissues within Voxels

In modern ultrasound systems, the information displayed in each pixel about the corresponding voxel depends on the selection of 10 factors: (1) the frequency of the ultrasound pulse transmitted into tissue—"ultrasound frequency," (2) the shape and duration of the ultrasound pulse transmitted into tissue—"ultrasound bandwidth," (3) the measurements made on the echo that come from the voxel—"demodulation method," (4) the number of times that similar pulse-echo cycles are from the voxel—"ensemble length," (5) the time interval between the pulse-echo cycles—"pulse repetition interval" (the

inverse of the pulse repetition frequency, PRF), (6) the filter method, (7) the analysis method, (8) the display method, (9) the time required to update the other pixels on the screen—"frame interval" (the inverse of frame rate), and (10) averaging between times and/or between pixels. The basic modes of ultrasound imaging can be characterized by the alternative choices between the possibilities of each of these factors.

The process of voxel interrogation has two parts: an analog part and a digital part. In modern ultrasound scanners, most of the processing is done digitally. In old instruments everything was done with analog electronics. Figure 3–17 diagrams the analog signal portion of a modern instrument. This Figure is the basis for describing the methods.

The ultrasound transmit pulse consists of a selected number of cycles. Transmit voltages applied to the transducer range from 4 to 400 V. The echo is segmented into pixels that are equal in length to the transmit pulse. In modern ultrasound imaging systems, the radio frequency oscillations in each pixel are converted to a digital signal. The voltages along the oscillation are measured, four times for each cycle, and the measured numbers are combined to form the digital signal. This process is called digitization. In modern instruments, each measurement has a dynamic range of 16 bits (binary digits). Each operating mode has a different pulse protocol and computation method.

Each of the following modes will be described using the same format. The number of cycles in the transmit pulse will be specified; this number will be called m. The duration of each received pixel is equal to the transmit pulse duration. The oscillations in each received pixel will be digitized at a frequency equal to four times the transmitted frequency, so there will be $4m$ sampled measurements digitized. Each of those sampled voltages will be identified by number. In the case in Figure 3–17 with two cycles transmitted, there are two cycles in each received pixel and 4×2 or 8 samples in each pixel. The sampled voltages are called V_1, V_2, V_3, V_4, V_5, V_6, V_7, and V_8. Finally, we may need to transmit along the ultrasound beam line more than once to determine if the tissue is moving. The number of times that we transmit, called ensemble length, will be called k. From here, the method is as simple as an income tax form.

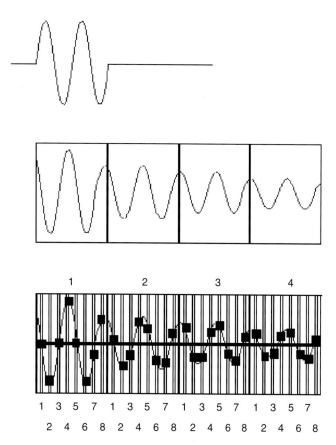

FIGURE 3–17. Ultrasound echo signals and demodulation. Upper: ultrasound transmit pulse. Middle: radio frequency ultrasound echo segmented into pixels. Lower: pixels parsed for digitization.

B-Mode Imaging at 5 MHz

The length of the transmit pulse is short to create the best depth resolution, therefore $m = 1$. At 5 MHz, one cycle lasts just 0.2 μs. The echo digitizing rate is four times the transmit frequency or 20 MHz. The pixel is short, containing just one cycle, so we digitize just four voltages, called V_1, V_2, V_3, and V_4. Now we calculate the energy in that 0.2-μs segment of the echo.

TABLE 3–12. Conversion of time gain compensation adjusted received voltages into a brightness scale.[a]

0	1	2	3	5	7	11	15	22	31	45	63	90	127	181	255
0	1	2	3	4	6	8	12	16	23	32	46	64	91	128	182
0	**1**	**2**	**3**	**4**	**5**	**6**	**7**	**8**	**9**	**10**	**11**	**12**	**13**	**14**	**15**

[a]Upper row: upper bound of voltage range. Middle row: lower bound of voltage range. Lower row: corresponding brightness level.

$$\text{Echo energy for each pixel} = V_1^2 + V_2^2 + V_3^2 + V_4^2$$

The pixels with the highest energies are displayed as white on the screen and the pixels with the lowest energies are displayed as black. An inverted gray scale or colorized scale may also be used.

Before display, time gain compensation is applied. For a pixel representing depth d from a tissue with attenuation rate A in dB/cm/MHz and ultrasound frequency F, the measured pixel voltage (square root of energy) is multiplied by $1.26^{A \times d \times F}$.

The eye can see only 16 levels of gray. Video screens display about the same. To convert 256 possible brightness levels into 16 levels of gray, the brightness levels are usually converted by postprocessing into a logarithmic brightness scale using Table 3–12.

Digitizing for Flow Measurement

To prepare for the flow imaging methods, we should show how to determine the amplitude and phase of the echo oscillation in the pixel. It is equal to the square root of the energy. The computation requires two numbers, I and Q.

$$I = V_1 - V_3$$

and

$$Q = V_2 - V_4$$

With algebra you can show that

$$\text{Energy} = I^2 + Q^2$$

if

$$V_1 \times V_3 + V_2 \times V_4 = 0$$

which is true in the absence of harmonics that result from high ultrasound intensities or the presence of ultrasound contrast agents.

I and Q can be used to form a diagram (Figure 3–18) that shows both the phase and the amplitude of the wave. The amplitude is shown as distance from the origin of the plot and the phase is shown as angle. This phase map forms the basis of the flow imaging methods.

Autocorrelation Doppler

For all Doppler methods, the length of the transmit pulse is long, about 5 cycles or 1 μs at 5 MHz to ensure that the phase measurement is accurate. The echo digitizing rate

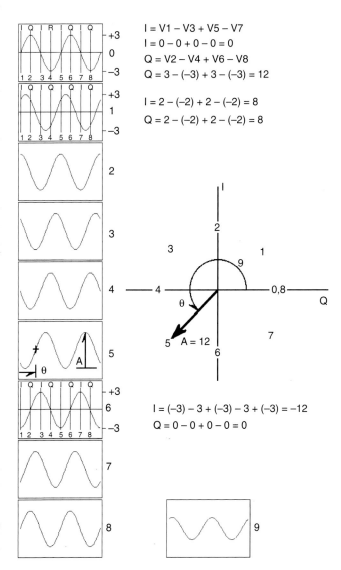

$I = V1 - V3 + V5 - V7$
$I = 0 - 0 + 0 - 0 = 0$
$Q = V2 - V4 + V6 - V8$
$Q = 3 - (-3) + 3 - (-3) = 12$

$I = 2 - (-2) + 2 - (-2) = 8$
$Q = 2 - (-2) + 2 - (-2) = 8$

$I = (-3) - 3 + (-3) - 3 + (-3) = -12$
$Q = 0 - 0 + 0 - 0 = 0$

FIGURE 3–18. Formation of a phase diagram from an ultrasound echo pixel.

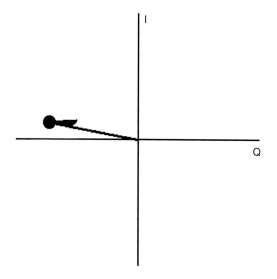

FIGURE 3–19. *I/Q* plot for one pulse-echo cycle.

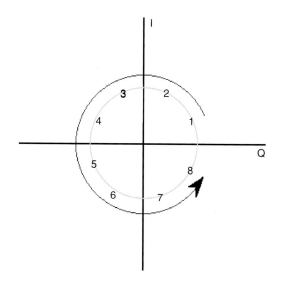

FIGURE 3–20. *I/Q* plot for eight pulse-echo cycles from tissue moving through the sample volume.

is 20 MHz. The pixel is long containing five cycles, so 20 voltage values are digitized to represent the voxel, V_1 to V_{20}. Then the phase of the echo in the voxel is calculated by computing the components *I* and *Q*.

$$I = V_1 - V_3 + V_5 - V_7 + V_9 - V_{11} + V_{13} - V_{15} + V_{17} - V_{19}$$

and

$$Q = V_2 - V_4 + V_6 - V_8 + V_{10} - V_{12} + V_{14} - V_{16} + V_{18} - V_{20}$$

The measurement produces a single value on the *I* vs. *Q* phase plane (Figure 3–19). From the value, the amplitude can be determined, but the phase has little meaning. The amplitude is the distance from the origin to the measurement. The energy is the square of the amplitude. By the Pythagorean theorem, the echo energy is $I^2 + Q^2$.

If the process of transmitting a pulse along a beam pattern and receiving an echo from the selected depth is repeated eight times, the resulting echo samples from the voxel under investigation can be compared. If the tissue in the voxel has neither moved nor changed, then over the period of the sampling, all samples are identical. If, however, all the tissue in the sample volume is moving toward the ultrasound transducer, then the magnitude will stay constant, but the phase of the echo will progressively change and each of the echoes will contribute a point to a circle of rotation around the origin (Figure 3–20). The number of samples collected from each voxel, to form this circle, is called the ensemble length.

In Figure 3–20, in each pulse repetition interval (PRI = 1/PRF), the phase of the echo has moved 1/8 cycle toward the transducer. The velocity component toward

the transducer is

$$V_D = dp \times \lambda/(2 \times PRI) = dp \times \lambda \times PRF/2$$
$$= (dp/PRI) \times (C/F) \times (1/2)$$

where = *dp* is the fraction of a complete cycle that the phase has shifted between one echo to another, λ is the ultrasound wavelength (*C/F*), 2 accounts for the round trip of the ultrasound, PRI is the time between echo samples, and PRF is the number of echo samples per second.

The component of the blood velocity measured by the Doppler is the leg of a right triangle. A right triangle can be circumscribed with a semicircle with the hypotenuse (the real velocity vector) shown in Figure 3–21. The com-

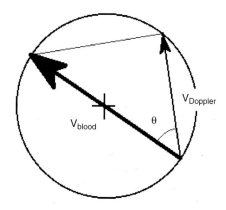

FIGURE 3–21. Component of blood velocity measured by Doppler.

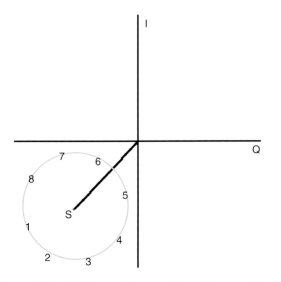

FIGURE 3–22. *I/Q* phase diagram with stationary echo *S*.

ponent velocity is represented by a cord of the circle formed by the blood velocity as diameter.

$$V_D \times \cos \theta = V_D = (dp/\mathrm{PRI}) \times (C/F) \times (1/2)$$
$$= (f/2) \times (C/F)$$

This is the well-known Doppler equation where (dp/PRI) is known as the Doppler frequency and happens, by fortunate chance, to be in the audible frequency range.

Unfortunately, in many cases, the interrogated Voxel contains echogenic solid tissue as well as moving blood so the phase diagram usually looks like Figure 3–22. The phase circle is rotating in a counterclockwise direction so the velocity component is away from the transducer. The stationary echo *S* makes analysis more difficult. If only

two pulse-echo cycles were taken, then an incorrect velocity measurement would result. Although the direction of rotation appears to be counterclockwise, as indicated by the arrow suggesting flow away from the transducer in Figure 3–23, the flow could be aliased, twice as fast toward the transducer.

In a color flow image, flow toward the transducer indicated by clockwise rotation on the *I/Q* diagram is usually shown as a red pixel on the image and flow away from the transducer indicated by counterclockwise rotation on the *I/Q* diagram is usually shown as a blue pixel on the image. If the points do not form a uniform circle on the *I/Q* phase diagram, then the signal contains variance; cardiac color Doppler systems show high variance as a green pixel on the image.

Color Power Angiography

Blood vessels usually are parallel to the skin and Doppler ultrasound beams are nearly perpendicular to the skin and vessels. Therefore, the Doppler examination angle is usually greater than 45° to the vessel axis. For convenience and consistency, many examiners use a Doppler examination angle of 60° between the ultrasound beam pattern and the vessel axis. However, the normal blood flow in a blood vessel is helical, converging into stenoses and diverging downstream. Therefore, color Doppler images usually contain intriguing color changes that can be confusing. To avoid the confusion of "too much information" some instruments provide a feature called "color power angiography," which shows pixels with blood motion in color without showing direction. These systems are based on an ensemble of pulse-echo cycles plotted on a phase diagram such as Figure 3–24.

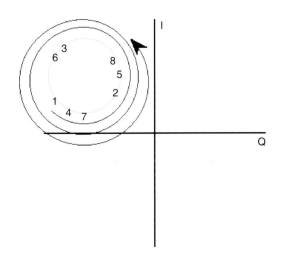

FIGURE 3–23. *I/Q* phase diagram with stationary echo *S* and high velocity flow.

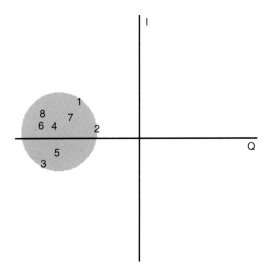

FIGURE 3–24. *I/Q* diagram for color power angiography.

In the example, data from a voxel acquired by eight pulse-echo cycles are shown. All of the echoes fall within the shaded region. The area of the shaded region on the *I/Q* diagram is the "Doppler power."

Fast Fourier Transform Spectral Waveform

The fast fourier transform (FFT) spectral waveform is created from the same kind of data as shown in Figures 3–18 through 3–23. The FFT spectrum uses 128 pulse-echo cycles for input data from a single voxel in tissue for each spectrum. A waveform is a collection of 100 spectra per second. Each *I/Q* phase diagram contains 128 points. The period of data gathering is about 10 ms (for a PRF of 12.8 kHz). The voxel (sample volume) is about 1 mm across. If the blood velocity is 100 cm/s (1000 mm/s), a cluster of red blood cells will cross the voxel in 1 ms; during the 10-ms data acquisition period, the blood in the voxel will be completely exchanged 10 times. There is no relationship between the phase of the echo of one cluster of red blood cells and another. Therefore every millisecond (13 pulse-echo cycles) the point on the phase diagram is unrelated to the prior phase. This introduces transit time spectral broadening into the spectral waveform.[3] Spectral broadening also occurs because of fluctuations in the blood velocity and because of system noise. The spectral broadening can be manipulated by adjusting the voxel size. It can also be used to measure "transverse velocity." Spectral broadening and spectral shape, however, are most useful for figuring out complex flow dynamics because they show all of the velocities all of the time.

A spectral waveform from a voxel shows the detailed time history of the flow through that voxel. Two-dimensional color flow imaging shows a single velocity for each voxel between 10 and 30 times per second (frame rate). Hemodynamic eddies can oscillate at frequencies of 50 Hz or greater. The FFT waveform, displayed 100 times per second, can show those eddies.

Conclusion

Over the past half century noninvasive examination of vascular disease has advanced greatly as Doppler methods were augmented with B-mode imaging to form duplex scanners. Duplex pulse Doppler spectral waveform analysis has become the standard noninvasive method for evaluating arterial stenoses, venous obstruction, and venous valve incompetence. The evolution has benefited from contributions by both manufacturers and clinical examiners. Confusions and disagreements are a natural part of that process. One of those disagreements is over the visualization of lesions and plaques in ultrasound B-mode images. Many examiners have classified plaque as "hard," "soft," "heterogeneous," "homogeneous," or "intimal thickening." In our experience, B-mode imaging of vascular structures has not provided clinically useful information. Another disagreement is the question of choice of Doppler examination angle. Because the geometry of arteries and veins prevents the use of coaxial ultrasound beams (which are possible when examining the aortic and mitral valves), some examiners believe that the cosine of the examination angle can be used to "correct" the velocity measurement taken at the poor angles permitted by anatomical restrictions. Other examiners believe that the definition of velocity is obscure, that a consistent examination angle should be used, and that the resultant velocity value should be used only in comparison with an empirical standard. We subscribe to the latter view.

All examiners hope that new examination methods such as color flow imaging can improve diagnostic accuracy. This is an elusive goal because each examination method has strengths and weaknesses. Comparison between methods yields surprises and increased understanding. A comparison between velocity measurements taken with color flow imaging and taken with Doppler spectral waveform (Figure 3–25) demonstrates the disagreement in results that invite resolution.

To ensure that the different modes of Doppler display work in concert, the methods of two-dimensional color Doppler imaging, color Doppler M-mode imaging and spectral waveform imaging should be combined (Figure 3–26). This permits an exact comparison between the Doppler FFT spectral waveform velocity information and the autocorrelation color display. Note that the two methods of velocity determination occur in different sections of the ultrasound system and use different ensemble lengths. Therefore, the velocity ranges and baseline shift can be set differently.

Ultrasound instruments are passing through a new rapid evolution, plunging in cost and size. It is now possible for a patient to buy an ultrasound system to wear and obtain constant examination.[4] It is also possible to obtain a correct velocity measurement from peripheral blood vessels without assumptions about the examination angle[5–8] and to measure tissue pulsations and vibrations as small as 0.05 μm. The depth derivative of displacement is pulsatility. It is possible to measure pulsatility due to capillary filling and display this information in ultrasound images.[9–11] This method has been used by Robert Pretlow to show that cancerous tissues in breast have pulse amplitudes three times as high as normal tissues. It has also been used by

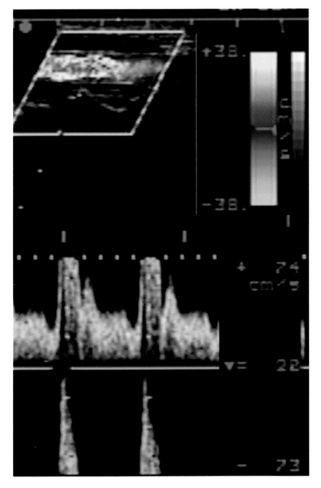

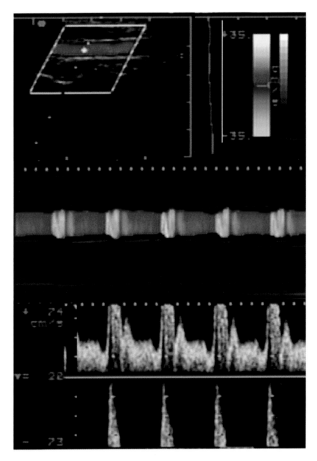

FIGURE 3–26. Combined spectral waveform and color M-mode imaging.

FIGURE 3–25. Comparison between Doppler color velocity and spectral waveform velocity. The peak systolic velocity according to the aliased color flow image is 38 + 30 or 68 cm/s. The peak systolic velocity according to the aliased spectral waveform is 74 + 70 or 144 cm/s. The difference in measured values could be a difference in angle adjustment and/or a difference in the processing of color flow data vs. spectral waveform data. In spite of the high velocity, which is localized in the middle of the color flow image, no stenosis is present in this artery. Arterial systole occurred by chance as the color flow data for the center of the image were being acquired.

John Kucewicz to show maternal and fetal pulsations in the placenta.

With access to internet information services, it is easy to keep track of the latest advancements in the medical literature[12] and the most recent patents.[13]

Acknowledgments. This work was supported by the Defense Research Projects Administration (DARPA) and the Office of Naval Research (ONR) N00014-96-1-0630.

References

1. Comess KA, Beach KW, Hatsukami T, Strandness DE Jr, Daniel-W. Pseudocolor displays in B-mode imaging applied to echocardiography and vascular imaging: An update. J Am Soc Echocardiogr 1992;5(1):13–32.
2. Vandeman FN, Meilstrup JW, Nealy PA. Acoustic prism causing sonographic duplication artifact in the upper abdomen. Invest Radiol 1990;25:658–63.
3. McArdle A, Newhouse VL, Beach KW. Demonstration of three-dimensional vector flow estimation using bandwidth and two transducers on a flow phantom. Ultrasound Med Biol 1995;21(5):679–92.
4. http://www.dxu.com/pci5000_f.html.
5. Papadofrangakis E, Engeler WE, Fakiris JA. Measurement of true blood velocity by an ultrasound system. U.S. Patent 4265126: Assignees: General Electric Company, Schenectady, NY; Issued: May 5, 1981; Filed: June 15, 1979.
6. Beach K, Overbeck J. Vector Doppler medical devices for blood velocity studies. U.S. Patent 5409010: Board of Regents of the University of Washington, Seattle, WA; Issued: April 25, 1995; Filed: May 19, 1992.
7. Overbeck J, Beach KW, Strandness DE Jr. Vector Doppler: Accurate measurement of blood velocity in two dimensions. Ultrasound Med Biol 1992;18(1):19–31.

8. Beach KW, Dunmire B, Overbeck JR, Waters D, Billeter M, Labs KH, Strandness DE Jr. Vector Doppler systems for arterial studies, Part I: Theory. J Vasc Invest 1996;2(4):155–65.

9. Beach KW, Phillips DJ, Kansky J. Ultrasonic plethysmograph. U.S. Patent 5289820: Assignees: The Board of Regents of the University of Washington, Seattle, WA; Issued: March 1, 1994; Filed: November 24, 1992.

10. Beach KW, Phillips DJ, Kansky J. Ultrasonic plethysmograph. U.S. Patent 5183046: Assignees: Board of Regents of the University of Washington, Seattle, WA; Issued: February 2, 1993; Filed: November 15, 1991.

11. Beach KW, Phillips DJ, Kansky J. Ultrasonic plethysmograph. U.S. Patent 5088498: Assignees: The Board of Regents of the University of Washington, Seattle, WA; Issued: February 18, 1992; Filed: January 18, 1991.

12. http://www.ncbi.nlm.nih.gov/entrez/.

13. http://www.uspto.gov/.

Section III
Cerebrovascular Diagnosis

4
Overview of Cerebrovascular Disease

Ali F. AbuRahma

Stroke is the third leading cause of death in the United States, and the second leading cause of death for women in the United States. It is the cause of death in approximately 150,000 to 200,000 Americans annually. The morbidity of those who survive a stroke has a significant socioeconomic impact on our society. It is estimated that strokes account for the disability of two million Americans. The cost of medical bills, hospitalization, and rehabilitation was estimated to be around $40 billion in 1996.

It has been reported that 75% of patients suffering a stroke have surgically accessible extracranial vascular disease.[1] Ischemic strokes constitute 80–85% of all strokes, and the remaining 15–20% are caused by cerebral hemorrhage.[2,3] It has been estimated that ≥50% carotid stenosis may be responsible for up to 25% of all ischemic strokes. Large population studies using carotid ultrasound estimate the prevalence of ≥50% carotid artery stenosis to be 3–7%. This emphasizes the importance of early detection for stroke prevention.

Significant changes in our thinking and treatment of this disease have occurred over the past 50 years, but this has been a topic fraught with controversy since the first carotid endarterectomy was reported. Eastcott et al.[4] performed a carotid resection with reanastomosis of a diseased vessel in a patient who suffered a transient ischemic attack. This was published in 1954, but DeBakey[5] reported a successful performance of this procedure earlier.

Today, carotid endarterectomy is the most commonly performed vascular surgical procedure, however, it is still controversial. The debate over medical versus surgical treatment for carotid artery disease has been extensively analyzed in the medical literature over the past 10 years. The CASSANOVA, Asymptomatic Carotid Atherosclerosis Study (ACAS), Veteran's Administration (VA) Cooperative study, and Asymptomatic Carotid Surgery Trial (ACST) have looked at medical versus surgical therapy in asymptomatic carotid stenosis.[6–9] The VA Cooperative study, the North American Symptomatic

Carotid Endarterectomy Trial Collaborators (NASCET) study, and the European Carotid Surgery Trialists' Collaborative Group (ECST) looked at symptomatic carotid disease.[10–12] Regardless of which criteria are used to determine whether operative intervention is warranted, a surgeon must stay within the accepted perioperative stroke rate of 3–7% (depending on indication) as recommended by the Ad Hoc Committee of the Stroke Council of the American Heart Association. What is generally agreed upon, however, is that early and accurate detection of stroke-prone patients remains one of the most important problems in medicine, since stroke has an immediate mortality of 20–25% within 30 days. Of the survivors of a first stroke, 25–50% will have an additional stroke.

Anatomy

The aortic arch gives off, from right to left, the innominate (brachiocephalic trunk), the left common carotid, and the subclavian arteries (Figure 4–1). The innominate artery passes beneath the left innominate vein before it branches into the right subclavian and the right common carotid arteries. The vertebral arteries branch off the subclavian arteries 2 or 3 cm from the arch, but many variations may occur (Figure 4–1). The left common carotid artery may arise from the innominate (bovine arch) in 16% of patients and cross to a relatively normal position on the left side. The left vertebral artery may arise directly from the aortic arch instead of from the left subclavian arteries (Figure 4–2). The right vertebral artery may arise as part of a trifurcation of the brachiocephalic trunk into subclavian, common carotid, and vertebral arteries (Figure 4–3). Occasionally, both subclavian arteries originate together as a single trunk off of the arch, or the right subclavian may arise distal to the left subclavian artery and cross to the right side.[13]

The common carotid arteries on each side travel in the carotid sheath up to the neck before branching into

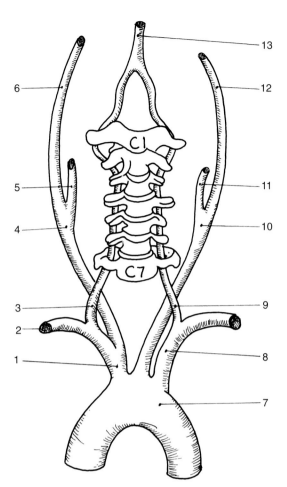

FIGURE 4–1. An illustration showing the aortic arch and its branches: (1) brachial-cephalic trunk, (2) right subclavian artery, (3) right vertebral artery, (4) right common carotid artery, (5) right external carotid artery, (6) right internal carotid artery, (7) aortic arch, (8) left subclavian artery, (9) left vertebral artery, (10) left common carotid artery, (11) left external carotid artery, (12) left internal carotid artery, (13) the basilar artery.

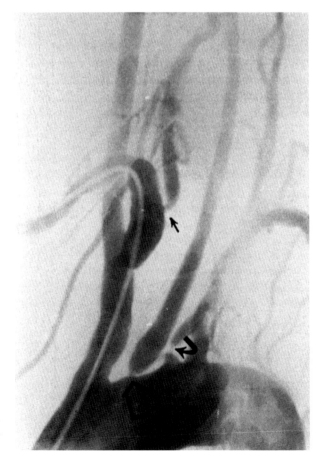

FIGURE 4–2. Arch aortogram showing the left vertebral artery originating from the arch of the aorta with tight stenosis at its origin (curved arrow) and the right vertebral artery (coming off the right subclavian artery) with a tight stenosis at its origin (straight arrow).

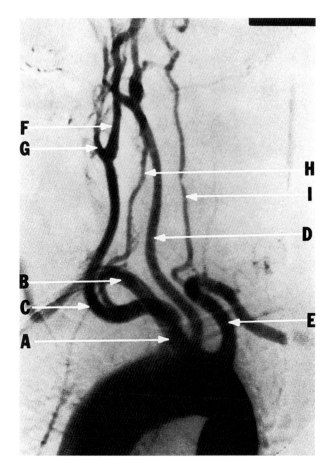

FIGURE 4–3. Abnormal origin of the vertebral artery (H) from the right common carotid artery (C) in a patient with a retroesophageal right subclavian artery (B). (Courtesy of Springer-Verlag, *Surgery of the Arteries to the Head*, 1992, by Ramon Berguer and Edouard Kieffer, eds.)

internal and external carotid arteries just below the level of the mandible. The external carotid artery supplies the face. Important branches of the external carotid artery include the superior thyroid, which can actually arise from the common carotid artery, and is important in that it accompanies the external branch of the superior laryngeal nerve, the ascending pharyngeal, and the lingual and occipital arteries that have a close association with the hypoglossal nerve (Figure 4–4). No branches of the internal carotid artery occur in the neck.

The carotid sinus, a baroreceptor, is located in the crotch of the bifurcation of the internal and external carotid artery. It is innervated by the nerve of Hering, which branches from the glossopharyngeal nerve. The carotid body is a very small structure that also lies in the crotch of the bifurcation and functions as a chemoreceptor, responding to low oxygen or high carbon dioxide levels in the blood. It is also innervated by the glossopharyngeal nerve via the nerve of Hering.

The corticotympanic artery and the artery to the pterygoid canal are branches of the internal carotid artery in its petrous portion. The cavernous, hypophyseal, semilunar, anterior meningeal, and ophthalmic arteries are branches of the cavernous portion of the internal carotid artery. The ophthalmic artery is clinically important since it communicates with the external carotid system, which is the basis of the periorbital Doppler study. The remaining branches of the internal carotid artery arise from the cerebral portion, i.e., the anterior and middle cerebral, posterior communicating, and chorioidal branches (Figure 4–5).

The vertebral artery leaves the subclavian artery and pushes upward through the foramina of the transverse processes of the cervical vertebrae into the cranium through the foramen magnum (Figure 4–6). The neck spinal branches enter the vertebral canal through the intervertebral foramen, and muscular branches are given off to the deep muscles of the neck. These latter branches anastomose with branches of the external carotid artery. Intracranially, the vertebral arteries give off the posterior inferior cerebellar and spinal arteries before they are united at the pontomedullary junction to form the basilar artery. The basilar artery terminates as the posterior cerebral artery after giving off the anterior inferior, superior cerebellar, pontine, and internal auditory arteries.

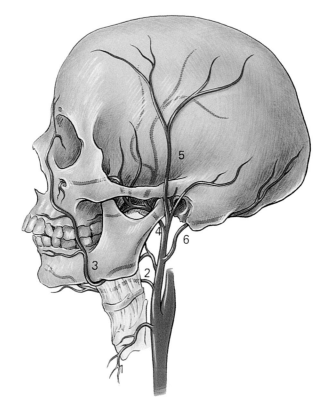

FIGURE 4–4. Main branches of the external carotid artery: (1) superior thyroid, (2) lingual, (3) facial, (4) internal maxillary artery, (5) superficial temporal artery, (6) occipital artery. (Courtesy of Springer-Verlag, *Surgery of the Arteries to the Head*, 1992, by Ramon Berguer and Edouard Kieffer, eds.)

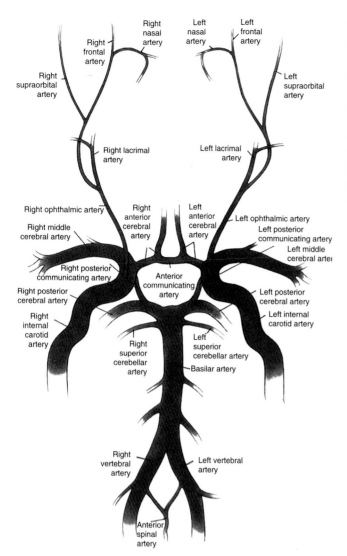

FIGURE 4–5. Major branches of the internal carotid artery (i.e., middle cerebral, anterior cerebral, posterior communicating, and ophthalmic artery) and vertebrobasilar arteries.

Blood flows through each internal carotid artery at about 350 ml/min, accounting for approximately 85% of the blood supply to the brain, and the vertebral arteries account for about 15% of the total blood supply to the brain.[14] Therefore, the carotid arteries, both from the standpoint of accessibility and functioning, become the system of importance for noninvasive testing.

Morphologic Variations of the Internal Carotid Artery

Tortuosity of the internal carotid artery (or loop) is generally defined as an S- or C-shaped elongation or curving in the course of the artery (Figure 4–7C). Coiling is a term used to describe an exaggerated, redundant S-shaped curve, or a complete circle, in the longitudinal axis of the artery (Figure 4–7A). Tortuosity and coiling are thought to be congenital developmental abnormalities that may become exaggerated with aging. They usually do not produce clinical symptoms.

Kinking is a sharp angulation with stenosis of segments of the internal carotid artery, (Figure 4–7B) and appears to be somewhat different than tortuosity and coiling. Kinking is less frequently bilateral and usually affects a few centimeters or more above the carotid bifurcation. Poststenotic dilatation may be present. Frequently, an atherosclerotic plaque on the concave side of the kink further narrows the lumen.

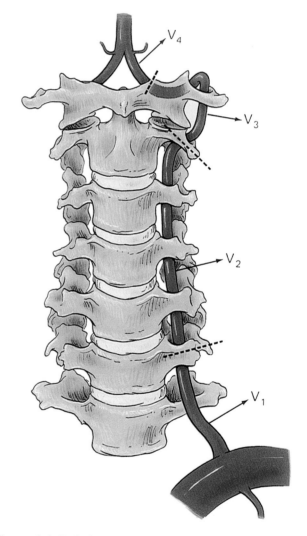

FIGURE 4–6. Relation of the vertebral artery and cervical spine. The dotted line indicates the level at which the vertebral artery becomes intradural. As noted, the vertebral artery is divided into four portions (V-1, V-2, V-3, and V-4). V-1 is the segment between its origin and the level where it enters the transverse process of the sixth cervical vertebra. V-2 is the segment of the artery through the foramina of the transverse processes of the cervical spines until the dotted line. V-3 is the segment between C-2 and C-1. V-4 is the segment prior to joining the other vertebral artery to form the basilar artery.

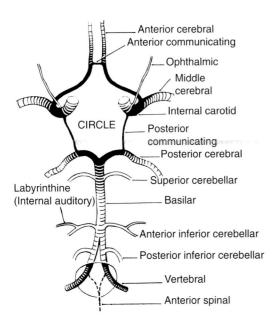

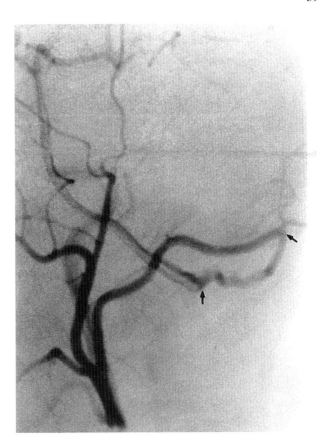

FIGURE 4–12. The Circle of Willis demonstrating rudimentary posterior communicating branches.

FIGURE 4–14. Occipital collateral may enter the vertebral artery at the level of C-1, as seen in this selective external carotid injection.

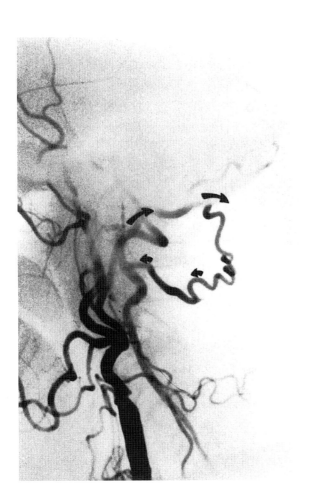

FIGURE 4–13. Occipital connection of the vertebral artery. In this patient with an occluded internal carotid artery, the collaterals from the occipital artery fill the vertebral artery anterograde toward the basilar artery and retrogradely toward the base of the neck, where the vertebral artery is occluded.

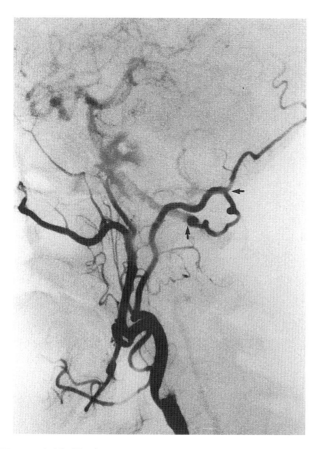

FIGURE 4–15. The importance of the occipital collateral is seen in this patient with an occluded internal carotid.

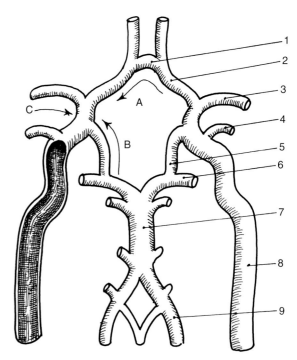

FIGURE 4–17. Illustration of a patient with an internal carotid artery occlusion. The flow to the corresponding cerebral hemisphere is maintained by flow from the opposite internal carotid artery (A), the vertebral basilar system (B), and the ophthalmic artery via the periorbital branches of the external carotid artery of the same side (C): (1) anterior communicating artery, (2) anterior cerebral artery, (3) middle cerebral artery, (4) ophthalmic artery, (5) posterior communicating artery, (6) posterior cerebral artery, (7) basilar artery, (8) internal carotid artery, (9) vertebral artery.

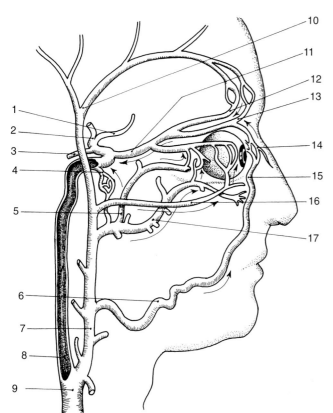

FIGURE 4–16. A patient with an occluded internal carotid artery with a reversal of flow through the ophthalmic artery via periorbital branches of the external carotid artery: (1) anterior cerebral artery, (2) middle cerebral artery, (3) posterior communicating artery, (4) caroticotympanic branch of the internal carotid artery, (5) middle meningeal artery, (6) fascial artery, (7) external carotid artery, (8) occluded internal carotid artery, (9) common carotid artery, (10) superficial temporal artery, (11) ophthalmic artery, (12) supraorbital artery, (13) supratrochlear artery, (14) dorsal nasal artery, (15) angular artery, (16) transverse fascial artery, (17) internal maxillary artery.

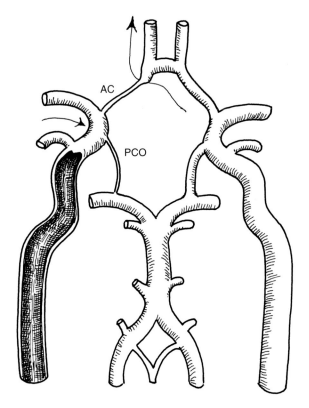

FIGURE 4-18. A patient with an internal carotid artery occlusion where the collateral flow may be reduced by the incomplete Circle of Willis [rudimentary right posterior communi-cating artery (PCO) and anterior cerebral artery (AC)].

bulbous portion of the internal carotid artery on its posterior lateral wall. The atherosclerosis appears as a fatty strip subintimally with a collection of fat cells that progresses to a fibrous plaque in the subendothelial layer, causing gradually decreasing flow. These plaques can enlarge in several ways. They may just continue to slowly enlarge from an accumulation of cholesterol and fibroblasts, leading to a central necrosis and rupture of the intimal lining of the vessel. This will lead to discharge of athromatous debris into the lumen of the vessel, which can embolize. The exposed necrotic core of the lesion can then become a nidus for platelet deposition and further embolization to the brain. Progressive accumulation of the arteriosclerotic process, often with thrombotic debris, may result in stenosis or total occlusion in the carotid artery, with subsequent thrombosis of the internal carotid artery distal to the lesion (Figure 4–19). Another mechanism by which there may be sudden plaque enlargement is intraplaque hemorrhage.[19] Intraplaque hemorrhage may produce acute narrowing of the lumen. If the intima overlying the site of the plaque hemorrhage ulcerates, the necrotic contents of the atheromas escape into the lumen and cause cerebral embolization with transient

arteries. Figures 4–16, 4–17, and 4–18 summarize the important collateral pathways in patients with an occluded internal carotid artery.

Pathology

Numerous theories exist as to the mechanism by which atherosclerosis develops in the carotid arteries, but whether you prescribe to the mechanical, sheer stress, chemical injury, or infectious theory,[18] the basic lesion is essentially the same. Atherosclerosis accounts for approximately 90% of extracranial cerebrovascular disease, with the remaining 10% being attributed to such disease processes as fibromuscular dysplasia, traumatic or spontaneous dissection, aneurysms, and arteritis, including Takayasu's arteritis.

The carotid plaque of atherosclerosis consists of cholesterol deposition in the arterial intima and an associated inflammatory reaction that results in fibroblast proliferation. These plaques occur preferentially at areas of vessel bifurcations and the process is similar to that seen with coronary artery disease. It can begin in the

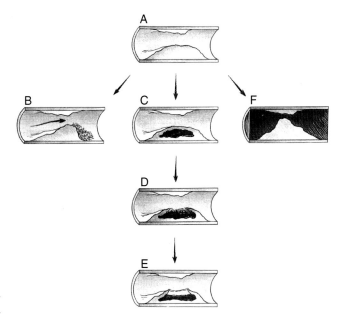

FIGURE 4-19. (A) Development of pathologic features in a plaque. (B) Partial obstruction created by a plaque may result in accumulation of a fibrin-platelet thrombus downstream from the obstruction. (C) The plaque may "soften" in its core. (D) This softening may break through to the surface, exposing the contents of the soft core to the bloodstream. (E) An ulceration may become covered by a fibrin deposit and even heal. (F) The increased size of the obstruction created by the plaque may result in thrombosis of the vessel lumen. (Courtesy of Springer-Verlag, *Surgery of the Arteries to the Head*, 1992, by Ramon Berguer and Edouard Kieffer, eds.)

ischemic attacks (TIAs) or cerebral infarcts. Nonulcerated lesions may alter flow and produce mural thrombi, which may fragment, causing embolization (Figure 4–20). The friability of these lesions is often not appreciated until seen by the vascular surgeon (Figure 4–21).

Blaisdell et al. and Hass et al.[20,21] studied the distribution of the atherosclerotic lesions involved in cerebrovascular disease and found that approximately one-third of responsible lesions occurred in the intracranial distribution that were surgically inaccessible. The remaining two-thirds of the lesions were in extracranial locations.

The common carotid bifurcation and the proximal internal carotid artery account for 50% of the lesions. Vertebral artery lesions account for 20%, left subclavian arterial lesions account for 10–15%, and lesions of the innominate and right subclavian arteries account for 15%. More than one lesion may be present (Figure 4–22).

Generally, the most common cause of cerebral ischemic events is embolic phenomena, primarily arterial in origin (carotid) and secondary to cardiac sources. The irregular plaque surface produces turbulence, which will act as a stimulus for platelet aggregation. If the platelet aggregates become large enough and embolize to an important vessel in the brain, symptoms will occur. If the platelet aggregates break up quickly from mechanical forces or from the effect of arterial prostacyclin, the symptoms will be transient, i.e., TIAs. If the embolic fragment persists, however, it can lead to focal infarction (Figure 4–23). As noted in Figure 4–24, the end result of the atherosclerotic plaque might be an internal carotid artery thrombosis. When an arteriosclerotic plaque

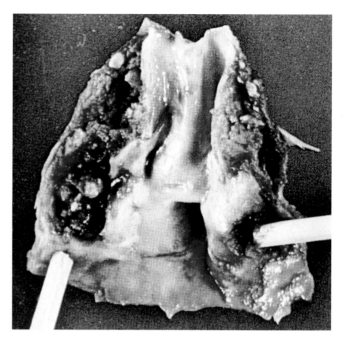

FIGURE 4–21. Carotid endarterectomy plaque.

expands to produce a critical reduction in blood flow, the vessel will ultimately undergo thrombosis. In the case of the internal carotid artery, this column of thrombus stops at the ophthalmic artery and remains stable, and if there is sufficient collateral circulation via the Circle of Willis, the thrombotic event may be entirely asymptomatic (Figure 4–24). However, if small thrombi rather than a thrombotic column form and are subsequently carried to the intracranaial vessels by continuous blood flow, then the patient will experience cerebral symptoms that can vary from transient amaurosis fugax or hemispheric events to a profound hemiplegia, depending upon the extent of the propagated thrombus or embolus (Figure 4–25). In addition, if the collateral circulation to the Circle of Willis is inadequate, the sudden loss of blood flow through a diseased internal carotid artery may induce a sudden drop in flow to the cerebral hemisphere, resulting in ischemic infarction as a consequence of inadequate proximal blood flow.

A less common cause of cerebrovascular ischemia is fibromuscular dysplasia (FMD), which is usually more distally located in the internal carotid artery. The most common form of the disease is characterized by hyperplasia of the media producing alternating bands of thinned areas, leading to a beady appearance on angiography. Often the internal carotid artery is involved at long lengths. Always look for evidence of fibromuscular dysplasia elsewhere. It will involve both internal carotid arteries in 65% of patients.[22]

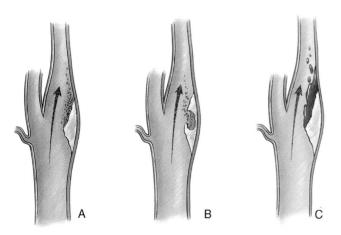

FIGURE 4–20. (A–C) Three mechanisms for thromboembolization from an internal carotid plaque. (A) Fibrin-platelet aggregates associated with an obstructing plaque. (B) Atheromatous contents. (C) Thrombus forming on the surface. (Courtesy of Springer-Verlag, Surgery of the Arteries to the Head, 1992, by Ramon Berguer and Edouard Kieffer, eds.)

FIGURE 4–22. Sites of atheroclerosis of brachiocepahalic vessels: (1) aortic arch, (2) left subclavian artery, (3) innominate artery, (4) right subclavian artery, (5) right and left vertebral arteries, (6) right and left common carotid arteries, (7) right internal carotid artery, (8) right external carotid artery (note atherosclerosis at the left subclavian, left vertebral, innominate with proximal right common carotid and subclavian arteries, and left carotid bifurcation).

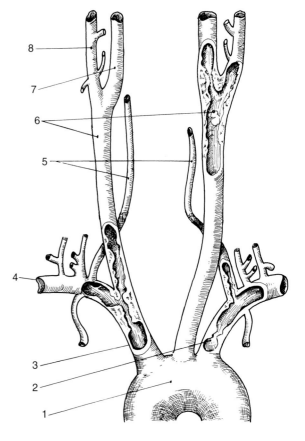

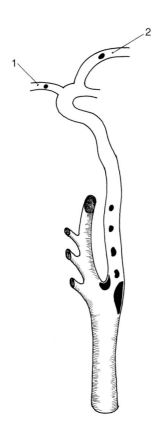

FIGURE 4–23. Embolization from an internal carotid artery stenotic lesion to the ophthalmic artery (1) and middle cerebral artery (2).

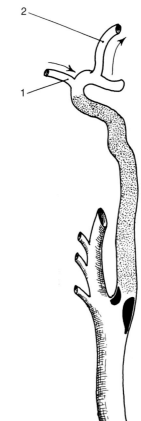

FIGURE 4–24. Internal carotid artery thrombosis with retrograde flow via the ophthalmic artery (1) to the terminal internal carotid artery and middle cerebral artery (2).

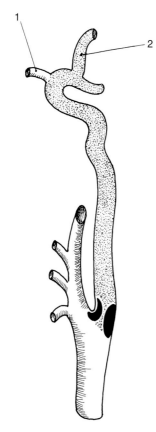

FIGURE 4–25. Internal carotid artery thrombosis that extends to the ophthalmic artery (1) and terminal internal carotid artery and middle cerebral artery (2).

Pathophysiology

It has been stated that a 70–80% reduction of the cross-sectional area of the arterial lumen must be present to produce a hemodynamically significant drop in the usual flow rate in the cerebrovascular system.[23] However, this may not always be the case. Important mechanisms of collateral flow and hemodynamic events that decrease cardiac output or systemic blood pressure, such as postural hypotension and cardiac arrhythmia, may produce transient episodes of ischemia. Embolization has been a documented cause of TIAs by proven ophthalmologic examination. Intraluminal particles of platelet fibrin aggregates, cholesterol fragments, and small clots have been noted. Most TIAs are probably caused by this mechanism. There is a permanent neurologic deficit as a result of permanently disrupted flow. A pale infarct occurs with focal cell necrosis and cerebral softening. The blood vessels lose integrity at the periphery of the infarct at a relatively ischemic spot. However, where neural death has not occurred, neurologic function may be altered and blood flow, while slow, may still be present.

Clinical Syndromes

The following well-defined syndromes of cerebrovascular ischemia have emerged:

1. TIAs are focal neurologic symptoms or deficits that usually clear completely within 2 h. Some last for only a few moments, and others last for a few hours, but no longer than 24 h.
2. Reversible ischemic neurologic deficits (RIND) are focal findings that clear over a period of days.
3. Minor stroke, which is defined as a neurologic deficit that clears completely in less than a week.
4. Major stroke, which is defined as a major neurologic deficit that lasts longer than a week.
5. Stroke in evolution or progressing stroke.
6. Complete stroke is a stroke with a significant return of function.
7. Diffuse cerebral ischemia or "low flow" syndrome.

Each of these syndromes requires a thorough history, physical, and neurologic evaluation with close attention to the severity of associated cardiovascular disease, hypertension, diabetes, neurologic aid, and diagnostic testing.

Over two-thirds of patients who have strokes have had prior TIAs. The mechanism by which TIAs occur is usually an embolic process. The source for these emboli can be from a number of sources—intracranial lesions, extracranial carotid, extracranial arch vessel lesions, primary cardiac thrombus, or even paradoxical emboli. The majority of TIAs will come from carotid bifurcation lesions, and this must be the site that is worked up first in these patients. When taking a history from patients who present with TIAs, it is important to obtain information as to previous episodes. Patients with a carotid source for their TIA will generally report having identical previous neurologic deficits, in contrast to cardiac TIAs that may vary; this is based on the principles of laminar flow within the carotid vessels that send the embolus to the same area each time.

The carotid TIA manifestations include transient ipsilateral blindness or visual impairment (amaurosis fugax) and contralateral sensory or motor deficit. There may be a degree of altered consciousness. Speech deficit may be present if the dominant hemisphere is affected.

The patient with amaurosis fugax will describe these episodes as someone pulling a shade over one of their eyes, which quickly resolves. A funduscopic inspection of these patients may reveal Hollenhorst plaques, bright yellow spots on the retina that represent cholesterol crystals. These may be present in asymptomatic patients with atherosclerotic disease as well.

Nonhemispheric TIAs present a dilemma to the vascular surgeon. These patients will present with symptoms of dizziness, ataxia, vertigo, bilateral neurologic or visual events, or even syncope. These symptoms may be related to an embolic event from primary atherosclerotic lesions involving the vertebrobasilar system, resulting in an ischemic event to the posterior brain or brain stem. Another mechanism for this may be a significantly diminished blood flow to the brain, or diffuse cerebral ischemia. To have this situation, the patient must have severe stenoses involving the majority of the extracranial vessels, incomplete Circle of Willis, or an altered flow state, i.e., subclavian steal syndrome.

Other clinical syndromes include reversible ischemic neurologic event (RIND). RIND is a focal neurologic deficit that takes several days to completely resolve. The mechanism by which RIND occurs is poorly understood. It is generally felt that these patients actually suffer focal cerebral infarctions, but these areas are very small and surrounding tissue compensates for the loss. Another syndrome is crescendo TIAs. These are hemispheric deficits that resolve within minutes, but occur with increasing frequency. Stroke in evolution is where initial neurologic symptoms may not completely resolve and subsequent neurologic events are progressive.

A completed stroke is a neurologic deficit that occurs and does not have a complete resolution of symptoms. This may be the result of a large embolus, a small embolus to an end vessel with surrounding vessel thrombosis, or thrombosis of the internal carotid artery.

Physical Examination

With a good history and thorough physical examination, it is possible to diagnose the nature and location of the vascular lesions with reasonable certainty, and the diagnosis can usually be confirmed by the noninvasive techniques to be described. The physical examination includes examining or checking the pulses of the superficial temporal artery, the carotid artery, both high and low in the neck, the subclavian artery above the mid-portion of the clavicle, and the radial artery. One side of the body should be compared with the other. The blood pressures in each arm should be compared. A 15–20 mm Hg difference in blood pressure may indicate a significant lesion of the subclavian or innominate arteries. Bruits in the neck, indicating turbulence in stenotic arteries, should be carefully evaluated. Listening for a bruit is also important. Remember that a near or total occlusion of the internal carotid artery has no bruit at all. A good pulsation may be felt under the mandible when a totally occluded internal carotid artery is present due to the palpation of the common carotid artery and the external carotid artery. These cannot be differentiated on a physical examination. It is sometimes difficult to palpate the subclavian arteries in obese or heavy-set individuals, and it is necessary to determine that cervical bruits are not really aortic ejection murmurs. A carotid bruit, heard louder at the level of the mandible than in the lower part of the neck, would probably indicate a stenosis of the internal carotid artery. This could also represent a stenosis of the innominate artery. Moderate stenosis may result in a systolic bruit, whereas more severe stenosis results in a systolic bruit that ends in diastole. A complete neurologic examination should be done.

Investigations

The work-up of patients presenting with asymptomatic carotid bruits or TIAs has changed over recent years. These changes have occurred because of recently published recommendations and improved noninvasive diagnostic tools. Initial screening in all of these patients must include carotid duplex scanning; and based on the findings of this study, the patient can take one of several routes. First, the patient may have no significant disease by duplex. These patients with classical hemispheric TIAs will require a cardiac work-up and, if negative, a systemic disease work-up, or possibly an arteriogram. Second, the patient may have a severe or tight stenosis or ulcerative plaque. In this situation, depending on the patient's operative risk, the surgeon's skill, the accuracy of the duplex, and the radiologist's complication rates, this patient could undergo magnetic resonance angiography or conventional arteriography, or surgery, without further work-up. Third, in patients with hemispheric TIAs and only mild to moderate disease by duplex, other sources should be explored, as well as carotid magnetic resonance angiography or arteriography. Again, many factors must be considered when working up patients for TIAs, and each patient must be individualized. A practical approach is described in Chapter 16.

Arteriography

Intraarterial injection is usually performed according to the Seldinger technique. The most commonly used artery is the common femoral artery, and to a lesser extent, the axillary or brachial arteries. Digital subtraction angiography (DSA) uses real-time digital video processing to detect the small amount of contrast medium that has been injected into the artery (Figures 4–26, 4–27, 4–28, and 4–29).

Interpretation of Stenosis

There are several methods of estimating stenoses. One of the most common methods described is the one

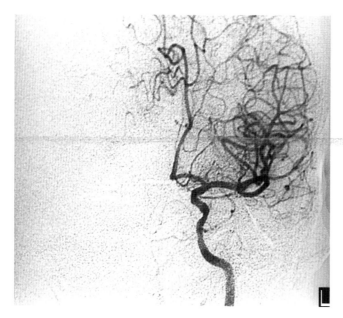

FIGURE 4–26. Carotid arteriogram showing a normal distal internal carotid artery and its two major branches: anterior and middle cerebral arteries.

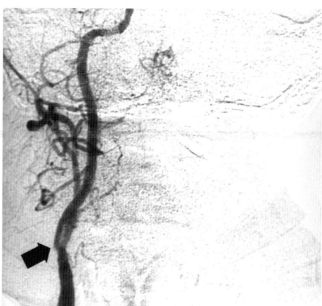

FIGURE 4–28. Carotid arteriogram showing severe stenosis of the carotid bifurcation and proximal internal carotid artery (arrow).

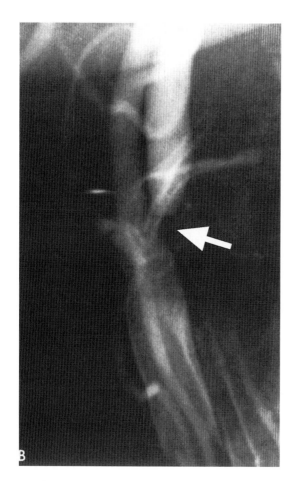

FIGURE 4–27. Carotid arteriogram showing tight stenosis of the proximal internal carotid artery (arrow).

used by the NASCET trial,[11] where the percentage of stenosis is calculated as a diameter reduction. The percentage of stenosis is determined by comparing the least transverse diameter at the stenosis to the diameter of the distal uninvolved internal carotid artery where the arterial walls become parallel (Figure 4–30). The percentage may then be expressed as the function of either the diameter or the cross-sectional area as follows.

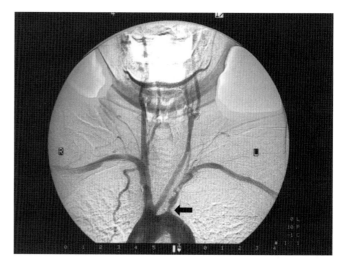

FIGURE 4–29. Four vessel arch aortogram showing severe stenosis of the proximal left subclavian artery (arrow).

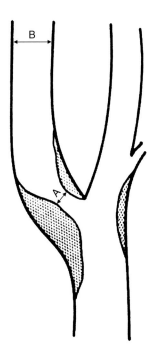

FIGURE 4–30. Information required for calculating the percentage of internal carotid artery stenosis. See text for details.

Percentage of Stenosis Calculation— Diameter Reduction

Percentage of stenosis equals 1 minus A divided by B multiplied by 100, i.e.

$$[1 - (A/B)] \times 100$$

Percentage of Stenosis Calculation— Area Reduction

To calculate the percentage of stenosis on the basis of the vessel cross-sectional area, and assuming the lesion is symmetrical, as seen in Figure 4–30, the percentage of stenosis (area reduction) will equal (1 minus A^2 divided by B^2) multiplied by 100, i.e.

$$[1 - (A^3/B^2)] \times 100$$

The third method of calculating the percentage of stenosis is to divide the area of residual lumen (A) by the area of the true lumen at the level of the stenosis (C), as adapted by the ECST, i.e.

$$\frac{C - A}{C} \times 100$$

This calculation will require a transverse view of the vessel in question.

Generally speaking, a stenosis that reduces the vessel diameter by 50% (which is equal to a 75% area reduction) is considered hemodynamically significant.

Treatment

Medical therapy generally includes control of risk factors, e.g., weight, a low-cholesterol diet that may enhance a normal endothelial cell metabolism, antihypertensive drugs for hypertensive patients to decrease shear forces on the endothelialized cells, and cessation of smoking. Specific medical therapy includes antiplatelet agents, such as aspirin, dipyridamole (Persantine, Boehringer), or combined aspirin and extended release dipyridamole (25 mg/200 mg capsule, Aggrenox, Boehringer), or clopidogrel (Plavix, Sanofi-Synthelabo).

Surgical intervention, a carotid endarterectomy, is indicated in patients with significant carotid artery stenosis (at least 50%) associated with TIA symptoms or strokes with a good recovery, as recommended by the NASCET study.[11] The NASCET study concluded, after analyzing 659 patients with TIAs or nondisabling strokes occurring within 6 months preceding presentations and with ipsilateral carotid stenosis of 70–99%, that the cumulative risk of an ipsilateral stroke occurring by the 18 month follow-up was 26% for 331 patients who were treated medically and 9% for 328 patients who were treated surgically. This yielded an absolute risk reduction of 17% ($p < 0.001$). The corresponding incidence of major or fatal ipsilateral stroke was 13% and 3% for medically and surgically treated groups, respectively. This translates into an absolute risk reduction of 11%, or a greater than 5 to 1 benefit in favor of operation ($p < 0.001$). The NASCET investigators concluded that carotid endarterectomy was highly beneficial for patients with recent hemispheric or retinal TIAs, or those with nondisabling stroke in the presence of ipsilateral high-grade carotid stenoses. The NASCET study also concluded that carotid endarterectomy was highly beneficial for symptomatic patients with 50% to <70% carotid artery stenosis.[24]

Patients with stenoses of >60% can be candidates for carotid endarterectomy if they are good risk patients.[7] The ACAS study also concluded that carotid endarterectomy was superior to medical therapy in good risk patients, and it reduced stroke by 55% over a 5-year period when surgical therapy was compared to medical therapy (5% versus 11%). Recently, the ACST Collaborative Group reported on the results of carotid endarterectomy in the prevention of stroke for ≥70% asymptomatic stenosis. Their conclusions were somewhat similar to the American study (the ACAS): in asymptomatic patients younger than 75 years of age with a carotid diameter reduction of 70%, immediate carotid endarterectomy decreased the net 5-year stroke risk by one-half, from 12% to 6% (including the 3% perioperative hazard).[9]

Recently, carotid angioplasty/stenting (CAS) has been recommended as an alternative to carotid endarterectomy. Several randomized and nonrandomized prospective trials have been conducted over the past few years to evaluate the efficacy of CAS in the prevention of strokes for both symptomatic and asymptomatic patients. Two of these studies are randomized prospective controlled trials. One of these, the SAPPHIRE study, just reported their early results comparing CAS to carotid endarterectomy in high-risk patients. The SAPPHIRE study was a randomized trial that compared carotid stenting using the angioguard emboli protection device to carotid endarterectomy in patients at increased risk for carotid surgery. Symptomatic patients with ≥50% stenosis and asymptomatic patients with ≥80% stenosis by ultrasound, who had one or more of the comorbidity criteria that placed them at increased risk for surgery, were included. The primary endpoints were death, stroke, and myocardial infarction at 30 days postprocedure, and ipsilateral stroke and death at 1 year. The composite endpoint of death, stroke, and myocardial infarction at 30 days was 5.8% for the stent group and 12.6% for the surgery group ($p = 0.047$). The trial concluded that carotid stenting in high-risk patients was comparable or somewhat favorable to carotid endarterectomy when combined death, stroke, and myocardial infarction were considered.[25]

The CREST (Carotid Revascularization Endarterectomy versus Stent trial), which compares the efficacy of carotid endarterectomy and carotid artery stenting in symptomatic patients in a randomized fashion, is presently being conducted. Recent data on the lead-in cases demonstrated a 30-day stroke and death rate of 3.6%. An update on 500 lead-in cases has demonstrated a 30-day stroke and death rate of 2.1% for asymptomatic patients and 5% for symptomatic patients with carotid artery stenting.[26]

References

1. Fields WS, North RR, Hass WK, *et al.* Joint study of extracranial arterial occlusion as a cause of stroke. I. Organization of study and survey of patient population. JAMA 1968;203:955–960.
2. Sherman DG, Dyken ML, Fisher M, *et al.* Antithrombotic therapy for cerebrovascular disorders. Chest 1989;95 (Suppl.):140S–155S.
3. Feldmann E. Intracerebral hemorrhage. In: Fisher M (ed). *Clinical Atlas of Cerebrovascular Disorders,* pp. 11.1–11.7. London: Mosby-Year Book Europe, 1994.
4. Eastcott HHG, Pickering GW, Robb CG. Reconstruction of internal carotid artery in a patient with intermittent attacks of hemiplegia. Lancet 1954;2:994–996.
5. DeBakey ME. Successful carotid endarterectomy for cerebrovascular insufficiency. Nineteen-year follow-up. JAMA 1975;233:1083–1085.
6. The CASSANOVA Study Group. Carotid surgery vs. medical therapy in asymptomatic carotid stenosis. Stroke 1991;22:1229–1235.
7. Asymptomatic Carotid Atherosclerosis Study Group. Study design for randomized prospective trial of carotid endarterectomy for asymptomatic atherosclerosis. Stroke 1989;20:844–849.
8. Hobson RW II. Management of symptomatic and asymptomatic carotid stenosis: Results of current randomized clinical trials. In: Bernstein EF (ed). *Vascular Diagnosis,* 4th ed., pp. 446–451. St. Louis, MO: Mosby, 1993.
9. MRC, Asymptomatic Carotid Surgery Trial (ACST) Collaborative Group. Prevention of disabling and fatal stroke by successful carotid endarterectomy in patients without recent neurological symptoms: Randomized controlled trial. Lancet 2004;363:1491–1500.
10. Mayberg MR, Wilson SE, Yatsu F. For the Veterans Affairs cooperative study program 309 trialist group. Carotid endarterectomy and prevention of cerebral ischemia in symptomatic carotid stenosis. JAMA 1991;266:3289–3294.
11. North American Symptomatic Carotid Endarterectomy Trial Collaborators. Beneficial effect of carotid endarterectomy in symptomatic patients with high-grade carotid stenosis. N Engl J Med 1991;325:445–453.
12. European Carotid Surgery Trialists' Collaborative Group, MRC European Carotid Surgery Trial. Interim results for symptomatic patients with severe (70–99%) or with mild (0–29%) carotid stenosis. Lancet 1991;337:1235–1243.
13. Anson BJ, McVay CB. *Surgical Anatomy,* Vol. 1, pp. 3–6. Philadelphia, PA: WB Saunders Co., 1971.
14. Larson CP Jr. Anesthesia and control of the cerebral circulation. In: Wylie EJ, Ehrenfeld WK (eds). *Extracranial Cerebrovascular Disease: Diagnosis and Management,* pp. 152–183. Philadelphia, PA: WB Saunders Co., 1970.
15. Reivich M, Hooling HE, Roberts B, *et al.* Reversal of blood flow through the vertebral artery and its effect on cerebral circulation. N Engl J Med 1961;265:878–885.
16. Connolly JE, Stemmer EA. Endarterectomy of the external carotid artery: Its importance in the surgical management of extracranial cerebrovascular occlusive disease. Arch Surg 1973;106:799–802.
17. Ehrenfeld WK, Lord RSA. Transient monocular blindness through collateral pathways. Surgery 1969;65:911–915.
18. Cook PJ, Honeybourne D, LIP GY, *et al.* Chlamydia pneumoniae antibody titers are significantly associated with stroke and transient cerebral ischemia: The West Birmingham Stroke Project. Stroke 1998;29(2):404–410.
19. Sillesen H, Nielsen T. Clinical significance of intraplaque hemorrhage in carotid artery disease. J Neuroimaging 1998;8(1):15–19.
20. Blaisdell FW, Hall AD, Thomas AN, *et al.* Cerebrovascular occlusive disease. Experience with panarteriography in 300 consecutive cases. Calif Med 1965;103:321–329.
21. Hass WK, Fields WS, North RR, *et al.* Joint study of extracranial arterial occlusion. II. Arteriography, techniques, sites, and complications. JAMA 1968;203:961–968.
22. AbuRahma AF. Overview of Cerebrovascular disease. In: AbuRahma AF, Diethrich EB (eds). *Current Noninvasive*

Vascular Diagnosis, pp. 1–7. Littleton, MA: PSG Publishing, 1988.

23. Strandness DE Jr, Sumner DS. *Hemodynamics for Surgeons,* pp. 512–524. New York: Grune & Stratton, Inc., 1975.

24. Barnett HJM, Taylor DW, Eliasziw MA, *et al.* For the NASCET collaborators: Benefits of carotid endarterectomy in patients with symptomatic, moderate, or severe stenosis. N Engl J Med 1998;339:1415–1425.

25. Yadav JS, Wholey MH, Kuntz RE, *et al.* Protected carotid artery stenting versus endarterectomy in high-risk patients. N Engl J Med 2004;351:1493–1501.

26. Hobson RW II, Howard VJ, Roubin GS, Brott TG, Ferguson RD, Popma JJ, Graham DL, Howard G, CREST Investigators. Carotid artery stenting is associated with increased complications in octogenarians: 30-day stroke and death rates in the CREST lead-in phase. J Vasc Surg 2004;40:1106–1111.

5
Overview of Various Noninvasive Cerebrovascular Techniques

Ali F. AbuRahma

Contrast cerebrovascular arteriography has been the definitive diagnostic technique for evaluation of cerebrovascular disease; however, its limitations and complications played a great role in the drive to develop accurate, reliable noninvasive diagnostic procedures. Although arteriography serves to define anatomic lesions and is indispensable for most vascular surgery, it provides little objective data regarding physiologic disability, nor is it without risk.

Most complications of cerebral arteriography can be assigned to technical error, embolic events, or neurotoxic effects of the contrast material. Catheter-related injuries at the puncture site are near 0.2%, with mortality estimated at 0.02%.[1] Allergic reactions to the contrast medium occur in about 2% of cases, while the overall incidence of neurologic deficits is around 1% if the transfemoral approach is used (the figure is slightly higher with the transaxillary route). Both the North American Symptomatic Carotid Endarterectomy Trial Collaborators (NASCET) and the Asymptomatic Carotid Atherosclerosis Study Group (ACAS) reported stroke rates of around 1%.[2,3] Recent literature reported major complication rates of 5.9% and 9.1% for cerebral angiography.[4,5]

A technical shortcoming of cerebral arteriography is its failure to delineate shallow, superficially ulcerating lesions. Because of this, a potential source of cerebral emboli could be overlooked. If we add to these risks the disadvantages of patient discomfort, the need for hospitalization, and expense, there is little wonder that many physicians are reluctant to subject their patients to cerebral arteriography. This makes the noninvasive vascular diagnostic techniques highly desirable and cost-effective alternatives.

In the past 30 years extensive research has been done in the field of cerebrovascular diagnosis, resulting in the development of a broad range of noninvasive diagnostic tools, extending even to the use of radioactive isotope scanning. While these nuclear studies have been useful in detecting intracranial lesions, they have not been as effective as the noninvasive techniques in localizing extracranial disease, the main site of pathology in the carotid tree.

Ultrasound was first applied to the study of the carotid circulation as early as 1954,[6] but it was not until 1967 that its clinical application in velocity detection was reported.[7] Brockenbrough, in 1970, further refined the technique and popularized the flowmeter.[8]

In 1971, D. E. Hokanson, working in Eugene Strandness' laboratory at the University of Washington in Seattle, was able to piece together all the elements necessary to provide the first noninvasive visualization of an arterial segment using pulsed Doppler methods.[9] The concept was quite simple. If one knew the size and location of the Doppler transducer, the position of the pulsed Doppler sample volume, and could transfer this to a cathode ray tube, it should be possible to paint a picture containing all points within an arterial segment where flow was occurring. This led to the development of ultrasonic arteriography, which was successfully applied to the study of carotid artery disease. Although this method worked, there were significant limitations: (1) it was time-consuming, (2) an experienced technologist was required, (3) the image was distorted by the patient's movement, (4) arterial wall calcification blocked the transmission of ultrasound, and (5) the arterial wall and plaque were not visualized. Because of these limitations, Strandness and colleagues began exploring the use of B-mode ultrasound to visualize the arterial wall. Very early in their application of this method they studied a patient whose internal carotid artery appeared patent by ultrasonic imaging but was found to be occluded by arteriography. This led to the obvious conclusion that thrombus may have acoustic properties similar to flowing blood and, thus, would be missed by imaging alone. The solution appeared to be the addition of a Doppler probe to the ultrasonic imaging to permit assessment of the presence or absence of flow. It was this combination of imaging plus Doppler that led to the term ultrasonic duplex scanner.[10] When real-time fast

Fourier transform (FFT) spectrum analysis was added, the basic components of the systems that are in widespread use today became available.

Another breakthrough came in 1974, when Gee et al.[11] introduced the use of the oculopneumoplethysmograph for carotid disease screening.

Due to the propensity for atherosclerotic disease to attack the extracranial (vs. intracranial) carotid network, noninvasive testing has concentrated on this area.

Generally speaking, there are two types of noninvasive approaches to extracranial circulation: direct, which examines flow changes in the cervical portion of the carotid artery near the bifurcation (site of the majority of lesions); and indirect, which detects significant stenotic lesions by assessing flow changes at locations distal to the bifurcation.

Duplex with color flow imaging systems using pulsed wave Doppler signals are now the most common direct methods for carotid evaluation; indirect methods such as continuous wave Doppler technique, periorbital Doppler,[8,12] and oculopneumoplethysmography[11,13,14] are outdated and are no longer used in the modern vascular laboratory for the diagnosis of carotid artery disease.

Indirect Methods

From a historical perspective, oculopneumoplethysmography (OPG/Gee) detects the ophthalmic artery pressure by suction ophthalmodynamometry. The main indication for OPG/Gee is the identification of carotid artery stenosis,[11,13,14] however, it can also be used in measuring ophthalmic artery pressure during external compression of the common carotid artery, reflecting the collateral pressure of the ipsilateral internal carotid artery. It may also be helpful in determining the safety of ligating or resecting the carotid artery.

This procedure has some limitations in common with all other types of oculoplethysmography, such as it cannot be used with certain types of eye disease and cannot be applied to some patients with severe hypertension if the systolic endpoint cannot be measured (fewer than 2% of patients). Also, it cannot distinguish between total occlusion and severe stenoses cannot detect subcritical stenoses or locate the exact site of the stenoses, and is not useful in documenting the progression of disease.

OPG/Gee measures the ophthalmic arterial systolic pressure by applying a vacuum to the eye. As the vacuum distorts the shape of the globe, intraocular pressure increases to the point at which it obliterates the arterial inflow. Strip chart recordings are then made as the vacuum is slowly decreased. The pulse wave reappears when the ophthalmic arterial pressure exceeds the intraocular pressure. A vacuum of 300 or 500 mm Hg is applied according to the patient's baseline blood pressure. Since the pressure in the ophthalmic artery reflects the pressure in the distal internal carotid artery, the measurement of ophthalmic arterial pressure using this test can be useful in detecting hemodynamically significant carotid stenoses.

Abnormal findings are ophthalmic systolic pressures that differ by equal to or more than 5 mm Hg and/or an abnormal ratio of ophthalmic-to-systolic pressure.

Another indirect test that was used in the past is the periorbital Doppler examination (ophthalmosonometry), the principle of which is based on evaluating the Doppler velocity flow pattern in the accessible branches of the ophthalmic artery and assessing the response to compression of the branches of the external carotid. The identification of advanced internal carotid stenosis by examination of the periorbital flow patterns with the Doppler detector was first described by Brockenbrough in 1969.[8] The original technique described by Brockenbrough used a nondirectional velocity detector to examine the signal obtained from the supraorbital artery and the response to the compression of the superficial temporal artery.[8] Further refinement became possible with the development of the directional Doppler detector, which permitted the documentation of reverse flow in the branches of the ophthalmic artery.[15,16]

Direct Methods

Several direct methods that were used in the past are now outdated, including pulsed Doppler arteriography,[17] carotid phonoangiography,[18] color-coded echoflow,[19] radionuclide arteriography, and carotid scanning.[20,21]

Real-Time B-Mode Carotid Imaging

B-mode ultrasound imaging has been used extensively for visualizing soft tissue structures. Carotid arteries, however, could not be seen properly until the advent of real-time techniques that have overcome the problem of visualization. With B-mode imaging alone, variations in the acoustic properties of different tissues reflect ultrasound waves and generate an image of the tissues being examined. These variations in acoustic reflectance are represented visually by shades of gray on the image, which facilitates identification of different tissues. The vessel wall, because of its high reflectively, may thus be visualized. Yet it is this tissue interaction with ultrasound that has imposed severe limitations on techniques that use this method for visualizing atherosclerotic plaques and occluded arteries.

Unfortunately, methods currently used for processing the reflected ultrasound waves are often incapable of differentiating flowing blood, thrombus, and noncalcified

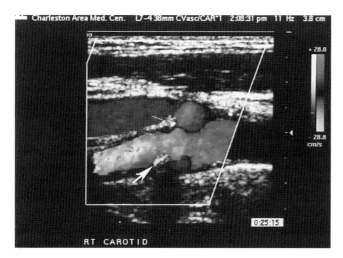

FIGURE 5–1. Color duplex ultrasound image of an internal carotid artery showing calcified plaque where a very dense acoustic signal is registered (arrow) with acoustic shadowing (underneath the arrow).

plaques. Thus, vessels that are completely occluded may appear patent. Likewise, noncalcified plaques may be entirely missed or, at best, only partly visualized. In addition, when atherosclerotic disease at the carotid bifurcation exists, calcium is a common component of the plaque and prevents the passage of ultrasound waves through this area. Thus, if there is a calcified plaque on the anterior wall of the vessel a very dense acoustic signal will be registered, but there will be no information concerning the lumen beneath the calcified segment. This is commonly referred to as acoustic shadowing (Figure 5–1). These limitations are largely overcome by combining B-mode imaging with flow detection techniques using Doppler, such as spectral waveform analysis and color flow imaging. Experience with B-mode imaging techniques for the classification of carotid artery disease has generally shown that interpretation of the image is most accurate for lesions of a minimal to moderate degree of stenosis, and least accurate for high-grade stenoses or occlusions. It is often difficult to estimate the size of the arterial lumen from a B-mode image because the interface between the arterial wall and flowing blood is not clearly seen. Calcified atherosclerotic plaque, which is extremely echogenic, results in bright echoes with acoustic shadows (Figure 5–1).

Continuous Wave and Pulse Doppler Wave Analysis

Nonimaging Doppler techniques can directly interrogate the common carotid, the internal carotid, and the external carotid arteries to detect a hemodynamically significant stenosis. Since these are nonimaging techniques, they provide only physiologic information and cannot differentiate a tight stenosis from occlusion. Information from more than one vessel along the path of the beam may also be included. A collateralized external carotid artery may be mistaken for an internal carotid artery when the internal carotid artery is actually occluded. These techniques require an experienced technologist.

Principles and Instrumentation

Either continuous wave Doppler or pulse Doppler can be used. Continuous wave Doppler emits ultrasound continuously and receives reflected wave continuously. The difference between the transmitted and received signals falls within the hearing range. The received signals can then be distinguished by their auditory characteristics. In addition, the signal can be evaluated visually on a strip chart recorder or with a spectral analysis. In pulse Doppler the beam of pulse Doppler ultrasound is not continuously transmitted and received. Range-gating allows signals only from specific depths to be processed, thereby controlling sample size and range resolution. Two vessels located directly above one another can be evaluated separately, and vessels can also be followed as their course changes.

Doppler Signal Displays

The display can be done using the following methods. (1) auditory—achieved by simply displaying the Doppler-shifted frequencies as an audible sound. (2) Analog recording—Doppler-shifted frequencies can be displayed on a strip chart recorder that incorporates a zero-crossing detector. The circuitry counts every time the input signal crosses the 0 baseline within a specific time span. Because the number of times the sound waves oscillate each second varies, for example, high-frequency waves have many oscillations while low-frequency waves have few, and because the direction of flow varies during the cardiac cycle, the machine estimates the frequency of the reflected signal and displays it.

The vertical access represents the amplitude of the Doppler-shifted frequencies while the horizontal axis represents time. Analog recording has the following limitations: it works poorly in the presence of background noise, it is amplitude dependent, it does not display two peak frequencies, and its poor directional resolution may cause a venous and arterial signal to be added together. (3) Spectrum analysis—the FFT method makes it possible to display the individual frequencies that make up the return signal. Information related to the intensity of the spectrum is also possible: for example, a narrow well-defined spectrum is displayed when a limited number of frequencies is evident in a laminar flow. Spectral broadening represents a variety of frequencies and is often associated with turbulent flow. The velocity profile shows various frequency shifts on the vertical axis and time on the horizontal axis.

Technique

The patient is positioned supine with the head on a pillow. Optimal signals are usually obtained with the neck slightly hyperextended and the head slightly rotated away from the side being examined. Acoustic coupling gel is applied to the area to be examined. Pointing cephalad and maintaining a 45° to 60° angle of insonation, the continuous wave Doppler probe is placed on one side of the trachea and just above the clavicle to investigate the common carotid artery. As the examiner moves the probe cephalad, a change in the Doppler arterial signal signifies the bifurcation of the common carotid artery into the external carotid artery, which usually courses medially, and the internal carotid artery, which usually courses laterally.

Interpretation

Normal Findings

The external carotid artery supplies blood to the vascular bed that has high peripheral resistance. Therefore, its signal is more pulsatile and very similar to the signal from peripheral arteries, such as the common femoral artery. As shown in Figure 5–2 the external carotid artery has a rapid upstroke and downstroke with a very low diastolic

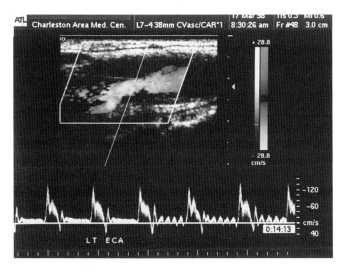

FIGURE 5–2. Color duplex ultrasound image of an external carotid artery. Note that the external carotid artery has a rapid upstroke and downstroke with a very low diastolic component. The diastolic notch is clearly seen and tapping of the superficial temporal artery causes oscillations in the waveform (bottom right).

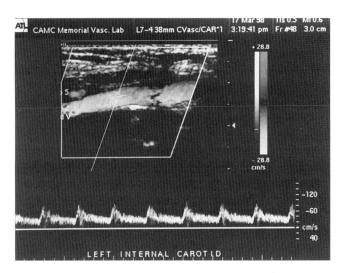

FIGURE 5–3. Color duplex ultrasound image of the internal carotid artery. Note that the waveform of the internal carotid artery has a rapid upstroke and downstroke with a high diastolic component. The diastolic notch may not be evident.

component. The diastolic notch is clearly seen and tapping the superficial temporal artery causes oscillations in the waveform (Figure 5–2).

The internal carotid artery signal is slightly more high-pitched and continuous than the signal from the external carotid artery. The blood flow in the internal carotid artery is less pulsatile since the brain is a low-resistance vascular bed, with increased flow during diastole. As shown in Figure 5–3, the waveform of the internal carotid artery has a rapid upstroke and downstroke with a high diastolic component. A diastolic notch may not be evident. The common carotid artery, meanwhile, has a flow characteristic of both the internal and external carotid arteries (Figure 5–4).

In a pulsed Doppler tracing, and because the sample volume would be more precisely placed in a center stream, the signals will have a narrow band of frequencies in systole with a blank area under that narrow band. The narrow band is called the spectral envelope; the blank area is called the frequency window or spectral window. The presence of these features is generally seen in laminar flow (Figure 5–5). In contrast, in continuous wave Doppler, because of the inability to regulate sample size or depth, a frequency window is not clear (Figure 5–6).

Abnormal Findings

The auditory signal from a stenotic vessel is characterized by a higher than normal pitch, with a very high-pitched hissing or squealing type of signal evident at significant stenosis. The waveform from a stenotic vessel has a higher than normal amplitude because of the accelerated flow through

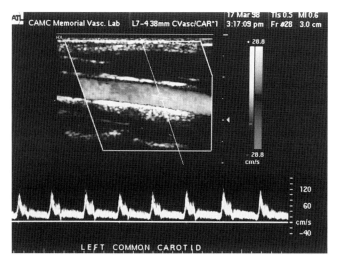

FIGURE 5–4. A color duplex ultrasound image of the common carotid artery. The common carotid artery signal has a flow characteristic of both the internal and external carotid arteries.

the stenosis (Figure 5–7). The very high-pitched hissing signal that is evident at a significant stenosis has a higher than normal amplitude in systole and diastole. In a spectral analysis, the band evident along the top of the waveform during systole may fill in the spectral window to create the spectral broadening that is consistent with turbulent flow (Figure 5–7). As seen in Figure 5–7, the more significant the stenosis, the greater the increase in systolic and diastolic frequencies. In severe stenoses there will be complete loss of the window. Distal to a stenosis, disturbed flow patterns are evident, i.e., damped monophasic flow (turbulence). It should be noted that an absent signal may suggest occlusion; however, a tight stenosis cannot be ruled out since blood flow may be difficult to detect with velocities of less than 6 cm/s.

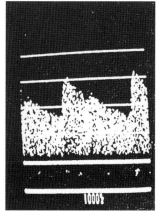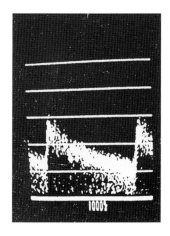

FIGURE 5–6. Left: continuous wave Doppler signal. Note the absence of a frequency window. Right: in contrast the pulse wave Doppler signal has a frequency window.

Occlusion of the internal carotid artery (Figure 5–8) is usually associated with a loss of the diastolic component in the ipsilateral common carotid artery. If the contralateral common carotid and internal carotid arteries are serving as collateral pathways, increased systolic and diastolic velocities may be evident in these arteries. If a carotid siphon stenosis is present, high resistance flow patterns may be evident in the extracranial internal carotid artery. Flow characteristics from one side must be compared with those on the other, as well as those in proximal to distal segments of the ipsilateral carotid system. Generally, this test is somewhat limited in patients with poor cardiac output or stroke volume, which may result in bilaterally diminished common carotid artery velocities. Unilateral reduction of velocities may

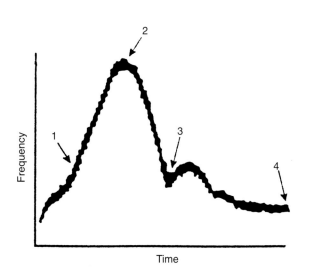

FIGURE 5–5. Spectral analysis of pulse Doppler waveform: 1, spectral envelope; 2, peak systole; 3, frequency window; 4, dicrotic notch; 5, diastole.

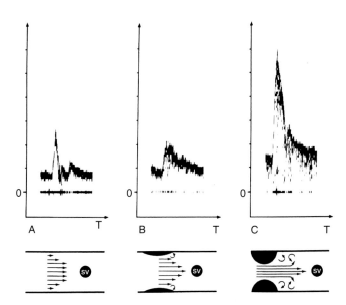

FIGURE 5–7. Waveforms from a normal vessel (A) in contrast to a mildly stenotic vessel (B) and a severely stenotic vessel (C). See text for a more detailed description.

based primarily on an analysis of the pulsed Doppler spectral waveforms.

Duplex Ultrasound Components

B-Mode Imaging

B-mode imaging has been used with varying degrees of success to evaluate carotid plaque morphology at the level of the carotid bifurcations, and to assess the histologic features of the plaques. Calcified atherosclerotic plaque, which is very echogenic, results in bright echoes and acoustic shadows (Figure 6–1). The ultrasonic carotid plaque morphology may correlate qualitatively with its histological composition, however, the clinical relevance of this information is somewhat controversial.[6–9] The B-mode characteristic of the carotid plaque that appears to correlate most closely with the clinical outcome is heterogeneity. This is generally defined as a plaque that has a mixture of hyperechoic, hypoechoic, and isoechoic plaques, a feature that may be attributed to the presence of intraplaque hemorrhage. This feature has been noted more frequently in patients with neurological events than in asymptomatic carotid stenoses. The size of the arterial lumen or the degree of stenosis may be difficult to evaluate using B-mode ultrasound only, because the interface between the arterial wall and the flow in blood is not always clearly seen. Acoustic shadowing from calcified plaques may also prevent thorough visualization of the arterial wall and lumen. These limitations are largely overcome by adding Doppler flow sampling, i.e., duplex technology. Generally speaking, B-mode imaging has been helpful in determining lesions of minimal to mod-

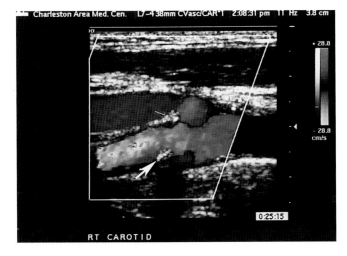

FIGURE 6–1. A color duplex ultrasound image of the carotid artery showing a calcified plaque (arrow) with acoustic shadowing underneath (under the arrow).

erate severity, but least accurate for high-grade stenoses or occlusion.

Doppler Spectral Waveform Analysis

A valuable adjunct to B-mode imaging is the use of spectral analysis to analyze the backscattered Doppler signal. Spectral analysis, as applied to Doppler ultrasound, is merely a method of determining the frequency content of the backscattered signal and the relative strengths or amplitude of these component frequencies. The original technique was utilized off line and employed a Kay sonograph, which although providing more information than was previously available with analog displays, was time-consuming and did not depict forward and reverse flow. Real-time spectral analysis was introduced using fast Fourier transform analysis. This has the advantages of saving time and detecting both forward and reverse flow. This method of signal processing was particularly suitable because pulsed Doppler beams were being utilized in the echo component. Other techniques of spectral analysis, including multiple bandpass filter analysis and time compression analysis, have been used, but have not achieved widespread acceptance.

The availability of the pulsed Doppler technique made it possible to obtain velocity information from a known location and, depending on the sample volume size, from a finite volume of the flow stream. The continuous-wave (CW) instruments utilized widely at that time for the detection of disease in the lower extremity were known to have a large sample volume that traversed the whole width of the vessel being insonated, and were really most suitable for determining the mean velocity in the forward or reverse direction. Also, the data analyzed by CW instruments were obtained not only from the vessel of interest, but also from other vessels in close proximity. With the pulsed instrument, the examiner could be certain that the data were being obtained from the vessel of interest. It was also possible, because of the finite sample volume, to interrogate a segment of the velocity profile and, perhaps, to detect changes that would not otherwise be apparent with a CW device.

A series of animal studies were conducted to determine the relationship between varying degrees of stenosis and spectral changes as identified by pulsed Doppler and fast Fourier spectrum analysis.[10] In these studies, artificial stenoses in the canine thoracic aorta were constructed using a snare loop technique, and the severity of stenosis was confirmed by arteriography. Validation that concentric stenoses were constructed was obtained by endoscopy under experimental perfusion pressures. A high-frequency (20-mHz) pulsed Doppler instrument was used to obtain center stream velocity samples at one, two, and three diameters distal to the areas of artificially created stenosis. The signals were subsequently analyzed

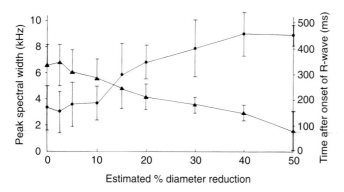

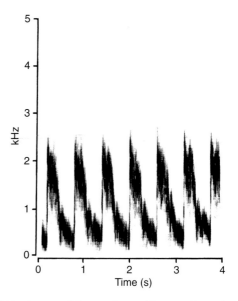

FIGURE 6–2. Results of an experimental study in canine thoracic aorta depicting the relationship between peak spectral width and percent diameter stenosis. The two graphs represent the maximum spectral width values obtained during the study as depicted by values on the left side and time after the onset of the R wave at which these values occurred as depicted on the right. Maximum spectral width increased gradually from a 15% diameter reducing stenosis to a 50% diameter reducing stenosis, while the time at which the maximum spectral width occurred appeared earlier in the cycle as this value increased.

FIGURE 6–3. A normal internal carotid artery Doppler spectra.

by spectral analysis and a computer program that measured peak spectral width as defined by the upper and lower frequency plots 8 dB on either side of the mode frequency. The time in the cycle at which maximum spectral broadening occurred could be determined, as an ECG timing device was utilized during the studies. The relationship between maximum spectral width and percent stenosis, and the time of maximum spectral width were determined and are depicted in Figure 6–2.

As noted, spectral broadening was present in normal vessels, and those with minimal degrees of stenosis up to a 15% diameter reduction, at which point this parameter gradually increased reaching a maximum value at 50% diameter-reducing stenosis. Statistical analysis of these results confirmed that this parameter could be utilized to differentiate between stenoses of 15% diameter and increments between 15% and 50% diameter reducing stenosis. In addition, it should be noted that maximum spectral width in normal or minimally stenotic arteries occurred late in the pulse cycle and, as the stenosis became more severe, occurred earlier in the cycle. While the velocity profile in the canine thoracic aorta differs from that seen in the human internal carotid artery, this study provided validation of the relationship between spectral broadening and nonhemodynamically significant stenoses.

The Doppler spectral waveform analysis is a signal processing technique that displays the complete frequency and amplitude content of the Doppler signal. This Doppler-shifted frequency is directly proportional to blood cell velocity, and the amplitude of the Doppler signal depends on the number of cells moving through the pulsed Doppler sample volume. The signal amplitude becomes stronger as the number of cells producing

Doppler frequency shift increases. This spectral information is usually presented graphically with time on the horizontal axis and frequency or velocity on the vertical axis; and amplitude is indicated by shades of gray (Figure 6–3).

The following is an explanation of these findings as it applies to the flow patterns within vessels. The center stream flow pattern in a normal artery is uniform or laminar, and a spectral waveform taken with the pulsed Doppler sample volume in the center of the lumen shows a relatively narrow band of frequency. It appears that even relatively mild degrees of stenosis are capable of producing deviations from laminar flow (as zones of vorticeal shedding) in the area distal to the stenosis (Figure 6–4), with the magnitude of these disturbances being

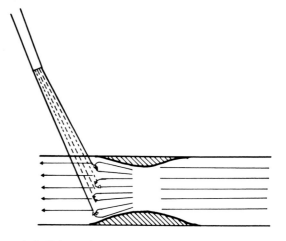

FIGURE 6–4. Schematic representation of a minor flow disturbance generated by nonhemodynamically significant stenosis with production of vorticeal shedding immediately beyond the area of the stenosis with resumption of a normal laminar flow pattern further downstream.

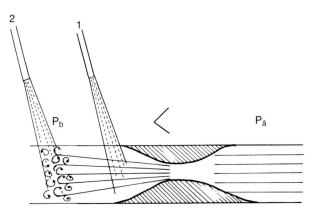

FIGURE 6–5. Schematic representation of major flow disturbance produced by hemodynamically significant stenosis with both increases in peak velocity in and immediately beyond the stenosis with decay of laminar flow to turbulent flow occurring at a maximum two diameters distal to the stenosis.

depicted by the magnitude of change in spectral width (spectral broadening). With hemodynamically significant stenoses, not only is spectral broadening present, which is produced by a major decay in the laminar flow pattern, but there is also a marked elevation in peak frequency or peak velocity at systole as a result of the high-speed jet of blood passing through and immediately beyond the stenosis (Figure 6–5). High-grade stenoses can, therefore, be recognized by the presence of both elevations in peak frequency at systole and diffuse spectral broadening.[5]

The end diastolic frequency or velocity is also increased in very severe stenoses. The Doppler spectral waveform criteria for classifying severity of carotid artery stenosis will be described in detail later.

The current application of duplex scanning in the detection of carotid artery disease utilizes this principle of identification of flow disturbance patterns by Doppler velocity detection instrumentation, with the emphasis in later years being on technical improvements in instrument design. A variety of duplex scanning instruments are available, the major differences among them being in the Doppler component. These are of two types: those utilizing CW Doppler and those utilizing pulsed Doppler beams. The outline below applies to the instrumentation available that currently uses pulsed Doppler beams for velocity detection and image generation.

Instrumentation

Originally, three fixed-focus 5-mHz transducers, mounted in a rotating wheel, generated a two-dimensional soft tissue image with 16 levels of gray, for characterization at

a rate of 30 frames per second. The image information is digitized, as a result of which the image can be frozen, and one of the transducers is used solely as a pulsed Doppler source. The axis of the Doppler beam is superimposed on the image with the location of the sample volume depicted by a prominent white dot (Figure 6–6). The backscattered Doppler signal is processed using fast Fourier transform spectral analysis with display of the spectra on an oscilloscope screen. Hard copy reproduction is obtained using either a Polaroid camera or light-sensitive paper.

The most significant changes in instrumentation have occurred in scan head design. The shape of the pulsed Doppler beam, and therefore its sample volume, has been modified using either medium-focus or short-focus scan heads. The medium-focus scan head, operating at 5 mHz, has a 40-mm focal point, while the short-focus scan head, at a transmitting frequency of 5 mHz, has a 20-mm focal point. The beam width of the medium-focus scan head is most narrow at 35–45 mm depth, whereas that of the short-focus scan head is most narrow at 20–30 mm. The medium-focus scan head is, therefore, more appropriate for evaluating blood flow in vessels deeper than 30 mm, while the short-focus scan head is ideal for evaluating flow in vessels located close to the surface, 2–3 cm from the skin. Because the carotid arteries lie within 30 mm of the skin surface in the majority of human subjects, the short-focus scan head, at least theoretically, is ideal for evaluating these vessels.

These features are not only important in a consideration of the depths of the vessels studied, but also in understanding the effects of the sample volume size on the velocity profile being evaluated. If a large sample volume

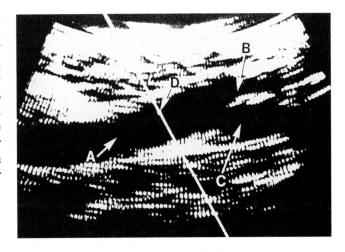

FIGURE 6–6. Oscilloscope screen depiction of the pulsed echo image generated by the duplex scanner with the Doppler beam axis depicted by the continuous white line and the location of the sample volume depicted by the bright white dot(D).

size is used in the evaluation of small-diameter vessels, a wide range of velocities will be detected under normal circumstances, which on spectral analysis will appear as spectral broadening. In these circumstances, this finding is normal and is similar to the spectra generated by CW instruments. Conversely, if a small sample volume is used in a large vessel, particularly if flow is axisymmetric, the velocities in the sample volume are likely to be similar, and on spectral analysis, will not display spectral broadening. At a range of 25 mm, the beam widths for the medium- and short-focus scan heads are 5.5 mm and 2 mm, respectively, at the 20 dB level. At this range, the sample volumes have been calculated at 3 mm^3 and 24 mm^3 for the short- and medium-focus scan heads, respectively. If spectral broadening, therefore, is an important feature in the evaluation, it is apparent that a short-focus scan head should be more sensitive than a medium-focus scan head.

An additional feature of the current instruments is the dedicated use of the pulsed signal to the Doppler component, which avoids the problem of aliasing encountered in the original prototypes. In the latter, the signal was shared between the echo and Doppler components and resulted in a limited peak frequency detection capability that could be exceeded when severe disease was present. With the pulsed echo component nonoperative, the usual pulse repetition frequency available to the Doppler component is doubled, increasing the frequency response of the 5-mHz instrument at 60° to 9.5 kHz, which is more than adequate to detect the frequencies associated with severe disease.

The quadrature outputs of the pulsed Doppler signal are then analyzed using an on-line fast Fourier transform spectral analyzer, providing a full-scale frequency display of 10 kHz, with 7 kHz usually being used for forward frequencies and 3 kHz for reverse frequencies. The amplitude of the component frequencies in the signal is depicted in gray-scale format on the oscilloscope screen.

To improve the signal-to-noise ratio on the spectral display, the signal in many instruments is "normalized," a principle that increases the highest amplitude of each analysis in the spectrum to a particular reference level with the subsequent same scaling factor being applied to all other amplitudes. Following this normalizing process, a variable amount of signal is then displayed depending on the dynamic range used with the Doppler signal. The use of a wide dynamic range enhances the likelihood that in addition to the Doppler backscattered signal, noise will also be displayed. Narrow dynamic range is ideal for evaluating the Doppler signal only.

The addition of high definition imaging (HDI) technology revolutionized the front end of the ultrasound image formation process. The extended signal processing, or ESP technology (Advanced Technology Laboratories/Phillips System), extends the momentum into the area of signal processing. The result is a substantial reduction in speckle noise, allowing a higher level of clarity and detail than has ever been seen in ultrasound images. Tissue differentiation and resolution of fine anatomical detail, already hallmarks of HDI images, are enhanced even further through the addition of ESP technology.

The technology developments that make high HDI and extended signal processing possible are many and complex. Perhaps the most appropriate place to begin is with the acoustic information that is returned to the ultrasound system from the body.

Each tissue within the body responds to ultrasound energy of different frequencies in a characteristic way, which is often referred to as the tissue signature. The tissue signature information is carried within the spectrum of ultrasound frequencies returning from the tissue. This band of frequencies is referred to as the frequency spectrum bandwidth, or simply, bandwidth.

HDI preserves the quantity and quality of tissue signature through the capture and preservation of the entire bandwidth. This results in more sonographic information with better detail and definition.

The ultrasound beamformer, together with the scanhead, determines the ultimate contrast resolution, spatial resolution, penetration, and consistency of the image. If the acoustic information containing the tissue signature is reduced in quantity, or distorted in the beamformer, there is no way of recovering it.

Beam formation is accomplished by pulsing the transducer elements in the scanhead to insonify the target. Sound waves reflected by the target return to the elements of the transducer, generating signals that are essentially separated in time. The beamformer delays these signals so when all the channels are summed together, the time variations in the signals are compensated for and the exact tissue definition is obtained.

The critical design requirements of the beamformer are to preserve the entire bandwidth, which contains all of the acoustic information and to prevent distortion of the signal during delay.

More recently, SonoCT real-time compound imaging was incorporated into duplex technology. Using up to nine "lines of sight," SonoCT imaging dramatically enhances image quality by providing up to nine times more information than conventional two-dimensional imaging. The resulting real-time image is a more realistic representation of actual tissue.

The clinical benefits of SonoCT real-time compound imaging include improved visualization of plaque border delineation, allows better assessment of plaque morphology, reduction of clutter artifacts seen in difficult-to-image patients, and reduction of posterior plaque shadowing to reveal the full extent of vascular disease.

The new HDI 5000 SonoCT systems (Advanced Technology Laboratories, Phillips) have a breakthrough pro-

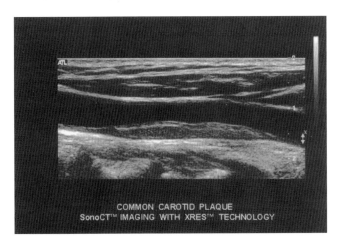

FIGURE 6–7. A SonoCT image showing tissue texture, borders, and margins.

cessing technology that optimizes image quality down to the pixel level. It displays a SonoCT image with unprecedented visualization of tissue texture, borders, and margins, almost free of image-degrading artifacts (Figure 6–7).

Carotid Examination Technique

The examination is conducted with the patient supine and the head slightly extended and turned slightly away from the side being examined and supported to eliminate lateral movement. Copious quantities of water-soluble acoustic gel are applied along the anterior border of the sternomastoid muscle and the scan head is applied to the skin surface. A 7.5- or 5-mHz transducer is usually used. Presently, we are using the HDI 5000 system, Advanced Technology Laboratory, Bothell, WA (Figure 6–8). If color flow imaging is used, Doppler information is displayed on the image after it is evaluated for its phase (i.e., direction toward or away from the transducer) and its frequency content (i.e., a hue or shade of color). The sample volume of the pulsed Doppler should be kept as small as possible and placed in the center of the vessel or the flow channel. A Doppler angle of 45–60° should be maintained to obtain consistent results in velocity measurements. The vessels are examined both in longitudinal (Figure 6–9) and transverse views (Figure 6–10), and followed from the clavicle to the mandible with anterior oblique, lateral, and posterior oblique projections to identify and evaluate any carotid plaques or pathology.

The scan head is then moved cephalad with the B-mode imaging display activated, and with frequent sampling of the center stream velocity signal. Audible interpretation alone is usually used during this phase of the examination. The region of the carotid bifurcation is identified by the presence of two vessels and visualization of the superior thyroid artery branch of the external carotid artery. This may be confirmed by sampling in the center stream just distal to the origin of these vessels and identifying the characteristic differences between the two arteries.

It is recommended that the dynamic range be set to 40–50 dB to optimize the gray-scale image and the time gain compensation (TGC) as needed, in regards to the depth of the carotid and vertebral arteries examined.

The external carotid signal is recognized by the presence of flow reversal, while the internal carotid signal is identified by the absence of flow reversal and the presence of forward flow during diastole. The scan head is moved further cephalad to insonate the proximal few centimeters of the internal carotid artery, which is the common site of disease. Abnormalities in the velocity spectra displayed on the screen are noted for subsequent reference. Once the general anatomy has been outlined, a detailed examination is performed. The initial quick scanning of the vessels provides a reference for deter-

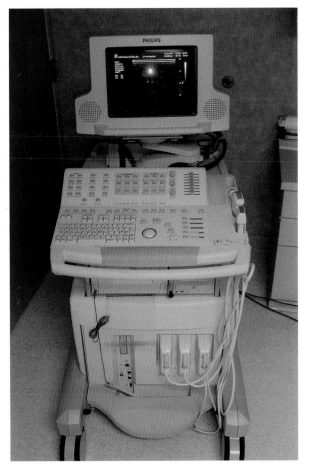

FIGURE 6–8. A duplex ultrasound machine, HDI 5000 system, Advanced Technology Laboratory/Phillips, Bothell, WA.

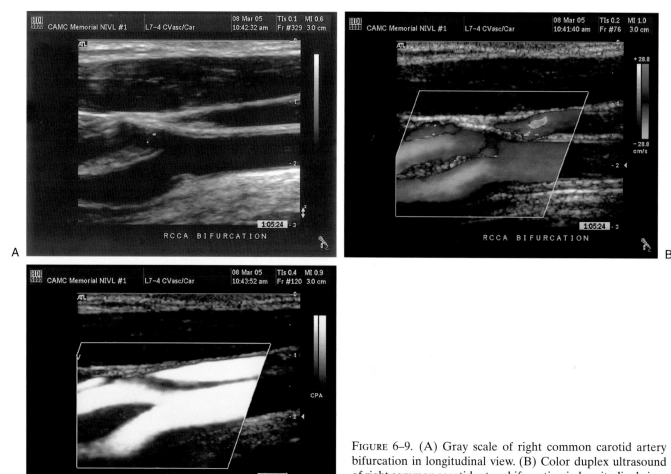

FIGURE 6–9. (A) Gray scale of right common carotid artery bifurcation in longitudinal view. (B) Color duplex ultrasound of right common carotid artery bifurcation in longitudinal view. (C) Power Doppler image of right common carotid artery bifurcation in longitudinal view.

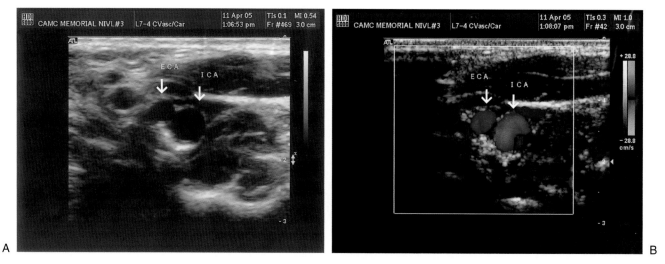

FIGURE 6–10. (A) Common carotid artery bifurcation in transverse view (grayscale). (B) Common carotid artery bifurcation in transverse view (color flow).

mining whether disease is present and, if so, its severity. It is likely that these areas will require more detailed interrogation than areas that are normal.

Following the preliminary scan, the scan head is returned to the base of the neck over the anterior border of the sternomastoid muscle, and the common carotid artery is again visualized. Note is taken of the presence or absence of calcification in the wall represented by dense acoustic shadows and a deeper acoustic window. Representative spectra are then obtained from the center stream with the Doppler beam axis at 60° and the signals recorded on videotape for subsequent analysis. During this part of the examination, the peak frequency or velocity should be noted and whether the velocity is always in the forward direction throughout the whole of the cycle.

Low peak systolic frequencies or velocities suggest occlusions of the internal or external carotid arteries, while frequencies approaching zero are suggestive of either high-grade stenosis or occlusion of the internal carotid artery. Other variations in the waveform may occur as a result of significant aortic disease.

The scan head is again moved cephalad with a second center stream sample being obtained just proximal to the region of the bulb. With rapid shifting from B-mode to Doppler mode imaging, the evaluation is continued through and into the proximal internal carotid artery, looking for abnormal spectral displays. Care must always be taken during sampling to ensure that the sample volume cursor is located in the center stream of the vessel, and the incident angle of the Doppler beam to the long axis of the vessel is as close as possible to 60°. The presence of disease is suspected by echogenic shadows impinging on the lumen of the vessel associated with either changes in spectral broadening or fluctuations in peak systolic and diastolic frequencies or velocities. It is frequently necessary to obtain multiple spectra along the center stream axis of the internal carotid artery to determine the location at which the most abnormal spectra occur. These should be recorded on videotape for future reference.

Attention is then directed to the subclavian artery in the posterior triangle of the neck and the vessel is visualized. Scanning proceeds proximally with identification of the origin of the vertebral artery and subsequent sampling with the Doppler component of the orifice in the proximal centimeter of the first portion of this vessel, as this is the usual site of stenotic disease.

With a clear view of the common carotid artery, the probe is slowly angled more posterior-laterally to identify the vertebral artery. This artery will have vertical shadows running through it from the spinous processes of the vertebrae, giving it the appearance of a series of Hs (Figure 6–11). Vertebral flow is documented, either antegrade or retrograde flow. Major elevations in peak frequency are characteristic of high-grade orifice steno-

sis. The contralateral side of the neck is then evaluated in a similar manner and representative recordings from the common carotid, external, and internal carotid arteries are obtained.

The following considerations are generally helpful in optimizing color flow setup and value. The appropriate color pulse repetition frequency (PRF) must be chosen by setting the color velocity scale for the expected velocities in the examined vessel. The scale should be adjusted to avoid systolic aliasing (low PRF) or diastolic flow gaps (high PRF) in normal vessels. Every effort should be made to avoid using large wider color boxes, which may slow down frame rates and resolution of the imaged vessel. It is recommended that color boxes that cover the entire vessel diameter and are approximately 1–2 cm of its length be used. The color, power, and gain should be optimized so that flow signals are recorded throughout the lumen of the examined vessel with no bleeding of color into the adjacent tissues.

The zero baseline of color bar (BRF) is set at approximately two-thirds of the range with the majority of frequencies allowed in the red direction for flow toward the brain, which will display higher arterial mean frequency shifts without aliasing artifacts. The color PRF and zero baseline may also need to be readjusted throughout the examination to allow for changes in velocity that may occur if carotid tortuosity or stenosis is present. Adjustments in the PRF are generally needed in the examination of the carotid bulb where the color differentiation scale should be set to visualize the slower flow in the boundary separation zone. The PRF range is generally adjusted higher to detect increased velocity in the region adjacent to the flow divider. Similarly, the color PRF should be increased to display higher velocities detected in the presence of carotid stenosis and to avoid aliasing. In the poststenotic zone, the color PRF should be decreased to observe the lower velocities and flow direction changes in the region of turbulent flow just distal to the stenosis. Color PRF should also be decreased when occlusion is suspected to detect the preocclusive, low velocity, high resistant signal associated with tight stenosis or carotid occlusion, and to confirm absence of flow at the sight of the occlusion. The color PRF should also be decreased in the presence of a carotid bruit to detect the lower frequencies associated with a bruit.

Color sensitivity (ensemble length) should be around 12 in systems where there is an adjustable control. The ensemble length can be increased in regions where more sensitive color representation is needed. Keep in mind that the frame rate will decrease when the ensemble length is increased. The color wall filter should also be set as low as possible, and you may need to decrease the wall filter manually when decreasing the color PRF. The color wall filter may automatically increase as the PRF is increased.

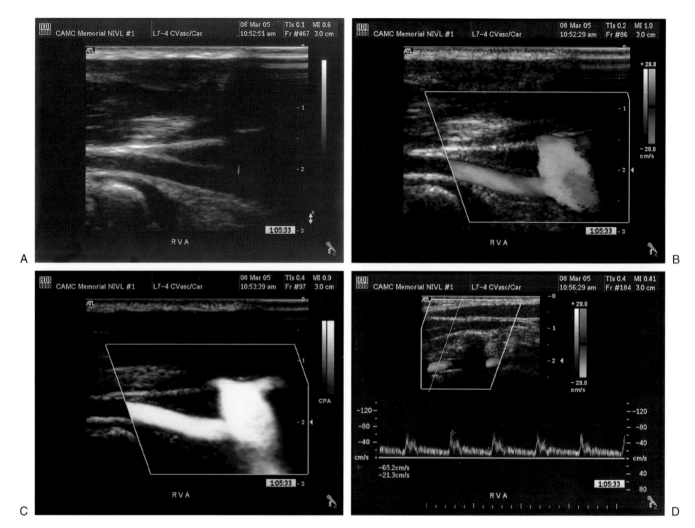

FIGURE 6–11. (A) Origin of right vertebral artery in grayscale. (B) Origin of right vertebral artery using color duplex ultrasound. (C) Origin of right vertebral artery using power Doppler. (D) Mid right vertebral artery (series of H appearance).

The angle of the color box should also be changed to obtain the most accurate Doppler angle between the scan lines and the direction of the blood flow. This will yield a better color display, secondary to better Doppler angle. The color box should be kept to a size that is adequate for visualizing the area of interest, and should be kept small enough to keep the frame rate at a reasonable number. The color gain should be adjusted throughout the examination to detect the changing signal strength. If this is not properly adjusted, too much color may be displaced or some color information may be lost, which may result in seeing color in areas where there is no flow. In patients with very low flow or questionable carotid occlusion, an overgained level may be advantageous to show any flow that may be present.

The desaturation of the color from darker to lighter hues on the color bar indicates increasing velocities. The colors are darkest close to the zero baseline, and as the velocities increase, the colors become lighter. Color should be selected so that the highest frequency shifts in each direction are of high contrast to each other so that you can easily detect aliasing, e.g., the color selection can be set so that low to high velocities are seen as dark blue to light green to aqua in one direction and red to orange to yellow in the opposite direction. Aliasing in these circumstances would appear as aqua, adjacent to yellow.

Since the frame rate is affected by the PRF, ensemble length, depth, and width of the color box, it should be kept as high as possible to capture the rapid change in flow dynamics that occurs with carotid stenosis, particularly in the carotid bulb region. The frame rate decreases with decreasing PRF and increasing the color ensemble length will also decrease the frame rate. Increased color box width and deep insonation will also decrease the frame rate.

Limitations of Duplex Technology

Duplex technology of the carotid arteries may be adversely affected by the following: acoustic shadowings from calcification, soft tissue edema or hematoma, the depth or course of the vessel, the size of the neck, and the presence of sutures or skin staples.

Duplex ultrasonography may also overestimate or underestimate the degree of stenoses or plaquing. Underestimation of disease can be noted if it fails to appreciate very low level echoes of soft plaque, or the examiner does not carefully interrogate the vessel and misses accelerated flow; or in patients with long, smooth plaque formation, which does not have the accelerated, turbulent flow pattern usually associated with the hemodynamically significant stenoses, or if an inappropriate Doppler angle is used (e.g., above 60°). Stenoses can also be overestimated when an artifact is mistaken for a carotid plaque, if accelerated flow is mistakenly attributed to stenosis, if there is vessel tortuosity or kinking, and in the presence of significant stenoses or occlusion on the contralateral side.

Due to the varying filling phases of the cardiac cycle, cardiac arrhythmia makes it more difficult to evaluate the flow spectra. Also, the flow velocity will be lower in a wider vessel and higher in a narrower vessel at the same flow intensity. Therefore, the flow in a wide carotid sinus can easily be disturbed, and may incorrectly suggest pathological findings.

Interpretation and Determination of Disease Severity

A complete extracranial carotid duplex examination should include the following data.

1. The peak systolic and end diastolic velocities of common carotid, internal carotid, and external carotid arteries, right and left subclavian arteries, and vertebral arteries.
2. The internal carotid artery to common carotid artery peak systolic velocities ratio.
3. Flow direction of the vertebral artery (antegrade or retrograde).
4. Analysis of the Doppler spectral waveform of the examined vessels.
5. The presence or absence of plaque and description of its morphology.

B-Mode Imaging Interpretation

An echoic area should be evident between the walls of the vessel, indicating the absence of pathology, i.e.,

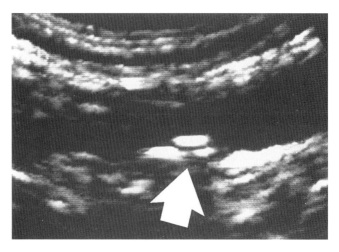

FIGURE 6–12. Duplex ultrasound image of the carotid artery showing homogeneous plaque (arrow).

plaquing, whose density usually differs from that of the blood. An echoic line indicating the endothelium may be evident at the vessel lumen. The following abnormalities can be noted on B-mode imaging:

1. Fatty streaks, low level echoes of similar appearance (homogeneous) can be detected.
2. Fibrous soft plaque (homogeneous): low to medium level echoes of similar appearance (Figure 6–12).
3. Complex plaque (heterogeneous): low, medium, and high level echoes indicating soft and dense areas (Figure 6–13). This plaque is a mixture of isoechoic, hyperechoic, or hypoechoic plaque.
4. Calcification: very bright, highly reflected echoes are noted. The acoustic shadowing from calcifications prevents a thorough evaluation of the vessel and may result in the calculation of an erroneous percentage of stenosis (Figure 6–1).
5. Vessel thrombosis: fresh carotid thrombosis may not be detected without using Doppler flow sampling since fresh thrombus has the same echogenicity of flowing blood.

Carotid plaque morphology is generally characterized into smooth (Figure 6–14) or irregular plaques (Figure 6–15) according to surface, and homogeneous (Figure 6–12) versus heterogeneous (Figure 6–13) according to plaque structure. An ulcerative plaque is usually an irregular plaque with a cleft within the plaque that can be seen on B-mode imaging (Figure 6–16).

Estimation of Stenosis Based on B-Mode Imaging

Ideally, carotid plaque should be visible from at least two of the longitudinal, or sagittal projections, and in the transverse view to give a rough estimate of stenosis.

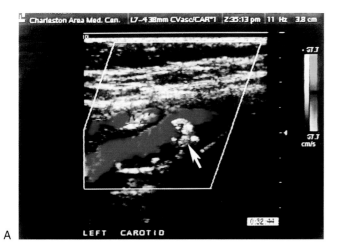

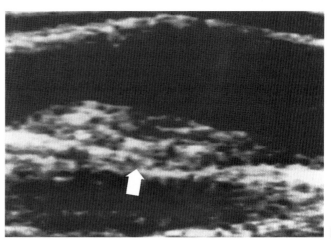

FIGURE 6–13. (A) Color duplex ultrasound image of the carotid bifurcation showing a complex heterogeneous plaque at the origin of the internal carotid artery (arrow). (B) A duplex ultrasound image of the carotid artery showing a heterogeneous plaque (arrow).

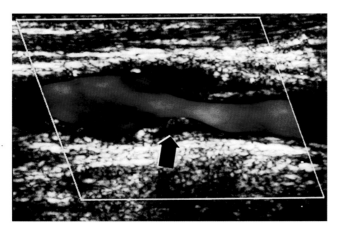

FIGURE 6–14. A color duplex ultrasound image of the carotid artery showing a smooth heterogeneous plaque (arrow). The dark center of the plaque may represent intraplaque hemorrhage.

Percent diameter stenosis equals the ratio of the residual diameter to vessel lumen diameter minus 1 multiplied by 100. Percentage of area of stenosis is calculated similarly, except you substitute the area for the diameter. The vessel lumen diameter (in longitudinal view) or area (in transverse view) is measured from intima to intima. Then the residual lumen diameter, or area, is measured (Figure 6–17). The percent reduction is calculated using the above formula. The approximate relationship between diameter and area of stenosis is shown in Table 6–1. These values are applicable to circular geometry.

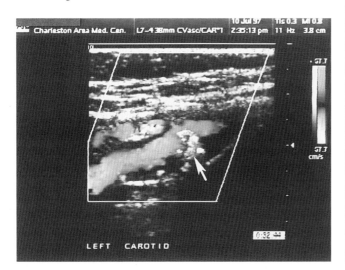

FIGURE 6–15. A carotid color duplex ultrasound image showing an irregular plaque of the proximal internal carotid artery (arrow).

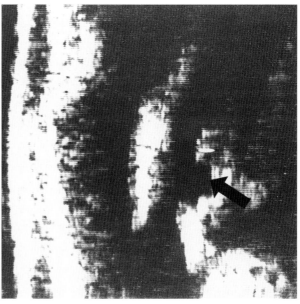

FIGURE 6–16. A duplex ultrasound image of the carotid bifurcation showing an ulcerative lesion of the proximal internal carotid artery (arrow).

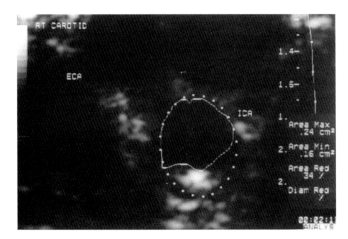

FIGURE 6–17. Calculation of area reduction percent stenosis. This image reflects the greatest stenosis in transverse diameter. An elliptical measurement of the arterial lumen is taken. Then an elliptical trace of the residual lumen is made. The percent area reduction is calculated by the duplex machine. To calculate the diameter reduction percent stenosis, a similar calculation is performed with the vessel in longitudinal view.

A chronic arterial occlusion may be diagnosed using B-mode imaging, although Doppler interrogation is essential to this diagnosis. Depending on the type of occlusive process, the artery may be filled with highly echogenic material or be anechoic.

Determination of Disease Severity Using Doppler Spectral Analysis

Identification of disease in the carotid system uses both qualitative and quantitative data. Careful attention to

TABLE 6–1. % Diameter stenosis vs. % area stenosis.[a,b]

% Stenosis by	
Diameter stenosis	Area reduction
0	0
10	19
11	36
30	51
40	64
50	75
60	84
70	91
80	96
90	99
100	100

[a]% Diameter stenosis (%Ds) = 100 × [1 − (inner diameter/outer diameter)]. % Area stenosis (%As) = 100 × [1 − (inner area/outer area)]. %As = 100 − 100 × [1 − %Ds/100)]².
[b]Assuming concentric circle.

unusual echoes on the image serves as a qualitative guide to the presence of disease at sites where careful scrutiny with a Doppler component should be performed. The changes in spectra obtained from the common, internal, and external carotid arteries provide quantitative information for the determination of the severity of disease in these locations. This is probably best considered by describing the normal and abnormal spectra generated in various anatomical locations by disease of varying severity, according to the University of Washington criteria.[11]

These original criteria by the University of Washington are described in the following sections since they are still commonly used in the United States, and they have been the foundation for interpretation of carotid artery stenosis. However, later is this chapter you will find that other authorities modified these criteria to be compatible with the indication for carotid endarterectomy as proposed by the North American Symptomatic Carotid Endarterectomy Trial (NASCET) and Asymptomatic Carotid Artherosclerosis Study (ACAS) trials.

Normal Internal Carotid Spectra or Minimal Disease (0–15% Stenosis)

The characteristic features of normal internal carotid artery spectra are shown in Figure 6–3. The peak frequency at systole is less than 4 kHz (a peak systolic velocity of <125 cm/s) with minimal degrees of spectral broadening during the initial deceleration phase of systole, followed by mild spectral broadening during diastole. The velocities are always in the forward direction and, therefore, the frequencies depicted on the scale are always above the zero line. The velocity envelope during systole is relatively narrow and displays a large clear window area under the systolic curve. Correlation with arteriographic findings has supported the view that this type of waveform may also be generated with minimal disease up to 15–20% diameter reduction and, therefore, identification of this type of waveform confirms the presence of either a normal vessel or one in which only minimal disease is present. Figure 6–18 is a color duplex imaging of a normal common carotid artery, an internal carotid artery, and an external carotid artery.

Mild Stenosis (16–<50%)

As noted in the discussion regarding findings with animal studies, it is over the range of mild stenosis that spectral broadening changes in both magnitude and timing, and it is the presence of spectral broadening in systole, particularly during the deceleration phase, which is characteristic of the spectra generated by the presence of mild disease. As shown in Figures 6–19 and 6–20, the peak

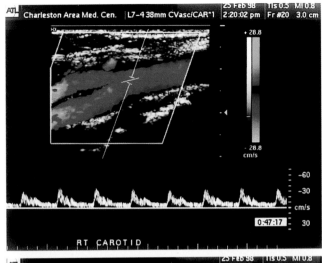

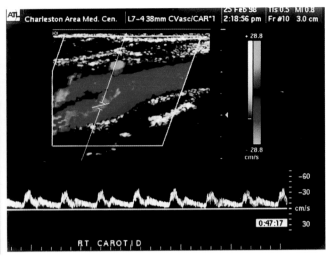

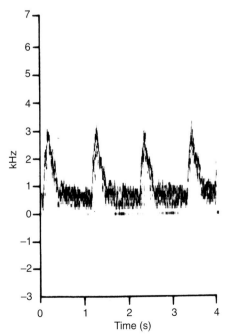

FIGURE 6–18. (A) A color duplex ultrasound image showing a normal common carotid artery with a normal Doppler spectra (bottom of figure). (B) A color duplex ultrasound image of the carotid bifurcation showing a normal internal carotid artery with a normal Doppler spectra (bottom of figure). (C) A color duplex ultrasound image of the carotid bifurcation showing a normal external carotid artery with a normal Doppler spectra (bottom of figure).

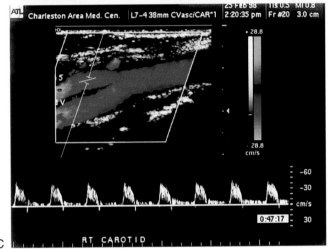

FIGURE 6–19. Internal carotid artery Doppler spectra associated with mild stenosis (15% to <50%).

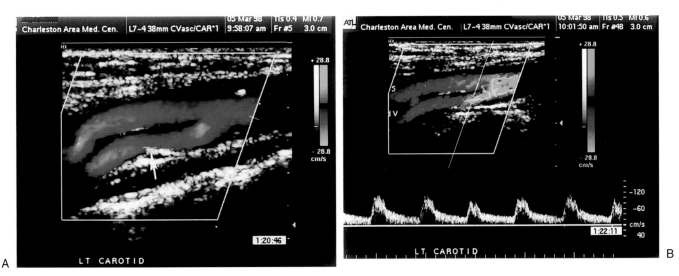

FIGURE 6–20. (A) A color duplex ultrasound image showing mild plaquing (15% to <50% stenosis) of the internal carotid artery (arrow). (B) The same patient in (A) showing internal carotid artery Doppler spectra associated with mild stenosis.

frequency remains below 4 kHz (a peak systolic velocity of <125 cm/s) and spectral broadening is also present during diastole, although it may be of greater magnitude than seen in the normal. Again, velocity is always in the forward direction, and therefore the frequencies, even during diastole, are above the zero frequency line.

Moderate to Severe Disease (50–<80% Stenosis)

As the lesion becomes progressively more occlusive (50–<80% diameter reduction), the velocity of the red blood cells traversing the stenosis increases, producing an increase in peak frequency or velocity at systole (Figures 6–21 and 6–22). Frequencies above 4 kHz in systole (a peak systolic velocity of >125 cm/s and an end diastolic velocity of <125 cm/s) are characteristic of this stenosis.

Tight Stenosis (80–99%)

With the development of high-grade lesions in excess of 80% diameter reduction, the end diastolic frequency increases (>4 kHz, or a peak systolic velocity of ≥125 cm/s and an end diastolic velocity of ≥125 cm/s) so that the ratio between peak frequency at systole and peak frequency at diastole falls, providing an accurate method of identifying these high-grade lesions. Diffuse spectral broadening is also present during the whole of the cycle, and with these lesions, the diastolic velocity at the lower frequencies approaches zero (Figures 6–23 and 6–24).

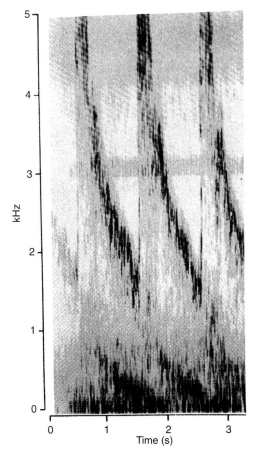

FIGURE 6–21. Internal carotid artery Doppler spectra of severe stenosis (50% to <80%).

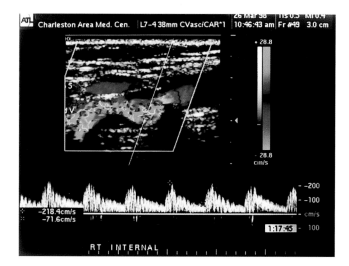

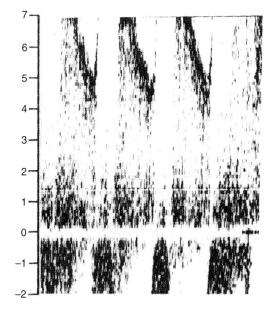

FIGURE 6–22. A color duplex ultrasound image of an internal carotid artery showing Doppler spectra of severe stenosis (50% to <80%). The peak systolic velocity on this patient was 218.4 cm/s with an end diastolic velocity of 71.6 cm/s.

FIGURE 6–23. Internal carotid artery Doppler spectra of tight stenosis (80–99%).

Internal Carotid Occlusion

Occlusion of the internal carotid artery (Figure 6–25) is recognized by imaging a vessel in the characteristic anatomical location of the internal carotid artery with no detectable Doppler signal. It is important to ensure that the internal carotid artery is being examined, and as part of this evaluation, visualization of the external carotid artery is mandatory. The differentiation between the internal and external carotid arteries is made by visualization of the superior thyroid artery branch. Changes in the real-time spectra produced by compression of the superficial temporal artery that increases the outflow resistance usually result in a decrease in peak systolic frequency. Other features characteristic of occlusion are the presence of frequencies to the zero baseline, or even

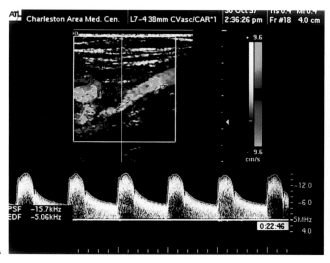

A

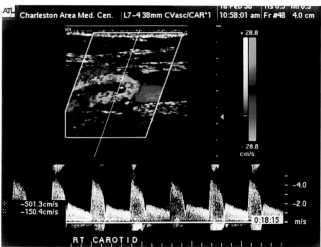

B

FIGURE 6–24. (A) A color duplex ultrasound image of the internal carotid artery showing Doppler spectra of tight stenosis (80–99%). The peak systolic frequency was 15.7 kHz with an end diastolic frequency of 5.06 kHz. (B) A color duplex ultrasound image of an internal carotid artery showing Doppler spectra of tight stenosis (80–99%). The peak systolic velocity was 501.3 cm/s with an end diastolic velocity of 150.4 cm/s.

negative frequencies, indicative of flow reversal obtained from the common carotid artery low in the neck.[12] When the internal carotid artery is occluded, the ipsilateral common carotid artery assumes a velocity pattern similar to that of the external carotid artery and the external carotid artery may assume flow characteristics of the internal carotid artery, i.e., high diastolic component.

Common carotid artery occlusion can also be diagnosed by color duplex ultrasound. Figure 6–26 shows retrograde flow of the external carotid artery and antegrade flow of the internal carotid artery.

Occlusions are periodically missed due to changes in physiologic parameters attendant upon the presence of internal carotid artery occlusions. Figure 6–27 shows the arteriogram and spectra obtained from a patient in whom

internal carotid occlusion was missed because the external carotid artery was a major source of collateral blood flow to the middle cerebral artery, and, as such, developed the spectral changes characteristic of a high-grade internal carotid stenosis. Errors such as this can be avoided by careful evaluation of the image for the presence of branches originating from the vessel being examined and the change in the velocity profile induced by superficial temporal artery compression.

The Role of Power Doppler and Carotid Artery Occlusion

Power Doppler ultrasound displays an estimate of the entire power contained in that part of the received radio

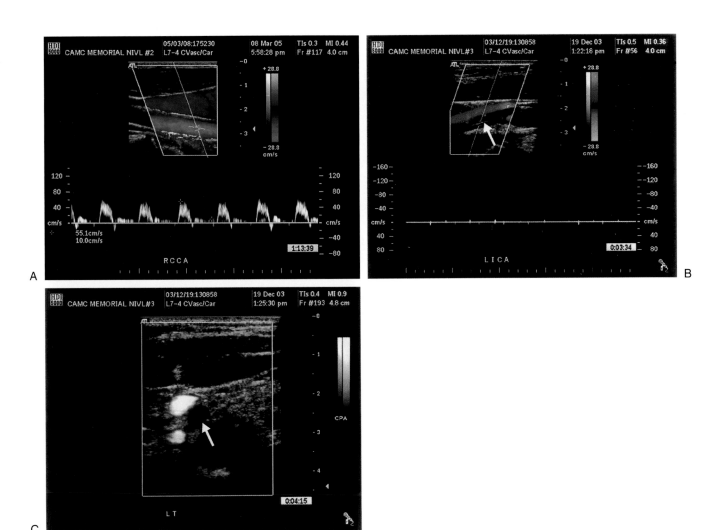

FIGURE 6–25. (A) A common carotid artery Doppler spectra produced by occlusion of the ipsilateral internal carotid artery. Peak frequency is not abnormally high, but the characteristic feature is the presence of reverse flow in diastole. (B) Internal carotid artery occlusion in longitudinal view (no color flow). (C) Internal carotid artery occlusion in transverse view [no color flow in power Doppler (arrow); color flow is seen in the external carotid artery].

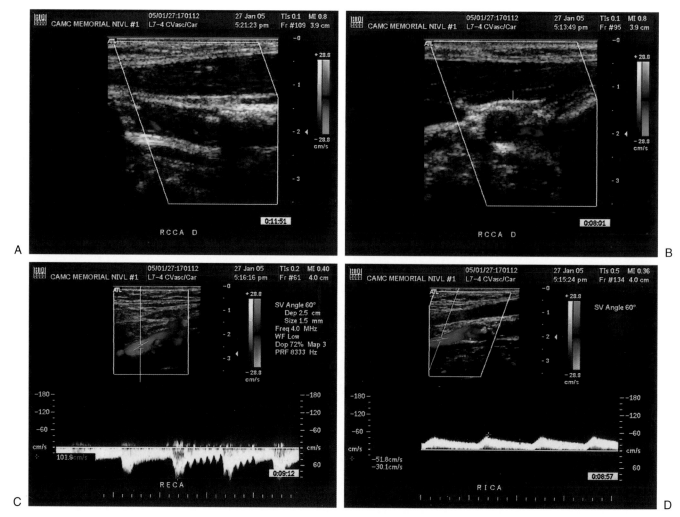

FIGURE 6–26. (A) Right common carotid artery occlusion in longitudinal view. (B) Right common carotid artery occlusion in transverse view. (C) Retrograde flow in external carotid artery. (D) Antegrade flow in internal carotid artery.

frequency ultrasound signal for which a phase shift corresponding to motion of the target is detected; in contrast, conventional color Doppler imaging displays Doppler frequency shift information. In a recent study by us,[13] five out of six patients (83%) who were felt to have total carotid occlusion by conventional color duplex were confirmed to have subtotal occlusion by adding power Doppler imaging (Figure 6–28).

External Carotid Artery Disease (High-Grade Stenosis)

Lesions producing a greater than 50% diameter reduction of the external carotid artery are identified by the presence of peak frequencies in excess of 4.5 kHz associ-

ated with diffuse spectral broadening (Figure 6–29). The overall shape of the waveform with frequencies in the negative range remains normal.

Proposed New Duplex Classification for Threshold Stenoses Used in Various Symptomatic and Asymptomatic Carotid Endarterectomy Trials[14]

Based on the duplex criteria, many laboratories, including our own, classified internal carotid artery stenosis into categories patterned after those used at the University of Washington:[11] normal, 1–15% stenosis, 16–49% stenosis, 50–79% stenosis, 80–99% stenosis, and total

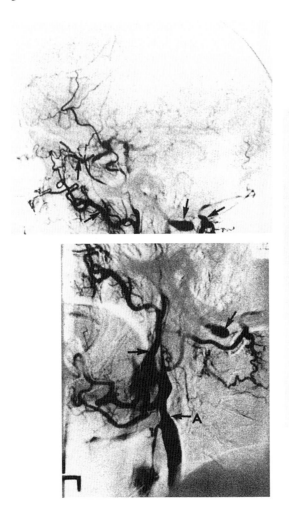

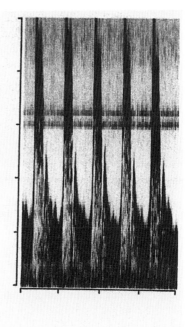

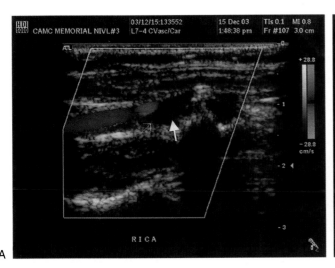

FIGURE 6–27. Arteriogram (left) and Doppler spectra (right) obtained from a missed internal carotid occlusion showing the external carotid artery functioning as a major collateral to the middle cerebral vessels. The spectra show peak frequencies in excess of 4.5 kHz in association with spectral broadening and no flow reversal. This appearance is produced by the low resistance outflow bed of the external carotid into the middle cerebral artery.

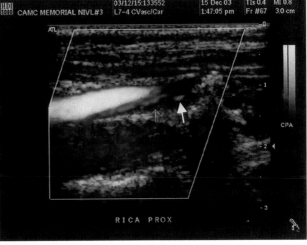

FIGURE 6–28. (A) Color duplex imaging of a right internal carotid artery suggesting total occlusion. (B) Power Doppler image of same artery showing string sign (arrow), i.e., subtotal occlusion.

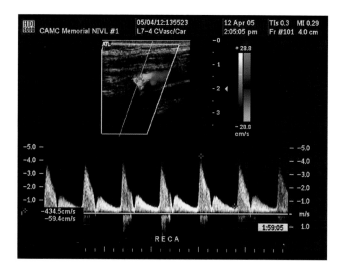

FIGURE 6–29. Doppler spectra produced by high-grade stenosis of external carotid arteries. This patient has a peak systolic velocity of 434.5 cm/s. Flow in diastole reaches the zero baseline.

occlusion. While these classifications have been useful clinically in the past, they do not correlate with threshold stenoses utilized in the recent trials investigating symptomatic (NASCET)[15] and asymptomatic (ACAS[16] and Veteran's Administration Asymptomatic Carotid Stenosis Trial Investigators[17]) carotid artery disease. With the publication of the NASCET findings showing conclusive benefit of carotid endarterectomy for symptomatic patients with 70–99% stenosis, several recent studies have attempted to develop duplex criteria to identify patients with ≥70% carotid stenosis.[18–21] With the subsequent report from the ACAS group[22] showing significant benefit of carotid endarterectomy in asymptomatic patients with ≥60% stenosis, others[23–26] reported optimal duplex criteria for detecting ≥60% stenosis.

It should be noted that the 5-year absolute risk reduction rate for ipsilateral stroke in the ACAS study was only 5.8%. Therefore, the duplex criteria for screening ≥60% internal carotid artery stenosis should have a high positive predictive value since these patients are likely to undergo invasive carotid angiography and/or carotid endarterectomy. This, along with increasing reports advocating carotid endarterectomy based on carotid duplex results alone, without preoperative arteriography,[27,28] prompted us to identify and evaluate new duplex velocity criteria for threshold stenoses used in various symptomatic and asymptomatic carotid endarterectomy trials (NASCET, ACAS, and VA studies). In addition, we identified the best duplex criteria that yielded a high positive predictive value (≥95%) for the threshold level of asymptomatic internal carotid artery stenosis of ≥60%, there-

fore minimizing unnecessary arteriography with its associated risk of stroke. We also identified the best duplex criteria that provided a high negative predictive value for the threshold level of symptomatic internal carotid artery stenosis of ≥70% to minimize missing patients who would benefit the most from a carotid endarterectomy.

Patient Population and Methods

Two hundred and thirty-one patients (462 arteries) who underwent both carotid color duplex scanning and arteriography from January 1992 to December 1994 were studied. Carotid color duplex scanning was performed using high-resolution real-time imaging (7.5 mHz) and a pulsed Doppler (5.0 mHz) duplex scanner (Ultramark-9, HDI system, Advanced Technology Laboratories, Bothel, WA) in standard fashion.[29]

Results

Four hundred and four carotid arteries had systolic and diastolic velocity measurements available for comparison with arteriography results.

Data derived from receiver operator curves were used to calculate the sensitivity, specificity, positive predictive value, negative predictive value, and overall accuracy of selected internal carotid artery peak systolic velocities, internal carotid artery end-diastolic velocities, and ratio of the peak systolic velocity of the internal carotid artery to the peak systolic velocity of the common

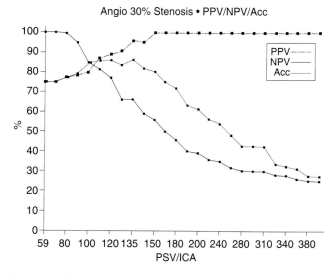

FIGURE 6–30. Response curve illustrating the positive predictive value, negative predictive value, and overall accuracy of various peak systolic velocities of the internal carotid artery in diagnosing ≥30% angiographic internal carotid artery stenosis.

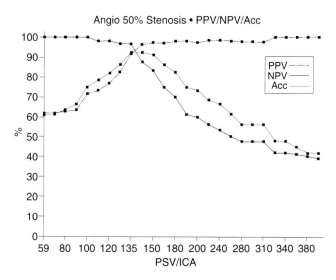

FIGURE 6–31. Response curve illustrating the positive predictive value, negative predictive value, and overall accuracy of various peak systolic velocities of the internal carotid artery in diagnosing ≥50% angiographic internal carotid artery stenosis.

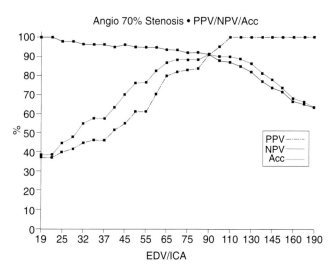

FIGURE 6–33. Response curve illustrating the positive predictive value, negative predictive value, and overall accuracy of various end diastolic velocities of the internal carotid artery in diagnosing ≥70% angiographic internal carotid artery stenosis.

carotid artery in detecting ≥30%, ≥50%, ≥60%, and ≥70–99% angiographic internal carotid artery stenosis. Figures 6–30 through 6–34 show the response curves for the positive predictive value, negative predictive value, and the overall accuracy for diagnosing various angiographic internal carotid artery stenoses for various internal carotid artery peak systolic velocities or end diastolic velocities.

Table 6–2A and B correlates the results obtained with the new proposed criteria to the percentage of angiographic stenoses in 404 carotid arteries.

The optimal duplex values that provide the best positive predictive value (≥95%) and have a good overall accuracy in detecting ≥60–99% and ≥70–99% internal carotid artery stenoses are listed in Table 6–3A and the optimal duplex values that provide the best negative pre-

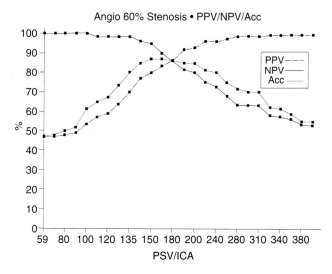

FIGURE 6–32. Response curve illustrating the positive predictive value, negative predictive value, and overall accuracy of various peak systolic velocities of the internal carotid artery in diagnosing ≥60% angiographic internal carotid artery stenosis.

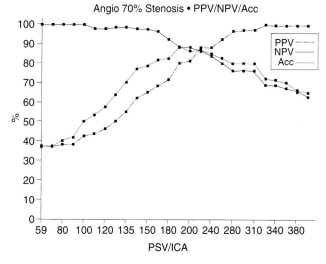

FIGURE 6–34. Response curve illustrating the positive predictive value, negative predictive value, and overall accuracy of various peak systolic velocities of the internal carotid artery in diagnosing ≥70% angiographic internal carotid artery stenosis.

TABLE 6–2A. Carotid duplex velocity criteria versus angiography: sensitivity, specificity, PPV, NPV, and overall accuracy according to the newly proposed categories of ICA stenosis.[a]

Duplex criteria (cm/s)	% Stenosis per angiogram					Total
	0–29%	30–49%	50–59%	60–69%	>70–99%	
ICA PSV <120	68	19	0	0	1	88
ICA PSV ≥ 120	32	30	13	4	1	80
ICA PSV ≥ 140	1	5	39	16	12	73
ICA PSV ≥ 150 and EDV ≥ 65	0	0	4	12	8	24
ICA PSV ≥ 150 and EDV ≥ 90	0	2	1	9	127	139
Total	101	56	57	41	149	404

[a]Kappa = 0.58 ± 0.03, perfect agreement = 68.32%. ICA, internal carotid artery; PSV, peak systolic velocity; EDV, end diastolic velocity.

TABLE 6–2B. Accuracy of color duplex ultrasound based on the new criteria.[a]

Duplex criteria overall	% Stenosis				
	Sensitivity	Specificity	PPV	NPV	Accuracy
ICA PSV > 120 cm/s (<30% vs. ≥30% stenosis)	93%	67%	90%	77%	87%
ICA PSV ≥ 140 cm/s (<50% vs. ≥50% stenosis)	92%	95%	97%	89%	93%
ICA PSV > 150 and EDV ≥ 65 cm/s (<60% vs. ≥ 60% stenosis)	82%	97%	96%	86%	90%
ICA PSV > 150 and EDV ≥ 90 cm/s (<70% vs. ≥70% stenosis)	85%	95%	91%	92%	92%

[a]ICA, internal carotid artery; PSV, peak systolic velocity; EDV, end diastolic velocity.

TABLE 6–3A. Selected optimal criteria with best PPV (> or equal to 95%) and overall accuracy in detecting > or equal to 60–99% and 70–99% ICA stenosis.[a]

Best PPV for ≥60% ICA stenosis	PPV	Overall accuracy	Sensitivity	Specificity	NPV
ICA PSV ≥220 cm/s	96%	82%	64%	98%	76%
ICA EDV ≥80 cm/s	96%	87%	79%	97%	84%
ICA/CCA PSV ratio ≥4.25	96%	71%	41%	99%	65%
ICA PSV and EDV 150 and 65[b]	96%	90%	82%	97%	86%
Best PPV for ≥70% ICA stenosis					
ICA PSV ≥300 cm/s	97%	80%	48%	99%	76%
ICA EDV ≥110 cm/s[b]	100%	91%	75%	100%	87%
ICA/CCA PSV ≥ none	—	—	—	—	—
ICA PSV and EDV 150, 110[b]	100%	91%	75%	100%	87%

[a]PPV, positive predictive value; NPV, negative predictive value; ICA, internal carotid artery; PSV, peak systolic velocity; CCA, common carotid artery; EDV, end diastolic velocity.
[b]These values have the best PPV and overall accuracy.

TABLE 6–3B. Selected optimal criteria with best NPV (> or equal to 95%) and overall accuracy in detecting > or equal to 60–99% and 70–99% ICA stenosis.[a]

Best NPV for ≥60% stenosis	NPV	Overall accuracy	Sensitivity	Specificity	PPV
ICA PSV ≥135 cm/s[b]	99%	80%	99%	64%	71%
ICA EDV—none	—	—	—	—	—
ICA/CCA PSV ratio ≥1.62	95%	71%	97%	47%	62%
ICA PSV and EDV—none	—	—	—	—	—
Best NPV for ≥70% ICA stenosis					
ICA PSV ≥150 cm/s[b]	99%	80%	99%	69%	65%
ICA EDV ≥60 cm/s	96%	83%	94%	77%	71%
ICA/CCA PSV ≥ none	—	—	—	—	—
ICA PSV and EDV—none	—	—	—	—	—

[a]NPV, negative predictive value; PPV, positive predictive value; ICA, internal carotid artery; PSV, peak systolic velocity; CCA, common carotid artery; EDV, end diastolic velocity.
[b]These values have the best NPV and overall accuracy.

dictive value (≥95%) and a good overall accuracy in detecting ≥60–99% and≥70–99% internal carotid artery stenoses are shown in Table 6–3B.

In choosing our criteria for peak systolic velocity and end diastolic velocity, we chose the values that gave the highest overall accuracy. Which criteria to use is, therefore, dependent on the "outcome" desired by the clinician. Although some surgeons have advocated carotid endarterectomy based on duplex criteria alone,[27,28] the decision to proceed with an arteriogram is based on the duplex findings in the majority of patients. The mortality and morbidity of arteriography vary from institution to institution, but can be significant.[22,30] We propose that vascular laboratories at institutions with significant mortality and morbidity in relation to carotid arteriography use duplex criteria with a ≥95% positive predictive value and the best overall accuracy in order to minimize the number of patients undergoing unnecessary arteriography (Table 6–3A). These criteria can also be utilized when carotid endarterectomy is performed without preoperative arteriography. In those institutions where arteriography does not significantly add to the mortality and morbidity of the overall treatment of carotid disease, we suggest using the criteria described in Table 6–3B. These criteria have the highest negative predictive value to ensure that only a minimum number of patients with ≥60% or ≥70% stenoses is missed.

The new classification that we are proposing would consist of lesions <30%, ≥30–49%, ≥50–59%, ≥60–69%, and ≥70%. This new duplex classification would fit into the existing trials (NASCET, ACAS, and VA), and may be of benefit as new conclusions are released. By reporting results using these criteria, the clinician will be better able to make decisions regarding the need for carotid endarterectomy or arteriogram based on the risks and benefits for individual patients. With the added risks of arteriography, decisions to operate would be better based on duplex findings alone. Having positive predictive values ranging from 90 to 97% and accuracies of 87–93% can eliminate many unnecessary arteriograms.

It is important to note that the data obtained by individual vascular laboratoriess will vary across the country. Differences in equipment, abilities and consistencies of vascular technicians, and reader interpretations will cause variabilities from laboratory to laboratory.[31] Therefore, each laboratory must adapt a method that employs the equipment it uses and has validated its method when using proposed new duplex criteria.

Other studies have sought to reconcile these trials [NASCET, European Carotid Surgery Trialists (ECST), and ACAS] with duplex criteria.[18–21] A summary of these studies can be found in Table 6–4. As noted in this table, different overall accuracies were reported according to each technique and according to specific duplex criteria. This can be partially explained by the differences in scanning techniques, technologists' experience, angle of insonation, or different ultrasound systems. It has been shown that linear array transducers may overestimate peak systolic velocity in a flow phantom.[32]

Consensus Panel on Diagnostic Criteria for Grading Carotid Artery Stenosis Using Color Duplex Ultrasound

A multidisciplinary panel of experts was invited by the Society of Radiologists and Ultrasound in 2002 to attend a consensus conference on diagnostic criteria to grade carotid artery stenosis using duplex ultrasound. The consensus panel agreed on a specific set of criteria that would be helpful in grading focal proximal internal carotid artery stenosis, which is noted in Table 6–5. These criteria were to be used for new laboratories requesting applicable criteria for prospective validation. It was also recommended for established laboratories, which had previously developed their own criteria that were outdated.

Validation of ultrasound criteria can be difficult since different scanners are used in various laboratories. Therefore, it is important for each laboratory to validate its own criteria, and use these accordingly.

Accuracy of Duplex Scanning in the Detection of Carotid Disease

Various clinical studies have reported an overall accuracy of 80–97% in diagnosing carotid artery stenosis.[14,18–21,33–40] Table 6–4A and B summarizes some of these studies.

Effect of Contralateral Stenosis or Occlusion on Ipsilateral Carotid Stenosis Duplex Criteria

A number of studies in the recent literature have reported decreased accuracy of duplex scanning in predicting the degree of ipsilateral internal carotid stenosis in the presence of contralateral high-grade stenosis or carotid occlusion.[29,41–46] When conventional standard criteria[11] were applied in this circumstance, the result was an overestimation of the degree of iplsilateral stenosis (up to 48%),[45] often resulting in incorrect assignment to a higher category of disease and thus creating a false-positive interpretation.[29,41–46] It has been proposed that this phenomenon occurs because of a compensatory increase in flow velocity in the ipsilateral carotid system to maintain a stable cerebral circulation via the Circle of Willis.[42]

TABLE 6–4A. Comparison of several studies correlating angiographic 50–69%, 60–99%, and 70–99% ICA stenosis with duplex scanning.[a]

Criteria (reference)	Number of ICAs	Ultrasound System	Accuracy (%)	Sensitivity (%)	Specificity (%)	PPV (%)	NPV (%)
30–49% stenosis							
PSV ≥120 cm/s[14]	462	ATL, UM9 (HDI)	87	93	67	90	77
50–69% stenosis							
PSV >140 cm/s[14]	462	ATL, UM9 (HDI)	93	92	95	97	89
PSV ≥130 cm/s and EDV ≤100 cm/s[18]	120	Acuson 128	97	92	97	93	99
60–99% stenosis							
PSV ≥150 cm/s and EDV ≥65 cm/s[14]	462	ATL, UM9 (HDI)	90	82	97	96	86
PSV ≥130 cm/s and EDV ≥40 cm/s[19]	120	Acuson 128	80	97	72	62	98
PSV ≥260 cm/s and EDV ≥70 cm/s[23]	352	Acuson 128, ATL, UM9	90	84	94	92	88
PSV ≥290 cm/s and EDV ≥80 cm/s[23]			88	78	96	95	84
70–99% stenosis							
PSV ≥150 cm/s and EDV ≥90 cm/s[14]	462	ATL, UM9 (HDI)	92	85	93	91	92
PSV ≥130 cm/s and EDV ≥100 cm/s[18]	770	QAD 1, QAD 2000	95	81	98	89	96
PSV ≥270 cm/s and EDV ≥110 cm/s[19]	120	Acuson 128	93	96	91	—	—
PSV ≥325 cm/s[20]	184	Acuson 128	88	83	91	80	92
ICA/CCA PSV ratio ≥4.0[20]			88	91	87	76	96
PSV ≥130 cm/s and EDV ≥100 cm/s[21,b]	914	QAD 2000 Phillips P700	95	87	97	89	96
PSV ≥130 cm/s and EDV ≥100 cm/s[21,c]			93	78	97	88	94

[a]PPV, positive predictive value; NPV, negative predictive value; PSV, peak systolic velocity; ICA, internal carotid artery; CCA, common carotid artery; EDV, end diastolic velocity.
[b]Prospective validation of criteria developed in Faught et al.,[18] including ICA occlusions.
[c]Analysis of criteria developed in Faught et al.,[18] excluding ICA occlusion.

TABLE 6–4B. Accuracy of carotid duplex ultrasound compared to arteriography in recent series.

Author	Year	Carotids/patients	Stenosis (%)	Sensitivity/specificity (%)	PPV/NPV (%)	Overall accuracy (%)
Patel[33]	1995	176/88	70–99	94/83		86
Hood[21]	1996	457/457	70–100	87/97	89/96	95
Huston[34]	1998	100/50	70–99	97/75	67/98	83
AbuRahma[14]	1998	462/231	70–99	85/95	91/92	92
Belsky[35]	2000	92/46	0–100	79/96	94/87	89
Anderson[36]	2000	80/40	50–69	35/87	50/78	73
			70–99	82/71	38/95	73
Back[37]	2000	74/40	50–100	100/72	88/100	91
			75–100	90/74	72/91	81
Johnston[38]	2001	452	50–99	87	46/73	68
Nederkoorn[39]	2002	313/313	70–90	88	76/75	88
MacKenzie[40]	2002	375/192	70–99	81/89	66/95	87

TABLE 6–5. Ultrasound consensus criteria for carotid stenosis.[a]

Stenosis range	ICA PSV	ICA EDV	ICA/CCA PSV ratio	Plaque
Normal	<125 cm/s	<40 cm/s	<2.0	None
<50%	<125 cm/s	<40 cm/s	<2.0	<50% diameter reduction
50–69%	125–230 cm/s	40–100 cm/s	2.0–4.0	≥50% diameter reduction
70—near occlusion	>230 cm/s	>100 cm/s	>4.0	≥50% diameter reduction
Near occlusion	May be low or undetectable	Variable	Variable	Significant, detectable lumen
Occlusion	Undetectable	Not applicable	Not applicable	Significant, no detectable lumen

[a]ICA, internal carotid artery; PSV, peak systolic velocity; EDV, end diastolic velocity; CCA, common carotid artery.

Fujitani et al.[45] were the first to recommend modification of the standard duplex criteria in patients with contralateral internal carotid occlusion. However, in this study, only the effect of the contralateral total carotid occlusion was studied. Patients with less than total occlusion of the contralateral artery were excluded from the study population.

The recognition of this phenomenon as consistent and clinically significant led us to undertake a retrospective study to compare the accuracy of various existing duplex criteria [standard,[11] Fujitani,[45] internal carotid/common carotid artery ratio (ICA/CCA)[47]] used in grading ipsilateral carotid stenosis in patients with contralateral high-grade stenosis or occlusion. In addition, we propose a new modified duplex criteria that we believe to be superior to the existing criteria in terms of overall accuracy.

These new criteria were developed because of our dissatisfaction with the results of the standard method in grading ipsilateral stenosis in the presence of severe contralateral disease. We had observed that most patients with ≥50% stenosis on arteriography had a peak systolic frequency of the internal carotid artery of ≥4.5 kHz in the presence of severe contralateral disease.

Patient Population and Methods

From January 1992 to December 1993, 178 patients (356 arteries) were identified as having significant (>50%) internal carotid artery stenosis by carotid duplex ultrasonography, and they subsequently underwent carotid arteriography within 6 weeks.

Criteria for duplex ultrasonography classification of the degree of stenosis are shown in Table 6–6. Four different sets of criteria for each patient were analyzed: (1) the standard criteria (University of Washington),[11] (2) Fujitani criteria,[45] (3) ICA/CCA ratio criteria,[47] and (4) the new revised criteria that we are proposing. These criteria were used to assign each artery to one of five

TABLE 6–6. Doppler frequency spectral or velocity criteria for carotid artery stenosis.[a]

Classification	Arteriographic lesion	Spectral criteria
Standard method		
Grade I	1–15% diameter reduction	PSF <4 kHz (<125 cm/s), minimal SB
Grade II	16–49% diameter reduction	PSF <4 kHz (<125 cm/s), increased SB
Grade III	50–79% diameter reduction	PSF ≥4 kHz (≥125 cm/s)
		EDF <4.5 kHz (<140 cm/s)
Grade IV	80–99% diameter reduction	PSF >4 kHz (>125 cm/s)
		EDF >4.5 kHz (>140 cm/s)
Grade V	Occlusion	No internal carotid flow signal
		Low or reversed diastolic component in common carotid artery
New method (AbuRahma) similar to standard method except for the following		
Grade II	16–49% diameter reduction	PSF <4.5 kHz (<140 cm/s)
		EDF <4.5 kHz (<140 cm/s)
Grade III	50–79% diameter reduction	PSF ≥4.5 kHz (≥140 cm/s)
		EDF <4.5 kHz (<140 cm/s)
Grade IV	80–99% diameter reduction	PSF >4.5 kHz (>140 cm/s)
		EDF >4.5 kHz (>140 cm/s)
Fujitani method—same as standard method except for the following		
Grade II	16–49% diameter reduction	PSF >4 kHz (>125 cm/s)
		EDF <5 kHz (<155 cm/s)
Grade III	50–79% diameter reduction	PSF >4.5 kHz (>140 cm/s)
		EDF <5 kHz (<155 cm/s)
Grade IV	80–99% diameter reduction	PSF >4.5 kHz (>140 cm/s)
		EDF >5 kHz (>155 cm/s)
ICA/CCA ratio method		
Grade I and II	1–49% diameter reduction	SVR <1.5
Grade III	50–79% diameter reduction	SVR ≥1.5, PEDV <100 cm/s
Grade IV	80–99% diameter reduction	SVR ≥1.8, PEDV >100 cm/s
Grade V	Occlusion	No internal carotid artery flow signal

[a]PSF, peak systolic frequency; EDF, end diastolic frequency; SB, spectral broadening; SVR, systolic velocity ratio (ICA/CCA peak systolic velocity ratio); PEDV, peak end diastolic velocity.

TABLE 6–7. Comparison of duplex grades to arteriogram grades.

	Arteriogram grades					
Duplex grades	Grade I (%)	Grade II (%)	Grade III (%)	Grade IV (%)	Grade V (%)	Total
Standard method						
Grade I	38 (100)	0	0	0	0	38
Grade II	0	17 (100)	0	0	0	17
Grade III	2 (1)	52 (30)	111 (64)	8 (5)	0	173
Grade IV	0	0	0	87 (100)	0	87
Grade V	0	0	0	2 (5)	39 (95)	41
($k = 0.760$, 95% confidence interval = 0.708–0.812)						
New method						
Grade I	38 (100)	0	0	0	0	38
Grade II	2 (3)	63 (93)	3 (4)	0	0	68
Grade III	0	6 (5)	108 (88)	8 (7)	0	122
Grade IV	0	0	0	87 (100)	0	87
Grade V	0	0	0	2 (5)	39 (95)	41
($k = 0.923$, 95% confidence interval = 0.891–0.955, $p < 0.001$)						
Fujitani method						
Grade I	38 (64)	20 (34)	1 (2)	0	0	59
Grade II	2 (4)	43 (78)	9 (16)	1 (2)	0	55
Grade III	0	6 (4)	101 (58)	66 (38)	0	173
Grade IV	0	0	0	28 (100)	0	28
Grade V	0	0	0	2 (5)	39 (95)	41
($k = 0.608$, 95% confidence interval = 0.547–0.668)						
ICA/CCA ratio method[a]						
Grades I and II	27 (48)	21 (38)	4 (7)	1 (2)	3 (5)	56
Grade III	13 (8)	48 (30)	93 (58)	7 (4)	0	161
Grade IV	0	0	14 (14)	87 (86)	0	101
Grade V	0	0	0	2 (5)	36 (95)	38
Total	40	69	111	97	39	356
($k = 0.642$, 95% confidence interval = 0.542–0.742)						

[a]ICA, internal carotid artery; CCA, common carotid artery.

categories: grade I, 1–15% stenosis; grade II, 16–49% stenosis; grade III, 50–79% stenosis; grade IV, 80–99% stenosis; and grade V, total occlusion.

Results

The standard method overestimated 56 (16%) of 356 stenoses in contrast to 3% for the new method ($p < 0.001$), and this effect was most evident in the 50% to <80% stenosis category (30%). The Fujitani method underestimated 97 (27%) of 356 stenoses, and the ICA/CCA ratio overestimated stenoses in 77 (22%) of 356. The overall exact correlation was 94, 82, 70, and 75% for the new, standard, Fujitani, and ICA/CCA ratio, respectively. The x^2 statistic and corresponding confidence intervals for the new method ($x^2 = 0.923$, ±0.016) are significantly higher ($p < 0.001$) than those for the standard method ($x^2 = 0.760$, ±0.027), the Fujitani method ($x^2 = 0.608$, ±0.031), and the ICA/CCA ratio method ($x^2 = 0.642$, ±0.051). The overall accuracy in diagnosing ≥50% ipsilateral stenosis in the whole series was 85% for the standard method, 97% for the new method, 95% for the Fujitani method, and 81% for the ICA/CCA ratio. The new method was superior to the standard and ICA/CCA ratio methods ($p < 0.001$) and the Fujitani method ($p = 0.024$).

Table 6–7 compares the results of duplex grades with those of arteriography on the basis of four different criteria. Tables 6–8 to 6–10 summarize the results of the study.

The new proposed criteria fared very well in the analysis, with only 3% overall overestimation of the disease and 3% overall underestimation of the disease. The overall exact correlation between duplex and arteriographic grading was 94% and was superior to the other criteria in each case ($p < 0.001$).

The new criteria yielded sensitivity, specificity, positive and negative predictive values, and overall accuracy values superior to those of the other three criteria in predicting ≥50% ipsilateral stenosis, when all patients with 0–100% contralateral stenosis were included ($p < 0.001$) in each case. When divided into 50% to <80% contralateral stenosis and 80–99% contralateral stenosis or total occlusion, the new criteria proved once again to be

TABLE 6–8. Comparison of duplex methods versus arteriography for sensitivity/specificity in diagnosis of > or equal to 50% ipsilateral stenosis in patients with arteries of 50% to <80% stenosis on contralateral side.[a]

Carotid arteriogram	<50% stenosis (%)	>50% stenosis (%)	Total	Sensitivity (%)	Specificity (%)	PPV (%)	NPV (%)	Overall accuracy (%)
Standard method[b]								
<50% stenosis	24 (100)	0	24	100	56	78	100	83
≥50% stenosis	19 (22)	68 (78)	87					
New method								
<50% stenosis	42 (95)	2 (5)	44	97	98	99	95	97
≥50% stenosis	1 (1)	66 (99)	67					
Fujitani method[c]								
<50% stenosis	42 (91)	4 (9)	46	94	98	98	91	96
≥50% stenosis	1 (1)	64 (99)	65					
ICA/CCA ratio method[d]								
<50% stenosis	19 (86)	3 (14)	22	96	44	73	86	76
≥50% stenosis	24 (27)	65 (73)	89					
Total	43	68	111					

[a]PPV, positive predictive value; NPV, negative predictive value; ICA, internal carotid artery; CCA, common carotid artery.
[b]New method versus standard method, $p < 0.001$ (Z statistics for proportion).
[c]New method versus Fujitani method, $p > 0.05$ (Z statistics for proportion).
[d]New method versus ICA/CCA ratio method, $p < 0.001$ (Z statistics for proportion).

superior to the standard and ICA/CCA ratio criteria ($p < 0.001$). The differences between the new criteria and Fujitani criteria in these patients did not reach statistical significance. This finding is not surprising, because the Fujitani criteria were developed from a study in which the contralateral artery was totally occluded and were designed to be used in such cases, rather than to be applied to all vessels studied, as they were in this series.

Some clinicians believe that the most important clinical issue is accuracy in detecting stenoses of greater than or less than 80%, contralateral to a tight stenosis or occlusion. The standard method results were very comparable to the new method and somewhat comparable to the ICA/CCA ratio method in all parameters examined, including overall accuracy. This finding is not surprising, because both the standard and new methods require an end diastolic frequency of the internal carotid artery of

TABLE 6–9. Comparison of duplex methods versus arteriography for sensitivity/specificity in diagnosis of >50% ipsilateral stenosis in patients with arteries with 80–99% stenosis of the contralateral side.[a]

Carotid arteriogram	<50% stenosis (%)	>50% stenosis (%)	Total	Sensitivity (%)	Specificity (%)	PPV (%)	NPV (%)	Overall accuracy (%)
Standard method								
<50% stenosis	26 (100)	0	26	100	53	68	100	76
≥50% stenosis	23 (32)	48 (68)	71					
New method								
<50% stenosis	45 (100)	0	45	100	92	92	100	96
≥50% stenosis	4 (8)	48 (92)	52					
Fujitani method								
<50% stenosis	45 (96)	2 (4)	47	96	92	92	96	94
≥50% stenosis	4 (8)	46 (92)	50					
ICA/CCA ratio method								
<50% stenosis	23 (92)	2 (8)	25	96	47	64	92	71
≥50% stenosis	26 (36)	46 (64)	72					

[a]PPV, positive predictive value; NPV, negative predictive value; ICA, internal carotid artery; CCA, common carotid artery.
[b]New method versus standard method, $p < 0.001$ (Z statistics for proportion).
[c]New method versus Fujitani method, not significant (Z statistics for proportion).
[d]New method versus ICA/CCA ratio method, $p < 0.001$ (Z statistics for proportion).

TABLE 6–10. Comparison of duplex methods versus arteriography for sensitivity/specificity in diagnosis of equal to or >50% stenosis in patients with total occlusion on contralateral side.[a]

Carotid arteriogram	<50% stenosis (%)	>50% stenosis (%)	Total	Sensitivity (%)	Specificity (%)	PPV (%)	NPV (%)	Overall accuracy (%)
Standard method[b]								
<50% stenosis	5 (100)	0	5	100	33	71	100	74
≥50% stenosis	10 (29)	24 (71)	34					
New method								
<50% stenosis	15 (94)	1 (6)	16	96	100	100	94	97
≥50% stenosis	0	23 (100)	23					
Fujitani method[c]								
<50% stenosis	15 (83)	3 (17)	18	88	100	100	83	92
≥50% stenosis	0	21 (100)	21					
ICA/CCA ratio method[d]								
<50% stenosis	6 (100)	0	6	100	40	73	100	77
≥50% stenosis	9 (27)	24 (73)	33					

[a]PPV, positive predictive value; NPV, negative predictive value; ICA, internal carotid artery; CCA, common carotid artery.
[b]New method versus standard method, $p < 0.01$ (Z statistics for proportion).
[c]New method versus Fujitani method, $p = 0.15$ (Z statistics for proportion).
[d]New method versus ICA/CCA ratio method, $p < 0.01$ (Z statistics for proportion).

>4.5 kHz for the diagnosis of ≥80% stenosis. However, the Fujitani method had a poorer sensitivity and an overall accuracy of only 85% in contrast to an overall accuracy of 98% for the new and standard methods in this group of patients (80–99% contralateral stenosis). This finding can be explained by the requirement of an end diastolic frequency of the internal carotid artery of >5 kHz for the

diagnosis of ≥80% stenosis for the Fujitani method. Similar observations were noted in patients with a total contralateral occlusion. Our results were comparable to data previously reported by others.[41–46]

Table 6–11 summarizes the duplex accuracy of various criteria in the presence of contralateral stenosis or occlusion.

TABLE 6–11. Accuracy of duplex criteria with contralateral severe stenosis or occlusion.[a]

Criteria and reference	Accuracy (%)	Sensitivity (%)	Specificity (%)	PPV (%)	NPV (%)
>50% stenosis					
Fujitani[45]	74	97	57	62	96
AbuRahma[29]					
Fujitani	92	88	100	100	83
Standard	74	100	33	71	100
AbuRahma	97	96	100	100	94
Ratios	77	100	40	73	100
50–79% stenosis					
Fujitani: PSV >140 cm/s, EDV <155 cm/s[45]	71	84	70	28	97
AbuRahma[29]					
Fujitani: PSV >140 cm/s, EDV <155 cm/s	97	99	98	98	95
Standard: PSV >125 cm/s, EDV <140 cm/s	83	100	56	78	100
AbuRahma: PSV ≥140 cm/s, EDV <140 cm/s	97	97	98	99	95
Ratios: ICA/CCA ratio ≥1.5, EDV <100 cm/s	76	96	44	73	86
80–99% stenosis					
Fujitani: PSV >140 cm/s, EDV >155 cm/s[45]	96	91	97	89	98
AbuRahma[29]					
Fujitani: PSV >140 cm/s, EDV >155 cm/s	94	96	92	92	96
Standard: PSV >125 cm/s, EDV >140 cm/s	76	100	53	68	100
AbuRahma: PSV >140 cm/s, EDV >140 cm/s	96	100	92	92	100
Ratios: ICA/CCA ratio ≥1.8, EDV >100 cm/s	71	96	47	64	92

[a]PPV, positive predictive value; NPV, negative predictive value; PSV, peak systolic velocity; EDV, end diastolic velocity; ICA, internal carotid artery; CCA, common carotid artery.

Clinical Use of Carotid Duplex Scanning

Carotid duplex ultrasound reports routinely include flow velocities and the degree of stenoses. However, several carotid reports, particularly those from nonaccredited vascular laboratories, have several inconsistencies that can be extremely critical in clinical decision making. A carotid duplex ultrasound examination should be termed "inconclusive" if the findings are uncertain, and it cannot be ensured that the carotid artery does not have significant carotid artery disease.[48,49] Calcification and shadowing, high bifurcation, short neck, or any other circumstances that prevent adequate interrogation of the carotid artery can result in an inconclusive examination. In this scenario, other diagnostic modalities must be recommended to delineate the proper pathology. Inconsistent carotid examination is used when the imaging and velocity determination of the color duplex ultrasound are not consistent with each other, and additional tests are also required in these circumstances. Significant carotid artery stenosis may be present without associated increased flow velocities. This can be partially explained by complex or calcified lesions or dampened flow by an extremely high-grade lesion.

The accuracy of duplex scanning in the examination of the carotid artery bifurcation has resulted in its use in symptomatic patients for the detection of disease, the evaluation of patients with neck bruits, postoperative studies of endarterectomized vessels, and the sequential examination of asymptomatic patients to document progression of disease.[50] Other clinical implications include carotid endarterectomy without angiography, intraoperative assessment of carotid endarterectomy, long-term follow-up after carotid endarterectomy, plaque morphology and outcome, and carotid duplex scanning following trauma. The clinical implications of duplex ultrasound technology will be discussed in detail in Chapter 16.

References

1. Kossoff G. Gray Scale Echography in Obstetrics and Gynecology. Report No. 60. Sydney, Australia, Commonwealth Acoustic Laboratories, 1973.
2. Olinger CP. Ultrasonic carotid echoarteriography. Am J Roentgenol 1969;106:282–295.
3. Hartley DJ, Strandness DE Jr. The effects of atherosclerosis on the transmission of ultrasound. J Surg Res 1969;9:575–582.
4. Barber FE, Baker DW, Nation AWC, et al. Ultrasonic duplex echo-Doppler scanner. IEEE Trans Biomed Eng 1974;81:109–113.
5. Blackshear WM, Phillips DJ, Chikos RM, et al. Carotid artery velocity patterns in normal and stenotic vessels. Stroke 1980;11:67–71.
6. Reilly LM. Importance of carotid plaque morphology. In: Bernstein EF (ed). Vascular Diagnosis, 4th ed., pp. 333–340. St. Louis, MO: Mosby-Year Book, 1993.
7. AbuRahma AF, Kyer PR, Robinson P, et al. The correlation of ultrasonic carotid plaque morphology and carotid plaque hemorrhage: Clinical implications. Surgery 1998;124:721–726.
8. AbuRahma AF, Thiele S, Wulu J. Prospective controlled study of the natural history of asymptomatic 60% to 69% carotid stenosis according to ultrasonic plaque morphology. J Vasc Surg 2002;36:437–442.
9. Gronholdt M, Nordestgaard B, Schroeder T, et al. Ultrasonic echolucent carotid plaques predict future strokes. Circulation 2001;104:68–73.
10. Thiele BL, Hutchison KJ, Green RM, et al. Pulsed Doppler waveform patterns produced by smooth stenosis in the dog thoracic aorta. In: Taylor DEM (ed). Blood Flow Theory and Practice, pp. 85–104. New York: Academic Press, 1983.
11. Zierler RE, Strandness DE Jr. Noninvasive dynamic and real-time assessment of extracranial cerebrovasculature. In: Wood JH (ed). Cerebral Blood Flow: Physiologic and Clinical Aspects, pp. 311–323. New York: McGraw-Hill, 1987.
12. Bodily KC, Phillips DJ, Thiele BL, et al. Noninvasive detection of internal carotid artery occlusion. Angiology 1981;32:517–521.
13. AbuRahma AF, Jarrett K, Hayes JD. Clinical implications of power Doppler three-dimensional ultrasonography. Vascular 2004;12:293–300.
14. AbuRahma AF, Robinson, PA, Stickler, DL, et al. Proposed new duplex classification for threshold stenoses used in various symptomatic and asymptomatic carotid endarterectomy trials. Ann Vasc Surg 1998;12:349–358.
15. North American Symptomatic Carotid Endarterectomy Trial Collaborators. Beneficial effect of carotid endarterectomy in symptomatic patients with high-grade carotid stenosis. N Engl J Med 1991;325:445–453.
16. Asymptomatic Carotid Atherosclerosis Study Group. Study design for randomized prospective trial of carotid endarterectomy for asymptomatic atherosclerosis. Stroke 1989;20:844–849.
17. Veteran's Administration Cooperative Study. Role of carotid endarterectomy in asymptomatic carotid stenosis. Stroke 1986;17:534–539.
18. Faught WE, Mattos MA, van Bemmelen PS, et al. Color-flow duplex scanning of carotid arteries: New velocity criteria based on receiver operator characteristic analysis for threshold stenoses used in the symptomatic and asymptomatic carotid trials. J Vasc Surg 1994;19:818–828.
19. Neale ML, Chambers JL, Kelly AT, et al. Reappraisal of duplex criteria to assess significant carotid stenosis with special reference to reports from the North American Symptomatic Carotid Endarterectomy Trial and the European Carotid Surgery Trial. J Vasc Surg 1994;20:642–649.
20. Moneta GL, Edwards JM, Chitwood RW, et al. Correlation of North American Symptomatic Carotid Endarterectomy Trial (NASCET) angiographic definition of 70% to 99% internal carotid artery stenosis with duplex scanning. J Vasc Surg 1993;17:152–159.

21. Hood DB, Mattos MA, Mansour A, et al. Prospective evaluation of new duplex criteria to identify 70% internal carotid artery stenosis. J Vasc Surg 1996;23:254–262.
22. Executive Committee for the Asymptomatic Carotid Atherosclerosis Study. Endarterectomy for asymptomatic carotid artery stenosis. JAMA 1995;273:1421–1428.
23. Moneta GL, Edwards JM, Papanicolaou G, et al. Screening for asymptomatic internal carotid artery stenosis: Duplex criteria for discriminating 60% to 99% stenosis. J Vasc Surg 1995;21:989–994.
24. Carpenter JP, Lexa FJ, Davis JT. Determination of sixty percent or greater carotid artery stenosis by duplex Doppler ultrasonography. J Vasc Surg 1995;22:697–705.
25. Burnham CB, Liguish J Jr, Burnham SJ. Velocity criteria redefined for the 60% carotid stenosis. J Vasc Technol 1996;20(1):5–11.
26. AbuRahma AF, Pollack JA, Robinson, PA, et al. New duplex criteria for threshold stenoses used in the asymptomatic carotid atherosclerosis study (ACAS). Vasc Surg 1999;33:23–32.
27. Marshall WG Jr, Kouchoukos NT, Murphy SF, et al. Carotid endarterectomy based on duplex scanning without preoperative arteriography. Circulation 1988;78(Suppl I):I-1–I-5.
28. Geuder JW, Lamparello PJ, Riles TS, et al. Is duplex scanning sufficient evaluation before carotid endarterectomy? J Vasc Surg 1989;9:193–201.
29. AbuRahma AF, Richmond BK, Robinson PA, et al. Effect of contralateral severe stenosis or carotid occlusion on duplex criteria of ipsilateral stenoses: Comparative study of various duplex parameters. J Vasc Surg 1995;22:751–762.
30. AbuRahma AF, Robinson PA, Boland JP, et al. Complications of arteriography in a recent series of 707 cases: Factors affecting outcome. Ann Vasc Surg 1993;7:122–129.
31. Haynes B, Thorpe K, Raylor W, et al. Poor performance of ultrasound in detecting high-grade carotid stenosis (Abstract). Can J Surg 1992;35:446.
32. Daigle RJ, Stavros AT, Lee RM. Overestimation of velocity and frequency values by multi-element linear array Dopplers. J Vasc Tech 1990;14:206–213.
33. Patel MR, Kuntz KM, Klufas RA, et al. Preoperative assessment of the carotid bifurcation: Can magnetic resonance angiography and duplex ultrasonography replace contrast arteriography? Stroke 1995;26:1753–1758.
34. Huston J, Nichols DA, Luetmer PH, et al. MR angiographic and sonographic indications for endarterectomy. AJNR 1998;19:309–315.
35. Belsky M, Gaitini D, Goldsher D, et al. Color-coded duplex ultrasound compared to CT angiography for detection and quantification of carotid artery stenosis. Eur J Ultrasound 2000;12:49–60.
36. Anderson GB, Ashforth R, Steinke DE, et al. CT angiography for the detection and characterization of carotid artery bifurcation disease. Stroke 2000;31:2168–2174.
37. Back MR, Wilson JS, Rushing G, et al. Magnetic resonance angiography is an accurate imaging adjunct to duplex ultrasound scan in patient selection for carotid endarterectomy. J Vasc Surg 2000;32:429–440.
38. Johnston DC, Goldstein LB. Clinical carotid endarterectomy decision-making. Neurology 2001;56:1009–1015.
39. Nederkoorn PJ, Mali WP, Eikelboom BC, et al. Preoperative diagnosis of carotid artery stenosis: Accuracy of noninvasive testing. Stroke 2002;33:2003–2008.
40. MacKenzie KS, French-Sherry E, Burns K, et al. B-mode ultrasound measurement of carotid bifurcation stenoses: Is it reliable? Vasc Endovasc Surg 2002;36:123–135.
41. Spadone DP, Barkmeier LD, Hodgson KJ, et al. Contralateral internal carotid artery stenosis or occlusion: Pitfall of correct ipsilateral classification. A study performed with color flow imaging. J Vasc Surg 1990;11:642–649.
42. Forconi S, Johnston KW. Effect of contralateral internal carotid stenosis on the accuracy of continuous wave Doppler spectral analysis results. J Cardiovasc Surg 1987;28:715–718.
43. Hayes AC, Johnston KW, Baker WH, et al. The effect of contralateral disease on carotid Doppler frequency. Surgery 1988;103:19–23.
44. Beckett WW Jr, Davis PC, Hoffman JC Jr. Duplex Doppler sonography of the carotid artery: False positive results in an artery contralateral to an artery with marked stenosis. AJR 1990;155:1091–1095.
45. Fujitani RM, Mills JL, Wang LM, et al. The effect of unilateral internal carotid arterial occlusion upon contralateral duplex study: Criteria for accurate interpretation. J Vasc Surg 1992;16:459–468.
46. Fisher M, Alexander K. Influence of contralateral obstructions on Doppler-frequency spectral analysis of ipsilateral stenoses of the carotid arteries. Stroke 1985;16:846–848.
47. Bluth EI, Stavros AT, Marich KW, et al. Carotid duplex sonography: A multicenter recommendation for standardized imaging and Doppler criteria. RadioGraphics 1988;8:487–506.
48. Lovelace TD, Moneta GL, Abou-Zamzam AM Jr, Edwards JM, Yeager RA, Landry GJ, Taylor LM Jr, Porter JM. Optimizing duplex follow-up in patients with an asymptomatic internal carotid artery stenosis of less than 60%. J Vasc Surg 2001;33:56–61.
49. Lavensen GS. The carotid artery ultrasound reports: Considerations in evaluation and management. J Vasc Ultrasound 2004;28:15–19.
50. Roederer GO, Langlois MD, Jager MD, et al. The natural history of carotid arterial disease in asymptomatic patients with cervical bruits. Stroke 1984;15:605–613.

7
The Role of Color Duplex Scanning in Diagnosing Diseases of the Aortic Arch Branches and Carotid Arteries

Clifford T. Araki, Bruce L. Mintz, and Robert W. Hobson II

Introduction

Extracranial cerebrovascular disease is most commonly diagnosed at the carotid bifurcation/proximal internal carotid artery. While ultrasound is excellent at detecting the bifurcation lesion, it has been limited in its application to disease in other cerebrovascular segments.

Atherosclerotic disease in the truncal branches of the aortic arch typically occurs at the origin of the branch vessels. The clinical consequences of these lesions include hypoperfusion and thromboembolic events that can impact the anterior or posterior cerebrovascular circulation and circulation to the upper extremities. Their potential for atheroembolic strokes in the anterior circulation and subclavian steal from the posterior circulation is sufficient for surgeons to consider intervention when significant lesions are detected.[1]

The incidence of atherosclerotic disease in the branches of the arch is much lower than it is for the carotid bifurcation but is not well documented. Studies performed in the 1960s and 1970s estimated disease in the arch branches to account for no more than 17% of symptomatic extracranial cerebrovascular disease.[2–4] In 1968, Hass *et al.* reported a severe lesion in one or more of the aortic arch branches in one-third of patients examined by cerebrovascular arteriography. In 101 autopsy patients, a similar percentage was ascribed to ulcerative disease in the arch branches, second only to the carotid sinus.[6]

The incidence of arch lesions has not been systematically evaluated by arteriography and ultrasound has not been considered sufficient to evaluate the arch and its branches. The lack of an adequate assessment has made the natural history of these lesions unclear and indications for repair have not been well established. With endovascular surgery poised to treat these once difficult lesions, the availability of a reliable noninvasive assessment of the arch lesion now becomes clinically significant.

There are no data available to indicate how many arch lesions are missed in a typical carotid ultrasound examination and yet the perceived limitations of ultrasound testing may be due to technique more than hardware. New ultrasonic approaches to these poorly assessed structures should be made to extend the characterization of the extracranial cerebrovascular examination for the potential benefit of this subset of patients.

Anatomy of the Aortic Arch and Brachiocephalic Veins

Aortic Arch

To ultrasonically evaluate the arch and its branches, the orientation of the arch has to be recognized as it projects from the left ventricle to the descending aorta. The aorta ascends to the right of midline as it leaves the left ventricle. The pericardium attaches to the ascending aorta and pulmonary artery as they leave the heart, just beyond their origination. The arch itself becomes an extrapericardial structure. The aorta ascends from the heart to the right of the pulmonary artery. It arches around and above the right branch of the pulmonary artery, anterior to the trachea; it then forms an oblique trajectory from the right anterior mediastinum to the left posterior mediastinum. It forms the descending thoracic aorta to the left of the trachea and esophagus. As the descending aorta, it continues its course along the posterior wall of the chest, toward the left side of the vertebral column.

The aortic arch is approximately 4.5 cm in length. At 2.5–3 cm, it has a slightly larger diameter than the abdominal aorta that we are accustomed to seeing. Three truncal branches arise from the arch: innominate (brachiocephalic trunk), the left common carotid artery, and the left subclavian artery (Figure 7–1). All arise perpendicular to the flow axis of the arch and ascend through the mediastinum to carry blood to the upper extremities and head.

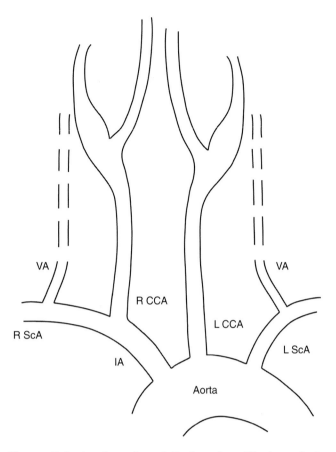

FIGURE 7–1. Aortic arch and its branches. IA, innominate artery; R ScA, right subclavian artery; VA, vertebral artery; R CCA, right common carotid artery; L CCA, left common carotid artery; L ScA, left subclavian artery.

The innominate artery is the first and largest arch branch. It arises near midline, anterior to the trachea, and courses gently to the right. Just below the base of the right neck, it bifurcates to form the right subclavian and right common carotid arteries.

The left common carotid artery is typically the second branch from the aortic arch. Arising immediately after the innominate artery, it also originates in front of the trachea and curves gently toward the left side of the neck. Both the innominate and left common carotid arteries start near midline, then curve gently laterally. The common carotid arteries course to the right and left of midline, where both right and left common carotid arteries approach the carotid bifurcation in a posterior position on either side of the trachea.

The left subclavian artery is the third arch branch, ascending toward the neck but bending laterally to course through the thoracic outlet. In some, the right subclavian artery may originate from the innominate slightly higher in the chest to take a more downward projection to enter the thoracic outlet.

The arch rises in the superior mediastinum fairly high in the chest but lies protected by the sternum. The truncal

branches also arise behind the sternum and sternoclavicular joints at about the level of the third and fourth thoracic vertebra. This protected position makes a direct transthoracic ultrasonic approach to the arch impossible.

The basic branch anatomy is shared by two-thirds (65%) of the population.[7] The remaining one-third has a variant anatomy. The most frequent variant lies in a common origin shared by the innominate and left common carotid arteries, the so-called brachiocephalic branch or bovine configuration. This occurs in 27% of the population. Much less frequently, the vertebral artery originates from the aorta between the left common carotid and the left subclavian arteries (2–6% of cases). Rarely (less than 1%), the right subclavian artery originates from the arch distal to the left subclavian or the right vertebral originates from the right common carotid artery or the arch.

Brachiocephalic Veins

The central veins demonstrate greater symmetry than the supraaortic arteries (Figure 7–2). The internal jugular

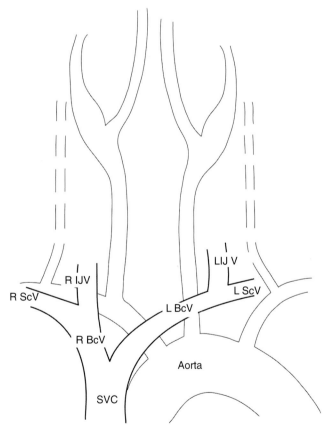

FIGURE 7–2. Brachiocephalic veins and superior vena cava. RScV, right subclavian vein; R IJV, right internal jugular vein; R BcV, right brachiocephalic vein; LBcV, left brachiocephalic vein; L ScV, left subclavian vein; L IJV, left internal jugular vein; SVC, superior vena cava.

veins of the neck and subclavian veins from the upper extremities are confluent, forming the right and left brachiocephalic veins. The external jugular veins also drain into the subclavian veins bilaterally, near the originations of the brachiocephalic veins. The right and left brachiocephalic veins converge to form the superior vena cava (SVC) at about the level of the aortic arch. The SVC lies to the right of the arch, causing a bit of asymmetry. The right brachiocephalic vein descends directly into the SVC as a short venous segment but the left brachiocephalic vein is longer and sharply angulated because of the position of the SVC. The left brachiocephalic vein courses obliquely from the left internal jugular (IJ) vein to the right chest, lying anterior to the branch arteries of the arch. Both brachiocephalic veins converge to form the SVC. Approximately 7 cm in length, the SVC is in contact with the pleura of the right lung, the trachea, and aorta. There are no valves in the brachiocephalic trunks or SVC.

Imaging the Aortic Arch and Brachiocephalic Veins

The arch and branches are a neglected area that is seldom imaged with ultrasound because of dense ultrasound reflections produced by bone and lung air. It is, however, described as part of a standard echocardiographic assessment made through a suprasternal approach.[8]

The suprasternal notch is the midline depression that lies at the base of the neck, between the sternum and larynx. Echocardiography uses the notch to visualize the ascending aorta, arch, and descending thoracic aorta as a means for evaluating the aorta for valvular insufficiency, dissection, aneurysm, or coarctation.[9] Though it is described as a standard echo approach, the image is often less than satisfactory, and is seldom used in adult echocardiography.

The echocardiographer uses a 2- to 5-MHz transducer to visualize the ascending aorta, arch, and descending aorta. The transducer produces a small footprint for the more superficial arch branches and is less suited for branch vessel assessment. For the neck, vascular sonographers use high-frequency (5–10 MHz) linear probes to image the extracranial cerebrovascular branches at the carotid bifurcation. The examination approaches the cervical carotid arteries from the lateral neck, alongside the sternocleidomastoid muscle. The scan typically ends centrally at the right common carotid origin and left common carotid artery at the neck base.

As a compromise, the midline, suprasternal approach should be our approach to the supraaortic vessels, using a low-frequency curvilinear probe rather than the small footprint echo or the high-frequency linear probe. The obvious drawbacks to imaging the arch and its branches from this angle include (1) interference from the sternum and claviculae that severely limits access. The ultrasound beam is projected downward through a narrow acoustic window that limits the anterior–posterior projection by the sternum and neck; (2) the truncal arteries project directly toward the probe and veins project directly away from the probe. The resulting B-mode echoes are weakly reflective and poorly illuminate the walls of the central branches; (3) color Doppler compensates for the weak B-mode image, but the number of large vessel flows and color artifacts picked up from the bright echo-reflective surfaces of the mediastinum and pleura produces a confusing image with large swaths of color.

To overcome these problems, recognizing the anatomy of the arch and brachiocephalic veins is important to scanning the central vessels. It is also important to maintain an orientation that is based upon the known ultrasonic anatomy. The examination can be performed by first placing the curvilinear transducer above the sternum and positioning the probe to produce a panoramic view of both common carotid arteries and IJ veins at the base of the neck (Figure 7–3). With this view as the reference point, the scan can be extended centrally by grayscale and color. The right common carotid artery will be seen to rapidly converge with the subclavian artery to become the innominate artery. On the left, the common carotid artery will be seen to simultaneously continue uninterrupted toward the arch. As the probe is projected centrally, both innominate and left common carotid artery will approach one another. The larger innominate artery will approach midline from the patient's right and the left common carotid artery will course obliquely from the left. From further left, the left subclavian artery will course toward the arch from the clavicle.

The arteries and veins of interest lie in front of the trachea. Because the arch projects obliquely from right to left, anterior to posterior, the probe, positioned for a transverse view of the innominate and left common carotid artery, will also capture the aorta in near transverse. The aorta will be seen in grayscale as a 2–3 cm pulsatile mass. By color, flow in the aorta will be notably disturbed. Flow in the innominate and left common carotid will be much more uniform and easily traced as tracks of color flow directed toward the probe. Both arteries can be interrogated by spectral Doppler as they approach the aorta.

Once the relative positions of the arteries are identified, the innominate artery (Figure 7–4) and left common carotid artery (Figure 7–5) may be imaged individually in longitudinal view by rotating the ultrasound probe on the neck base to the left of midline.

The left subclavian artery may be the most difficult to follow. To visualize the subclavian, the transducer probe will be positioned above the clavicle, projecting the heel of the probe toward the left posterior aspect of the notch (Figure 7–6). Ultrasound reflections will capture bright

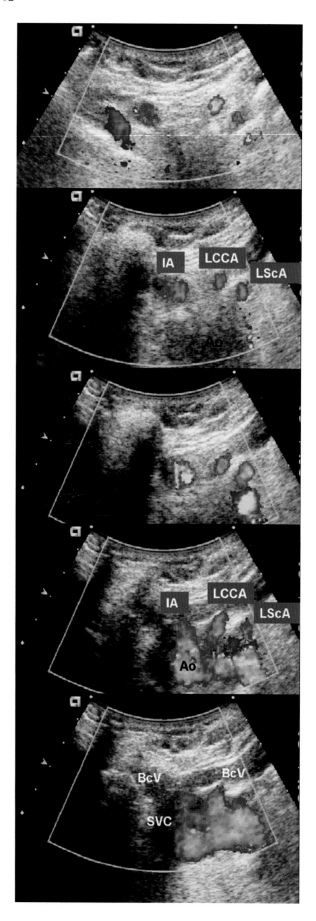

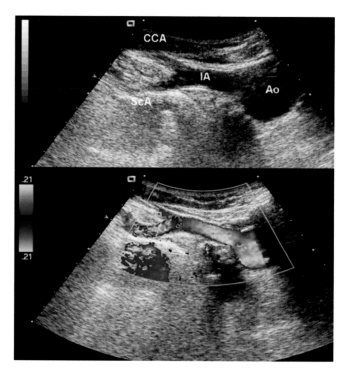

FIGURE 7–3. Imaging the aortic arch and its branches. Branches of the arch from the neck base (top) to aorta (bottom) are scanned with a 4-MHz curvilinear probe placed horizontally above the suprasternal notch. The innominate artery (IA), left common carotid artery (LCCA), and left subclavian artery (LScA) are shown in oblique slices. Scanning centrally, the supraaortic branches enter the aorta (Ao). With greater probe angulation (bottom), the convergence of the right and left brachiocephalic veins (BcV) can be imaged to form the superior vena cava (SVC). The right sternoclavicular joint produces an acoustic shadow alongside the SVC.

reflections from the pleura and left lung. Artifactual duplication of the left subclavian artery by B-mode and color could then result from mirror imaging reverberation (Figure 7–6).

The subclavian artery should be identified as the color flow pattern that lies superficial to any color artifact. To avoid further confusion, the left subclavian artery could be followed from the axillary artery, below the clavicle, through the thoracic outlet to the subclavian artery.

Difficulties in imaging may be associated with configuration of the arch. The arch has been described in coiled and uncoiled configurations with the supraaortic trunks

FIGURE 7–4. Longitudinal view of the innominate artery from the aorta (Ao) to the innominate artery (IA), right common carotid artery (CCA), and right subclavian artery (ScA), using a 4-MHz curvilinear probe. The probe is placed toward the left of midline. A shadow is cast from the left clavicle at the sternoclavicular joint. A mirror imaging reverberation artifact can be noted below the bright reflector and right subclavian artery.

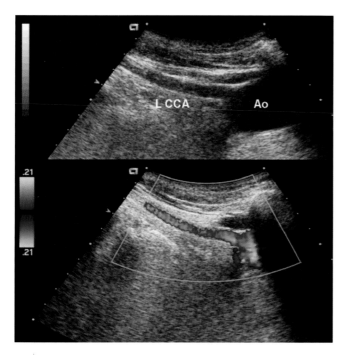

FIGURE 7–5. Longitudinal view of the left common carotid artery (L CCA) and aorta (Ao) scanned with a 4-MHz curvilinear probe, demonstrating the origin of the left common carotid artery, internal jugular vein, and shadowing from the sternoclavicular joint.

Brachiocephalic Veins

Imaging the brachiocephalic veins follows the same reference points as the arterial scan, with a view of the IJ veins bilaterally at the base of the neck. From that point both veins can be followed to their confluence with the subclavian veins and traced to the SVC (Figures 7–3 and 7–7). The left brachiocephalic vein lies anterior to the left common carotid and innominate arteries as it approaches the SVC. Visualization requires a greater anterior angulation, and may be more difficult than visualizing the truncal arterial branches.

The SVC lies to the right of the aorta. This causes some dissymmetry between the right and left brachiocephalic veins that join to form the SVC. The right brachiocephalic vein is short and descends vertically to the SVC. The left brachiocephalic vein will be seen to curve from the patient's left to right as it descends centrally. It is approximately 6 cm in length and will be seen coursing anterior to the branch arteries of the arch. Because the right brachiocephalic vein and SVC are in contact with the pleura of the right lung, there may be substantial color artifact that must be sorted out to identify the confluence.

originating from different points of the arch.[10] The better configuration positions the innominate on the right edge of the apex and the left subclavian artery on the left edge. The take-off points, located on the superior wall of the arch, are optimally positioned for ultrasound imaging and endovascular cannulation. The more difficult imaging configuration occurs when the innominate artery arises from the aorta, before the apex, and its origin lies below the level of the apex. In this "uncoiled" position the left common carotid and subclavian arteries may be similarly displaced to the right. The deeper take-off of the innominate artery may prevent adequate ultrasonic visualization as well as increase the difficulty of endovascular cannulation.

Difficulties caused by anomalous anatomy and inaccessible origination of any arch branch due to coiling or confusing color artifacts may be overcome by continually backtracking the scan to familiar territory at the neck base. Retracing the path of each branch should then allow normal anatomy to be separated from variants and artifacts. The lack of branches central to the innominate, left common, and left subclavian arteries should allow indirect spectral Doppler evidence of a hemodynamically significant stenosis or occlusion when the orificial lesion is not accessible.

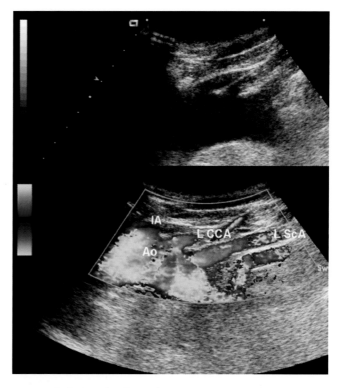

FIGURE 7–6. Longitudinal view of the left subclavian artery (LScA) and originations of the left common carotid artery (LCCA) and innominate artery (IA) from the aorta (Ao). A mirror imaging reverberation artifact can be noted below the bright reflector and left subclavian artery.

94 C.T. Araki et al.

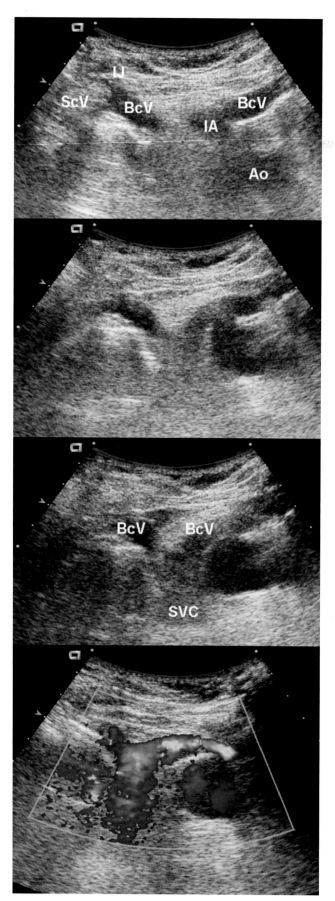

FIGURE 7–7. Imaging the brachiocephalic veins and superior vena cava. From the neck base (top), the right subclavian vein (ScV) and right internal jugular vein (IJ) can be seen to enter the right brachiocephalic vein (BcV). The left brachiocephalic vein crosses from left to right anterior to the innominate artery (IA), above the aorta (Ao). When scanning centrally (bottom), the confluence of both brachiocephalic veins (BcV) can be seen to form the superior vena cava (SVC).

Using Color Flow to Assess the Central Vessels

B-mode imaging does not provide an optimal view of the great vessels and color imaging is important for confirming the relevant structures and guiding the spectral Doppler interrogation. Advantages and limitations of color flow imaging are worth discussing.

Color Doppler technology is the main form of color flow imaging used in commercial instrumentation. Activation of the color Doppler mode displays flow-related color within the borders of a box that is superimposed on the B-mode image. Color Doppler slows the frame rate. While B-mode information can be acquired from single pulses, color Doppler information for a scan line requires multiple insonation pulses. The number of pulses required to collect the Doppler information is called a pulse train or packet.[11] More pulses in a packet provide a better estimate of flow velocities but requires more time. Hence, turning color on decreases the frame rate.

The frame rate also decreases because the color is written within a large number of color gates that are present in the color box. While spectral Doppler uses one gate in one scan line to sample the Doppler shifted frequencies, color Doppler packs the color box with multiple gates in multiple scan lines to display colorized flow anywhere within the box. The vertical dimension of the box determines the number of sample gates along each scan line and the lateral dimension determines the number of scan lines.[12] The frame rate decreases because the same calculation is made for all gates in the box, whether color is applied to the pixel or not. The operator is able to select the color box size and, to a certain extent, the number of gates in a scan line and the number of scan lines. This affects the size of the color pixel and allows the operator to trade-off color resolution for frame rate.[13]

Color Doppler

Color adds an obvious advantage to standard B-mode/spectral Doppler duplex if it rapidly identifies blood flow and guides the placement of the spectral Doppler. Limitations in color may hinder diagnosis and extend the examination time if it is used as a crutch rather than an aid. Color may do the following:

- Overwhelm subtle grayscale shadings of the B-mode image that may be more important than the color information.
- Slow the frame rate to below real-time imaging. Scan times will improve if most of the scan is performed in B-mode and color is activated only when necessary.
- Mislead the inexperienced sonographer. Color sensitivity adjustments are subjective, experience based, and instrument specific. Color registration may be difficult to achieve.
- Have difficulty demonstrating the presence of flow. Echoes received from moving red blood cells are much weaker than the reflections returned for the B-mode image. A relatively good B-mode image of an artery may not be matched by a good velocity signal by color or spectral Doppler simply because of a lack of adequate signal strength. Overreliance on the presence or absence of color may be misleading.
- Overflow the edge of the vessel. The size of a color pixel is variable and can be much larger than the grayscale pixel. Color overflowing the vessel edge may misrepresent the tightness of a stenosis.
- Demonstrate flow where there is none. Mirror image reverberation artifact can occur when a bright reflector lies below the insonated vessel. The result is a false duplication of flow by spectral and color Doppler below the bright interface. A reverberation color artifact may also occur within bright stationary reflectors with the vibration of stiff calcified surfaces.

To the inexperienced sonographer, who does not recognize the potential pitfalls and the necessary adjustments for optimization, color can be a major frustration. This is particularly true when the dependence on color has limited the person's recognition of grayscale morphology and spectral Doppler waveform characteristics. However, once the limits are recognized, there is a distinct advantage to using color to guide the examination. Among the benefits are the following:

- Setting the pulse repetition frequency (PRF) about the expected average velocity will provide good luminal color fill.
- Higher velocity flows produce color aliasing that displays a mixture of hues in adjacent pixels. Within the area of aliasing, color mixing occurs over the top of the color bar scale. There is a scattering of color progressions from light red to light blue that occurs through the unsaturated hues, passing through white. Aliasing can be distinguished from physiologic flow reversals, which cause the color to change in adjacent pixels from uniformly saturated reds to saturated blues, passing through black rather than white.

- Turbulence can produce a color bruit. Flow turbulence produces a high-frequency vibration in the vessel wall. This vibration is transmitted to the skin surface as an audible bruit or palpable thrill and is also picked up by color Doppler as intense speckling of color that spills over the wall of the vessel around the point of greatest turbulence.
- If a stenosis is suspected, possibly with color aliasing or bruit, the point of highest velocity can be located by increasing the PRF. With a tight stenosis or arteriovenous fistula, it is not unusual to find a color hotspot in a tight stenosis or arteriovenous fistula that is continuously lit, indicating continuous forward flow across the stenosis. This is presumably the result of a pressure drop that is maintained throughout the cardiac cycle, indicating that the pressure distal to the stenosis remains lower than the diastolic pressure.
- Color is helpful for distinguishing ulcerations from hypoechoic plaque. For this purpose, it would be worth increasing spatial resolution over frame rate to increase the number of sample gates and decrease the size of the color pixel. It is also advisable to decrease the PRF, increase the filter, and increase persistence. The latter adjustments will detect the slower flows filling the ulcerations and smooth the color fill throughout the cardiac cycle.

Through these characteristics, color flow imaging provides an excellent adjunctive modality for assessing the central vessels of the chest. The relatively simple branch anatomy of the large vessels and the lack of potential small branch collaterals and the assessment made distal to an arterial stenosis or occlusion make the evaluation more straightforward.

Conclusions

The prevalence and clinical significance of arch branch disease will be recognized only through routine evaluation. Unfortunately, suprasternal ultrasonic imaging of the aortic arch and brachiocephalic veins will probably not be a routine part of the standard carotid evaluation. It can, however, prove especially useful in identifying an arch lesion that is suggested by flow disturbances in the common carotid artery, flow reversals in the vertebral artery, or asymmetrical brachial pressures. Identifying these lesions at the time of a cerebrovascular ultrasound examination can be especially important now that catheter-based intervention may be an easy next step.

Suprasternal imaging of the brachiocephalic veins may also be a valuable tool for an upper extremity venous examination, which tends to be limiting above the clavicle. Ultrasonic imaging may even be useful in determining the placement of central venous catheters.

Used correctly, color Doppler is capable of greatly improving the scan time for a cerebrovascular examination and can be critical for the examination of the aortic arch branches and the quality of a difficult examination. It is still an adjunctive component of the examination and for the typical patient, color flow imaging may not add to the final outcome.

References

1. Berguer R. Reconstruction of the supraaortic trunks and vertebrobasilar system. In: Moore WS (ed). *Vascular Surgery: A Comprehensive Review*, 6th ed., pp. 627–642. Philadelphia: WB Saunders Co, 2002.
2. Tyras DH, Barner HB. Coronary-subclavian steal. Arch Surg 1977;112:1125–1127.
3. Fields WS, Lemak NA. Joint study of extracranial arterial occlusion. Subclavian Steal—a review of 168 cases. JAMA 1972;222:1139–1143.
4. Hadjipetrou P, Cox S, Piemonte T, Eisenhauer A. Percutaneous revascularization of atherosclerotic obstruction of aortic arch vessels. J Am College Cardiol 1999;33:1238–1245.
5. Hass WK, Fields WS, North RR, *et al.* Joint study of extracranial arterial occlusion-II: arteriography, techniques, sites, and complications. JAMA 1968;203:159–164.
6. Khatibzadeh M, Sheikhzadeh A, Gromoll B, Stierle U. Topographic pattern of advanced atherosclerotic lesions in carotid arteries. Cardiology 1998;89:235–240.
7. Uflacker R. Thoracic aorta and arteries of the trunk. In: Uflacker R (ed). *Atlas of Vascular Anatomy: An Angiographic Approach*, pp. 143–188. Baltimore: Williams & Wilkins, 1997.
8. Allen MN. The transthoracic exam. In: Allen MN (ed). *Echocardiography*, 2nd ed., pp. 181–206. London: Lippincott, Williams & Wilkins, 1999.
9. Peters PJ. Echocardiographic evaluation of the aorta in echocardiography. In: Allen MN (ed). *Echocardiography*, 2nd ed., pp. 599–614. London: Lippincott, Williams & Wilkins, 1999.
10. Eisenhauer AC. Subclavian and innominate revascularization: Surgical therapy versus catheter-based intervention. Curr Interv Cardiol Rep 2000;2:101–110.
11. Zagzebski JA. Color Doppler and color flow imaging. In: *Essentials of Ultrasound Physics*, pp. 109–122. St Louis, MO: Mosby, 1996.
12. Hedrick WR, Hykes DL, Starchman DE. *Color-Flow Imaging in Ultrasound Physics and Instrumentation*, 3rd ed., pp. 162–177. St. Louis, MO: Mosby, 1995.
13. Miele FR. Doppler. In: Miele FR (ed). *Ultrasound Physics and Instrumentation*, Vol. 2, pp. 7-1–7-28. Miele Enterprises, LLC, 2003.

8
Vertebral Artery Ultrasonography

Marc Ribo and Andrei V. Alexandrov

Introduction

Although the vertebrobasilar system accounts for up to 20% of the total cerebral blood flow and a proportionate share of strokes,[1] many cases of vertebrobasilar disease remain undiagnosed or diagnosed incorrectly. Some common symptoms, such as dizziness or transient loss of consciousness, do not always prompt detailed examination of the posterior circulation vessels. A simple, fast, noninvasive ultrasound examination of the extra- and intracranial portions of the vertebrobasilar system can yield valuable information for diagnosis and treatment.[2–10]

Noninvasive ultrasound can differentiate normal from diseased arteries, identify all categories of stenosis, localize the disease process including occlusions, detect progression of the disease, detect and quantify cerebral embolism, and assess collateral circulation to maintain cerebral blood flow.

Mastering cerebrovascular ultrasound requires knowledge of anatomy, physiology of cardiovascular and nervous systems, fluid dynamics, pathological changes in a variety of cerebrovascular disorders,[11–21] as well as basic ultrasound physics and instrumentation.[22–28]

The aim of this chapter is to describe the methods of cerebrovascular ultrasound testing of the vertebrobasilar system, practical criteria for interpretation, and relevance of these findings to patient management. Rapid bedside evaluation by an expert sonographer with a portable ultrasound unit is an excellent screening test that can provide an immediate impact on patient management at a lower cost and no time delays compared to other imaging methods.

Anatomy of the Vertebrobasilar Arterial System

When performing a vascular ultrasound examination, it is necessary to think about generated images with respect to transducer position, i.e., a sonographer should "think in 3-D" or three dimensions about the vessel being investigated. A sonographer should further imagine how this arterial segment would look on an angiogram. We strongly encourage those learning and interpreting ultrasound to be familiar with cerebral angiograms[11] since invasive angiography is the gold standard for assessment of accuracy of ultrasound testing.

The vertebral arteries arise from the subclavian arteries and pass cephalad in the neck to enter the bony canal at the C6 vertebrae. They course through the transverse processes of the vertebrae (Figure 8–1), and enter the base of the skull through the foramen magnum. At this point, the right and left vertebral arteries join together to form the basilar artery. The trunk of the basilar artery courses for about 3 cm or more before terminating in the posterior cerebral arteries (Figure 8–1), which make up the posterior portion of the circle of Willis.

Extracranial Duplex Ultrasound Examination Technique and Scanning Protocol

The extracranial vertebrobasilar duplex examination includes longitudinal B-mode scans of the vertebral artery mid-cervical portion followed by the origin and the most distal portion accessible on the neck. To optimize the grayscale image, set the dynamic range to 40–50 dB and the time-gain compensation (TGC) as appropriate to the depth of the vertebral arteries.

Duplex ultrasound allows segmental assessment of the vertebral artery flow between transverse processes in 96–100% of cases (Figure 8–2), and visualization of the vertebral artery origins in 65–90% of the patients. These segments should be thoroughly evaluated in patients with strokes or transient ischemic attacks in the posterior circulation. Vertebral duplex provides not only

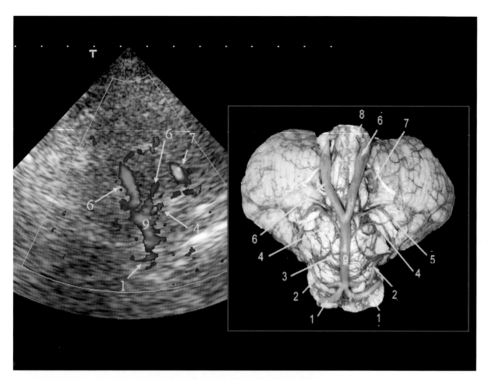

FIGURE 8–1. Anatomy of the vertebrobasilar system. Comparison between the display observed by transcranial color-coded duplex and an anatomopathologic specimen.1: Left posterior cerebral artery; 4: anterior inferior cerebellar artery; 6: vertebral arteries; 7: posterior inferior cerebellar artery.

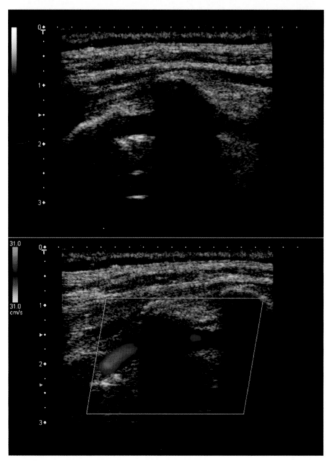

FIGURE 8–2. (A) Longitudianal view of the vertebral artery between the vertebral "shadows" on B-mode. (B) Superimposed color flow image.

information about the portion insonated directly, but indirect information about the proximal and distal vessel segments. The spectrum of vertebral pathology detectable by duplex scanning includes

1. vertebral artery stenosis (origin, V2, V3, and V4 segments) (Figure 8–3),
2. vertebral artery occlusion or absence of flow due to congenital aplasia,
3. hypoplastic vertebral artery, and
4. subclavian steal (Figure 8–4).

Unfortunately there are no established criteria for grading various degrees of extracranial vertebral artery stenosis, however, normal peak systolic velocity is approximately 40–50 cm/s. The velocity may be low in a subdominant or hypoplastic vertebral artery. If duplex shows a significant, i.e., ≥50% vertebral stenosis, the velocity doubles compared to prestenotic or poststenotic segments or the contralateral side. A greater than 70% stenosis will triple the velocity. Generally, most significant focal stenoses in the vertebral artery produce a peak systolic velocity elevation above 100 cm/s. Large vessel atheromatous disease that could be responsible for posterior circulation symptoms usually presents with vertebral artery stenosis or occlusion with preexisting plaque formation (Figure 8–3).

Infrequently, duplex examination may show findings consistent with vertebral artery dissection,[28] and further testing needs to be done to determine if it is an isolated vertebral dissection or an extension of aortic arch dissection. Further consideration should be given as to whether this dissection is spontaneous or trauma related.

Finally, the finding of subclavian steal (Figure 8–4), often a harmless hemodynamic phenomenon, indicates the presence of atherosclerotic stenosis or occlusion in the subclavian artery.[29] Occasionally, subclavian steal can produce symptoms related to transient hypoperfusion in the basilar artery.[29,30] Latent subclavian steal can be demonstrated by early systolic deceleration and the arrival of highest velocities in late systole. The "hyperemia test" can provoke flow reversal in patients with latent steal. A blood pressure cuff is inflated in the ipsilateral arm to suprasystolic values and the patient is asked to perform physical exercise of that arm to increase metabolic demand and vasodilation. Upon sudden cuff release a systolic flow reversal with low diastolic antegrade flow is seen (Figure 8–4).

The so-called alternating flow signal or a total reversal of flow at rest represents different stages of the subclavian steal phenomenon. It is called a syndrome if clinical symptoms of posterior circulation ischemia develop.

Imaging in the Longitudinal Plane

Optimize the image so that the normal linear reflectivity of the arterial wall is apparent. To find the vertebral

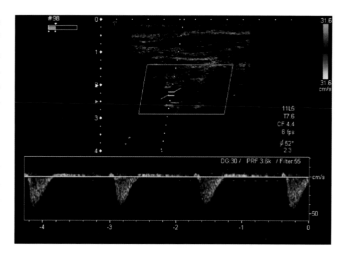

FIGURE 8–4. Subclavian steal; reversed systolic flow in the cervical portion of the vertebral artery with very low antegrade diastolic velocity.

artery, visualize the common carotid artery (longitudinal view, transducer position anterior to the sternocleidomastoid muscle). Steer the color beam toward the proximal common carotid artery (CCA). Rock the probe slightly to the lateral aspect of the neck to image the vertebral artery as it courses through the transverse processes of the vertebrae ("shadows"). "Heel-toe" the probe above the clavicle to image the origin of the vertebral artery as it arises from the subclavian artery. Confirm that the direction of flow in the vertebral artery is the same as the CCA.

Color Flow Ultrasound Evaluation of Flow Dynamics

Choose the appropriate color pulse repetition frequency (PRF) by setting the color velocity scale for the expected velocities in the vessel. For normal adult arteries, the peak systolic velocity range is usually around or under 40–50 cm/s. Adjust the scale further to avoid systolic aliasing (low PRF) or diastolic flow gaps (high PRF or filtering) in normal vessels.

Optimize the color power and gain so that flow signals are recorded throughout the lumen of the vessel with no "bleeding" of color into the surrounding tissues.

Avoid using large or wide color boxes since this will slow down frame rates and resolution of the imaging system. Use color boxes that cover the entire vessel diameter and 1–2 cm of its length. Align the box, i.e., select an appropriate color flow angle correction, according to the vessel geometry and course.

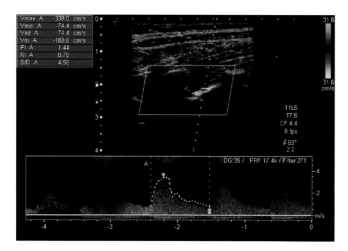

FIGURE 8–3. Vertebral stenosis in its cervical portion. Angle corrected velocity measurement shows a peak systolic velocity of 339 cm/s.

Doppler Spectral Evaluation of Flow Dynamics

Display the longitudinal image of the vertebral artery. Use color flow image as a guide for Doppler examination (Figure 8–2). Begin the examination using a Doppler sample volume size of 1.5 mm positioned in the middle of the vessel. Consistently follow one of the choices for angle correction: parallel to the vessel walls or to the color flow jet. Adjust the Doppler spectral power and gain to optimize the quality of the signal return. Slowly sweep the sample volume throughout the different intervertebral visualized segments. Identify regions of flow disturbance or where flow is absent. Additionally, include Doppler spectral waveforms proximal, within, and distal to all areas where flow abnormalities were observed. Locate the origin or proximal segment of the vertebral artery. Record flow patterns paying careful attention to flow direction. Follow accessible cervical segments of the vertebral artery. Change angulation of the color box and Doppler sample along with the course of the artery.

Extracranial Duplex Examination Should Provide the Following Data

1. Peak systolic velocity in all vessel segments.
2. End diastolic velocity in all vessel segments.
3. Flow direction and peak systolic velocity of both vertebral arteries.
4. Views demonstrating the presence and location of pathology.

Tips to Improve Accuracy

1. Consistently follow a standardized scanning protocol.
2. Always perform a complete examination of the vertebral arteries after the carotid examination.
3. Sample velocity signals throughout all arterial segments accessible.
4. Use multiple scan planes.
5. Take time to optimize the B-mode, color, and spectral Doppler information.
6. Videotape or create a digital file of the entire study including sound recordings.
7. Always use the highest imaging frequencies to achieve higher resolution.
8. Account for any clinical conditions or medications that might affect velocity.
9. Integrate data from the right and left carotid and vertebral arteries.
10. Do not hesitate to admit uncertainty and list all causes for limited examinations.
11. Expand the Doppler examination to the intracranial vessels when possible (see Chapter 9).

Tips for Optimizing Color Flow Set-up

According to standardized protocols, the patient's head should be to the left of the image. This orientation should then clearly indicate the appropriate direction of flow in the vertebral arteries. The arterial and venous flow directions are then given color assignments with respect to flow toward or away from the transducer. Traditionally, flow toward the transducer is assigned red while flow away from the probe is assigned blue. The direction of flow relative to the probe will change if the probe is rotated 180° or if the color box is steered in the opposite direction, i.e., the vein will appear red while the artery will appear blue. When this occurs, the color should be changed back to the original assignment to avoid confusion. It must also be noted that the color will change along the course of an artery if the flow direction varies throughout the cardiac cycle (triphasic, to-from) or if the vessel changes direction relative to the orientation of the sound beam.

The zero baseline of the color bar (PRF) is set at approximately two-thirds of the range with the majority of frequencies allowed in the red direction (for flow towards the brain). This setting allows you to display higher arterial mean frequency shifts (velocities) without aliasing artifacts. Allowance should be made for some flow in the reverse (blue) direction to allow for changes in flow direction (i.e., subclavian steal). When the transducer is rotated 180°, the color will change, and the zero baseline will shift with the color changes to accommodate for flow in the forward direction. You will need to adjust both the color assignment and the zero baseline to the initial setup for consistency. The color PRF and zero baseline may need to be readjusted throughout the examination to allow for the changes in velocity that occur with tortuosity and stenosis. When bruits are encountered, the color PRF should be decreased to detect the lower frequencies associated with a bruit. Usually, the frequency of these bruits is less than 1 kHz.

When occlusion is suspected, the color PRF should be decreased to detect the preocclusive, low-velocity, high-resistance signal associated with critical stenosis or occlusion and to confirm absence of flow at the site of occlusion.

The color wall filter should be set as low as possible. Note that the color wall filter may automatically increase as you increase the PRF. You may need to decrease the wall filter manually when you decrease the color PRF.

The angle of the color box should be changed to obtain the most acute Doppler angles between the scan lines and the direction of blood flow. This will result in a better color display because of more suitable Doppler angles. The angle should always be equal or less than 60°. Because linear array transducers are steered at angles of 90° and 70° from the center of the array, this may require a "heel-toe" maneuver with the transducer on the surface of the skin to adjust the position of the vessel within the color box. An alternative would be to physically change the orientation of the transducer 180°.

The desaturation of color from darker to lighter hues on the color bar indicates increasing Doppler frequency shifts, i.e., increasing velocities. Note that close to the zero baseline, the colors are the darkest. As the velocity increases, the color becomes lighter. You should select colors so that the highest frequency shifts in each direction are of high contrast to each other so that aliasing can be readily detected. For example, you could set the color selections so that low to high velocities are seen as dark blue to light green to aqua in one direction and red to orange to yellow in the opposite flow direction. Aliasing would then appear as aqua adjacent to yellow.

The frame rate should be kept as high as possible to capture the very rapid change in flow dynamics that occurs with stenosis. Remember that frame rate is affected by

1. PRF—frame rate decreases with decreasing PRF;
2. Ensemble length—increasing the color ensemble length will decrease the frame rate;
3. Width of the color box—increased width will decrease the frame rate;
4. Depth—deep insonation decreases the frame rate.

The color box should be kept to a size that is adequate for visualizing the area of interest and yet small enough to keep the frame rate at a reasonable number, approximately 15 or more to ensure adequate filling of the vessel. The frame rate is usually displayed in Hertz on the monitor.

The color gain should be adjusted throughout the examination to detect the changing signal strength. If the color gain is not properly adjusted, some color information may be lost or too much color may be displayed. In this case, you will see color in areas where there should be no flow. The gain should initially be adjusted to an "overgained" level, with color displayed in the tissue and then turned down until the tissue noise just disappears or is minimally present. This is the level at which all color images should be assessed. In situations where there is very low flow, or questionable occlusion, an "overgained" level may be advantageous to show any flow that might be present, e.g., total occlusion versus a near occlusion or critical stenosis.

References

1. Savitz SI, Caplan LR. Vertebrobasilar disease. N Engl J Med. 2005;352:2618–26.
2. Strandness DE, McCutcheon EP, Rushmer RF. Application of a transcutaneous Doppler flowmeter in evaluation of occlusive arterial disease. Surg Gynecol Obstet 1966; 122(5):1039–45.
3. Spencer MP, Reid JM, Davis DL, Paulson PS. Cervical carotid imaging with a continuous-wave Doppler flowmeter. Stroke 1974;5(2):145–54.
4. Barber FE, Baker DW, Nation AW, Strandness DE, Reid JM. Ultrasonic duplex echo-Doppler scanner. IEEE Trans Biomed Eng 1974;21(2):109–113.
5. Budingen HJ, von Reutern GM, Freund HJ. Diagnosis of cerebro-vascular lesions by ultrasonic methods. Int J Neurol 1977;11(2–3):206–18.
6. Aaslid R, Markwalder TM, Nornes H. Noninvasive transcranial Doppler ultrasound recording of flow velocity in basal cerebral arteries. J Neurosurg 1982;57(6):769–74.
7. Spence JD, Coates RK, Pexman JA. Doppler flow maps of the carotid artery compared with the findings on angiography. Can J Surg 1983;26(6):556–8.
8. Bogdahn U, Becker G, Schlief R, Reddig J, Hassel W. Contrast-enhanced transcranial color-coded real-time sonography. Stroke 1993;24:676–684.
9. Rubin JM, Bude RO, Carson PL, Bree RL, Adler RS. Power Doppler US: A potentially useful alternative to mean frequency-based color Doppler US. Radiology 1994;190(3): 853–6.
10. Burns PN. Harmonic imaging with ultrasound contrast agents. Clin Radiol 1996;51:50–55.
11. Krayenbuehl H, Yasargil MG. *Cerebral Angiography,* 2nd ed. Stuttgart: Thieme, 1982.
12. Bernstein EF. *Vascular Diagnosis,* 4th ed. St. Louis: Mosby-Year Book, 1993.
13. Polak JF. *Peripheral Vascular Sonography: A Practical Guide.* Baltimore: Williams & Wilkins, 1992.
14. Strandness DE. *Duplex Scanning in Vascular Disorders,* 2nd ed. New York: Raven Press, 1993.
15. Zweibel WJ. *Introduction to Vascular Ultrasonography,* 4th ed. St. Louis: Harcourt Health Sciences, 2000.
16. von Reutern GM, Budingen HJ. *Ultrasound Diagnosis in Cerebrovascular Disease.* Stuttgart: Thieme, 1993.
17. Tegeler CH, Babikian VL, Gomez CR. *Neurosonology.* St. Louis: Mosby, 1996.
18. Hennerici M, Neuerburg-Heusler D. *Vascular Diagnosis with Ultrasound. Clinical Reference with Case Studies.* Stuttgart: Thieme, 1998.
19. Hennerici M, Mearis S. *Cerebrovascular Ultrasound: Theory, Practice, and Future Developments.* Cambridge: Cambridge University Press, 2001.
20. Bartels E. *Color-Coded Duplex Ultrasonography of the Cerebral Arteries: Atlas and Manual.* Stuttgart: Schattauer, 1999.
21. Babikian VL, Wechsler LR (eds). *Transcranial Doppler Ultrasonography,* 2nd ed. Woburn, MA: Butterworth Heinemann, 1999.
22. Edelman SK. *Understanding Ultrasound Physics,* 2nd ed. The Woodlands: ESP, Inc., 1997.
23. Kremkau FW. *Diagnostic Ultrasound: Principles and Instruments,* 5th ed. New York: Harcourt Health Sciences, 1998.
24. *Zagzebski JA. Essentials of Ultrasound Physics.* St. Louis: Mosby, 1997.
25. Alexandrov AV. *Cerebroavascular Ultrasound in Stroke Prevention and Treatment.* New York: Blackwell, 2004.
26. Bartels E, Fuchs HH, Flugel KA. Duplex ultrasonography of vertebral arteries: Examination, technique, normal values, and clinical applications. Angiology 1992;43(3 Pt 1): 169–80.

27. Bartels E. *Color-Coded Duplex Ultrasonography of the Cerebral Vessels*. Stuttgart: Schattauer, 1999.
28. Bartels E, Flugel KA. Evaluation of extracranial vertebral artery dissection with duplex color-flow imaging. Stroke 1996;27(2):290–5.
29. Bornstein NM, Norris JW. Subclavian steal: A harmless haemodynamic phenomenon? Lancet 1986;2(8502):303–5.
30. Toole JF. *Cerebrovascular Disorders*, 4th ed. New York: Raven Press, 1990.

9
Transcranial Doppler Sonography

Marc Ribo and Andrei V. Alexandrov

The Principles of Transcranial Doppler

Transcranial Doppler sonography (TCD) was first introduced by Rune Aaslid and colleagues in 1982 to non-invasively measure blood flow velocities in the major branches of the Circle of Willis through the intact skull.[1] A 2-MHz frequency pulse wave ultrasonic beam penetrates the skull and allows returned echo signals to be detected. The frequency shift of the returned echoes is calculated using the Doppler equation $f_D = 2 f_o v \cos\theta / (c - \cos\theta)$, where f_D is Doppler shift, f_o is the emitting frequency, v is the scatterer speed, θ is the Doppler angle, and c is the sound propagation speed. The average speed of sound in soft tissues is 1540 m/s and the Doppler angle for TCD examination is assumed to be 0° for all arteries ($\cos 0° = 1$). Therefore the Doppler equation is rearranged to calculate the velocity of moving blood in basal cerebral arteries: $v(\text{cm/s}) = 77 f_D(\text{kHz})/f_o(\text{MHz})$, where the 77 coefficient is valid for the frequency and velocity units shown in parentheses.

TCD allows the depth and the direction of flow relative to the transducer position and the ultrasonic beam direction to be located. The depth of insonation displayed in centimeters or millimeters is manually adjusted. This is accomplished by changing the pulse repetition frequency, which is based on the average speed of sound in soft tissues. Thus to locate the signals originating at a depth of 5 cm, the machine emits the pulse and waits for the time period necessary for ultrasound to make a round trip to and from this depth [i.e., $(0.05/1540) \times 2 = 0.00006\,\text{s}$]. The direction of flow depends on the angle at which the ultrasonic beam intercepts an artery. The flow moving toward the transducer (i.e., the angle of interception is less than 90°) will increase the frequency of the returned signal compared to the emitted frequency. The flow intercepted at 90° will produce no detectable Doppler shift. And if the arterial flow is directed away from the probe (i.e., the angle >90°), the frequency of the returned signal will be less than the emitted one. Therefore the Doppler shifts are coded as positive or negative and the direction of flow is determined accordingly.

Power Motion Mode

Transcranial power motion mode Doppler (PMD) was recently invented by Mark Moehring and Merrill Spencer.[2] In its current configuration, PMD, or M-mode, uses 33 overlapping Doppler samples to simultaneously display flow signal intensity and direction over 6 cm of intracranial space. PMD provides a color-coded display of all flow signals detectable at a given position and direction of the transducer in real time (Figure 9–1). The brighter PMD colors reflect stronger intensities, and this "road map" can serve as a guide for more complete spectral analysis. PMD promises to make a standard TCD examination[1-3] easy even for an inexperienced person. Instead of lengthy acquisition of skills to find windows of insonation with a single-channel spectral TCD, a clinician can search for a window of insonation relying less on sound recognition and arm coordination and not be locked into a single spectrum depth. Furthermore, PMD flow patterns, or signatures, may have their own diagnostic significance, and these flow changes can be observed over large segments of intracranial vasculature in real time. PMD may prove helpful for thrombolysis monitoring and embolus detection by tracking the time–space path of high-intensity signals traveling simultaneously to several major intracranial vessels.

Transcranial Color Duplex

There is an increasing number of reports on the use of transcranial color coded duplex (TCCD) for intracranial vascular studies[4-6] (Figure 9–1). TCCD offers a two-dimensional B-mode image that permits the brain structures to be identified. It is particularly useful in the

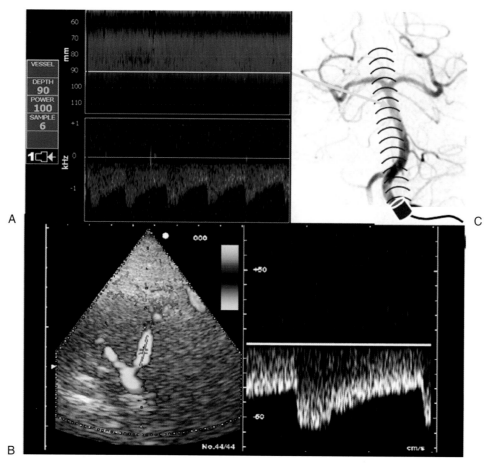

FIGURE 9–1. PMD and TCCD imaging of a normal basilar artery. On PMD display (A) the blue ribbon represents the existence of a flow away from the probe in depths between 65 and 100 mm. TCCD display (B) shows convergence of both vertebral arteries into the proximal basilar artery. (C) Insonation of vertebral and basilar arteries using a transforaminal approach.

detection of distal arterial lesions allowing angle correction in those branches parallel to the skull.[7] At bedside, B-mode imaging is able to demonstrate the midline shifting in malignant middle cerebral artery (MCA) infarctions[8] or hematoma growth with intracerebral bleeds. Duplex technology is now used in the development of brain perfusion assessment techniques with gaseous microbubble contrast agents for ultrasound imaging.[9–11]

Examination Technique

There are four "windows" for insonation (Figure 9–2): temporal, orbital, foraminal, and submandibular.[1,3] The transtemporal approach allows insonation of the middle (MCA), anterior (ACA), posterior (PCA), and communicating arteries. The transorbital approach is used to insonate the ophthalmic artery (OA) and internal carotid artery (ICA) siphon. The transforaminal approach allows the terminal vertebral and basilar arteries to be insonated

through the foramen magnum. The submandibular approach is used to obtain ICA velocities as they enter the skull. To shorten the time necessary to find the window and different arterial segments, the examination should begin with the maximum power and gate settings (i.e., power 100%, gate 15 mm). Identify and store the highest velocity signals and any abnormal or unusual waveforms.

Transtemporal insonation steps:

1. Set the depth at 50 mm (distal M1-MCA) or 56 mm (mid M1-MCA).
2. Place the probe above the zygomaticus arch and aim it slightly upward and anterior to the contralateral ear/window.
3. Find any flow signal and avoid too anterior and too posterior angulation.
4. Find a flow signal directed toward the probe that resembles MCA flow.
5. Follow the signal until is disappears at shallow (40–45 mm) and deep (65–70 mm) depths.

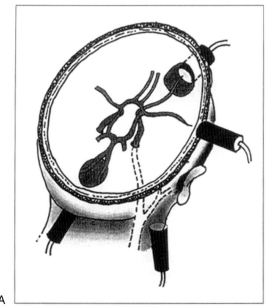

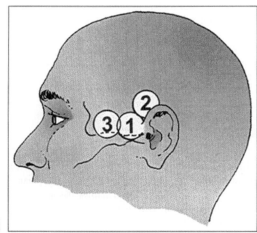

FIGURE 9–2. (A) Windows of insonation *(left to right)*: transforaminal, submandibular, temporal, and transorbital. (B) The temporal window for insonation may be found above the zygomatic arch at the middle (1), posterior (2), and anterior (3) positions.

6. Find the ICA bifurcation at 65 mm and obtain both MCA and ACA signals.
7. Find the terminal ICA signal just inferior to the bifurcation at 60–65 mm.
8. Return to the bifurcation and follow the ACA signal to 70–75 mm depths.
9. Return to the bifurcation, set the depth at 63 mm, and slowly turn the transducer posteriorly by 10–30°(usually there is a flow gap between the bifurcation and PCA signals).
10. Find PCA signals directed toward (P1) and away (P2) from the probe.

Transorbital insonation steps:

1. Decrease power to a minimum or 10%.
2. Set the depth at 52 mm and place the transducer over the eyelid and angle it slightly medially.
3. Determine flow pulsatility and direction in the distal ophthalmic artery.
4. Confirm these findings at 55–60 mm.
5. Set the depth at 60–64 mm and find the ICA siphon flow signals (usually located medially).

Transforaminal insonation steps:

1. Use full power, set the depth at 75 mm, place the transducer at midline an inch below the edge of the skull and aim it at the bridge of the nose, and identify a flow directed away from the probe.
2. Increase the depth to 80 mm [proximal basilar artery (BA)], 90 mm (mid BA), and >100 mm (distal BA).
3. Confirm these findings while decreasing the depth of insonation.
4. Set the depth at 60 mm and place the probe laterally aiming at the uni- or contralateral eye.
5. Find the vertebral artery (VA) flow directed away from the probe and follow it at 40–50 mm and 70–80 mm depths and repeat the examination on the contralateral side.

Submandibular insonation steps:

1. Set the depth at 50–60 mm, place the probe laterally under the jaw, and aim it upward and slightly medially.
2. Find a low resistance flow directed away from the probe.

The TCD interpretation consists of the assessment of (1) **velocity** changes (focal or global), (2) **asymmetry** of flow parameters (side-to-side, segmental), (3) **pulsatility** (high or low resistance), and (4) **waveform/sound** pattern recognition of flow changes. A normal transcranial Doppler examination may reveal a wide range of depths of insonation, velocity values and waveforms.

Criteria for normal TCD findings:

1. Good windows of insonation; all proximal arterial segments were found.
2. Direction of flow and depths of insonation are given in Table 9–1.
3. The difference between flow velocities in the homologous arteries is less than 30%.
4. A normal MCA mean flow velocity (MFV) does not exceed 170 cm/s in children[12] and 80 cm/s in adults.[13]
5. A normal velocity ratio: MCA > ACA ≥ siphon ≥ PCA ≥ BA > VA.
6. A positive end-diastolic flow velocity (EDV) of 20–40% of the peak systolic velocity (PSV) values and a low resistance pulsatility index (PI) of 0.6–1.1 are present in all intracranial arteries while breathing room air. A

TABLE 9–1. Normal depth, direction, and mean flow velocities in the arteries of the Circle of Willis.[a]

Artery[b]	Depth (mm)	Direction	Children	Adults
M1-MCA	45–65	Toward	<170 cm/s	32–82 cm/s
A1-CA	62–75	Away	<150 cm/s	18–82 cm/s
ICA siphon	60–64	Bidirectional	<130 cm/s	20–77 cm/s
OA	50–62	Toward	Wide range	Wide range
PCA	60–68	Bidirectional	<100 cm/s	16–58 cm/s
BA	80–100+	Away	<100 cm/s	12–66 cm/s
VA	45–80	Away	<80 cm/s	12–66 cm/s

[a]Mean flow velocity values are modified from Adams et al.[12] and Hennerici et al.[21]
[b]MCA, middle cerebral artery; ACA, anterior cerebral artery; ICA, internal carotid artery; OA, ophthalmic artery; PCA, posterior cerebral artery; BA, basilar artery; VA, vertebral artery.

high resistance flow pattern (PI ≥ 1.2) is seen in the OAs only.

7. High resistance flow patterns (PI ≥ 1.2) can be found in all arteries during hyperventilation.

Cerebrovascular Resistance and Hemodynamic Indexes

Cerebrovascular resistance (CVR) is determined by several factors that impede cerebral blood flow (CBF) and thus determine MFV: *the vessel radius, length*, and *blood viscosity*. The changes in flow resistance are mostly accomplished by arterial-arteriolar constriction/dilatation or intracranial pressure (ICP) dynamics. Under normal conditions the brain is a low-resistance arterial system and the ICA branches have considerably greater end-diastolic flow than the external carotid artery (ECA) branches. The resistance to flow is described by the PI and the resistance (RI) indexes. PI (Gosling-King) = PSV – EDV/MFV (normal values for MCA are 0.6–1.1). RI (Pourcelot) = PSV – EDV/PSV (normal values for MCA are 0.49–0.63[14]).

These indexes quantitatively reflect CVR and depend greatly on the strength of the signal recorded as well as the envelope and time averaging software. Therefore "weak signals," "poor" windows, incomplete examination, and individual variations may produce substantial drawbacks. Additional information can be gained by visual flow pattern recognition (Figure 9–3).

Pathologically increased PIs (>1.2) are seen with ICP and decreased cerebral perfusion pressure (CPP) due to decreased EDV. Pathologically low PIs (<0.5) are mainly seen in the arteries feeding arteriovenous malformations (AVM) since direct shunting of blood into the venous system results in abnormally low CVR.[15] Very low PIs may also be seen distal to a severe extra- or intracranial stenosis indicating compensatory vasodilation.[16]

Although these indexes per se may not be sufficient to diagnose extracranial disease, they should be used in a battery of TCD parameters allowing integrated assessment of intracranial circulation.[17]

Other useful indexes include the pulsatility transmission index (PTI), flow acceleration (FA), delta-MCA (δ-MCA), hemispheric index (HI), and the arterial velocities ratios.

PTI (Lindegaard) = PI (study vessel) / PI(reference vessel) × 100%; normal MCA/ICA: 93–107.[11]

FA = PSV – EDV/time differential; normal MCA: 392–592 cm/s^2.[18]

δ-MCA = Ipsi-MCA PSV – contralat-MCA PSV; normal MCA: 8.7 ± 5.9 cm/s.[19]

HI (Lindegaard) = MFV MCA/MFV ICA (normal values 1.76 ± 0.1, pathologic value ≥3).[20]

Arterial velocities ratio = VMCA/VACA (normal values 1.27 ± 0.12).[13]

PTI makes it possible to avoid the influence of changing cardiac output in patients with normal pulsatility of flow in the reference vessel. PTI is usually increased with elevated ICP and in the presence of MCA stenosis (the intracranial PI is compared to the extracranial vessel).[14,17]

The MCA flow acceleration index decreases in the presence of a severe ipsilateral extracranial carotid stenosis (229 ± 115 cm/s^2 in patients with 75–100% ICA stenosis.[14,18]

Delta-MCA also changes with increasing severity of carotid stenosis. Canthelmo et al. showed that if the ICA residual lumen diameter is greater than 1 mm, δ-MCA is 16.4 ± 11.7; and if the residual lumen diameter is ≤1 mm, δ-MCA is 26.6 ± 25.4; if a complete ICA occlusion is present, δ-MCA is 38.7 ± 19.4.[19] Again, note the large standard deviations that reflect between-individual differences and affect the diagnostic accuracy of these indexes if taken separately from other flow data. These indexes may be used cautiously to unmask extracranial distal ICA or siphon stenosis if other TCD and carotid duplex findings are unremarkable.

HI compares MCA MFV to the ipsilateral ICA and may help to differentiate an MCA FV increase due to spasm and/or hyperperfusion. The M1-MCA vasospasm after subarachnoid hemorrhage (SAH) is usually associated with HI values >3, while a severe (<1 mm residual lumen) M1-MCA vasospasm has been shown to correlate with HI values greater than 6.[20]

The arterial velocity ratios help to find MCA branch occlusion since higher velocities in the ACA may indicate the diversion of blood volume to the ACA due to higher resistance and/or decreased flow in the M2-MCA segment. The increased ACA velocities may reflect collateralization of flow via transcortical collaterals. However, ACA FVs can also be increased in the presence of the atretic contralateral A1-ACA segment, functioning anterior communicating artery (AComA), and the stenosis of the terminal ICA and/or unilateral A1-ACA.

Other factors that affect CBF, MFV, and the hemodynamic indexes include age, gender cardiac function, hematocrit and fibrinogen, carbon dioxide, and vasodilatory or constricting medications.[14]

TCD measurement of flow velocities, however, does not allow calculation of CBF in ml/min because of the variable and unknown arterial diameter and peripheral resistance.[9] However, the area under the waveform envelope, intensity of the signal, and relative change in the MFVs determined with the same angle of insonation are usually proportional to regional CBF changes.[10] For example, MFV changes due to vasomotor reactivity with different vasodilatory stimuli reflect CBF changes assuming that the perfused territory remains constant during investigation.[11] The use of TCD for monitoring physiological responses to vasodilatory substances is based on the concept of cerebral vasomotor reactivity (VMR) in order to identify patients at a particular risk for cerebral ischemic events.

Vasomotor Reactivity Assessment with Transcranial Doppler

The North American Symptomatic Carotid Endarterectomy Trial (NASCET), European Carotid Surgery Trialists (ECST), and Asymptomatic Carotid Atherosclerosic Study (ACAS) trials data[21–24] indicate that both hemodynamic and thromboembolic mechanisms of stroke are important in patients with carotid atherosclerosis,[25] and the emphasis is now made on identifying patients with asymptomatic severe carotid stenosis at the highest risk of stroke.[26] Therefore VMR as an index of intracranial collateralization capacity may have a prognostic value in predicting the symptomatic or asymptomatic course of carotid occlusive disease and stroke recurrence.[27]

Vasomotor reactivity assessed by TCD using vasodilating or constricting stimuli is not a measure of autoregulation. The brain autoregulation maintains CBF constant with physiological variations in blood pressure. The changes in CO_2 concentration induce a vasomotor response, which changes CBF paralleled by the velocity changes.[28] Thus, FV changes on TCD during normo-, hyper-, and hypocapnia may prove a useful index of VMR and the capacity of smaller cerebral arteries to adapt to various stimuli (Figure 9–3). Patients with ICA stenosis may be at an increased risk for stroke due to exhausted vasomotor reserve capacity on TCD.

CO_2 Reactivity

The FV modulation is most reliably and reproducibly measured by TCD at the M1-MCA segment during inhalation of different CO_2 concentrations. The end-expiratory CO_2 is measured by an infrared gas analyzer and expressed as volume percentage. The baseline TCD recording should be obtained under normocapnia, or when breathing room air, and then during steady states when air is inhaled with CO_2 concentrations ranging from 6% to 2% given for 2–3 min each. A voluntary hyperventilation is used to produce hypocapnia. TCD measurements of flow velocities should be made during each steady state and several (up to 20) cardiac cycles should be averaged to minimize variations in mean FVs. The baseline MFV is considered 100% and is compared to hyper- and hypocapnia states. VMR is expressed as percent changes of M1-MCA mean FV from hypercapnia to hypocapnia.

In normal volunteers free of cerebrovascular disease mean VMR was 86 ± 16%, $n = 40$, mean age 51 years.[29,30] On average, mean MCA FVs increased by 52% during hypercapnia and decreased by 35% during hypocapnia.[30]

Decreased VMR was observed in patients with ICA occlusions and symptomatic carotid artery disease in many studies, however, normal VMR could also be seen in these patients.[30] In the study reported by Ringelstein, VMR on the occluded or affected side was decreased on average by 20–25% compared to the nonoccluded side or to the normal controls.[30] The most important observation was that patients with low flow infarctions, ischemic ophthalmopathy, and hypostatic transient ischemic attacks (TIAs) had VMR of less than 38%, which is less than three standard deviations below the normal controls.[30]

VMR also decreases with the severity of carotid stenosis and increases after carotid endarterectomy on average by 20–25%, however, relatively large standard deviations allow for a considerable overlap between the subgroups of patients.[30] The most dramatic improvement of VMR was reported by Ringelstein in patients with preoperatively very low values, i.e., less than 50%. Decreased VMR may potentially identify patients with asymptomatic carotid stenosis, which carries the highest risk of stroke, and this parameter should be verified in prospective studies.[27,30,31]

Assessment of CO_2 reactivity requires special equipment that may not necessarily be available. A simpler method of VMR assessment uses voluntary breath-holding.[32] VMR is represented by the breath-holding index (BHI), which is the ratio of the percent MFV increase during hypercapnia over the time (seconds) of breath-holding. Baseline FVs are obtained during inhalation of room air followed by a 30s breath-holding followed by a 4-s recording of the highest FVs. The efficacy of breath-holding can be assessed by a respiratory activity monitor.[32]

In normal subjects, BHI is usually greater than 1 (1.12 ± 0.3, $n = 10$, mean age 63 ± 11 years).[33] In

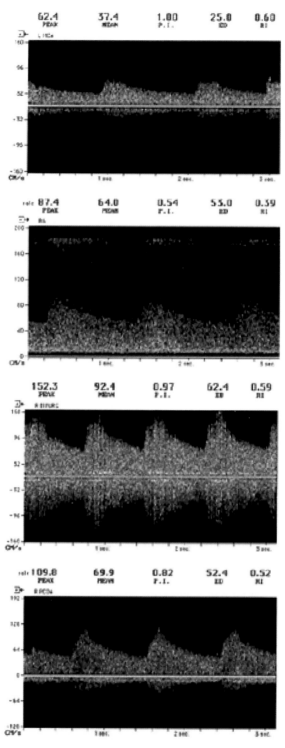

FIGURE 9–3. (A) Normal low-resistance flow in the Ml-MCA segment has sharp systolic flow acceleration, slow deceleration, and an end-diastolic velocity of 40% (range 20–50%) of the peak systolic values. The pulsatility index (PI) is 1.0 (range 0.6–1.1). End-diastolic flow may decrease and PI may increase with slower heart rate, hypertension, and decreased end-diastolic blood pressure (top image). Abnormally low flow resistance results in elevated velocities above age-expected limits, end-diastolic flow velocity exceeding 50% of peak systolic values, and a decreased pulsatility index of 0.54. This waveform can be seen during hypercapnia, poststenotic vasodilatation, and in partial arteriovenous malformation feeders (second image). Hyperemia typically produces abnormally high flow velocities, low-resistance PI values, and nonharmonic murmurs in the MCA and ACA as well as other intracranial arteries. The Lindegaard ratio is calculated to confirm the parallel increase in mean flow velocity in the insonated and feeding vessels (i.e., MCA/ICA < 3) (third image). Collateral flow via PComA may have elevated velocities, low resistance, a rounded shape of the peak systolic component, and a soft "wind-blowing" sound. A similar waveform may be observed in the MCA when it receives collateral flow from the posterior circulation (fourth image).

Waveform

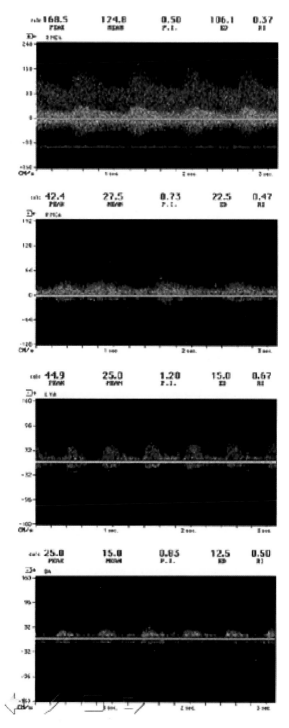

B

FIGURE 9–3. (B) Arterial stenosis produces a focally significant increase in flow velocities (>30% compared with other arterial segments). The "double" waveform recording shows the stenotic flow and a low-velocity, low-resistance poststenotic flow detected simultaneously using a large (>11mm) gate of insonation (top image). Arterial near occlusion has a residual flow detected by transcranial Doppler as a "blunted" waveform. This recording shows the delayed minimal systolic flow acceleration and decreased velocities typically seen due to a flow volume decrease with near occlusion. Note the normal pulsatility of flow due to a patent vessel distal to the site of insonation (second image). Arterial occlusion distal to the site of insonation may produce increased resistance to flow in the absence of a bifurcation between these arterial segments. This high resistance (PI ~ 1.2) waveform was obtained just proximal to the basilar artery occlusion at the origin. It may be the only focal sign of a distal arterial obstruction (third image). Minimal flow signals may be a source of error responsible for false-positive and false-negative transcranial Doppler studies. False-positive results are usually obtained with poor windows of insonation, uncooperative patients, and incomplete examination. True signals have very low velocities, almost absent end-diastolic flow, and are found together with other signs of occlusion (fourth image).

Waveform

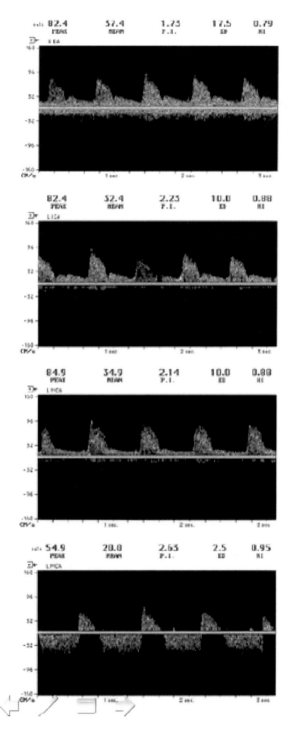

C

Figure 9–3. (C) Under normal conditions, only the ophthalmic artery (OA) has a high-resistance flow pattern with PI values 1.2 and greater. This artery carries the flow away from the brain and forms anastomoses with a high-resistance system of the external carotid artery branches. The OA velocities may vary substantially (top image). Hyperventilation induces vasoconstriction that also increases resistance to flow. The systolic component sharpens, the diacrotic notch becomes more pronounced, and the end-diastolic flow decreases. Often the triphasic waveform is observed similar to the peripheral arteries. The decrease in mean flow velocity may be proportional to the flow volume decrease caused by vasoconstriction (second image). Increased intracranial pressure decreases cerebral perfusion pressure and affects the end-diastolic flow, since blood pressure is lowest during this part of the cardiac cycle with sharp late-systolic deceleration resulting in a shorter transsystolic time (third image). When intracranial pressure exceeds cerebral perfusion pressure, reverberating flow can be detected that indicates systolic flow propagation toward the brain followed by diastolic flow reversal. If found in both MCAs and the BA for 30 min, this flow pattern indicates cerebral circulatory arrest and correlates with absent brain perfusion on a nuclear brain scan (fourth image).

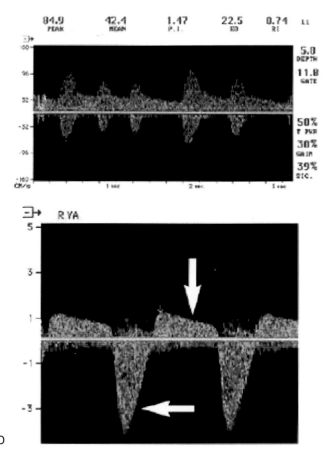

D

FIGURE 9–3. (D) Microembolic signals (MES) on transcranial Doppler appear as high-intensity transient signals that are primarily unidirectional (*arrow*). MES have short duration and occur randomly through the cardiac cycle. MES may be found during routine transcranial Doppler in patients with atrial fibrillation, carotid stenosis, or dissection, and may point to the pathogenetic mechanism of stroke (top image). Subclavian steal occurs when a flow-limiting lesion in the proximal subclavian artery causes flow reversal in the vertebral artery. Transcranial Doppler detects alternating flow at the junction of vertebral arteries. High-resistance flow toward the probe (*horizontal arrow*) is the reversed vertebral right artery, which now supplies a high-resistance system of the arm. Low-resistance flow (*vertical arrow*) is seen during late systole–diastole and has a normal direction since less pressure is necessary to perfuse the brain vasculature (bottom image).

asymptomatic individuals, BHI was 0.8 ± 0.4 on the stenotic side before and 1.09 ± 0.2 after carotid endarterectomy (CEA). In symptomatic individuals, BHI was 0.4 ± 0.2 on the stenotic side before and 1.06 ± 0.2 after CEA.[33] Recently, a BHI threshold of <0.69 was established in controlled prospective studies that predicts an increased risk of stroke in patients with asymptomatic severe ICA stenosis and risk of recurrent stroke in patients with symptomatic ICA stenoses or occlusion.[29]

Interpretation of CO_2 reactivity testing should be individualized with particular attention paid to the procedure employed since it requires patient cooperation and relies on the sonographer's experience. Abnormally low VMR ($<50\%$ CO_2 reactivity, or <0.5 BHI) may indicate maximal vasodilation at rest and therefore poor collateral capacity of the Circle of Willis and potentially higher risk of stroke distal to the extracranial lesion due to exhausted cerebral vasomotor reserve.[30,33] These findings, however, need to be validated in prospective outcome studies.

Vasomotor Reactivity Testing with Diamox

Diamox is a potent and reversible inhibitor of carbonic anhydrase, however, the mechanism by which it increases CBF is still disputable since cerebral metabolic rate of oxygen and arterial blood pressure remain unaffected while arterial PCO_2 increases only slightly.[27]

When administered intravenously, the effect of 1000 mg diamox (acetazolamide) bolus can be observed within 3 min with FVs reaching maximum values in 10 min, which lasts for 20 min. In normal subjects, a 35% increase in FVs is usually observed during hypercapnia.[31] Administration of diamox may be associated with minor and transient side effects: dizziness, oral dysesthesia, tinnitus, and nausea.[34] Since diamox belongs to the sulfanilamide group, any known allergy to the sulfa drugs would be a contraindication for its use.

Using xenon-133 and technetium-99 HMPAO tracers, a 30% increase in CBF was observed in normal subjects following administration of 1000 mg of diamox as well as a high dependency of CBF changes on the degree of carotid stenosis.[35,36] A good correlation was found between mean FVs on TCD and changes in CBF on SPECT or PET.[37,38] Significantly reduced VMR was seen in patients with high grade carotid stenosis suggesting that at baseline the cerebral resistance vessels are maximally dilated to maintain CBF. VMR testing with diamox shows the reduction in or even abolition of the extent to which the resistance vessels can further dilate to compensate for it.[27] However, in spite of uni- or bilateral carotid occlusion some patients have good VMR indicating a sufficient collateral capacity of the Circle of Willis and sufficient cerebral autoregulation. Therefore, VMR testing with diamox may help to differentiate patients with carotid artery disease at high and low risk of stroke and may assist in patient selection for CEA prior to cardiopulmonary bypass (CABG).

Application of Vasomotor Reactivity Testing

Major vascular risk factors for stroke have a chronic effect on the cerebral vasculature that often precedes cerebral ischemic symptoms.[31] Thus diabetes and familial hypercholesterolemia are associated with greater FV increase to vasodilatory stimuli, while chronic hypertension increases the pulsatility of flow.[39–41]

Although the degree of carotid stenosis is the strongest predictor of subsequent stroke risk,[22–24] the impaired VMR can help identify patients at a particularly high risk of stroke.[29,42]

VMR can also be impaired in patients with subarachnoid hemorrhage (SAH).[43] With increased severity of vasospasm there is a gradual reduction of VMR in response to changes in arterial CO_2.[44] Although VMR changes often parallel the course of vasospasm, nimodipine has no effect on CO_2 reactivity.[45] Whether impaired VMR has an independent prognostic value in patients with SAH and other pathologies is still unclear.[31]

Diagnostic Criteria for Transcranial Doppler

The diagnostic criteria for TCD required by the Intersocietal Commission of Accreditation of Vascular Laboratories include arterial stenosis, arterial spasm and hyperemia, collateral patterns and flow direction, cerebral embolization, cerebral circulatory arrest, increased ICP, arterial occlusion, and steal syndrome. When applying for accreditation, each laboratory should accept diagnostic criteria that may include application of published criteria or the use of internally generated criteria. *Whether published or internally generated, normal values and criteria for abnormal findings have to be internally validated.*

This section provides a summary of various criteria, both previously published by other investigators[3,12–15,17,20,21] and generated internally by the STAT Neurosonology Service, University of Texas Houston Medical School.

Intracranial Arterial Stenosis

Middle Cerebral Artery

A focally significant velocity increase MFV ≥ 100 cm/s, and/or a PSV ≥ 140 cm/s, and/or an interhemispheric MFV difference of >30 cm/s in adults free of abnormal circulatory conditions are characteristic (Figure 9–4). If anemia, congestive heart failure, and other circulatory conditions associated with elevated or decreased velocities are present, then a focal MFV difference >30% between arterial segments should be applied. In general, a greater than 50% M1-MCA stenosis should double the prestenotic or homologous contralateral MCA velocity values. In children with sickle cell disease MCA MFV > 170 cm/s is considered abnormal.

Additional findings may include turbulence, or disturbed flow distal to the stenosis; increased unilateral A1-

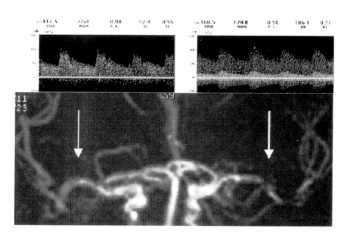

FIGURE 9–4. Left M1-MCA stenosis. A 70-year-old woman with multiple left hemispheric transient ischemic attacks. Transcranial Doppler showed a focally significant increase in the left M1-MCA flow velocities, a "double" waveform showing the stenotic flow insonated with a wide >11-mm gate. MRA shows decreased flow signals in the left mid-to-distal M1-MCA.

ACA MFVs (flow diversion/compensatory increase or ICA bifurcation stenosis) with a side-to-side ACA MFV ratio >1.2; a low-frequency noise produced by nonharmonic covibrations of the vessel wall; and musical murmurs due to harmonic covibrations producing pure tones (rare).

If FVs are increased throughout MCA mainstem, the differential diagnosis includes MCA stenosis, terminal ICA or siphon stenosis, hyperemia or compensatory flow increase in the presence of contralateral ICA stenosis, ACA occlusion, and incorrect vessel identification.

MCA near-occlusion or "blunted" MCA waveform presents as a focal decrease in mean flow velocities with slow systolic acceleration, slow flow deceleration, and MFV MCA < ACA or any other intracranial artery (Figure 9–5).

The decreased or minimal flow velocities with slow systolic acceleration can be due to a tight elongated MCA stenosis or thrombus causing near occlusion, or a proximal ICA obstruction. The "blunted" waveform is common in patients with acute ischemic stroke particularly presenting with hyperdense MCA on noncontrast CT scan or a flow gap on MRA (Figure 9–5).

Anterior Cerebral Artery

A focally significant ACA FV increase (ACA > MCA), and/or an ACA MFV > 80 cm/s, and/or a >30% difference between proximal and distal ACA segments, and/or a >30% difference compared to contralateral ACA with no evidence of collateralization via AcomA are characteristic. The differential diagnosis includes anterior crossfilling due to a proximal carotid artery disease. Additional

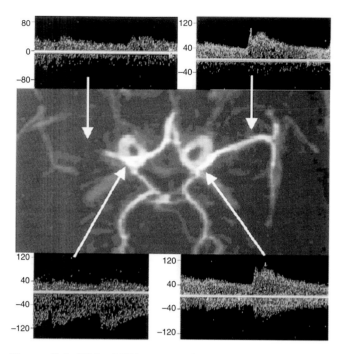

FIGURE 9–5. Right MCA near-occlusion. A 65-year-old man presented with recurrent right MCA ischemic strokes. Transcranial Doppler showed a "blunted" MCA flow signal with decreased flow velocities at the M1 origin and increased velocities in the A1-ACA indicating compensatory flow diversion. Note the decreased systolic flow acceleration in the right MCA and ACA > MCA ratio compared with the contralateral side.

findings may include turbulence and a flow diversion into MCA and/or compensatory flow increase in the contralateral ACA.

The decreased or minimal flow velocities at the A1-ACA origin may indicate a suboptimal angle of insonation from the unilateral temporal window, an atretic or tortuous A1-ACA segment, and A1-ACA near occlusion.

Common errors include incorrect vessel identification (ICA versus ACA) and velocity underestimation (suboptimal angle of insonation, poor window, weak signals).

Terminal Internal Carotid Artery/Siphon Stenosis

A focally significant FV increase in the terminal ICA bifurcation (temporal window), and/or an ICA siphon (transorbital window) resulting in an MFV ICA > MCA, and/or an MFV ICA > 70 cm/s (adults), and/or a >30% difference between arterial segments are characteristic.

The differential diagnosis includes moderate proximal ICA stenosis and/or compensatory flow increase with contralateral ICA stenosis. Additional findings may include turbulence, blunted MCA, OA MFV increase, and/or flow reversal with low pulsatility. The ICA siphon

MFVs may decrease due to siphon near-occlusion (a blunted siphon signal) or distal obstruction (i.e., MCA occlusion or increased ICP).

Posterior Cerebral Artery

A focally significant FV increase presenting as an MFV PCA > ACA or ICA and/or an MFV PCA > 50 cm/s are characteristic. The differential diagnosis includes collateral flow via PcomA and siphon stenosis. Additional findings may include turbulence and a compensatory flow increase in MCA. Common sources of error include unreliable vessel identification without transcranial duplex imaging or the presence of an arterial occlusion and the top-of-the-basilar stenosis.

Basilar Artery

A focally significant FV increase presenting as an MFV BA > MCA or ACA or ICA, and/or an MFV BA > 60 cm/s, and/or a >30% difference between arterial segments are characteristic. The differential diagnosis includes the terminal VA stenosis.

Basilar artery near-occlusion is a focal FV decrease (<30% and/or BA < VA) resulting in a blunted waveform (differential with fusiform basilar with or without thrombus) or absent end-diastolic flow (differential with occlusion).

Additional findings may include turbulence, a compensatory flow increase in VAs and PICAs indicating cerebellar collateralization, and a collateral supply via PComA(s) to PCA(s) with a reversed flow in the top of the basilar artery. Common sources of error include a tortuous basilar ("not found" does not mean obstructed), elongated or distal BA stenosis, collateral flow from the posterior to anterior circulation enhancing flow changes with mild stenosis and/or tortuosity.

Terminal Vertebral Artery

A focally significant FV increase presenting as an MFV VA >> BA, and/or an MFV VA > 50 cm/s (adults), and/or a >30% difference between VAs or its segments are characteristic. The terminal VA stenosis may also present as a high resistance (PI ≥ 1.2) flow in one VA and/or a blunted or minimal flow signal. The differential diagnosis includes proximal BA or contralateral terminal VA stenoses and a compensatory flow increase in the presence of a contralateral VA occlusion. Additional findings may include turbulence, a compensatory flow increase in the contralateral vertebral artery or its branches (cerebellar collaterals), low BA flow velocities (hemodynamically significant lesion, hypoplastic contralateral VA). Common sources of error include a compensatory flow increase due to hypoplastic contralateral VA, low velocities in both VAs due to a suboptimal angle of insonation, extracranial VA stenosis or occlusion with well-developed muscular collaterals, and elongated VA stenosis/hypoplasia.

TCD can reliably detect stenoses located in M1-MCA, ICA siphon, terminal vertebral, proximal basilar arteries, and P1 PCA. The sensitivity is 85–90%, specificity 90–95%, PPV 85%, and NPV 98% with lower accuracy parameters for the posterior circulation.[3,12,15,17,20,21] TCD sensitivity is limited in patients with deep (>65 mm) stenoses due to low PRF; stenoses of M2, A2, P2 segments due to a suboptimal angle or unknown location; low flow elongated stenoses that resemble normal or low flow velocities; subtotal stenosis due to a drop in flow volume producing weak signals; tortuous vessels due to the changing angle of insonation; and collaterals and hyperemia that may mimic the stenotic flow.

Arterial Vasospasm and Hyperemia

Arterial vasospasm (VSP) is a complication of SAH, and it becomes symptomatic in more than 25% of patients by producing ischemic brain damage and delayed neurological deficit (DID). DID usually occurs when VSP results in a severe (≤1 mm) intracranial arterial narrowing producing flow depletion with extremely high velocities. It may affect the proximal stem and distal branches of intracranial arteries. VSP may co-exist with hydrocephalus, edema, and infarction. The differential diagnosis with TCD should always include hyperemia, and the possibility that both spasm and hyperemia may coexist since most SAH patients routinely receive hypertension–hemodilution–hypervolemia (HHH) therapy.

Although quantitative criteria have been studied extensively,[20,46] grading VSP severity is difficult, and the interpretation of TCD findings should be individualized. Daily TCDs may detect considerable velocity/pulsatility changes that should be related to the patient's condition, medications, BP, time after onset, etc.

Proximal vasospasm in any intracranial artery results in a focal or diffuse elevation of mean flow velocities without a parallel FV increase in the feeding extracranial arteries (intracranial/extracranial vessel ratio >3).

Distal vasospasm in any intracranial artery may produce a focally pulsatile flow (PI ≥ 1.2) indicating increased resistance distal to the site of insonation. No MFV increase may be found.

Additional findings may include daily changes in velocity, ratio, and PIs anytime during the first 2 weeks but particularly pronounced during the critical 3–7 days after the onset of SAH.

MCA-specific criteria: see Table 9–2. The differential diagnosis includes hyperemia, a combination of

TABLE 9–2. Criteria for grading M1-MCA vasospasm with or without hyperemia.[a]

Velocity	MCA/ICA ratio[b]	Interpretation
<120	≤3	Hyperemia
>80	3–4	Hyperemia + possible mild spasm
≥120	3–4	Mild spasm + hyperemia
≥120	4–5	Moderate spasm + hyperemia
>120	5–6	Moderate spasm
≥180	6	Moderate-to-severe spasm
≥200	≥6	Severe spasm
>200	4–6	Moderate spasm + hyperemia
>200	3–4	Hyperemia + mild (often residual) spasm
>200	<3	Hyperemia

[a]Optimized criteria were developed using the data from Bragoni et al.,[14] De Chiara et al.,[39] and Sugimari et al.[40]
[b]MCA, middle cerebral artery; ICA, internal carotid artery.

vasospasm and hyperemia in the same vessel, residual vasospasm, and hyperemia.

Prognostically unfavorable signs include an early appearance of MCA MFV ≥ 180 cm/s, a rapid (>20% or + >65 cm/s) daily MFV increase during critical days 3–7, an MCA/ICA ratio ≥6, and the abrupt appearance of high pulsatility (PI > 1.5) of flow in two or more arteries indicating increased ICP and/or distal vasospasm.[20,46]

Other intracranial arteries: see Table 9–3. Grading VSP severity in the arteries other than MCA is difficult. Sloan suggested reporting VSP as possible, probable, and definite.[46] The differential diagnosis includes hyperemia and its combination with vasospasm in these arteries.

An individual correlation of baseline angiography with same day TCD findings may improve the accuracy of TCD in detecting further VSP onset. A focal increase in MFVs and an increase in MFVs disproportionate to therapy will indicate the development of vasospasm. For example, an MCA MFV increase by +50 cm/s may indicate a 20% diameter reduction of the vessel[47] and since FV is inversely proportionate to the vessel radius, a 30% diameter reduction usually doubles the velocity on TCD.

TABLE 9–3. Optimized criteria for grading vasospasm (VSP) in intracranial arteries.

Artery/MFV[a]	Possible VSP[b]	Probable VSP[b]	Definite VSP[b]
ICA	>80	>110	>130
ACA	>90	>110	>120
PCA	>60	>80	>90
BA	>70	>90	>100
VA	>60	>80	>90

[a]MFV, mean flow velocity; ICA, internal carotid artery; ACA, anterior cerebral artery; PCA, posterior cerebral artery; BA, basilar artery; VA, vertebral artery.
[b]After hyperemia has been mostly ruled out by the focality of the velocity increase and by an intracranial artery/extracranial ICA ratio >3 except posterior circulation vessels. Optimized criteria were modified from Sloan MA et al.[46]

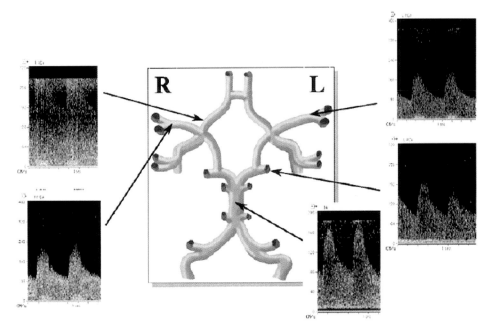

FIGURE 9–6. Severe ACA, PCA, and BA vasospasm. Arterial vasospasm. A 55-year-old woman had a subarachnoid hemorrhage and surgically clipped left PCA aneurysm. Transcranial Doppler showed an MFV/PI of 222/0.5 in the right A1-ACA with an ACA/ICA MFV ratio >6; 131/0.9 in the right M1-MCA with an MCA/ICA MFV ratio = 4; 109/0.9 in the basilar artery; 130/0.8 in the left PCA; and 103/1.0 in the left M1-MCA with an MCA/ICA MFV ratio <3. The interpretation was severe right A1-ACA vasospasm with moderate basilar and left PCA vasospasm. Digital subtraction angiography confirmed these findings.

Therefore TCD is more sensitive to changes in intracranial artery diameter than angiography. Since TCD is a screening tool, the criteria should be adjusted toward a higher sensitivity to detect any degree of vasospasm in order to institute HHH therapy. At the same time, a higher specificity threshold should be used for severe vasospasm to minimize the number of false-negative angiograms. TCD may also help to guide angiography toward the affected vessel and to select the best projection to demonstrate the lesion (Figure 9–6). Angioplasty with papaverine can be performed to restore the patency of the vessel affected by VSP (Figure 9–7).[48]

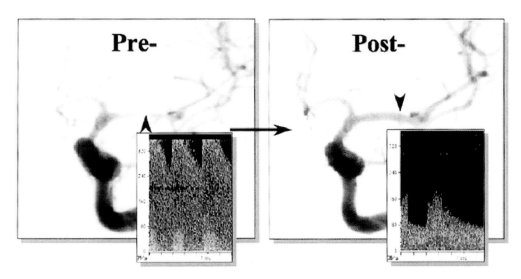

FIGURE 9–7. Angioplasty for severe vasospasm and the velocity changes on transcranial Doppler. A 51-year-old woman with subarachnoid hemorrhage developed severe MCA vasospasm detected by transcranial Doppler as an MFV/PI of 302/0.3 and an MCA/ICA MFV ratio >10. After angioplasty with papaverine the velocity decreased to 106/1.0 with an MCA/ICA MFV ratio of 3.

Hyperemia often results in elevated MFVs in intracranial and feeding extracranial vasculature (Table 9–2). Hyperemia is common in patients with SAH receiving HHH therapy, and early in the postoperative period after CEA or CABG. Hyperperfusion syndrome after CEA includes headache and seizures and usually produces a >30% increase in MCA MFV unilateral to the reconstructed carotid artery.

Collateral Patterns and Flow Direction

The intracranial collateral channels are dormant under normal circulatory conditions. A collateral channel opens when a pressure gradient develops between the two arterial systems that have anastomoses. TCD can detect some of these collateral pathways: reversed OA, anterior crossfilling via AComA, and PComA flow either to or from the anterior circulation. Flow direction will depend on the direction of collateralization. When present, a collateral flow rarely implies an anatomic variant, but most often implies the presence of a flow-limiting lesion proximal to the recipient arterial system and the origin of the collateral channel detected.

The direction of flow determines which arterial system is the donor (the source of flow) and which is the recipient (the collateral flow destination). TCD can therefore provide information on whether any collateral channel is functioning and in which direction it is working. This information should be used to estimate the level of the arterial obstruction and to refine the extracranial duplex ultrasound or MRA findings. For example, a severe extracranial ICA stenosis with >70% diameter reduction is hemodynamically significant and is almost always accompanied by abnormal TCD findings.[17] A battery of TCD parameters may be used to decide on the severity of ICA lesions, particularly when the applicability of other tests is limited.

Reversed Ophthalmic Artery

A low pulsatility flow is primarily directed away from the probe with transorbital insonation at 50–62 mm. The differential diagnosis includes siphon flow and/or low velocity OA flow signals. Additional findings may include no substantial difference in MFVs detected in OA and siphon, high velocities in the ICA siphon suggesting either a high grade proximal ICA and/or siphon stenosis, and no flow signals at depths ≥60 mm suggesting ICA occlusion.

Interpretation

If the reversed OA is the only abnormal finding, this indicates possible proximal ICA stenosis. Occasionally, this

may be the only sign of ICA dissection or occlusion. If the reversed OA is found with a blunted MCA signal, there is a probable proximal ICA and/or siphon stenosis or occlusion. If the reversed OA is found with at least one other collateral channel (anterior crossfilling, or PComA) there is a definite proximal ICA high-grade stenosis or occlusion.

Common sources of error include ICA dissection, terminal ICA occlusion distal to the OA origin, and retrograde filling of the ICA siphon with a normal OA direction. Furthermore, a normal OA direction does not rule out proximal ICA stenosis.

Anterior Communicating Artery

The collateral flow through AComA cannot be distinguished from the neighboring ACAs due to the smaller AComA length and diameter and a large gate of insonation. Therefore, we report anterior crossfilling via AComA as opposed to the velocity and direction of flow in AComA itself.

Anterior Crossfilling

Elevated A1-ACA MFVs on the donor side present as ACA > MCA and/or donor ACA MFVs more than 1.2 times greater than contralateral ACA, possible stenotic-like flow at depths 72–78 mm directed away from the donor side, and a normal or low MFV in A1-ACA of the recipient side with or without A1 flow reversal. The differential diagnosis includes distal A1-ACA stenosis and compensatory flow increase if one A1 segment is atretic. The finding of a reversed A1 segment and vessel identification is operator dependent.

Interpretation

If only elevated donor ACA velocities are found, the differential diagnosis includes A1-ACA stenosis and atresia of the contralateral A1 segment. With the latter, the donor A1 segment supplies both A2 segments (may be present in normal individuals as well as in patients with ICA or MCA stenoses). If an elevated donor ACA velocity is found with a stenotic flow at midline depths, the differential includes the distal A1 stenosis, ICA siphon stenosis, and crossfilling via AComA. If an elevated donor ACA MFV is found with a reversed contralateral A1, this indicates probable proximal ICA stenosis. If an elevated donor ACA MFV is found with the stenotic-like flow at midline depths and a reversed contralateral A1 ACA, there is a definite proximal ICA stenosis or occlusion.

Posterior Communicating Artery

PComA connects the posterior and anterior cerebral arterial systems and may be detected by TCD since it usually has a length >5 mm and a favorable angle of insonation. When functioning, it can be detected as a flow signal consistently present at varying depths from 60 to 75 mm via a transtemporal approach. Under normal conditions, this area has no detectable flow when the sonographer switches from ICA bifurcation posteriorly to locate PCA. The direction of flow in PComA corresponds to collateralization: the anterior-to-posterior collateral flow is directed away from the probe, whereas the posterior-to-anterior collateral flow is directed toward the probe. The vessel identification is difficult since the PComA is prone to anatomic variations.

Collateralization via PComA

The flow signals directed either away from or toward the probe with posterior angulation of the transducer over the temporal window are consistently found at 60–75 mm. The velocity range is similar to or higher then those detected in M1-MCA and ICA bifurcation (anterior-to-posterior collateral flow) or basilar artery (posterior-to-anterior collateral flow). A possible stenotic-like flow may be found at depths of 60–75 mm with a similar probe direction. The differential diagnosis includes terminal ICA or PCA stenoses.

Interpretation

PComA identification is operator dependent. If found, PComA implies arterial obstruction in one of the following arteries. If a posterior-to-anterior collateral flow is found, a probable proximal ICA stenosis is present. If an anterior-to-posterior collateral flow is found, a probable BA or dominant VA stenosis is present.

Reversed Flow in the Basilar Artery

If an occlusion develops in the proximal basilar artery, a pressure gradient develops between the carotid circulation and posterior cerebral arteries, superior cerebellar arteries, and perforating vessels. If a thrombus or embolus in the proximal basilar artery does not completely occlude the vessel immediately, the patient may be able to recruit posterior communicating arteries and deliver blood from the carotids via the reversed basilar stem to parts of the cerebellum and smaller distal basilar branches. This collateral flow reaches the low-resistance system of cerebellar anastomoses and the brainstem parenchyma. This is why patients may have neurological dysfunction of variable clinical severity and good diastolic velocities on Doppler. Identification of low-resistance flow moving toward the probe, i.e., reversed basilar flow at 80–100 mm, may indicate continuing perfusion of vital brain structures and often explains the good level of consciousness and partial neurological deficits despite the presence of a proximal basilar obstruction.[49]

Cerebral Embolization

TCD can detect microembolization of cerebral vessels in real time. As an investigational tool, TCD is used to monitor CEA, CABG, angioplasty/stenting, as well as stroke patients with presumed cardiac or arterial sources for brain embolization. All microembolic signals (MES) detected by TCD are asymptomatic since the size of the particles producing them is comparable to or even smaller then the diameter of the brain capillaries. However, the MES cumulative count is related to the incidence of the neuropsychological deficit after CABG, and its significance as a risk factor for stroke is under investigation.[50,51] During surgery or intraarterial procedures microembolic signals can be of different composition, either solid or gaseous. Identification of embolic material is important since air bubbles have a lower pathogenic impact. Recently, multifrequency TCD had shown promising results in differentiating the nature of the embolus.[52]

Nevertheless, it is important to know how to detect and identify MES because occasionally the TCD examiner may be the only witness to cerebral microembolization and this finding may suggest a vascular origin of the neurological event and allow clinicians to investigate potential sources of embolism (heart chambers and septum, aortic arch, arterial stenosis or dissection).

The gold standard for MES identification is an on-line interpretation of video- or digitally taped flow signals. The spectral recording should be obtained with minimal gain at a fixed angle of insonation. The probe should be maintained with a fixation device for at least 0.5–1 h monitoring. The use of two-channel simultaneous registration and a prolonged time of monitoring may improve the yield of the procedure. Multigated or multiranged registration at different insonation depths may improve differentiation of embolic signals from artifacts.[51]

According to the International Cerebral Hemodynamics Society definition,[53] MES have the following:

1. Random occurrence during the cardiac cycle.
2. Brief duration (usually <0.1 s).
3. High intensity (>3 dB over background).
4. Primarily unidirectional signals (if fast Fourier transformation is used).
5. Audible component (chirp, pop).

To avoid discrediting this promising method, the research studies should report the following 14 parameters: ultrasound device, transducer type and size, insonated artery, insonation depth, algorithms for signal intensity measurement, scale settings, detection threshold, axial extension of sample volume, fast Fourier transform (FFT) size (number of points used), FFT length (time), FFT overlap, transmitted ultrasound frequency, high-pass filter settings, and the recording time.[54] No current system of automated embolus detection seems to have the required sensitivity and specificity for clinical use.[54]

In 2004 Mackinnon et al. presented the first ambulatory TCD system (like a "Holter" monitor for MCA flow velocity) able to offer good-quality recordings of >5h. In view of the demonstrated temporal variability in embolization, this technique is likely to improve the predictive value of recording for asymptomatic embolic signals and may be particularly useful in patients in whom embolic signals are relatively infrequent, such as those with asymptomatic carotid stenosis and atrial fibrillation.[55]

Increased Intracranial Pressure

A normal intracranial waveform is detected by TCD when the brain acts as a low-resistance vascular system at normal or low ICP values (Figure 9–3). When ICP increases up to the diastolic pressure of the resistance vessels, the EDV decreases and flow deceleration occurs more rapidly. If ICP is greater than diastolic but less than systolic pressures, the result is either a triphasic waveform as in the peripheral arteries or a sharp-peak systolic flow with an absent end-diastolic component. A further increase in ICP may lead to cerebral circulatory arrest.

Increased ICP may result in high resistance waveforms: PI ≥ 1.2, decreased or absent EDV, or triphasic or reverberating flow. The following algorithm may help to differentiate the mechanisms of increased resistance to flow.

If PI ≥ 1.2 and a positive end-diastolic flow is present in

1. All arteries: hyperventilation; hypertension; increased ICP.
2. Unilateral: compartmental ICP increase; stenoses distal to the site of insonation; intracranial hemorrhage with mass effect or hydrocephalus.[56]
3. One artery: distal obstruction (spasm, stenosis, edema).

If PI ≥ 2.0 and end-diastolic flow is absent in

1. All arteries: extremely high ICP; possible arrest of cerebral circulation.
2. Unilateral: compartmental ICP increase, occlusion distal to the insonation site.
3. One artery: distal obstruction (occlusion, severe spasm, edema).

Cerebral Circulatory Arrest

A progressive elevation of ICP to extreme levels due to brain edema and mass effect can lead to stepwise compression of small to large intracranial arteries causing cerebral circulatory arrest. A prolonged absence of brain perfusion will eventually lead to brain death.

If cerebral circulatory arrest is suspected, use the following algorithm:

1. Positive MCA or BA end-diastolic flow = no cerebral circulatory arrest.
2. Absent end-diastolic flow = uncertain cerebral circulatory arrest (too early or too late).
3. Reversed minimal end-diastolic flow = possible cerebral circulatory arrest (continue monitoring).
4. Reverberating flow = probable cerebral circulatory arrest (confirm in both MCAs at depths of 50–58mm and BA at 80–90mm, then monitor arrest for 30min).

TCD cannot be used to diagnose brain death since this is a clinical diagnosis. It can be used to confirm cerebral circulatory arrest except in infants less than 6 months old.[57] TCD can be used to monitor the progression to cerebral circulatory arrest. Once the reverberating flow is found it should be monitored for at least 30min in the three major intracranial arteries to avoid false-positive findings. For example, a transient cerebral circulatory arrest can occur in patients with SAH and head trauma due to A-waves of ICP.[58] TCD can also be used to determine the appropriate time for other confirmatory tests (i.e., to minimize studies with residual CBF), and to discuss the upcoming issues with the patient's family.

The criteria and accuracy for TCD testing for cerebral circulatory arrest were addressed in an International Consensus statement.[59]

Steal Syndrome

Subclavian "steal" is a hemodynamic condition of a reversed flow in one vertebral artery to compensate for a proximal hemodynamic lesion in the unilateral subclavian artery. Thus blood flow is diverted or "stolen" from the brain to feed the arm (Figure 9–8). The subclavian steal usually represents an accidental finding since it rarely produces neurological symptoms. If asymptomatic it is called a "subclavian steal phenomenon." If symptoms of vertebrobasilar ischemia are present, it is called a "subclavian steal syndrome."[60]

The main findings include a difference in BP between arms >20mm Hg and usually systolic flow reversal with PI ≥ 1.2 in one vertebral artery (Figures 9–3 and 9–8) as well as a low resistance flow in the donor artery. Right to left subclavian steal is found in 85% of cases.[60]

SUBCLAVIAN STEAL

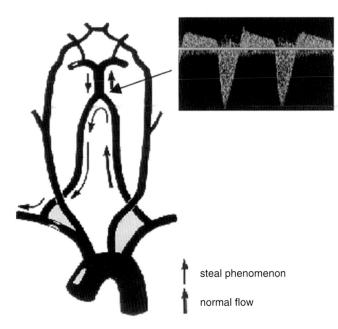

FIGURE 9–8. Subclavian steal. Subclavian steal results in a reversed flow direction in one of the vertebral arteries *(scheme)*, an alternating flow pattern on transcranial Doppler, and retrograde filling of the reversed vertebral artery.

If the difference in BP between the arms is 10–20 mm Hg and the steal waveforms are not present at rest, or flow reversal is incomplete, the hyperemia test should be performed either to provoke the steal or to augment flow reversal. The cuff should be inflated to oversystolic BP values and flow reduction to the arm should be maintained for at least 0.5–1 min. The cuff should be quickly released and any augmentation of flow should be monitored by TCD.

Transcranial Doppler in Acute Stroke

TCD may facilitate the diagnosis of cerebral arterial occlusion and can improve outcomes. First, it can be used to identify the presence and location of an obstructive intracranial thrombus confirming the vascular origin of the patient's neurological symptoms.[61] Second, it provides valuable information about the collateral flow to the vascular territory distal to the artery occlusion, and helps in selecting patients for intraarterial interventions.[62] Third, it provides real-time bedside monitoring of thrombolysis. And finally, it augments residual flow and speeds up thrombolysis, allowing patients to recover from stroke more rapidly and completely.

Arterial Occlusion

The diagnosis of an intracranial arterial occlusion with TCD is difficult. The operator must be experienced and the best results are usually obtained for M1-MCA, ICA siphon, and BA. The main prerequisite is a good window of insonation and to prove this, other arteries should be identified through the same approach. The main finding is no detectable signals from the location where the artery is expected to be.

The specific findings for **MCA** include no signal at any depth of 40–65 mm via a transtemporal approach. Secondary findings are a flow diversion/compensatory increase in ACA and/or PCA, no signals from ACA and ICA with PCA flow identified, and proximal M1-MCA high-resistance flow. The findings need to be confirmed by insonation across the midline from the contralateral temporal window.

The specific findings for **ICA siphon** include no signals at 62–70 mm via a transorbital approach. Secondary findings include a collateral flow in PComA and/or crossfilling via AComA, a blunted MCA flow signal, and a contralateral ICA compensatory flow/velocity increase.

The specific findings for **BA** include no signals at any depth of 80–100+ mm via a transforaminal approach. Secondary findings include a flow velocity increase in one or both VAs indicating cerebellar collateral flow; a high resistance flow signal in one or both VAs indicating proximal BA occlusion; a high resistance flow signal at the origin of the BA indicating distal BA occlusion; retrograde flow toward the probe at the top of the basilar artery (proximal BA occlusion collateralized via PcomAs); functional PComA(s) with flow directed away from the probe via the temporal window; and low BA velocities with the top-of-the-basilar occlusion.

In 2001 Demchuck *et al.* developed the thrombolysis in brain ischemia (TIBI) classification by using TCD to noninvasively monitor intracranial vessel residual flow signals (Figure 9–9). The TIBI classification correlates with initial stroke severity, clinical recovery, and mortality in IV-tissue plasminogen activator (t-PA)-treated stroke patients. In addition, a flow-grade improvement correlated with clinical improvement. The real advantage of TCD is lost if only flow velocity differences are reported and other hemodynamic findings are ignored. TIBI flow grades show information that can be obtained through waveform analysis providing qualitative and quantitative information of the flow status.[63]

Patient Management Optimization

Although TCD does not provide estimates of brain parenchymal perfusion[64,65] or transcortical collateralization of flow, it offers information about collateral flow

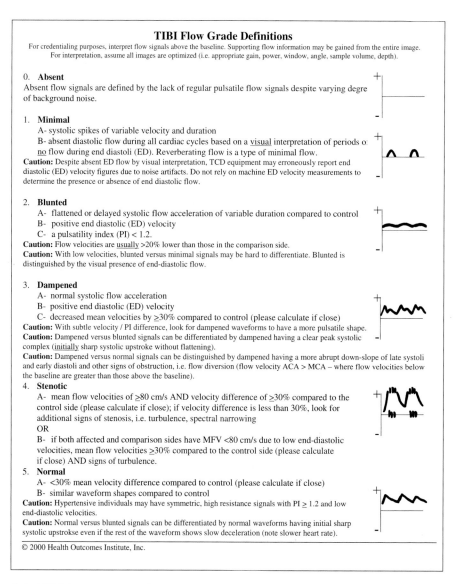

TIBI Flow Grade Definitions

For credentialing purposes, interpret flow signals above the baseline. Supporting flow information may be gained from the entire image. For interpretation, assume all images are optimized (i.e. appropriate gain, power, window, angle, sample volume, depth).

0. **Absent**
Absent flow signals are defined by the lack of regular pulsatile flow signals despite varying degree of background noise.

1. **Minimal**
    A- systolic spikes of variable velocity and duration
    B- absent diastolic flow during all cardiac cycles based on a <u>visual</u> interpretation of periods o: <u>no</u> flow during end diastoli (ED). Reverberating flow is a type of minimal flow.
    Caution: Despite absent ED flow by visual interpretation, TCD equipment may erroneously report end diastolic (ED) velocity figures due to noise artifacts. Do not rely on machine ED velocity measurements to determine the presence or absence of end diastolic flow.

2. **Blunted**
    A- flattened or delayed systolic flow acceleration of variable duration compared to control
    B- positive end diastolic (ED) velocity
    C- a pulsatility index (PI) < 1.2.
    Caution: Flow velocities are <u>usually</u> >20% lower than those in the comparison side.
    Caution: With low velocities, blunted versus minimal signals may be hard to differentiate. Blunted is distinguished by the visual presence of end-diastolic flow.

3. **Dampened**
    A- normal systolic flow acceleration
    B- positive end diastolic (ED) velocity
    C- decreased mean velocities by $\geq$30% compared to control (please calculate if close)
    Caution: With subtle velocity / PI difference, look for dampened waveforms to have a more pulsatile shape.
    Caution: Dampened versus blunted signals can be differentiated by dampened having a clear peak systolic complex (<u>initially</u> sharp systolic upstroke without flattening).
    Caution: Dampened versus normal signals can be distinguished by dampened having a more abrupt down-slope of late systoli and early diastoli and other signs of obstruction, i.e. flow diversion (flow velocity ACA > MCA – where flow velocities below the baseline are greater than those above the baseline).

4. **Stenotic**
    A- mean flow velocities of $\geq$80 cm/s AND velocity difference of $\geq$30% compared to the control side (please calculate if close); if velocity difference is less than 30%, look for additional signs of stenosis, i.e. turbulence, spectral narrowing
    OR
    B- if both affected and comparison sides have MFV <80 cm/s due to low end-diastolic velocities, mean flow velocities $\geq$30% compared to the control side (please calculate if close) AND signs of turbulence.

5. **Normal**
    A- <30% mean velocity difference compared to control (please calculate if close)
    B- similar waveform shapes compared to control
    Caution: Hypertensive individuals may have symmetric, high resistance signals with PI $\geq$ 1.2 and low end-diastolic velocities.
    Caution: Normal versus blunted signals can be differentiated by normal waveforms having initial sharp systolic upstrokse even if the rest of the waveform shows slow deceleration (note slower heart rate).

© 2000 Health Outcomes Institute, Inc.

FIGURE 9–9. TIBI flow grade definitions. Permission requested from Health Outcomes Institute, Inc.

supply at the level of the Circle of Willis and major proximal branches[66,67] as described above. Information about the perfusion status of the affected brain tissue may help optimize and individualize patient management. For example, in the setting of an acute vertebrobasilar occlusion, identification of the reversed basilar artery flow indicates good collaterals through the posterior communicating arteries, associated with favorable outcomes.[49] In the last year, the development of new software for TCCD able to detect perfusion defects after echocontrast administration is very promising.[50] Finally information obtained from an acute neurovascular ultrasound examination has shown significant potential as a screening tool for intravenous/intraarterial lysis protocols.[62]

Monitoring Thrombolytic Therapy with Ultrasound

Once the arterial occlusion is located, the ultrasound probe can be fixated with a head frame allowing monitoring of the blood flow in the affected artery during t-PA infusion. The first noticeable improvement of flow to the brain occurs at a median time of 17 min after t-PA bolus. Median time to completion of recanalization is 35 min after bolus,[68] and those patients who complete recanalization before the end of 1 h t-PA infusion are 3.5 times more likely to achieve favorable outcome at 3 months. An average rate of spontaneous complete recanalization of the MCA occlusion appears to be about 6% per hour during the first 6 h after symptom onset.[69–71]

Systemic t-PA increases the complete recanalization rate to 12.7%/h. Early complete recanalization is closely associated with dramatic clinical recovery.[72]

However, one-third of early complete recanalizations do not result in immediate clinical improvement. Despite this, one-third of patients with silent recanalizations recover completely at 3 months, indicating the existence of a stunned brain syndrome.[73]

Continuous TCD monitoring of the affected artery shows persistence of the occlusion, thrombus migration, partial or complete recanalization, and reocclusion. Also, visualization of microembolic signals during thrombolysis may indicate thrombus degradation or imminent recanalization. After recanalization, early arterial reocclusion affects up to 25% of t-PA-treated patients, more commonly those with partial or incomplete initial recanalization. Arterial reocclusion accounts for two-thirds of patients who experience deterioration following improvement with t-PA therapy.[74] TCD demonstration of frequent arterial reocclusion with intravenous t-PA has fostered interest in combination therapies, i.e., a thrombolytic drug with anticoagulants, GP IIb IIIa antagonists, or a direct thrombin inhibitor.[75–77]

Ultrasound Enhanced Thrombolysis

In the past 30 years numerous scientists showed in experimental models that ultrasound facilitates the activity of fibrinolytic agents within minutes of its exposure to thrombus and blood-containing drugs.[78–84] The mechanisms of ultrasound-enhanced thrombolysis include improved drug transport, reversible alteration of fibrin structure, and increased t-PA binding to fibrin[78–86] for frequencies ranging from kHz to those used in diagnostic ultrasound.[83,84] Although kHz frequencies penetrate better with less heating, a combination of t-PA with an experimental kHz delivery system resulted in excessive risk of intracerebral hemorrhage (ICH) in stroke patients.[87–89] We used diagnostic 2 MHz transcranial Doppler to evaluate acute stroke patients and reported an unexpectedly high rate of complete recanalization and dramatic clinical recovery when t-PA infusion was continuously monitored with TCD for diagnostic purposes. The CLOTBUST trial (Combined Lysis of Thrombus in Brain ischemia using transcranial Ultrasound and Systemic t-PA) was a phase II multicenter randomized clinical trial (Houston, Barcelona, Edmonton, Calgary).[90] The CLOTBUST trial demonstrated that in stroke patients treated with intravenous t-PA, continuous TCD monitoring of intracranial occlusion safely augments t-PA-induced arterial recanalization (38% vs. 13% of sustained complete MCA recanalization at 2 h after TPA bolus). This early boost in recanalization resulted in a trend toward clinical recovery at 3 months (42% vs. 29%), the

subject of a properly powered phase III trial. TCD has a positive biological activity that aids systemic thrombolytic therapy in patients with acute ischemic stroke. The phase II CLOTBUST trial provides clinical evidence for the existence of ultrasound-enhanced thrombolysis in humans that can amplify the existing therapy for ischemic stroke. Early brain perfusion augmentation, complete recanalization, and dramatic clinical recovery are feasible goals for ultrasound-enhanced thrombolysis. A further increase of this effect is being tested with eco-contrast agents that seem to multiply the energy delivered to the clot by ultrasound and by enhancing the lytic effects.[91]

Other Clinical Applications

There are several established clinical applications of TCD that were recently evaluated by an international group of experts (Table 9–4).[92,93] TCD provides a bedside tool for detection of intracranial stenosis, occlusion, collateral channels, and microembolic activity,[49] including testing for the right-to-left shunts, like patent foramen ovale or pulmonary fistulas.[95]

TCD has a pivotal role in predicting the risk of ischemic stroke in children with sickle cell disease. In a prospective study by Adams et al., mean velocities greater than 170–200 cm/s were associated with a 44% increase in relative risk of ischemic stroke over 5 years.[12,96–98] A subsequent randomized trial showed a 90% relative stroke risk reduction when blood transfusion was administered in children with TCD findings of MFV $\geq$ 200 cm/s.[99]

TCD has an established role in detecting and monitoring arterial vasospasm in patients with SAH.[20,46–48] TCD helps to decide when to start, enforce, and continue HHH therapy, when to perform DSA with angioplasty and papaverine to combat severe vasospasm, and when to transfer patients from the intensive care unit after vasospasm has subsided.[46,48]

TCD offers a quick bedside test to detect markedly elevated ICP, thus providing an opportunity for decompression or hyperventilation to be performed before clinical deterioration.[57,58] TCD also allows detection of a combination of vasospasm and hydrocephalus as well as progression of ICP to cerebral circulatory arrest.

The capacity of TCD to monitor both brain perfusion and embolization in real time has led to numerous applications of TCD during surgical and interventional procedures. Stump et al. showed that 58% of microembolic signals during cardiopulmonary bypass are associated with surgical maneuvers or time intervals while the cumulative embolic count was predictive of postoperative neuropsychological deficit.[100] Spencer reported that when surgeons responded to TCD information during CEA monitoring, the incidence of permanent deficits

TABLE 9–4. Accuracy of TCD ultrasonography by indication.[a]

Indication	Sensitivity, %	Specificity, %	Reference standard	Evidence/class
Sickle cell disease	86	91	Conventional angiography	A/I
Right-to-left cardiac shunts	70–100	≥95	Transesophageal echocardiography	A/II
Intracranial stenoocclusive disease			Conventional angiography	
Anterior circulation	70–90	90–95		B/II–III
Posterior circulation	50–80	80–96		B/III
Occlusion				
MCA	85–95	90–98		B/III
ICA, VA, BA	55–81	96		B/III
Extracranial ICA stenosis			Conventional angiography	
Single TCD variable	3–78	60–100		C/II–III
TCD battery	49–95	42–100		C/II–III
TCD battery + carotid duplex	89	100		C/II–III
Vasomotor reactivity testing				
≥70% extracranial ICA stenosis/occlusion			Conventional angiography, clinical outcomes	B/II–III
Carotid endarterectomy			EEG, MRI, clinical outcomes	B/II
Cerebral microembolization			Experimental model, pathology, MRI, neuropsychological tests	
General				B/II–IV
Coronary artery bypass graft surgery microembolization				B/II–III
Prosthetic heart valves				C/III
Cerebral thrombolysis			Conventional angiography, MR angiography, clinical outcome	B/II–III
Complete occlusion	50	100		
Partial occlusion	100	76		
Recanalization	91	93		
Vasospasm after spontaneous subarachnoid hemorrhage			Conventional angiography	I–II
Intracranial ICA	25–30	83–91		
MCA	39–94	70–100		
ACA	13–71	65–100		
VA	44–100	82–88		
BA	77–100	42–79		
PCA	48–60	78–87		
Vasospasm after traumatic subarachnoid hemorrhage			Conventional angiography	I–III
Cerebral circulatory arrest and brain death	91–100	97–100	Conventional angiography, EEG, clinical outcome	II

[a]Permission requested from the Therapeutics and Technology Assessment Subcommittee of the American Academy of Neurology (Neurology 2004;62:1468–1481).
[b]TCD, transcranial Doppler; MCA, middle cerebral artery; ICA, internal carotid artery; VA, vertebral artery; BA, basilar artery; ACA, anterior cerebral artery; PCA, posterior cerebral artery.

decreased from 7% to 2% for 500 operations.[101] As shown by TCD, cerebral embolization was present in 54%, hypoperfusion in 29%, and combined embolism plus hypoperfusion in 17% of these complications.[100] During CEA TCD can provide useful information.[100] It can show microembolization during skin preparation suggesting fragile plaque structure. If MCA MFV does not recover from <30% of precrossclamping values, a shunt may be needed. TCD detection of flow changes through ECA collaterals can help avoid embolization/hypoperfusion with ECA manipulations. An MCA MFV drop during plaque removal indicates a drop in BP or a kink in a shunt. TCD shows microembolism during release of carotid crossclamps. Finally, a prolonged >30s MCA MFV increase to greater than 1.5 times precrossclamp values after the CEA indicates hyperperfusion syndrome, which can be treated with TCD monitoring.[94,101]

Conclusions

Transcranial Doppler is a portable and inexpensive tool that is widely used. However, TCD requires intense and in-depth training as well as experience in both performing the test and interpreting the results. The absence of temporal windows is present in 5–15% of all patients when the ultrasound beam cannot penetrate the skull.[1,3] Due to these limitations and the failure to change the management plan in patients screened for carotid artery disease, Comerota *et al.* advised not incorporating TCD as part of the routine noninvasive cerebrovascular examination.[102,103] However, the technology has improved rapidly. The contrast agents, such as stabilized gaseous microbubbles, overcome the absent windows.[97] Detection of multigated bilateral emboli and compatibility of TCD with other monitoring modalities are realities. Very portable and sensitive units are available to serve as a "neurological stethoscope" to the brain vasculature at the bedside. At the same time, clinicians need to identify the best responders for acute stroke therapies, patients at high risk of stroke with asymptomatic and moderate carotid stenoses, and decide on surgical procedure selection (i.e., CABG+CEA) and stenting. A neurovascular ultrasound examination that combines urgent bedside carotid duplex and TCD is becoming a valuable source of diagnostic information in acute stroke patients, helping in decision making [61] and even enhancing the effects of fibrinolytic drugs.[90]

References

1. Aaslid R, Markwalder TM, Nornes H. Noninvasive transcranial Doppler ultrasound recording of flow velocity in basal cerebral arteries. J Neurosurg 1982;57:769–774.
2. Moehring MA, Spencer MP. Power M-mode transcranial Doppler ultrasound and simultaneous single gate spectrogram. Ultrasound Med Biol 2002;28:49–57.
3. Otis SM, Ringelstein EB. The transcranial Doppler examination: Principles and applications of transcranial Doppler sonography. In: Tegeler CH, Babikian VL, Gomez CR (eds). *Neurosonology*, pp. 140–155. St. Louis: Mosby, 1996.
4. Postert T, Braun B, Meves S, Koster O, Przuntek H, Weber S, Buttner T. Contrast-enhanced transcranial color-coded sonography in acute hemispheric brain infarction. Stroke 1999;30:1819–1826.
5. Bartels E, Flugel KA. Quantitative measurements of blood flow velocity in basal cerebral arteries with transcranial duplex colorflow imaging. A comparative study with conventional transcranial Doppler sonography. J Neuroimag 1994;4:77–81.
6. Gerriets T, Seidel G, Fiss I, Modrau B, Kaps M. Contrast enhanced transcranial color-coded duplex sonography: Efficiency and validity. Neurology 1999;52:1133–1137.
7. Hennerici MMS. *Cerebrovascular Ultrasound: Theory, Practice and Future Developments*. Cambridge: Cambridge University Press, 2001.
8. Gerriets T, Stolz E, Modrau B, Fiss I, Seidel G, Kaps M. Sonographic monitoring of midline shift in hemispheric infarctions. Neurology 1999;52:45–49.
9. Kontos HA. Validity of cerebral arterial blood flow calculations from velocity measurements. Stroke 1989;20:1–3.
10. Giller CA, Bowman G, Dyer H, Mootz L, Krippner W. Cerebral arterial diameters during changes in blood pressure and carbon dioxide during craniotomy. Neurosurgery 1993;32:737–742.
11. Aaslid R, Lindegaard KF, Sorteberg W, Nornes H. Cerebral autoregulation dynamics in humans. Stroke 1989;20: 45.
12. Adams RJ, McKie V, Nichols F, et al. The use of transcranial ultrasonography to predict stroke in sickle cell disease. N Engl J Med 1992;326:605–610.
13. Babikian V, Sloan MA, Tegeler CH, DeWitt LD, Fayad PB, Feldmann E, Gomez CR. Transcranial Doppler validation pilot study. J Neuroimag 1993;3:242–249.
14. Bragoni M, Feldmann E. Transcranial Doppler indicies of intracranial hemodynamics. In: Tegeler CH, Babikian VL, Gomez CR (eds). *Neurosonology*, pp. 129–139. St. Louis: Mosby, 1996.
15. Lindegaard KF, Gromilund P, Aaslid R, et al. Evaluation of cerebral AVMs using transcranial Doppler ultrasound. J Neurosurg 1986;65:335–344.
16. Lindegaard KF, Bakke SJ, Gromilund P, et al. Assessment of intracranial hemodynamics in carotid artery disease by transcranial Doppler ultrasound. J Neurosurg 1985;63: 890–898.
17. Wilterdink JL, et al. Transcranial Doppler ultrasound battery reliably identifies severe internal carotid artery stenosis. Stroke 1997;28:133–136.
18. Kelley RE, et al. Transcranial Doppler ultrasonography of the middle cerebral artery in the hemodynamic assessment of internal carotid artery stenosis. Arch Neurol 1990;49:960–964.
19. Canthelmo NL, et al. Correlation of transcranial Doppler and noninvasive tests with angiography in the evaluation of extracranial carotid disease. J Vasc Surg 1990;11: 786–792.
20. Lindegaard KF, Nornes H, Bakke SJ, et al. Cerebral vasospasm diagnosis by means of angiography and blood velocity measurements. Acta Neurochir (Wien) 1987;100: 12–24.
21. Hennerici M, Neuerburg-Heusler D. *Vascular Diagnosis with Ultrasound: Clinical References with Case Studies*, p. 96. Stuttgart: Thieme, 1998.
22. North American Symptomatic Carotid Endarterectomy Trial Collaborators. Beneficial effect of carotid endarterectomy in symptomatic patients with high grade carotid stenosis. N Engl J Med 1991;325:445–453.
23. European Carotid Surgery Trialists' Collaborative Group. MRC European carotid surgery trial: Interim results for symptomatic patients with severe (70–99%) stenosis and with mild (0–29%) stenosis. Lancet 1991;337:1235–1244.
24. Executive Committee for the Asymptomatic Carotid Atherosclerosis Study. Endarterectomy for asymptomatic carotic artery stenosis. JAMA 1995;273:1421–1428.
25. Fischer M. Carotid plaque morphology in symptomatic and asymptomatic patients. In: Caplan LR, Shifrin EG, Nicolaides AN, Moore WS (eds). *Cerebrovascular Ischemia: Investigation and Management*, pp. 19–24. London: Med-Orion, 1996.
26. Thomas DJ. The Asymptomatic Carotid Surgery Trial: a neurologist's view. In: Caplan LR, Shifrin EG, Nicolaides

AN, Moore WS (eds). *Cerebrovascular Ischemia: Investigation and Management*, pp. 411–421. London: Med-Orion, 1996.

27. Bornstein NM, Gur AY, Shifrin EG, Morag BA. The value of a combined transcranial Doppler and Diamox test in assessing intracerebral hemodynamics. In: Caplan LR, Shifrin EG, Nicolaides AN, Moore WS (eds). *Cerebrovascular Ischemia: Investigation and Management*, pp. 143–148. London: Med-Orion, 1996.

28. Bishop CCR, Insall M, Powell S, Rutt D, Browse NL. Effect of internal carotid artery occlusion on middle cerebral artery blood flow at rest and in response to hypercapnia. Lancet 1986;29:710.

29. Silvestrini M, Vernieri F, Pasqualetti P, Matteis M, Passarelli F, Troisi E, Caltagirone C. Impaired cerebral vasoreactivity and risk of stroke in patients with asymptomatic carotid artery stenosis. JAMA 2000;283:2122–2127.

30. Ringelstein EB. CO_2-reactivity: dependence from collateral circulation and significance in symptomatic and asymptomatic patients. In: Caplan LR, Shifrin EG, Nicolaides AN, Moore WS (eds). *Cerebrovascular Ischemia: Investigation and Management*, pp. 149–154. London: Med-Orion, 1996.

31. Babikian VL, Schwarze JJ. Cerebral blood flow and cerebral physiology. In: Tegeler CH, Babikian VL, Gomez CR (eds). *Neurosonology*, pp. 140–155. St. Louis: Mosby, 1996.

32. Markus HS, Harrson MJG. Estimation of cerebrovascular reactivity using transcranial Doppler, including the use of breath-holding as the vasodilatory stimulus. Stroke 1992;23:668–673.

33. Silvestrini M, Troisi E, Matteis M, Cupini LM, Caltagirone C. Transcranial Doppler assessment of cerebrovascular reactivity in symptomatic and asymptomatic carotid stenosis. Stroke 1996;27:1970–1973.

34. Kleiser B, Scholl D, Widder B. Assessment of cerebrovascular reactivity by Doppler CO_2 and Diamox testing: Which is the appropriate method? Cerebrovasc Dis 1994;4:134.

35. Burt RW, Witt RM, Cikrit DF, Carter J. Increased retention of HMPAO following acetazolamide administration. Clin Nucl Med 1991;16:568.

36. Hojer-Pedersen E. Effect of acetazolamide on cerebral blood flow in subacute and chronic cerebrovascular disease. Stroke 1987;18:887.

37. Dahl A, Lindegaard KF, Russel D, Nyberg-Hansen, Rootwelt K, Sorteberg W, Nornes H. A comparison of transcranial Doppler and cerebral blood flow studies to assess cerebrovascular reactivity. Stroke 1992;23:15.

38. Dahl A, Russel D, Nyberg-Hansen R, Rootwelt K, Bakke SJ. Cerebral vasoreactivity in unilateral carotid artery disease. Stroke 1994;25:621.

39. De Chiara S, *et al.* Cerebrovascular reactivity by transcranial Doppler ultrasonography in insulin-dependent diabetic patients. Cerebrovasc Dis 1993;3:11:111–115.

40. Sugimori H, *et al.* Cerebral hemodynamics in hypertensive patients compared with normotensive volunteers. Stroke 1994;25:1384–1389.

41. Rubba P, *et al.* Cerebral blood flow velocity and systemic vascular resistance after acute reduction of low-density lipoprotein in familial hypercholesterolemia. Stroke 1993;24:1154–1161.

42. Kleiser B, Widder B. Course of carotid artery occlusions with impaired cerebrovascular reactivity. Stroke 1992;23: 171–174.

43. Shinoda J, *et al.* Acetazolamide reactivity on cerebral blood flow in patients with subarachnoid hemorrhage. Acta Neurochir (Wien) 1991;109:102–108.

44. Hassler W, Chioffi F. CO_2 reactivity of cerebral vasospasm after aneurysmal subarachnoid hemorrhage. Acta Neurochir (Wien) 1989;98:167–175.

45. Seiler RW, Nirkko A. Effect of nimodipine on cerebrovascular response to CO_2 in asymptomatic individuals and patients with subarachnoid hemorrhage: A transcranial Doppler ultrasound study. Neurosurgery 1990;27: 247–251.

46. Sloan MA. Transcranial Doppler monitoring of vasospasm after subarachnoid hemorrhage. In: Tegeler CH, Babikian VL, Gomez CR (eds). *Neurosonology*, pp. 156–171. St. Louis: Mosby, 1996.

47. Newell DW, *et al.* Distribution of angiographic vasospasm after subarachnoid hemorrhage: Implications for diagnosis by TCD. Neurosurgery 1990;27:574–577.

48. Piepgras A, *et al.* Reliable prediction of grade of angiographic vasospasm by transcranial Doppler sonography. Stroke 1994;25:260.

49. Ribo M, Garami Z, Uchino K, Song J, Molina CA, Alexandrov AV. Detection of reversed basilar flow with power-motion doppler after acute occlusion predicts favorable outcome. Stroke 2004;35:79–82.

50. Wiesmann M, Meyer K, Albers T, Seidel G. Parametric perfusion imaging with contrast-enhanced ultrasound in acute ischemic stroke. Stroke 2004;35:508–513.

51. Markus H. Doppler embolus detection: stroke treatment and prevention. In: Tegeler CH, Babikian VL, Gomez CR (eds). *Neurosonology*, pp. 239–251. St. Louis: Mosby, 1996.

52. Russell D, Brucher R. Online automatic discrimination between solid and gaseous cerebral microemboli with the first multifrequency transcranial doppler. Stroke 2002;33: 1975–1980.

53. The International Cerebral Hemodynamics Society Consensus Statement. Stroke 1995;26:1123.

54. Ringlestein EB, *et al.* Consensus on microembolus detection by TCD. Stroke 1998;29:725–729.

55. Mackinnon AD, Aaslid R, Markus HS. Long-term ambulatory monitoring for cerebral emboli using transcranial Doppler ultrasound. Stroke 2004;35:73–78

56. Marti-Fabregas J, Belvis R, Guardia E, Cocho D, Marti-Vilalta JL. Relationship between transcranial Doppler and CT data in acute intracerebral hemorrhage. AJNR Am J Neuroradiol 2005;26:113–118.

57. Hennerici M, Neuerburg-Heusler D. *Vascular Diagnosis with Ultrasound: Clinical References with Case Studies*, p. 120. Stuttgart: Thieme, 1998.

58. Newell D. Trauma and brain death. In: Tegeler CH, Babikian VL, Gomez CR (eds). *Neurosonology*, pp. 189–199. St. Louis: Mosby, 1996.

59. Ducrocq X, Braun M, Debouverie M, Junges C, Hummer M, Vespignani H. Brain death and transcranial doppler:

Experience in 130 cases of brain dead patients. J Neurol Sci 1998;160:41–46.

60. Toole JF. *Cerebrovascular Disorders*, 4th ed., pp. 199–123. New York: Raven Press, 1990.

61. Chernyshev OY, Garami Z, Calleja S, Song J, Campbell MS, Noser EA, Shaltoni H, Chen CI, Iguchi Y, Grotta JC, Alexandrov AV. Yield and accuracy of urgent combined carotid/transcranial ultrasound testing in acute cerebral ischemia. Stroke 2005;36:32–37.

62. Saqqur M, Shuaib A, Alexandrov AV, Hill MD, Calleja S, Tomsick T, Broderick J, Demchuk AM. Derivation of transcranial Doppler criteria for rescue intra-arterial thrombolysis. Multicenter experience from the interventional management of stroke study. Stroke 2005;36: 865.

63. Demchuk AM, Burgin WS, Christou I, Felberg RA, Barber PA, Hill MD, Alexandrov AV. Thrombolysis in brain ischemia (TIBI) transcranial Doppler flow grades predict clinical severity, early recovery, and mortality in patients treated with intravenous tissue plasminogen activator. Stroke 2001;32:89–93.

64. Wiesmann M, Meyer K, Albers T, Seidel G. Parametric perfusion imaging with contrast-enhanced ultrasound in acute ischemic stroke. Stroke 2004;35:508–513.

65. Wilterdink JL, Feldmann E, Furie KL, Bragoni M, Benavides JG. Transcranial Doppler ultrasound battery reliably identifies severe internal carotid artery stenosis. Stroke 1997;28:133–136.

66. Christou I, Felberg RA, Demchuk AM, Grotta JC, Burgin WS, Malkoff M, Alexandrov AV. A broad diagnostic battery for bedside transcranial Doppler to detect flow changes with internal carotid artery stenosis or occlusion. J Neuroimag 2001;11:236–242.

67. von Reutern GM. *Ultrasound Diagnosis of Cerebrovascular Disease: Doppler Sonography of the Extra- and Intracranial Arteries Duplex Scanning.* Stuttgart: Thieme, 1993.

68. Alexandrov AV, Burgin WS, Demchuk AM, El-Mitwalli A, Grotta JC. Speed of intracranial clot lysis with intravenous tissue plasminogen activator therapy: Sonographic classification and short-term improvement. Circulation 2001; 103:2897–2902.

69. Molina CA, Montaner J, Abilleira S, Ibarra B, Romero F, Arenilla JF, Alvarez-Sabin J. Timing of spontaneous recanalization and risk of hemorrhagic transformation in acute cardioembolic stroke. Stroke 2001;32:1079–1084.

70. Furlan A, Higashida R, Wechsler L, Gent M, Rowley H, Kase C, Pessin M, Ahuja A, Callahan F, Clark WM, Silver F, Rivera F. Intra-arterial prourokinase for acute ischemic stroke. The proact II study: A randomized controlled trial. Prolyse in acute cerebral thromboembolism. JAMA 1999;282:2003–2011.

71. Uchino KMC, Saqqur M, Demchuk AM, Felberg RA, Calleja S, Wojner AW, Alexandrov AV. Likelihood of early arterial recanalization with intravenous tpa and its predictors: A multicenter transcranial doppler study. Stroke 2003;34:347(abstract).

72. Molina CA RM, Rubiera M, Montaner J, Arenillas JF, Santamarina E, Alvarez-Sabin J. Predictors of early arterial reocclusion after tpa-induced recanalization. Stroke 2004;35:250(abstract).

73. Alexandrov AV, Hall CE, Labiche LA, Wojner AW, Grotta JC. Ischemic stunning of the brain: Early recanalization without immediate clinical improvement in acute ischemic stroke. Stroke 2004;35:449–452.

74. Alexandrov AV, Grotta JC. Arterial reocclusion in stroke patients treated with intravenous tissue plasminogen activator. Neurology 2002;59:862–867.

75. Schmulling S, Rudolf J, Strotmann-Tack T, Grond M, Schneweis S, Sobesky J, Thiel A, Heiss WD. Acetylsalicylic acid pretreatment, concomitant heparin therapy and the risk of early intracranial hemorrhage following systemic thrombolysis for acute ischemic stroke. Cerebrovasc Dis 2003;16:183–190.

76. Straub S, Junghans U, Jovanovic V, Wittsack HJ, Seitz RJ, Siebler M. Systemic thrombolysis with recombinant tissue plasminogen activator and tirofiban in acute middle cerebral artery occlusion. Stroke 2004;35:705–709.

77. Sugg R, Pary JK, Uchino K, Shaltoni HM, Gonzales NR, Alexandrov AV, Ford SR, Shaw SG, Mathern DE, Grotta JC. Tpa argatroban stroke study (tarts). International Stroke Conference 2005 (abstract).

78. Trubestein G, Engel C, Etzel F, Sobbe A, Cremer H, Stumpff U. Thrombolysis by ultrasound. Clin Sci Mol Med Suppl 1976;3:697s–698s.

79. Lauer CG, Burge R, Tang DB, Bass BG, Gomez ER, Alving BM. Effect of ultrasound on tissue-type plasminogen activator-induced thrombolysis. Circulation 1992;86(4):1257–1264.

80. Blinc A, Francis CW, Trudnowski JL, Carstensen EL. Characterization of ultrasound-potentiated fibrinolysis *in vitro*. Blood 1993;81(10):2636–2643.

81. Kimura M, Iijima S, Kobayashi K, Furuhata H. Evaluation of the thrombolytic effect of tissue-type plasminogen activator with ultrasonic irradiation: *In vitro* experiment involving assay of the fibrin degradation products from the clot. Biol Pharm Bull 1994;17(1):126–130.

82. Akiyama M, Ishibashi T, Yamada T, Furuhata H. Low-frequency ultrasound penetrates the cranium and enhances thrombolysis *in vitro*. Neurosurgery 1998;43(4): 828–832; discussion 832–833.

83. Suchkova V, Siddiqi FN, Carstensen EL, Dalecki D, Child S, Francis CW. Enhancement of fibrinolysis with 40-kHz ultrasound. Circulation 1998;98(10):1030–1035.

84. Behrens S, Daffertshofer M, Spiegel D, Hennerici M. Low-frequency, low-intensity ultrasound accelerates thrombolysis through the skull. Ultrasound Med Biol 1999;25(2):269–273.

85. Behrens S, Spengos K, Daffertshofer M, Schroeck H, Dempfle CE, Hennerici M. Transcranial ultrasound-improved thrombolysis: Diagnostic vs. therapeutic ultrasound. Ultrasound Med Biol 2001;27(12):1683–1689.

86. Spengos K, Behrens S, Daffertshofer M, Dempfle CE, Hennerici M. Acceleration of thrombolysis with ultrasound through the cranium in a flow model. Ultrasound Med Biol 2000;26(5):889–895.

87. Daffertshofer M, Hennerici M. Ultrasound in the treatment of ischaemic stroke. Lancet Neurol 2003;2(5): 283–290.

88. Alexandrov AV, Demchuk AM, Burgin WS, Robinson DJ, Grotta JC. Ultrasound-enhanced thrombolysis for acute ischemic stroke: Phase I. Findings of the CLOTBUST trial. J Neuroimag 2004;14(2):113–117.

89. Alexandrov AV, Wojner AW, Grotta JC. CLOTBUST: Design of a randomized trial of ultrasound-enhanced thrombolysis for acute ischemic stroke. J Neuroimag 2004;14(2):108–112.

90. Alexandrov AM, Grotta JC, Ford SR, Garami Z, Montaner J, Alvarez-Sabin J, Saqqur M, Demchuk AM, Chernyshev OY, Moye LA, Hill MD, Wojner AW, for the CLOTBUST Investigators. A multi-center randomized trial of ultrasound-enhanced systemic thrombolysis for acute ischemic stroke. N Engl J Med 2004;351:2170–2178.

91. Cintas P, Nguyen F, Boneu B, Larrue V. Enhancement of enzymatic fibrinolysis with 2-MHz ultrasound and microbubbles. J Thromb Haemost 2004;2(7):1163–1166.

92. Babikian VL, Feldmann E, Wechsler LR, Newell DW, Gomez CR, Bogdahn U, Caplan LR, Spencer MP, Tegeler CH, Ringelstein EB, Alexandrov AV. Transcranial Doppler ultrasonography: 1997 update. Neurology 1998;50(Suppl. 4).

93. Sloan MA, Alexandrov AV, Tegeler CH, Spencer MP, Caplan LR, Feldmann E, Wechsler LR, Newell DW, Gomez CR, Babikian VL, Lefkowitz D, Goldman RS, Armon C, Hsu CY, Goodin DS. Assessment: Transcranial Doppler ultrasonography: Report of the therapeutics and technology assessment subcommittee of the American Academy of Neurology. Neurology 2004;62: 1468–1481.

94. Alexandrov AV, Babikian VL, Adams RJ, Tegeler CH, Caplan LR, Spencer MP. The evolving role of transcranial Doppler in stroke prevention and treatment. J Stroke Cerebrovasc Dis 1998;7:101–104.

95. Jauss M, Zanette E. Detection of right-to-left shunt with ultrasound contrast agent and transcranial Doppler sonography. Cerebrovasc Dis 2000;10:490–496.

96. Bendixen BH, Adams HP, Leira EC, Change KC, Hanson MD, Woolson RF, Clarke WR. Responses to treatment with a low molecular weight heparinoid or placebo among persons with acute ischemic stroke secondary to large atherosclerosis. Neurology 1998;50:A345 (abstract).

97. Nabavi DG, Droste DW, Kemeny V, Schulte-Altendorneburg G, Weber S, Ringelstein EB. Potential and limitations of echocontrast-enhanced ultrasonography in acute stroke patients: A pilot study. Stroke 1998;29:949–954.

98. Adams RJ, McKie VC, Carl EM, et al. Long-term stroke risk in children with sickle cell disease screened with transcranial Doppler. Ann Neurol 1997;42:699–704.

99. The STOP Trial. NIH Alert. October, 1997.

100. Stump DA, Newman SP. Embolus detection during cardiopulmonary bypass. In: Tegeler CH, Babikian VL, Gomez CR (eds). Neurosonology, pp. 252–255. St. Louis: Mosby, 1996.

101. Spencer MP. Transcranial Doppler monitoring and causes of stroke from carotid endarterectomy. Stroke 1997; 28:685–691.

102. Comerota AJ, Katz ML, Hosking JD, Hashemi HA, Kerr RP, Carter AP. Is transcranial Doppler a worthwhile addition to screening tests for cerebrovascular disease? J Vasc Surg 1995;21:90–97.

103. Ries F. Echocontrast agents in transcranial Doppler sonography. In: Tegeler CH, Babikian VL, Gomez CR (eds). Neurosonology, pp. 221–228. St. Louis: Mosby, 1996.

10
Ultrasonic Characterization of Carotid Plaques

Andrew N. Nicolaides, Maura Griffin, Stavros K. Kakkos, George Geroulakos,
Efthyvoulos Kyriacou, and Niki Georgiou

Introduction

The multidisciplinary approach combining angiography, high-resolution ultrasound, thrombolytic therapy, plaque pathology, histochemistry, coagulation studies, and more recently molecular biology has led to the realization that carotid plaque rupture is a key mechanism underlying the development of cerebrovascular events.[1–3]

Plaques with a large extracellular lipid-rich core, thin fibrous cap, reduced smooth muscle density, and increased numbers of activated macrophages and mast cells appear to be most vulnerable to rupture.[3,4] Fibrous caps may rupture because of reduced collagen synthesis as well as increased matrix degradation or in response to extrinsic mechanical or hemodynamic stresses.[5] Plaques at the carotid bifurcation coincide with points at which stresses produced by biomechanical and hemodynamic forces are maximal.[6]

Histological studies on the vascular biology of symptomatic and asymptomatic carotid plaques have recently been reviewed by Golledge et al.[7] They showed that the features of unstable plaques removed from symptomatic patients were surface ulceration and plaque rupture (48% of symptomatic versus 31% of asymptomatic, $p < 0.001$), thinning of the fibrous cap, and infiltration of the cap by a greater number of macrophages and T-lymphocytes.

The identification of unstable plaques *in vivo* and subsequent plaque stabilization may prove to be an important modality for a reduction in the lethal consequences of atherosclerosis.[8,9] This putative concept of plaque stabilization, although attractive, has not yet been rigorously validated in humans. Indirect data from clinical trials involving lipid lowering/modification and lifestyle/risk factor modification provide strong support for this new approach.[10]

Conventional angiography has been used for several decades to investigate the presence and severity of internal carotid artery stenosis, but its invasive nature means that it cannot be repeated frequently and carries a risk of stroke of 1.2%. In addition, angiography provides little information on plaque structure. In contrast, high-resolution ultrasound has enabled us to study the presence, rate of progression or regression of plaques, and most importantly their consistency.

Ultrasonic characteristics of unstable (vulnerable) plaques have been determined[11–13] and populations or individuals at increased risk for cardiovascular events can now be identified.[14] In addition, high-resolution ultrasound has enabled us to identify the different ultrasonic characteristics of unstable carotid plaques associated with amaurosis fugax, transient ischemic attacks (TIAs), stroke, and different patterns of computed tomography (CT) brain infarction.[12,13] This information has provided new insight into the pathophysiology of the different clinical manifestations of extracranial atherosclerotic cerebrovascular disease using noninvasive methods.

The aim of this chapter is to highlight the advances in ultrasonic plaque characterization and their potential applications in clinical practice.

Ultrasonic Plaque Classification

High-resolution ultrasound provides information not only on the degree of carotid artery stenosis but also on the characteristics of the arterial wall including the size and consistency of atherosclerotic plaques. Several studies have indicated that "complicated" carotid plaques are often associated with ipsilateral neurological symptoms and share common ultrasonic characteristics, being more echolucent (weak reflection of ultrasound and therefore containing echo-poor structures) and heterogeneous (having both echolucent and echogenic areas). In contrast, "uncomplicated" plaques, which are often asymptomatic, tend to be of uniform consistency (uniformly hypoechoic or uniformly hyperechoic) without evidence of ulceration.[11,15,16]

TABLE 10–1. Design of published studies on carotid plaque characterization in relation to risk for neurologic events.

Reference	Carotid bifurcations n	Follow-up in years	Type of patients A = asymptomatic S = symptomatic	Plaque characteristics studied
O'Holleran et al., 1987[18]	296	3.8	A	Calcified, dense, soft
Sterpetti et al., 1988[25]	238	2.8	A and S	Homogeneous, heterogeneous
Langsfeld et al., 1989[26]	419	1.8	A	Plaque types 1 to 4
Bock et al., 1993[27]	242	2.3	A	Echolucent, echogenic
Polak et al., 1998[22]	270	3.3	A	Hypo-, iso-, hyperechoic
Mathiesen et al., 2001[28]	223	3.0	A	Plaque types 1 to 4
Grønholdt et al., 2001[29]	111	4.4	A	Grayscale median
	135	4.4	S	Grayscale median
Liapis et al., 2001[30]	442	3.7	A and S	Plaque types 1 to 4
AbuRahma et al., 1998[31]	391	3.1	A	Homogeneous, heterogeneous
Carra et al., 2003[32]	291	2.7	A	Homogeneous, heterogeneous

Different classifications of plaque ultrasonic appearance have been proposed. Reilly classified[15] carotid plaques as homogeneous and heterogeneous, defining as homogeneous plaques those with "uniformly bright echoes" that are now known as uniformly hyperechoic (type 4) (see below). Johnson classified plaques as dense and soft,[17,18] Widder as echolucent and echogenic based on the their overall level of echo patterns,[19] while Gray-Weale described four types: type 1, predominantly echolucent lesions, type 2, echogenic lesions with substantial (>75%) components of echolucency, type 3, predominately echogenic with small area(s) of echolucency occupying less than a quarter of the plaque, and type 4, uniformly dense echogenic lesions.[20] Geroulakos subsequently modified the Gray-Weale classification by using a 50% area cut-off point instead of 75% and by adding a fifth type, which as a result of heavy calcification on its surface cannot be correctly classified.[11]

In an effort to improve the reproducibility of visual (subjective) classification, a consensus conference has suggested that echodensity should reflect the overall brightness of the plaque with the term hyperechoic referring to echogenic (white) and the term hypoechoic referring to echolucent (black) plaques.[21] The reference structure, to which plaque echodensity should be compared, should be blood for hypoechoic, the sternomastoid muscle for isoechoic, and bone for hyperechoic plaques. More recently, a similar method has been used by Polak.[22]

In the past a number of workers had confused echogenicity with homogeneity.[15] It is now realized that measurements of texture are different from measurements of echogenicity. The observation that two different atherosclerotic plaques may have the same overall echogenicity but frequently have variations of texture within different regions of the plaque was made as early as 1983.[23] The term homogeneous should therefore refer to plaques of uniform consistency irrespective of whether they are predominantly hypoechoic or hyperechoic. The

term heterogeneous should be used for plaques of nonuniform consistency, i.e., having both hypoechoic and hyperechoic components (Gray-Weale[20] types 2 and 3). Although O'Donnnell had proposed this otherwise simple classification in 1985[16] and Aldoori in 1987,[24] there has been considerable diversity in terminology used by others, as shown in Table 10–1.[18,22,25–32] Because of this confusion, frequently plaques having intermediate echogenicity or being complex are inadequately described. For example, echolucent plaques have been considered as heterogeneous.[26] A reflection of this confusion is a report from the committee on standards for noninvasive vascular testing of the Joint Council of the Society for Vascular Surgery and the North American Chapter of the International Society for Cardiovascular Surgery proposing that carotid plaques should be classified as homogeneous or heterogeneous.[33]

Regarding the clinical significance of carotid plaque heterogeneity, it seems that the heterogeneous plaques described in the three studies published in the 1980s (Table 10–1) include hypoechoic plaques. Also heterogeneous plaques in all studies listed in Table 10–1 contain hypoechoic areas (large or small) and appear to be the plaques that are associated with symptoms or if found in asymptomatic individuals they are the plaques that subsequently tend to become symptomatic.

Correlation with Histology

Reilly has shown for the first time that carotid plaque characteristics on B-mode ultrasound performed before operation correlate with carotid plaque histology.[15] As indicated above, by evaluating visually the sonographic characteristics of carotid plaques, two patterns were identified: a homogeneous pattern containing uniform hyperechoic echoes corresponding to dense fibrous tissue and a heterogeneous pattern containing a mixture of hyperechoic areas representing fibrous tissue and anechoic areas that represent intraplaque hemorrhage or lipid.[33] Thus, it was realized early that ultrasound could not distinguish between hemorrhage and lipid. Because most heterogeneous lesions contained intraplaque hemorrhage and ulcerated lesions, it was thought at the time that the presence of a plaque hemorrhage reflected the potential for plaque rupture and development of symptoms. However, it was subsequently realized that plaque hemorrhage was very common and was found in equal frequency in both symptomatic and asymptomatic plaques[34] and that ultrasound was highly sensitive in demonstrating plaque hemorrhage (27/29, 93%), as well as specific (84%).[16,31,35] It was both sensitive and specific in demonstrating calcification in carotid endarterectomy specimens.[36]

Aldoori reported that plaque hemorrhage was seen histologically in 21 patients, 19 (78%) of whom were diagnosed preoperatively as having echolucent heterogeneous plaques on ultrasound imaging.[24] Gray-Weale[20] also validated his plaque classification by demonstrating a statistically significant relationship ($p < 0.001$) between ultrasound appearance of type 1 and 2 plaques (echolucent appearance) and the presence of either intraplaque hemorrhage or ulceration in the endarterectomy specimen. It is now apparent from those ultrasound-histology correlations that Reilly's heterogeneous plaques correspond closely to Gray-Weale's echolucent (types 1 and 2) plaques.

The above findings were confirmed by studies performed in the 1990s using the new generation of ultrasound scanners with their improved resolution. Van Damme[37] reported that fibrous plaques (dense homogeneous hyperechoic lesions) were detected with a specificity of 87% and a sensitivity of 56%. Recent intraplaque hemorrhage was echographically apparent as a hypoechoic area in 88% of cases, corresponding to a specificity of 79% and a sensitivity of 75%. Kardoulas,[38] in another study, confirmed Van Damme's results on fibrous plaques, with fibrous tissue being significantly greater (73%) in plaques with an echogenic character compared with those with an echolucent morphology (63%; $p = 0.04$).

More recently the European carotid plaque study group that performed a multicenter study confirmed that plaque echogenicity was inversely related to hemorrhage and lipid ($p = 0.005$) and directly related to collagen content and calcification ($p < 0.0001$).[39]

Plaque shape (mural vs. nodular) on ultrasound has been shown to be associated with histology features characteristic of unstable plaques. Weinberger[40] demonstrated that mural plaques propagating along the carotid wall had a 72% frequency of recent organizing hemorrhage. In contrast, nodular plaques causing local narrowing of the vessel had only a 23% incidence of organizing hemorrhage ($p < 0.01$).

We now know that stable atherosclerotic plaques have on histological examination a thick fibrous cap, a small lipid core, are rich in smooth muscle cells (SMC) that produce collagen, and have a poor content of macrophages. In contrast, unstable plaques that are prone to rupture and development of symptoms have a thin fibrous cap, a large lipid core, few SMC, and are rich in macrophages.[3] Macrophages are responsible for the production of enzymes, matrix metaloproteinases (stromelysins, gelatinases, collagenases) that play an important role in remodeling the plaque matrix and erosion of the fibrous cap.[41] Recently, Lammie[42] reported a highly significant association between a thin fibrous cap and a large necrotic core ($p < 0.002$) in carotid endarterectomy specimens and a good agreement between ultrasound and pathological measurements of fibrous cap thickness (thick vs. thin fibrous cap, kappa = 0.53).

There is considerable debate on the question of whether thrombosis on the surface of the plaque, being an otherwise significant feature of complicated plaques, can discriminate between symptomatic and asymptomatic plaques. Acute thrombosis on ultrasound appears as a completely echolucent defect adjacent to the lumen[43] and it is almost certain that by the time the operation is performed (usually several weeks after the event) the thrombus has undergone remodeling.

Natural History Studies

Johnson did the first study, which has shown the value of ultrasonic characterization of carotid bifurcation plaques in asymptomatic patients, in the early 1980s.[17,18] In that study, hypoechoic carotid plaques in comparison to hyperechoic or calcified ones increased the risk of stroke during a follow-up period of 3 years; this effect was prominent in patients with carotid stenosis more than 75% (as estimated by cross-sectional area calculations and spectral analysis), as stroke occurred in 19% of them. None of the patients with calcified plaques developed a stroke.

A second study performed in the 1980s by Sterpetti[25] has shown that the severity of stenosis (lumen diameter reduction greater than 50%) and the presence of a heterogeneous plaque were both independent risk factors for the development of new neurological deficits (TIA and stroke). Twenty-seven percent of the patients with heterogeneous plaques and hemodynamically significant stenosis developed new symptoms. Unfortunately, their study had mixed cases as 37% of the patients had a history of previous neurologic symptoms, mainly hemispheric ones. History of these neurological symptoms was a risk factor for the development of new neurological symptoms during the follow-up period, although this was found only in the univariate analysis. Because no subgroup analysis was performed, no conclusion can be drawn regarding asymptomatic or symptomatic patients.

In a similar study of patients with asymptomatic carotid stenosis AbuRahma[31] reported that the incidence of ipsilateral strokes during follow-up was significantly higher in patients having heterogeneous plaques than in those having homogeneous ones: 13.6% versus 3.1% ($p = 0.0001$; odds ratio: 5). Similarly, the incidence rate of all neurological events (stroke or TIA) was higher in patients with heterogeneous than in those with homogeneous plaques: 27.8% versus 6.6% ($p = 0.001$; odds ratio, 5.5). Heterogeneous plaques were defined as those composed of a mixture of hypoechoic, isoechoic, and hyperechoic lesions, and homogeneous plaques as those that consisted of only one of the three components. Similar results indicating an increased risk in patients with heterogeneous plaques were reported by Carra[32] (Table 10–2).

The study published in the 1980s by Langsfeld[26] confirmed that patients with *hypoechoic plaques* (type 1, predominantly echolucent raised lesion, with a thin "eggshell" cap of echogenicity and type 2, echogenic lesions with substantial areas of echolucency) had a twofold risk of stroke: 15% in comparison to 7% in those having *hyperechoic plaques* [type 3, predominately echogenic with small area(s) of echolucency deeply localized and occupying less than a quarter of the plaque and type 4, uniformly dense echogenic lesions]. A confounding factor was that patients with greater than 75% stenosis were also at increased risk. However, the overall incidence of new symptoms was low, in contrast with the previous studies, perhaps because only asymptomatic patients were included in that study. Based on their results, the authors proposed an aggressive approach in those patients with greater than 75% stenosis and heterogeneous plaques. There is some confusion regarding the interchangeable use of the terms heterogeneous and hypoechoic in that article. The authors raised the point that it is important for each laboratory to verify its ability to classify plaque types. The same group in another study published 4 years later reported a 5.7% annual vessel event rate (TIA and stroke) for echolucent carotid plaques versus 2.4% for the echogenic ones ($p = 0.03$).[27]

Given the fair interobserver reproducibility for type 1 plaques, the use of reference points was proposed: anechogenicity to be standardized against circulating blood, isoechogenicity against sternomastoid muscle, and hyperechogenicity against bone (cervical vertebrae). This method was used in the late 1990s by Polak,[22] who investigated the association between stroke and internal carotid artery plaque echodensity in 4886 asymptomatic individuals aged 65 years or older, who were followed up prospectively for 48 months. Some 68% of those had carotid artery stenosis, which exceeded 50% in 270 patients. In this study plaques were subjectively characterized as hypoechoic, isoechoic, or hyperechoic in relation to the surrounding soft tissues. Hypoechoic plaques causing 50–100% stenoses were associated with a significantly higher incidence of ipsilateral, nonfatal stroke than iso- or hyperechoic plaques of the same degree of stenosis (relative risk 2.78 and 3.08, respectively). The authors of this study suggested that quantitative methods of grading carotid plaque echomorphology such as computer-assisted plaque characterization might be more precise in determining the association between hypoechoic (echolucent) plaques and the incidence of stroke. Subsequent studies[28–30] have supported the finding that

TABLE 10–2. Results of prospective studies of plaque characterization in relation to risk for neurologic events.

Reference	Endpoint	Stenosis	Findings
O'Holleran *et al.*, 1987[18]	Stroke, transient ischemic attack (TIA)	>75%	Cumulative 5 year stroke risk was 80% for soft (echolucent plaques) 10% for dense (echogenic and calcified plaques)
Sterpetti *et al.*, 1988[25]	Stroke, TIA	>50%	Events: 27% for heterogeneous plaques 9% for homogeneous plaques
Langsfeld *et al.*, 1989[26]	Neurological symptoms	>75%	Events: 15% for echolucent plaques 9% for echogenic plaques
Bock *et al.*, 1993[27]	Stroke, TIA	—	Annual event rate: 5.7% for echolucent plaques 2.4% for echogenic plaques
Polak *et al.*, 1998[22]	Stroke	>50%	RR for ipsilateral stroke was 2.78 in hypoechoic plaques
Mathiesen *et al.*, 2001[28]	Neurological	>35%	RR for cerebrovascular events was 4.6 in subjects with echolucent plaques
Grønholdt *et al.*, 2001[29]	Ipsilateral stroke	>80%	RR for ischemic stroke was 7.9 in subjects with echolucent plaques
Liapis *et al.*, 2001[30]	Stroke, TIA	>70%	RR was 2.96 for stroke and 2.02 for TIA in echolucent plaques
AbuRahma *et al.*, 1998[31]	Stroke, TIA	—	Ipsilateral stroke occurred in 13.6% of heterogeneous plaques 3.1% of homogeneous plaques
Carra *et al.*, 2003[32]	Stroke, TIA	>70%	Ipsilateral event occurred in 5% of heterogeneous plaques 1.3% of homogeneous plaques

hypoechoic plaques are associated with an increased risk when compared with hyperechoic plaques (see below). We now know that echolucent and heterogeneous plaques are not mutually exclusive and the risk is increased in both. Type 2 plaques, which are associated with the highest incidence of neurological events, are by definition included in both echolucent and heterogeneous groups (see the section on plaque types below).

The Need for B-Mode Image Normalization

Ultrasound examination and plaque characterization have been until now highly subjective. When the examination is performed in a dimly lit room the gain is usually reduced by the operator; when it is performed in a brightly lit room the gain is increased. Although the human eye can adjust to the image brightness to a certain extent, reproducible measurements of echodensity are not possible. Ultrasonic image normalization, which was introduced in the late 1990s, has enabled us to overcome this problem.

Computer-assisted plaque measurements of echodensity were initially made from digitized B-mode images of plaques taken from a duplex scanner with fixed instrument settings including gain and time control. The median of the frequency distribution of gray values of the pixels within the plaque (grayscale median—GSM, scale 0–255, 0 = black, 255 = white) was used as the measurement of echodensity. Early work had demonstrated that plaques with a GSM of less than 32, i.e., echolucent plaques had a 5-fold increase in the prevalence of silent brain infarcts on CT brain scans.[44] Other teams found similar results but the cut-off point was different from 32.[45] Soon it became apparent that ultrasonic image normalization was necessary, so that images captured under different instrument settings, from different scanners, by different operators, and through different peripherals such as video or magnetooptical disk could be comparable.

As a result a method has been developed to normalize images by means of digital image processing using blood and adventitia as the two reference points.[46] With the use of commercially available software (Adobe Photoshop version 3.0 or later, Adobe Systems Inc.) and the "histogram" facility, the GSM of the two reference points (blood and adventitia) in the original B-mode image was determined. Algebraic (linear) scaling of the image was performed with the "curves" option of the software so that in the resultant image the GSM of blood was equal to 0 and that of the adventitia to 190. Thus brightness of all pixels in the image including those of the plaque became adjusted according to the two reference points. This resulted in a significant improvement in the comparability of the ultrasonic tissue characteristics.

Appropriate areas of blood and adventitia for image normalization and the avoidance of areas of acoustic

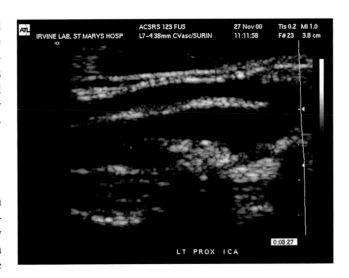

FIGURE 10–1. Image obtained for plaque analysis. The ultrasound beam is at right angles to the adventitia; the time gain compensation curve (TGC) is vertical through the vessel lumen; a bright segment of adventitia is visible adjacent to the plaque.

shadow in the selection of the plaque area are imperative. The duplex settings recommended are as follows: maximum dynamic range, low persistence, and high frame rate. A high-frequency linear array transducer ideally 7–10 MHz should be used. A high dynamic range ensures a greater range of grayscale values. High frame rate ensures good temporal resolution. In addition to these presets the time gain compensation curve should be positioned vertically through the lumen of the vessel, as there is little attenuation of the beam at this point. This ensures that the adventitia of the anterior wall has the same brightness as the adventitia of the posterior wall. The overall gain should be adjusted to give optimum image quality (bright echoes with minimum noise in the blood). A linear postprocessing curve should also be used and finally where possible the ultrasound beam should be at 90° to the arterial wall (Figure 10–1).

The previously discussed guidelines should result in the following: an area of noiseless blood, an echodense piece of adventitia in the vicinity of the plaque, and visualization of the extent and borders of the plaque. It is here that color images can provide further information about plaque outline.

Two major reproducibility studies have been performed in order to establish the validity of the method of image normalization and the value of GSM measurements.[47,48] These studies have demonstrated that GSM after image normalization is a highly reproducible measurement that could be used in natural history studies of asymptomatic carotid atherosclerotic disease, aiming to identify patients at higher risk of stroke. A key issue for the successful reproducibility of normalized images is that only the inner half of the

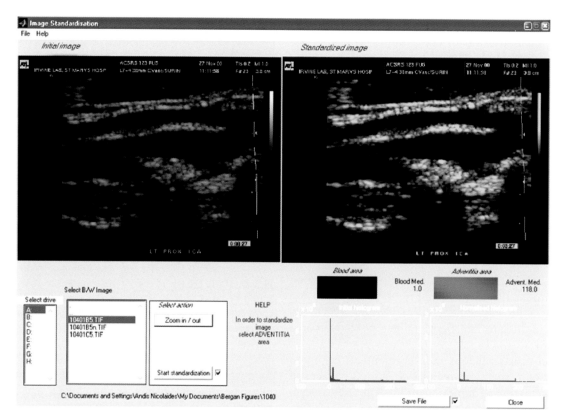

FIGURE 10–2. A user-friendly method of image normalization. Original image is on the left. By sampling pixels representing blood and pixels of center of adventitia after magnification, the normalized image is produced on the right. This image can be saved in a database.

brightest section of adventitia should be sampled for normalization.

Adequate training is essential if the level of reproducibility reported above is to be achieved. It is necessary not only in the use of the software but also in the appropriate scanning technique.

The authors have developed a research software package, now commercially available, that can be used to analyze ultrasonic images of plaques. This package has five main modules. The first provides a user-friendly way to normalize images (Figure 10–2). A zooming facility allows enlargement of the image so that the middle half of the adventitia can be selected accurately. The second provides a means of calibration and of making measurements of distance or area in mm and mm², respectively. The third provides a method of normalizing images to a standard pixel density (20 pixels per mm). This is because a number of texture features are pixel density dependent and various degrees of image magnification even on the same scanner do alter the pixel density (see section on "Texture Features"). The fourth provides the user with a means of selecting the area of interest (plaque) and saving it as a separate file (Figure 10–3). An image enhancement facility allows clearer visualization of the edges of the plaque. The fifth classifies plaques according to the Geroulakos classification[11] and extracts a number of texture features and saves them on a file for subsequent statistical analysis. In addition, images are color contoured. Pixels with a grayscale value in the range of 0–25 are colored black. Pixels with values 26–50, 51–75, 76–100, 101–125, and greater than 125 are colored blue, green, yellow, orange, and red, respectively (Figure 10–4). In addition, this module allows printing of the plaque images and selected features or saving the latter in a file (Figure 10–5). For the purpose of automatic classification by computer, the Geroulakos classification has been redefined in terms of pixels and gray levels. Examples of plaque types 1–4 are shown in Figure 10–6. For plaque type 5 only the calcified or visible bright areas of the plaque should be selected ignoring the areas of acoustic shadows where information on plaque texture is lacking.

Type 1. Uniformly echolucent (black): (less than 15% of the plaque area is occupied by colored areas, i.e., with pixels having a grayscale value greater than 25). If the fibrous cap is not visible, the plaque can be detected as a black filling defect only by using color flow or power Doppler.

Type 2. Mainly echolucent: (colored areas occupy 15–50% of the plaque area).

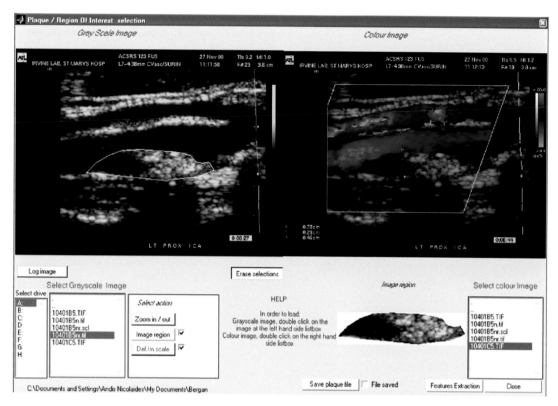

FIGURE 10–3. This module provides the facility for outlining the plaque and saving it as a separate file in the database. The color image on the right provides some indication of the extent of hypoechoic areas near the lumen.

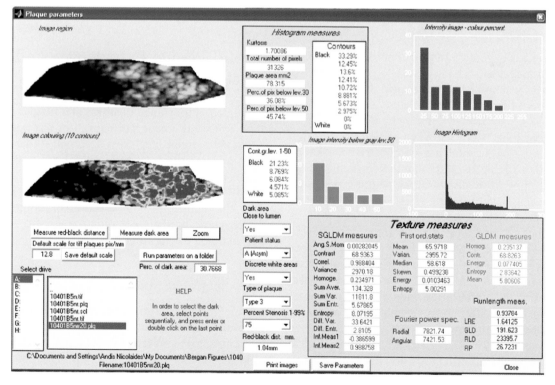

FIGURE 10–4. This module extracts a large number of well-established standard first-order and second-order statistical features used in image analysis. The program determines the type of plaque automatically and allows input from the operator about the presence of a dark area adjacent to the lumen, presenting symptoms and percent carotid stenosis.

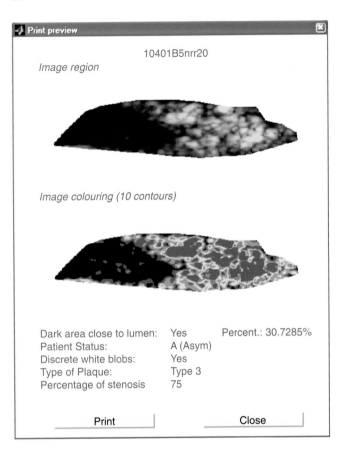

FIGURE 10–5. Printout of normalized grayscale image of plaque and color contoured image with selected plaque characterization features.

Type 3. Mainly echogenic: (colored areas occupy 50–85% of the plaque area).

Type 4 and 5. Uniformly echogenic: (colored areas occupy more than 85% of the plaque area).

A reproducibility study between visual classification and computer classification has demonstrated a kappa statistic of 0.61 (Table 10–3). It should be noted that the computer cannot distinguish between plaque types 4 and 5. This is because the operator selects only the calcified area of plaque type 5. However, this is not a major drawback since both plaque types 4 and 5 are associated with low risk. The high event rate associated with plaque types 1–3 and low event rate with plaques 4 and 5 found after image normalization and visual classification is also found after image normalization and typing by computer (Table 10–4). In fact, after image normalization and computer classification the group of patients with plaque types 1–3 contains 99 (93.5%) of all 106 neurological events. When compared with type 4 and 5 plaques the relative risk is 3.3 (95% CI 1.56–7.00). Also, after image normalization and computer classification plaque types 1–3 contain 44 (93.6%) of all 46 strokes (RR 3.4 with 95% CI 1.07–10.9).

Carotid Plaque Echodensity and Structure in Normalized Images

The clinical importance of ultrasonic plaque characterization following image normalization has been focused on two main areas: first, cross-sectional studies aiming at better understanding of the pathophysiology of carotid disease and second, natural history studies seeking to identify high- and low-risk groups for stroke in order to refine the indications on selection of symptomatic or asymptomatic patients not only for carotid endarterectomy but also for stenting.

Cross-Sectional Studies

The use of image normalization and computer analysis has resulted in the identification of differences in carotid plaque structure—in terms of echodensity and degree of stenosis—not only between symptomatic and asymptomatic plaques in general but also between plaques associated with retinal or hemispheric symptoms.[49] In a series of asymptomatic and symptomatic patients presenting with amaurosis fugax, TIAs, and stroke with good

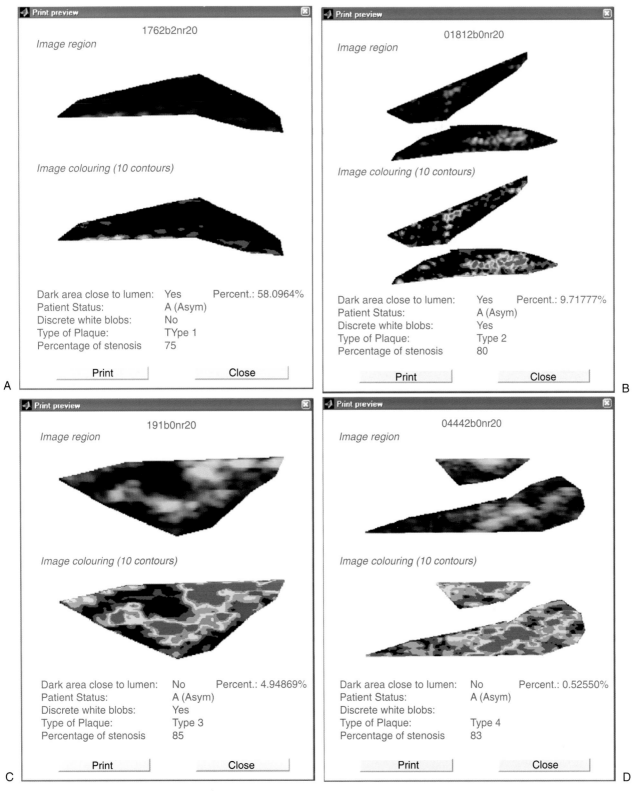

FIGURE 10–6. Examples of plaque types: (A) type 1, (B) type 2, (C) type 3, (D) type 4.

TABLE 10–3. Relationship between plaque visual classification after image normalization and plaque classification by computer (kappa = 0.61).[a]

Plaque type: visual classification after image normalization	Plaque type classification by computer after image normalization				
	1	2	3	4/5	Total
1	57 (51%)	53 (47%)	2 (1.8%)	0	112 (100%)
2	6 (1.6%)	251 (68%)	110 (30%)	3 (0.8%)	370 (100%)
3	0	9 (3%)	281 (91%)	20 (6.5%)	310 (100%)
4/5	0	0	92 (34%)	178 (66%)	270 (100%)
Total	63 (6%)	313 (29%)	486 (46%)	201 (19%)	1062 (100%)

[a]Because of the low event rate in plaque types 4 and 5 and because the computer cannot distinguish between them these plaques have been grouped together.

recovery having 50–99% stenosis on carotid duplex scan, plaques associated with symptoms were significantly more hypoechoic, with higher degrees of stenosis than those not associated with symptoms (mean GSM = 13.3 versus 30.5 and mean degree of stenosis = 80.5% versus 72.2%). Furthermore, plaques associated with amaurosis fugax were hypoechoic (mean GSM = 7.4) and severely stenotic (mean stenosis 85.6%). Plaques associated with TIAs and stroke had a similar echodensity and a similar degree of stenosis (mean GSM = 14.9 versus 15.8 and degree of stenosis = 79.3% versus 78.1%).[50] These findings confirm previous reports, which have shown that hypoechoic plaques are more likely to be associated with symptoms. In addition, they support the hypothesis that amaurosis fugax has a pathophysiological mechanism different from that of TIAs and stroke.

Our group has found that GSM separates echomorphologically the carotid plaques associated with silent nonlacunar CT-demonstrated brain infarcts from plaques that are not so associated. The median GSM of plaques associated with ipsilateral nonlacunar silent CT-demonstrated brain infarcts was 14, and that of plaques that were not so associated was 30 (p = 0.003).[48] Additionally, emboli counted on transcranial Doppler (TCD) in the ipsilateral middle cerebral artery were more frequent in the presence of low-plaque echodensity (low GSM), but not in the presence of a high degree of stenosis. These data support the embolic nature of cerebrovascular symptomatology.[49]

There are several biological findings that can explain the association of hypoechoic plaques with symptoms. Our group has found that hypoechoic plaques with a low GSM have a large necrotic core volume.[51] In addition, hypoechoic plaques have increased macrophage infiltration on histological examination of the specimen after endarterectomy.[52]

The role of biomechanical forces in the induction of plaque fatigue and rupture has been emphasized.[53–55] In our group of patients, carotid plaques associated with amaurosis fugax were hypoechoic and were associated with very high-grade stenoses. It may well be that the plaques that are hypoechoic and homogeneous undergo low internal stresses and therefore do not rupture but progress to tighter stenosis with poststenotic dilatation, turbulance, and platelet adhesion in the poststenotic area resulting in the eventual production of showers of small platelet emboli. Such small platelet emboli may be too small to produce hemispheric symptoms but are detected by the retina. In contrast, plaques associated with TIAs and stroke were less hypoechoic and less stenotic than those associated with amaurosis fugax. These plaques are hypoechoic but more heterogeneous and may undergo stronger internal stresses. Therefore, they may tend to

TABLE 10–4. The ipsilateral AF, TIAs, and strokes that occurred during follow-up in patients with different types of plaque after image normalization and classification by computer.[a]

Plaque type classified by computer	Events absent	AF	TIAs	Stroke	All events	Total
1	56 (88.9%)	2 (3.2%)	1 (1.6%)	4 (6.3%)	7 (11.1%)	63 (100%)
2	271 (86.6%)	6 (1.9%)	17 (5.4%)	19 (6.1%)	42 (13.4%)	313 (100%)
3	435 (89.7%)	10 (2.1%)	19 (3.9%)	21 (4.3%)	50 (10.3%)	485 (100%)
4/5	194 (97.1%)	0	5 (2.5%)	2 (1.5%)	7 (3.5%)	201 (100%)
Total	956 (90.0%)	18 (1.7%)	42 (3.8%)	46 (4.4%)	106 (10.0%)	1062 (100%)

[a]AF, amaurosis fugax; TIAs, transient ischemic attacks.

rupture at an earlier stage (lower degrees of stenosis), producing larger particle debris (plaque constituents or thrombi) that deprive large areas of the brain of adequate perfusion.

Prospective Studies

The Tromsø study conducted in Norway involving 223 subjects with carotid stenosis > 35% has found that subjects with echolucent atherosclerotic plaques have increased risk of ischemic cerebrovascular events independent of degree of stenosis.[28] The authors give no details on the patient's neurological history. The adjusted relative risk for all cerebrovascular events in subjects with echolucent plaques was 4.6 (95% CI 1.1–18.9), and there was a significant linear trend (p = 0.015) for higher risk with increasing plaque echolucency. Ipsilateral neurological events were also more frequent in patients with echolucent or predominantly echolucent plaques (17.4% and 14.7%, respectively). The authors concluded that evaluation of plaque morphology in addition to the grade of stenosis might improve clinical decision making and differentiate treatment for individual patients and that computer-quantified plaque morphology assessment, being a more objective method of ultrasonic plaque characterization, may further improve this.

This method has been recently used by Grønholdt,[29] who found that echolucent plaques causing >50% diameter stenosis were associated with increased risk of future stroke in symptomatic (n = 135) but not asymptomatic (n = 111) individuals. Echogenicity of carotid plaques was evaluated with high-resolution B-mode ultrasound and computer-assisted image processing. The mean of the standardized median grayscale values of the plaque was used to divide plaques into echolucent and echorich. Relative to symptomatic patients with echorich 50–79% stenotic plaques, those with echorich 80–99% stenotic plaques, echolucent 50–79% stenotic plaques, and echolucent 80–99% stenotic plaques had relative risks of ipsilateral ischemic stroke of 3.1 (95% CI, 0.7–14), 4.2 (95% CI, 1.2–15), and 7.9 (95% CI, 2.1–30), equivalent to absolute risk increase of 11%, 18%, and 28%, respectively. The authors suggested that measurement of echolucency, together with the degree of stenosis, might improve selection of patients for carotid endarterectomy. The relatively small number of asymptomatic individuals was probably the reason why plaque characterization was not helpful in predicting risk in the asymptomatic group.

Ultrasonic Plaque Ulceration

Several studies have indicated a strong association between macroscopic plaque ulceration and the development of embolic symptoms (amaurosis fugax, TIAs,

stroke) and signs such as silent infarcts on CT brain scans.[56–60] However, the ability of ultrasound to identify plaque ulceration is poor.[15,19,61–67] The sensitivity is low (41%) when the stenosis is greater than 50% and moderately high (77%) when the stenosis is less than 50%. This is because ulceration is much easier to detect in the presence of mild stenosis, when the residual lumen and plaque surface are more easily seen, than with severe stenosis, when the residual lumen and the surface of the plaque are not easily defined because they are not always in the plane of the ultrasound beam.

Two studies have investigated plaque surface characteristics and the type of plaque in relation to symptoms. The first one was a retrospective analysis of 578 symptomatic patients (242 with stroke and 336 with TIAs) recruited for the B-scan Ultrasound Imaging Assessment Program. A matched case-control study design was used to compare brain hemispheres with ischemic lesions to unaffected contralateral hemispheres with regard to the presence and characteristics of carotid artery plaques. Plaques were classified as smooth when the surface had a continuous boundary, irregular when there was an uneven or pitted boundary, and pocketed when there was a crater-like defect with sharp margins. The results demonstrated an odds ratio of 2.1 for the presence of an irregular surface and of 3.0 for hypoechoic plaques in carotids associated with TIAs and stroke.[68]

The second study included 258 symptomatic and 65 asymptomatic patients. Carotid plaque morphology was classified according to Gray-Weale,[20] and plaque surface features were assessed. The results demonstrated that plaque types 1 and 2 were more common in symptomatic patients. The incidence of ulceration was 23% in the symptomatic and 14% in the asymptomatic group (p = 0.04).[69]

In the absence of any prospective natural history studies in which ultrasound has been used for identifying plaque ulceration, the finding of plaque ulceration cannot be used for making clinical decisions.

Stenosis: A Confounding Factor

Natural history studies have demonstrated that the risk of developing ipsilateral symptoms including stroke increases with increasing severity of internal carotid artery stenosis (Table 10–5). In addition, a number of important messages have emerged recently. One is that the different methods used on either side of the Atlantic to express the degree of stenosis have a different relationship to risk. Another is the realization that a considerable number of events occur in patients with low grade asymptomatic carotid stenosis. Also, the relationship between risk and degree of internal carotid stenosis depends on the methodology used. Finally, both the

TABLE 10–5. Natural history studies of patients with asymptomatic internal carotid artery stenosis in which grades of stenosis up to 99% have been included.[a]

Publication	Grading of stenosis			n	Mean follow-up (years)	Events			Event rate (annual)		
	Area	N%	E%			TIAs +AF[b]	Stroke	TIAs+ stroke	TIAs +AF	Stroke	TIAs+ Stroke
Johnson et al., 1985[6]	**<75**	<50%	<70%	176	3	12	3	15	2.3%	0.6%	1.7%
	>75	>50%	>70%	121		57	12	69	15.7%	3.3%	19%
Chambers and Norris, 1986[8]	**<75**	<50%	<70%	387	2	8	6	14	1.0%	0.1%	1.8%
	>75	>50%	>70%	113		16	6	22	7.0%	2.6%	9.7%
Hennerici et al., 1987[9]		**<80%**	<88%	119	2.5	15	4	19	5.0%	1.3%	6.4%
		>80%	>88%	36		2	3	5	2.2%	3.3%	5.5%
Norris et al., 1991[10]		**<50%**	<70%	303	3.4	11	13	24	1.1%	1.3%	2.3%
		50–75%	72–85%	216		28	5	33	3.8%	0.6%	4.5%
		75–99%	85–99%	177		36	11	47	6.0%	1.8%	7.8%
Zhu and Norris, 1991[11]		**<50%**	<72%	734[c]	4	12	10	22	0.4%	0.3%	0.7%
		50–74%	72–85%	172[c]		12	2	14	1.7%	0.3%	2.0%
		75–99%	85–99%	94[c]		23	6	29	6.1%	1.6%	7.7%
MacKey et al., 1997[12]	<12%	**<50%**		358	3.6	5	5	10	0.4%	0.4%	0.8%
	12–65%	**50–79%**		207		3	6	9	0.4%	0.8%	1.2%
	65–99%	**79–99%**		113		12	7	19	2.9%	1.7%	4.7%
Nadareishvili et al., 2002[13]		**<50%**	<72%	108	10	—	—	10	—	—	0.9%
		50–99%	72–99%	73		—	—	12	—	—	7.7%
ECST (asymptomatic side) 1995[14]		<47%	**0–69%**	2113	4.5	—	54	—	—	0.5%	—
		47–99%	**70–99%**	127		—	13	—	—	2.3%	—
NASCET (asymptomatic side)		**<50%**	<72%	1496	5	—	116	—	—	1.5%	—
		50–74%	72–85%	172		—	31	—	—	2.8%	—
Inzitary et al., 2000[15]		**75–99%**	85–99%	73		—	12	—	—	3.3%	—
		<60%	<77%	1604		—	128	—	—	1.6%	—
		60–99%	77–99%	73		—	34	—	—	3.1%	—
ACSRS Nicolaides et al., 2005[84]	12–49%	**50–69%**		194	3.5	7	3	10	0.4%	0.4%	1.5%
	50–82%	**70–89%**		593		31	23	54	1.5%	1.1%	2.6%
	82–99%	**90–99%**		328		24	20	44	2.1%	1.7%	3.8%

[a]The method used to grade the stenosis in each study (area, N% = NASCET or E% = ECST) is shown in bold.
[b]AF, amaurosis fugax; TIAs, transient ischemic attacks.
[c]Indicates carotid arteries rather than patients.

severity of internal carotid stenosis and plaque characterization texture features are independent predictors of risk and can complement each other. Thus, plaque characterization cannot be considered independent of stenosis.

Two main methods are currently used to express percent diameter stenosis. The first one defines the residual lumen as a percentage of the normal distal internal carotid artery (ICA). It has been used in North America since the late 1960s and more recently the North American Symptomatic Carotid Endarterectomy Trial (NASCET)[70] and the Asymptomatic Carotid Atherosclerosis Study (ACAS).[71] It has become known as the North American, "NASCET," or "N" method.[72] The second method expresses the residual lumen as a percentage of the diameter of the carotid bulb and has been used in the European Carotid Surgery Trial (ECST).[73] It has become known as the European or "ECST" or "E" method.[74] The relationship between both methods is shown in Figure 10–7.

Several natural history studies[17,27,75–82] indicate that the risk of stroke in asymptomatic patients is low (0.1–1.6% per year) for NASCET stenosis less than 75–80% and higher (2.0–3.3% per year) with greater degrees of stenosis (Table 10–5). Different cut-off points, ranges, and methods of grading stenosis have been used in these natural history studies[17,27,75–82] and randomized controlled trials.[70,71,73,83] Universal agreement as to the best method for grading ICA stenosis and optimum cut-off points in relation to risk have not yet been established.

The NASCET randomized controlled study has used angiography and a cut-off point of 70% stenosis in relation to the distal internal carotid, which is equivalent to 83% stenosis in relation to the bulb (Figure 10–7). The ECST randomized controlled study has used angiography also, but a cut-off point of 70% stenosis in relation to the bulb, which is equivalent to 47% stenosis in relation to the distal ICA. Many vascular surgeons are under the impression that these cut-off points are similar! The only similarity is the value of 70%. In reality the difference in terms of plaque size or residual lumen is considerable. However, with increasing degrees of stenosis the values of the two methods converge and the discrepancy decreases (Figure 10–7).

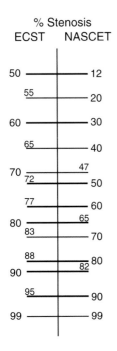

% Stenosis
ECST   NASCET

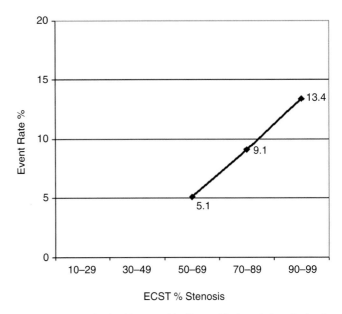

ECST % Stenosis

FIGURE 10–7. The relationship between ECST and NASCET percentage stenosis. The conversion scale is based on the following equations: NASCET stenosis = (ECST stenosi − 43) × (100/57) and ECST stenosis = [NASCET stenosis × (57/100) + 43]. Note: a 43% stenosis of the bulb reduces the lumen to the diameter of the lumen of the normal distal internal carotid artery. (Reproduced from Nicolaides *et al.*, 2005. Eur J Vasc Endovasc Surg 30, 275–284, with permission.)

FIGURE 10–8. The incidence of ipsilateral ischemic hemispheric events in relation to the ECST percentage stenosis of the internal carotid artery in the ACSRS study. (Reproduced from Nicolaides *et al.*, 2005. Eur J Vasc Endovasc Surg 30, 275–284, with permission.)

The results of the Asymptomatic Carotid Stenosis and Risk of Stroke (ACSRS) prospective natural history study have demonstrated that the risk of ipsilateral ischemic hemispheric events has a linear relationship with ECST stenosis (Figure 10–8) but not with NASCET stenosis (Figure 10–9).[84]

Natural history studies including the ACSRS that have included patients with asymptomatic carotid stenosis up to 99% (Table 10–5) have demonstrated that a considerable number of events occur at low grades of stenosis. In fact, in the ACSRS study 37 (34%) of 108 ipsilateral ischemic hemispheric events including 16 (35%) of the 46 strokes (Table 10–6) occurred in patients with stenosis less than 60% NASCET (<77% ECST), the selection criterion for carotid endarterectomy in asymptomatic patients as indicated from the findings of the ACAS trial. Only 10 (9%) of the events including 3 (3%) strokes occurred in patients with stenosis less than 70% ECST, equivalent to approximately 50% NASCET. The question that has been posed is whether plaque characterization can improve the selection of patients at increased risk in the range of 50–70% NASCET (equivalent to 72–83% ECST).

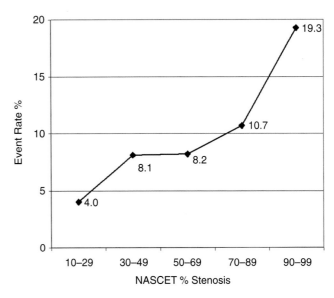

NASCET % Stenosis

FIGURE 10–9. The incidence of ipsilateral ischemic hemispheric events in relation to the NASCET percentage stenosis of the internal carotid artery in the ACSRS study. (Reproduced from Nicolaides *et al.*, 2005. Eur J Vasc Endovasc Surg 30, 275–284, with permission.)

TABLE 10–6. The number of different ipsilateral ischemic hemispheric neurological events in relation to less than 60% and 60–99% NASCET internal carotid artery stenosis (chi square 4.6; $p = 0.21$).[a]

% NASCET stenosis	AF	TIA	Stroke	All events	All patients
<60	6 (1.2%)	15 (3.0%)	16 (3.2%)	37 (7.4%)	499
60–99	12 (1.9%)	29 (4.6%)	30 (4.7%)	71 (11.2%)	636
Total	18 (1.6%)	44 (3.9%)	46 (4.1%)	108 (9.7%)	1115

[a]AF, amaurosis fugax; TIAs, transient ischemic attacks.

Plaque Type and Risk

As pointed out above, most natural history studies performed in the past have used different methods of plaque classification without prior image normalization. It is now realized that image normalization results in marked change in the appearance of plaques with reclassification of a large number. The relationship between plaque classification before image normalization and after image normalization in patients admitted to the ACSRS study is shown in Table 10–7.[85] Before image normalization 131 plaques were classified as type 1, 288 as type 2, 319 as type 3, 166 as type 4, and 188 as type 5. It can be seen that after image normalization 66% of type 1, 49% of type 2, 46% of type 3, 66% of type 4, and 82% of type 5 were reclassified as a different plaque type (kappa statistic 0.22) demonstrating that there was a poor agreement between plaque classification before and after image normalization. After image normalization 652 (60%) of the plaques changed category. This marked change in plaque category is found in all plaque types including type 5. Before image normalization plaques with a calcified cap that had more than 15% of the plaque obscured by an acoustic shadow were classified as type 5. After image normalization the area of plaque adjacent to the calcification and acoustic shadow could be seen and outlined more easily in relation to blood. This area changed considerably in many plaques and explains why a large number of plaques initially classified as type 5 changed to type 4, 3, and even 2 after image normalization (Table 10–7).

The ipsilateral neurological events (amaurosis fugax, TIAs, and stroke) that occurred in the ACSRS study during follow-up in patients with different types of plaque before and after image normalization are shown in Tables 10–8 and 10–9, respectively. It can be seen that after image normalization the incidence of events in relation to different plaque types has changed. After image normalization there was a decreased incidence in patients with plaque types 4 and 5 with the vast majority of events occurring in plaque types 1, 2, and 3. Before image normalization only 82 (71%) of the 116 neurological events occurred in plaque types 1–3, but after image normalization the number increased to 109 (94%).

When plaque types 1–3 are compared with plaque types 4 and 5 before image normalization the relative risk of having an event is 1.12 (95% CI 0.76 to 1.66) (chi square, $p = 0.45$). Also, 37 (73%) of the 51 ischemic strokes have occurred in patients with plaque types 1–3 (Table 10–8). When plaque types 1–3 are compared with plaque types 4 and 5 after image normalization the relative risk of having an event is 4.8 (95% CI 2.27–10.28) (chi square, $p = 0.0001$). Also, 49 (96%) of the 51 ischemic strokes have occurred in patients with plaque types 1–3 (Table 10–9).

When echolucent plaques (types 1 and 2) are compared with echogenic (types 3 and 4) plaques the incidence of ipsilateral neurological events is 61 (14.9%) out of 409 in the former and 53 (8.3%) out of 635 in the latter (Table 10–9) (RR 1.6 95% CI 1.16–2.32) (chi square, $p = 0.003$).

TABLE 10–7. The relationship between plaque classification before and after image normalization (kappa = 0.22).

Plaque type before image normalization	Plaque type after image normalization					
	1	2	3	4	5	Total
1	44 (34%)	54 (41%)	22 (17%)	11 (7%)	0	131 (100%)
2	23 (8%)	148 (51%)	97 (34%)	16 (6%)	4 (1.4%)	288 (100%)
3	10 (3%)	68 (21%)	173 (54%)	54 (17%)	14 (4%)	319 (100%)
4	0	35 (21%)	62 (37%)	57 (34%)	12 (7%)	166 (100%)
5	0	27 (19%)	96 (51%)	47 (25%)	18 (10%)	188 (100%)
Total	77 (7%)	332 (31%)	450 (41%)	185 (17%)	48 (6%)	1092 (100%)

TABLE 10–8. The ipsilateral AF, TIAs, and strokes that occurred during follow-up in patients with different types of plaque before image normalization.[a]

Plaque type	Events absent	AF	TIAs	Stroke	All events	Total
1	125 (95.4%)	1 (0.8%)	4 (3.1%)	1 (0.8%)	6 (4.6%)	131 (100%)
2	243 (84.4%)	3 (1.0%)	19 (6.6%)	23 (8.0%)	45 (15.6%)	288 (100%)
3	288 (90.3%)	5 (1.6%)	13 (4.0%)	13 (4.0%)	31 (9.7%)	319 (100%)
4	146 (88.0%)	6 (3.6%)	4 (2.4%)	10 (6.0%)	20 (12%)	166 (100%)
5	174 (92.5%)	4 (2.1%)	6 (3.2%)	4 (2.6%)	14 (7.5%)	188 (100%)
Total	976 (89.4%)	19 (1.7%)	46 (4.2%)	51 (4.7%)	116 (10.6%)	1092 (100%)

[a]AF, amaurosis fugax; TIAs, transient ischemic attacks.

When heterogeneous plaques (types 2 and 3) are compared with homogeneous plaques (types 1 and 4) the incidence of ipsilateral neurological events is 102 (13%) out of 782 in the former and 12 (4.6%) out of 262 in the latter (Table 10–5) (RR 2.8 95% CI 1.59–5.10) (chi square, $p = 0.0001$).

Before image normalization the ipsilateral neurological event rate was high in all plaque types (Table 10–8). After image normalization the event rate was high in plaque types 1–3 and low in types 4 and 5 (Table 10–9). This justifies grouping plaques 1–3 as high risk and 4 and 5 as low risk (see below).

Several research teams have indicated that the risk for stroke is higher with echolucent plaques (types 1 and 2) when compared with echogenic plaques (types 3 and 4) (Table 10–2). Others have claimed that heterogeneous plaques are associated with a higher risk for stroke than homogeneous plaques (Table 10–2). As pointed out earlier the results of the ACSRS study are compatible with both findings. This is because type 2 plaques that are associated with the highest stroke risk (Table 10–9) are included by most authors in both the echolucent and heterogeneous groups. The low risk associated with type 4 plaques can be explained by the fact that these plaques contain a large amount of collagen that is uniformly distributed, giving them stability. With decreasing amounts of collagen that is not uniformly distributed, the plaques may become increasingly unstable reaching a maximum risk in type 2 plaques that have a large lipid core and relatively little unevenly distributed collagen. It is now believed that type 2 and 3 plaques are unstable and tend to rupture because they are of nonuniform consistency and have nonuniform stresses within them during each pulsation. This is in contrast to type 1 plaques that have a uniform consistency and tend to progress without early rupture presenting with symptoms only when the stenosis becomes severe.[48]

Plaque Type, Stenosis, and Risk

The relationship between plaque type, stroke, and ipsilateral internal carotid stenosis (mild, moderate, and severe) has been explored in the ACSRS natural history study.[85] In this study the relationship between stenosis expressed as percentage stenosis of the bulb (ECST method) and stroke is shown in Figure 10–10. As in all other natural history studies the stroke rate increases with increasing degrees of internal carotid stenosis.

Table 10–10 shows the incidence of ipsilateral ischemic stroke in relation to both plaque type and severity of stenosis. For stenosis in the 50–69% range the incidence of stroke is low irrespective of plaque type (Table 10–10: cells a and e). For stenosis in the 70–89% range the stroke rate was 5.7% in patients with plaque types 1–3 and 0.8% in patients with plaque types 4 and 5 (Table 10–10: cells b and f). For stenosis in the 90–99% range the stroke rate is 7.7% in patients with plaque types 1–3 and zero in patients with plaque types 4 and 5 (Table 10–10: cells c and g).

TABLE 10–9. The ipsilateral AF, TIAs, and strokes that occurred during follow-up in patients with different types of plaque after image normalization.[a]

Plaque type	Events absent	AF	TIAs	Stroke	All events	Total
1	70 (91.0%)	2 (2.6%)	1 (1.3%)	4 (5.2%)	7 (9.1%)	77 (100%)
2	278 (84.1%)	7 (2.1%)	23 (6.7%)	24 (7.1%)	54 (15.9%)	332 (100%)
3	419 (93.1%)	10 (2.2%)	17 (3.8%)	21 (4.7%)	48 (10.7%)	450 (100%)
4	180 (97.3%)	0	3 (1.6%)	2 (1.1%)	5 (2.7%)	185 (100%)
5	46 (95.8%)	0	2 (4.2%)	0	2 (4.2%)	48 (100%)
Total	976 (89.4%)	19 (1.7%)	46 (4.2%)	51 (4.7%)	116 (10.6%)	1092 (100%)

[a]AF, amaurosis fugax; TIAs, transient ischemic attacks.

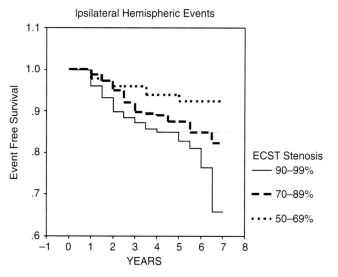

FIGURE 10–10. The ipsilateral hemispheric event-free cumulative survival rate in relation to the ECST percentage stenosis of the internal carotid artery (50–69% group: *n* = 101; 70–89% group: *n* = 593; 90–99% group: *n* = 328). Overall log rank: 11.7, *p* = 0.0026; 50–69 vs. 70–89%, *p* = 0.045; 70–89 vs. 90–99%, *p* = 0.020; 50–69 vs. 90–99%, *p* = 0.0014. (Reproduced from Nicolaides *et al.*, 2005. Eur J Vasc Endovasc Surg 30, 275–284, with permission.)

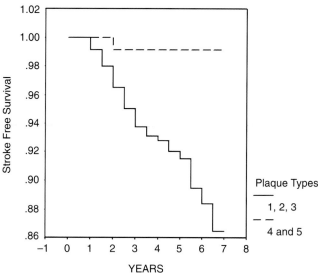

FIGURE 10–11. Kaplan–Meier estimates of the ipsilateral stroke free survival rate in 905 patients with greater than 70% stenosis (percentage stenosis in relation to the bulb: ECST method) for plaque types: 1, 2, 3 (*n* = 724) vs. 4, 5 (*n* = 181). Log rank *p* = 0.0028. (Reproduced from Nicolaides *et al.*, 2005. Vascular 13, 211–221, with permission.)

Thus, for the 905 patients with stenosis in the range of 70–99% (cells b, c, f, and g in Table 10–10) the incidence of stroke was (47/724) 6.5% (cells b and c) in plaque types 1, 2, and 3 and only (1/181) 0.55% (cells f and g) in plaque types 4 and 5 (RR 11.7 with 95% CI 1.63–84.5) (chi square with Yates correction 9.0; *p* = 0.003). The cumulative stroke-free survival rate in these 905 patients with greater than 70% stenosis for plaque types 1–3 and 4 and 5 is shown in Figure 10–11. For patients with plaque types 1–3 the cumulative stroke rate is 14% at 7 years (2% per year) and for patients with plaque types 4 and 5 the cumulative event rate is 1% at 7 years (0.14% per year).

The results of the ACSRS study indicate that for asymptomatic patients with internal carotid stenosis less than 70%, the annual risk of stroke is low (1.6%)

irrespective of plaque type (Table 10–10). It is 4.6% for grades of stenoses 70–89% and 6.5% for 90–99%. The incidence of stroke in the ACSRS study is also very low (0.9%) for plaque types 4 and 5 irrespective of the degree of stenosis and increases to 5.7% with plaque types 1–3. Thus, it appears that the lesions that are associated with greater than 70% stenosis that are types 1–3 (cells b and c in Table 10–6) (RR 11.7 with 95% CI 1.63–84.5) identify a higher risk group. This higher risk group has a cumulative annual stroke rate of 2% per year in contrast to plaques types 4 and 5 producing greater than 70% stenosis that have a cumulative annual stroke rate of 0.14% per year (Figure 10–11).

The results of the ACAS randomized controlled trial[71] have suggested that surgery is beneficial in those patients who have an asymptomatic greater than 60% internal

TABLE 10–10. The incidence of ipsilateral ischemic stroke in relation to plaque type after image normalization and severity of stenosis.

Plaque type after image normalization	Grade of stenosis (ECST)			
	50–69%	70–89%	90–99%	Total
1, 2 and 3	2/135 (1.5%)	26/453 (5.7%)	21/271 (7.7%)	**49/859 (5.7%)**
	a	**b**	**c**	**d**
4 and 5	1/52 (1.9%)	1/129 (0.8%)	0/52	**2/235 (0.9%)**
	e	**f**	**g**	**h**
Total	**3/187 (1.6%)**	**27/582 (4.6%)**	**21/323 (6.5%)**	**51/1092 (4.7%)**
	i	**j**	**k**	**l**

carotid stenosis as measured by the NASCET method, which is equivalent to 77% ECST stenosis (Table 10–7). Similar results have been produced by the ACST randomized controlled study,[83] but in the publication of the latter study it has not been stated whether the cut-off point of 70% stenosis based on duplex is meant to be in relation to the distal internal carotid (NASCET method) or the bulb (ECST method). Plaque characterization was not performed in the ACAS study. Plaque classification into echolucent or echogenic plaques was attempted in the ACST study but no significant difference was found. In the ACST study plaque classification was performed locally without image normalization and without recording of images for assessment at the coordinating center and for enhanced quality control.

The results of the ACSRS study suggest that asymptomatic patients with plaque types 4 and 5 classified as such after image normalization and taking into consideration not only the calcified area but also the area of the plaque adjacent to the calcification not affected by acoustic shadow are at low risk even when they produce a severe stenosis. In the ACSRS study 181 (20%) of the 905 plaques with greater than 70% ECST stenosis fell into this category (Table 10–10). Also, patients with plaque types 1–3 with ECST stenosis in the range of 70–83%, which is approximately equivalent to 50–70% NASCET, are at increased risk and may need prophylactic carotid endarterectomy.

Texture Features Other Than Grayscale Median

With the exception of GSM, very few studies have investigated the association between textural features of carotid plaque ultrasonic images and patient symptoms.[86–88] The use of a GSM cut-off point of 40, by demonstrating an odds ratio of approximately four, has achieved only partial separation of symptomatic from asymptomatic carotid plaques.[89] Thus, it has been suggested that the additional use of textural features might improve the identification of high-risk plaques.[90,91] Ultrasonic texture characterization using computer algorithms has been successfully applied to liver images.[92,93]

Several of the texture features offered by the fifth module of the image analysis software have been found to be associated with plaques of different symptomatology. Many of these features measure similar parameters and good results have been obtained with several combinations. One example is given below. The value of these texture features was tested in a cross-sectional study of 409 patients referred to the vascular laboratory for diagnostic duplex scanning. Of these 242 were asymptomatic, 40 presented with amaurosis fugax, 72 with TIAs, and 55 with stroke. Plaques were classified into three main

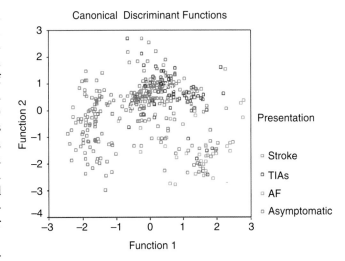

FIGURE 10–12. Discriminant function analysis of 409 plaques after image normalization (242 asymptomatic, 40 presenting with AF, 72 with TIAs, and 55 with stroke and good recovery). Three main groups of plaques are displayed.

groups (Figure 10–12) on the basis of image normalization and six features, two (homogeneity and angular second movement) based on the spatial gray level dependence matrix method (SGLDM), Runlength-SRE, plaque type (1–5), GSM, and black area close to the lumen using discriminant function analysis. Black area close to the lumen was defined as an area with gray scale pixels in the range of 0–25 that is greater than 15% of the total plaque area. The discriminant function classified plaques into three groups (Figure 10–12). The group on the left in Figure 10–12 consisted of asymptomatic plaques, the group at the top of plaques that were asymptomatic or were associated with TIAs or stroke, and the group at the bottom right of plaques that were asymptomatic or associated with amaurosis fugax. It can be argued that because all plaques start by being asymptomatic, it is very likely that the group at the top of the figure is that of unstable plaques that tend to produce TIAs or stroke. Similar arguments can be produced for the other groups. This methodology is being tested in the ACSRS natural history study and features shown to be associated with symptomatic plaques in the cross-sectional study above are proving to be good predictors of stroke.

Schulte-Altedorneburg reported that thrombosis at the plaque surface was often seen in "completely echolucent" plaques ($p < 0.001$).[94] It is likely that the echolucent plaque component represents the thrombus or its combination with the lipid core. A recent study has demonstrated a strong association between symptomatic plaques and intraluminal thrombus attached to the plaque.[95] It may well be that the presence of a black area adjacent to the lumen identifies many plaques associated with thrombus formation. This needs to be tested in future studies.

TABLE 10–11. The incidence of ipsilateral ischemic hemispheric events in relation to black area near the lumen after image normalization and severity of stenosis in the first 1098 patients admitted to the ACSRS.

| | | Black area adjacent to lumen | | | | |
| | | Absent | | Present | | |
Stenosis	Number	Events	No events	Events	No events	OR (95% CI)
50–69%	304	5 (3.4%)	140	18 (11%)	141	3.57 (1.29 to 9.89)
70–89%	655	6 (2.2%)	260	61 (16%)	328	8.10 (3.43 to 18.93)
90–99%	139	2 (4.6%)	41	25 (26%)	71	7.21 (1.62 to 32.05)

Future Perspectives—The Asymptomatic Carotid Stenosis and Risk of Stroke Study

The methodology of computer-assisted carotid plaque characterization after image normalization is now being applied in a prospective multicenter international natural history study of asymptomatic carotid stenosis with stroke as the primary end-point. The aim of the ACSRS study[84,85,95] is to identify a high-risk subgroup that has an ipsilateral stroke rate greater than 4% (ideally greater than 7%), based on clinical risk factors and the findings of the noninvasive investigations, mainly ultrasonic carotid plaque characterization (echodensity and texture) in addition to degree of stenosis. In addition, a low-risk subgroup with an ipsilateral stroke rate of less than 1% should be identified.

The ACSRS study is still in progress and the results of texture analysis of plaques have not yet been published. Only preliminary analyses with limited resuls are available.

As indicated above a number of texture features can be used in the successful identification of a high-risk group.[96–98] One of the most powerful features is the presence of a black area adjacent to the lumen. This feature has been suggested by Pedro et al.[99] and has also been shown to be associated with symptomatic plaques in the author's cross-sectional study (Figure 10–12). When applied to the ACSRS study this feature alone can identify a high-risk group for symptoms (Table 10–11). The increased risk is present across all grades of stenosis (Figures 10–13–10–15).

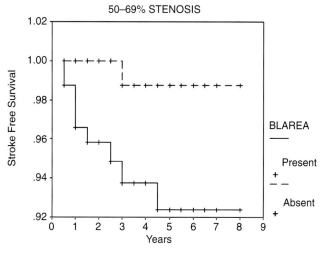

FIGURE 10–13. Kaplan–Meier estimates of the ipsilateral stroke free survival rate in patients admitted to the ACSRS study with 50–69 ECST percentage stenosis for plaques with (n = 159) and without (n = 145) a black area adjacent to the lumen after image normalization. Log rank p = 0.018.

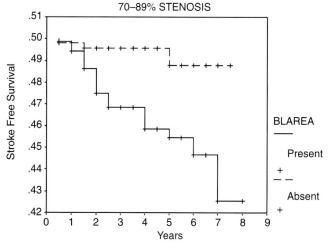

FIGURE 10–14. Kaplan–Meier estimates of the ipsilateral stroke free survival rate in patients admitted to the ACSRS study with 70–89 ECST percentage stenosis for plaques with (n = 389) and without (n = 266) a black area adjacent to the lumen after image normalization. Log rank p = 0.002.

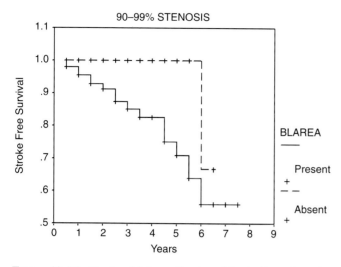

FIGURE 10–15. Kaplan–Meier estimates of the ipsilateral stroke free survival rate in patients admitted to the ACSRS study with 90–99 ECST percentage stenosis for plaques with ($n = 112$) and without ($n = 43$) a black area adjacent to the lumen after image normalization. Log rank $p = 0.02$.

Conclusions

Ultrasound, apart from being a valuable diagnostic tool, provides useful information on the natural history of carotid artery atherosclerosis. The high resolution of modern equipment and our ability to normalize images have provided the basis for reproducible plaque characterization features that can identify unstable plaques. The identification of a high-risk group of patients based on ultrasound features other than stenosis is becoming a reality. It should lead to a better selection of patients for carotid endarterectomy. Innovations such as algorithms and software identifying patients at high risk for stroke are expected to become available on duplex scanners in the near future.

References

1. Libby P. Molecular basis of acute coronary syndromes. Circulation 1995;91:2844–2850.
2. Clinton S, Underwood R, Hayes L, et al. Macrophage-colony stimulating factor gene expression in vascular cells and human atherosclerosis. Am J Pathol 1992;140:301–316.
3. Davies MJ, Richardson PD, Woolf N, Katz DR, Mahn J. Risk of thrombosis in human atherosclerotic plaques: Role of extracellular lipid, macrophage and smooth muscle cell content. Br Heart J 1993;69:377–381.
4. Falk E. Why do plaques rupture. Circulation 1992;86(6): 30–42.
5. Glagov S, Bassiouny HS, Sakaguchi Y, Goudet CA, Vito RP. Mechanical determinants of plaque modeling, remodeling and disruption. Atherosclerosis 1997;131:3–4.
6. Shah PK. Role of inflammation and metalloproteinases in plaque disruption and thrombosis. Vasc Med 1998;3: 199–206.
7. Golledge J, Greenhalgh RM, Davies AH. The symptomatic carotid plaque. Stroke 2000;31(3):774–781.
8. Shah PK. Pathophysiology of plaque rupture and the concept of plaque stabilization. Cardiol Clin 1996;14(1): 17–29.
9. Muller WD, Faust M, Kotzka J, Krone W. Mechanisms of plaque stabilization. Herz 1999;24:26–31.
10. Rabbani R, Topol EJ. Strategies to achieve coronary arterial plaque stabilization. Cardiovasc Res 1999;41:402–417.
11. Geroulakos G, Ramaswami G, Nicolaides A, James K, Labropoulos N, Belcaro G, Holloway M. Characterisation of symptomatic and asymptomatic carotid plaques using high-resolution real time ultrasonography. Br J Surg 1993; 80:1274–1277.
12. Sabetai MM, Tegos TJ, Nicolaides AN, et al. Hemispheric symptoms and carotid plaque echomorphology. J Vasc Surg 2000;31:39–49.
13. Tegos TJ, Sabetai MM, Nicolaides AN, El-Atrozy TS, Dhanjil S, Stevens JM. Patterns of brain computed tomography infarction and carotid plaque echogenicity. J Vasc Surg 2001;33:334–339.
14. Belcaro G, Nicolaides AN, Laurora G, et al. Ultrasound morphology classification of the arterial wall and cardiovascular events in a 6-year follow-up study. Arterioscler Thromb Vasc Biol 1996;16:851–856.
15. Reilly LM, Lusby RJ, Hughes L, Ferrell LD, Stoney RJ, Ehrenfeld WK. Carotid plaque histology using real-time ultrasonography: Clinical and therapeutic implications. Am J Surg 1983;146:188–193.
16. O'Donnell TF Jr, Erdoes L, Mackey WC, Mc Cullough J, Shepard A, Heggerick P, Isner J, Callow AD. Correlation of B-mode ultrasound imaging and arteriography with pathologic findings at carotid endarterectomy. Arch Surg 1985; 120:443–449.
17. Johnson JM, Kennelly MM, Decesare D, Morgan S, Sparrow A. Natural history of asymptomatic carotid plaque. Arch Surg 1985;120:1010–1012.
18. O'Holleran LW, Kennelly MM, Decesare D, McClurken M, Johnson JM. Natural history of asymptomatic carotid plaque. Five year follow-up study. Am J Surg 1987;154: 659–662.
19. Widder B, Paulat K, Hachspacher J, et al. Morphological characterization of carotid artery stenoses by ultrasound duplex scanning. Ultrasound Med Biol 1990;16:349–354.
20. Gray-Weale AC, Graham JC, Burnett JR, Burne K, Lusby RJ. Carotid artery atheroma: Comparison of preoperative B-mode ultrasound appearance with carotid endarterectomy specimen pathology. J Cardiovasc Surg 1988;29: 676–681.
21. deBray JM, Baud JM, Dauzat M for the Consensus Conference. Concensus on the morphology of carotid plaques. Cerebrovasc Dis 1997;7:289–296.
22. Polak JF, Shemanski L, O'Leary DH, et al. for the Cardiovascular Health Study. Hypoechoic plaque at US of the carotid artery: An independent risk factor for incident stroke in adults aged 65 years or older. Radiology 1998; 208:649–654.

23. Wolverson MK, Bashiti HM, Peterson GJ. Ultrasonic tissue characterization of atheromatous plaques using a high resolution real time scanner. Ultrasound Med Biol 1983; 9:599–609.

24. Aldoori MI, Baird RN, Al-Sam SZ, et al. Duplex scanning and plaque histology in cerebral ischaemia. Eur J Vasc Surg 1987;1:159–164.

25. Sterpetti AV, Schultz RD, Feldhaus RJ, et al. Ultrasonographic features of carotid plaque and the risk of subsequent neurologic deficits. Surgery 1988;104:652–660.

26. Langsfeld M, Gray-Weale AC, Lusby RJ. The role of plaque morphology and diameter reduction in the development of new symptoms in asymptomatic carotid arteries. J Vasc Surg 1989;9:548–557.

27. Bock RW, Gray-Weale AC, Mock PA, Robinson DA, Irwig L, Lusby RJ. The natural history of asymptomatic carotid artery disease. J Vasc Surg 1993;17:160–171.

28. Mathiesen EB, Bønaa KH, Joakimsen O. Echolucent plaques are associated with high risk of ischemic cerebrovascular events in carotid stenosis. The Tromsø Study. Circulation 2001;103:2171–2175.

29. Grønholdt M-LM, Nordestgaard BG, Schroeder TV, Vorstrup S, Sillesen H. Ultrasonic echolucent carotid plaques predict future strokes. Circulation 2001;104:68–73.

30. Liapis CD, Kakisis JD, Kostakis AG. Carotid stenosis. Factors affecting symptomatology. Stroke 2001;32:2782–2786.

31. AbuRahma AF, Kyer PD III, Robinson PA, Hannay RS. The correlation of ultrasonic carotid plaque morphology and carotid plaque hemmorhage: Clinical implications. Surgery 1998;124:721–728.

32. Carra G, Visona A, Bonanome A, Lusiani L, Pesavento R, Bortolon M, Pagnan A. Carotid plaque morphology and cerebrovascular events. Int Angiol 2003;22:284–289.

33. Thiele BL, Jones AM, Hobson RW, Bandyk DF, Baker WH, Sumner DS, Rutherford RB. Standards in non-invasive cerebrovascular testing. Report from the committee on standards for non-invasive vascular testing of the Joint Council of the Society for Vascular Surgery and the North American Chapter of the International Society for Cardiovascular Surgery. J Vasc Surg 1992;15:995–1003.

34. Fisher CM, Ojemann RG. A clinicopathologic study of carotid endarterectomy plaques. Rev Neurol (Paris) 1986; 142:573–576.

35. Bluth EI, Kay D, Merritt CR, et al. Sonographic characterization of carotid plaque: detection of hemorrhage. Am J Roentgenol 1986;146:1061–1065.

36. Bendick PJ, Glover JL, Hankin R, et al. Carotid plaque morphology: Correlation of duplex sonography with histology. Ann Vasc Surg 1988;2:6–13.

37. Van Damme H, Trotteur G, Vivario M, et al. Echographic characterization of carotid plaques. Acta Chir Belg 1993; 93:233–238.

38. Kardoulas DG, Katsamouris AN, Gallis PT, et al. Ultrasonographic and histologic characteristics of symptom-free and symptomatic carotid plaque. Cardiovasc Surg 1996;4: 580–590.

39. European Carotid Plaque Study Group. Carotid artery plaque composition—Relationship to clinical presentation and ultrasound B-mode imaging. Eur J Vasc Endovasc Surg 1995;10:23–30.

40. Weinberger J, Marks SJ, Gaul JJ, et al. Atherosclerotic plaque at the carotid artery bifurcation. Correlation of ultrasonographic imaging with morphology. J Ultrasound Med 1987;6:363–366.

41. Shah PK, Falk E, Badimon JJ, et al. Human monocyte–derived macrophages induce collagen breakdown in fibrous caps of atherosclerotic plaques. Potential role of matrix degrting metaloproteinases and implications for plaque rapture. Circulation 1995;92:1565–1569.

42. Lammie GA, Wardlaw J, Allan P, et al. What pathological components indicate carotid atheroma activity and can these be identified reliably using ultrasound? Eur J Ultrasound 2000;11:77–86.

43. Urbano LA, Perren F, Rossetti AO, et al. Thrombus in the internal carotid artery complicating an "unstable" atheromatous plaque. Circulation 2003;107:e19–20.

44. El-Barghouty NM, Nicolaides A, Bahal V, Geroulakos G, Androulakis A. The identification of high risk carotid plaque. Eur J Vasc Surg 1996;11:470–478.

45. Biasi GM, Sampaolo A, Mingazzini P, de Amicis P, El-Barghouti N, Nicolaides AN. Computer analysis of ultrasonic plaque echolucency in identifying high risk carotid bifurcation lesions. Eur J Vasc Endovasc Surg 1999;17:476–479.

46. El-Atrozy T, Nicolaides A, Tegos T, Zarka AZ, Griffin M, Sabetai M. The effect of B-mode image standardisation on the echodensity of symptomatic and asymptomatic carotid bifurcation plaques. Int Angiol 1998;17:179–186.

47. Tegos TJ, Sabetai MM, Nicolaides AN, et al. Comparability of the ultrasonic tissue characteristics of carotid plaques. J Ultrasound Med 2000;14:399–407.

48. Sabetai MM, Tegos TJ, Nicolaides AN, Dhanjil S, Pare GJ, Stevens JM. Reproducibility of computer-quantified carotid plaque echogenicity. Stroke 2000;31:2189–2196.

49. Tegos TJ, Sabetai MM, Nicolaides AN, et al. Correlates of embolic events detected by means of transcranial Doppler in patients with carotid atheroma. J Vasc Surg 2001;33:131–138.

50. Sabetai MM, Tegos TJ, Nicolaides AN, El-Atrozy TS, Dhanjil S, Griffin M, Belcaro G, Geroulakos G. Hemispheric symptoms and carotid plaque echomorphology. J Vasc Surg 2000;31:39–49.

51. Sabetai MS, Coker J, Sheppard M, Tegos T, Belcaro G, Stansby G, Nicolaides AN. The association of carotid plaque necrotic core volume and echogenicity with ipsilateral hemispheric symptoms. Circulation 2001;104(Suppl 2):671 (abst).

52. Gronholdt M-LM, Nordestgaard BG, Bentzon J, Wiebe BM, Zhou J, Falk E, Sillesen H. Macrophages are associated with lipid-rich carotid artery plaques, echolucency on B-mode imaging, and elevated plasma lipid levels. J Vasc Surg 2002;35:137–145.

53. Richardson PD, Davies MJ, Born GVR. Influence of plaque configuration and stress distribution and fissuring of coronary atherosclerotic plaque. Lancet 1989;ii:941–944.

54. Ku DN, McCord BN. Cyclic stress causes rupture of the atherosclerotic plaque cap. Circulation 1993;88(Suppl 1):1362 (abst).

55. Glagov S, Bassiouny HS, Sakaguchi Y, Goudet CA, Vito RP. Mechanical determinants of plaque modeling, remodeling and disruption. Atherosclerosis 1997; 131(Suppl):S13–S14.

56. Zukowski AJ, Nicolaides AN, Lewis RT, Mansfield AO, Williams MA, Helmis E, Malouf GM, Thomas D, Al-Kutoubi A, Kyprianou P, et al. The correlation between carotid plaque ulceration and cerebral infarction seen on CT scan. J Vasc Surg 1984;1:782–786.

57. Persson AV, Robichaux WT, Silverman M. The natural history of carotid plaque development. Arch Surg 1983;118:1048–1052.

58. Seager JM, Klingman N. The relationship between carotid plaque composition and neurological symptoms. J Surg Res 1987;43:78–85.

59. Sterpetti AV, Hunter WJ, Schulz RD. Importance of ulceration of carotid plaque. J Cardiovasc Surg 1991;32:154–158.

60. Eliasziw M, Streifler JY, Fox JA. Significance of plaque ulceration in symptomatic patients with high-grade stenosis. Stroke 1994;25:305–308.

61. Fisher GG, Anderson DC, Farber R, Lebow S. Prediction of carotid disease by ultrasound and digital subtraction angiography. Arch Neurol 1985;42:224–227.

62. O'Leary DH, Holen J, Ricotta JJ Roe S, Schenk EA. Carotid bifurcation disease: Prediction of ulceration with B-mode ultrasound. Radiology 1987;162:523–525.

63. Comerota AJ, Katz ML, White JV, Grosh JD. The preoperative diagnosis of the ulcerated carotid atheroma. J Vasc Surg 1990;11:505–510.

64. Farber R, Bromer M, Anderson D, Loewenson R, Yock D, Larson D. B-mode real-time ultrasonic carotid imaging: Impact on decision-making and prediction of surgical findings. Neurology 1984;34:541–544.

65. Ricotta JJ. Plaque characterization by B-mode scan. Surg Clin North Am 1990;70:191–199.

66. Goodson SF, Flanigan DP, Bishara RA, Schuler JJ, Kikta MJ, Meyer JP. Can carotid duplex scanning supplant arteriography in patients with focal carotid territory symptoms? J Vasc Surg 1987;5:551–557.

67. Rubin JR, Bondi JA, Rhodes RS. Duplex scanning versus conventional arteriography for the evaluation of carotid artery plaque morphology. Surgery 1987;102:749–755.

68. Iannuzzi A, Wilcosky T, Mercuri M, Rubba P, Bryan FA, Bond G. Ultrasonographic correlates of carotid atherosclerosis in transient ischemic attack and stroke. Stroke 1995;26:614–619.

69. Golledge J, Cuming R, Ellis M, Davies AH, Greenhalgh RM. Carotid plaque characteristics and presenting symptom. Br J Surg 1997;84:1697–1701.

70. North American Symptomatic Carotid Endarterectomy Trial Collaborators. Beneficial effect of carotid endarterectomy in symptomatic patients with high-grade carotid stenosis. N Engl J Med 1991;325:445–453.

71. Executive Committee for the Asymptomatic Carotid Atherosclerosis Study. Endarterectomy for asymptomatic carotid artery stenosis. J Am Med Assoc 1995;273:1421–1428.

72. Nicolaides AN, Shifrin EG, Bradbury A, Dhanjil S, Griffin M, Belcaro G, Williams M. Angiographic and duplex grading of internal carotid stenosis: Can we overcome the confusion? J Endovasc Surg 1996;3:158–165.

73. European Carotid Surgery Trialists Collaborative Group. MRC European carotid surgery trial: Interim results for symptomatic patients with severe (70–99%) or with mild (0–29%) carotid stenosis. Lancet 1991;337:1235–1243.

74. De Bray JM, Glatt B. Quantification of atheromatous stenosis in the extracranial internal carotid artery. Cerebrovasc Dis 1995;5:414–426.

75. Chambers BR, Norris JW. Outcome in patients with asymptomatic neck bruits. N Engl J Med 1986;315:860–865.

76. Hennerici M, Hulsbomer HB, Hefter H, Lammerts D, Rautenberg W. Natural history of asymptomatic extracranial arterial disease. Results of a long-term prospective study. Brain 1987;110:777–791.

77. Norris JW, Zhu CZ, Bornstein NM, Chambers BR. Vascular risks of asymptomatic carotid stenosis. Stroke 1991;22:1485–1490.

78. Zhu CZ, Norris JW. A therapeutic window for carotid endarterectomy in patients with asymptomatic carotid stenosis. Can J Surg 1991;34:437–440.

79. Mackey AE, Abrahamowicz M, Langlois Y, Battista R, Simard D, Bourque F, et al. Outcome of asymptomatic patients with carotid disease. Neurology 1997;48:896–903.

80. Nadareishvili ZG, Rothwell PM, Beletsky V, Pagniello A, Norris JW. Long-term risk of stroke and other vascular events in patients with asymptomatic carotid artery stenosis. Arch Neurol 2002;59:1162–1166.

81. The European Carotid Surgery Trialists Collaborative Group. Risk of stroke in the distribution of an asymptomatic carotid artery. Lancet 1995;345:209–212.

82. Inzitari D, Eliasziw M, Gates P, Sharpe BL, Chan RKT, Meldrum HE, et al. The causes and risk of stroke in patients with asymptomatic internal-carotid-artery stenosis. N Engl J Med 2000;342:1693–1700.

83. MRC Asymptomatic Carotid Surgery Trial (ACST) Collaborative Group. Prevention of disabling and fatal strokes by successful carotid endarterectomy in patients without recent neurological symptoms: Randomized controlled trial. Lancet 2004;363:1491–1502.

84. Nicolaides AN, Kakkos SK, Griffin M, Sabetai M, Dhanjil S, Tegos T, Thomas DJ, Giannoukas A, Geroulakos G, Georgiou N, Francis S, Ioannidou E, Dore CJ, and the Asymptomatic Carotid Stenosis and Risk of Stroke (ACSRS) Study Group. Severity of asymptomatic carotid stenosis and risk of ipsilateral hemispheric ischaemic events: Results from the ACSRS Study. Eur J Vasc Endovas Surg 2006;31:336.

85. Nicolaides A, Kakkos SK, Griffin M, Sabetai M, Dhanjil S, Thomas DJ, Geroulakos G, Georgiou N, Francis S, Ioannidou E, Doré CJ. Effect of image normalization on carotid plaque classification and risk of ipsilateral hemispheric events: Results from the ACSRS study. Vascular 2005;13:211–221.

86. Mazzone AM, Urbani MP, Picano E, Paterni M, Borgatti E, De Fabritiis A, et al. In vivo ultrasonic parametric imaging of carotid atherosclerotic plaque by video densitometric technique. Angiology 1995;46:663–672.

87. Elatrozy T, Nicolaides A, Tegos T, Griffin M. The objective characterisation of ultrasonic carotid plaque features. Eur J Vasc Endovasc Surg 1998;16:223–230.

88. Tegos TJ, Mavrophoros D, Sabetai MM, Elatrozy TS, Dhanjil S, Karapataki M, *et al*. Types of neurovascular symptoms and carotid plaque ultrasonic textural characteristics. J Ultrasound Med 2001;20:113–121.

89. Elatrozy T. Preoperative characterisation of carotid plaques. Ph.D. thesis. Imperial College, University of London, 2000.

90. Christodoulou CI, Pattichis CS, Pantziaris M, Tegos T, Nicolaides A, Elatrozy T, *et al*. Multi-feature texture analysis for the classification of carotid plaques. In: *IJCNN '99. Proceedings of International Joint Conference on Neural Networks*, 1999 July 10–16, Washington DC. 1999;5:3591–3596.

91. Kyriacou E, Pattichis MS, Christodoulou CI, Pattichis CS, Kakkos S, Griffin M, Nicolaides A. Ultrasound imaging in the analysis of carotid plaque morphology for the assessment of stroke. In: Suri JS, Yyan C, Wilson DL, Laxminarayan S (eds). *Advanced Plaque Imaging: Pixel to Molecular*. Studies in Health Technology and Informatics. IOS Press, 2005;113:241–75 (ISBN:1-58603-516-9).

92. Wu Q. Automatic tumor detection for MRI liver images. Ph.D. thesis. London, England: Imperial College, 1996;48–59.

93. Jirák D, Dezortová M, Tamir P, Hájek M. Texture analysis of human liver. J Magn Reson Imaging 2002;15:68–74.

94. Schulte-Altedorneburg G, Droste DW, Haas N, Kemeny V, Nabavi DG, Fuzesi L, Ringelstein EB. Preoperative B-mode ultrasound plaque appearance compared with carotid endarterectomy specimen histology. Acta Neurol Scand 2000;101:188–194.

95. Fisher M, Paganini-Hill A, Martin A, Cosgrove M, Toole JF, Barnett HJM, Norris J. Carotid plaque pathology. Thrombosis, ulceration and stroke pathogenesis. Stroke 2005;36: 253–257.

96. Nicolaides AN, Griffin M, Kakkos SK, Geroulakos G, Kyriakou E. In: Mansour MA, Labropoulos N (eds). *Evaluation of Carotid Plaque Morphology in Vascular Diagnosis*, pp. 131–148. Philadelphia: Elsevier Saunders, 2005.

97. Nicolaides AN. Asymptomatic carotid stensosis and risk of stroke. Identification of a high risk group (ACSRS). Int Angiol 1995;14:21–23.

98. Nicolaides A, Kakkos S, Sabetai M, Griffin M, Ioannidou E, Francis S, Kyriakou E. Asympomatic carotid stenosis and risk of stroke: Natural history study. Stroke 2005;36:424 (abst).

99. Pedro LM, Fernandes e Fernandes J, Pedro MM, Goncalves I, Dias NV, Fernandes e Fernandes R, Caneiro TF, Balsinha C. Ultrasonographic risk score of carotid plaques. Eur J Vasc Endovasc Surg 2002;24:492–498.

11

Carotid Plaque Echolucency Measured by Grayscale Median Identifies Patients at Increased Risk of Stroke during Carotid Stenting. The Imaging in Carotid Angioplasty and Risk of Stroke Study

A. Froio, G. Deleo, C. Piazzoni, V. Camesasca, A. Liloia, M. Lavitrano, and G. M. Biasi

Stenting of carotid artery disease has emerged as a potential alternative to carotid endarterectomy (CEA), the current gold standard treatment for carotid artery lesions.[1-4] After the initial experience with an unacceptably high rate of neurologic complications, the results have now improved, and, as a consequence, several trials have been planned to compare carotid angioplasty/stenting (CAS) with CEA.[5]

Even though it is generally accepted that the composition and the characteristics of the plaque may influence the outcome of CEA and CAS, especially in the case of CAS in which the plaque is not removed but remodeled, indications for either one of the two procedures are mostly based (both in trial and in clinical practice) on the percentage of stenosis and the presence or absence of preprocedural neurologic symptoms, whereas the features of the plaque are somehow disregarded if not ignored. The reason for this is related to the fact that the percentage of stenosis, as well as the presence or absence of symptoms, is easy to identify and quantify, whereas the plaque is usually defined as soft, lipidic, fibrolipidic, hemorrhagic, colliquated, ulcerated, pretty homogeneous, etc., which makes the parameter rather undetermined and unreliable.[6]

But the advent of high-resolution B-mode scanners and the use of a quantitative, computer-assisted index of echogenicity [such as grayscale median (GSM)] introduced by our team have greatly improved the correlation between plaque characterization and clinical features.[7, 8]

The aim of the Imaging in Carotid Angioplasty and Risk of Stroke (ICAROS) registry was to determine the preprocedural echographic criteria, which can identify the carotid plaque related to a higher risk of stroke during CAS so that a better selection of candidates for CAS may be made.[9,10]

Echographic Evaluation of Carotid Plaque

The study of carotid plaque morphology by ultrasonography, which usually relies on visual characterization based on subjective and qualitative evaluation of the B-mode images, has created controversies concerning the clinical importance of some characteristics of the plaque observed with duplex scan (i.e., ulceration or intraplaque hemorrhage and their correlation with the presence or absence of neurologic symptoms).[11]

Ulceration and hemorrhage are frequently defined according to subjective criteria, which is liable to create some confusion. Carr and colleagues demonstrated this because, in their study, they found both a significant and a nonsignificant correlation between neurologic symptoms and the presence of ulceration and hemorrhage, using different definitions of ulceration (gross ulceration versus microscopic ulceration: correlation only with gross ulceration; $p = 0.02$) and hemorrhage (plaque hemorrhage versus intraplaque hemorrhage: borderline correlation only with intraplaque hemorrhage; $p = 0.06$).[12] As a consequence of this, Greenhalgh wrote: "The fact that it has taken so long for plaque type to be shown to relate to stroke risk in asymptomatic severely stenosed carotid arteries can mean one of two things: it can mean plaque type never has and never will relate to stroke risk or second, that the precise combination of findings has not been clearly recognized."

To overcome the unreliability related to the morphologic characteristics of carotid plaques, we should keep in mind that echography means detection of echoes, that is, detection of echogenicity. Echography can reliably register areas with a lot of echoes (hyperechoic or echogenic) and areas with few echoes (hypoechoic or echolucent).

Echogenicity could be assessed according to the Gray-Weale/Geroulakos classification.[13,14] Only through the advent of high-resolution B-mode scanners did a more reliable analysis of echogenicity became available.

Barnett and colleagues recently wrote: "Modern ultrasound done in well-equipped and closely supervised laboratories can distinguish between echodense (echogenic) and echolucent carotid lesions . . . however, such sophisticated technology did not exist when NASCET was launched in 1987; at that time it was an inadequate method to evaluate both the degree of stenosis and the nature of the carotid lesion causing the symptoms."[15]

The improvement in ultrasonography allowed several authors to assess the relationship between echogenicity and neurologic events. In the Cardiovascular Health Study, 4886 individuals aged 65 years or older without symptoms of cerebrovascular diseases were followed for an average of 3.3 years.[16] Hypoechoic plaques were associated with a risk of stroke. Liapis and colleagues found evidence that in a cohort of patients with carotid stenosis followed for an average of 3.6 years, the presence of echolucent plaques was related to the development of neurologic events.[17] Gronholdt and colleagues and Mathiesen and colleagues performed prospective studies to assess the relationship between plaque morphology and the risk of ischemic stroke.[18,19] In the Tromso Study, subjects with echolucent plaques have an increased risk of ischemic cerebrovascular events, independent of the degree of stenosis and cardiovascular risk factors. Gronholdt and colleagues found evidence that echolucent plaques causing greater than 50% stenosis are associated with a risk of future stroke. Thus, echolucency is now recognized as an important factor in determining future neurologic events.

Further improvement in carotid echographic evaluation has been achieved through the introduction of a computer-assisted *objective* grading of the echogenicity of carotid plaques, namely the GSM.

Grayscale Median Calculation

The GSM is a computer-assisted grading of the echogenicity of carotid plaques. It is a measure of overall plaque echogenicity, which is a quantitative index of the echoes registered from the plaque.

The following conditions are needed to ensure the reliability of the GSM.

Duplex Scanner Setup

Every duplex scanner makes it possible to collect images with the characteristics required for the computer-assisted analysis of echogenicity. For GSM calculation there are no unsuitable duplex scanners.

A 7-MHz linear array single or multifrequency transducer should be used. The dynamic range is the range in acoustic power (in decibels) between the faintest and the strongest signals that can be displayed on the screen. The decrease of the dynamic range increases the apparent contrast in the image. For GSM calculation the maximum dynamic range should be used in order to have the greatest possible display of gray scale values (grayer and flatter image).

The frame rate, which means the number of scannings that the probe does producing the images, must be positioned at the maximum level, ensuring good temporal resolution.

The persistence is the number of frames that are mathematically added to produce each image. Higher persistence tends to suppress noise, but it is always done at the expense of time resolution, and it may blur real targets. The persistence is displayed on the screen device as a series of numbers from 1 to 5 and the right persistence would be 2 or 3 (medium to low level).

A linear postprocessing curve is used because image normalization is achieved with linear scaling.

The overall gain should be increased until the plaque can be easily recognized and noise appears within the lumen. It should then be decreased to obtain a lumen free of noise (black).

The time gain compensation (TGC) curve is adjusted (gently sloping) with the aim of obtaining images where the far and near walls of the artery produce the same echogenicity. At the level of the arterial lumen no gains of the TGC curve must be done. This is essential for normalization of carotid plaques with anterior and posterior components. The consequence of this is that the ultrasound beam should be at 90° to the arterial wall, with a horizontal adventitia.

Image Recording

The patient should be in supine position. The carotid vessels are analyzed using different longitudinal views (anterolateral, lateral, and posterolateral). The minimum depth should be used, so that the plaque occupies a large part of the image. Excessive magnification is not required.

In case of acoustic shadow the image can be analyzed only if >50% of the area depicts acoustic information. The GSM cannot be calculated in plaques without any ultrasound information due to acoustic shadowing. The larger the section of plaque that can be visualized, the more accurate is the information provided by GSM.

Before image recording, the following criteria should be fulfilled:

1. Blood: a noiseless vessel lumen in the vicinity of the plaque.

2. Adventitia: in the proximity of the plaque it should be bright, thick, and horizontal.
3. Plaque: well defined and with the maximum thickness.
4. Anterior and posterior walls of the carotid artery should be visible.

The following images (in longitudinal projections) should be recorded:

1. The B-mode (grayscale) image.
2. The color image: may help in the delineation of the luminal margin of the plaque (especially with hypoechoic dark plaques).

Attention should be paid in order to have B-mode and color image in the same plane.

Digital storage media (magnetooptical disk and compact disk) are preferred to analogic video tape requiring a video grabber card.

Image Normalization and Grayscale Median Calculation

GSM is calculated using Adobe Photoshop (5.0 or higher).

In Adobe Photoshop both the B-mode and the color image should be open. In the B-mode image the color information should be discarded: from the "Image" menu, click on "Mode," then "Grayscale."

Using the "Lasso" tool, drag the pointer to outline the plaque. Then, click on "Histogram" in the "Image" menu. The "median" value shown in the panel is the GSM.

Hypoechoic dark (echolucent) regions are associated with a GSM that tended to approach 0, whereas hyperechoic bright (echogenic) regions are associated with a GSM that tended to approach 255.

The GSM calculated in this manner is not standardized and consequently the GSM is influenced by duplex scanner settings. The lack of reproducibility of nonstandardized GSM has been demonstrated by our group and by others: the GSM cut-off point for the identification of carotid plaques at increased risk of producing stroke was 50 in Milan and 32 in London.[7,20]

Normalization (standardization) allows comparison of images from different scanners by different ultrasonographers. Due to normalization, GSM is a highly reproducible index of echogenicity.

Image normalization is a grayscale transformation using linear scaling: grayscale values of all pixels in an image are adjusted according to two reference points, blood and adventitia. Blood and adventitia were selected (instead of muscles, vertebrae, intima-media complex, etc.) because they are easily and clearly recognizable in the vicinity of the plaque and constitute the two distinct ends of grayscale (blood = dark, adventitia = bright). The process modifies the image such that in the resultant

image the GSM of the blood is in the range of 0–5 and the GSM of the adventitia in the range of 185–195.

Several steps are required for image normalization.

Using the "Lasso" tool, drag the pointer to select an area in the blood that should be free of noise. To check this, in the "Image" menu click on "Histogram." The "median" value shown in the panel is the GSM. The GSM of the selected area in the blood should be 0. If not, the gain of duplex scanner is not set properly (see above).

Similarly, using the "Lasso" tool, the brightest part of the adventitia on the same arterial wall of the plaque should be selected. It is important to note the following:

- Image magnification should be performed before adventitia outlining.
- The selected area should not be too small (area, not a point!).
- The selected area should be horizontal.

The GSM of adventitia should then be obtained using the "Histogram" function. Unlike the GSM of blood, every GSM value measured in the adventitia is accepted.

To normalize the image, click on "Image" menu then "Adjustments" and finally "Curves." The straight line shown in the panel represents the relationship between the grayscale of the input (x-axis) image and that of the output (y-axis). Each axis has a black and a white edge: this is the grayscale, ranging from 0 (completely black) to 255 (completely white).

The aim of normalization is to modify the subjectivity related to the echographic examination. This purpose can be achieved using the brightest (adventitia) and the faintest (blood) area of the image: in particular conditions (the duplex scanner settings described above) these areas are independent of the type of duplex scanner and the ultrasonographer. Normalizing the image the faintest point remains unchanged with a GSM value of 0 before and 0 after standardization (a proper gain adjustment is essential for this purpose). On the other hand, the GSM value of the brightest area (adventitia) drives all the normalization process: the adventitial GSM value measured before (input value) is converted arbitrarily to a GSM value of 190 (output value). In the normalized image the GSM value of blood and adventitia is 0 and 190, respectively, independent of the type of duplex scanner and the ultrasonographer.

In Adobe Photoshop, the straight line shown in the panel should be modified so that the new line crosses a new point with the input value corresponding to the measured adventitial GSM value and the output value corresponding to 190.

The image is now standardized. Using the "Lasso" tool the plaque should be outlined. In the "Histogram" panel the following measurements are obtained:

1. GSM, defined as the median of overall gray shades of the pixels in the plaque.

2. Total percentage of echolucent pixels, defined as the percentage of pixels with GSM < 25 (PEP25).

The reproducibility of this method is high.[21,22]

If you need help in measuring the GSM, please feel free to contact us at gsm@unimib.org.

Embolic Burden and Stroke Risk in Carotid Stenting

The embolic risk during CAS is well documented. Markus and colleagues showed that, during angioplasty, multiple embolic signals were detected immediately after balloon inflation in 90% of cases. Embolic signals were common immediately after the procedure (80% of cases) but thereafter became less frequent.[23]

Coggia and colleagues developed an *ex vivo* human model to study the embolic potential of carotid bifurcation angioplasty and stenting. The studies showed that carotid angioplasty and stenting generate embolic particles after each stage of the procedure and that the size of most embolic particles generated was less than 120 μm, with many platelet or cholesterol microthrombi. The maximum size of particles detected in the last phase, i.e., during the balloon angioplasty, was between 1000 and 2100 μm.[24]

Jordan and colleagues showed that CAS, compared with CEA, is accomplished with more than eight times the rate of microemboli when evaluated with transcranial Doppler ultrasonography (8.8 versus 74.0; $p = 0.0001$).[25]

Ohki and colleagues showed that echolucent plaques ($p < 0.05$) and plaques with stenosis of 90% or more ($p < 0.05$) generated a higher number of embolic particles following balloon angioplasty and stenting. Multiple regression analysis revealed that echogenicity and severity of stenosis were significant independent risk factors.[26]

Henry and colleagues showed that the number of particles released during CAS and collected by means of a distal balloon occlusion device was higher in echolucent plaques with a low GSM.[27]

Several studies analyzed the impact of emboli on the brain. Using transcranial Doppler ultrasonography, Ackerstaff and colleagues studied the effect of the total number of particles detected during CEA on perioperative neurologic events. It was demonstrated that microemboli (more than 10) noted during the procedure were related to both intraoperative and postoperative cerebral complications. Isolated microemboli never resulted in new morphologic changes on postoperative cerebral computed tomographic (CT) scans. On the other hand, the detection of more than 10 microemboli was significantly related to new lesions on magnetic resonance imaging (MRI).[28]

Tübler and colleagues analyzed the relationship between particles collected by means of a distal balloon occlusion and the occurrence of neurologic complications during CAS. The maximum area, the maximum diameter, and the number of captured particles were higher in patients with cerebrovascular accidents than in those with uncomplicated procedures.[29]

These studies showed that the incidence of neurologic complications during CAS is related to embolization from carotid plaque: it appears clear that the reduction of embolic particles from the carotid plaque is essential to decrease neurologic deficits.

Based on these assumptions, our group suggested that plaque echogenicity measured by the GSM can be a useful indicator of embolic potential in the carotid arteries.[6,9]

The Imaging in Carotid Angioplasty and Risk of Stroke ICAROS Study

ICAROS was a registry of carotid angioplasty and stenting procedures that reported any cerebral event following the procedure and correlated the risk of cerebral embolization with the echographic characteristics of the carotid plaque. The aim of the ICAROS study was to determine the preprocedural echographic criteria, which can identify the carotid plaque related to a higher risk of stroke during CAS, so that a better selection of candidates for CAS may be performed.

The study was open to all interventionalists performing carotid endovascular procedures. Participants were free to apply their own endovascular techniques and devices, including cerebral protection mechanisms (percutaneous femoral or cervical approach, minimal surgical dissection of the common carotid artery, primary stenting, preliminary and/or postdeployment dilation, etc.), but techniques and instrumentation were precisely documented.

All cerebral ischemic events following the procedure were reported and investigated in detail with physical examination by an independent neurologist and with cerebral CT or MRI. The degree of stenosis was calculated based on the ratio of the peak systolic velocity of the internal carotid artery to that of the common carotid artery. A complete angiographic evaluation of supraaortic trunks, carotid arteries, and intracranial circulation was performed.

Several training courses on how to set up the duplex scanner for the collection of the images were organized worldwide for ultrasonographers from the participating centers. Duplex scanning images were then sent to the coordinating center (Bassini Teaching Hospital), where the optimal color and B-mode images were transferred onto a personal computer. Image normalization and calculation of the GSM were performed by the same operator (who was blinded to clinical data and outcome) by means of Adobe Photoshop 5.0 software, as previously described. The overall rate of neurological complications was 6.7% (28/418), with transient ischemic attack 3.1% (13/418), minor strokes 2.2% (9/418), and major strokes 1.4% (6/418), while no deaths were observed.[10]

The GSM value in complicated patients was significantly lower than in uncomplicated cases, both in the stroke ($p < 0.005$) and in the stroke plus transient ischemic attack (TIA) ($p < 0.005$) subset. A receiver operating characteristic (ROC) curve was used to choose the best GSM cut-off value: the most successful threshold value was 25. The prevalence of a GSM value of less than 25 (echolucent plaques) was high 155/418 (37%) patients. Eleven out of 155 patients with GSM $\leq$ 25 had a stroke (7.1%) compared to 4 out of 263 patients with GSM > 25 (1.5%, $p = 0.005$). The event rates increased to 12.9% and 3.0%, respectively, when both stroke and TIA were counted ($p = 0.002$).

There were 5/219 (2.3%) strokes in protected and 10/199 (5.0%) in unprotected procedures ($p = 0.18$). However, protection gave different results in the GSM subgroups: in patients with GSM $\leq$ 25 a brain protection device tended to increase the risk of stroke (12.5% vs. 5.2%, $p = 0.15$), whereas it had a protective value in the echogenic subgroup (0% vs. 4.8%, $p = 0.01$).

The overall neurological complication rate was higher in primary lesions than in restenoses (5.2% vs. 2.2%, $p =$ ns). This difference was observed also in GSM > 25 patients (4.0% vs. 0%, $p < 0.05$) but not in GSM $\leq$ 25 patients (6.6% vs. 7.8%, $p =$ ns).

The stroke rate was 2.8% for asymptomatic and 5.3% for symptomatic patients ($p =$ ns), with a similar trend in GSM subsets. The neurological complication rate was 1.5% (3/202) in <85% carotid stenosis rate subset and 5.6% (12/216) in $\geq$85% ($p < 0.05$). The neurological complication rate was significantly higher in patients with positive cerebral CT than in those with negative CT (7.7% vs. 2.4%, $p < 0.05$).

A multivariate regression analysis revealed that GSM (OR = 7.11, $p = 0.0019$) and degree of stenosis (OR = 5.76, $p = 0.010$) are significant independent predictors of stroke alone, while preprocedural symptomatology (OR = 2.92, $p = 0.061$) and preprocedural brain CT (OR = 2.54, $p = 0.099$) are borderline significant. Similar results were found in the analysis of stroke plus TIA as endpoints.

Conclusions

The clinical impact of GSM relies on the ability to identify a vast number of patients at higher risk of stroke during CAS and to distinguish subsets of patients (with restenosis or with the protected procedure) in which the rate of neurological complications is different from the overall population.

A computer-assisted echogenicity evaluation through image normalization and measurement of GSM is a simple method to identify preprocedurally high- risk carotid plaques, in which endovascular treatment could be burdened with a higher risk. GSM is one of the parameters that should be mandatory for indication to treatment in order to quantify the individual risk related to the specific procedure. A low GSM value is not an absolute contraindication to CAS, but an index related to a higher risk for the procedure.

Echographic evaluation of carotid plaque through GSM should therefore always be included in the planning of any clinical trial on the endovascular treatment of carotid lesions.

References

1. Ferguson GG, Eliasziw M, Barr HW, et al. The North American Symptomatic Carotid Endarterectomy Trial: Surgical results in 1415 patients. Stroke 1999;30:1751–8.
2. MRC European Carotid Surgery Trial. Interim results for symptomatic patients with severe (70–99%) or with mild (0–29%) carotid stenosis. European Carotid Surgery Trialists' Collaborative Group. Lancet 1991;337:1235–43.
3. Executive Committee for the Asymptomatic Carotid Atherosclerosis Study. Endarterectomy for asymptomatic carotid artery stenosis. JAMA 1995;273:1421–8.
4. Halliday A, Mansfield A, Marro J, et al. Prevention of disabling and fatal strokes by successful carotid endarterectomy in patients without recent neurological symptoms: Randomised controlled trial. Lancet 2004;363:1491–502.
5. Roubin GS, New G, Iyer SS, et al. Immediate and late clinical outcomes of carotid artery stenting in patients with symptomatic and asymptomatic carotid artery stenosis: A 5-year prospective analysis. Circulation 2001;103:532–7.
6. Biasi GM. Is it time to reconsider the selection criteria for conventional or endovascular repair of carotid artery stenosis in the prevention of cerebral ischemia? J Endovasc Ther 2001;8:339–40.
7. Biasi GM, Mingazzini PM, Baronio L, et al. Carotid plaque characterization using digital image processing and its potential in future studies of carotid endarterectomy and angioplasty. J Endovasc Surg 1998;5:240–6.
8. Biasi GM, Sampaolo A, Mingazzini P, De Amicis P, El-Barghouty N, Nicolaides AN. Computer analysis of ultrasonic plaque echolucency in identifying high risk carotid bifurcation lesions. Eur J Vasc Endovasc Surg 1999;17:476–9.
9. Biasi GM, Ferrari SA, Nicolaides AN, Mingazzini PM, Reid D. The ICAROS registry of carotid artery stenting. Imaging in Carotid Angioplasties and Risk of Stroke. J Endovasc Ther 2001;8:46–52.
10. Biasi GM, Froio A, Diethrich EB, et al. Carotid plaque echolucency increases the risk of stroke in carotid stenting: The Imaging in Carotid Angioplasty and Risk of Stroke (ICAROS) study. Circulation 2004;110:756–62.

11. European Carotid Plaque Study Group. Carotid artery plaque composition—relationship to clinical presentation and ultrasound B-mode imaging. Eur J Vasc Endovasc Surg 1995;10:23–30.

12. Carr S, Farb A, Pearce WH, Virmani R, Yao JS. Atherosclerotic plaque rupture in symptomatic carotid artery stenosis. J Vasc Surg 1996;23:755–65; discussion 765–6.

13. Geroulakos G, Ramaswami G, Nicolaides A, et al. Characterization of symptomatic and asymptomatic carotid plaques using high-resolution real-time ultrasonography. Br J Surg 1993;80:1274–7.

14. Gray-Weale AC, Graham JC, Burnett JR, Byrne K, Lusby RJ. Carotid artery atheroma: Comparison of preoperative B-mode ultrasound appearance with carotid endarterectomy specimen pathology. J Cardiovasc Surg (Torino) 1988; 29:676–81.

15. Barnett HJ, Eliasziw M, Meldrum H. Plaque morphology as a risk factor for stroke. JAMA 2000;284:177.

16. Polak JF, Shemanski L, O'Leary DH, et al. Hypoechoic plaque at US of the carotid artery: An independent risk factor for incident stroke in adults aged 65 years or older. Cardiovascular Health Study. Radiology 1998;208: 649–54.

17. Liapis CD, Kakisis JD, Kostakis AG. Carotid stenosis: Factors affecting symptomatology. Stroke 2001;32:2782–6.

18. Mathiesen EB, Bonaa KH, Joakimsen O. Echolucent plaques are associated with high risk of ischemic cerebrovascular events in carotid stenosis: The Tromso study. Circulation 2001;103:2171–5.

19. Gronholdt ML, Nordestgaard BG, Schroeder TV, Vorstrup S, Sillesen H. Ultrasonic echolucent carotid plaques predict future strokes. Circulation 2001;104:68–73.

20. el-Barghouty N, Geroulakos G, Nicolaides A, Androulakis A, Bahal V. Computer-assisted carotid plaque characterisation. Eur J Vasc Endovasc Surg 1995;9:389–93.

21. Elatrozy T, Nicolaides A, Tegos T, Zarka AZ, Griffin M, Sabetai M. The effect of B-mode ultrasonic image standardisation on the echodensity of symptomatic and asymptomatic carotid bifurcation plaques. Int Angiol 1998;17:179–86.

22. Sabetai MM, Tegos TJ, Nicolaides AN, Dhanjil S, Pare GJ, Stevens JM. Reproducibility of computer-quantified carotid plaque echogenicity: Can we overcome the subjectivity? Stroke 2000;31:2189–96.

23. Markus HS, Clifton A, Buckenham T, Brown MM. Carotid angioplasty. Detection of embolic signals during and after the procedure. Stroke 1994;25:2403–6.

24. Coggia M, Goeau-Brissonniere O, Duval JL, Leschi JP, Letort M, Nagel MD. Embolic risk of the different stages of carotid bifurcation balloon angioplasty: An experimental study. J Vasc Surg 2000;31:550–7.

25. Jordan WD Jr, Voellinger DC, Doblar DD, Plyushcheva NP, Fisher WS, McDowell HA. Microemboli detected by transcranial Doppler monitoring in patients during carotid angioplasty versus carotid endarterectomy. Cardiovasc Surg 1999;7:33–8.

26. Ohki T, Marin ML, Lyon RT, et al. Ex vivo human carotid artery bifurcation stenting: Correlation of lesion characteristics with embolic potential. J Vasc Surg 1998;27:463–71.

27. Henry M, Henry I, Klonaris C, et al. Benefits of cerebral protection during carotid stenting with the PercuSurge GuardWire system: Midterm results. J Endovasc Ther 2002; 9:1–13.

28. Ackerstaff RG, Jansen C, Moll FL, Vermeulen FE, Hamerlijnck RP, Mauser HW. The significance of microemboli detection by means of transcranial Doppler ultrasonography monitoring in carotid endarterectomy. J Vasc Surg 1995;21:963–9.

29. Tubler T, Schluter M, Dirsch O, et al. Balloon-protected carotid artery stenting: Relationship of periprocedural neurological complications with the size of particulate debris. Circulation 2001;104:2791–6.

12
Duplex Ultrasound in the Diagnosis of Temporal Arteritis

George H. Meier and Courtney Nelms

Giant cell arteritis is the most common primary arteritis diagnosed, with an average incidence of 15–25 cases per 100,000 population over the age of 50.[1] Giant cell arteritis can be subclassified into at least three main types: cranial, affecting the arteries of the face, head, and posterior cerebral circulation; large vessel, involving the axillary and subclavian arteries; and aortic, leading to aneurysmal degeneration of the ascending aorta or aortic valve insufficiency. Of these, the most common presentation is the cranial form, traditionally referred to as temporal arteritis. In this form, the arteritis involves the superficial temporal arteries as well as the facial artery branches. Involvement of the ophthalmic artery can lead to retinal ischemia and is the second leading cause of acquired blindness in the United States.[2]

In the temporal arteritis form of giant cell arteritis, the diagnosis can often be challenging. The American College of Rheumatology developed clinical criteria for the diagnosis of giant cell arteritis in 1990[3] (Table 12–1). Using these criteria, three of the five criteria must be present to define the diagnosis of temporal arteritis. The presence of a positive biopsy demonstrating giant cell arteritis is only one of the five criteria and is therefore insufficient alone to diagnose giant cell arteritis. Additionally, giant cell arteritis may not involve the artery evenly along its course, resulting in areas of normal artery interspersed with areas of abnormality. In fact, the irregular distribution of arterial involvement is common in temporal arteritis,[4] risking a false negative biopsy if too small a segment of artery is biopsied. Current recommendations suggest that bilateral biopsy should be done even in cases of unilateral symptoms,[5,6] and at least 5cm of artery should be biopsied on either side. In spite of this approach, a substantial number of temporal artery specimens miss the areas of active disease.[7–10] For these reasons, the absence of histologic evidence of giant cell arteritis is insufficient to rule out the disease and many patients require treatment even in the absence of a positive biopsy.

The pathologic findings resulting in a positive biopsy consist of three dominant findings in temporal arteritis: the presence of a halo of edema around or within the artery wall, usually associated with giant cell formation; stenosis secondary to narrowing after the inflammation abates; or occlusion of the artery due to obliterative arteritis. Therefore, any of these may represent a positive biopsy depending on the stage of the arteritis and the duration of symptoms or treatment. For any diagnostic modality to replace biopsy, these findings must be apparent.

High-resolution duplex ultrasound is a common test for many vascular disorders and the easy access to the superficial temporal artery makes it an obvious modality to consider for the diagnosis of temporal arteritis. Its use in temporal arteritis has two potential utilities. First, the mapping of areas of arterial involvement for biopsy may allow a positive biopsy rate higher than currently seen with blind biopsy. If abnormalities on duplex ultrasound are seen (halo, stenosis, or occlusion), then directed biopsy may produce a higher yield, avoiding the false-negative biopsy discussed above. The second benefit of duplex ultrasound in temporal arteritis may be the benefit of avoiding biopsy completely. If the clinical suspicion is high based on the American College of Radiology (ACR) criteria, then an ultrasound indicating arterial pathology may provide sufficient accuracy to avoid open surgical biopsy altogether. The presence of halo, stenosis, or occlusion on ultrasound evaluation may not need correlation with open biopsy, but in selected patients may warrant treatment without biopsy. While this use of ultrasound has not been established as a standard, the potential is enticing and the avoidance of open biopsy should be the ultimate goal in the diagnosis of temporal arteritis.

TABLE 12–1. Diagnostic criteria for temporal arteritis (American College of Rheumatology[3]).

Age greater than or equal to 50 years
New headache
Temporal artery abnormality on physical examination
Elevated ESR[a] ≥ 50 mm/h
Abnormal findings on temporal artery biopsy

[a]ESR, erythrocyte sedimentation rate.

Ultrasound Protocol

Duplex ultrasound permits localization of inflammation or stenosis of the temporal arteries and their branches. The presence of significant tenderness along the course of the superficial temporal artery may alter the examination, but generally ultrasound interrogation can be achieved along the full length of the temporal artery and its branches.

Patients are placed in a supine position with the head slightly elevated. The head is turned away from the side to be scanned. Color duplex ultrasound is performed bilaterally on the temporal arteries with a high-resolution linear transducer (L 10–5 MHz). The common superficial temporal arteries are established as a landmark medial to the ear and then followed inferiorly and superiorly to the frontal and parietal branches of the temporal artery. The vessels should be followed in longitudinal and transverse planes throughout the examination, with and without color flow, looking for the "halo" effect (Figures 12–1 and 12–2), arterial stenosis (Figure 12–3), and arterial occlusion. This can be challenging in many patients since the tortuosity of the artery may mean that keeping it in a single plane for visualization is difficult. Color flow imaging is used to facilitate following the anatomic course and branching of the artery and to define areas of flow disturbance or luminal narrowing. Color flow will allow for easier identification of the "halo" effect with the color settings adjusted appropriately. Care should be taken to prevent the color from "bleeding" over into the outer walls of the arteries and possibly obscuring the

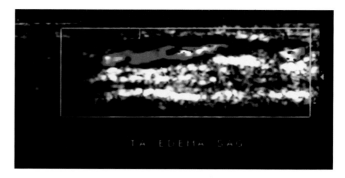

FIGURE 12–2. Halo seen in longitudinal cross-section.

inflammation. This examination can be tedious due to the small size of the vessels, frequent tortuosity, and location of the arterial segments below the scalp above the hairline. Peak systolic velocities and end diastolic velocities should be obtained throughout the temporal arteries and branches, including the superficial temporal artery medial to the ear prior to the bifurcation, common temporal artery inferior to the ear, parietal branch coursing toward the scalp, and the frontal branch coursing toward the forehead. Care is taken to use appropriate angle correction between 45–60° with respect to the blood flow vector. A stenosis is defined as at least a two-fold increase of the peak systolic velocity accompanied by poststenotic turbulence.

B-mode imaging can define the areas of inflammation that represent edema within the arterial wall. The wall of the arterial segments affected with arteritis appears to be acoustically homogeneous and presents a "halo" around the lumen of the artery. These areas may be intermittent

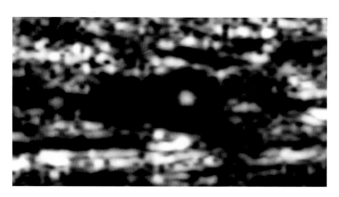

FIGURE 12–1. Halo seen in transverse.

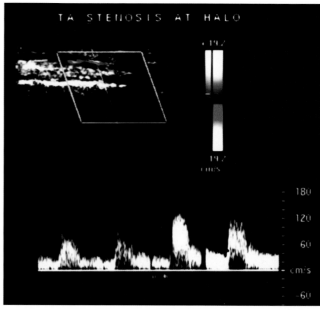

FIGURE 12–3. Spectral Doppler evaluation for stenosis.

or focal within the branches; therefore a thorough evaluation of all branches is necessary. More echogenic, diffuse plaque is probably atherosclerosis, not inflammation, but may also represent areas of "burned out" arteritis. Elevations in peak systolic velocities may be noted in these areas. Alternatively, occlusions of segments of the artery may represent similar issues and should also be noted for reporting.

Once the arteries are fully interrogated, a map should be generated for each side imaged. This map of pathologic findings on ultrasound should be used as a guide by the surgeon to allow accurate biopsy of the areas of concern. If no abnormalities are noted, then conventional blind biopsy is warranted.

Results of Duplex Ultrasound for Temporal Arteritis

While the diagnosis of temporal arteritis is clinical based on the ACR criteria outlined in Table 12–1, the presence of a biopsy consistent with giant cell arteritis is an important adjunct to reassure the patient and clinician of the diagnosis, justifying the initiation of steroid therapy to prevent progression or blindness. Unfortunately, biopsy is inexact, as temporal arteritis has a propensity for skip lesions with normal artery in the intervening segments as discussed earlier. Therefore, the challenge in diagnosis is in defining the inflammatory lesions in the artery responsible for the clinical consequences. Duplex ultrasound holds great promise in this regard since high-resolution ultrasound of the superficial temporal artery can often provide information about the likelihood of disease involvement as well as the extent of disease seen. Duplex ultrasound for directed biopsy was first proposed as early as 1982.[11] Unfortunately, no series using this strategy of ultrasound-directed biopsy has yet demonstrated efficacy, although some benefit has been suggested.[6] While this information has not yet been fully incorporated into the diagnostic algorithm for temporal arteritis, it seems likely that with further study and technical refinements, this noninvasive modality may ultimately be able to replace open biopsy in the diagnosis of temporal arteritis.

The halo effect seen around the artery correlates with areas of edema and giant cell formation surrounding the lumen. In these areas the artery appears enlarged clinically, with the bulk of the enlargement due to inflammation and edema. The main underlying pathology behind the clinical syndrome of temporal arteritis is small vessel ischemia. Therefore, the clinical consequences of temporal arteritis are associated with stenosis or occlusion rather than the halo formation associated with acute periarterial inflammation. Only as the inflammation progresses to fibrosis does the ischemic component begin, resulting in the symptoms associated with temporal

arteritis. For this reason, the halo may not be as important as the presence of arterial stenosis or occlusion in the risk of visual changes associated with temporal arteritis.

One of the earliest reports suggesting utility of high-resolution color flow duplex ultrasound in temporal arteritis was by Williamson in 1992.[12] In this patient serial evaluation of ophthalmic artery blood flow was correlated with the changes in visual symptoms, showing return of blood flow and resolution of visual symptoms associated with increased immunosuppressive therapy. The fact that these changes in small artery blood flow could be qualitatively assessed noninvasively promised a new diagnostic modality for temporal arteritis.

Aburahma and Thaxton[13] reviewed their experience with duplex ultrasound in temporal arteritis in 21 patients, 19 of whom underwent temporal artery biopsy. In this series duplex was performed prebiopsy in only 8 of the patients, but the authors concluded that the use of duplex ultrasound might be beneficial in guiding the location and side of temporal artery biopsy in these patients.

The next step in evaluation of duplex ultrasound was a paper published by Schmidt in the *New England Journal of Medicine* in 1997.[14] This prospective evaluation of 30 patients, only 21 of whom had positive biopsies, evaluated three criteria: halo formation (a marker of inflammatory edema of the artery), arterial stenosis, and arterial occlusion. Using these three criteria, 28 of the 30 patients had a positive ultrasound evaluation. These results were compared to 30 age- and sex-matched controls, with any of the three ultrasound criteria demonstrated in only two patients.

While further research in duplex ultrasound for the diagnosis of temporal arteritis was clearly warranted, our group undertook a slightly different study published in 2002.[15,16] In this paper, we evaluated all patients referred to our practice for temporal artery biopsy by duplex ultrasound prior to biopsy. In these 32 patients only 7 met the criteria for the diagnosis of temporal arteritis. In this first attempt at applying duplex ultrasound diagnostic criteria to patients being evaluated for temporal arteritis, no positive biopsy was seen in any patient without one of the three criteria mentioned above. Therefore, we felt that temporal artery biopsy should be undertaken only on patients with ultrasound abnormalities, either halo or stenosis/occlusion.

Since these initial studies, multiple other studies have been published.[17–27] While the conclusions reached have often been contradictory (Table 12–2), ultrasound can clearly demonstrate abnormalities in the superficial temporal artery associated with temporal arteritis. The most recent meta-analysis published in 2005 attempted to review the world literature on ultrasound and temporal arteritis and reach conclusions based on the studies available. Karassa and his colleagues reviewed 23 studies

TABLE 12–2. Summary of studies using duplex ultrasound to diagnose temporal arteritis.

Study	Number of patients	Ultrasound findings evaluated			Conclusions
		Halo formation	Stenosis	Occlusion	
Schmidt[14]	30	+	+	+	May replace biopsy
Venz[28]	20	+			Halo alone not specific enough
LeSar[15]	32	+	+	+	May limit need for biopsy if negative
Nesher[27]	32	+			May limit need for biopsy if negative
Salvarani[26]	86	+			Did not improve upon physical examination
Murgatroyd[23]	26	+	+	+	May be helpful
Pfadenhauer[29]	67	+	+	+	Cannot replace biopsy
Reinhard[30]	48	+		+	May limit the need for biopsy if positive

totaling 2036 patients written in 5 different languages.[18] Their conclusions were that ultrasound may be helpful, but guidelines to its use and application were absent based on this heterogeneous collection of studies. Thus, we are left at this moment with more questions than answers, with great variability in the application of ultrasound techniques from site to site and no current potential for resolving these issues.

Future Directions

For us to define how better to use ultrasound for the diagnosis of giant cell arteritis, specifically temporal arteritis, we have to define what types of trials will be needed to demonstrate benefit. These trials are designed to embellish and define prospectively what can be done to diagnose temporal arteritis. While all of the strategies carry some risk, the overall benefit to patients with temporal arteritis may subsume the individual risk.

There are three basic approaches to trials to better define the use of ultrasound in the diagnosis of temporal arteritis. First is the use of duplex ultrasound to guide biopsy. For this strategy to be effective, a prospective predictive duplex ultrasound must be performed and then correlated with biopsy findings. The key to this study would be the interrogation of only those segments of the temporal artery appropriate for biopsy and the surgeon's focus on complete biopsy of those segments for correlation. Generally, this would include the common superficial temporal artery as well as the proximal portion of the parietal and frontal branches. A predictive score derived from the prebiopsy temporal artery duplex ultrasound would need to be correlated with carefully controlled biopsies with special attention to the anatomic location of disease. The anatomic correlations of biopsy and ultrasound would hopefully demonstrate the specific abnor-

malities seen on both. Areas of abnormality outside of the biopsy specimen would be excluded from this analysis. In this way accurate correlation of biopsy pathology in temporal arteries could be analyzed versus ultrasound findings in the same segment. Currently no series has accurately defined the abnormalities within the biopsy zone, and correlated this directly with ultrasound of the corresponding areas. In this study the only risk is the possibility of a positive ultrasound finding outside of the zone of biopsy, equivalent to the current risk when duplex ultrasound is used prior to biopsy. In this scenario, a decision to treat independent of biopsy would need to be reached.

The second approach is defining the criteria to help avoid unnecessary biopsies. In this study, all patients would undergo preprocedure duplex ultrasound scanning. If abnormalities were defined on the ultrasound scan in the zone of routine biopsy, then biopsy would be performed. If no abnormalities were seen in areas accessible for biopsy, then treatment would be based on clinical criteria and no biopsy would be performed. Using this strategy prospectively, patients would be followed for treatment outcomes, biopsy results, and the subsequent development of temporal arteritis. This study assumes that arterial pathology is present both in temporal arteritis and in degenerative atherosclerosis. Biopsy results would be used to refine the group of patients treated for temporal arteritis, excluding those patients with degenerative atherosclerosis alone. A negative ultrasound evaluation would be assumed to rule out either temporal arteritis or degenerative atherosclerosis, eliminating the need for biopsy. The risk of this study is the possibility of missing temporal arteritis in a patient with a false-negative duplex ultrasound evaluation. While in most series the risk of a false-negative ultrasound evaluation is quite small, it is not zero. In these patients the routine use of the five clinical criteria would be necessary to avoid undertreatment of patients with negative biopsies or ultrasounds.

A third approach to defining the value of duplex ultrasound in temporal arteritis would be its value as an indicator of positive biopsy results. Again, an ultrasound evaluation of the temporal arteries in the area of biopsy would be performed. If significant arterial pathology were found, then this would be viewed as a positive biopsy and the patient would be treated based on the diagnostic criteria outlined in Table 12–1. Instead of using surgical biopsy as one of the five criteria, either an abnormal duplex ultrasound or a positive surgical biopsy would be assumed to be equivalent. Since two additional criteria would be necessary for the diagnosis of temporal arteritis, this decreases the severity of a false-positive ultrasound study and requires additional criteria for the clinical diagnosis of temporal arteritis. By prospective assessment, the benefits of this diagnostic strategy could be objectively defined. Unfortunately since in most series the rate of positive biopsy is only about 25%, 75% of the patients would still require a biopsy to rule out the disease. Only in that less than 25% of patients with a positive ultrasound would biopsy be avoided and in those patients the risk of steroid therapy would be assumed. This strategy would result in every patient being exposed to either a biopsy or steroid therapy, both of which carry additional risk.

From our perspective and experience, either of the first two strategies seem to be the best next step in the use of ultrasound for temporal arteritis. In our opinion the third strategy exposes the patients to too much risk without adequate benefit. Ideally, the study should be undertaken as multicenter trials using a common protocol. Only in this manner can these data be generalized to the wider population of patients presenting with possible temporal arteritis to the clinician. In spite of these concerns ultrasound remains a viable diagnostic tool in the management of temporal arteritis.

References

1. Weyand CM, Goronzy JJ. Giant-cell arteritis and polymyalgia rheumatica. Ann Intern Med 2003;139(6):505–15.
2. Gonzalez-Gay MA, et al. Visual manifestations of giant cell arteritis. Trends and clinical spectrum in 161 patients. Medicine (Baltimore) 2000;79(5):283–92.
3. Hunder GG, et al. The American College of Rheumatology 1990 criteria for the classification of giant cell arteritis. Arthritis Rheum 1990;33(8):1122–8.
4. Lie JT. Illustrated histopathologic classification criteria for selected vasculitis syndromes. American College of Rheumatology Subcommittee on Classification of Vasculitis. Arthritis Rheum 1990;33(8):1074–87.
5. Pless M, et al. Concordance of bilateral temporal artery biopsy in giant cell arteritis. J Neuroophthalmol 2000;20(3):216–8.
6. Ponge T, et al. The efficacy of selective unilateral temporal artery biopsy versus bilateral biopsies for diagnosis of giant cell arteritis. J Rheumatol 1988;15(6):997–1000.
7. van der Straaten D, et al. A case of biopsy-negative temporal arteritis—diagnostic challenges. Surv Ophthalmol 2004;49(6):603–7.
8. Hoffman GS. Giant cell arteritis: Biopsy may not be diagnostic. Cleve Clin J Med 1998;65(4):218.
9. Lie JT. Temporal artery biopsy diagnosis of giant cell arteritis: Lessons from 1109 biopsies. Anat Pathol 1996;1:69–97.
10. Hall S, et al. The therapeutic impact of temporal artery biopsy. Lancet 1983;2(8361):1217–20.
11. Barrier J, et al. The use of Doppler flow studies in the diagnosis of giant cell arteritis. Selection of temporal artery biopsy site is facilitated. JAMA 1982;248(17):2158–9.
12. Williamson TH, et al. Colour Doppler ultrasound in the management of a case of cranial arteritis. Br J Ophthalmol 1992;76(11):690–1.
13. AbuRahma AF, Thaxton L. Temporal arteritis: Diagnostic and therapeutic considerations. Am Surg 1996;62(6):449–51.
14. Schmidt WA, et al. Color duplex ultrasonography in the diagnosis of temporal arteritis. N Engl J Med 1997;337(19):1336–42.
15. LeSar CJ, et al. The utility of color duplex ultrasonography in the diagnosis of temporal arteritis. J Vasc Surg 2002;36(6):1154–60.
16. Nelms CR, Carter KA, Meier GH, et al. Diagnosis of temporal artery pathology using duplex ultrasonography. J Vasc Ultrasound 2002;26(4):273–7.
17. Schmidt WA, Blockmans D. Use of ultrasonography and positron emission tomography in the diagnosis and assessment of large-vessel vasculitis. Curr Opin Rheumatol 2005;17(1):9–15.
18. Karassa FB, et al. Meta-analysis: Test performance of ultrasonography for giant-cell arteritis. Ann Intern Med 2005;142(5):359–69.
19. Butteriss DJ, et al. Use of colour duplex ultrasound to diagnose giant cell arteritis in a case of visual loss of uncertain aetiology. Br J Radiol 2004;77(919):607–9.
20. Schmidt WA, Gromnica-Ihle E. Duplex ultrasonography in temporal arteritis. Ann Intern Med 2003;138(7):609; author reply 609–10.
21. Schmidt D, et al. Comparison between color duplex ultrasonography and histology of the temporal artery in cranial arteritis (giant cell arteritis). Eur J Med Res 2003;8(1):1–7.
22. Nicoletti G, et al. Colour duplex ultrasonography in the management of giant cell arteritis. Clin Rheumatol 2003;22(6):508–9.
23. Murgatroyd H, et al. The use of ultrasound as an aid in the diagnosis of giant cell arteritis: A pilot study comparing histological features with ultrasound findings. Eye 2003;17(3):415–9.
24. Hetzel SD, Reinhard M, Haedrich-Auw C. Comparison between color duplex ultrasonography and histology of the temporal artery in cranial arteritis. Eur J Med Res 2003;8(2):91.
25. Schmidt WA, Gromnica-Ihle E. Incidence of temporal arteritis in patients with polymyalgia rheumatica: A

prospective study using colour Doppler ultrasonography of the temporal arteries. Rheumatology (Oxford) 2002;41(1): 46–52.

26. Salvarani C, *et al.* Is duplex ultrasonography useful for the diagnosis of giant-cell arteritis? Ann Intern Med 2002; 137(4):232–8.

27. Nesher G, *et al.* The predictive value of the halo sign in color Doppler ultrasonography of the temporal arteries for diagnosing giant cell arteritis. J Rheumatol 2002;29(6): 1224–6.

28. Venz S, *et al.* [Use of high resolution color Doppler sonography in diagnosis of temporal arteritis.] Rofo 1998;169(6): 605–8.

29. Pfadenhauer K, Weber H. Duplex sonography of the temporal and occipital artery in the diagnosis of temporal arteritis. A prospective study. J Rheumatol 2003;30(10): 2177–81.

30. Reinhard M, Schmidt D, Hetzel A. Color-coded sonography in suspected temporal arteritis—experiences after 83 cases. Rheumatol Int 2004;24(6):340–6.

13
Duplex Ultrasound Velocity Criteria for Carotid Stenting Patients

Brajesh K. Lal and Robert W. Hobson II

Introduction

Stroke is the third leading cause of death in the United States with over 783,000 strokes reported annually.[1] Over one-third of patients die and another one-third are severely disabled. The annual economic cost exceeds $30 billion.[2] Randomized trials have established the efficacy of carotid endarterectomy (CEA) in the prevention of stroke for patients with high-grade carotid stenosis (CS).[3-7] The advent of newer technologies and a desire for less invasive treatment have encouraged investigators to propose carotid artery stenting (CAS) as an alternative to CEA.[1,8-10] Our institution[1, 8,11-17] (Figure 13–1), along with others,[18-22] has demonstrated that CAS is technically feasible and safe in patients with restenosis after CEA, surgically inaccessible lesions, previous radiation, or significant medical comorbidities. The 30-day stroke and death rate in 190 CAS procedures at our institution was 4.15%, indicating a competitive alternative to CEA.[14] However, due to the proven efficacy of CEA, current indications for CAS have been limited to situations where CEA yields suboptimal results.[13,23]

Two randomized trials have compared CAS and CEA. The SAPPHIRE (Stenting and Angioplasty with Protection in Patients at High Risk for Endarterectomy) investigators randomized 334 high-risk patients to CAS or CEA.[24] The 30-day composite stroke, death, and myocardial infarction rate was not different between the two groups (CAS 12.2% vs. CEA 20.1%). The European CAVATAS (Carotid and Vertebral Artery Transluminal Angioplasty Study) investigators also reported comparable 30-day combined stroke and death rates (CEA 5.9% vs. CAS 6.4%).[25] The authors concluded that CAS was not inferior to CEA.

These trials were not powered to identify a difference between CAS and CEA. The NIH/NINDS-supported CREST (Carotid Revascularization Endarterectomy versus Stent Trial) is currently underway to make that determination.[26] In the lead-in phase of the trial, the combined stroke and death rate was 5.6% for symptomatic and 2.4% for asymptomatic patients undergoing CAS.[27] These preliminary results indicate low complication rates with CAS. The results of CREST may determine the role of CAS in future years. However, current data suggest clinical equipoise between CEA and CAS based on the three clinical end points of stroke, myocardial infarction (MI) and death. As a result of this information, the Food and Drug Administration (FDA) has approved the use of CAS in selected high-risk patients (significant medical comorbidities, post-CEA restenosis, anatomically inaccessible lesions above C_2, and radiation-induced stenoses).

In-Stent Restenosis: The Rationale for Post-Carotid Artery Stenting Surveillance

The incidences of in-stent restenosis (ISR) after bare metal stenting of the coronary and renal arteries have been reported as 20–35% and 15–25%, respectively.[13] It was therefore thought that ISR rates would be high with CAS too. Indeed, early reports noted post-CAS ISR in the ranges of 1–50%.[13] However, the reported rate of ISR depends on the definition of restenosis utilized, the duration of follow-up, and the methods of diagnosis and calculation used. Most studies have relatively short follow-up periods (≤12 months), and report absolute recurrence rates weighting each procedure equally regardless of the length of follow-up. This results in an underreporting of ISR rates. With longer follow-up (1–74 months) and the use of lifetable analysis, we reported more meaningful data on ISR after CAS. The majority of restenoses ≥40% occurred within 18 months (13/22, 60%) and the majority of clinically significant restenoses ≥80% occurred within 15

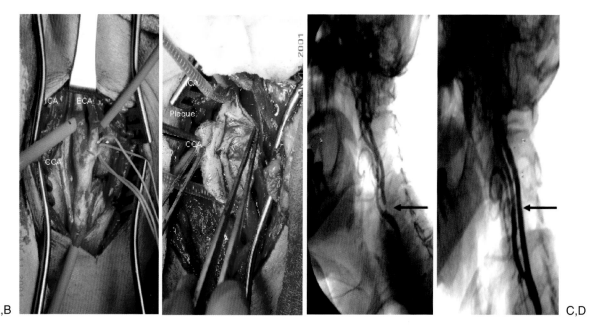

FIGURE 13–1. Methods of carotid revascularization practiced at our institution. (A, B) Carotid endarterectomy. Exposure and dissection of the plaque. CCA, common carotid artery; ICA, internal carotid artery; ECA, external carotid artery. (C, D) Carotid artery stenting. (B) Prestenting angiogram, arrow at stenosis in ICA; (C) poststenting angiogram, arrows at distal and proximal ends of stent.

months (3/5, 60%) of their intervention (Figure 13–2). The incidence of ISR ≥ 40 and ≥60% was 42.7% and 16.4%, respectively, at 48 months of follow-up. Our data also noted that hemodynamically significant (≥80%) ISR after CAS was 6.4% at 5 years (Figure 13–3). It is clear that a significant number of patients will develop moderate ISR after CAS, of which some will progress to high-grade stenosis. There is additional evidence that the placement of a stent induces continuing arterial remod-

eling. Nitinol self-expanding stents can continue to expand over a 2-year period poststenting.[28] Conversely, neointimal thickening has been reported to occur up to 1 year poststenting; further thickening may overwhelm positive remodeling of the arterial diameter from the stent and result in hemodynamically significant in-stent restenosis. This provides conclusive evidence that continued surveillance of patients is essential once CAS has been performed.

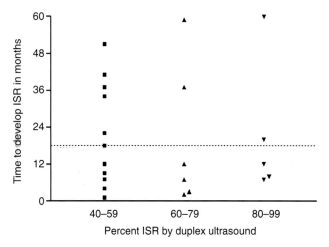

FIGURE 13–2. Distribution of in-stent restenosis cases based on time of diagnosis from initial carotid artery stenting procedure. Note that the majority of restenoses occurred within 18 months of the initial carotid artery stenting procedure. The dotted line identifies the 18 month postprocedure mark. ISR, in-stent restenosis. [Adapted from Lal B K, Hobson RW 2nd, Goldstein J, et al. In-stent recurrent stenosis after carotid artery stenting: Life table analysis and clinical relevance. J Vasc Surg 2003;38(6): 1162–8.]

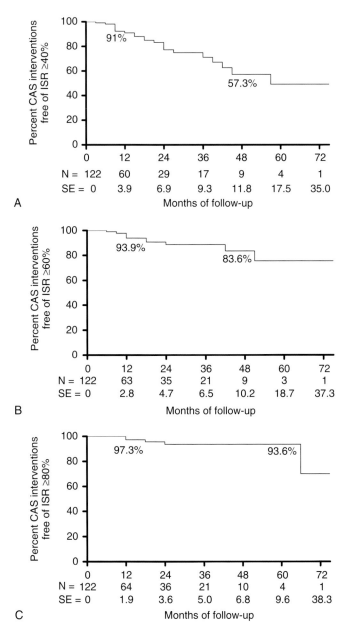

FIGURE 13–3. Kaplan–Meier cumulative event-free rates for clinically significant in-stent restenosis after CAS. (A) Event-free rate for ISR ≥ 80%. (B) Event-free rate for ISR ≥ 60%. (C) Event-free rate for ISR ≥ 40%. CAS, carotid artery stenting; ISR, in-stent restenosis; N, number at risk; SE, standard error. [Adapted from Lal BK, Hobson RW 2nd, Goldstein J, et al. In-stent recurrent stenosis after carotid artery stenting: Life table analysis and clinical relevance. J Vasc Surg 2003;38(6):1162–8.]

Duplex Ultrasonography: The Ideal Method for Post-Carotid Artery Stenting Surveillance

The characteristics of the ideal follow-up technique for CAS patients remain generally similar to that for CEA patients. The technique must be able to reliably identify changes in arterial diameter and stent morphology in an objective manner and be readily available, inexpensive, and associated with low observer variability. Computed tomography and magnetic resonance imaging may be considered: they are both expensive modalities and are associated with significantly reduced accuracy in determining diameter estimates of the carotid arteries. Therefore duplex ultrasonography (DU) remains the optimal imaging modality for post-CAS surveillance. It is non-invasive, safe, free of complications, readily available in vascular laboratories around the country, and is associated with a large experience with primary and recurrent carotid stenosis of the native carotid artery.

The utility of DU scanning in the detection of native carotid artery disease is well documented. Ultrasound velocities correlate with angiographic percent stenosis in the native unstented carotid artery.[29] The appropriate threshold velocities signifying different degrees of stenoses have been intensively analyzed and identified leading to the use of peak systolic velocity (PSV), end diastolic velocity (EDV), PSV/EDV ratio, or internal/common carotid artery (ICA/CCA) ratio, alone or in combination, to define normal and increasingly stenosed ICAs.[30] While thousands of carotid stents have been placed worldwide and in the United States, DU velocity criteria have not been well established for patients undergoing CAS. Robbin et al.[31] studied the use of DU in the follow-up of stented carotid arteries and noted that velocity measurements were unreliable after stenting. Similarly, Ringer et al.[32] reviewed their experience immediately after carotid stent placement and concluded that strict velocity criteria for restenosis were unreliable. Both groups applied limited, randomly selected velocity criteria to their data, and did not perform a systematic analysis to confirm their findings.

At our institution, we initially applied Intersocietal Commission for the Accreditation of Vascular Laboratories (ICAVL) accredited cutoff PSV and EDV criteria developed for native (unstented) carotid arteries to the follow-up of our first 90 CAS procedures.[17] Of these, 38 demonstrated a mean PSV ≥ 130 cm/s on postprocedure DU performed within 3 days. Using the velocity criteria established in our laboratory for unstented arteries, these patients would be characterized as technical failures of the procedure, having in-stent residual stenoses in the range of 20–49%. However, only six procedures demonstrated true angiographically proven residual stenosis ≥20%. We therefore concluded that stenting resulted in an elevation in measured DU velocities despite normal luminal diameters. Based on receiver operating characteristic (ROC) analysis of our data we found that a PSV ≥150 cm/s in combination with an ICA/CCA ratio ≥2.16 provides optimal sensitivity (100%), specificity (97.6%), positive predictive value (PPV) (75%), negative predictive value (NPV) (100%), and accuracy (97.7%) for differentiating 0–19% and ≥20% ICA in-stent residual stenosis after CAS[17] (Figure 13–4).

Compliance, a measure of arterial stiffness, is the relationship between strain (fractional deformation of wall) and stress (force per unit area of wall).[33] In an artery, it is described by the change in volume of a segment of artery in relation to pulsatile change in blood pressure. We reported, for the first time, a significant decrease in the compliance of the ICA after placement of a carotid stent (Figure 13–5). The enhanced stiffness of the stent-arterial wall complex renders the flow–pressure relationship of the carotid artery closer to that observed in a rigid tube[34] so that the energy normally applied to dilate the artery results in an increased velocity.

The new DU velocity criteria above define procedural success (<20% residual stenosis) and will most reliably discriminate normal from in-stent residual stenosis (≥20%) immediately after CAS. These proposed criteria can form the basis for additional prospective validation

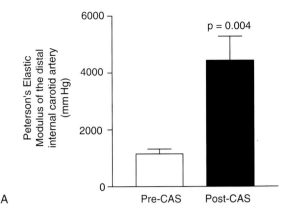

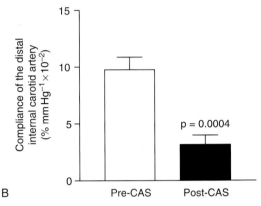

FIGURE 13–5. Measurement of elastic modulus (A) and compliance (B) demonstrates increased stiffness of the stented distal internal carotid artery post-CAS versus the native distal internal carotid artery (pre-CAS) ($n = 20$ for each measurement). Pre-CAS, prior to carotid artery stenting; post-CAS, after carotid artery stenting. [Adapted from Lal BK, Hobson RW 2nd, Goldstein J, Chakhtoura EY, Duran WN. Carotid artery stenting: Is there a need to revise ultrasound velocity criteria? J Vasc Surg 2004;39(1):58–66.]

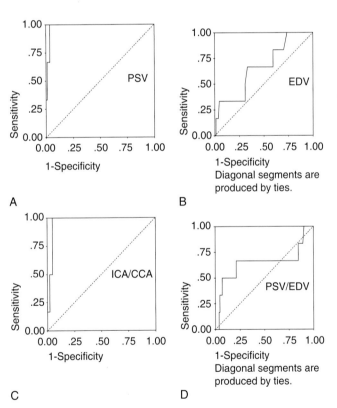

FIGURE 13–4. Receiver operating characteristics curves of various ultrasound velocity measurements (in cm/s) for differentiating between ≥20% or <20% angiographic in-stent residual stenosis immediately after carotid stenting. (A) In-stent PSV. (B) In-stent EDV. (C) In-stent PSV/EDV ratio. (D) In-stent PSV of ICA/CCA ratio. [Adapted from Lal BK, Hobson RW 2nd, Goldstein J, Chakhtoura EY, Duran WN. Carotid artery stenting: Is there a need to revise ultrasound velocity criteria? J Vasc Surg 2004;39(1):58–66.]

studies to further develop criteria identifying post-CAS ISR of higher grades. Until these revised criteria are available, we recommend early registration of baseline velocity measurements after CAS against which future results should be compared.

While velocity criteria are being developed, increasing resolution of B-mode imaging is improving our ability to visualize the stent and luminal morphology. Further studies are required to establish the accuracy of luminal diameter measurements obtained by B-mode alone. However, it is possible that additional information derived from current B-mode imaging and spectral broadening may be used to supplement velocity measurements. For instance, in the presence of a PSV ≥ 150 cm/s and an ICA/CCA ratio ≥2.16, B-mode imaging may show no evidence of luminal encroachment in the stent, or there may be no spectral broadening. These data may therefore supplement the velocity criteria for determination of severity of in-stent stenosis.

Recommendations

1. All patients undergoing CAS must be placed in a regular follow-up protocol involving DU and clinical evaluation. The current risk of hemodynamically significant ISR is 6.4% over 4 years. Most ISR appears to occur early after CAS (18 months). Therefore follow-up must occur at baseline, 6 months, and annually thereafter.

2. The first follow-up DU after CAS must occur as soon after the procedure as possible, preferably during the same admission. Velocity criteria used to define residual stenosis ≥20% had to be revised to include a PSV ≥150 cm/s and an ICA/CCA ratio ≥2.16 in our laboratory. These values must be used as a guide to revise velocity criteria in individual vascular laboratories.

3. B-mode imaging of the arterial lumen and spectral waveform analysis must be used to supplement and enhance the accuracy of velocity criteria.

4. Revised velocity criteria defining higher grades of ISR are still under development; early registration of baseline velocities to compare subsequent follow-up velocities is the optimal surveillance protocol currently available. Elevations in PSV and/or ICA/CCA ratios may be indicative of developing ISR, which must then undergo angiographic evaluation and appropriate management.

References

1. Lal BK, Hobson IR. Carotid artery occlusive disease. Curr Treat Options Cardiovasc Med 2000;2(3):243–54.
2. Matcher DB, Duncan PW. Cost of Stroke. Stroke Clin Updates 1994;5:9–12.
3. Hobson RW 2nd, Weiss DG, Fields WS, et al. Efficacy of carotid endarterectomy for asymptomatic carotid stenosis. The Veterans Affairs Cooperative Study Group. N Engl J Med 1993;328(4):221–7.
4. North American Symptomatic Carotid Endarterectomy Trial Collaborators. Beneficial effect of carotid endarterectomy in symptomatic patients with high-grade carotid stenosis. N Engl J Med 1991;325(7):445–53.
5. Executive Committee for the Asymptomatic Carotid Atherosclerosis Study. Endarterectomy for asymptomatic carotid artery stenosis. JAMA 1995;273(18):1421–8.
6. Barnett HJ, Taylor DW, Eliasziw M, et al. Benefit of carotid endarterectomy in patients with symptomatic moderate or severe stenosis. North American Symptomatic Carotid Endarterectomy Trial Collaborators. N Engl J Med 1998; 339(20):1415–25.
7. Halliday A, Mansfield A, Marro J, et al. Prevention of disabling and fatal strokes by successful carotid endarterectomy in patients without recent neurological symptoms: Randomised controlled trial. Lancet 2004;363(9420):1491–502.
8. Hobson RW 2nd, Goldstein JE, Jamil Z, et al. Carotid restenosis: Operative and endovascular management. J Vasc Surg 1999;29(2):228–35; discussion 35–8.
9. Dorros G. Complications associated with extracranial carotid artery interventions. J Endovasc Surg 1996;3(2): 166–70.
10. Ferguson RD, Ferguson JG. Carotid angioplasty. In search of a worthy alternative to endarterectomy. Arch Neurol 1996;53(7):696–8.
11. Hobson RW 2nd, Lal BK, Chakhtoura E, et al. Carotid artery stenting: Analysis of data for 105 patients at high risk. J Vasc Surg 2003;37(6):1234–9.
12. Hobson RW 2nd, Lal BK, Chakhtoura EY, et al. Carotid artery closure for endarterectomy does not influence results of angioplasty-stenting for restenosis. J Vasc Surg 2002; 35(3):435–8.
13. Lal BK, Hobson RW 2nd, Goldstein J, et al. In-stent recurrent stenosis after carotid artery stenting: Life table analysis and clinical relevance. J Vasc Surg 2003;38(6):1162–8; discussion 9.
14. Cuadra S, Hobson R, Lal B, et al. Carotid artery stenting: Does the outcome depend on the indication? Abstract presented at the Vascular 2005, Annual conference of the Society for Vascular Surgery, Society for Vascular Technology, and Society for Vascular Medicine and Biology, Chicago, IL, 2005.
15. Choi HM, Hobson RW, Goldstein J, et al. Technical challenges in a program of carotid artery stenting. J Vasc Surg 2004;40(4):746–51; discussion 51.
16. Hobson RW 2nd. Carotid artery stenting. Surg Clin North Am 2004;84(5):1281–94, vi.
17. Lal BK, Hobson RW 2nd, Goldstein J, Chakhtoura EY, Duran WN. Carotid artery stenting: Is there a need to revise ultrasound velocity criteria? J Vasc Surg 2004;39(1):58–66.
18. Al-Mubarak N, Roubin GS, Vitek JJ, New G, Iyer SS. Procedural safety and short-term outcome of ambulatory carotid stenting. Stroke 2001;32(10):2305–9.
19. Roubin GS, New G, Iyer SS, et al. Immediate and late clinical outcomes of carotid artery stenting in patients with symptomatic and asymptomatic carotid artery stenosis: A 5-year prospective analysis. Circulation 2001;103(4):532–7.
20. Vitek JJ, Roubin GS, New G, Al-Mubarek N, Iyer SS. Carotid angioplasty with stenting in post-carotid endarterectomy restenosis. J Invasive Cardiol 2001;13(2):123–5; discussion 58–70.
21. Wholey MH, Wholey M, Mathias K, et al. Global experience in cervical carotid artery stent placement. Catheter Cardiovasc Interv 2000;50(2):160–7.
22. Ohki T, Veith FJ. Carotid artery stenting: Utility of cerebral protection devices. J Invasive Cardiol 2001;13(1): 47–55.
23. Veith FJ, Amor M, Ohki T, et al. Current status of carotid bifurcation angioplasty and stenting based on a consensus of opinion leaders. J Vasc Surg 2001;33(2 Suppl): S111–6.
24. Yadav JS, Wholey MH, Kuntz RE, et al. Protected carotid-artery stenting versus endarterectomy in high-risk patients. N Engl J Med 2004;351(15):1493–501.

25. Endovascular versus surgical treatment in patients with carotid stenosis in the Carotid and Vertebral Artery Transluminal Angioplasty Study (CAVATAS): A randomised trial. Lancet 2001;357(9270):1729–37.

26. Hobson RW 2nd. Update on the Carotid Revascularization Endarterectomy versus Stent Trial (CREST) protocol. J Am Coll Surg 2002;194(1 Suppl):S9–14.

27. Hobson RW 2nd, Howard VJ, Roubin GS, *et al.* Carotid artery stenting is associated with increased complications in octogenarians: 30-day stroke and death rates in the CREST lead-in phase. J Vasc Surg 2004;40(6):1106–11.

28. Willfort-Ehringer A, Ahmadi R, Gruber D, *et al.* Arterial remodeling and hemodynamics in carotid stents: A prospective duplex ultrasound study over 2 years. J Vasc Surg 2004;39(4):728–34.

29. Alexandrov AV, Brodie DS, McLean A, Hamilton P, Murphy J, Burns PN. Correlation of peak systolic velocity and angiographic measurement of carotid stenosis revisited. Stroke 1997;28(2):339–42.

30. Faught WE, Mattos MA, van Bemmelen PS, *et al.* Color-flow duplex scanning of carotid arteries: New velocity criteria based on receiver operator characteristic analysis for threshold stenoses used in the symptomatic and asymptomatic carotid trials. J Vasc Surg 1994;19(5):818–27; discussion 27–8.

31. Robbin ML, Lockhart ME, Weber TM, *et al.* Carotid artery stents: Early and intermediate follow-up with Doppler US. Radiology 1997;205(3):749–56.

32. Ringer AJ, German JW, Guterman LR, Hopkins LN. Follow-up of stented carotid arteries by Doppler ultrasound. Neurosurgery 2002;51(3):639–43; discussion 43.

33. Wilson KA, Hoskins PR, Lee AJ, Fowkes FG, Ruckley CV, Bradbury AW. Ultrasonic measurement of abdominal aortic aneurysm wall compliance: A reproducibility study. J Vasc Surg 2000;31(3):507–13.

34. Green JF. *Mechanical Concepts in Cardiovascular and Pulmonary Physiology,* 2nd ed. Philadelphia, PA: Lea & Febiger, 1977.

14
Use of Transcranial Doppler in Monitoring Patients during Carotid Artery Stenting

Mark C. Bates

Introduction

It has been over 20 years since Aaslid first described the technique of middle cerebral artery range gated Doppler interrogation via a low-frequency ultrasound transducer stationed just above the zygomatic arch.[1] Since that time insonation techniques with probe fixation headgear have made continuous real-time imaging much easier and advances in Doppler technology including "power Doppler" have improved signal clarity.[2] A detailed review of the physics and utility of transcranial Doppler (TCD) is eloquently presented in Chapter 9. The objective of this chapter is to expose the reader to some of the lessons learned from adjuvant transcranial Doppler during carotid stent-supported angioplasty.

Carotid endarterectomy has been proven in large randomized trials to reduce the risk of stroke or future neurologic events in patients with symptomatic and asymptomatic extracranial cerebrovascular disease.[3,4] The carotid endarterectomy techniques have matured and through the years we have learned that in the hands of experienced surgeons, the risk of a periprocedural neurologic event is very low.[5,6] The inherent risk of transcatheter interaction with the typical friable internal carotid artery lesion and resultant embolization of material to the brain was recognized early on as a limitation to carotid artery stenting.[7–10] The development of cerebral protection devices including distal occlusive balloons, distal filter systems, and proximal occlusive systems has rekindled enthusiasm about carotid artery stenting as an alternative to endarterectomy.[11–20]

Carotid artery stenting remains very controversial in many countries and currently there are no well-controlled randomized clinical trials that have shown clinical equipoise between carotid artery stenting and carotid endarterectomy.[21] There does appear to be a subgroup of patients that may benefit from this technology. These patients have been categorized as "high risk" for surgery based on anatomic and clinical criteria. At present there is one well-designed randomized trial evaluating carotid endarterectomy versus stenting in high-risk patients for endarterectomy.[22] While the SAPPHIRE trial did not show a statistically significant reduction in risk of periprocedural stroke in patients undergoing stenting versus surgery, there did seem to be an overall lower risk of serious adverse events when also considering myocardial infarction as an endpoint.[22] There have also been multiple registries of high-risk patients who have undergone carotid stenting with outcomes compared to historical controls. These studies also suggest carotid stenting may be a safe alternative to surgery in high-risk patients.[23–26] The recent approval by the United States Food and Drug Administration (FDA) for carotid artery stenting in patients that are considered high risk for surgery underscores the importance of better understanding the embolic risk of carotid artery stenting and TCD has given considerable insight to investigators on that front. In fact, TCD has provided early carotid stent pioneers with important feedback on embolic risks during different stages of the procedure and also significant insight into the physiology of the reperfusion syndrome.

Transcranial Doppler, Periprocedural Setup

The patient is placed in the normal supine position on the angiographic table. The TCD headgear (Figure 14–1A) is placed in a position such that the lateral Doppler transducer fixation gaits can be aligned just above the zygomatic arch along the temporal window. This allows for the continuous sampling of pulse wave Doppler signals from the middle cerebral distribution, as detailed in Figure 14–1B. Fortunately, the headgear is radiolucent, except for the lateral brackets and tightening apparatus as shown in Figure 14–2. Thus, digital subtraction intracerebral angiography can be performed without removal of the headgear. The patient is then prepped and

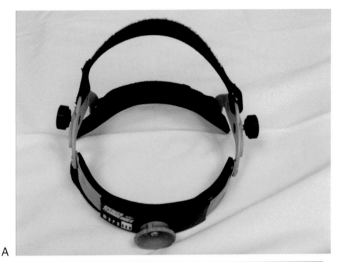

A

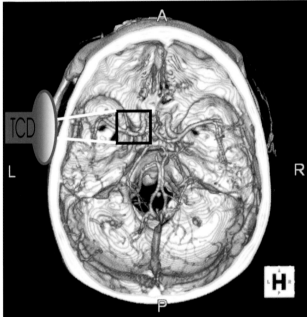

B

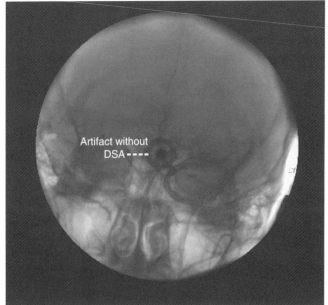

A

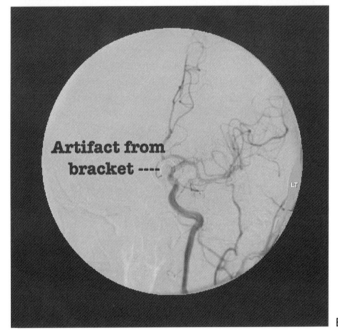

B

FIGURE 14–1. (A) The Spencer technologies headgear utilized for securing the transcranial Doppler probe for periprocedural imaging. The torque device in the front tightens the harness depending on the patient's cranial circumference. The lateral devices allow for positioning of the transcranial Doppler in a position appropriate for ideal insonation of the middle cerebral system. (B) A CT angiogram of a patient who subsequently underwent carotid artery stenting. The "TCD" represents the positioning of the probe and the square is the insonation window or area being monitored during carotid stenting.

FIGURE 14–2. (A) A nonsubtracted image illustrating an artifact in the midline related to the ratchet device used to harness the transcranial Doppler. (B) During digital subtraction angiography the artifact silhouette persists but it is still possible to define the intracranial cerebral anatomy in the AP view without removing the transcranial Doppler harness.

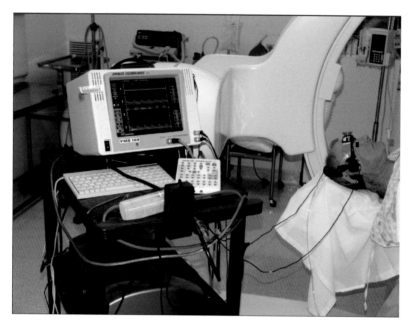

FIGURE 14–3. The typical setup during transcranial Doppler monitoring in the angiographic suite. The patient is placed in a supine position and the transcranial Doppler bracket is fixed to the head prior to baseline angiography.

draped in standard sterile fashion and baseline TCD interrogation is performed (Figure 14–3). Ideally, bilateral continuous pulse flow Doppler insonation of the middle cerebral arteries is monitored and digitally recorded throughout the procedure. It should be noted that anywhere from 9 to 16% of patients might not have an ideal window for accurate insonation of the middle cerebral artery.[27,28] In the case of an inadequate image of a window hand positioning of the probe and continuous monitoring are utilized versus continued attempts at repositioning the probe at different stages in the procedure.[27]

Preprocedural "Baseline" Transcranial Doppler Observations

The baseline TCD pattern may show blunting of the peak systolic wave in patients with severe extracranial disease.[28] More importantly, the TCD may give some insight into the collateral support via the Circle of Willis.[29,30] This information will help the operator better understand the patient's ability to tolerate cerebral protection systems that may arrest or even reverse ipsilateral internal carotid artery flow. Niesen et al. reported the utilization of baseline ratio between the peak systolic velocity in the ipsilateral middle cerebral vessel compared to the contralateral middle cerebral system as a reference for collateral support.[31] Also, the baseline intracranial flow characteristics could be important in predicting patients who are at risk for postprocedural reperfusion syndrome and intracranial hemorrhage. Mori et al. suggested the possibility of utilizing further hemodynamic testing in

patients who are at increased risk for intracranial hemorrhage prior to placing them on the table.[32] This may include utilization of carbon dioxide reactivity or VMR testing with Diamox prior to interaction with the lesion.

Periprocedural Transcranial Doppler Observations

Transcranial Doppler provides two important parameters for continuous monitoring during carotid artery stenting. The first is related to ensuring preserved middle cerebral flow velocity and pulse volume. The utilization of a proximal or distal occlusive device for cerebral protection does result in interruption or reversal of flow in the ipsilateral internal carotid artery.[33] During internal carotid artery flow arrest or reversal a dramatic drop in middle cerebral flow velocity on TCD may precede the clinical hemispheric symptoms in patients with severe contralateral disease or inadequate collateral support due to an incomplete Circle of Willis. This provides the operator with additional insight as to how balloon occlusion will be tolerated and whether the procedure will need to be staged. Currently, the most widely tested distal occlusion balloon protection system is the guard wire (previously known as Percusurge). This device is a low-pressure balloon on a 0.014-inch wire that can be navigated across the lesion and then inflated to occlude the internal carotid artery during transcatheter intervention.[20] Utilization of this type of distal balloon occlusion system has proven to be effective in reducing the risk of embolization. However, Al-Mubarak et al. have shown with TCD

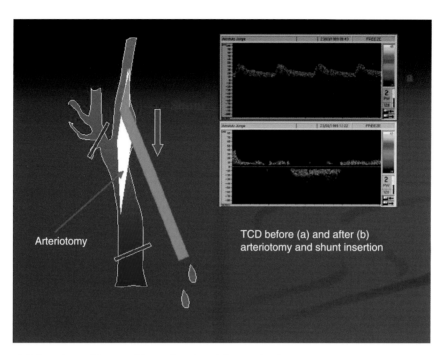

FIGURE 14–4. Transcranial Doppler evidence of intentional middle cerebral artery flow reversal during carotid endarterectomy. (Compliments of Dr. Juan Parodi.)

release of particles during balloon deflation that is likely related to inadequate particle retrieval from the cul-de-sac around the balloon.[34]

Parodi and Bates have shown with TCD the ability to completely reverse flow in the middle cerebral artery by transcatheter occlusion of the ipsilateral common and external carotid artery, while at the same time creating negative pressure at the tip of the guiding sheath as noted in Figure 14–4.[35] This may have significant implications for optimizing cerebral protection during carotid stenting and ultimately even facilitate clot retrieval during transcatheter treatment of acute stroke.

In patients with an intact Circle of Willis undergoing carotid stenting with a protection system that preserves flow (i.e., filter) the sudden interruption of flow to the ipsilateral middle cerebral artery could be an ominous finding suggesting a large embolic event or spasm in the internal carotid artery proper. Also, filter systems do have a threshold of particulate debris based on the filtered design and size.[36] If the volume of embolic debris exceeds the filter threshold then occlusion can occur and this may be heralded by changes on TCD. Similar changes can occur if there is spasm in the ipsilateral internal carotid artery system related to the distal protection filter.[27]

The second variable that is monitored by TCD during carotid artery stenting is the occurrence of microemboli signals (MESs). The reflective properties of microembolic material as it passes through the middle cerebral artery are translated into sudden signal shifts that are depicted as high velocity transient spikes on the continuous Doppler recording.[37–39] These high intensity signals may represent the egress of small particles or microembolic

debris into the ipsilateral hemisphere.[40] It is difficult to differentiate artifact from small air bubbles from true embolic debris and that is one of the limitations of this technology.[41–43] *Ex vitro* studies by Coggia *et al.* and Ohki *et al.* have provided significant insight into when particles are released during different stages of the procedure.[44,45] The peak embolic risk during angioplasty in the *ex vitro* model appears to be during balloon deflation.[44] Similar findings are seen *in vivo* with continuous TCD during carotid stenting at the time of balloon deflation.[46,47] In our experience MESs are seen during all stages of carotid stenting with or without protection even with navigation of a 0.014-inch wire across the lesion (Figure 14–5).

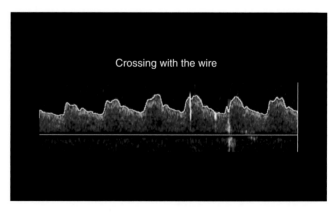

FIGURE 14–5. Small subtle microembolic signals (MESs) coincident with advancing the wire through the lesion. These MESs are shown as bright signals with the most prominent seen in the fourth complete Doppler pulse sequence.

Postprocedural Transcranial Doppler Observations

Some authors have followed TCD with serial interval studies during the first 12h following carotid stenting.[48,49] Our center believes that this may be particularly important in patients who are at increased risk for intracranial hemorrhage. The preprocedural risk factors for reperfusion syndrome and/or intracranial hemorrhage include contralateral severe carotid disease or occlusion, baseline high-grade stenosis or "string sign" with slow flow, hypertension during the carotid stenting procedure, and baseline decrease of vasoreactivity.[50] Figure 14–6 details the TCD hemodynamic sequence of a patient who developed the typical reperfusion syndrome complicated by intra-

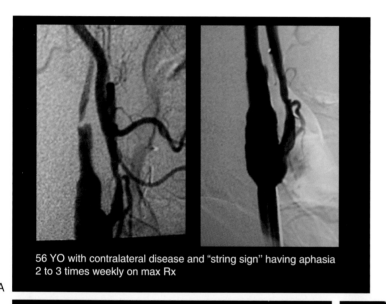

56 YO with contralateral disease and "string sign" having aphasia 2 to 3 times weekly on max Rx

A

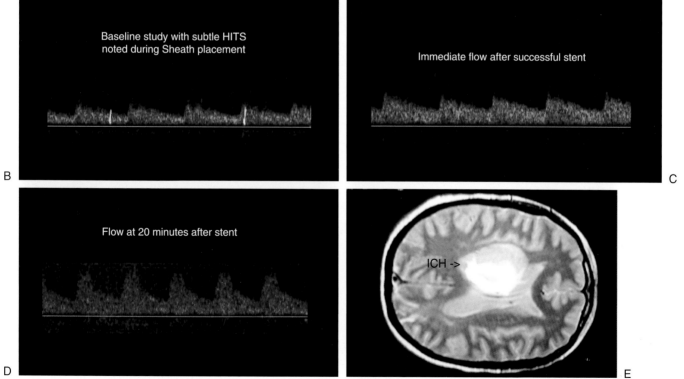

Baseline study with subtle HITS noted during Sheath placement

Immediate flow after successful stent

B

C

Flow at 20 minutes after stent

ICH ->

D

E

FIGURE 14–6. (A) Baseline angiography and follow-up angiography after carotid stenting in a patient with multiple risk factors for postprocedural intracranial hemorrhage. (B) Baseline low pulse volume middle cerebral artery Doppler in the patient illustrated in (A). (C) Immediate flow after carotid stent placement in the patient presented in (A). Note that the flow velocity has increased by approximately 30%. (D) The flow pattern in the same patient depicted in (A). This is 20min following stent placement and note the flow velocity is now three times greater than the baseline velocity. (E) CT scan confirming a large intracranial hemorrhage depicted as an intracerebral hemorrhage (ICH) 12h after stent placement.

cranial hemorrhage during our early experience with unprotected carotid stenting 10 years ago.

Few studies have actually reported continuous TCD in the early postoperative period after carotid stenting. However, it seems that MESs are uncommon during the recovery period after carotid stenting.[51]

Significance of Microemboli during Carotid Artery Stenting

Microembolic signals detected during carotid endarterectomy have been associated with a decrease in cognitive function.[52] Similarly, MESs with so-called "embolic storms" during different stages of carotid stent procedures are associated with ipsilateral defects on early follow-up diffusion weighted magnetic resonance imaging (MRI) scan.[53–57] Currently, there are very few data with regard to cognitive function in patients following protected carotid artery stenting, and this is a concern. Interestingly, in a small subgroup analysis of patients during the Carotid and Vertebral Artery Transluminal Angioplasty Study (CAVATAS) there were similar outcomes on neurologic testing in both the carotid endarterectomy and carotid stenting groups in spite of a higher number of MESs in the latter.[58]

The threshold or "safe" size for microemboli has not been clearly defined. Early work suggests that any particles more than 50 μm in size will not circulate to the venous cerebral system and thus by definition will cause some arteriolar occlusions.[59] Significant work on this front has been done to better understand the decrease in cognitive function that is seen after coronary artery bypass surgery. Based on a postmortem study by Moody *et al.* it appears that the particles causing decreased cognitive function after coronary artery bypass surgery are less than 70 μm in size.[60] This is particularly important to understand since most distal protection filters have a pore size of 100–120 μm.

Differentiating Microemboli from Air Bubbles

The differentiation of air bubbles from true atheroemboli has been very difficult. Several techniques have been described including a defined threshold of greater than 10 hits in a sequence.[27] Different mathematical sequences have also been defined through the years, however, there currently is no ideal way to differentiate these *in vivo*.[41–44]

There are certain stages of the procedure where contamination from an air artifact would be less likely. For example, crossing the lesion with the wire as noted in Figure 14–5 should not be associated with air emboliza-

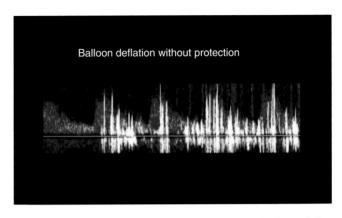

FIGURE 14–7. Multiple MESs in a patient after balloon deflation in our early experience before cerebral protection was available.

tion and is likely true microemboli. Also, many centers have reported that the highest numbers of emboli occur with predilatation or postdilatation as the balloon is deflated and it is also unlikely there is significant trapped air or artifact during this time as depicted in Figure 14–7. However, scattered MESs are typically seen during contrast injections, which is related to microbubbles in the contrast (Figure 14–8).

Most of the carotid stents used today are self-expanding stents made of nickel titanium with an outer constraining sheath. There is always a high volume of MES with retracting of the sheath housing the self-expanding stent and some authors have suggested that this is related to the shear force of a stent against the plaque.[27] However, we feel this is related to trapped air within the fabric of the stent and, thus, is less likely to be of pathologic concern (Figure 14–9).

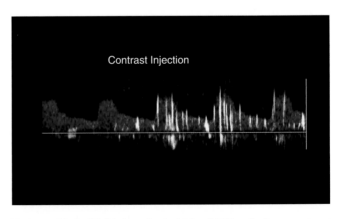

FIGURE 14–8. Multiple air bubble MESs during contrast injection.

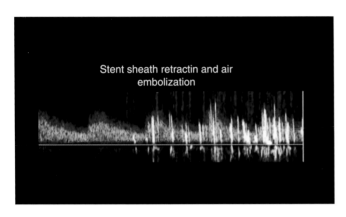

Figure 14–9. Fairly impressive air bubble microemboli during sheath retraction at the time of stent deployment.

Conclusions

Currently, TCD has not been declared mandatory for periprocedural adjuvant monitoring in patients undergoing carotid artery stenting based on consensus documents.[61] Many centers believe that transcranial Doppler is more of an academic tool to help understand the benefits and failure modes of current protection systems. Periprocedural transcranial Doppler is clearly indicated in patients who are at high risk for reperfusion syndrome and may also give additional insight into the long-term issues of decreased cerebral flow reserve and/or worsening cognitive function after carotid stenting. Obviously, there is much more to learn in terms of better understanding microemboli and the long-term consequences MESs have on the patients after carotid stenting. We believe TCD provides invaluable information during the procedure and should be applied to all patients undergoing carotid stenting. Clearly, the argument could be made that patients at high risk for reperfusion syndrome or those undergoing carotid stenting with internal carotid artery flow arrest or flow reversal should have TCD guidance. Only future studies will help us understand the importance of MESs in predicting issues related to cognitive function.

References

1. Aaslid R, Markwalder TM, Nornes H. Noninvasive transcranial Doppler ultrasound recording of flow velocity in basal cerebral arteries. J Neurosurg 1982;57(6):769–74.
2. Bogdahn U, Becker G, Winkler J, et al. Transcranial color-coded real-time sonography in adults. Stroke 1990;21:1680–88.
3. North American Symptomatic Carotid Endarterectomy Trial Collaborators. Beneficial effect of carotid endarterectomy in symptomatic patients with high-grade carotid stenosis. N Engl J Med 1991;325:445–53.
4. European Carotid Surgery Trialists' Group. MRC European carotid surgery trial: Interim results for symptomatic patients with severe or with mild carotid stenosis. Lancet 1991;337:1235–43.
5. AbuRahma AF, Hannay RS. A study of 510 carotid endarterectomies and a review of the recent carotid endarterectomy trials. WV Med J 2001;97(4):197–200.
6. Bond R, Rerkasem K, AbuRahma AF, Naylor AR, Rothwell PM. Patch angioplasty versus primary closure for carotid endarterectomy. Cochrane Database Syst Rev 2004;(2):CD000160.
7. Diethrich EB. Indications for carotid artery stenting: A preview of the potential derived from early clinical experience. J Endovasc Surg 1996;3:132–9.
8. Naylor AR, Bolia A, Abbott RJ, Pye IF, Smith J, Lennard N, Lloyd AJ, London NJ, Bell PR. Randomized study of carotid angioplasty and stenting versus carotid endarterectomy: A stopped trial. J Vasc Surg 1998;28(2):326.
9. Leisch F, Kerschner K, Hofman R, Bibl D, Engleder C, Bergmann H. Carotid stenting: Acute results and complications. Z Kardiol 1999;88:661–68.
10. Bettman MA, Katzen BT, Whisnant J, Brant-Zawadski MB, Broderick JP, Furlan AJ, Hershey LA, Howard V, Kuntz R, Loftus CM, Pearce W, Roberts A, Roubin G. Cartoid Stenting and Angioplasty. A statement for healthcare professionals from the councils on cardiovascular radiology, stroke, cardio-thoracic and vascular surgery, epidemiology and prevention, and clinical cardiology, American Heart Association. Stroke 1998;29:336–48.
11. Theron JG, Peyelle GG, Coskun O, et al. Carotid artery stenosis: Treatment with protected balloon angioplasty and stent placement. Radiology 1996;201:627–36.
12. Wholey MH, Al-Mubarak N, Wholey MH. Updated review of the global carotid artery stent registry. Catheter Cardiovasc Interv 2003;60:259–66.
13. Ohki T, Feith FJ. Carotid artery stenting: Utility of cerebral protection devices. J Invasive Cardiol 2001;13:47–55.
14. Henry M, Amor M, Klonaris C, et al. Angioplasty and stenting of the extracranial carotid arteries. Tex Heart Inst J 2000;27:150–58.
15. Reimers B, Corvaja N, Moshiri S, et al. Cerebral protection with filter devices during carotid artery stenting. Circulation 2001;104:12–15.
16. Parodi JC, Mura RL, Ferreira LM, et al. Initial evaluation of carotid angioplasty and stenting with three different cerebral protection devices. J Vasc Surg 2000;32:1127–36.
17. Al-Mubarak N, Colombo A, Gaines PA, et al. Multicenter evaluation of carotid artery stenting with a filter protection system. J Am Coll Cardiol 2002;39:841–46.
18. Mathur A, Roubin GS, Iyer SS, et al. Predictors of stroke complicating carotid artery stenting. Circulation 1998;97:1239–45.
19. Yadav JS, Roubin GS, Iyer S, et al. Elective stenting of the extracranial carotid arteries. Circulation 1997;95:376–81.
20. Al-Moubarak N, Roubin GS, Vitek JJ, et al. Effect of the distal-balloon protection system on microembolization during carotid stenting. Circulation 2001;104:199–200.
21. Zarins CK. Carotid endarterectomy: The gold standard. J Endovasc Surg 1996;3:10–15.
22. Yadav JS, WholeyMH, Kuntz RE, Fayed, P, Katzen, BT, Mishkel GJ, Bajwa TK, Whitlow P, Strickman NE, Jaff MR,

Popma JJ, Snead DB, Cutlilp DE, Firth BG, Ouriel K. Stenting and Angioplasty with Protection in Patients at High Risk for Endarterectomy Investigators. N Engl J Med 2004;351(15):1493–501.

23. Ireland JK, Chaloupka JC, Weigele JB, *et al.* Potential utility of carotid stent assisted percutaneous transluminal angioplasty in the treatment of symptomatic carotid occlusive disease in patients with high neurological risk. Stroke 2003;34:308.

24. Qureshi AI, Boulos AS, Kim SH, *et al.* Carotid angioplasty and stent placement using the Filterwire for distal protection: An international multicenter study. Stroke 2003;34:307.

25. Roubin GS, New G, Iyer SS, *et al.* Immediate and late clinical outcomes of carotid artery stenting in patients with symptomatic and asymptomatic carotid artery stenosis: A 5-year prospective analysis. Circulation 2001;103: 532–37.

26. MacDonald S, Venables GS, Cleveland TJ, *et al.* Protected carotid stenting: Safety and efficacy of the MedNova NeuroSheild filter. J Vasc Surg 2002;35:966–72.

27. Benichou H, Bergeron P. Carotid angioplasty and stenting: Will periprocedural transcranial Doppler monitoring be important? J Endovasc Surg 1996;3:217–23.

28. (a) Hartmann A, Mast H, Thompson JL, Sia RM, Mohr JP. Transcranial Doppler waveform blunting in severe extracranial carotid artery stenosis. Cerebrovasc Dis 2000;10(1): 33–8. (b) Gomez CR, Brass LM, Tegeler CH, *et al.* The transcranial Doppler standardization project. J Neuroimaging 1993;3:190–92.

29. Visser GH, Wieneke GH, van Huffelen AC, Eikelboom BC. The use of preoperative transcranial Doppler variables to predict which patients do not need a shunt during carotid endarterectomy. Stroke 2003;34:813–9.

30. Reinhard M, Muller T, Roth M, Guschlbauer B, Timmer J, Hetzel A. Bilateral severe carotid artery stenosis or occlusion—-cerebral autoregulation dynamics and collateral flow patterns. Acta Neurochir (Wien) 2003;145(12):1053–9.

31. Niesen WD, Rosenkranz M, Eckert B, Meissner M, Weiller C, Sliwka U. Hemodynamic changes of the cerebral circulation after stent-protected carotid angioplasty. AJNR Am J Neuroradiol 2004;25(7):1162–7.

32. Mori T, Fukuoka M, Kazita K, Mima T, Mori K. Intraventricular hemorrhage after carotid stenting. J Endovasc Surg 1999;6(4):337–41.

33. Tan W, Bates MC, Wholey M. Cerebral protection systems for distal emboli during carotid artery interventions. J Intervent Cardiol 2001;14(4):1–9.

34. Al-Mubarak N, Roubin GS, Vitek JJ, Iyer SS. Microembolization during carotid artery stenting with the distal-balloon antiemboli system. Int Angiol 2002;21(4):344–8.

35. Parodi JC, Bates MC. Angioplasty and stent with reversal of internal carotid flow as a cerebral protection device. In: Greenhalgh RM (ed). *ATLAS: Vascular and Endovascular Surgical Techniques*, 4th ed., pp. 198–213. Philadelphia: Saunders, 2001.

36. Kindel M, Spiller P. Transient occlusion of an Angioguard protection system by massive embolization during angioplasty of a degenerated coronary saphenous vein graft. Catheter Cardiovasc Interv 2002;55:2501–4.

37. Moehring MA, Ritcey JA. Microembolus sizing in a blood mimicking fluid using a novel dual-frequency pulsed Doppler. Echocardiography 1996;13(5):567–71.

38. Moehring MA, Ritcey JA. Sizing emboli in blood using pulse Doppler ultrasound—II: Effects of beam refraction. IEEE Trans Biomed Eng 1996;43(6):581–88.

39. Moehring MA, Klepper JR. Pulse Doppler ultrasound detection, characterization and size estimation of emboli in flowing blood. IEEE Trans Biomed Eng 1994;41(1):35–44.

40. Crawley F, *et al.* Comparison of hemodynamic cerebral ischemia and microembolic signals detected during carotid endarterectomy and carotid angioplasty. Stroke 1997; 28(12):2460–64.

41. Devuyst G, Darbellay GA, Vesin JM, Kemeny V, Ritter M, Droste DW, Molina C, Serena J, Sztajzel R, Ruchat P, Lucchesi C, Dietler G, Ringelstein EB, Despland PA, Bogousslavsky J. Automatic classification of HITS into artifacts or solid or gaseous emboli by a wavelet representation combined with dual-gate TCD. Stroke 2001;32(12): 2803–9.

42. Georgiadis D, Uhlmann F, Lindner A, Zierz S. Differentiation between true microembolic signals and artifacts using an arbitrary sample volume. Ultrasound Med Biol 2000; 26(3):493–6.

43. Rodriguez RA, Giachino A, Hosking M, Nathan HJ. Transcranial Doppler characteristics of different embolic materials during in vivo testing. J Neuroimaging 2002;12(3): 259–66.

44. Ohki T, Roubin GS, Veith FJ, *et al.* The efficacy of a filter in preventing embolic events during carotid artery stenting. An ex-vivo analysis. J Vasc Surg 1999;30:1034–44.

45. Coggia M, Goeau-Brissonniere O, Duval JL, *et al.* Embolic risk of the different stages of carotid bifurcation balloon angioplasty: An experimental study. J Vasc Surg 2000;31: 550–57.

46. Antonius Carotid Endarterectomy, Angioplasty, and Stenting Study Group. Transcranial Doppler monitoring in angioplasty and stenting of the carotid bifurcation. J Endovasc Ther 2003;10(4):702–10.

47. Orlandi G, Fanucchi S, Fioretti C, Acerbi G, Puglioli M, Padolecchia R, Sartucci F, Murri L. Characteristics of cerebral microembolism during carotid stenting and angioplasty alone. Arch Neurol 2001;58(9):1410–3.

48. Abou-Chebl A, Yadav JS, Reginelli JP, Bajzer C, Bhatt D, Krieger DW. Intracranial hemorrhage and hyperperfusion syndrome following carotid artery stenting: Risk factors, prevention, and treatment. J Am Coll Cardiol 2004;43(9): 1596–601.

49. Dalman JE, Beenakkers IC, Moll FL, Leusink JA, Ackerstaff RG. Transcranial Doppler monitoring during carotid endarterectomy helps to identify patients at risk of postoperative hyperperfusion. Eur J Vasc Endovasc Surg 1999; 18(3):222–7.

50. Morrish W, Grahovac S, Douen A. Intracranial hemorrhage after stenting and angioplasty of extracranial carotid stenosis. AJNR Am J Neuroradiol 2000;21:1911–16.

51. Censori B, Camerlingo M, Casto L, Partziguian T, Caverni L, Bonaldi G, Mamoli A. Carotid stents are not a source of microemboli late after deployment. Acta Neurol Scand 2000;102(1):27–30.

52. Gaunt ME, Martin PJ, Smith JL, Bell PR. Clinical relevance of intraoperative embolization detected by transcranial Doppler ultrasonography during carotid endarterectomy: A prospective study of 100 patients. AR Br J Surg 1994;81: 1435–9.

53. van Heesewijk HP, Vos JA, Louwerse ES, Van Den Berg JC, Overtoom TT, Ernst SM, Mauser HW, Moll FL, Ackerstaff RG. Carotid PTA and Stenting Collaborative Research Group. New brain lesions at MR imaging after carotid angioplasty and stent placement. Radiology 2002;224(2): 361–5.

54. Jaeger H, Mathias K, Drescher R, Hauth E, Bockisch G, Demirel E, Gissler HM. Clinical results of cerebral protection with a filter device during stent implantation of the carotid artery. Cardiovasc Intervent Radiol 2001;24(4): 249–56.

55. Wilkinson ID, Griffiths PD, Hoggard N, Cleveland TJ, Gaines PA, Macdonald S, McKevitt F, Venables GS. Short-term changes in cerebral microhemodynamics after carotid stenting. AJNR Am J Neuroradiol 2003;24(8): 1497–9.

56. Jaeger HJ, Mathias KD, Drescher R, Hauth E, Bockish G, Demirel E, Gissler HM. Diffusion-weighted MR imaging after angioplasty or angioplasty plus stenting of arteries supplying the brain. AJNR Am J Neuroradiol 2001;22(7): 1234–5.

57. Schluter M, Tubler T, Steffens JC, Mathey DG, Schofer J. Focal ischemia of the brain after neuroprotected carotid artery stenting. J Am Coll Cardiol 2003;42(6):1014–6.

58. Crawley F, Stygall J, Lunn S, et al. Comparison of microembolism detected by transcranial Doppler and neuropsychological sequelae of carotid surgery and percutaneous transluminal angioplasty. Stroke 2000;31:1329–34.

59. Sadoshima S, Heistad DD. Regional cerebral blood flow during hypotension in normotensive and stroke-prone spontaneously hypertensive rats: Effect of sympathetic denervation. Stroke. 1983;14(4):575–9.

60. Moody DM, Brown WR, Challa VR, Stump DA, Reboussin DM, Legault C. Brain microemboli associated with cardiopulmonary bypass: A histologic and magnetic resonance imaging study. Ann Thorac Surg 1995;59(5):1304–7.

61. Bettman MA, Katzen BT, Whisnant J, Brant-Zawadzki M, Broderick JP. Carotid stenting and angioplasty: A statement for healthcare professionals from the Councils on Cardiovascular Radiology, Stroke, Cardio-Thoracic and Vascular Surgery, Epidemiology, and Prevention, and Clinical Cardiology, American Heart Association. Circulation 1998;97(1): 121–3.

15
Use of an Angle-Independent Doppler System for Intraoperative Carotid Endarterectomy Surveillance

Manju Kalra, Todd E. Rasmussen, and Peter Gloviczki

Carotid Imaging

For the first few decades following the development and refinement of carotid endarterectomy in the 1950s through 1970s cerebral arteriography was the sole preoperative diagnostic modality and was considered the gold standard for carotid artery imaging. Cerebral arteriography, however, carries a risk of cerebrovascular events of 4% and permanent neurological deficit of approximately 1%.[1] Noninvasive techniques such as oculoplethysmography (OPG), Doppler waveform analysis, and supraorbital directional flow were extensively studied, showed poor or no correlation with arteriography, and were deemed unreliable for surgical decision making.[2,3] The Echoflow (Diagnostic Electronic Corp., Lexington, MA), a continuous wave directional Doppler velocity flowmeter that provided a velocity-sensitive color-coded computer-generated image of the extracranial carotid arteries developed in the 1970s was evaluated by several authors and showed merit as a screening tool for carotid stenosis.[3–7] It was not until the development of duplex ultrasonography (DUS) in the 1980s, however, that the supremacy of arteriography for surgical planning was seriously challenged.[8–12] DUS has become the most widely used screening tool for the detection of carotid stenosis, and in the majority of patients preoperative imaging with DUS alone is accurate, safe, and cost effective.[9,13–16]

Intraoperative Carotid Imaging

Assessment of technical perfection in the operating room is a necessary part of carotid endarterectomy. Historically, such assessment was limited to palpation of the reconstructed carotid artery. Continuous wave Doppler provides an audible assessment of arterial flow that is more sensitive than palpation and less invasive than arteriography, but it does not provide a quantitative measure

and is therefore limited in its reliability and applicability.[17] The use of intraoperative contrast arteriography improves the ability to detect technical problems following endarterectomy and remains a common method for this evaluation. The routine use of intraoperative angiography has been shown to impact the results of carotid endarterectomy favorably by reducing operative mortality (2.9–1%), the permanent stroke rate (1.9–0.9%), and the temporary neurological deficit rate (6.3–1%) as well as the incidence of residual and recurrent stenotic lesions.[18] However, this technique is invasive and cumbersome and carries risk associated with vessel puncture and contrast injection.[18,19] It is routinely performed in a single projection and provides no functional assessment of flow within the reconstructed artery. Furthermore very few, if any, arterial reconstructions are followed with routine repeat arteriography in the months and years following the operation. These limitations of arteriography have accelerated the acceptance of duplex ultrasound for the intraoperative assessment of arterial reconstructions, especially in the carotid circulation.

The use of duplex ultrasonography in the operating room following carotid endarterectomy represents a significant advance that is less invasive than arteriography and provides more objective information than continuous wave Doppler and arteriography.[20,21] Duplex provides not only a grayscale or B-mode image of the vessel, but also a functional assessment of flow through the carotid artery using pulsed Doppler spectral analysis. Schwartz et al. in 1988 identified technical errors in 22% of patients undergoing intraoperative duplex scanning during carotid endarterectomy, with immediate corrective measures undertaken in 11%.[20] DUS has been shown to compare favorably with arteriography for the intaroperative assessment of carotid endarterectomy with false negative rates of 3.4% and 2.1%, respectively.[22] Panneton et al. reported abnormalities on intraoperative duplex examination in 41% of patients undergoing carotid endarterectomy; 30% of these defects were classified as minor and

11% major hemodynamically significant based on the absence or presence of elevated peak systolic velocities, visible residual plaque-producing stenosis, thrombus, or intimal flap/dissection.[23] Ipsilateral perioperative neurological events occurred in two of three patients with unrevised significant defects identified on intraoperative duplex with none occurring following revision of the remaining 14 significant defects. In addition to improved immediate results, normal intraoperative duplex examination has been associated with improved late patency.[24] Even minor defects appeared to be associated with an increased incidence of late restenosis in this study.[24] Therefore, the sensitivity of intraoperative duplex has been shown to be similar to arteriography, it is safer and less cumbersome, and its routine use may decrease restenosis rates following carotid endarterectomy.[22–27]

Despite the usefulness of duplex ultrasound following carotid endarterectomy, this modality has limitations. Duplex requires B-mode imaging of the vessel in order to set or determine the angle of ultrasound insonation and perform pulsed Doppler sampling of arterial velocity. Such imaging requires training and experience in order to acquire accurate, reproducible readings, a skill that in some centers may necessitate a technologist or radiologist. Furthermore interpretation of the B-mode image in the operating room is often subjective and small defects are of unknown consequence and may be misleading. These facts combined with the cost of the duplex ultrasound equipment and the radiologist/technologist time may prohibit its use in the majority of centers performing carotid endarterectomy.

Angle-Independant Doppler System

Recent development and refinement of diffractive ultrasonic transducers have facilitated measurement of blood velocity independent of a B-mode image.[28–30] Thus a functional assessment of blood flow can be obtained with simpler, compact equipment that is easier to use and less expensive than conventional duplex. Traditionally only hemodynamically significant defects detected with duplex scanning have been routinely repaired.[20,23,24] The sensitivity of duplex scanning permits identification of even minor residual abnormalities, the significance of which remains unknown. Identification of elevated peak systolic velocities without a B-mode image with an angle-independent ultrasound would potentially enable detection of hemodynamically significant defects.

Concept of Angle-Independent Ultrasound

Based on the Doppler equation (Figure 15–1) an angle of insonation must be determined or known with a high degree of accuracy in order to determine the velocity of

$$\Delta f = \frac{2 f_0 V \cos \theta}{C}$$

FIGURE 15–1. Doppler equation calculating the magnitude of frequency shift (Δf) where f_o = frequency of transmitted sound, V = velocity of blood, θ = the angle of insonation between the axis of the ultrasound beam and the direction of blood flow, and C = velocity of sound in tissue (~1.56×10^5 cm/s). (Reproduced from J Vasc Surg 2003;37:374–80. Copyright © 2003, with permission from Society of Vascular Surgery.)

flowing blood. Standard duplex ultrasound combines a pulsed Doppler system with a B-mode scanner to allow the insonating beam to be aligned to the vessel at a desired or defined angle. The angle of insonation is set manually by the operator and requires training and experience to perform measurements in a reproducible manner.

The angle-independent ultrasound technology is based on a diffractive transducer that consists of a series of linear piezoelectric elements spaced a fraction of a wavelength apart. The diffracting conditions can be altered to generate multiple ultrasonic beams from a single insonating probe.[28–31] This diffractive transducer technology has led to the development of a new ultrasonic Doppler system that forms two ultrasound beams to insonate vessels and thereby functions to sample arterial velocities without an operator-determined angle (e.g., angle-independent) of insonation (Figure 15–2).

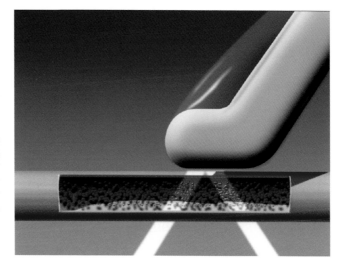

FIGURE 15–2. The diffractive transducer creates two continuous wave ultrasound beams that insonate the blood vessel and facilitates measurement of blood velocity without the need to set an angle of insonation.

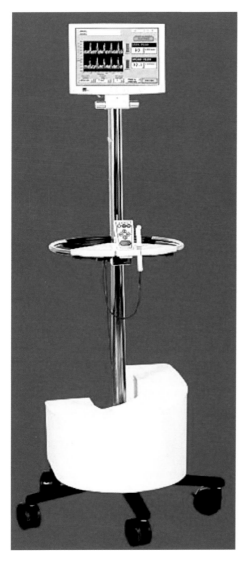

FIGURE 15–3. EchoFlow BVM-1 blood velocity meter (EchoCath, Inc, Princeton, NJ) with elevated display, remote control, printer capability, and mobile console. (Reproduced from J Vasc Surg 2003;37:374–80. Copyright © 2003, with permission from Society of Vascular Surgery.)

The commercially available EchoFlow BVM-1 blood velocity meter (EchoCath, Inc, Princeton, NJ) is a diffractive transducer-based technology that uses two ultrasonic beams and a 10-MHz probe to record blood velocity (Figure 15–3). The diffracting transducer in the EchoFlow device generates two beams to insonate the vessel at two distinct angles. The first ultrasound beam is at an unknown angle of insonation and the second beam differs from the first by a known degree. The two frequency measurements taken from the different ultrasound beams produce two Doppler shift equations with two unknowns (velocity and θ).[28–31] These equations can be solved to determine θ and ultimately blood velocity based on the mathematical equation or principle of two unknowns described by Daigle.[32] Thereby analysis of the two ultrasound beams and their respective Doppler equations allows the EchoFlow system to provide blood velocity measurements without the need to preset an angle of insonation as is necessary with standard duplex ultrasound.

In addition, based on velocity measured and the size of the vessel insonated this flowmeter also allows flow to be measured independently of the angle of insonation. Its use was initially reported in animal studies.[33] Skladany et al. made 65 flow determinations in the carotid arteries of five pigs. Flow measurements were obtained in arteries bled into a calibrated vessel and compared with the true volume of the blood captured. The flowmeter measured flow-volume rates in milliliters per minute were found to be within ± 15% of the cylinder captured volume.[33]

Clinical Evaluation of the Angle-Independent Doppler System

The small size and portability, low operator dependency, and low cost of this ultrasonic flowmeter suggested potential for widespread clinical applicability. There is no need for the operator to hold the probe at a predetermined angle to measure flow velocity in the carotid artery. The system is therefore easier to use, does not require a technologist or a radiologist, and is less expensive than conventional duplex scan. To measure velocity intraoperatively in the carotid artery, one probe can be used for all patients and all size vessels. The probe is placed over the surface of the vessel and a single switch is pushed to obtain a measurement (Figure 15–2). The waveform and velocity measurements are displayed on an LCD screen (Figure 15–4).

The EchoFlow angle-independent ultrasonic Doppler system was evaluated by us for intraoperative surveillance following carotid endarterectomy in 65 consecutive patients (36 female, 29 male; mean age, 71 years). Velocity measurements of the common, internal, and external carotid arteries were performed in 65 patients after carotid endarterectomy Three velocity measurements were obtained by the vascular surgeon from each of the arteries with the EchoFlow device and compared with the velocity measurements obtained with the duplex ultrasound scan performed by a radiologist.[34]

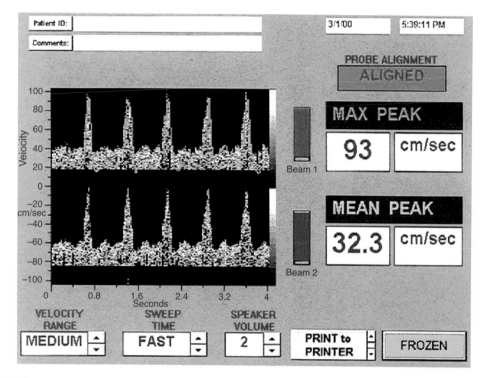

FIGURE 15–4. EchoFlow system projects the arterial Doppler waveform on the left of the display screen and the velocity readings on the right. It also provides an audible Doppler signal and has the capability to send readings to a printer.

Reliability of Angle-Independent Velocity Measurement

Velocity measurements obtained using the angle-independent system were reproducible in the common, internal, and external carotid arteries with intrapatient correlation coefficients of 0.95, 0.96, and 0.95, respectively (Table 15–1).

Comparison to Duplex Ultrasound

Mean velocity measurement difference (bias) between EchoFlow and duplex was −12 cm/s for the common carotid artery, −8 cm/s for the internal carotid artery, and −11 cm/s for the external carotid artery (Table 15–2). Intraclass correlation coefficients were 0.60, 0.69, and 0.73 for the common, internal, and external carotid arteries, respectively. Within-patient differences showed a significant correlation with increasing velocity measurements in each of the three arteries measured ($p < 0.05$).

The vast majority of velocity measurements from the common, internal, and external carotid arteries fell within two standard deviations of the mean differences between EchoFlow and duplex. The majority of velocity measurements from each of the three carotid arteries with

EchoFlow were within an error of ±25 cm/s compared to velocity measurements obtained by duplex ultrasound (Figure 15–5). Seventy-five percent of common, 88% of internal, and 78% of external carotid velocity measurements obtained with the angle-independent ultrasound scan device were within 25 cm/s of the velocities measured with duplex ultrasound scan. Differences between the EchoFlow device and duplex scan velocity measurements correlated with increasing arterial velocities in each of the three arteries measured ($p < 0.05$).

When interpreting these results, it is important to recall the limitations of the study. Only peak systolic velocity was

TABLE 15–1. Intrapatient reliability of EchoFlow carotid velocity measurements.

Vessel[a]	Within patient standard deviation (cm/s)	Intraclass correlation coefficient
CC	4.65	0.95
IC	4.42	0.96
EC	6.81	0.95

[a]CC, common carotid; IC, internal carotid; EC, external carotid.

TABLE 15–2. Comparison of carotid velocity measurements between EchoFlow and duplex.

Vessel[a]	Mean difference (bias) (Echoflow-duplex)	Standard deviation of differences (Echoflow-duplex)	Limits of agreement (95%)	Diff ≤25 cm/s (%)	Intraclass correlation coefficient
CC	−11.91	22.0	−55 to 31	75.4	0.60
IC	−8.33	20.0	−47 to 31	87.5	0.69
EC	−11.35	30.6	−71 to 49	77.5	0.73

[a]CC, common carotid; IC, internal carotid; EC, external carotid.

measured; the study included only a limited number of patients and an assessment on outcome was not reported. Also, the specific point of insonation on the artery from which velocities were sampled may have varied between the EchoFlow and duplex scan probes, making agreement between these two methods difficult to confirm.[34]

Based on the results of this preliminary study application of the angle-independent ultrasound system should be viewed as a supplement to and not a replacement for standard duplex ultrasound at the present time. This new system represents an initial or screening modality available in the operating room to assess arterial reconstruction or bypass much like continuous wave Doppler is currently used. If a technical defect is suspected duplex ultrasound or intraoperative arteriography should continue to be performed.

The noninvasive and compact nature of the angle-independent ultrasound device combined with its simple operating system make its potential application broad. The manufacturing cost of this unit has been contained and is less than $10,000 for a fully equipped unit, significantly less expensive than the standard duplex ultrasound machine.[33] Furthermore, elimination of the need for a specially trained person to operate the device substantially reduces the operating cost of the unit.

By providing an objective velocity measurement with an audible Doppler signal this technology significantly extends continuous wave Doppler yet is nearly as

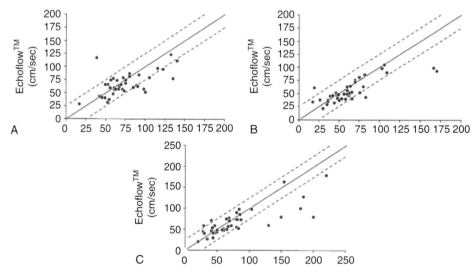

FIGURE 15–5. (A) Comparison of peak systolic velocity measurements between EchoFlow (y-axis) and duplex (x-axis) from the common carotid artery. Dashed reference lines represent error of ±25 cm/s. (Reproduced with permission from J Vasc Surg 2003;37:374–80). (B) Comparison of peak systolic velocity measurements between EchoFlow (y-axis) and duplex (x-axis) from the internal carotid artery. Dashed reference lines represent error of ±25 cm/s. (Reproduced with permission from J Vasc Surg 2003;37:374–80). (C) Comparison of peak systolic velocity measurements between EchoFlow (y-axis) and duplex (x-axis) from the external carotid artery. Dashed reference lines represent error of ± 25 cm/s. (Reproduced from J Vasc Surg 2003;37:374–80. Copyright © 2003, with permission from Society of Vascular Surgery.)

simple to use. This technology may provide surgeons who do not otherwise have access to duplex ultrasound machines and the expertise necessary to use them with a comparable means of assessing arterial velocity in the operating room. It has potential broad applicability in the intraoperative assessment of arterial velocities following reconstruction or bypass.

References

1. Hankey GJ, Warlow CP, Sellar RJ. Cerebral angiographic risk in mild cerebrovascular disease. Stroke 1990;21(2):209–22.
2. Lefemine AA, Broach J, Woolley TW. Comparison of arteriography and noninvasive techniques for the diagnosis of carotid artery disease. A statistical analysis of 140 patients. Am Surg 1986;52(10):526–31.
3. Persson AV, O'Leary DH, Kovacs A, Dyer VE. Clinical use of noninvasive evaluation of the carotid artery. Surg Clin North Am 1980;60(3):513–26.
4. Curry GR, White DN. Color coded ultrasonic differential velocity arterial scanner (Echoflow). Ultrasound Med Biol 1978;4(1):27–35.
5. Oliva L, Gemma GB, Bertoglio C, Rezzo R, Stabilini L. [Doppler ultrasonic arteriography with colorimetric morpho-function analysis of frequency (Echoflow). Preliminary trials]. Minerva Med 1981;72(37):2465–71.
6. Schain FB, Balzer K, Carstensen G. Non-invasive studies of the extra-cranial cerebral arteries: Indication for angiography and operation. Thorac Cardiovasc Surg 1982;30(1):2–6.
7. Torvaldsen S, McCauley J, Patel AS, Chakera TM. Assessment of cervical carotid artery disease. A comparison between the Doppler "Echoflow" and conventional angiography. Med J Aust 1985;142(10):542–5.
8. Hames TK, Humphries KN, Ratliff DA, Birch SJ, Gazzard VM, Chant AD. The validation of duplex scanning and continuous wave Doppler imaging: A comparison with conventional angiography. Ultrasound Med Biol 1985;11(6):827–34.
9. Dawson DL, Zierler RE, Strandness DE Jr, Clowes AW, Kohler TR. The role of duplex scanning and arteriography before carotid endarterectomy: A prospective study. J Vasc Surg 1993;18(4):673–80; discussion 680–3.
10. Taylor DC, Strandness DE Jr. Carotid artery duplex scanning. J Clin Ultrasound 1987;15(9):635–44.
11. Londrey GL, Spadone DP, Hodgson KJ, Ramsey DE, Barkmeier LD, Sumner DS. Does color-flow imaging improve the accuracy of duplex carotid evaluation? J Vasc Surg 1991;13(5):659–63.
12. Bray JM, Galland F, Lhoste P, Nicolau S, Dubas F, Emile J, et al. Colour Doppler and duplex sonography and angiography of the carotid artery bifurcations. Prospective, double-blind study. Neuroradiology 1995;37(3):219–24.
13. Wagner WH, Treiman RL, Cossman DV, Foran RF, Levin PM, Cohen JL. The diminishing role of diagnostic arteriography in carotid artery disease: Duplex scanning as definitive preoperative study. Ann Vasc Surg 1991;5(2):105–10.
14. McKittrick JE, Cisek PL, Pojunas KW, Blum GM, Ortgiesen P, Lim RA. Are both color-flow duplex scanning and cerebral arteriography required prior to carotid endarterectomy? Ann Vasc Surg 1993;7(4):311–6.
15. Chervu A, Moore WS. Carotid endarterectomy without arteriography. Ann Vasc Surg 1994;8(3):296–302.
16. Shifrin EG, Bornstein NM, Kantarovsky A, Morag B, Zelmanovich L, Portnoi I, et al. Carotid endarterectomy without angiography. Br J Surg 1996;83(8):1107–9.
17. Seifert KB, Blackshear WM Jr. Continuous-wave Doppler in the intraoperative assessment of carotid endarterectomy. J Vasc Surg 1985;2(6):817–20.
18. Courbier R, Jausseran JM, Reggi M, Bergeron P, Formichi M, Ferdani M. Routine intraoperative carotid angiography: Its impact on operative morbidity and carotid restenosis. J Vasc Surg 1986;3(2):343–50.
19. Blaisdell FW, Lim R Jr, Hall AD. Technical result of carotid endarterectomy. Arteriographic assessment. Am J Surg 1967;114(2):239–46.
20. Schwartz RA, Peterson GJ, Noland KA, Hower JF Jr, Naunheim KS. Intraoperative duplex scanning after carotid artery reconstruction: A valuable tool. J Vasc Surg 1988;7(5):620–4.
21. Bandyk DF, Mills JL, Gahtan V, Esses GE. Intraoperative duplex scanning of arterial reconstructions: Fate of repaired and unrepaired defects. J Vasc Surg 1994;20(3):426–32; discussion 432–3.
22. Dilley RB, Bernstein EF. A comparison of B-mode real-time imaging and arteriography in the intraoperative assessment of carotid endarterectomy. J Vasc Surg 1986;4(5):457–63.
23. Panneton JM, Berger MW, Lewis BD, Hallett JW Jr, Bower TC, Gloviczki P, et al. Intraoperative duplex ultrasound during carotid endarterectomy. Vasc Surg 2001;35(1):1–9.
24. Baker WH, Koustas G, Burke K, Littooy FN, Greisler HP. Intraoperative duplex scanning and late carotid artery stenosis. J Vasc Surg 1994;19(5):829–32; discussion 832–3.
25. Coelho JC, Sigel B, Flanigan DP, Schuler JJ, Spigos DG, Tan WS, et al. An experimental evaluation of arteriography and imaging ultrasonography in detecting arterial defects at operation. J Surg Res 1982;32(2):130–7.
26. Seelig MH, Oldenburg WA, Chowla A, Atkinson EJ. Use of intraoperative duplex ultrasonography and routine patch angioplasty in patients undergoing carotid endarterectomy. Mayo Clin Proc 1999;74(9):870–6.
27. Papanicolaou G, Toms C, Yellin AE, Weaver FA. Relationship between intraoperative color-flow duplex findings and early restenosis after carotid endarterectomy: A preliminary report. J Vasc Surg 1996;24(4):588–95; discussion 595–6.
28. Vilkomerson DL, Lyons D, Chilipka T. Diffractive transducers for angle-independant velocity measurements. *Proceedings of the 1994 Ultrasonics Symposium*, pp. 1677–1682. Piscataway: IEEE Press, 1994.
29. Vilkomerson D, Chilipka T, Lyons D. Higher-order diffracting-grating transducers. Med Imaging (SPIE) 1997;3037:206–12.
30. Palachon PV, Lyons D, Chilipka T, Shung K. Improved diffracting grating transducers. Med Imaging (SPIE) 1999;3664:155–60.

31. Vilkomerson DL, Lyons D, Domagala P, Chilipka T. Considerations in design of angle-independent Doppler instruments using diffracting-grating transducers. *Proceedings of the 1999 Ultrasonics Symposium,* pp. 1459–1464. Piscataway: IEEE Press, 1999.

32. Daigle R. Aortic flow sensing using an ultrasonic esophageal probe. Doctoral thesis, Colorado State University, 1974.

33. Skladany M, Vilkomerson D, Lyons D, Chilipka T, Delamere M, Hollier LH. New, angle-independent, low cost Doppler system to measure blood flow. Am J Surg 1998; 176(2):179–82.

34. Rasmussen TE, Panneton JM, Kalra M, Hofer JM, Lewis BD, Rowland CM, *et al.* Intraoperative use of a new angle-independent Doppler system to measure arterial velocities after carotid endarterectomy. J Vasc Surg 2003;37(2):374–80.

16
Clinical Implications of the Vascular Laboratory in the Diagnosis of Cerebrovascular Insufficiency

Ali F. AbuRahma

Various noninvasive tests for the evaluation of cerebrovascular insufficiency have been described in previous chapters. Most forms of noninvasive testing pose less stress and less expense to the patient than angiography. While early forms of noninvasive testing depended on the presence of severe disease, the current techniques, especially carotid artery imaging, demonstrate the opposite characteristic. Carotid imaging is able to detect minimal disease that is not hemodynamically significant; in fact, overestimation of the degree of stenosis in these cases has been a consistent problem. Nevertheless, any test intended for screening must have a high degree of sensitivity to be used appropriately in the initial assessment of disease. Noninvasive assessment, therefore, combines low risk, low cost, and high sensitivity.

Although we agree that patients should be evaluated by careful history and physical examination, our policy tends to rely on noninvasive vascular testing as an initial step in the diagnosis of carotid artery disease. The results of noninvasive tests may also help in obtaining optimal angiograms. An example is the patient with noninvasive evidence of severe stenosis who has no significant stenosis demonstrated in standard views of the carotid artery bifurcation. The results of the noninvasive tests indicate the need for additional projections, and if the bifurcation region does not show the expected lesion, there is a strong indication for obtaining adequate siphon views.

Prior to the advent of digital techniques, standard angiograms were routinely used in the evaluation of patients with cerebral ischemic attacks in order to determine whether vascular reconstructive surgery was indicated. Standard angiography was of limited clinical value, particularly as a means of diagnostic screening in asymptomatic patients, because of prohibitive costs, poor patient acceptance, and the risk of arterial catheterization. As a result, noninvasive vascular tests became established as the preferred means of diagnostic screening in asymptomatic patients, because they provided an objective method of determining the hemodynamic signifi-

cance of carotid disease in a safe and relatively cost-efficient manner.

Recent studies have questioned the role of arteriography as the "gold standard" in the evaluation of carotid artery occlusive disease.[1-5] Contrast arteriography has also been noted to have an 1–4% incidence of neurologic complications with about a 1% incidence of stroke reported in the Asymptomatic Carotid Atherosclerosis Study (ACAS).[6] Other complications of arteriography that were reported include complications at the arterial puncture site (5%), and contrast-induced renal dysfunctions in 1–5%. With this in mind, it would be beneficial and cost-effective if these patients could be safely evaluated without invasive arteriography. Color duplex ultrasonography of the carotid arteries and magnetic resonance angiography (MRA) are two noninvasive modalities that can detect and grade carotid artery stenosis.

Carotid Angiography, Magnetic Resonance Angiography, and/or Color Duplex Ultrasound in the Diagnosis of Carotid Artery Disease (Single or Combined)

Carotid duplex ultrasound (DUS) is readily available, noninvasive, inexpensive, fast, repeatable with good resolution of carotid plaque morphology, and has excellent accuracy in most experienced medical centers. One of its limitations is that there is no suitable acoustic access to certain vessels of interest in the body. For example, it cannot directly visualize the origin of the left carotid artery, the distal internal carotids, or the Circle of Willis (Figure 16–1). Therefore, a screening examination based on ultrasound alone may be incomplete for certain surgical patients. Ultrasound is also highly operator

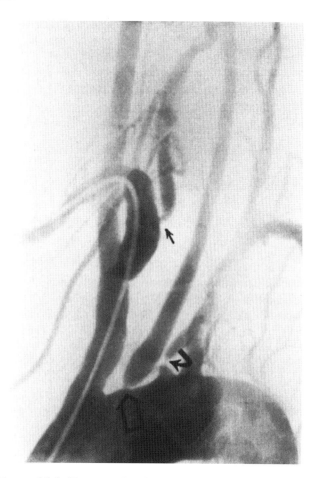

FIGURE 16–1. Four vessel arch aortogram showing tight stenosis at the origin of the left common carotid artery (open arrow), a tight stenosis of the right vertebral artery (straight arrow), and a tight stenosis of the left vertebral artery (curved arrow) which originates from the arch of the aorta.

dependent, with a skilled technologist providing more reliable information than the novice.

The weaknesses of color DUS as a noninvasive screening examination are complemented by MRA. MRA is also a noninvasive modality and can access almost any place in the body, e.g., the carotid artery from the arch to the Circle of Willis, and is not obscured by overlying bone or dense vascular calcification. It is repeatable and less costly than conventional angiography with excellent resolution for severe to total occlusion or minimal carotid artery disease. It can display vessel anatomy as a rotating three-dimensional angiogram that can be readily interpreted by those who did not perform the study (Figure 16–2). Severe or tight stenoses (≥70%) are usually seen as a flow gap (Figure 16–3). Like ultrasound, it can be used to measure blood flow volumes and blood velocity, although it lacks the temporal resolution of Doppler devices. MRA can also be combined with cerebral magnetic resonance imaging at the same time. Since it is noninvasive, it can be applied safely on patients with compromised renal functions or severe contrast allergies.

There is no danger of thromboembolic phenomena as might occur with catheter manipulation during conventional contrast angiography. However, there are several instances in which MRA is likely to be unsuccessful: patients who require intensive monitoring or mechanical respiration are difficult to study by MRA, patients who are claustrophobic will require sedation before the study, and patients who cannot hold still for approximately 4–8 min at a time will have images that are considerably degraded. The images are also degraded by the presence of small pieces of metal in the body near the vessel of interest, e.g., surgical clips and small fragments from surgical instruments. Patients with intracranial aneurysms, clips, or cardiac pacemakers are excluded from having a magnetic resonance angiogram. Other disadvantages of MRA include poor plaque morphology and overestimation of stenoses in certain patients (Figure 16–4). MRA is extremely sensitive to the presence of vascular stenosis. When there is a difficulty, it is usually in specificity, i.e., the stenosis may be overestimated, but rarely missed or underestimated. This overestimation may result from turbulence. Whenever there is a mixing flow or chaotic flow (blood flow that is accelerating and decelerating rapidly), the vascular signal may be lost, and this loss of signal may be misinterpreted as a stenosis.

Cerebral arteriography, on the other hand, has the following advantages: it is relatively accurate and is capable of describing the extent of the lesion or the pathology (Figure 16–1). However, as indicated earlier, it is invasive with a definite small risk of neurologic complications, expensive, with only a fair description of the plaque morphology, and it may also underestimate the pathology or stenosis if proper filming is not undertaken (Figure 16–5).

Several studies have reported satisfactory results of carotid endarterectomy performed with color DUS alone or in combination with MRA.[7–15] Jackson et al. prospectively evaluated carotid MRA and compared its accuracy with color-flow duplex.[16] Fifty patients were prospectively evaluated with conventional angiography and MRA after clinical and color-flow duplex findings indicated the need for carotid angiography. Using receiver-operating characteristic (ROC) curves, the probability of correctly predicting a ≥60% stenosis using various color-flow duplex thresholds and MRA was assessed. Sensitivity, specificity, positive predictive value (PPV), and negative predictive value (NPV) in determining ≥60% stenoses were estimated. For MRA the sensitivity was 85% [95% confidence interval (CI) = 69–94%], specificity 70% (CI = 56–81%), PPV 68% (CI = 53–80%), and NPV 86% (CI = 72–94%). For color-flow duplex, the sensitivity was 89% (CI = 74–96%), specificity 93% (CI = 82–98%), PPV 89% (CI = 74–96%), and NPV 93% (CI = 82–98%). When MRA and color-flow duplex results were concordant (n = 64), the sensitivity was 100% (CI = 89–100%), specificity 95% (CI = 81–99%), PPV 94% (CI = 77–99%), and NPV 100% (CI = 92–100%).

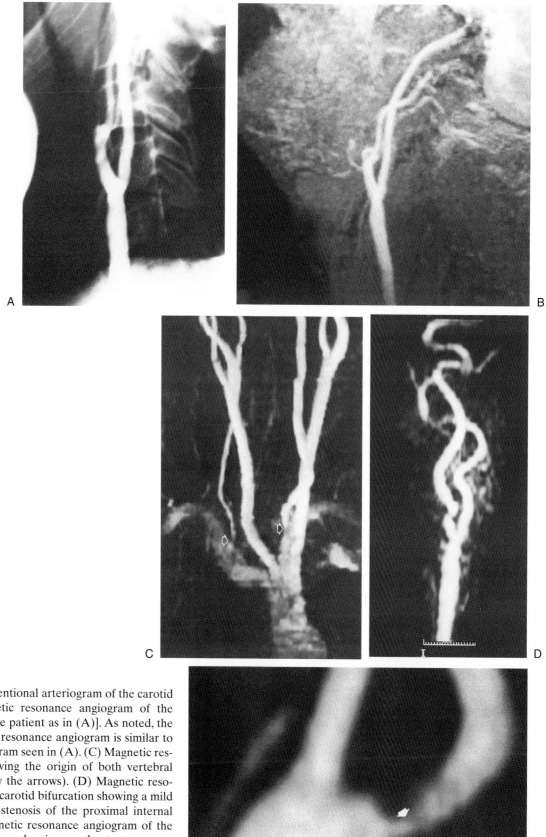

FIGURE 16–2. (A) Conventional arteriogram of the carotid bifurcation. (B) Magnetic resonance angiogram of the carotid bifurcation [same patient as in (A)]. As noted, the quality of this magnetic resonance angiogram is similar to the conventional angiogram seen in (A). (C) Magnetic resonance angiogram showing the origin of both vertebral arteries (as indicated by the arrows). (D) Magnetic resonance angiogram of the carotid bifurcation showing a mild to moderate degree of stenosis of the proximal internal carotid artery. (E) Magnetic resonance angiogram of the carotid artery bifurcation showing moderate to severe stenosis of the internal carotid artery (white arrow).

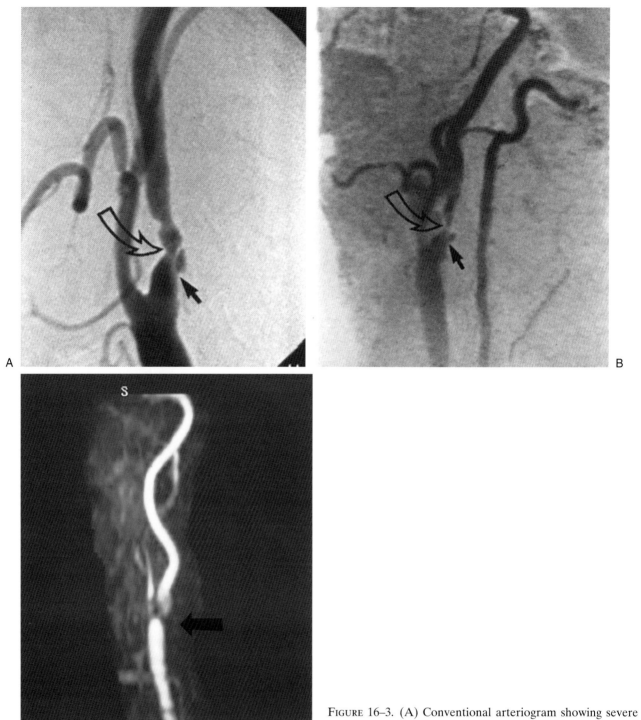

Figure 16–3. (A) Conventional arteriogram showing severe to tight stenosis of the proximal internal carotid artery (curved white arrow) with associated ulceration (black arrow). (B) Three-dimensional TOF magnetic resonance angiogram of the same patient showing the same tight stenosis with ulceration. (C) Carotid magnetic resonance angiogram showing severe to tight stenosis of the internal carotid artery without ulceration as indicated by flow gap (black arrow).

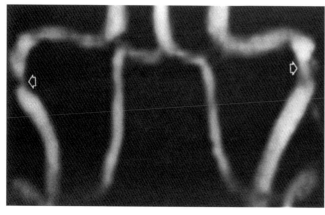
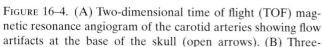

A

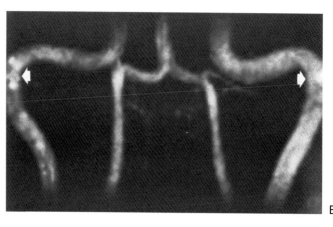

B

FIGURE 16–4. (A) Two-dimensional time of flight (TOF) magnetic resonance angiogram of the carotid arteries showing flow artifacts at the base of the skull (open arrows). (B) Three-dimensional TOF magnetic resonance angiogram of the same patient showing that the narrowing is no longer evident (white arrows).

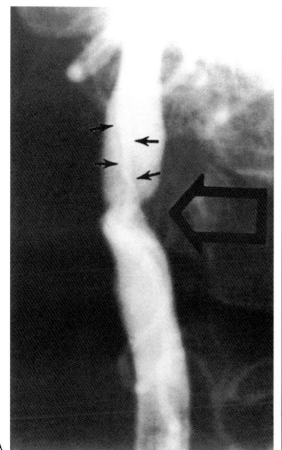

A

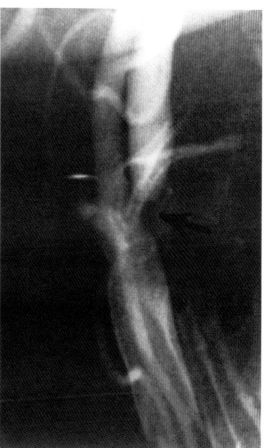

B

FIGURE 16–5. (A) Frontal projection of the carotid artery bifurcation showing minimal disease of the internal carotid artery (large arrow). (B) The same patient on oblique projection showing tight stenosis of the origin of the internal carotid artery (solid black arrow).

The area under the ROC curve for color-flow duplex was 95%, compared to 83% for MRA ($p = 0.0005$). They concluded that the low specificity of MRA precludes its use as the definitive imaging modality for carotid stenosis. The 93% specificity of color-flow duplex alone warrants its consideration as a definitive carotid imaging study. By ROC curve analysis, color-flow duplex offers superior accuracy to MRA. The data of Jackson et al. support non-invasive preoperative carotid imaging for detecting a threshold stenosis of ≥60% whether color-flow duplex is used alone, or in combination with the selective use of MRA.

In a prospective diagnostic study, Nederkoorn et al.[13] investigated the accuracy of noninvasive testing compared with digital subtraction angiography (DSA). They performed DUS, MRA, and DSA on 350 consecutive symptomatic patients. Separate and combined test results of DUS and MRA were compared with the reference standard DSA. DUS had a sensitivity of 87.5% (95% CI, 82.1–92.9%) and a specificity of 75.7% (95% CI, 69.3–82.2%) in identifying severe 70–99% internal carotid artery stenosis. MRA yielded a sensitivity of 92.2% (95% CI, 86.2–96.2%) and a specificity of 75.7% (95% CI, 68.6–82.5%). When MRA and DUS results were combined, agreement between these two modalities (84% of patients) gave a sensitivity of 96.3% (95% CI, 90.8–99.0%) and a specificity of 80.2% (95% CI, 73.1–87.3%) for identifying severe stenosis. It was concluded that MRA showed a slightly better accuracy than DUS in the diagnosis of carotid artery stenosis, however, to achieve the best accuracy, both tests should be performed subsequently.

Westwood et al.[15] conducted a study to determine if sufficient evidence exists to support the use of MRA as a means of selecting patients with recently symptomatic severe carotid stenosis for carotid endarterectomy (CEA). A systematic review of published research on the diagnostic performance of MRA was analyzed. One hundred and twenty-six potentially relevant articles were identified, but many articles failed to examine the performance of MRA as a diagnostic test at the surgical decision thresholds used in major clinical trials on CEA. Twenty-six articles were included in a meta-analysis that showed a maximal joint sensitivity and specificity of 99% (95% CI, 98–100%) for identifying 70–99% stenosis and 90% (81–99%) for identifying 50–99% stenosis. Only four articles evaluated contrast-enhanced MRA. They concluded that MRA was accurate for selecting patients for CEA at the surgical decision thresholds established in the major endarterectomy trials, but the evidence was not very robust because of the heterogeneity of the studies included.

Recently, Nederkoorn et al.[14] performed a systematic review of published studies retrieved through PUBMED, from bibliographies of review papers, and from experts. The English-language medical literature (between 1994 and 2001) was searched for studies that met the selection criteria: (1) DUS and/or MRA was performed to estimate the severity of carotid artery stenosis, (2) DSA was used as the standard of reference, and (3) the absolute numbers of true positives and negatives and false positives and negatives were available or derivable for at least one definition of disease (degree of stenosis).

Sixty-three publications on DUS, MRA, or both were included in the analysis, yielding the test results of 64 different patient series on DUS and 21 on MRA. For the diagnosis of 70–99% versus <70% stenosis, MRA had a pooled specificity of 90% (95% CI, 86–93) and a pooled sensitivity of 95% (95% CI, 92–97). These numbers were 87% (95% CI, 84–90) and 86% (95% CI, 84–89) for DUS, respectively. For recognizing occlusion, MRA yielded a sensitivity of 98% (95% CI, 94–100) and a specificity of 100% (95% CI, 99–100), and DUS had a sensitivity of 96% (95% CI, 94–98) and a specificity of 100% (95% CI, 99–100). A multivariable summary ROC curve analysis for diagnosing 70–99% stenosis demonstrated that the type of MR scanner predicted the performance of MRA, whereas the presence of verification bias predicted the performance of DUS. For diagnosing occlusion, no significant heterogeneity was found for MRA; for DUS, the presence of verification bias and type of DUS scanner were explanatory variables. MRA had a significantly better discriminatory power than DUS in diagnosing 70–99% stenosis (regression coefficient, 1.6; 95% CI, 0.37–2.77). No significant difference was found in detecting occlusion (regression coefficient, 0.73; 95% CI, –2.06–3.51). These results suggest that MRA has a better discriminatory power compared with DUS in diagnosing 70–99% stenosis and is a sensitive and specific test compared with DSA in the evaluation of carotid artery stenosis. For detecting occlusion, both DUS and MRA are very accurate.

Several other studies reported on the value of MRA[17–22] and CTA[23,24] in the diagnosis of carotid artery stenosis.

Doppler ultrasound is likely to remain the initial screening method of the carotid bifurcation in most centers. However, MRA may be used as a screening method in two situations: (1) when obtaining a magnetic resonance image of the brain to assess prior ischemic events, screening images of the bifurcation can easily be included with very little additional expense; and (2) MRA may be used for patients whose findings are equivocal by ultrasound, e.g., patients with unfavorable anatomy, such as high bifurcation, tortuous vessels that are difficult to identify, considerable overlying adipose tissue that may obscure the vessel, or dense vascular calcifications that cause acoustic shadowing. MRA can also provide a noninvasive assessment of those portions of the carotid that are not accessible to the ultrasound transducer, which can be manifested by an ultrasound showing a dampened waveform consistent with the presence of a tandem lesion or proximal stenosis or occlusion.

Specific application of any of these three modalities, i.e., color duplex ultrasonography, MRA, and conventional contrast angiography, are described in the following sections.

Asymptomatic Carotid Bruit

Although some asymptomatic carotid bruits radiate from the heart or the great vessels, a considerable proportion of them originate from the carotid artery bifurcations. Fell et al.[25] reported on 100 patients with 165 asymptomatic carotid bruits. Duplex scanning showed a normal internal carotid artery in 12 cases (7%), <50% stenosis in 83 (50%), ≥50% stenosis in 61 (37%), and occlusion in 9 (6%). Thus, although the majority of neck bruits were associated with some degree of carotid stenosis, only 43% had ≥50% stenosis, which may justify further work-up in selected patients. Noninvasive carotid testing permits separation of earlier, moderate atheromatous lesions from advanced, flow-reducing lesions. Most authorities agree that the early lesions require no treatment, but the patient should be followed at yearly intervals with repeat noninvasive testing to detect possible progression to more advanced stenosis. Identification of advanced stenosis of the internal carotid artery indicates a patient who is at an increased risk for subsequent stroke.

As indicated earlier, the ACAS study concluded that patients with ≥60% stenoses who were treated medically had a higher stroke rate over a 5-year period in comparison to patients who underwent a CEA. With this in mind, most authorities recommend screening for asymptomatic carotid stenoses, particularly in patients who are good candidates for a potential CEA. Figure 16–6 summarizes a practical approach in patients with asymptomatic carotid bruits or nonhemispheric symptoms. After the initial step of carotid DUS, if <60% stenosis was detected, it is recommended that the test be repeated in 6 months.

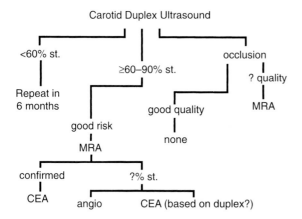

FIGURE 16–6. Management protocol for patients with asymptomatic carotid bruit or nonhemispheric symptoms. MRA, magnetic resonance angiography; CEA, carotid endarterectomy; st., stenosis.

If stenosis of ≥60–99% was detected and the patient is a good risk, a magnetic resonance angiogram can be done to complement the findings of the ultrasound, and if confirmed, a CEA is recommended. If the magnetic resonance angiogram was not conclusive or contradicted the ultrasound findings, then angiography may be considered in centers with a minimal stroke risk rate from angiography. However, in patients with a good quality carotid DUS, an endarterectomy may be considered based on ultrasound findings only. Several authorities would not recommend CEA in asymptomatic patients unless carotid stenosis exceeds 70–80%. In patients who had a good quality ultrasound showing total occlusion, no further follow-up is needed. However, if the quality of the ultrasound was limited, a magnetic resonance image is recommended to confirm occlusion.

Another indication for studying asymptomatic patients is to screen patients with advanced coronary artery disease or peripheral vascular diseases. Due to the diffuse nature of atherosclerosis, many of these patients have occult carotid bifurcation lesions with a resulting increased risk of stroke. This type of screening is carried out most often in patients who are being considered for cardiac or major peripheral arterial operations in order to detect carotid stenoses that may substantially increase the risk of intraoperative and postoperative stroke.

Patients with Atypical or Nonhemispheric Symptoms

Patients with atypical or nonhemispheric symptoms often do not have a clear indication for angiography. Some of these patients' symptoms include dizziness, blackouts, bilateral visual disturbances, or bilateral motor or sensory deficits. Since a variety of nonvascular causes, such as orthostatic hypotension, cardiac arrhythmias, and medications, may be responsible for these symptoms, noninvasive carotid testing is important in identifying these patients with hemodynamically significant carotid stenosis. Our management protocol for this group of patients is outlined in Figure 16–6.

Patients with Focal Neurologic Deficits (Transient Ischemic Attacks or Strokes)

A major proportion of transient ischemic attacks (TIAs) or permanent focal neurologic deficits in hemispheric distribution or with amaurosis fugax is caused by embolization from ulcerations and atheromatous plaques. Therefore, the purpose of carotid screening in patients with hemispheric neurologic symptoms is to identify lesions that could be the source of cerebral emboli or could reduce cerebral hemispheric blood flow. In the North American Symptomatic Carotid Endarterectomy Trial (NASCET) study,[26] carotid endarterectomy was highly beneficial for patients with

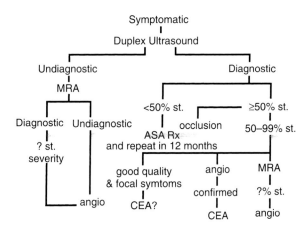

FIGURE 16–7. Management protocol for patients with suspected hemispheric symptoms (cerebrovascular disease). For <50% stenosis, repeat ultrasound in 12 months. MRA, magnetic resonance angiography; CEA, carotid endarterectomy; ASA Rx, acetylsalicylic acid treatment; st., stenosis.

recent hemispheric TIAs or mild strokes and >70–99% and 50–69% stenoses of the ipsilateral internal carotid artery. Based on these results, patients with symptoms of severe stenoses of the carotid artery should be treated by CEA unless their medical condition makes the risk of surgery prohibitive. Our management protocol for this group of patients is outlined in Figure 16–7. As noted in Figure 16–7, the initial step is to obtain a color DUS, and if the study is diagnostic and shows <50% stenosis, the patient is treated medically (e.g., aspirin therapy and repeat color DUS in 12 months). If the stenosis is ≥50%, the ultrasound is of good quality, and the patient has classical focal hemispheric

symptoms, a CEA can be done based on the carotid DUS findings alone; or MRA can be done to complement the ultrasound findings, and if the diagnosis is confirmed, surgery may be considered without angiography. Angiography is reserved for patients with a marginal quality DUS or magnetic resonance angiogram, or in patients with contradictory magnetic resonance angiogram and DUS results. If the DUS shows total occlusion and the ultrasound was of good quality, no further work-up is usually necessary. For patients with a DUS that is not diagnostic, an arteriogram or magnetic resonance angiogram is done, and if it is diagnostic and the severity of stenosis is established, surgery can be done accordingly. If the MRA is not diagnostic, angiography is recommended.

Specific Duplex Criteria for Specific Clinical Situations

In choosing our criteria for peak systolic velocity and end diastolic velocity, we chose the values that gave the highest overall accuracy. However, which criteria to use should depend on the "outcome" desired by the clinician. Although some surgeons have advocated CEA based on duplex criteria alone,[5,12,16] the decision to proceed with an arteriogram is based on the duplex findings in the majority of patients. The mortality and morbidity of arteriography vary from institution to institution, but can be significant.[6,27] We propose that vascular laboratories at institutions with significant mortality and morbidity in relation to carotid arteriography use duplex criteria

TABLE 16–1. Selected optimal criteria with best PPV (≥95%) and overall accuracy in detecting ≥60–99% and 70–99% ICA stenosis.[a]

Best PPV	PPV	Overall accuracy	Sensitivity	Specificity	NPV
For ≥60% ICA stenosis					
ICA PSV ≥ 220 cm/s	96%	82%	64%	98%	76%
ICA EDV ≥ 80 cm/s	96%	87%	79%	97%	84%
ICA/CCA PSV ratio ≥4.25	96%	71%	41%	99%	65%
ICA PSV and EDV 150 and 65[b]	96%	90%	82%	97%	86%
For ≥70% ICA stenosis					
ICA PSV ≥ 300 cm/s	97%	80%	48%	99%	76%
ICA EDV ≥ 110 cm/s[b]	100%	91%	75%	100%	87%
ICA/CCA PSV ≥ none	—	—	—	—	—
ICA PSV and EDV 150, 110[b]	100%	91%	75%	100%	87%

[a]PPV, positive predictive value; NPV, negative predictive value; ICA, internal carotid artery; PSV, peak systolic velocity; EDV, end diastolic velocity; CCA, common carotid artery.
[b]These values have the best PPV and overall accuracy.

TABLE 16–2. Selected optimal criteria with best NPV ($\geq$95%) and overall accuracy in detecting $\geq$60–99% and 70–99% ICA stenosis.[a]

Best NPV	NPV	Overall accuracy	Sensitivity	Specificity	PPV
For $\geq$60% ICA stenosis					
ICA PSV $\geq$ 135 cm/s[b]	99%	80%	99%	64%	71%
ICA EDV—none	—	—	—	—	—
ICA/CCA PSV ratio $\geq$ 1.62	95%	71%	97%	47%	62%
ICA PSV and EDV—none	—	—	—	—	—
For $\geq$70% ICA stenosis					
ICA PSV > 150 cm/s[b]	99%	80%	99%	69%	65%
ICA EDV $\geq$ 60 cm/s	96%	83%	94%	77%	71%
ICA/CCA PSV $\geq$ none	—	—	—	—	—
ICA PSV and EDV—none	—	—	—	—	—

[a]NPV, negative predictive value; PPV, positive predictive value; ICA, internal carotid artery; PSV, peak systolic velocity; EDV, end diastolic velocity; CCA, common carotid artery.
[b]These values have the best NPV and overall accuracy.

with 95% or greater PPV and the best overall accuracy in order to minimize the number of patients undergoing unnecessary arteriography (Table 16–1). These criteria can also be utilized when CEA is performed without preoperative arteriography. In those institutions where arteriography does not significantly add to the mortality and morbidity of the overall treatment of carotid disease, we suggest using the criteria described in Table 16–2. These criteria have the highest negative predictive value to ensure that only a minimum number of patients with equal to or greater than 60% or 70% stenoses are missed.

A new classification was proposed by us which would consist of lesions <30% stenosis, $\geq$30–49% stenosis, $\geq$50–59% stenosis, $\geq$60–69% stenosis, and $\geq$70% stenosis. This new duplex classification would fit into the existing trials [NASCET, ACAS, and Veteran's Administration Cooperative Study (VA)], and may be of benefit as new conclusions are released.[28] By reporting results using these criteria, the clinician will be better able to make decisions regarding the need for CEA or arteriogram based on the risks and benefits for individual patients. With the added risks of arteriography, decisions to operate would be better based on duplex findings alone. Having PPVs of 90–97% and accuracies of 87–93% can eliminate many unnecessary arteriograms.

It is important to note that the data obtained by individual vascular laboratories will vary as a result of differences in equipment, abilities, and consistencies of vascular technicians and reader interpretations.[28] Therefore, each laboratory must adapt a method that employs the equipment they use and has validated their method when using proposed new duplex criteria.

Intraoperative Assessment of Carotid Endarterectomy

Intraoperative use of the B-mode ultrasound imaging system for completion evaluation of the CEA has been advocated by Sigel et al.[29] The development of smaller scanning heads and probes together with techniques of sterilization has made this application feasible. The ultrasound examination can be performed quickly and, unlike angiography, requires no delay for film processing. Nor is it necessary to inject contrast material. Angiography is also associated with the risks of subintimal injections, thromboembolic complications, and allergic reactions.

Despite careful operative techniques, certain vascular defects can be missed, e.g., intimal flaps, luminal thrombus/platelet aggregation, stricture, etc. that occur in the course of carotid repair (Figure 16–8). These defects can escape visual inspection and palpation of the repair. If these defects are left undetected, they can result in stroke secondary to thrombus formation, platelet aggregation, or arterial thrombosis; or they may result in postoperative recurrent carotid stenoses. Blaisdell et al. reported the fallibility of clinical assessment by routine completion angiography, which revealed unsuspected defects in 25% of cases.[30] A number of investigators have subsequently confirmed the observations of Blaisdell et al. by using angiography, alone or in combination with various ultrasound techniques, such as continuous-wave Doppler examination, pulse Doppler spectral analysis, or duplex ultrasonography. Intraoperative monitoring has consistently documented severe defects in the internal carotid artery (ICA) or the common carotid artery (CCA) that warranted immediate correction in approximately

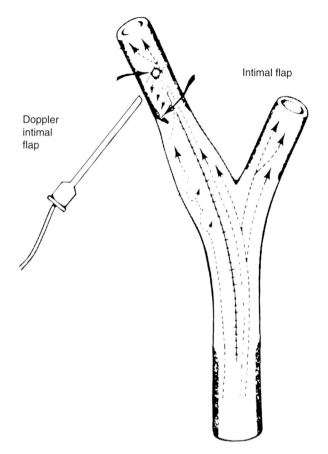

Doppler intimal flap

Intimal flap

FIGURE 16–8. The application of Doppler probe to detect defects of a repaired internal carotid artery (intimal flap).

2–10% of all repairs.[31–37] Although the percentage of patients with residual repair defects in whom a postoperative stroke would develop if the defects were left untreated is not known, prudent surgical practice dictates that detection and revision of these defects should be done at the primary operation, since the sequelae of an ICA thrombosis are frequently catastrophic.

Baker et al.[33] reported that recurrent stenoses (>75%) developed in 17% of patients with abnormal unrepaired CEAs by intraoperataive imaging compared with 4.3% in normal CEAs (p < 0.001). This suggests that abnormalities detected by intraoperative DUS, if not corrected, may contribute to recurrent carotid stenosis after CEA.

Kinney et al.[34] showed the importance of intraoperative scanning in a prospective study of 461 CEAs. They correlated the results of intraoperative assessment by clinical inspection, ultrasound, or arteriography with an end point of stroke. The CEA site was assessed by ultrasound and arteriography in 268 cases, by ultrasound and Doppler spectral analysis alone in 142 cases, and with clinical inspection in only 51 cases. Based on intraoperative assessment, 26 endarterectomies (6%) were revised

at the time of the surgery. Perioperative morbidity was similar in cases with normal, mildly abnormal, or no ultrasound. There were 12 temporary (3%) and six permanent (1%) neurologic deficits and six deaths (four strokes and two cardiac events). Based on life-table analysis, the incidence of >50% ICA stenosis or occlusions was increased (p < 0.007) in patients with residual flow abnormality or no study. However, patients with normal intraoperative studies had a significantly lower rate of late ipsilateral stroke compared with the other patients (p = 0.04). The incidence of stroke was increased (p = 0.00016) in patients with ICA restenosis or occlusion (3 of 35) compared with patients without recurrent stenosis (3 of 426) during a mean follow-up of 30 months. It was concluded that a normal intraoperative duplex scan may prevent recurrent stenosis as well as stroke after CEA in the long-term.

Most authorities rely on imaging or Doppler flow detection technique to exclude technical defects. The diagnostic signal analysis is highly sensitive and specific (>90%), particularly if pulse Doppler analysis is performed. This technique is simple, widely available, and relatively inexpensive. Although abnormalities of the Doppler flow signal are readily apparent by audible interpretation, quantitative spectral analysis is preferable. With flow and pressure reducing lesions, a spectral broadening is present throughout the pulse cycle, and a peak systolic velocity (PSV) exceeding 150cm/s is noted. Visual inspection of velocity spectra and calculation of PSV can be obtained by a high-frequency pulse Doppler probe or duplex scanning, which permits classification of flow patterns into three categories: normal flow, mild to moderate flow disturbance, and severe flow disturbance.[31] When a significant residual flow abnormality is identified, angiography is usually recommended to delineate the abnormality before reexploration of the repair.

Recently, intraoperative duplex ultrasonography has been advocated because of its ability to provide both anatomic and hemodynamic information.[35–38] Improvements in linear ray scan head design and electronic signal processing, including color-coded velocity display, have made duplex scanning feasible in the operating room and an ideal modality for intraoperative assessment of CEA. Duplex scanning has an advantage over Doppler flow analysis alone, in that the structure of the anatomic defects associated with severe flow disturbance can usually be determined. B-mode imaging is sensitive in detecting small intimal defects in flaps, however, most authorities have not repaired these minor lesions, and the outcome of the procedure has not been adversely influenced.[37]

A comparison of intraoperative and early postoperative duplex findings after CEA indicated that a majority of these abnormalities identified by duplex scanning

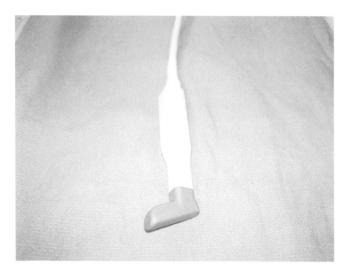

FIGURE 16–9. Transducer covered by sterile disposable plastic sleeve that contains acoustic gel.

within 3–6 months of CEA represent residual rather than recurrent stenoses.[36]

Recently, Ascher *et al.*[39] reported on the value of intraoperative carotid artery duplex scanning in a modern series of 650 consecutive primary endarterectomy procedures (April 2000 to April 2003). Major technical defects at intraoperative duplex scanning (>30% luminal ICA stenosis, free-floating clot, dissection, arterial disruption with pseudoaneurysm) were repaired. CCA residual disease was reported as wall thickness and percent stenosis (16–67%; mean 32% ± 8%) in all cases. Postoperative 30-day TIA, stroke, and death rates were analyzed. There were no clinically detectable postoperative thromboembolic events in this series. All 15 major defects (2.3%) identified with duplex scanning were successfully revised. These included seven intimal flaps, four free-floating clots, two ICA stenoses, one ICA pseudoaneurysm, and one retrograde CCA dissection. Diameter reduction ranged from 40% to 90% (mean, 67 ± 16%), and peak systolic velocity ranged from 69 to 497 cm/s (mean, 250 ± 121 cm/s). Thirty-one patients (5%) with the highest residual wall thickness (>3 mm) in the CCA and 19 (3%) with the highest CCA residual diameter reduction (>50%) did not have postoperative stroke or TIA. Overall postoperative stroke and mortality rates were 0.3% and 0.5%, respectively; combined stroke and mortality rate was 0.8%. One stroke was caused by hyperperfusion, and the other occurred as an extension of a previous cerebral infarct. It was concluded that intraoperative duplex scanning had a major role in these improved results, because it enabled detection of clinically unsuspected significant lesions. Residual disease in the CCA does not seem to be a harbinger of stroke or TIA.

Color duplex scanning with a 7.5- to 10-MHz linear ray transducer has been used for intraoperative studies.

These studies are conducted with the transducer covered by a sterile disposable plastic sleeve that contains acoustic gel (Figure 16–9). The probe is generally positioned in the cervical incision directly over the exposed carotid repair. A sterile solution is instilled into the incision for acoustic coupling. As the surgeon scans the arterial repair, the technologist adjusts the instrument to optimize the Doppler angle, sample volume, color-coded image, and recorded velocity spectra. Vessel walls are imaged at 90°, but blood flow patterns should be evaluated at Doppler angles of <60°.

For CEAs with primary closure, the entire CEA segment should be examined with duplex ultrasound. The point in the CCA at which the lesion is transected should be examined. Normally, this should leave a distinct shelf, which can be appreciated on B-mode imaging. This can be easily visualized in both transverse and longitudinal views. The velocity data proximal to, in, and distal to the endarterectomy site should also be done in longitudinal view and sampling of the PSVs in the endarterectomy site should be obtained. Similarly, scanning of the proximal ICA in the bulb and beyond it should be done and attention should be called to the point of the transaction of the plaque or the end of the plaque distally. The external carotid artery should also be examined for the first few centimeters, looking for residual plaques or areas of thrombus. In patients who have CEAs closed with a patch, either polytetrafluoroethylene (PTFE) or Dacron, it is impossible to scan through the patch itself because of the air within the wall of the patch. However, it is possible to scan along the side of the artery, either posterior or anterior to the patch, which may yield the necessary information (Figures 16–10 and 16–11).

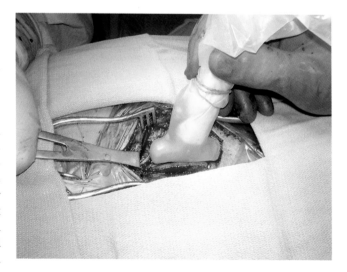

FIGURE 16–10. Probe scanning position for carotid endarterectomy closed with a patch. It is impossible to scan through the PTFE patch, but the operator can scan along the side of the artery, either posterior or anterior to the patch.

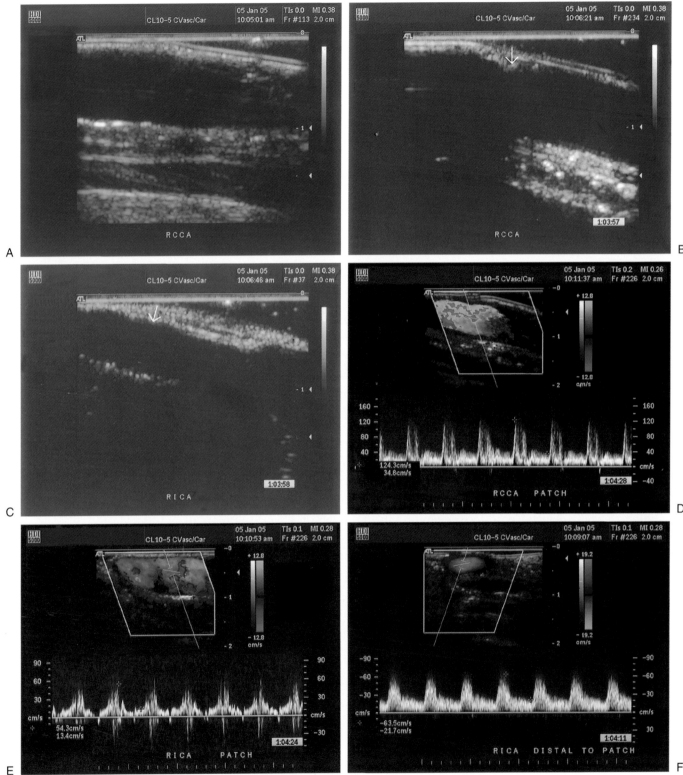

Figure 16–11. Intraoperative duplex ultrasound of carotid endarterectomy: (A) common carotid artery in grayscale. Note the shelf of the proximal end of carotid endarterectomy (arrow), (B) common carotid artery bifurcation in grayscale (arrow), (C) internal carotid artery in grayscale, (D) common carotid artery with color flow, (E) internal carotid artery with patch with color flow, and (F) distal internal carotid artery with color flow.

The limitations of this technique are largely related to lack of experience, correct measurement of duplex derived flow velocities, recognition of abnormal flow patterns, and transducer size. Intraoperative duplex imaging has the following advantages over angiography: comparable or higher accuracy, safety, ease of repeated use after reexploration, and low cost. Color duplex scanning is also sensitive to variations in anatomy and minor vascular defects that may alter blood flow streamlines. Certain flow patterns produced by carotid patch angioplasty should be noted and should not be regarded as abnormal. Some authorities have reported vascular defects in as many as one-third of their repairs, but only one-third of these appear to justify reexploration.

Intraoperative Monitoring of Carotid Endarterectomy with Transcranial Doppler Sonography

Transcranial Doppler (TCD) sonography has the advantage of allowing monitoring of both hemodynamic and embolic events, primarily in the middle cerebral artery distribution during CEA. The middle cerebral artery cannot be insonated in 5–15% of patients, most commonly because of the lack of a window for Doppler signal penetration of the skull. Severe cerebral ischemia is considered present in the first minute after carotid occlusion if the middle cerebral artery velocity decreases to 15% of the baseline or lower, and mild ischemia if it drops to 15–40% of the baseline. An adequate perfusion is present if the velocity is >40% of the baseline.[40] Following insertion of the shunt or upon declamping, a brisk recovery in middle cerebral artery velocity should be seen, usually >80%. Absolute mean velocities of 15 cm/s or even 30 cm/s have been alternatively suggested. A middle cerebral artery velocity of 30 cm/s has correlated roughly with a carotid artery stump blood pressure of 50 mm Hg. Some authorities reported that TCD detects critically low flow that results in neurologic deficits, even in the absence of electroencephalographic changes. The converse is also true: a pronounced drop in mean velocity has been observed in conjunction with a normal EEG and no resultant cerebral infarction, the cortex surviving from the other cerebral and laptomeningeal vessels.

In a recent study, Ackerstaff et al.[41] concluded that in CEA, TCD-detected microemboli during dissection and wound closure, ≥90% middle cerebral artery velocity decrease at cross-clamping, and ≥100% pulsatility index increase at clamp release are associated with operative stroke. In combination with the presence of preoperative cerebral symptoms and ≥70% ipsilateral ICA stenosis, these four TCD monitoring variables can reasonably discriminate between patients with and without operative stroke. This supports the use of TCD as a potential intraoperative monitoring modality to alter the surgical technique by enhancing a decrease of the risk of stroke during or immediately after the operation.

TCD can also be used in the postoperative period to detect early thrombosis of the carotid artery, continued embolization, or the hyperperfusion syndrome. It has been reported that markedly increased mean velocity (150% of the baseline) may herald an intracranial hemorrhage. The use of TCD monitoring during CEA has led some surgeons to modify their operative techniques based on hearing a distressing frequency of emboli while operating with the continuously audible TCD.

Patients Who Develop a Neurologic Deficit After Leaving the Operating Room

If patients wake up well after CEA and then develop a neurologic deficit, emergent reexploration is indicated. If the deficit proves to be a TIA as symptoms resolve prior to the return to the operating room, heparin anticoagulation followed by duplex scan is preferred. A thrombosed ICA may be treated operatively or medically (anticoagulation), particularly in patients with dense deficits. A patent carotid without apparent pathology is immediately followed by CT scanning to identify intracranial hemorrhage or other pathology. If negative, an angiogram should be done to confirm the duplex findings and assess the intracranial vasculature. If negative, oral anticoagulation is started. Thromboembolism of inaccessible intracranial vasculature has been treated with selective catheterization and lytic therapy, although this is still considered investigational. Blood clots found at the endarterectomy site are treated by emergency reexploration.

Post-Carotid Endarterectomy Surveillance

Restenosis is a known entity that occurs after CEA and may vary between 12 and 36%, but the frequency of restenosis varies depending on the diagnostic method used and the frequency of follow-up examinations.[42–52] Several studies have reported on the value of postoperative carotid duplex surveillance, but no consensus has been reached.[42–52] The advantages that have been cited are detection of significant restenosis prior to the onset of neurologic events, which aids in the prevention of potential strokes, and follow-up on the contralateral carotid artery to document the development of surgically correctable stenosis. Opponents of routine postoperative carotid duplex surveillance claim that restenosis is benign in nature, therefore, a large number of strokes may not be prevented by this surveillance.[45,46,48,49,52] Despite the high rate of restenosis, symptoms attributed to restenoses are rare, therefore several authorities have suggested that routine surveillance of patients after CEA is not efficacious.[44–46,49]

Mattos et al.[46] described their experience with postoperative carotid duplex surveillance and found an equal stroke-free survival at 5 years between patients with or without >50% restenosis. In addition, only one of 380 patients suffered a stroke in their study, suggesting a benign clinical significance of recurrent carotid artery stenosis. Mackey et al. claim a low rate of clinically significant restenosis.[45] Their retrospective series of 258 patients (348 arteries) show a potential 4% incidence of late strokes, but this included all patients who underwent repeat CEA for asymptomatic restenosis. They also noted that the majority of restenoses (53%) remained asymptomatic and did not progress to occlusion throughout follow-up. Of 10 documented late occlusions, eight did not result in stroke. Eight patients with operable restenosis had TIAs and underwent reoperation. They found that even patients with 75–99% restenosis most often remained asymptomatic (37%) or had TIAs (32%). Only two (11%) of 19 patients with 75–99% restenosis had an unheralded stroke. They felt that postoperative carotid duplex surveillance was not justified due to the low incidence of symptomatic restenosis.

In spite of these findings, investigators have been reluctant to advise that postoperative carotid duplex surveillance be abandoned because the cost-effectiveness of this surveillance has not been formally investigated. Others have reported that high-grade stenosis (>75%), whether caused by myointimal hyperplasia of the CEA site or progressive atherosclerosis of the contralateral carotid artery, is associated with an increased risk of late stroke.[34,52]

Ouriel et al. reported an 11% incidence of restenotic lesions greater than 80%. Although the incidence of symptoms with restenotic lesions was low (12%), the onset of symptoms at the time of occlusion was significant.[47] Forty-two percent of patients became symptomatic at the time of occlusion, with 33% resulting in a stroke. This led to the observation that critical restenoses are precursors to stroke, even if asymptomatic, and, therefore, the detection of >80% restenosis allows future stroke prevention, if operative intervention is undertaken.[47] Mattos et al. also described the outcome for >80% restenosis. In their group, one of three patients with >80% restenosis suffered a stroke, one

had a TIA, and one remained asymptomatic. This suggests a more serious course once restenosis reaches >80%.[46]

So far, a consensus has not yet been reached in the surgical literature regarding the usefulness, cost-effectiveness, or timing of postoperative carotid duplex surveillance.

Timing of Postoperative Carotid Duplex Surveillance

Several authors have recommended an initial surveillance duplex on the operative carotid system within the first 6 months[43,46–48,52] to detect residual stenosis from the operative procedure or early restenosis.[47] For example, Roth et al.[52] recently recommended an initial DUS to ensure a technically successful CEA, with subsequent postoperative carotid duplex surveillance at 1–2 years, as long as restenosis and contralateral stenoses remain <50%. More frequent follow-up (every 6 months) is warranted if >50% stenosis is noted, or with the onset of symptomatic disease.[52]

Several studies have reported that the majority of restenoses occurs during the first 1–2 years after CEA. Mattos et al.[43] noted that 70% of restenoses were detected within 1 year after the CEA, and 96% developed within 15 months. Thomas et al.[42] reported that 70% of restenoses in their study occurred within 1 year of the CEA. Similar observations were noted by us previously.[50]

Ricco et al.[53] reported on the need for follow-up duplex scan 1 year after CEA was performed with prosthetic patching and intraoperative completion arteriography. A total of 605 CEA procedures with prosthetic patch closure and intraoperative completion arteriography were performed in 540 patients. All patients underwent duplex scan at 4 days and then yearly after the procedure. Intraoperative completion arteriography showed abnormalities in 114 cases, including 17 involving the ICA and 73 involving the external carotid artery. Successful revision was achieved in all cases and confirmed by repeat arteriography. Postoperative duplex scans at 4 days detected three abnormalities involving the ICA (0.5%), including asymptomatic occlusion in one case and residual stenosis >50% in two cases. Ninety-eight percent of patients were stenosis-free at 1 year. Actuarial stroke-free survival was 98.3% at 3 years. Diameter reduction of the contralateral carotid artery progressed over 70% within 1 year after CEA in 22.9% of patients with contralateral carotid stenosis over 50% at the time of the initial intervention. The findings of this study indicate that duplex scan follow-up 1 year after CEA with intraoperative completion arteriography is unnecessary unless postoperative duplex scan demonstrates residual stenosis of the ICA. However, duplex scan at 1 year is beneficial for patients presenting with contralateral carotid artery disease with diameter reduction >50% at the time of CEA.

Lovelace et al.[54] conducted a study on optimizing duplex follow-up in patients with an asymptomatic ICA stenosis of <60%. All patients who underwent initial carotid duplex examination for any indication since January 1, 1995, with at least one patent, asymptomatic, previously nonoperated ICA with <60% stenosis; with 6 months or greater follow-up; and with one or more repeat duplex examinations were entered into the study. On the basis of the initial duplex examination, ICAs were classified into two groups: those with a PSV <175 cm/s and those with a PSV of 175 cm/s or more. Follow-up duplex examinations were performed at varying intervals to detect progression from <60% to 60–99%. A total of 407 patients (640 asymptomatic ICAs with <60% stenosis) underwent serial duplex scans (mean follow-up, 22 months). Three ICAs (0.5%) became symptomatic and progressed to 60–99% ICA stenosis at a mean of 21 months, whereas four other ICAs occluded without stroke during follow-up. Progression to 60–99% stenosis without symptoms was detected in 46 ICAs (7%) (mean, 18 months). Of the 633 patent asymptomatic arteries, 548 ICAs (87%) had initial PSVs <175 cm/s, and 85 ICAs (13%) had initial PSVs of 175 cm/s or more. Asymptomatic progression to 60–99% ICA stenosis occurred in 22 (26%) of 85 ICAs with initial PSVs of 175 cm/s or more, whereas 24 (4%) of 548 ICAs with initial PSVs <175 cm/s progressed ($p < 0.0001$). The Kaplan–Meier method showed freedom from progression at 6 months, 12 months, and 24 months was 95%, 83%, and 70% for ICAs with initial PSVs of 175 cm/s or more versus 100%, 99%, and 95%, respectively, for ICAs with initial PSVs <175 cm/s ($p < 0.0001$).

They concluded that patients with <60% ICA stenosis and PSVs of 175 cm/s or more on initial duplex examination are significantly more likely to progress asymptomatically to 60–99% ICA stenosis, and progression is sufficiently frequent to warrant follow-up duplex studies at 6-month intervals. Patients with <60% ICA stenosis and initial PSVs <175 cm/s may have follow-up duplex examinations safely deferred for 2 years.

Cost-Effectiveness of Postoperative Carotid Duplex Surveillance

There have been reports that postoperative carotid duplex surveillance is not cost-effective since there is such a low incidence of symptomatic restenosis. Patel et al. evaluated the cost-effectiveness of postoperative carotid duplex surveillance.[51] They concluded that postoperative carotid duplex surveillance after CEA has an unfavorable cost-effectiveness ratio. In the process of their analysis, they identified a subset of patients in which postoperative carotid duplex surveillance may be cost-effective. These included patients in whom the rate of progression to >80% stenosis exceeded 6% per year. In their analysis, they felt that some groups of patients could potentially have a rate of disease progression that approaches or exceeds the level at which postoperative carotid duplex surveillance becomes cost-effective. Some of these include patients with multiple risk factors, e.g., smoking, hypertension, hyperlipidemia, diabetes mellitus, coronary artery disease, female gender, and a young age. In addition, they concluded that with postoperative carotid duplex surveillance, the rate of carotid artery occlusion could be reduced by 15% per year. Our evaluation of the cost of postoperative carotid duplex surveillance agrees with these conclusions (see Our Clinical Experience).

Our Clinical Experience

Three hundred and ninety-nine CEAs were randomized into 135 with primary closure, 134 with PTFE patch closures, and 130 with vein patch closures and followed for a mean of 47 months. Postoperative carotid duplex surveillance was done at 1, 6, and 12 months, and every year thereafter (a mean of 4.0 studies/artery). A Kaplan–Meier analysis was used to estimate the rate of ≥80% restenosis over time and the time frame of progression from <50% to 50–79% and ≥80% stenosis.

Greater than or equal to 80% restenosis developed in 24 (21%) with primary closure and nine (4%) with patching. A Kaplan–Meier estimate of freedom from 50–79% restenosis at 1, 2, 3, 4, and 5 years was 92%, 83%, 72%, 72%, and 63% for primary closure and 99%, 98%, 97%, 97%, and 95% for patching A Kaplan–Meier estimate of freedom from ≥80% restenosis at 1, 2, 3, 4, and 5 years was 92%, 83%, 80%, 76%, and 68% for primary closure and 100%, 99%, 98%, 98%, and 91% for patching ($p < 0.01$).

Out of 56 arteries with 20–50% restenosis, 2/28 patch closures and 10/28 primary closures progressed to 50–<80% restenosis ($p = 0.02$) and 0/28 patch closures and 6/28 primary closures progressed to ≥80% ($p = 0.03$). In primary closures, the median time to progression from <50% to 50–79%, <50% to ≥80%, and 50–79% to ≥80% was 42, 46, and 7 months, respectively. Of the 24 arteries with ≥80% restenosis in primary closures, 10 were symptomatic. Thus, assuming that symptomatic restenosis would have undergone duplex examinations anyway, there were 14 asymptomatic arteries (12%)

that could have been detected only by postoperative carotid duplex surveillance (estimated cost of $139,200) and would have been candidates for redo CEA. Of the nine arteries with patch closures (three PTFE and six vein patch closures) with ≥80% restenosis, six asymptomatic arteries (four vein patch closure and two PTFE, 3%) could have been detected by postoperative carotid duplex surveillance. In patients with a normal duplex at the first 6 months, only 4/222 (2%) patched arteries (two asymptomatic) developed ≥80% restenosis versus 5/13 (38%) in patients with abnormal duplex examinations ($p < 0.001$).

Assuming a 5% stroke rate for the 14 repeat CEAs for asymptomatic ≥80% restenosis in the primary closure group in our series,[55] 0.7 strokes would be associated with the 14 repeat CEAs and approximately 4.7 strokes would have been prevented through surgical intervention prior to occlusion (assuming a similar outcome of ≥80% restenosis as described by Mattos et al.[46]). There was a net reduction of four strokes in patients with primary closure and an approximate cost of $56,150 per stroke prevented.

Also, assuming a similar outcome of >80% restenosis as described by Ouriel et al.,[47] and if one-half of these >80% restenosis would progress to total occlusion (7 patients), and assuming one-third of patients with total occlusion would suffer a stroke, then approximately 2.3 strokes would be prevented by doing the 14 redo CEAs. Since 0.7 strokes would result from repeating 14 CEAs,[55] the net effect would be prevention of 1.6 strokes at a cost of $224,600, i.e., $140,250 per stroke prevented. This analysis does not take into consideration the value of duplex screening of the contralateral nonoperated side.

The justification for this cost is unclear without a definite estimate of the economic burden for caring for these stroke victims. Considering the low incidence of >80% restenosis in patients with patch angioplasty closure, the cost-effectiveness of postoperative carotid duplex surveillance appears to be unfavorable and, therefore, should be limited to a single DUS to detect residual stenosis. Subsequent follow-up should be dictated by the results found on the initial scan and the onset of neurologic symptoms.

Our randomized prospective studies confirm that carotid restenosis is a known entity that follows a percentage of patients who undergo carotid surgery. In the past, the clinical significance of carotid restenosis has led some investigators to conclude that postoperative carotid duplex surveillance is not warranted. We showed that based on the incidence of >80% restenosis, postoperative carotid duplex surveillance may be beneficial in patients with primary closure with examinations at 6 months and at 1–2 year intervals for several years. For patients with patching, a 6-month postoperative duplex examination, if normal, is adequate.

Duplex Ultrasound Surveillance of Carotid Stents

Kupinski et al.[56] conducted a study to evaluate the DUS characteristics of carotid stents including comparing hemodynamic to B-mode and color-flow imaging data in 40 carotid stents placed in the common or internal carotid arteries of 37 patients. DUS examinations included PSV and end diastolic velocity (EDV) taken proximal to the stent (prestent), at the proximal, mid, and distal regions of the stent, and distal to the stent (poststent). The stents were evaluated at 1 day, and 3, 6, and 12 months postprocedure and yearly thereafter. The average follow-up interval was 6 ± 1 month. In 31 patient ICA stents, the PSV proximally within the stent was 92 ± 6 cm/s with an EDV of 24 ± 2 cm/s. The mid stent PSV was 86 ± 5 cm/s with an EDV of 24 ± 2 cm/s. The distal stent PSV was 90 ± 4 with an EDV of 26 ± 2 cm/s. Proximal to the stent, the PSV was 70 ± 3 cm/s with an EDV of 17 ± 1 cm/s. Distal to the stent, the PSV was 77 ± 4 cm/s with an EDV of 25 ± 2 cm/s. There were no defects observed on B-mode image and no areas of color turbulence. Three stents developed stenotic areas with PSVs of 251, 383, and 512 cm/s. The EDV was 50, 131, and 365 cm/s, respectively. Poststenotic turbulence was present in each of these stents. An elevated PSV of >125 cm/s was found in 32% of the stents (9 of 28) without evidence of stenosis on B-mode image of poststenotic turbulence. These data demonstrate that velocities within stented carotid arteries can be elevated above established ranges for normal. They concluded that velocity criteria may need to be adjusted when applied to stented carotid arteries. It has been suggested that focal velocity increase at the point of maximal narrowing >150 cm/s and a prestenotic (or prestent) to stenotic segment PSV ratio of 1:≥2 are suggestive of significant instent restenosis.[57]

Determination of Progression

It has now become clear that it is possible to determine major progression of disease in two different categories with duplex scanning technology. Progression of disease from a mild form (20–50% diameter reduction) to a severe form (50–99% diameter reduction) can be accurately detected based on significant changes in peak frequency.[58] In addition, in severe stenosis, it is possible to identify the development of extreme degrees of stenosis (>80% diameter reduction) by the changes in the ratio between peak systolic and end diastolic frequencies. The ability to identify such disease progression without invasive arteriographic studies will contribute to our understanding of the natural history of the disease process.

Natural History of Carotid Artery Stenosis, Contralateral to Carotid Endarterectomy

A few nonrandomized studies have reported on the natural history of carotid artery stenosis contralateral to CEA. Recently, we analyzed the natural history of carotid artery stenosis contralateral to CEA from two randomized prospective trials.[50,59]

The contralateral carotid arteries of 534 patients who participated in two randomized trials comparing CEA with primary closure versus patching were followed clinically and had DUSs at 1 month and every 6 months. Carotid artery stenoses were classified into <50%, ≥50–<80%, ≥80–99%, and occlusion. Late contralateral CEAs were done for significant carotid artery stenoses. Progression of carotid artery stenosis was defined as progress to a higher category of stenosis. A Kaplan–Meier life table analysis was used to estimate freedom from progression of carotid artery stenosis. The correlation of risk factors and carotid artery stenosis progression was also analyzed.

Out of 534 patients, 61 had initial contralateral CEAs, within 30 days of the ipsilateral CEA, and 53 had contralateral occlusions. Overall, 109/420 (26%) progressed at a mean follow-up of 41 months (range: 1–116 months). Progression of contralateral carotid artery stenosis was noted in 5/162 (3%) patients who had baseline normal carotids; 56/157 (36%) patients with <50% carotid artery stenosis progressed versus 45/95 (47%) patients with 50–<80% carotid artery stenosis ($p = 0.003$). The median time for progression was 24 months for <50% carotid artery stenosis and 12 months for ≥50–<80% carotid artery stenosis ($p = 0.035$). Freedom from progression for patients with baseline <50% and ≥50–<80% carotid artery stenosis at 1, 2, 3, 4, and 5 years was 95%, 78%, 69%, 61%, 48%; and 75%, 61%, 51%, 43%, and 33%, respectively ($p = 0.003$). Freedom from progression in patients with baseline normal carotid arteries at 1, 2, 3, 4, and 5 years was 99%, 98%, 96%, 96%, and 94%. Late neurologic events referable to the contralateral carotid artery were infrequent in the whole series (28/420, 6.7%) and included 10 strokes (2.4%) and 18 TIAs (4.3%) (28/258, 10.9% in patients with contralateral carotid artery stenosis); however, late contralateral CEAs were done in 62 patients (62/420, 15%, in the whole series, 62/258, 24%, in patients with contralateral carotid artery stenosis). The survival rates were 96%, 92%, 90%, 87%, and 82% at 1, 2, 3, 4, and 5 years.

We concluded that progression of contralateral carotid artery stenosis was noted in a significant number of patients with baseline contralateral carotid artery stenosis. Serial carotid DUSs every 6–12 months for patients with ≥50–<80% carotid artery stenosis and every 12–24 months for ≤50% carotid artery stenosis are adequate.

Carotid Endarterectomy Based on Carotid Duplex Ultrasonography Without Angiography

In many centers, carotid evaluation by angiography is no longer done routinely, even when planning for surgery, to eliminate the risk of neurologic events during angiography. The risk of stroke from angiography is around 1%.[6]

Although standard conventional angiography is still generally considered to be the definitive diagnostic test for carotid artery stenosis, there has been an increasing interest in performing CEA based on clinical evaluation and duplex scanning only.[3–5,7–12,60–63] This has been stimulated by improvement in the accuracy and reliability of color carotid duplex scanning, along with the increasing demands to minimize both the risk of carotid angiography and the cost of medical care. CEAs are generally indicated for high-grade stenoses of asymptomatic patients and in moderate to severe stenoses in patients with hemispheric neurologic events. These stenoses can usually be accurately detected by duplex scanning.

Dawson et al.[60] reviewed arteriograms and duplex scans in 83 patients and found that in 87% the clinical presentation and duplex findings were adequate for patient management. They concluded that arteriography was necessary in 13% that (1) showed an unusual or atypical pattern of disease, (2) had technically inadequate duplex scans, or (3) had an internal carotid artery stenosis of <50%. This group[7] completed a subsequent prospective evaluation of 94 cases that showed that arteriography affected clinical management in only one case (1%). Dawson et al.[7] indicated that while specific indications for CEA without angiography remain controversial, the results of angiography rarely alter the clinical treatment plan when a technically adequate duplex scan shows an 80–99% stenosis in asymptomatic patients or an ipsilateral 50–99% stenosis in patients with hemispheric neurologic symptoms.[7]

The duplex and arteriogram results of 85 patients were prospectively evaluated by Moore et al. with a panel of neurologists, neurosurgeons, and vascular surgeons.[3] The duplex scan results were prospectively compared with arteriography. One hundred and fifty-nine of 170 carotid arteries were correctly characterized (94%); hemodynamically significant stenoses were correctly characterized in 100%. Thirty-two CEAs were performed by these authors in 29 patients without angiography. All duplex-predicted lesions were confirmed at surgery, and there were no perioperative strokes.

If arteriography is not done, there is a potential to miss significant lesions in the carotid siphon or an intracranial aneurysm or tumor as the cause of TIAs. However, it is unlikely that carotid siphon disease will produce significant symptoms,[64,65] and, therefore, does not impact the decision to perform CEA. Intracranial aneurysms occur in approximately 1–2% of patients undergoing arteriography,[66] but most are small and unlikely to be affected by CEA.[66] With the advances in imaging techniques, the concern for occult brain tumors has become less relevant.

In addition, associated costs are significant with some institutions reporting charges for cerebrovascular arteriography as high as $5000 to $6000. Strandness[67] has suggested that wider use of duplex scanning as the sole preoperative test could result in substantial savings. For instance, if 150,000 CEAs are done annually, with an average cost of angiography of $3000, the total cost of angiography alone would be $750 million dollars (not counting the costs of an estimated 7500 TIAs, 1500 strokes, and 100 deaths). If these same patients had duplex scanning alone, the total costs would be approximately $37 million; this represents a savings annually in the United States alone of $712 million.[67] We have already begun to see a shift in the testing that is done for a preoperative diagnosis. A report from the University of Vermont stated that 87% of their last 130 CEAs were performed without arteriography, with acceptable rates of stroke and death.[68]

CEA should not be attempted without arteriography unless the following criteria are met:[7]

1. The distal ICA is free of significant disease (disease is localized to the carotid bifurcation).
2. The CCA is free of significant disease.
3. Vascular anomalies, kinks, or loops are not present.
4. The duplex scan is technically adequate.
5. Vascular laboratory duplex accuracy is known.

Some potential pitfalls include patients with nonhemispheric symptoms, recurrent stenosis, or ICA stenosis of <50%.[7,60,68] However, as experience grows, indications may be expanded.

Therefore, angiography is most likely to be useful when the duplex scan is not diagnostic, in patients with atypical lesions that appear to extend beyond the carotid bifurcation, and for stenoses of <50% in patients with classical hemispheric neurologic symptoms.

Carotid Endarterectomy Based on Duplex Ultrasonography with Minimal Angiographic Findings

We published a report on CEA for symptomatic carotid artery disease and failed medical treatment with plaque associated with <60% stenosis by DUS.[69] All patients in this study underwent arteriography, which showed normal to <20% stenosis. CEA was uneventful in these 14 patients, and their symptoms resolved.

We found that carotid DUS is superior to carotid arteriography in detecting irregular or ulcerative heterogeneous plaques associated with mild degrees of stenosis. These patients should also be worked up to exclude other noncarotid causes of the TIAs or strokes.

Ultrasonic Carotid Plaque Morphology and Carotid Plaque Hemorrhage: Clinical Implications

The lack of neurologic symptoms in many patients with significant carotid stenosis has perplexed many scientists. It has been proposed that the character of the plaque may be as, or more important, than significant stenosis in producing neurologic events.

We[70] examined the importance of ultrasonic plaque morphology and its correlation to the presence of intraplaque hemorrhage and its clinical implications. We studied 152 carotid plaques associated with ≥50% ICA stenoses in 135 patients who had CEAs and characterized them ultrasonographically into irregular/ulcerative, smooth, heterogeneous, homogeneous, or not defined. Heterogeneous plaques were defined as a mixture of hyperechoic, isoechoic, and hypoechoic plaques. In contrast, homogeneous plaques were defined as consisting of only one of the three types of echogenic plaques. An isoechoic plaque was defined as having the ecogenicity of a normal intima-media complex. A hyperechoic plaque was brighter than an isoechoic plaque, and a hypoechoic plaque was not as bright as an isoechoic plaque. An irregular plaque was defined as a plaque that lacks a smooth surface with or without an intimal layer. A smooth plaque was defined as a plaque without surface irregularities or ulcerations. All plaques were examined pathologically for the presence of intraplaque hemorrhage. The ultrasonic morphology of the plaques included 63 with surface irregularity (41%), 48 smooth (32%), 59 heterogeneous (39%), 52 homogeneous (34%), and 41 (27%) not defined. Intraplaque hemorrhage was present in 57 out of 63 (90%) irregular plaques and 53 out of 59 (90%) heterogeneous plaques, in contrast to 13 out of 48 (27%) smooth plaques and 17 out of 52 (33%) homogeneous plaques ($p < 0.001$). Fifty-three out of 63 (84%) irregular plaques and 47 out of 59 (80%) heterogeneous plaques had TIAs/stroke symptoms, in contrast to 9 out of 48 (19%) for smooth plaques and 15 out of 52 (29%) for homogeneous plaques ($p < 0.001$). Fifty-four percent of the irregular plaques and 57% of the heterogeneous plaques had ipsilateral cerebral infarcts, in contrast to 12% of the smooth plaques ($p < 0.001$) and 14% of the homogeneous plaques ($p < 0.001$). We concluded that irregular and/or heterogeneous carotid plaques are more often associated with intraplaque hemorrhage, neurologic events, and cerebral infarcts. Therefore, ultrasonic plaque morphology may be helpful in selecting patients for CEA.

In another recent study, we[71] analyzed the natural history of 60–<70% asymptomatic carotid stenosis according to ultrasonic plaque morphology and its implication on treatment.

Patients with 60–<70% asymptomatic carotid stenosis during a 2-year period entered into a protocol of carotid duplex surveillance/clinical examination every 6 months. Their ultrasonic plaque morphology was classified as heterogeneous (Group A, 162) or homogeneous (Group B, 229). CEA was done if the lesion progressed to ≥70% stenosis or became symptomatic.

Three hundred and eighty-two patients (391 arteries) were followed at a mean follow-up of 37 months. The clinical/demographic characteristics were similar for both groups. The incidence of future ipsilateral strokes was significantly higher in Group A than in Group B: 13.6% versus 3.1% ($p = 0.0001$, odds ratio 5). Similarly, the incidence of all neurologic events (stroke/TIAs) was higher in Group A than in Group B: 27.8% versus 6.6% ($p = 0.0001$, odds ratio of 5.5). Progression to ≥70% stenosis was also higher in Group A than in Group B: 25.3% versus 6.1% ($p = 0.0001$, odds ratio 5.2). Forty-four (27.2%) late CEAs were done in Group A (16 for stroke, 21 for TIAs, and seven for ≥70% asymptomatic carotid stenosis) versus 13 (5.7%) for Group B (five for stroke, seven for TIAs, and one for ≥70% asymptomatic carotid stenosis ($p = 0.0001$, odds ratio 6.2).

We concluded that patients with 60–<70% asymptomatic carotid stenosis with heterogeneous plaquing were associated with a higher incidence of late stroke, TIAs, and progression to ≥70% stenosis than patients with homogeneous plaquing. Prophylactic CEA for 60–<70% asymptomatic carotid stenosis may be justified if associated with heterogeneous plaquing.

In another study[72] of the correlation of ultrasonic carotid plaque morphology and the degree of carotid stenosis, 2460 carotid arteries were examined using color DUS during a 1-year period. Carotid stenoses were classified into <50%, 50–<60%, 60–<70%, and >70–99%.

Heterogeneous plaques were noted in 138 of 794 arteries with <50% stenosis, 191/564 with 50–<60% stenosis, 301/487 with 60–<70% stenosis, and 496/615 with 70–99% stenosis. The higher the degree of stenosis, the more likely it is to be associated with heterogeneous plaques. Heterogeneous plaques were present in 59% of ≥50% stenoses versus 17% for <50% stenoses, 72% of ≥60% stenoses versus 24% for <60% stenosis, and 80% of ≥70% stenoses versus 34% for <70% stenoses ($p <0.0001$ and odds ratios of 6.9, 8.1, and 8.0, respectively). Heterogeneous plaques were associated with a higher incidence of symptoms than homogeneous plaques in all grades of stenoses: 68% versus 16% for <50% stenosis;

76% versus 21% for 50–<60%; 79% versus 23% for 60–<70%, and 86% versus 31% for ≥70–99% ($p < 0.0001$ and odds ratios of 8.9, 11.9, 12.6, and 13.7, respectively). Heterogenosity of plaques was more positively correlated to symptoms than any degree of stenosis (regardless of plaque structure). Eighty percent of all heterogeneous plaques were symptomatic versus 58% for all ≥50% stenoses, 68% for all ≥60% stenoses, and 75% for all ≥70% stenoses ($p < 0.0001, p < 0.0001$, and $p = 0.02$, respectively).

We concluded that the higher the degree of carotid stenosis, the more likely it is to be associated with ultrasonic heterogeneous plaquing and cerebrovascular symptoms. Heterogenosity of the plaque was more positively correlated to symptoms than to any degree of stenosis. These findings suggest that plaque heterogenosity should be considered in selecting patients for CEA.[72]

Differentiating unstable from stable plaques by ultrasound has been hampered by the subjectiveness of interpreting such images.[73–76]

Biasi et al.[75] conducted a study to confirm that plaque echogenicity evaluated by computer analysis, as suggested by preliminary studies, can identify plaques associated with a high incidence of strokes. A series of 96 patients with carotid stenosis in the range of 50–99% were studied retrospectively (41 with TIAs and 55 asymptomatic). Carotid plaque echogenicity was evaluated using a computerized measurement of the median grayscale value (GSM). All patients had a CT brain scan to determine the presence of infarction in the carotid territory.

The incidence of ipsilateral brain CT infarctions was 32% for symptomatic plaques and 16% for asymptomatic plaques ($p = 0.076$). It was 25% for >70% stenosis and 20% for <70% stenosis ($p = 0.52$). It was 40% in those with a GSM of <50 and 9% for plaques with a GSM of >50 ($p < 0.001$) with a relative risk of 4.6 (95% CI 1.8–11.6).

It was concluded that a computer analysis of plaque echogenicity was better than the degree of stenosis in identifying plaques associated with an increased incidence of CT brain scan infarction and consequently useful for identifying individuals at high risk of stroke.

Kern et al.[74] investigated the value of real-time compound ultrasound imaging for the characterization of atherosclerotic plaques in the ICA. Thirty-two patients (22 men, 10 women; mean age, 75 years) with plaques of the ICA as identified by high-resolution B-mode scanning were investigated with real-time compound ultrasound imaging with the use of a 5- to 12-MHz dynamic range linear transducer on a duplex scanner. Two independent observers rated plaque morphology according to a standardized protocol. The majority of plaques were classified as predominantly echogenic and as plaques of irregular surface, whereas ulcerated plaques were rarely observed. The interobserver agreement for plaque surface characterization was good for both compound ultrasound (kappa = 0.72) and conventional B-mode ultrasound (kappa = 0.65). For the determination of plaque echogenicity, the reproducibility of compound ultrasound [kappa(w) = 0.83] was even higher than that of conventional B-mode ultrasound [kappa(w) = 0.74]. According to a semiquantitative analysis, real-time compound ultrasound was rated superior in the categories plaque texture resolution, plaque surface definition, and vessel wall demarcation. Furthermore, there was a significant reduction of acoustic shadowing and reverberations.

They concluded that real-time compound ultrasound was a suitable technique for the characterization of atherosclerotic plaques, showing good general agreement with high-resolution B-mode imaging. This advanced technique allows reduction of ultrasound artifacts and improves the assessment of plaque texture and surface for enhanced evaluation of carotid plaque morphology. This subject will be covered in depth elsewhere in this volume.

Intima-Media Thickness by Duplex Ultrasound

Poli et al.[76] reported on a study of ultrasonographic measurement of the CCA wall thickness in hypercholesterolemic patients, and they concluded that there was a correlation between the thickness of the carotid artery and the presence of cardiovascular risk factors. The measurement consists of determining the distance between the leading edge of the lumen-to-wall interface of the artery and the interface between the media and the adventitia on the artery wall. The combined width of this region is defined as intima-media thickness (IMT). It is believed that patients with larger IMTs had a greater number of cardiovascular risk factors than patients with thinner IMTs. O'Leary et al.[77] reported for the Cardiovascular Health Study Collaborative Research Group that thickening of the carotid wall was a marker for atherosclerosis in the elderly. This study clearly shows the strong cross-sectional relationships between risk factors and the thickness of the wall of both the ICA and the CCA. CCA wall thickening is a diffuse process whereas ICA wall thickness is a sonographic measurement of carotid plaque thickness and cholesterol deposition. Therefore, an increased internal carotid IMT corresponds to an increased degree of carotid artery stenosis, and the measurement of the ICA wall thickness correlates with the extent of subjectively graded percentage of stenosis.[78]

O'Leary et al.[79] showed a clear-cut scaling effect as well as excess risk with increasing thickening of the ICA and the CCA, as well as for a combined score adding measurement from the common and ICAs. IMT is felt to be a marker for future myocardial infarction as well as for stroke.

The Role of Carotid Duplex Scanning After Trauma

DUS can be used in evaluating vascular injuries of the neck. Although carotid trauma is not strictly a disease of the carotid bifurcation, developments in this area parallel the changes seen in surgery for atherosclerotic disease. Carotid duplex following cervical trauma was prospectively evaluated by Fry et al.[80] Fifteen patients had duplex scan and arteriography, and 11 of these had a region of interest in zone II and four in zone III. One injury was diagnosed by duplex scan in this group and this was confirmed by arteriography; both studies were normal in the remaining 14 patients. On the next 85 patients Fry et al. then performed duplex scan only, with arteriography reserved only for an abnormal duplex result. In this group, 62 patients had potential injuries in zone II and the remainder in zone III. Seven arterial injuries were identified by duplex scan and confirmed by arteriography. The remaining 76 patients had normal duplex scans and no sequelae up to 3 weeks postdischarge. It was concluded that DUS is a valuable tool in evaluating carotid injury.

Dissection of the Internal Carotid Artery

ICA dissection has been reported more often recently than was previously suspected. This disease can appear spontaneously, or may follow traumatic events accompanied by the fully developed picture of focal ischemia with facial and neck pain and Horner's syndrome (ptosis, miosis, and anhydrosis). It can also appear with very few symptoms, or may even be completely asymptomatic. Using a color flow DUS, the diagnosis can be made when the flow signal is carefully followed over the entire neck region. In the longitudinal section, forward and backward signal components in blue/red color coding are generally seen next to one another in the proximal ICA. Distally, an area free of flow signals marks the proximal end of the dissection. Corresponding Doppler signals characterize partial recanalization with systolic forward and backward signal components, but with diastolic forward flow preservation.[81–83] On angiography, proximally there is a thread-like occlusion/subtotal stenosis of the ICA without a connection to the intracranial vasculature (Figure 16–12). Monthly follow-up assessments are important, since the majority of the cases spontaneously recanalize.

Vertebrobasilar Insufficiency

During the 1970s and 1980s, there was limited clinical experience in regard to vertebrobasilar insufficiency, due in part to the difficulty in noninvasive study of vertebral artery flow. Furthermore, documented alterations in the

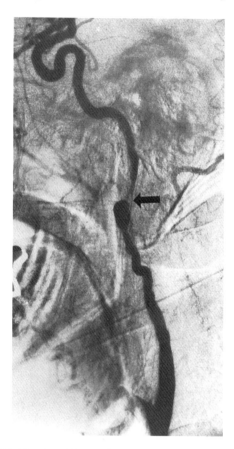

FIGURE 16–12. Carotid arteriogram showing internal carotid artery dissection of the higher cervical portion, as indicated by the black arrow.

vertebral flow may have little bearing on the clinical situation. Keller *et al.* studied vertebral artery flow using directional Doppler ultrasound in 90 patients, 40 of whom underwent subsequent arteriography.[84] The probe was positioned in the dorsal oropharynx after appropriate topical anesthesia, and the following four determinations were made: (1) the flow direction in each vertebral artery, (2) the related amplitude of both signals, (3) cessation of the flow in either vertebral artery during any part of the cardiac cycle, and (4) response of the vertebral flow to ipsilateral CCA compression. Under normal circumstances, the vertebral flow was always craniad and of equal amplitude in both vessels. It never reached zero during any phase diastole, and it did not change with CCA compression. Alteration of any of these normal observations was diagnostic of vertebral artery occlusive disease with a specificity of 82%. Kaneda *et al.*[85] simplified the previous technique by positioning the probe just below the mastoid process directed toward the contralateral eye. He reported a diagnostic accuracy of 92%. Others have found the mastoid approach unreliable, since spatial relationships between the probe and the vessel axis were poorly defined and more intervening structures were present.

Recent studies have shown that with adequate skill and patience on the operator's part, the innominate, sub-clavian, cervical, and prevertebral segment of the vertebral artery can be displayed with real-time, pulsed echo methods. Duplex scanning appears to be the most successful and accurate technique to diagnose atherosclerotic lesions of the vertebral arteries in the neck region. With this technique, the cervical segment of the vertebral artery can be visualized and the direction of the flow can be determined, whether antegrade or retrograde, which may be suggestive of subclavian steal. It has been reported that a reliable investigation of the prevertebral segment and the orifice of the vertebral artery is possible in more than 80% of cases (Figure 6–10 in Chapter 6). Some studies[85–87] claim more rapid identification and a higher success rate if color flow imaging is used. For detecting stenoses of ≥50% of the arch branches and at the site of the origin of the vertebral artery, duplex scanning has a high sensitivity, specificity, and overall accuracy. However, this technique still has several disadvantages, including the fact that satisfactory displays of the origin of the vertebral artery cannot be achieved in all patients. In addition, it is obvious that in those arteries in which the examination is successfully completed, only a limited spectrum of disease involvement can be identified. Accuracy of ultrasonic examination of the intradural segment of the vertebral artery can be improved by the use of simultaneous B-mode and color flow imaging. This subject will be covered in depth in another chapter in this volume.

Color Duplex Ultrasound in the Diagnosis of Temporal Arteritis

Temporal arteritis is sometimes diagnosed clinically, but a temporal artery biopsy is usually recommended to confirm the diagnosis.[88] The American College of Rheumatology requires three of the following five criteria to be met to establish the diagnosis: age ≥50 years, new onset of localized headache, temporal artery tenderness or decreased pulse, erythrocyte sedimentation rate ≥50 mm/h, and histologic findings. Schmidt *et al.*[88] examined the usefulness of color duplex ultrasonography in patients suspected of having temporal arteritis. In their prospective study, all patients seen in the departments of rheumatology and ophthalmology from January 1994 to October 1996 who had clinically suspected active temporal arteritis or polymyalgia rheumatica were examined by duplex ultrasonography. They examined both common superficial temporal arteries and the frontal and parietal rami as completely as possible in longitudinal and transverse planes to see if they were perfused, if there was a halo around the lumen, and (using simultaneous pulsed-wave Doppler ultrasonography) if there was a stenosis. Stenosis was considered to be present if blood flow velocity was more then twice the rate recorded in the area before the stenosis, perhaps with waveforms demonstrating turbulence and reduced velocity behind the area of stenosis. Two ultrasound studies were performed and read before the biopsies. Based on standard criteria, the final diagnoses were temporal arteritis in 30 patients, 21 with biopsy-confirmed disease; polymyalgia rheumatica in 37; and negative histologic findings and a diagnosis other than temporal arteritis or polymyalgia rheumatica in 15. They also studied 30 control patients matched for age and sex to the patients with arteritis.

Schmidt et al.[88] found that in 22 (73%) of the 30 patients with temporal arteritis, ultrasonography showed a dark halo around the lumen of the temporal arteries. The halos disappeared after a mean of 16 days (range: 7–56) of treatment with corticosteroids. Twenty-four patients (80%) had stenoses or occlusions of temporal artery segments, and 28 patients (93%) had stenoses, occlusions, or a halo. No halos were identified in the 82 patients without temporal arteritis; 6 (7%) had stenoses or occlusions. For each of the three types of abnormalities identified by ultrasonography, the interrater agreement was ≥95%.

They concluded that there are characteristic signs of temporal arteritis that can be visualized by color duplex ultrasonography. The most specific sign is a dark halo, which may be due to edema of the artery wall. In patients with typical clinical signs and a halo on ultrasonography, it may be possible to make a diagnosis of temporal arteritis and begin treatment without performing a temporal artery biopsy. This subject will be covered in depth in another chapter in this volume.

References

1. Cartier R, Cartier P, Fontaine A. Carotid endarterectomy without angiography: The reliability of Doppler ultrasonography and duplex scanning in preoperative assessment. Can J Surg 1993;36:411–421.

2. Polak JF. Noninvasive carotid evaluation: Carpe diem. Radiology 1993;186:329–331.

3. Moore WS, Ziomek S, Quinones-Baldrich WJ, et al. Can clinical evaluation and noninvasive testing substitute for arteriography in the evaluation of carotid artery disease? Ann Surg 1988;208:91–94.

4. Norris JW, Halliday A. Is ultrasound sufficient for vascular imaging prior to carotid endarterectomy? Stroke 2004;35: 370–371.

5. Moore WS. For severe carotid stenosis found on ultrasound, further arterial evaluation is unnecessary. Stroke 2003;34: 1816–1817.

6. Executive Committee for the Asymptomatic Carotid Atherosclerosis Study. Endarterectomy for asymptomatic carotid artery stenosis. JAMA 1995;273:1421–1428.

7. Dawson DL, Zierler RE, Strandness DE Jr, et al. The role of duplex scanning and arteriography before carotid endarterectomy: A prospective study. J Vasc Surg 1993; 18:673–683.

8. Horn M, Michelini M, Greisler HP, et al. Carotid endarterectomy without arteriography: The preeminent role of the vascular laboratory. Ann Vasc Surg 1994;8:221–224.

9. Chervu A, Moore WS. Carotid endarterectomy without arteriography. Ann Vasc Surg 1994;8:296–302.

10. Mattos MA, Hodgson KJ, Faught WE, et al. Carotid endarterectomy without angiography: Is color-flow duplex scanning sufficient? Surgery 1994;116:776–783.

11. Walsh J, Markowitz I, Kerstein MD. Carotid endarterectomy for amaurosis fugax without angiography. Am J Surg 1986;152:172–174.

12. Marshall WG, Jr., Kouchoukos NT, Murphy SF, et al. Carotid endarterectomy based on duplex scanning without preoperative arteriography. Circulation 1988;78(Suppl I):I-1–I-5.

13. Nederkoorn PJ, Mali WPTM, Eikelboom BC, Elgersma OEH, Buskens E, Hunink MGM, Kappell LJ, Buijs PC, Wust AFJ, Lugt van der Lugt A, van der Graaf Y. Preoperative diagnosis of carotid artery stenosis: Accuracy of noninvasive testing. Stroke 2002;33:2003–2008.

14. Nederkoorn PJ, van der Graaf Y, Hunink Y. Duplex ultrasound and magnetic resonance angiography compared with digital subtraction angiography in carotid artery stenosis. Stroke 2003;34:1324–1332.

15. Westwood ME, Kelly S, Berry E, Bamford JM, Gough MJ, Airey CM, Meaney JFM, Davies LM, Cullingworth J, Smith MA. Use of magnetic resonance angiography to select candidates with recently symptomatic carotid stenosis for surgery: A systematic review. BMJ 2002;324:1–5.

16. Jackson MR, Chang AS, Robles HA, et al. Determination of 60% or greater carotid stenosis: A prospective comparison of magnetic resonance angiography and duplex ultrasound with conventional angiography. Ann Vasc Surg 1998; 12:236–243.

17. Willinek WA, von Falkenhausen M, Born M, Gieseke J, Holler T, Klockgether T, Textor HJ, Schild HH, Urbach H. Noninvasive detection of steno-occlusive disease of the supra-aortic arteries with three-dimensional contrast-enhanced magnetic resonance angiography. A prospective, intra-individual comparative analysis with digital subtraction angiography. Stroke 2005;36:38–43.

18. Al-Kwifi O, Kim JK, Stainsby J, Huang Y, Sussman MS, Farb RI, Wright GA. Pulsatile motion effects on 3-D magnetic resonance angiography: Implications for evaluating carotid artery stenoses. Magn Reson Med 2004;52: 605–611.

19. van Bemmel CM, Elgersma OE, Vonken EJ, Fiorelli M, van Leeuwen MS, Niessen WJ. Evaluation of semiautomated internal carotid artery stenosis quantification from 3-dimensional contrast-enhanced magnetic resonance angiograms. Invest Radiol 2004;39:418–426.

20. Kim DY, Park JW. Computerized quantification of carotid artery stenosis using MRA axial images. Magn Reson Imaging 2004;22:353–359.

21. U-King-Im JM, Trivedi R, Cross J, Higgins N, Graves M, Kirkpatrick P, Antoun N, Gillard JH. Conventional digital subtraction x-ray angiography versus magnetic resonance angiography in the evaluation of carotid disease: Patient satisfaction and preferences. Clin Radiol 2004;59: 358–363.

22. Back MR, Rogers GA, Wilson JS, Johnson BL, Shames ML, Bandyk DF. Magnetic resonance angiography minimizes need for arteriography after inadequate carotid duplex ultrasound scanning. J Vasc Surg 2003;38:422–430.

23. Anderson GB, Ashforth R, Steinke DE, Ferdinancy R, Findlay JM. CT angiography for the detection and charac-

terization of carotid artery bifurcation disease. Stroke 2000; 31:2168–2174.

24. Koelemay MJ, Nederkoorn PJ, Reitsma JB, Majoie CB. Systematic review of computed tomographic angiography for assessment of carotid artery disease. Stroke 2004;35: 2306–2312.

25. Fell G, Breslau P, Know RA, et al. Importance of noninvasive ultrasonic Doppler testing in the evaluation of patients with asymptomatic carotid bruits. Am Heart J 1981;102: 221–226.

26. North American Symptomatic Carotid Endarterectomy Trial (NASCET) Investigators. Clinical alert: Benefit of carotid endarterectomy for patients with high-grade stenosis of the internal carotid artery. National Institute of Neurological Disorders and Stroke, Stroke and Trauma Division. Stroke 1991;22:816–817.

27. AbuRahma AF, Robinson PA, Boland JP, et al. Complications of arteriography in a recent series of 707 cases: Factors affecting outcome. Ann Vasc Surg 1993;7:122–129.

28. AbuRahma AF, Robinson PA, Stickler DL, et al. Proposed new duplex classification for threshold stenoses used in various symptomatic and asymptomatic carotid endarterectomy trials. Ann Vasc Surg 1998;12:349–358.

29. Sigel B, Coelho JC, Flanigan DP, et al. Detection of vascular defects during operation by imaging ultrasound. Ann Surg 1982;196:473–480.

30. Blaisdell FW, Lin R, Hall AD. Technical result of carotid endarterectomy—-arteriographic assessment. Am J Surg 1967;114:239–246.

31. Bandyk DF, Govostis DM. Intraoperative color flow imaging of "difficult" arterial reconstructions. Video J Color Flow Imaging 1991;1:13–20.

32. Hallett JW Jr, Berger MW, Lewis BD. Intraoperative color-flow duplex ultrasonography following carotid endarterectomy. Neurosurg Clin North Am 1996;7:733–740.

33. Baker WH, Koustas G, Burke K, et al. Intraoperative duplex scanning and late carotid artery stenosis. J Vasc Surg 1994;19:829–833.

34. Kinney EV, Seabrook GR, Kinney LY, et al. The importance of intraoperative detection of residual flow abnormalities after carotid artery endarterectomy. J Vasc Surg 1993;17: 912–922.

35. Coe DA, Towne JB, Seabrook GR, et al. Duplex morphologic features of the reconstructed carotid artery: Changes occurring more than five year after endarterectomy. J Vasc Surg 1997;25:850–857.

36. Cato R, Bandyk D, Karp D, et al. Duplex scanning after carotid reconstruction: A comparison of intraoperative and postoperative results. J Vasc Tech 1991;15:61–65.

37. Lane RJ, Ackroyd N, Appleberg M, et al. The application of operative ultrasound immediately following carotid endarterectomy. World J Surg 1987;11:593–597.

38. Sawchuk AP, Flanigan DP, Machi J, et al. The fate of unrepaired minor technical defects detected by intraoperative ultrasound during carotid endarterectomy. J Vasc Surg 1989;9:671–676.

39. Ascher E, Markevich N, Kallakuri S, Schutzer RW, Hingorani AP. Intraoperative carotid artery duplex scanning in a modern series of 650 consecutive primary endarterectomy procedures. J Vasc Surg 2004;39:416–420.

40. Halsey JH Jr. Risks and benefits of shunting in carotid endarterectomy. Stroke 1992;23:1583–1587.

41. Ackerstaff RGA, Moons KGM, van de Vlasakker CJW, Moll FL, Vermeulen FEE, Algra A, Spencer MP. Association of intraoperative transcranial Doppler monitoring variables with stroke from carotid endarterectomy. Stroke 2000;31:1817–1823.

42. Thomas M, Otis S, Rush M, et al. Recurrent carotid artery stenosis following endarterectomy. Ann Surg 1984;200: 74–79.

43. Mattos MA, Shamma AR, Rossi N, et al. Is duplex follow-up cost-effective in the first year after carotid endarterectomy? Am J Surg 1988;156:91–95.

44. Cook JM, Thompson BW, Barnes RW. Is routine duplex examination after carotid endarterectomy justified? J Vasc Surg 1990;12:334–340.

45. Mackey WC, Belkin M, Sindhi R, et al. Routine postendarterectomy duplex surveillance: Does it prevent late stroke? J Vasc Surg 1992;16:934–940.

46. Mattos MA, van Bemmelen PS, Barkmeier LD, et al. Routine surveillance after carotid endarterectomy: Does it affect clinical management? J Vasc Surg 1993;17:819–831.

47. Ouriel K, Green RM. Appropriate frequency of carotid duplex testing following carotid endarterectomy. Am J Surg 1995;170:144–147.

48. Ricotta JJ, DeWeese JA. Is route carotid ultrasound surveillance after carotid endarterectomy worthwhile? Am J Surg 1996;172:140–143.

49. Golledge J, Cuming R, Ellis M, et al. Clinical follow-up rather than duplex surveillance after carotid endarterectomy. J Vasc Surg 1997;25:55–63.

50. AbuRahma AF, Robinson PA, Saiedy S, et al. Prospective randomized trial of carotid endarterectomy with primary closure and patch angioplasty with saphenous vein, jugular vein, and polytetrafluoroethylene: Long-term follow-up. J Vasc Surg 1998;27:222–234.

51. Patel ST, Kuntz KM, Kent KG. Is routine duplex ultrasound surveillance after carotid endarterectomy cost-effective? Surgery 1998;124:343–353.

52. Roth SM, Back MR, Bandyk DF, et al. A rational algorithm for duplex scan surveillance after carotid endarterectomy. J Vasc Surg 1999;30:453–460.

53. Ricco JB, Camiade C, Roumy J, Neau JP. Modalities of surveillance after carotid endarterectomy: Impact of surgical technique. Ann Vasc Surg 2003;17:386–392.

54. Lovelace TD, Moneta GL, Abou-Zamzam AH, Edwards JM, Yeager RA, Landry GJ, Taylor LM, Porter JM. Optimizing duplex follow-up in patients with an asymptomatic internal carotid artery stenosis of less than 60%. J Vasc Surg 2001;33:56–61.

55. AbuRahma AF, Snodgrass KR, Robinson PA, et al. Safety and durability of redo carotid endarterectomy for recurrent carotid artery stenosis. Am J Surg 1994;168:175–178.

56. Kupinski AM, Khan AM, Stanton JE, Relyea W, Ford T, Mackey V, Khurana Y, Darling RC, Shah DM. Duplex ultrasound follow-up of carotid stents. J Vasc Ultrasound 2004;28:71–75.

57. Robbin ML, Lockhart ME, Weber TM, et al. Carotid artery stent: Early and intermediate follow-up with Doppler ultrasound. Radiology 1997;205:749–756.

58. Roederer GO, Langlois YE, Jager KA, et al. The natural history of carotid artery disease in asymptomatic patients with cervical bruits. Stroke 1984;15:605–613.

59. AbuRahma AF, Hannay RS, Khan JH, *et al.* Prospective randomized study of carotid endarterectomy with polytetrafluoroethylene versus collagen impregnated Dacron (Hemashield) patching: Perioperative (30-day) results. J Vasc Surg 2002;35:125–130.

60. Dawson DL, Zierler RE, Kohler TR. Role of arteriography in the preoperative evaluation of carotid artery disease. Am J Surg 1991;161:619–624.

61. Kuntz KM, Skillman JJ, Whittemore AD, *et al.* Carotid endarterectomy in asymptomatic patients: Is contrast angiography necessary? A morbidity analysis. J Vasc Surg 1995;22:706–716.

62. Kent KC, Kuntz KM, Patel MR. Perioperative imaging strategies for carotid endarterectomy: An analysis of morbidity and cost-effectiveness in symptomatic patients. JAMA 1995;274:888–893.

63. Campron H, Cartier R, Fontaine AR. Prophylactic carotid endarterectomy without arteriography in patients without hemispheric symptoms: Surgical morbidity and mortality and long-term follow-up. Ann Vasc Surg 1998;12:10–16.

64. Roederer GO, Langlois YE, Chan ARW, *et al.* Is siphon disease important in predicting outcome of carotid endarterectomy? Arch Surg 1983;118:1177–1181.

65. Mattos MA, van Bemmelen PS, Hodgson KJ, *et al.* The influence of carotid siphon stenosis on short and long-term outcome after carotid endarterectomy. J Vasc Surg 1993;17:902–911.

66. Lord RSA. Relevance of siphon stenosis and intracranial aneurysm to results of carotid endarterectomy. In: Ernst CB, Stanley JC (eds). *Current Therapy in Vascular Surgery*, 2nd ed., pp. 94–101. Philadelphia, PA: BC Decker, 1991.

67. Strandness DE Jr. Extracranial arterial disease, In: Strandness DR Jr (ed). *Duplex Scanning in Vascular Disorders*, 2nd ed., pp. 113–158. New York: Raven Press, 1993.

68. Pilcher DB, Ricci MA. Vascular ultrasound. Surg Clin North Am 1998;78:273–293.

69. AbuRahma AF, White JF III, Boland JP. Carotid endarterectomy for symptomatic carotid artery disease demonstrated by duplex ultrasound with minimal arteriographic findings. Ann Vasc Surg 1996;10:385–389.

70. AbuRahma AF, Kyer PD III, Robinson PA, *et al.* The correlation of ultrasonic carotid plaque morphology and carotid plaque hemorrhage: Clinical implications. Surgery 1998;124:721–728.

71. AbuRahma AF, Thiele SP, Wulu JT. Prospective controlled study of the natural history of asymptomatic 60% to 69% carotid stenosis according to ultrasonic plaque morphology. J Vasc Surg 2002;36:437–442.

72. AbuRahma AF, Wulu JT, Crotty B. Carotid plaque ultrasonic heterogeneity and severity of stenosis. Stroke 2002;33:1772–1775.

73. Choo V. New imaging technology might help prevent stroke. Lancet 1998;351:809.

74. Kern R, Szabo K. Hennerici M, Meairs S. Characterization of carotid artery plaques using real-time compound B-mode ultrasound. Stroke 2004;35:870–875.

75. Biasi GM, Sampaolo A, Mingazzini P, De Amicis P. El-Barghouty N, Nicolaides AN. Computer analysis of ultrasonic plaque echolucency in identifying high-risk carotid bifurcation lesions. Eur J Vasc Endovasc Surg 1999;17:476–479.

76. Poli A, Tremoli E, Colombo A, Sirtori M, Pignoli P, Paoletti R. Ultrasonographic measurement of the common carotid artery wall thickness in hypercholesterolemic patients. A new model for the quantitation and follow-up of preclinical atherosclerosis in living human subjects. Atherosclerosis 1988;70:253–261.

77. O'Leary DH, Polak JF, Kronmal RA, *et al.* Thickening of the carotid wall. A marker for atherosclerosis in the elderly? Cardiovascular Health Study Collaborative Research Group. Stroke 1996;27:224–231.

78. Polak JF, O'Leary DH, Kronmal RA, *et al.* Sonographic evaluation of carotid artery atherosclerosis in the elderly: Relationship of disease severity to stroke and transient ischemic attack. Radiology 1993;188:363–370.

79. O'Leary DH, Polak JF, Kronmal RA, Manolio TA, Burke GL, Wolfson SK Jr. Carotid-artery intima and media thickness as a risk factor for myocardial infarction and stroke in older adults. Cardiovascular Health Study Collaborative Research Group. N Engl J Med 1999;340:14–22.

80. Fry WR, Dort JA, Smith RS, *et al.* Duplex scanning replaces arteriography and operative exploration in the diagnosis of potential cervical vascular injury. Am J Surg 1994;168:693–696.

81. Steinke W. Schwartz A, Hennerici M. Doppler color flow imaging of common carotid artery dissection. Neuroradiology 1990;32(6):502–505.

82. Sturzenegger M. Ultrasound findings in spontaneous carotid artery dissection. The value of duplex sonography. Arch Neurol 1991;48(10):1057–1063.

83. Cals N, Devuyst G, Jung DK, Afsar N, de Freitas G, Despland PA, Bogousslavsky J. Uncommon ultrasound findings in traumatic extracranial dissection. Eur J Ultrasound 2001;12:227–231.

84. Keller HM, Meier WE, Kumpe DA. Noninvasive angiography for the diagnosis of vertebral artery disease using Doppler ultrasound (vertebral artery Doppler). Stroke 1976;7:364–369.

85. Kaneda H, Irino T, Minami T, *et al.* Diagnostic reliability of the percutaneous ultrasonic Doppler technique for vertebral arterial occlusive diseases. Stroke 1977;8:571–579.

86. Bartels E, Fuchs HH, Flugel KA. Color Doppler imaging of vertebral arteries: A comparative study with duplex ultrasonography. In: Oka M, *et al.* (eds). *Recent Advantages in Neurosonology.* Amsterdam: Elsevier Science Publishers, 1992.

87. De Bray JM. Le duplex des axes verebro-sous-claviers. J Echographie Med Ultrasons 1991;12:141–151.

88. Schmidt WA, Kraft HE, Vorpahl K, *et al.* Color duplex ultrasonography in the diagnosis of temporal arteritis. N Engl J Med 1997;337:1336–1342.

Section IV
Noninvasive Diagnosis of Peripheral Arterial Disease of the Extremities

17
Overview of Peripheral Arterial Disease of the Lower Extremity

Ali F. AbuRahma

Introduction

As the population continues to grow in average age, chronic lower extremity ischemia is becoming more prevalent. Recently, Dormandy et al.[1] reported the weighted mean incidence of intermittent claudication from five large population-based studies. The incidence ranged from two per 1000 men per year in the 30- to 54-year-old group to seven per 1000 in those over 65 years of age. In a recent summary of large population studies from Italy, Britain, Holland, and Finland, the prevalence of intermittent claudication increases gradually from <1% in 30-year-old men to 3% in 55- to 59-year-old men. The prevalence also increases starting at age 60, from 3% to over 7% in those 70 years old and older.[2] It is believed that the overall incidence and prevalence of peripheral arterial disease are likely to increase significantly with the aging of the population, and it has been estimated that the number of individuals aged ≥65 will grow by 70% in the United States between 2010 and 2030.[3]

Anatomy of the Lower Extremity Vascular System

The arterial anatomy relevant to the lower extremity circulation is demonstrated in Figure 17–1.

At its most distal aspect, the *aorta* branches to form paired *common iliac arteries*. These continue retroperitoneally to the pelvic brim, at which the common iliac vessels branch to form paired *internal* and *external iliac arteries*. The *internal iliac* (or hypogastric) *arteries* provide blood supply to the pelvic structures, while the *external iliac* courses inferior to the inguinal ligament to become the *common femoral artery*.

The common femoral artery then bifurcates early in its course to form the *profunda femoris artery*, which supplies the thigh musculature, and the *superficial femoral*

artery, which continues inferiorly to become the *popliteal artery* at its point of entry into the adductor canal.

The popliteal artery then continues below the knee, where the *anterior tibial artery* branches, piercing the interosseous membrane to supply the anterior compartment of the lower leg. The *tibioperoneal trunk* then continues briefly, where the *posterior tibial artery* branches to course in a plane deep to the soleus muscle. The vessel then continues inferiorly as the *peroneal artery*. The posterior tibial artery is divided into lateral and medial plantar arteries below the medial malleolus to supply the sole of the foot.

Ultimately, the anterior tibial artery continues on to the dorsum of the foot, where it becomes the *dorsalis pedis artery*. Here it anastomoses with branches of the posterior tibial and peroneal arteries to form the *plantar arch*.[4] On the dorsum of the foot, the dorsalis pedis artery forms two branches: the dorsal metatarsal and the deep plantar arteries. The deep plantar artery penetrates into the sole of the foot and joins the lateral plantar artery (branch of the posterior tibial artery) to form the plantar arch.

Collateral Circulation

In the event of chronic obstruction of major arterial vessels, collateral pathways exist that allow preservation of sufficient distal blood flow to maintain viability of the tissues distally. The degree of adequacy of these pathways determines what degree of functional disability results.

With obstruction at the level of the distal aorta and common iliac arteries, a variety of pathways for collateral circulation exist (Figure 17–2). Communications may exist between the lumbar and circumflex iliac or hypogastric arteries. Other communications may exist between the gluteal branches of the hypogastric arteries and recurrent branches of the common femoral or profunda femoris arteries. Visceral–parietal communications may also exist at this level between the inferior mesenteric

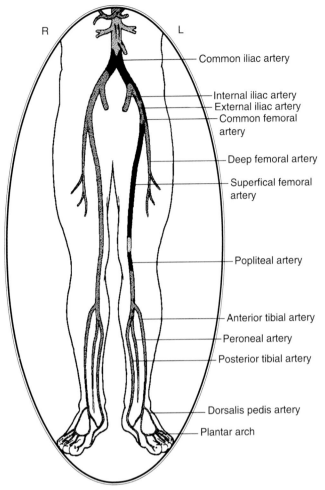

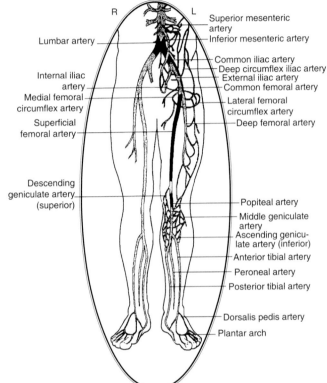

FIGURE 17–1. A normal right arterial tree (except for occlusion of the right common iliac artery) beginning with the common iliac artery down to the pedal branches. The *left side* shows occlusion of the left common iliac artery, stenosis of the left external iliac artery, and occlusion of the left superficial femoral artery, popliteal artery, and diseased tibioperoneal trunk.

FIGURE 17–2. (A) Collateral circulation of the left lower extremity secondary to occlusion of the major arterial segments as noted in Figure 17–1. (B) Arteriogram showing complete occlusion of the left common iliac artery (*arrow*). Note the collateral circulation around the obstruction. This also shows extensive disease of both right and left external iliac arteries.

and internal iliac vessels via hemorrhoidal branches at the level of the rectum.

More distally, with obstruction of the common femoral artery, collateral circulation around the hip is provided via communication of the inferior epigastric and deep circumflex branches of the external iliac arteries with the internal pudendal and obturator branches of the internal iliac arteries (Figure 17–2B).

With chronic obstruction of the superficial femoral artery, collateral circulation to the popliteal artery is provided by communications with the profunda femoris artery via the geniculate arteries, as well as descending branches of the lateral femoral circumflex arteries. With popliteal occlusion, it is these geniculate arteries that are responsible for the filling of the more distal tibial vessels as well (Figure 17–2B). More distally, branches of the peroneal, anterior tibial, and posterior tibial arteries all provide collateral supply to the plantar arch vessels.[4,5]

Normal Structure of the Arterial Wall

Before discussion of any pathologic process affecting the arterial wall, it is important to understand the basic structural anatomy of the normal blood vessel. The artery is composed of three major layers known as the *intima*, *media*, and *adventitia*.

The *intima*, the innermost layer, consists of a layer of endothelium that lines the luminal surface and overlies one or more layers of smooth muscle. These are then covered by a layer of connective tissue known as the *internal elastic lamina*.

Just beyond the internal elastic lamina begins the *media*, which is bounded by the internal and external elastic lamina. The media is composed of smooth muscle cells arranged in layers and lying in a matrix of proteoglycan substance. Collagen and elastin fibers are also present within this layer.

The *adventitia* is the outermost layer of the arterial wall and the layer responsible for the majority of the vessel's strength. It is composed of connective tissue, fibroblasts, capillaries, neural fibers, and occasional leukocytes. In large vessels a microvasculature known as the *vasa vasorum* is present within the adventitial layer, serving to nourish the adventitia and outermost layers of the media.[6]

Atherosclerosis

Pathophysiology

Intermittent claudication as a symptom of peripheral arterial disease can be caused by flow limiting stenosis, which is almost secondary to atherosclerosis. Whether or not a stenotic lesion is flow limiting depends on both flow velocities and the degree of stenosis.[7] Flow velocity at rest

has been estimated to be as low as 20 cm/s in the femoral artery. A diameter reduction of >90% would be required for a stenotic lesion at these rates to be considered hemodynamically significant. However, the metabolic requirements in the distal tissue of an exercising or active individual are higher, and the femoral artery velocities may increase up to 150 cm/s, and at this velocity level, a stenosis of 50% can cause significant pressure and flow gradient leading to inadequate oxygen delivery. In general, patients with mild intermittent claudication typically have a single segment disease, which is often associated with well-developed collateral circulation, in contrast to patients with severe claudication or critical limb ischemia, which is associated with multilevel disease.

The hemodynamic abnormalities of peripheral arterial occlusive disease reflected in ankle-brachial index (ABI) measurements or direct measurement of calf blood flow do not necessarily correlate with walking performance or severity of the claudication symptoms.[8] Biochemical changes and microcirculatory changes induced by the cycle of ischemia and reperfusion have been suggested as evidence of this observation. This may lead to skeletal muscle injury due to distal axonal degeneration, which, in turn, may cause muscle atrophy, further compromising exercise tolerance. This injury may be mediated at the cellular level through increased oxidative stress, generation of oxygen-free radicals, and lipid peroxidation that occurs during reperfusion of ischemic tissue. Several studies have demonstrated the accumulation of several metabolic intermediates, such as acylcarnitines, impaired synthesis of phosocreatinine, and supranormal levels of adenosine diphosphates.[9] Patients with advanced chronic peripheral arterial disease have an abundance of these antimetabolic compounds, which signify well-established metabolic myopathy. Increased acylcarnitine accumulation has been noted to correlate well with decreased treadmill exercise performance.[10]

The basic underlying disease process affecting the arterial wall, and the one responsible for the clinical manifestations of lower extremity peripheral arterial disease, is atherosclerosis. Simply put, atherosclerosis is a disease of medium to large arterial vessels that causes luminal narrowing, thrombosis, and occlusion resulting in ischemia of the end organ involved. The process of atherosclerosis is extremely complex and is the subject of continuous investigation within the medical and surgical community. In addition to lower extremity vascular disease, atherosclerosis is known to produce many other clinical events of importance including, but not limited to, myocardial infarction, stroke, mesenteric vascular insufficiency, and aortic aneurysm formation.[11]

Atherosclerosis is primarily a disease of the intima characterized by the proliferation of smooth muscle cells and the accumulation of lipid material. The earliest lesion appears to be that of the *fatty streak*. In this lesion, lipid accumulates within the vessel wall, either extracellularly or intracellularly, within macrophages known as *foam cells*. This lesion often forms quite early in the course of the disease and may even be found in the arterial system of young children.[12]

The *fibrous plaque*, the next phase of atherogenesis, is characterized histologically by a thick fibrous luminal cap composed of smooth muscle cells and connective tissue. This plaque typically overlies a core composed of necrotic debris and lipid material (the atheroma). Continued proliferation of smooth muscle cells and accumulation of lipid material results in the luminal narrowing characteristic of the disease.[13]

In some cases, although it is unclear why, the plaque may develop features of luminal ulceration and wall calcification or hemorrhage. These changes result in what is known as the *complicated lesion* of atherosclerosis. The nature of this lesion is far more unstable and is the source for the arterioarterial thromboembolic events observed in these patients.[14]

Risk Factors

Through epidemiologic data, a number of risk factors for the development of atherosclerosis have been reasonably well established. These factors include hypertension, hypercholesterolemia, cigarette smoking, obesity, diabetes mellitus, stress, sedentary lifestyle, and family history. Of these, hypertension, hypercholesterolemia [of the low-density lipoprotein (LDL) fraction], and cigarette smoking have demonstrated the greatest significance and are classified as "major" risk factors. Of these "major" risk factors, cigarette smoking appears to convey the greatest relative risk of developing atherosclerosis, as well as for accelerating the process once it has been established.[6,15,16]

The association between smoking and peripheral arterial disease is very firmly established.[17] Overall, smokers carry a three times higher relative risk of developing intermittent claudication and experience claudication symptoms an average of 10 years earlier than nonsmokers. The Framingham study showed that smokers are twice as likely to develop peripheral arterial disease as coronary artery disease.[18] Celermajer *et al.*[19] reported that abnormal endothelial/nitric oxide-dependent vasodilatation has been implicated as an explanation for the smoking-induced development and progression of atherosclerosis.

Several research studies have both supported and refuted the significance of total cholesterol as an independent risk factor for peripheral arterial disease.[2] However, the ratio of total to high-density lipoprotein cholesterol has been recognized as an accurate predictor of peripheral arterial disease. Cheng *et al.*[20] concluded that lipoprotein (a) is an independent risk factor for peripheral arterial disease.[20] It should be noted that the association between hypertriglyceridemia and the progression of coronary and carotid atherosclerosis is well-established.[21]

The presence of diabetes mellitus increases the risk of claudication by two-fold. There is strong evidence that better control of blood sugar delays the onset of microvascular diabetic retinopathy and nephropathy, however, the effect of such control in progression of macrovascular disease remains controversial.[22] Glucose intolerance, insulin resistance, and hyperinsulinemia have all been implicated as independent risk factors for peripheral arterial disease.

The role of hypertension in the development of peripheral arterial disease has been controversial, with the Framingham and the Finnish studies arriving at opposite conclusions. Hypertension may have both a cause and effect relation to peripheral arterial disease. Aggressive blood pressure control in newly diagnosed hypertensive patients occasionally decreases perfusion sufficiently to unmask and unrecognize hemodynamically significant stenotic lesions.

Hyperhomosysteinemia has been established as a risk factor for peripheral arterial disease with an odds ratio of above six.[23] This entity has been related to premature atherosclerosis and preferentially associated with peripheral arterial disease more often than coronary artery disease. Finally, a family history has not been found to be a significant independent risk factor in the development of peripheral arterial disease, in contrast to patients with coronary artery disease.

Association of Peripheral Arterial Disease, Coronary Artery Disease, and Cerebrovascular Disease

Pooling evidence from available studies such as the TransAtlantic Intersociety Consensus (TASC) concluded that approximately 60% of patients with peripheral arterial disease have significant coronary artery disease, cerebrovascular disease, or both, whereas about 40% of those with coronary artery or cerebrovascular disease also have peripheral arterial disease.[2] Murabito *et al.*[18] reported that the diagnosis of concomitant coronary artery disease can be established with a clinical history, physical examination, and EKG in 40–60% of all patients with intermittent claudication.

The relative risk for developing intermittent claudication increases by two- to three-fold for male versus female, and for each additional decade of life.[22]

Theories of Atherogenesis

The extreme complexity of the atherosclerotic process has resulted in the formulation of several theories to explain its pathogenesis. These theories are based on attempts to account for one or more aspects of the disease and are therefore not mutually exclusive. In general, three theories have emerged as the most reasonable: the response to injury hypothesis, the lipid hypothesis, and the monoclonal (or mutagenic cellular transformation) hypothesis.

The Response to Injury Hypothesis

The response to injury hypothesis is based on the marked similarity of atherosclerotic lesions to those occurring after experimental injury. The hypothesis states that some form of arterial injury (via the aforementioned risk factors) results in focal disruption of the endothelium, thus allowing interaction between the blood elements and the arterial walls. This then allows interaction of leukocytes and platelets with the disrupted surface. Platelet degranulation results, as does migration of macrophages into the injured intimal layer. One substance released from the platelet—platelet derived growth factor (PDGF)—is thought to induce the smooth muscle proliferation characteristic of the process.[24,25] This hypothesis may explain the marked tendency for atherosclerosis to develop in regions of increased turbulence such as that observed at major arterial bifurcations.

Lipid Hypothesis

The relatively simple lipid hypothesis states that the lipids within the atherosclerotic lesion are derived from circulating lipoproteins in the bloodstream. Support for this theory has been provided by the Association of Atherosclerosis with elevated levels of LDL.[26] This hypothesis, however, fails to account for other features of the lesion, including smooth muscle proliferation and thrombotic events.

The Monoclonal Hypothesis—Smooth Muscle Proliferation

The monoclonal hypothesis states that the smooth muscle proliferation characteristic of the plaque is similar to a benign neoplasm arising from a single progenitor cell from the monocyte–macrophage lineage. Evidence for this is provided by the observance of a monotypic enzyme pattern in the plaques of heterozygotic individuals, as opposed to the bimorphic pattern seen in the undiseased arterial wall.[27] The aforementioned risk factors function as theoretical mutagens.

This hypothesis considers events that cause smooth muscle proliferation as critical in atherogenesis. Actions of other growth factors may either stimulate or inhibit cell proliferation, depending on the circumstances, as well as on macrophage-derived cytokine activity, such as the finding of transforming growth factor-β receptors in human atherosclerosis[28] provides evidence for an acquired resistance to apoptosis. Resistance to apoptosis may lead to proliferation of a resistant cell subset associated with progression of stenotic lesions.

This theory once again focuses on the smooth muscle proliferation but fails to account for the other features of the lesion.

In summary, obviously no one theory provides an adequate explanation for all the pathologic changes observed in atherogenesis. This subject remains a focus of continual investigation worldwide and it is hoped that with improved understanding of the atherogenic process, better preventive strategies might be developed.

Hemodynamic Changes in Atherosclerosis

Atherosclerotic occlusive disease primarily affects circulatory flow through energy losses at fixed arterial stenoses. The reasons for this arise from knowledge of the physical properties of blood as a fluid. As blood flow enters an area of stenosis, its velocity increases across the stenosis to maintain constant flow. Energy is then lost with the change in velocity at both the entry to and exit from the stenotic area. The greater the degree of stenosis, the more severe the change in velocity and thus the greater the energy loss. In general, flow studies have demonstrated that significant changes in flow and velocity do not occur until the degree of stenosis approaches 50%, which in turn corresponds to an area reduction of approximately 75%. This is termed *critical stenosis*.

It is important to remember, however, that resistances in series are additive; thus multiple subcritical stenoses in series can produce significant hemodynamic changes and result in marked impairment of distal flow.[29,30]

Clinical Manifestations

The clinical manifestations of lower extremity atherosclerotic occlusive disease occur along a well-defined spectrum of severity, ranging from intermittent claudication to the observation of trophic changes suggesting impending limb loss.

Claudication is defined as pain (or discomfort) produced with brisk use of an extremity and relieved with rest. We have also observed that the location of the discomfort is typically experienced one joint distal to the stenotic area. For example, disease involving the superficial femoral artery manifests itself via calf claudication. Blood flow is adequate in the resting state, thus pain occurs only when the increased metabolic demand created by exercising muscle exceeds the supply available due to the degree of fixed arterial obstruction.[31] Aside from diminished distal pulses, significant physical findings are usually absent at this stage.

The differential diagnosis of intermittent claudication should include other conditions, which may be neurologic or musculoskeletal in origin. Calf claudication can be caused by venous claudication, chronic compartment syndrome, Baker's cyst, and nerve root compression. The tight bursting pain of compartment syndrome is generally typical and venous claudication is relieved by leg elevation. Hip or buttock claudication should be differentiated from pain related to hip arthritis and spinal cord compression. The persistent aching pain caused by variable amounts of exercise and associated symptoms in other joints may distinguish arthritis from claudication. Patients with spinal cord compression frequently present with a history of back pain and have symptoms on standing, but require a change in position as well as rest to obtain relief. Foot claudication should be distinguished from other causes related to arthritis or inflammatory processes.

Ischemic rest pain develops when the degree of circulatory impairment progresses to the point at which the blood supply is inadequate to meet the metabolic demand of the muscle even in the resting state. Frequently, the pain increases during periods of lower extremity elevation (lying in a bed) and is relieved with dependency. Physical findings at this stage typically include decreased skin temperature and delayed capillary refill, as well as Buerger's signs (dependent rubor and pallor on elevation).

Trophic changes represent the most severe manifestations of chronically impaired lower extremity circulation. In this stage of the disease, the lower extremity displays actual changes related to ischemia that are visible to the naked eye. These changes range from subtle signs such as dependent rubor, atrophy of skin and muscle, and loss of hair or nail substance to frank ulceration, cyanosis, and gangrene. The presence of trophic changes is suggestive of impending limb loss and necessitates urgent intervention for limb salvage to be possible.[32]

Natural History and Staging

Several studies over the past 40 years have concluded that approximately 75% of all patients with claudication experience symptom stabilization or improvement over their lifetime without the need for any intervention.[33,34] This clinical improvement or stabilization holds true, despite arteriographic evidence for disease progression in most of these patients. In 25% of claudicant patients, symptoms worsened, particularly during the first year, in approximately 8%, and subsequently at the rate of 2–3% per year. It has been estimated that around 5% of these

patients will undergo an intervention within 5 years of their initial diagnosis. Several large studies estimate that 2–4% of these patients will require a major amputation.[35,36] Diabetes and smoking are the most significant primary risk factors for disease progression and higher intervention and amputation rates. Dormandy and Murray[36] concluded that an ABI of 0.5 on initial diagnosis was the most significant predictor for peripheral arterial disease deterioration requiring intervention. They also observed that men were at higher risk for disease progression than women. Other studies have confirmed that the presence of peripheral arterial disease significantly increased the risk of myocardial infarction, stroke, ischemia of splanchnic organs, and the risk of cardiovascular death. Criqui et al.[37] noted a relative risk of 3.3 for total mortality and a relative risk of 5.8 for coronary artery disease mortality in men with peripheral arterial disease over a 10-year study. They also noted a two-fold higher relative risk of a total, coronary, and cardiovascular mortality in symptomatic versus asymptomatic peripheral artery disease patients. It has been estimated that the average life expectancy of patients with intermittent claudication was decreased by about 10 years.[33] A review of over 20 studies by TASC places the 5, 10, and 15 year mortality rate for patients with intermittent claudication at 30%, 50%, and 70%, respectively.[2]

Determination of the ABI has proven to be a powerful clinical tool. An ABI of <0.5 has been associated with more severe coronary artery disease and increased mortality.[38] It has been demonstrated that patients with an ABI of <0.3 had a significantly lower survival rate than those with a range of 0.31–0.9.[38]

After the initial diagnosis of chronic lower extremity ischemia is made, it is important to stage the severity of the process accurately. This is crucial because it is the stage of the disease and the natural history of each stage that ultimately determine which therapy is most appropriate.

The most common staging system used by vascular surgeons today is that devised by the Society of Vascular Surgery and the International Society of Cardiovascular Surgery (SVS/ISCVS). Rutherford et al.[39] defined claudication categories 0–3 as asymptomatic, mild, moderate, and severe (Table 17–1). Categories 4–6 encompass ischemic rest pain and minor and major tissue loss of patients with critical limb ischemia. Rutherford's classification is presently the recommended standard when describing clinical assessment and progress.[2] The other classification that is used by our medical colleagues is the Fontaine classification. In this classification, the stages of the disease are categorized into Class I–IV (I corresponds to 0 in Rutherford's classification and IV corresponds to stage III in Rutherford's classification).

TABLE 17–1. Classification of peripheral arterial disease (PAD): Rutherford categories.

Grade	Category	Clinical description
0	0	Asymptomatic
I	1	Mild claudication
I	2	Moderate claudication
I	3	Severe claudication
II	4	Ischemic rest pain
III	5	Minor tissue loss
III	6	Major tissue loss

Stage 0 (Asymptomatic)

In stage 0, the patient is symptom free. The natural history of stage 0 disease is such that few patients will progress to limb loss over a period of 5 years. For this reason, the only treatment recommended for this stage involves risk factor modification such as cessation of smoking, reduction of serum lipids, and improved control of diabetes mellitus. Close observation is also important since any progression to a more advanced stage necessitates a change in the treatment strategy.

Stage I (Claudication)

Stage I has been further subdivided into two groups based on the claudication distance. Stage IA disease is defined as claudication occurring at a distance of greater than 1/2 block, whereas stage IB disease is defined as claudication occurring at a distance of less than 1/2 block.

The natural history of patients with claudication is such that very few patients will progress to limb loss. The actual percentages in the literature vary somewhat, but the 5-year limb loss rate seems to average approximately 5%.[31,40]

Because of the relatively benign natural history of stage I disease, the cornerstone of therapy remains aggressive medical management, particularly for patients with stage IA disease. Stage IB disease may be considered a relative indication for invasive intervention if medical therapy fails or if the degree of disability is intolerable for the patient. Once again, progression to a more advanced stage necessitates a change in the treatment plan.

Stage II (Ischemic Rest Pain)

Stage II is generally viewed as the earliest phase of limb-threatening ischemia. The natural history at this stage carries a far worse prognosis. Patients with stage II disease are far more likely to have progression of their disease process and ultimately to suffer limb loss.[41] For this reason, invasive intervention is indicated at this stage.

Stage III (Trophic Changes)

The presence of trophic changes indicates the most severe underlying circulatory impairment, as evidenced by actual tissue loss or gangrenous changes. Untreated, most patients will progress to gangrene and limb loss. For this reason, an aggressive interventional approach is indicated to limit additional tissue loss and allow limb salvage.[41]

Diagnostic Investigation

History and Physical Examination

As with any condition, evaluation begins with a comprehensive history and physical examination prior to any objective testing.

The initial history should be directed toward the occurrence of pain in the lower extremities. As defined previously, claudication typically manifests itself as pain that occurs with brisk use of an extremity (via walking) and is relieved consistently by several minutes of rest. The location and character of the pain should be reproducible, as should be the claudication distance. Rest pain should also be inquired about and, once again, may be most prominent at night when the legs are elevated. Any history of ulceration, loss of hair, nail substance, or skin/muscle atrophy should be sought. The presence of impotence, frequently present in aortoiliac disease, should be carefully documented.

Because of the systemic nature of atherosclerosis, the possibility of multivessel involvement exists and should be considered in all patients. A careful history should be elicited regarding symptoms of coronary disease (angina or myocardial infarction), cerebrovascular disease (transient ischemic attacks or prior strokes), or previous vascular procedures.

Physical examination begins with a comprehensive head-to-toe assessment. When attention is directed toward the lower extremities, thorough visual inspection should reveal evidence of any trophic changes. It is important to look between the toes as well, to avoid missing subtle areas of skin loss. Skin temperature and capillary refill should be assessed and may be diminished with more advanced disease. Pulses should be palpated at all levels and their strength documented as follows: +2 (normal), +1 (diminished), 0 (no palpable pulse). Others classify pulses as 3+, 2+, 1+, and 0.

If the pulse is nonpalpable, a Doppler probe should be used to determine the presence or absence of flow in the vessel, and its flow characteristics (monophasic versus biphasic).

Noninvasive Tests

A variety of noninvasive tests are available for assessment of the lower extremity vascular system. These are discussed in detail in subsequent chapters.

Perhaps the most useful bedside noninvasive test available to the clinician is the ABI. This test may be performed with only a sphygmomanometer and a Doppler probe. To perform the test, Doppler systolic pressure measurements are taken at the level of the ankle (use the higher of posterior tibial or dorsalis pedis artery pressure) and compared with those in the brachial artery as follows:

$$ABI = \frac{Ankle\ pressure\ (mm\ HG)}{Brachial\ pressure\ (mm\ Hg)}$$

A ratio of less than 1 is abnormal. Generally, patients with claudication have indices of 0.5–0.8, whereas those with rest pain have indices of 0.5 or less. When trophic changes are present, the ABI is frequently less than 0.3.[42]

In general, noninvasive testing should precede the ordering of any more invasive evaluations.

Magnetic Resonance Angiography

Magnetic resonance angiography (MRA) is a technique used to study blood vessels using magnetic imaging technology. This technique is useful in the assessment of the peripheral vasculature including the aorta, upper and lower extremities, and carotid arterial systems. Advantages include the lack of need for contrast administration and the noninvasive nature of the test. These factors help to make MRA attractive; however, there are several disadvantages that must be considered. First, the patient is required to remain completely still within a confined space for several minutes, which may be intolerable for some people. The presence of any previously placed aneurysm clips within the brain or the presence of a pacemaker precludes the use of MRA due to the powerful magnetic forces generated. Finally, the presence of turbulent flow can result in signal loss, which may result in an overestimation of the degree of stenosis.[43]

Contrast Angiography

Contrast angiography has long been the gold standard for the assessment of the aorta and lower extremity vascular tree. The procedure involves arterial puncture, with subsequent passage of a catheter system to the area targeted for imaging. Contrast medium is then injected and radiographs are taken, preferably in more than one plane.

The resolution of angiography may be enhanced via the use of digital subtraction technology. This electronic technique permits digital processing of the video signal from a conventional signal image intensifier fluoroscopic system. In digital subtraction angiography (DSA), a time subtraction technique known as mask-mode radiography is utilized. With this technique, an initial fluoroscopic image is recorded and digitally processed. Contrast is then administered and additional images recorded. Finally the images are digitally "subtracted" from each other, resulting in radiographs of higher resolution than those obtained with conventional angiography, with smaller amounts of contrast media.[44]

Risks of angiography include the risks of arterial puncture, which may result in compromise of the distal circulation due to induction of thrombosis, embolism, or dissection, or in pseudoaneurysm formation, as well as the risks associated with contrast administration. Risks associated with contrast administration include allergic reactions, hypotension, systemic vasodilatation, stroke, and convulsions. Renal insufficiency may also be precipitated via contrast administration. This risk may be minimized via adequate hydration and the use of nonionic low-osmolarity contrast agents.[45] Overall, the morbidity related to angiography may be as high as 7%.[46] Recent studies have reported lower major complication rates for peripheral arteriography (2.1%).[47] Therefore, it is generally believed that arteriography should be performed only on those patients in whom invasive intervention is considered. Figures 17–3 to 17–7 illustrate some normal and abnormal findings.

Treatment Options

Discussions on the treatment of lower extremity peripheral vascular disease have filled volumes and are not the focus of this text. However, a brief discussion of the various treatment strategies is provided for completeness. Basically, the treatments may be classified into three major categories: (1) medical therapy, (2) surgical therapy, and (3) endovascular therapy.

Medical Therapy

Medical therapy is the treatment of choice for patients with SVS/ISCVS stage 0 (asymptomatic) or stage I (claudication) disease. This begins with identification and aggressive modification of risk factors. This includes improving control of hypertension and diabetes mellitus, reduction of serum lipids, dietary modification, and—most importantly—cessation of smoking.[15,16]

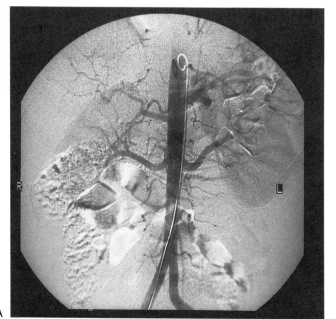

A

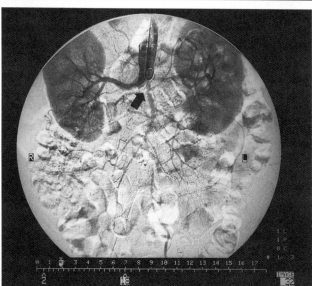

B

FIGURE 17–3. (A) Arteriogram of a normal aorta and right and left common iliac arteries. (B) Arteriogram showing complete occlusion of the infrarenal abdominal aorta (*arrow*) at the level of the renal artery.

Recent evidence suggests that the risk of developing new or worsening claudication can be reduced significantly by lipid-lowering agents.[48,49] The mechanism of action of these drugs can include plaque stabilization, preventing rupture, and favorable vasomotor effects. A low-density lipoprotein, cholesterol level of <100 mg/dl may be achieved through diet control or lipid-lowering agents if necessary.

The next essential facet of medical therapy should be institution of an exercise program. Although the mecha-

nism is not completely understood, exercise does result in improvement in the majority of claudicators willing to comply with the program. It was once thought that the exercise helped to facilitate development of collateral circulation, but this has not been supported by available data. Rather, it is more likely that exercise induces adaptive changes in the muscle, which result in more efficient extraction of oxygen from the blood.[50]

Overall, exercise commonly leads to increased claudication-free walking distance, the ability to better perform activities of higher intensity, and improved quality of life.[51,52] Other benefits of exercise include improved glucose utilization, a reduction in cholesterol

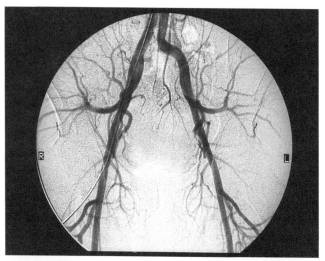

A

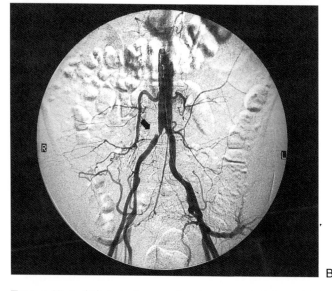

B

FIGURE 17–4. (A) Arteriogram showing normal right and left common iliacs, internal iliacs, external iliacs, and right and left common femoral arteries and bifurcation to the proximal superficial femoral artery and deep femoral artery. (B) Arteriogram showing tight stenosis of the right common iliac artery (*arrow*).

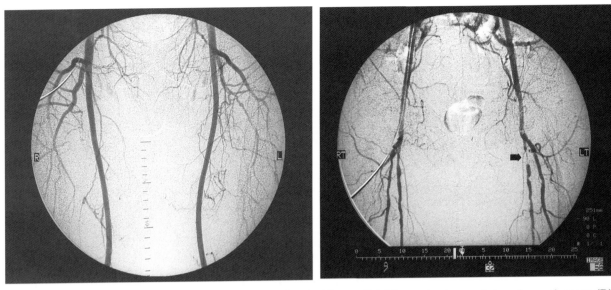

FIGURE 17–5. (A) Arteriogram showing a normal proximal and mid-superficial femoral artery and deep femoral artery. (B) Arteriogram showing almost total occlusion of the proximal left superficial femoral artery (*arrow*) and severe stenosis of the proximal right superficial femoral artery.

and triglyceride levels, and a higher rate of smoking cessation.[2]

Pharmacologic therapy is available for the treatment of claudication. To date only one agent, pentoxifylline (Trental), has been approved by the U.S. Food and Drug Administration for the treatment of peripheral vascular disease. This drug, classified as a *hemorrheologic agent*, is believed to improve microcirculatory blood flow by enhancing the flexibility of the erythrocyte membrane, thus decreasing blood viscosity.[53] In initial double-masked trials, pentoxifylline treatment yielded a 45% response rate, compared with 23% for placebo.[54] Although this is encouraging, it is obvious that not all patients will respond. We typically recommend a 6-week trial of the drug, at which time a decision is made regarding whether the agent should be continued.[55]

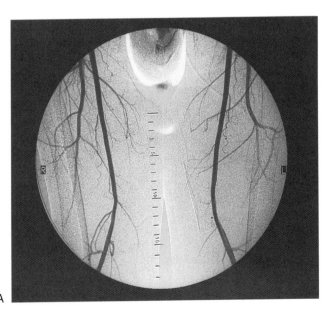
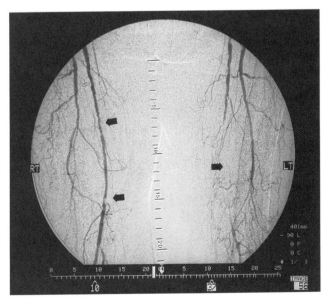

FIGURE 17–6. (A) Arteriogram of a normal proximal, mid and distal superficial femoral artery (right and left). (B) Arteriogram showing total occlusion of the distal left superficial femoral artery (*arrow*) and severe stenoses of the right distal superficial femoral artery (*arrows*).

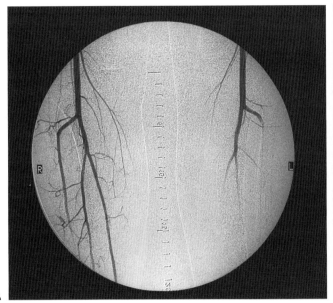

A

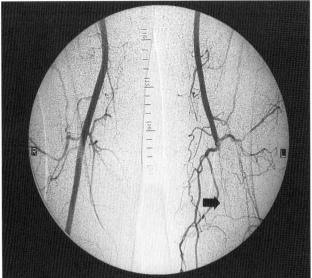

B

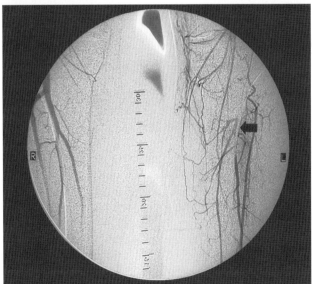

C

FIGURE 17–7. (A) Arteriogram of the right distal popliteal artery and its trifurcation vessel (anterior tibial, tibioperoneal trunk: peroneal artery and posterior tibial artery). (B) Arteriogram showing occlusion of the left popliteal artery (*arrow*). (C) Arteriogram of the same patient in (B) showing reconstitution of the distal portion of the tibioperoneal trunk with posterior tibial and peroneal runoff (*arrow*).

Recently, cilostazol (Pletal) has been introduced as a new treatment for patients with claudication. It appears to modestly benefit walking ability and it has other potential useful effects, including inhibition of platelet aggregation and beneficial effect on serum lipids. In a randomized, prospective, double-blind study examining walking ability in patients with peripheral arterial disease with moderate to severe claudication, cilostazol was superior to both placebo and pentoxifylline (Trental).[56]

Surgical Therapy

Surgical therapy remains the gold standard for treatment of limb-threatening ischemia and, in select cases, dis-abling claudication. Overall, two techniques predominate in the surgical treatment of peripheral vascular disease: endarterectomy and bypass.

Endarterectomy involves removal of the diseased intima and innermost media, leaving behind a smooth arterial surface. It is especially well suited to the treatment of short segmental or ostial lesions such as those seen at the carotid or aortic bifurcations.

Bypass, as the name implies, involves the routing of blood flow around a stenotic or occluded arterial segment using a conduit, typically either autogenous vein or prosthesis [polytetrafluoroethylene (PTFE) or Dacron]. This extremely versatile technique remains the most commonly utilized method in treating arterial occlusive disease of the lower extremity.

Operative therapy is recommended for patients with long segment and multisegmental disease, especially if total occlusion is present. Aortofemoral bypass is associated with a low operative mortality (2–3%) and an 80–85% 5-year patency rate. Iliac reconstruction is generally recommended for isolated unilateral iliac arterial disease, which can also be treated by a femoral artery to femoral artery crossover bypass graft. Infrainguinal arterial reconstruction is associated with a 60–80% 5-year patency rate, with better outcome noted for autogenous vein conduit than for prosthetic bypasses.[57]

Endovascular Therapy

Endovascular therapy is an evolving modality in which devices are introduced directly into the vascular lumen via an open or percutaneous approach. The stenotic areas are then addressed via several techniques.

1. *Balloon angioplasty*, in which a balloon is expanded across a stenotic area, thus fracturing the plaque and expanding the arterial lumen via a "controlled dissection."
2. *Atherectomy*, in which a specially designed catheter is used to shave a portion of the plaque from inside the vessel lumen.
3. *Stenting*, or stented endovascular grafting, which is an evolving technique involving the placement of an expandable metal stent across the stenotic area.

The application of percutaneous endovascular therapy for arterial occlusive disease of the lower extremities continues to increase. The long-term results of endovascular therapy are expected to improve with the progression of the technology supporting these therapeutic interventions. Overall, the initial technical success rates for open surgical procedures and percutaneous endovascular therapy are somewhat similar, however, surgery frequently provides greater long-term patency. On the other hand, angioplasty is often associated with lower morbidity and mortality rates, and late failure of percutaneous endovascular therapies can often be treated successfully with percutaneous reinterventions.[58]

References

1. Dormandy J, Heeck L, Vig S. Intermittent claudication: Understated risks. Semin Vasc Surg 1999;12:96–108.
2. TransAtlantic Inter-Society Consensus (TASC) Working Group. Management of peripheral arterial disease (PAD). J Vasc Surg 2000;31:S5–S44, S54–S74.
3. Stanley JC, Barnes RW, Ernst CB, Hertzer NR, Mannick JA, Moore WS. Work Force Issues Report of the Society for Vascular Surgery and the International Society for Cardiovascular Surgery, North American Chapter, Committee on Workforce Issues. J Vasc Surg 1996;23:172–181.
4. Crafts RC. Lower limb. In: Crafts RC (ed). *A Textbook of Human Anatomy*, pp. 397–517. New York: John Wiley, 1985.
5. Taylor LM, Porter JM, Winck T. Femoropopliteal occlusive disease. In: Greenfield LJ (ed). *Surgery: Scientific Principles and Practice*, 2nd ed., pp. 1810–1823. Philadelphia: JB Lippincott, 1997.
6. Zarins CK, Glagov S. Artery wall pathology in atherosclerosis. In: Rutherford RB (ed). *Vascular Surgery*, 4th ed., pp. 203–221. Philadelphia: WB Saunders, 1995.
7. Young DF, Cholvin NR, Kirkeeide RL, Roth AC. Hemodynamics of arterial stenosis at elevated flow rates. Circ Res 1977;41:99–107.
8. Arfvidsson B, Wennmalm A, Gelin J, Dahllof AG, Hallgren B, Lundholm K. Covariation between walking ability and circulatory alterations in patients with intermittent claudication. Eur J Vasc Surg 1992;6:642–646.
9. Hiatt WR. Nonoperative, nonpharmacologic management of lower extremity occlusive disease. In: Ernst CB, Stanley JC (eds). *Current Therapy in Vascular Surgery*, pp. 530–533. Philadelphia: Mosby, 2000.
10. Hiatt WR, Wolfel EE, Regensteiner JG, Brass EP. Skeletal muscle carnitine metabolism in patients with unilateral peripheral arterial disease. J Appl Physiol 1992;73:346–353.
11. Ross R, Glomset JA. The pathogenesis of atherosclerosis. N Engl J Med 1976;295:369–377.
12. Taylor KE, Glagov S, Zarins CK. Preservation and structural adaptation of endothelium over experimental foam cell lesions. Arteriosclerosis 1989;9:881–894.
13. Faggiotto A, Ross R. Studies of hypercholesterolemia in the nonhuman primate. II. Fatty streak conversion to fibrous plaque. Arteriosclerosis 1984;4:341–356.
14. Glagov S, Zarins CK, Giddens DP, et al. Atherosclerosis: What is the nature of the plaque? In: Strandness DE Jr, Didishiem P, Clowes AW, et al. (eds). *Vascular Diseases: Current Research and Clinical Application*, pp. 15–33. Orlando, FL: Grune & Stratton, 1987.
15. Pooling Project Research Group. Relationship of blood pressure, serum cholesterol, smoking habit, relative weight and EKG abnormalities to incidence of major coronary events. J Chronic Dis 1978;31:201–306.
16. Krupski WC, Rapp JH. Smoking and atherosclerosis. In: Goldstone J (ed). *Perspectives of Vascular Surgery*, Vol. 1, pp. 103–134. St. Louis, MO: Quality Medical Publishing, 1988.
17. Powel JT. Vascular damage from smoking: Disease mechanisms at the arterial wall. Vasc Med 1998;3:21–28.
18. Murabito JM, D'Agostino RG, Silbershatz H, Wilson WF. Intermittent claudication: A risk profile from the Framingham heart study. Circulation 1997;96:44–49.
19. Celermajer DS, Sorensen KE, Georgakopoulos D, Bull C, Thomas O, Robinson J, Deanfield JE. Cigarette smoking is associated with dose-related and potentially reversible impairment of endothelium-dependent dilation in healthy young adults. Circulation 1993;88:2149–2155.
20. Cheng SWK, Ting ACW, Wong J. Lipoprotein (a) and its relationship to risk factors and severity of atherosclerotic peripheral vascular disease. Eur J Vasc Endovasc Surg 1997;14:17–23.

21. Blauw GJ, Lagaay AM, Smelt AH, Westendorp RG. Stroke, statins and cholesterol: A meta-analysis of randomized, placebo-controlled, double-blind trials with HMG-CoA reductase inhibitors. Stroke 1997;28:946–950.

22. Dormandy J, Heeck L, Vig S. Predictors of early disease in the lower limbs. Semin Vasc Surg 1999;12:109–117.

23. Boushey CJ, Beresford SA, Omenn GS, Motulsky AG. A quantitative assessment of plasma homocysteine as a risk factor for vascular disease: Probable benefits of increasing folic acid intake. JAMA 1995;274:1049–1057.

24. A Coordination Group in China. A pathological survey of atherosclerotic lesions of coronary artery and aorta in China. Pathol Res Pract 1985;180:457–462.

25. Stevens SL, Hilgarth K, Ryan VS, et al. The synergistic effect of hypercholesterolemia and mechanical injury on intimal hyperplasia. Ann Vasc Surg 1992;6:55.

26. Steinberg D, Parthasarathy S, Carew T, et al. Modifications of low density lipoprotein that increase its atherogenicity. N Engl J Med 1989;320:915–924.

27. Benditt EP. Implications of the monoclonal character of human atherosclerotic plaques. Am J Pathol 1977;86:693–702.

28. McCaffrey TA, Du B, Fu C, et al. The expressions of TGF-beta receptors in human atherosclerosis: Evidence of acquired resistance to apoptosis due to receptor imbalance. J Mol Cell Cardiol 1999;31:162T.

29. Karayannacos PE, Talukder N, Nerem R, et al. The rule of multiple noncritical arterial stenoses in the pathogenesis of ischemia. J Thorac Cardiovasc Surg 1977;73:458–469.

30. Cronenwett JL. Arterial hemodynamics. In: Greenfield LJ (ed). Surgery—Scientific Principles and Practice, 2nd ed., pp. 1656–1667. Philadelphia: PA: JB Lippincott, 1997.

31. Imparato AM, Kim GE, Davidson T, et al. Intermittent claudication: Its natural course. Surgery 1975;78:795–799.

32. Boyd AM. The natural course of arteriosclerosis of lower extremities. Proc R Soc Med 1962;55:591–593.

33. Bloor K. Natural history of atherosclerosis of the lower extremities. Ann R Coll Surg Engl 1961;28:36–51.

34. Dormandy JA, Heeck L, Vig S. The natural history of claudication: Risk to life and limb. Semin Vasc Surg 1999;12:123–137.

35. Weitz JI, Byrne J, Clagett GP, Farkouh ME, Porter JM, Sackett DL, Strandness DE Jr, Taylor LM. Diagnosis and treatment of chronic arterial insufficiency of the lower extremities: A critical review. Circulation 1996;94:3026–3049.

36. Dormandy JA, Murray GD. The fate of the claudicant: A prospective study of 1969 claudicants. Eur J Vasc Surg 1991;5:131–133.

37. Criqui MH, Langer Rd, Fronek A, Feigelson HS, Klauber MR, McCann TJ, Browner D. Mortality over a period of ten years in patients with peripheral arterial disease. N Engl J Med 1992;326:381–386.

38. McDermott MM, Feinglass J, Slavensky R, Pierce WH. The ankle-brachial index as predictor of survival in patients with peripheral vascular disease. J Gen Intern Med 1994;9:445–449.

39. Rutherford RB, Baker JD, Ernst C, Johnston KW, Porter JM, Ahn S, Jones DN. Recommended standards for reports dealing with lower extremity ischemia: Revised version. J Vasc Surg 1997;26:517–538.

40. Peabody CN, Kannel WB, McNamara PM. Intermittent claudication: Surgical significance. Arch Surg 1974;109:693–697.

41. Veith FJ, Gupta SK, Wengerter KR, et al. Changing arteriosclerotic disease patterns and management strategies in lower-limb-threatening ischemia. Ann Surg 1990;212:402–414.

42. Yao JST. New techniques in objective arterial evaluation. Arch Surg 1973;106:600–604.

43. Masaryk TJ, Modic MT, Ruggieri PM, et al. Three dimensional (volume) gradient-echo imaging of the carotid bifurcation: Preliminary clinical experience. Radiology 1989;171: 801–806.

44. Turnipseed WD. Diagnosis of carotid artery disease by digital subtraction angiography. In: AbuRahma AF, Dietrich EB (eds). Current Noninvasive Vascular Diagnosis, pp. 337–355. Littleton, MA: PSG Publishing, 1988.

45. Katayama H, Yamaguchi K, Kozuka T, et al. Adverse reactions to ionic and nanianic contrast media: a report from the Japanese Committee on the saftey of contrast media. Radiology 1990;175:621–628.

46. AbuRahma AF, Robinson PA, Boland JP, et al. Complications of arteriography in a recent series of 707 cases: Factors affecting outcome. Ann Vasc Surg 1993;7:122–129.

47. Balduf LM, Langsfeld M, Marek JM, et al. Complication rates of diagnostic angiography performed by vascular surgeons. Vasc Endovasc Surg 2002;36:439–445.

48. Pedersen TR, Kjekshus J, Pyorala K, Olsson AG, Cook TJ, Musliner TA, Robert JA, Haghfelt T. Effect of simvastatin on ischemic signs and symptoms in the Scandinavian Simvastatin Survival Study (4S). Am J Cardiol 1998;81:333–338.

49. Gould AL, Rossouw JE, Santanello NC, Heyse JF, Furberg CD. Cholesterol reduction yields clinical benefit: Impact of statin trials. Circulation 1998;97:946–952.

50. Bylund AC, Hammarsten J, Holm J, et al. Enzyme activities in skeletal muscles from patients with peripheral arterial insufficiency. Eur J Clin Invest 1976;6:425–429.

51. Gardner AW, Poehlman ET. Exercise rehabilitation programs for the treatment of claudication pain: A meta-analysis. JAMA 1995;274:975–980.

52. Regensteiner JG, Steiner JF, Hiatt WR. Exercise training improves functional status in patients with peripheral arterial disease. J Vasc Surg 1996;23:104–115.

53. Muller R. Hemorrheology and peripheral vascular disease. A new therapeutic approach. J Med 1981;12:209–235.

54. Porter JM, Cutler BS, Lee BY, et al. Pentoxifylline efficacy in the treatment of intermittent claudication. Am Heart J 1982;104:66–72.

55. AbuRahma AF, Woodruff BA. Effects and limitations of pentoxifylline therapy in various stages of peripheral vascular disease of the lower extremity. Am J Surg 1990;160: 266–270.

56. Dawson DL. Comparative effects of cilostazol and other therapies for intermittent claudication. Am J Cardiol 2001;87:19D–27D.

57. Comerota AJ. Endovascular and surgical revascularization for patients with intermittent claudication. Am J Cardiol 2001;87:34D–43D.

58. Bates MC, AbuRahma AF. An update on endovascular therapy of the lower extremities. J Endovasc Therapy 2004; 11:II-107–II-127.

18
Overview of Noninvasive Vascular Techniques in Peripheral Arterial Disease

Ali F. AbuRahma

Various noninvasive vascular diagnostic techniques have been described in the past four decades to help the clinician in the management of vascular patients. Although many physicians still rely entirely upon arteriography as the main tool for evaluation of peripheral arterial occlusive disease, the role of the vascular laboratory cannot be denied. These techniques should remain as a valuable adjunct to the information gained from the complete history and physical examination. Noninvasive vascular tests help the physician to evaluate the presence or absence of significant arterial occlusive disease, severity of disease, location of disease, and, in the presence of multisegmental disease, which arterial segment is mostly affected.

There are other challenging questions for physicians dealing with patients with peripheral vascular disease: In patients with both arterial occlusive disease and neuropathy, which condition is more likely to be responsible for the pain or ulceration? Will an ulcer or amputation heal at a specific level? Is a patient's impotence hormonal, vascular, neurogenic, or physchogenic in nature? Since the traditional diagnostic tools of clinical history and vascular examination are often inadequate in answering some of these questions, and since arteriography is invasive, painful, and provides no physiological information, increasing attention has been focused on the value of the vascular laboratory in these diagnostic challenges. This chapter will emphasize methods that have clinical applications and that are commonly used. The techniques that are outdated or used only for research are only briefly mentioned.

General indications for obtaining noninvasive assessment of the peripheral arterial system include absence of normal pulses, suboptimal examiner reliability or experience, a clinical history or examination potentially consistent with peripheral arterial occlusive disease, and a planned vascular procedure. The subcommittee on peripheral vascular disease of the American Heart Association has suggested that instruments used in the clinical vascular laboratory be (1) simple, (2) reliable and reproducible, (3) easily used by paramedical personnel, (4) capable of intrinsic standardization, (5) suitable for measurement during and/or after exercise, and (6) adaptable to current recording devices. Various clinical applications of the vascular laboratory in patients with peripheral vascular disease are discussed in later chapters.

Several noninvasive diagnostic techniques have been used in the diagnosis of peripheral arterial disease: continuous-wave (CW) Doppler ultrasound, pulsed Doppler ultrasound, B-mode ultrasound, various plethysmographic techniques, including pulse volume recording, thermography, electromagnetic flowmeter, radionuclide angiography, and the use of radioisotopes. The most commonly used methods for diagnosis of peripheral vascular disease of the lower extremity at present are segmental Doppler pressures (with or without Doppler wave analysis) using CW Doppler, pulse volume recording, and Duplex ultrasonography.[1-5] These three commonly used methods will be described in detail in the next chapters.

Ultrasound

The use of ultrasound in the range of 1–10 MHz for medical diagnosis has become widespread since its introduction by Satomura in 1959.[6] Current instruments either use the Doppler effect to detect flow velocity or rely on tissue reflectance of transmitted sound waves (B-mode ultrasound) to produce acoustic images of blood vessels, or a combination of both Doppler and B-mode imaging (duplex ultrasound).

Doppler Ultrasound

Although Satomura[6] was credited for developing the first Doppler flow detector in 1959, its clinical application was pioneered by Strandness *et al.* in 1966.[7] Since then, the instrumentation has been further improved and refined. The principle of this device depends on the observation made by the Austrian physicist, Christian Doppler (1803–1853), who demonstrated that the frequency of light or sound emitted by a source moving toward the observer is higher (shorter wavelength) than the transmitted frequency, and lower (longer wavelength) when the source is moving away from the observer, e.g., the pitch of the train whistle sounds higher as the train approaches and lower as the train moves away.

The Doppler effect can be stated as

$$\overline{V} = \frac{C \Delta f}{2 fo \cos \theta}$$

where $\overline{V}$ = average flow velocity; C = velocity of sound in tissue; Δf = Doppler frequency shift; fo = transmitting frequency of ultrasound beam; and θ = angle of the incident sound beam to the blood vessel being examined. Since transmitting frequency, angle of incidence, and sound velocity in tissue can be kept constant, frequency shift (Δf) becomes proportional to the velocity of blood flow.

Continuous-Wave Doppler Ultrasound

There are two types of Doppler ultrasound detectors: CW Doppler ultrasound and pulsed Doppler ultrasound. Both instruments work on the principle of the Doppler effect.

The Principle of Doppler Ultrasound

The Doppler unit contains an oscillator, which vibrates at a specific frequency. The oscillator may be of varying frequencies from 2 to 10 MHz. The standard frequency used for peripheral arterial examination is 5–10 MHz. The oscillator causes a piezoelectric crystal to emit a beam of ultrasound. This piezoelectric crystal is in a hand-held probe. The beam of the ultrasound emitted from the probe does not readily pass through air; therefore, an acoustic gel is placed on the skin to permit uniform transmission of the beam. Moving blood cells in the path of the ultrasonic beam cause a frequency shift (magnitude of change in hertz) in the reflected ultrasound, which is proportional to the velocity of the blood flow. The backscattered ultrasound is received by a second receiving crystal in the hand-held probe. The pitch of the velocity signal will change if the angle between the beam and the vessel is changed. To produce a frequency shift detectable by the observer, the blood velocity must be

greater than 3–6 cm/s. Again, it should be noted that the lower the frequency of the ultrasound, the deeper the penetration; and the deeper the penetration, the wider the beam of ultrasound, and thereby the less the resolution.

There are various methods of displaying the Doppler velocity signals. The three most commonly used methods are the audio output, the analog waveform, and the sound spectrum analysis.

The received ultrasonic beam can be amplified and projected audibly through a loudspeaker or earphones. There are three acceptable methods of listening to the audio output: stereo earphones, stethoscopic earpieces, and a loudspeaker. The analog wave tracing, by means of a frequency-to-voltage converter (zero-crossing detector), and sound spectral analysis of the audio frequency spectrum are described in detail in Chapter 19.

There are now two commercially available types of Doppler ultrasound flow velocity meters utilizing CW ultrasound: the nondirectional and the directional type. The instruments with directional capacity detect flow away from and toward the probe (by detecting both negative and positive Doppler shifts). Thus, the position of the probe relative to the flow in the artery is important. The directional Doppler units may be equipped with two directional flowmeters, which read flow toward and away from the probe (Figure 18–1). Note in Figure 18–1, which is an example of readings from two such meters, that the arterial flow is oscillatory, i.e., at different times there are forward and reverse flow components. The net flow in this case is toward or away from the probe. Another method of determining the direction of the flow is by analyzing the analogue wave tracing. The forward and reverse flows are both sensed by the direction of the Doppler probe

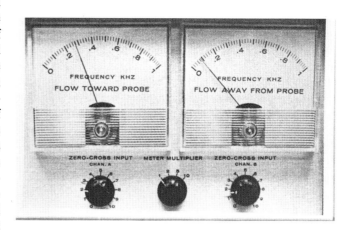

FIGURE 18–1. Directional Doppler unit.

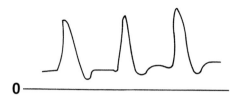

FIGURE 18–2. Directional analogue wave tracing. The net forward flow is above the zero line.

and both may be occurring simultaneously during the arterial pulse. The directional analogue wave tracing represents the average of the forward flow and the reverse flow at a given point in time. The net forward flow is presented above the zero line (Figure 18–2). The net reverse flow (or flow away from the probe) appears below the zero line. The higher pitched sounds will appear farther from the zero baselines on the analogue recording.

Pulsed Doppler Ultrasound

Pulsed Dopplers, unlike CW Dopplers, use the same piezoelectric crystal to alternately transmit and receive the backscattered signal. By sampling the reflected signals at discrete time intervals after transmission, they are capable of analyzing individual points along the course of the sound beam with resolution of approximately 1–1.5 mm. As the probe is moved across the blood vessel, two-dimensional velocity data can be collected for small volumes rather than mean cross-sectional areas as with CW Dopplers.

The pulsed Doppler instrument emits short bursts (0.5–1.0 μs) of ultrasound. The receiving crystal is time-gated to receive reflected Doppler-shifted ultrasound signals at variable intervals following the emitted bursts. The time required for ultrasound to travel to and from the site of detected flow is proportional to the distance of the flow stream from the transducer. The use of several gates allows simultaneous detection of flow from multiple points along the path of the sound beam. The pulsed Doppler detector permits determination of the depth of the flow signals, and this information, coupled to a transducer by a position-sensing arm, permits the unblanking of spots on the storage oscilloscope at the sites of detected flow. This will appear as a painted picture on the oscilloscope screen. Flow velocity can also be recorded in multiple longitudinal and transverse sections of the vessel. These recordings are not available through conventional arteriography.

Instrumentation

Many types of Doppler instruments are commercially available, varying from small, portable, pocket-sized models to more sophisticated instruments. The CW detectors emit an ultrasound beam without interruption. Such devices are not range-specific, i.e., they will detect blood flow at any depth within the range of the instrument up to several centimeters, depending upon the frequency of the instrumentation. The pulsed Doppler detectors transmit intermittent bursts of ultrasound that can be sampled for retained signals at various times after transmission, permitting range resolution of detected flow at a given point from the transducer. As mentioned earlier, CW Doppler units can be directional or nondirectional. Figure 18–3 shows a commonly used pocket Doppler unit (Meda-Sonics, Mountview, CA); Figure 18–4 shows commonly used directional Doppler units (Imex System, Golden, CO).

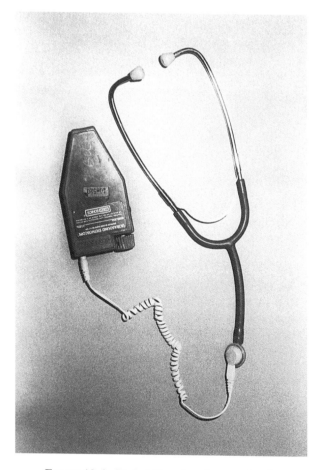

FIGURE 18–3. Pocket Doppler ultrasound unit.

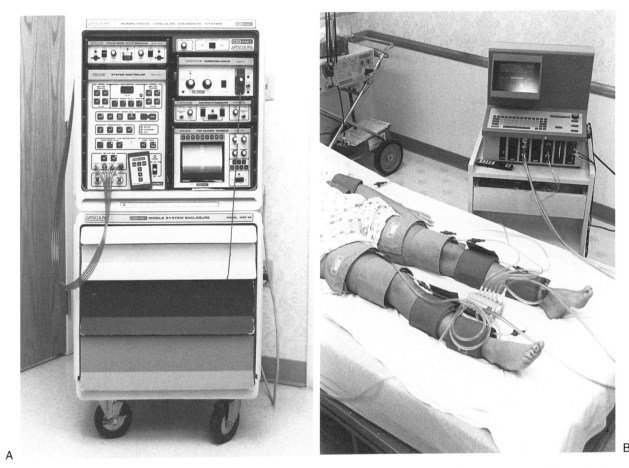

FIGURE 18–4. (A) The VascuLab system, which has a directional Doppler unit. (B) The Imex system, Golden, CO.

B-Mode Ultrasound

B-mode ultrasound graphically records cross-sectional mapping on the storage oscilloscope by detecting reflected echoes of ultrasound at various tissue interfaces within the range of the instrument. B-mode ultrasound application is not based on Doppler effect. Rather, the image it produces represents spatial differences in ultrasound reflectance from tissue interfaces of differing acoustic impedance. Modern B-mode scanners utilize brightness modulation and scan converter memory systems to permit display of a wide range of tissue densities in grayscale images. This refinement allows accurate definition of luminal thrombus contained within the blood vessels. The B-mode scanner has been further modified in the past 20 years by using multiple rotating transducers to produce real-time vessel images.[8] The standard units use 2 MHz (abdominal imaging) while special B-scan devices may operate at higher frequencies (5 MHz for carotid, 5–10 MHz for extremities). This modality will be described in detail in other chapters.

Duplex Ultrasound and Color Flow Imaging

When B-mode scanners and pulsed ultrasound Dopplers are combined, the resulting duplex scan is capable of not only imaging the vessel under study, but also of detecting blood flow velocity at multiple points within its lumen. Presently, color duplex ultrasonography is the most common modality used in modern vascular laboratories. This instrumentation will be described in detail in several other chapters. Color flow imaging provides the duplex information described above, i.e., combined real-time B-mode imaging (grayscale evaluation) and Doppler spectral analysis. In addition, it evaluates the Doppler flow information for its phase (direction toward or away from the transducer, and color is assigned on this basis) and its frequency content (which determines the hue or shade of the assigned color).

Plethysmography

Principle

The principle of plethysmography is based on graphic recordings of a change in dimension of a portion of the body in response to each heartbeat or in response to temporary obstruction of the venous system (venous occlusion plethysmography).[9] Most plethysmographs directly or indirectly record the change in column of a digit, limb, or other part of the body. An exception to this is the photoplethysmograph (PPG) that records the change in reflection of light from the change in number of red blood cells in the cutaneous microcirculation.

Instrumentation

In the past, the most commonly used plethysmographic device was the oscillometer. This instrument is simple, inexpensive, and portable. However, it is a nonstandardized instrument with poor sensitivity, and provides no pulse contour information or permanent record. It is no longer recommended for the evaluation of vascular patients. Various types of plethysmographs have been used in the past. Each type employs a different transducer principle for recording the changes in body dimension.

1. The water plethysmograph[10] is one of the oldest methods of recording limb or digit volume, using the displacement of water as a means of recording changes in limb girth. This technique has been widely used by physiologists, but the instrument is bulky, cumbersome, and impractical for routine clinical use.

2. The photoelectric or PPG[11] has been used for many years as a pulse sensor. This technique includes an infrared light-emitting diode[12] to transmit light into skin. Light reflected from blood cells is received by either a photocell or a phototransistor, which permits recording of the pulsatile cutaneous microcirculation. This technique was used in screening for peripheral arterial disease,[13] cerebrovascular disease,[14] and venous diseases.[15]

Recently, Bortolotto et al.,[16] in a study assessing vascular aging and atherosclerosis in hypertensive subjects using pulse wave velocity versus a second derivative of a photoplethysmogram, concluded that an index of the second derivative of photoplethysmography correlated with age and was useful in the evaluation of vascular aging in hypertensive patients.[16]

3. The strain-gauge plethysmograph (SGP), originally described by Whitney,[17] uses the principle of the change in the resistance of a column of mercury in an elastic gauge as a sensor of digit or limb volume. This technique is simple and versatile in screening for peripheral arterial and venous disease. Modifications of this instrument have permitted electrical calibration of the gauge *in situ* on the

limb[18] and automatic calculation of the limb flow from the excursion of a panel meter needle.[19] This technique is less cumbersome than standard volume plethysmography, and has been accepted for measuring limb blood flow.[20] It can also be used to obtain pulse volume waveforms, which have been proven to be valuable in the diagnosis of arterial occlusive disease.

4. The air plethysmograph has been used in a variety of instruments, including the oscillometer, Winsor plethysmograph,[21] and pulse volume recorder (PVR),[22] all of which have been used extensively in the evaluation of peripheral arterial occlusive disease and venous diseases. This technique is described in detail in Chapter 20. Volume or air plethysmography utilizes pneumatic cuffs placed at multiple levels around the extremity. By standardizing the injected volume of air and the pressure within the cuff, momentary volume changes of the limb result in pulsatile pressure changes within the air-filled bladder. These changes can be displayed as segmental pressure pulse contours, which correspond closely to a direct intraarterial recording at that level. By adding venous occlusion to plethysmography, indirect measurements of arterial flow are possible. This can be done by placing a pneumatic cuff on the proximal extremity, which is then inflated to a pressure that temporarily arrests venous outflow without impairing arterial inflow. Under these circumstances, the initial rate of volume change in the distal extremity, as measured by any of the plethysmographic techniques, is equal to the rate of arterial inflow. This is usually expressed as cubic centimeters flow per 100 ml tissue per minute. Since resting arterial flow is not reduced until an advanced degree of ischemia is present,[22] this technique has not found wide clinical application.

5. Quantitative air plethysmography measures volume changes of the entire lower leg by calibration with pressure changes and expresses these volume changes in absolute units. As shown in Figure 18–5, an air chamber that surrounds the lower leg is inflated to

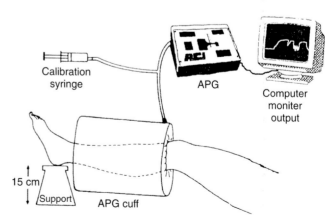

FIGURE 18–5. This is an air plethysmography [APG, (ACI Medical, San Marcos, CA)].

6 mm Hg, the lowest level at which good chamber/limb contact occurs with minimal venous compression. The leg blood flow is measured during venous occlusion. Calibration is performed by injecting 100 cm³ of air into the chamber and observing the pressure changes. A pneumatic occlusion tourniquet with an attached manometer is applied just proximal to the knee. After equilibration, the tourniquet is rapidly deflated to 50 mm Hg to occlude the venous outflow. The increasing leg volume is recorded for 20 s and represents the arterial inflow to the leg during that period. The arterial inflow in cubic centimeters/milliliter can be calculated from the slope of the volume/time curve during the 20 s. This technology has been reported to be reproducible, however because it is cumbersome, it is not presently widely used.[23]

Clinical Applications

Plethysmographic techniques permit evaluation of peripheral vascular disease by one of the following three techniques: pulse-wave analysis, determination of digit or limb blood pressure, and determination of arterial or venous blood flow. Pulse-wave analysis is particularly useful in peripheral arterial and carotid occlusive diseases. Assessment of digit or limb blood pressure permits semiquantitation of peripheral arterial occlusive disease, and the assessment of limb blood flow permits quantitation of peripheral arterial and venous diseases.

Pulse-Wave Analysis

The contour and amplitude of the plethysmographic pulsation with each heartbeat is a qualitative guide to the presence and degree of peripheral arterial occlusive disease.[24] Normally, the pulse wave has a steep upslope, a relatively narrow peak, and a dicrotic wave on the downslope, which is concave toward the baseline. In the presence of arterial occlusive disease, the pulse-wave contour is damped with a more gradual upslope, a broad rounded peak, and loss of the dicrotic wave on the downslope, which becomes convex away from the baseline. The amplitude or height of the pulse wave diminishes progressively with increasing arterial obstruction (Figure 18–6). The amplitude of the pulse wave will also decrease in response to sympathetic stimulation, such as that induced by a deep inspiration.

Recently, Kuvin et al.[25] concluded that finger arterial pulse-wave amplitude was helpful in the assessment of peripheral vascular endothelial function.

The digit and segmental limb systolic blood pressures can be determined by plethysmography. However, such determinations are more simply done by Doppler ultrasound. The measurement of systolic blood pressure usually requires a plethysmography transducer on the

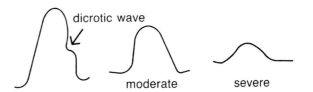

FIGURE 18–6. Pulse wave tracing. A normal pulse wave has a steep upslope, a relatively narrow peak, and a dicrotic wave on the downslope, which is concave toward the baseline. Note the contour and amplitude in the presence of moderate and severe arterial occlusion.

distal phalanx.[26] Photopulse, strain gauge, or air transducers are suitable for detecting the return of pulsations following deflation of a specially designed blood pressure cuff. Such digit pressure measurements are particularly useful in patients with diabetes mellitus, Raynaud's syndrome, and advanced peripheral arterial occlusive disease.

Determination of digit or limb blood flow by plethysmography provides an accurate quantitation of peripheral arterial or venous disease. The limb or digit blood flow may be determined by means of venous occlusion plethysmography from the rate of initial increase in limb or digit circumference in response to temporary venous occlusion with a proximal pneumatic cuff.[10] The limb blood flow may remain normal in peripheral arterial occlusive disease until the disease becomes far advanced. Thus, it is necessary to measure the abnormal attenuation of increase in limb blood flow during stress, such as that during reactive hyperemia or following limb exercise.[27] Normally, arterial blood flow increases by several times the resting level during hyperemia and rapidly returns to normal within a few seconds (reactive hyperemia) or in 1 or 2 min (postexercise hyperemia). In the presence of arterial occlusive disease, the hyperemia would be attenuated and prolonged in proportion to the degree of the circulatory obstruction.

Transcutaneous PO₂

This technology allows quantitative estimation of cutaneous oxygen delivery that is independent of arterial wall mechanical properties (e.g., medial calcinosis).[28] This monitoring device is a modification of the Clark polarographic oxygen electrode coupled to a servo/controlling heating coil and thermistor. It operates on the principle that vasodilation occurs when the skin heats. At skin temperatures higher than 43°C, the ratio of transcutaneous PO_2 (TCPO₂) to arterial PO_2 is constant and approximates 1. Conventional probes are, therefore, set between 43 and 45°C. The relationship is complex and affected by several factors, although the TCPO₂ is directly related to skin blood flow. Several attempts have been made to increase the accuracy of predictions based on $TCPO_2$ measurements, e.g., response to maneuvers including oxygen inhalation, postocclusion reactive hyperemia, exercise, and leg dependency. None of these maneuvers was found to significantly increase the overall accuracy. Other factors that may limit the accuracy and overall usefulness of this methodology include changes in skin temperature, sympathetic tone, age, edema, hyperkerotosis, and cellulitis.

The clinical application of absolute $TCPO_2$ measurement using this technology is limited by the broad overlap of values correlating with the clinical classification of arterial disease. Mild to moderate arterial occlusive disease is generally not detected by reduced $TCPO_2$ levels. The normal range in these patients is $\geq 40\,mm\,Hg$. $TCPO_2$ measurements have maximal sensitivity at critically low levels of tissue perfusion; therefore it is useful in predicting amputation or wound healing in an extremity with severe peripheral vascular occlusive disease. Generally speaking, most wounds or amputations will heal if the $TCPO_2$ is greater than $30\,mm\,Hg$ at that level. For $TCPO_2$ values between 20 and $30\,mm\,Hg$, the likelihood of healing is unpredictable. For $TCPO_2$ levels of $<20\,mm\,Hg$, most amputations or wounds will not heal.[29] This methodology will be described in detail in a later chapter.

Laser Doppler Measurements

This method uses a narrow monochromatic incident light source (laser) to interrogate particles [blood cells, red blood cells (RBCs)] moving in the dermal microcirculation. A pick-up system records the reflected light and the Doppler-shifted signal corresponds to the average velocity of the particles. These measurements can vary based on several factors, including significant scattering on both the incident and reflected light beams, anatomic variables including skin pigmentation, topography, epidermis thickness, random complexity of the microcirculation, and the number of RBCs in the sample volume. The term RBC-flux has been used to describe the measurement, as it represents neither velocity nor flow. The signal is a product of the number of moving RBCs in the sample volume and their mean velocity (flux = RBC volume fraction × mean velocity). This noninvasive technology provides continuous readout and it is easy to operate, however, it cannot be calibrated, its reproducibility is frequently problematic, and the data are not expressed in familiar or absolute units (velocity or flow rate).[30] Systolic skin pressure (SSP) can be measured using a blood pressure cuff applied directly over the sensor. This technique involves inflation of a cuff placed over the sensor until RBC-flux stops. The cuff is then deflated, and

the SSP is the point at which the recorded signal returns. Laser Doppler fluxometry has been used in association with various maneuvers to detect microangiopathy and predict clinical outcome. Loss of reactive hyperemia response following temporary arterial occlusion and failure to increase RBC-flux with skin healing are signs of microangiopathy in diabetic patients with compromised wound healing. In addition, loss of venoarteriolar response, a sympathetic axonal reflex of vasoconstriction when the foot is lowered below the heart level, occurs in the presence of advanced peripheral neuropathy in diabetic patients and may predict wound-healing difficulties.

Eicke et al.[31] conducted a study comparing CW Doppler ultrasound of the radial artery and laser Doppler flowmetry of the fingertips with sympathetic stimulation, and concluded that both methods were feasible to monitor flow changes due to sympathetic stimulation.

Kubli et al.,[32] in a study of the reproducibility of laser Doppler imaging of the skin blood flow as a tool to assess endothelial function, concluded that endothelium-dependent and -independent responses of dermal blood flow evaluated with laser Doppler imaging are highly reproducible from day to day, at least in healthy non-smoking young male subjects. These observations have implications for testing for endothelial function in clinical studies.

Radioisotope Techniques

Various radioisotope techniques have been described in the diagnosis of peripheral arterial occlusive diseases, e.g., radionuclide angiography, the xenon-133 washout technique, the use of radioactive microsphere assessment of regional blood flow, and arterial venous shunting. Other methods have been used for the diagnosis of venous disorders, e.g., iodine-125 fibrinogen leg scanning.

Radionuclide angiography using technetium-99m permits visualization of the major arteries using an Anger camera. This technique is particularly useful in screening for the presence of aortic aneurysms and carotid arterial occlusive disease.[33]

The ^{133}Xe washout technique is useful to determine discrete muscle compartment blood flow.[34] This technique involves injection of approximately $50\,\mu Ci$ of ^{133}Xe dissolved in saline into the muscle with subsequent recording of the rate of washout of the isotope from the site of injection. Xenon-133 freely crosses the capillary endothelium, and the rate of washout is directly proportional to capillary blood flow. This technique has been predominantly employed in clinical investigation of peripheral arterial disease and compartment compression syndromes. The use of radioactive microspheres[35] has permitted assessment of regional distribution of blood flow, particularly in patients with advanced arterial occlusive disease or ischemic ulceration. Radionuclide-tagged particles of albumin are injected intraarterially, and their distribution is determined by scanning of the extremity. This technique detects areas of poor perfusion. The degree of radioactivity of tissues surrounding an ischemic ulcer is an accurate guide to the healing potential of the lesion. Microspheres also permit assessment of the degree of arteriovenous (AV) shunting.[36]

Temperature Detection

Abnormalities in limb temperature may reflect changes in blood flow and the presence of arterial occlusive disease. Several techniques, such as thermometry, thermography, and calorimetry, were used in the past, but they are now outdated.

Electromagnetic Flowmeter

The electromagnetic flowmeter aids in measuring flow rates and is reasonably accurate in real time without interrupting or restricting the flow stream. When a fluid conductor moves at right angles through a magnetic field, an electrical potential is induced in the fluid perpendicular to both the magnetic field and the direction of the flow. The magnitude of the voltage depends on the spatially averaged velocity flow, the strength of the magnetic field, and the diameter of the blood vessel. The standard noncannulating electromagnetic flow probe consists of an electromagnet and two electrodes embedded in a C-shaped plastic device for easy application to the vessel. The electrodes are located opposite each other and at right angles to the poles of the electromagnets. A voltage proportional to the velocity of flow appears at the interface between the fluid and the vessel wall. In turn, this voltage is conducted across the vessel wall, where it is picked up by the electrodes and is amplified to drive a recording system. The volume flow (in cubic centimeters per second) is measured by a special formula. A supply of calibrated probes of varying diameters are gas-sterilized and made available in the operating room. It is important that the electrodes be kept clean and free of deposits of blood or other protein material, since such deposits can alter the electrical resistance and distort the flow recordings. A length of vessel about three times the width of the probe is dissected out to allow easy application and to prevent angulation of the probe. All electrical equipment, particularly the electrocautery, is disconnected prior to using the electromagnetic flowmeter. This is to prevent stray currents from passing through the ground electrodes of the flowmeter, where they could produce an electrical burn or shock. Also, it helps to eliminate troublesome electrical interference. After the probe has been positioned on the vessel, the distal vessel is momentarily occluded in order to adjust the zero. The resulting reactive hyperemia is allowed to subside for a few seconds to several minutes before pulsatile and mean flows are recorded. It is important to ensure that the vessel probe is surrounded by tissue fluids or by saline in order to duplicate the conditions of *in vitro* calibration. For a branched vessel, or in the case of an end-to-side graft where there are two or more outflow tracts, it is helpful to occlude each of the outflow tracts or branches in turn to obtain some idea of flow distribution.

The flow value (milliliters per minute) is recorded at rest and often following intraarterial injection of a vasodilating agent (papaverine hydrochloride). A flow value recorded after administration of a vasodilator is termed a stimulated or augmented flow. The electromagnetic flowmeter has been useful in detecting technical errors, such as intimal flaps, kinked or faulty anastomosis and twisted grafts, the presence of emboli or thrombi, and construction of a graft of inadequate size. These problems are detected during operation, are immediately corrected, and reoperation can be avoided.[37]

Conclusions

The most important function of the noninvasive vascular laboratory is the provision of diagnostic services for the evaluation of patients with clinical vascular diseases. This includes confirmation of the diagnosis, prediction of the therapeutic result, monitoring of surgical or medical therapy, and follow-up of the natural history or influence of therapy on peripheral vascular disease. Various noninvasive vascular diagnostic techniques have been used to detect peripheral vascular occlusive disease. Presently, the most commonly used methods are the measurement of segmental Doppler pressures, with or without Doppler waveform analyses, either alone or in combination with duplex ultrasonography (with color flow imaging).[1,2–5,38–42] These modalities are described in detail in the following chapters.

References

1. AbuRahma AF, Khan S, Robinson PA. Selective use of segmental Doppler pressures and color duplex imaging in the localization of arterial occlusive disease of the lower extremity. Surgery 1995;118:496–503.
2. Toursarkissian B, Mejia A, Smilanich RP, Schoolfield J, Shireman PK, Sykes MT. Noninvasive localization of infrainguinal arterial occlusive disease in diabetics. Ann Vasc Surg 2001;15:73–78.

3. Holland T. Utilizing the ankle brachial index in clinical practice. Ostomy Wound Manage 2002;48:38–40.

4. Adam DJ, Naik J, Hartshorne T, Bello M, London NJ. The diagnosis and management of 689 chronic leg ulcers in a single-visit assessment clinic. Eur J Vasc Endovasc Surg 2003;25:462–468.

5. Carser DG. Do we need to reappraise our method of interpreting the ankle brachial pressure index? J Wound Care 2001;10:59–62.

6. Satomura S, Kaneko Z. Ultrasonic blood rheograph. Proceedings of the Third International Conference on Medical Electronics, 1960, p. 254.

7. Strandness DE Jr, McCutcheon EP, Rushmer RF. Application of transcutaneous Doppler flow meter in evaluation of occlusive arterial disease. Surg Gynecol Obstet 1966;122:1039–1045.

8. Green PS, Marich KW. Real-time orthographic ultrasonic imaging for cardiovascular diagnosis. In: Harrison, DE, Sandler H, and Miller HA (eds). Cardiovascular Imaging and Image Processing: Theory and Practice, Vol. 72. Palos Verdes Estates, CA: Society of Photo-Optical Instrumentation Engineers, 1975.

9. Landowne M, Katz LN. A critique of the plethysmographic method of measuring blood flow in the extremities of man. Am Heart J 1942;23:644–675.

10. Brodie PE, Russell AE. On the determination of the rate of blood flow through an organ. J Physiol 1905;32:47P.

11. Hertzman AP. The blood supply of various skin area as estimated by the photoelectric plethysmograph. Am J Physiol 1938;124:328–340.

12. Barnes RW, Clayton JM, Bone GE, et al. Supraorbital photo-pulse plethysmography: Simple accurate screening from carotid occlusive disease. J Surg Rx 1977;22:319–327.

13. Eldrup-Jorgensen SV, Schwartz SI, Wallace JD. A method of clinical evaluation of peripheral circulation: Photoelectric hemodensitometry. Surgery 1966;59:505–513.

14. Barnes RW, Garrett WV, Slaymaker EE, et al. Doppler ultrasound and supraorbital photoplethysmography for noninvasive screening of carotid occlusive disease. Am J Surg 1977;134:183–186.

15. Barnes RW, Garrett WV, Hommel BA, et al. Photoplethysmography assessment of altered cutaneous circulation in the post-phlebitic syndrome. Proc Assoc Adv Med Instrum 1978;13:25–29.

16. Bortolotto LA, Blacher J, Kondo T, Takazawa K, Safar ME. Assessment of vascular aging and atherosclerosis in hypertensive subjects: Second derivative of photoplethysmogram versus pulse wave velocity. Am J Hypertens 2000;13:165–171.

17. Whitney RJ. The measurement of changes in human limb volume by means of mercury-in-rubber strain gauge. J Physiol 1949;109:5P.

18. Hokanson DE, Sumner DS, Strandness DE Jr. An electrically calibrated plethysmography for direct measurement of limb blood flow. IEEE Trans Biomed Eng 1975;BME–22:25–29.

19. Barnes RW, Hokanson DE, Wu KK, et al. Detection of deep vein thrombosis with an automatic electrically-calibrated strain gauge plethysmograph. Surgery 1977;82:219–223.

20. Yao JST, Needham TN, Gourmoos C, Irvine WT. A comparative study of strain-gauge plethysmography and Doppler ultrasound in the assessment of occlusive arterial disease of the lower extremities. Surgery 1972;71:4–9.

21. Winsor T. The segmental plethysmograph: Description of the instrument. Angiology 1957;8:87–101.

22. Darling RC, Raines VK, Brenner V, et al. Quantitative segmental pulse volume recorder. A clinical tool. Surgery 1972;72:873–877.

23. Nicholaides A. Quantitative air-plethysmography in management of arterial ischemia. In: Bernstein EF (ed). Vascular Diagnosis, 4th ed., pp. 544–546. St. Louis: Mosby, 1993.

24. Strandness DE Jr. Wave Form Analysis in the Diagnosis of Arteriosclerosis Obliterans and Peripheral Arterial Disease, a Physiologic Approach, pp. 92–113. Boston: Little Brown & Co., 1969.

25. Kuvin JT, Patel AR, Sliney KA, Pandian NG, Sheffy J, Schnall RP, Karas RH, Udelson JE. Assessment of peripheral vascular endothelial function with finger arterial pulse wave amplitude. Am Heart J 2003;146:168–174.

26. Gundersen J. Segmental measurement of systolic blood pressure in the extremities including the thumb and the great toe. Acta Chir Scand 1972 (Suppl. 426);1–90.

27. Hillestad LK. The peripheral blood flow in intermittent claudication. IV. The significance of claudication distance. Acta Med Scand 1963;173:467–478.

28. Rich K. Transcutaenous oxygen measurements: Implications for nursing. J Vasc Nurs 2001;19:55–59.

29. Kram HB, Appel PL, Shoemaker WC. Multisensor transcutaneous oximetric mapping to predict below-knee amputation wound healing: Use of a critical PO2. J Vasc Surg 1989;9:796–800.

30. Belcaro G, et al. Evaluation of skin blood flow and venoarteriolar response in patients with diabetes and peripheral vascular disease by laser Doppler flowmetry. Angiology 1989;40:953–957.

31. Eicke BM, Milke K, Schlereth T, Birklein F. Comparison of continuous wave Doppler ultrasound of the radial artery and laser Doppler flowmetry of the fingertips with sympathetic stimulation. J Neurol 2004;251:958–962.

32. Kubli S, Waeber B, Dalle-Ave A, Feihl F. Reproduciblity of laser Doppler imaging of skin blood flow as a tool to assess endothelial function. J Cardiovasc Pharmacol 2000;36:640–648.

33. Moss CM, Rudavsky AZ, Veith FJ. The value of scintiangiography in arterial disease. Arch Surg 1976;111:1235–1242.

34. Lassen NA. Muscle blood flow in normal man and in patient with intermittent claudication evaluated by simultaneous Xe-133 and Na-24 clearances. J Clin Invest 1964;43:1805–1812.

35. Siegel ME, Giargiana FA Jr., Rhodes BA, et al. Perfusion of ischemic ulcer of the extremity: A prognostic indicator of feeling after healing. Arch Surg 1975;110:265–268.

36. Rhodes BA, Rutherford RB, Lopez-Majano V, et al. Arteriovenous shunt measurements in extremities. J Nucl Med 1972;13:357–362.

37. Terry HJ. The electromagnetic measurement of blood flow during arterial surgery. Biomed Eng 1972;7:466–474.

38. Lee BY, Campbell JS, Berkowitz P. The correlation of ankle oscillometric blood pressures and segmental pulse volumes to Doppler systolic pressures in arterial occlusive disease. J Vasc Surg 1996;23:116–122.

39. Hatsukami TS, Primozich JF, Zierler RE. Color Doppler imaging of infrainguinal arterial occlusive disease. J Vasc Surg 1992;16:527–533.

40. Moneta GL, Yeager RA, Lee RW. Noninvasive localization of arterial occlusive disease: A comparison of segmental Doppler pressures and arterial duplex mapping. J Vasc Surg 1993;17:578–582.

41. Collier P, Wilcox, Brooks D. Improved patient selection for angioplasty utilizing color Doppler imaging. Am J Surg 1990;160:171–173.

42. Feigelson HS, Criqui MH, Fronek A. Screening for peripheral arterial disease: The sensitivity, specificity, and predictive value of noninvasive tests in a defined population. Am J Epidemiol 1994;140:526–534.

19
Segmental Doppler Pressures and Doppler Waveform Analysis in Peripheral Vascular Disease of the Lower Extremities

Ali F. AbuRahma and Kimberly S. Jarrett

The credit for first developing Doppler flow detectors belongs to Satomura, whose clinical report appeared in 1959.[1] However, until Strandness et al.[2] popularized the use of transcutaneous flow detection to study peripheral vascular occlusive disease, the diagnosis or objective assessment of limb ischemia was dependent upon clinical examination, arteriography, or plethysmography. The development of the continuous-wave or pulsed Doppler techniques opened a new field for the diagnosis of peripheral vascular occlusive disease.

Instrumentation and Physical Principles

A continuous-wave (CW) Doppler velocity detector is used to sense apparent changes in the reflected sound wave frequency produced by the movement of red blood cells relative to an ultrasound probe. An electric oscillator vibrates a piezoelectric crystal (ceramic) at 5–10 MHz. This produces an ultrasound wave that is transmitted via an acoustic coupling gel into the body. The ultrasonic beam is reflected back to a receiver in the probe by all the structures in its path, including the moving red blood cells. The movement of the blood cells causes a frequency shift (Doppler shift) in the reflected sound wave. The Doppler shift is proportional to the blood flow velocity. There is a Doppler effect whenever there is relative motion between the source and the receiver of the sound. Blood is the moving target and the transducer is the stationary source. Depending on the direction of the flow relative to the Doppler beam, the reflected frequency is higher or lower than the transmitted frequency (Doppler shift). The signal is electrically mixed with the transmitting frequency and processed to produce a frequency in the audible range. A received ultrasonic beam can be amplified and projected audibly through either a loudspeaker or earphones. A second method of displaying the Doppler velocity signal is by converting it to a visible analog waveform. With the analog waveform, the amplified signal is electronically converted and displayed on a channel recorder similar to an ECG (Figure 19–1).

Therefore, there are several types of Doppler velocimetry: (1) auditory: this processes the Doppler signal as sound. It has the advantage of containing all Doppler frequencies with the exception of those extreme frequencies removed by filtering. A trained technician or physician can easily distinguish normal signals from those received proximal to, within, or distal to a stenosis or occlusion. A higher pitched signal can mean that the probe angle is very acute to the vessel angle or it can indicate a significant arterial occlusion. (2) Analog wave tracing: this method employs a zero crossing frequency meter to display the signals graphically on a strip chart recorder. It has an acceptable overall accuracy, but it is not as sensitive as the spectral analysis and it also has the following drawbacks: noise and under- or overestimation of high and low velocities, respectively. (3) Spectral analysis: this method displays frequency on the vertical axis, time on the horizontal axis, and the amplitude of backscattered signals at any frequency and time (Figure 19–2). It has the advantage of displaying the amplitudes at all frequencies, but it is free of many of the disadvantages that were previously described for the analog wave tracing.

Indications for Testing

The arterial lower extremity Doppler examination is a useful tool in many aspects of peripheral vascular medicine. It validates the diagnosis of the presence, location, and severity of arterial occlusive disease, helping to differentiate true vascular claudication from pseudoclaudication that arises from neurologic or musculoskeletal disorders. Therefore, this test is indicated for patients with symptoms and signs of arterial occlusive disease, which vary from claudication and rest pain to skin changes suggestive of arterial insufficiency, e.g., nonhealing ulcers.[3–7]

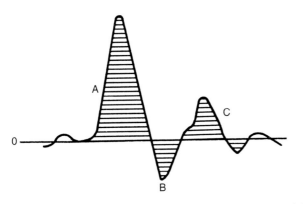

FIGURE 19–1. Normal arterial velocity tracing (multiphasic). (A) Systolic component; (B) early diastolic component; (C) late diastolic component.

TABLE 19–1. Indications for arterial Doppler examination.

1. Calf pain while walking (claudication).
2. Leg pain at rest, suggestive of ischemia.
3. Skin changes suggestive of arterial insufficiency.
4. Nonhealing ulcers.
5. Previous vascular reconstructive procedures—-follow-up.
6. Intraoperative application.
7. Determination of the level of amputation and the response after lumbar sympathectomy.
8. Assistance in the diagnosis of Raynaud's disease or phenomenon and arteriovenous fistula.
9. Detection of pulses in shock states or in trauma.

The arterial lower extremity Doppler study is also helpful in determining the level of leg amputation and the benefit from lumbar sympathectomy.[8–10] In addition, the Doppler examination is useful in screening patients with Raynaud's disease or syndrome,[11] or arteriovenous (AV) fistula,[12] and to rapidly assess patients who have suffered possible arterial trauma.

In the case of iatrogenic arterial injury, Doppler ultrasound is suitable for assessing postcatheterization arterial obstruction following femoral or brachial cardiac catheterization or peripheral arteriography. Similarly, any complication following insertion of indwelling arterial monitoring catheters can be readily screened with the Doppler detector. It is also helpful in patients with shock.

Intraoperative measurement of ankle pressures after completion of aortofemoral bypass or aortoiliac endarterectomy can be used to predict the results of the procedure. The determination of segmental pressure measurements in the postoperative period aids in quantitatively assessing the results of aortofemoral bypass (Table 19–1).

Methods and Interpretations

The complete arterial lower extremity Doppler examination consists of three components: (1) analysis of the arterial analog wave tracing, (2) measurement of the segmental systolic limb pressures, and (3) calculation of the ankle-brachial index (ABI).

After the history is taken, the patient is allowed to rest in the supine position on the examining table for 10–15 min to ensure the measurement of pressures in the resting state. The patient is placed in the supine position with the extremities at the level of the heart. The head of the bed can be elevated slightly, and the patient's head can rest on a pillow. The patient's hip is generally externally rotated with the knee slightly bent to facilitate the lower extremity evaluation. Alternative positions for the Doppler lower extremity examination include right or left lateral decubitus (patient on his or her side) or the prone position for access to the popliteal artery.

The Doppler probe (transducer) must be positioned on the long axis of the vessel. An angle of insonation of approximately 45–60° is usually used for this study. The leg pulses (femoral, popliteal, dorsalis pedis, and posterior tibial) are evaluated by palpation and by audible Doppler signals. The pulses are graded as II, I, or 0, and the Doppler signals are graded as normal (biphasic), abnormal (monophasic), or absent.

Qualitative Doppler Waveform Analysis

For the lower extremities, Doppler velocity waveforms are recorded from the following arteries bilaterally: (1) common femoral artery at the groin level, (2) superficial femoral artery, (3) popliteal artery, (4) posterior tibial

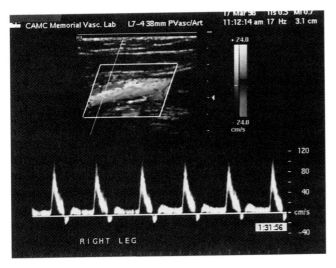

FIGURE 19–2. A spectral analysis of the right common femoral artery. This method displays frequency on the vertical axis, time on the horizontal axis, and the amplitude of back-scattered signals at any frequency and time. (This picture was taken by a color duplex ultrasound machine.)

artery (at the level of the medial malleolus), (5) dorsalis pedis artery (at the dorsum of the foot), and (6) occasionally the peroneal artery (at the level of the lateral malleolus). Auditory signals are obtained. If the examiner is using a headset, the right earphone provides forward (antegrade) flow signals, while the left earphone provides reverse (retrograde) flow signals. The qualities of the auditory signals and the waveforms are observed and analyzed.

The normal arterial velocity signal is multiphasic. That is, it is characterized by one systolic and one or more diastolic components (Figure 19–1). In the major peripheral arteries, the systolic component is a large positive deflection indicative of a high net forward flow velocity. This is followed by a brief period of net flow reversal. This flow reversal is then followed immediately by another positive deflection, the diastolic forward flow component. The brief period of flow reversal characteristic of the major peripheral arterial velocity signal is a function of the generally high resistance of the extremity vascular bed. Lowering resistance, via vasodilation, can eliminate the net flow reversal. The normal arterial velocity signal is also pulsatile, i.e., it cycles with each heartbeat. Thus, the normal nonpulsatile, phasic, low-pitch venous signal is easily differentiated from the pulsatile, multiphasic arterial signal.

Abnormal signals are generally monophasic (Figure 19–3), nonpulsatile, or absent. Biphasic signals can also be considered abnormal (Figure 19–3). It is imperative to observe for deterioration of the waveform, e.g., triphasic to biphasic or triphasic to monophasic of the Doppler signal quality from one level to the next level. A monophasic and dampened signal can be obtained proximal to an obstruction as well as distal to it. In the absence of additional obstructions, the distal signal can normalize.

The arterial velocity signal produced just before an occlusion is characteristically of short duration, i.e., a slapping signal of low amplitude. However, the arterial signal produced over a stenotic segment is a high-pitched signal with less prominent diastolic components. The signal from just beyond the stenotic segment is also characterized by dampened systolic and absent diastolic components, but it is not as high pitched as the stenotic signal. The signal beyond an occluded arterial segment is like a poststenotic signal, although the systolic component may be of even lower amplitude. The signal produced by the prominent collateral arterial signal is high pitched and almost continuous. These similarities among the abnormal arterial velocity signals make the differentiation difficult. Therefore, if there is difficulty in interpreting these signals, they can be called either normal or abnormal for practical purposes (Figure 19–3).

As noted in the abnormal wave tracing, a Doppler signal obtained from a common femoral artery that is diseased shows the poor quality of the signal (poor upslope

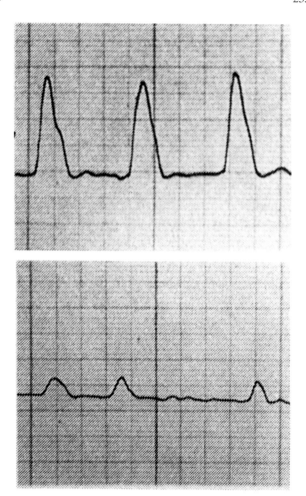

FIGURE 19–3. An abnormal arterial tracing of the lower extremity in a patient with stenosis of the common femoral artery. The upper tracing was recorded from the popliteal artery distal to the obstruction and the lower tracing was taken at the level of the posterior tibial artery. These signals are monophasic.

and downslope, with a somewhat rounded peak) (Figure 19–3). A similar waveform can be obtained from the common femoral artery distal to a proximal iliac artery obstruction. Similarly, the Doppler signals obtained from the posterior tibial artery at the level of the ankle distal to that occlusion is somewhat continuous with low pressure resistance secondary to a vasodilated arterial bed in the presence of proximal arterial obstruction.

Quantitative Interpretation Criteria of Doppler Waveform

1. *Pulsatility index (PI):* This is calculated by dividing the peak-to-peak frequency by the mean (average) frequency[13] as seen in Figure 19–4. This ratio is independent of the beam-to-vessel Doppler angle when using

hand-held Doppler equipment. As seen in Figure 19–4, the pulsatility index equals P1 to P2 divided by the mean frequency. Normally, the values of the PI increase from the central to peripheral arteries. A PI of >5.5 is normal for the common femoral artery, while a normal PI for the popliteal artery is approximately 8.0. These values decrease in the presence of proximal occlusive disease, e.g., a PI of <4 or 5 in the common femoral artery with a patent superficial femoral artery (SFA) indicates proximal aortoiliac occlusive disease. However, the same reduced PI is not diagnostic if the SFA is occluded.

2. *Inverse damping factor:* This is calculated by dividing the distal PI by the proximal PI of an arterial segment. It indicates the degree to which the wave is dampened as it moves through an arterial segment,[13] e.g., severe stenosis or occlusion of the SFA is usually present when the inverse femoral-popliteal dampening factor is less than 0.9 (a normal value = 0.9–1.1).

3. *Transient time:* Systole should be simultaneously evident at a specific site bilaterally. Delay on one side may indicate a more proximal occlusive disease. You must compare the signals bilaterally at the same site.

4. *Acceleration time or index:* This differentiates inflow from outflow disease. It is based on the principle that arterial obstruction proximal to the site of the Doppler probe prolongs the time between the onset of systolic flow to the point of maximum peak in waveforms at the probe site (Figure 19–5). Figure 19–5A shows a normal common femoral artery tracing. There is a quick systolic upslope representing a normal acceleration time, in contrast to Figure 19–5B, which shows a slower upslope from the onset of systole to maximum peak from an abnormal common femoral artery tracing. Acceleration time is not prolonged when there is disease distal to the probe. It is applied to those signals evaluated by spectral analysis because it is necessary to maximize sensitivity and minimize artifacts. Generally, an acceleration time of equal to

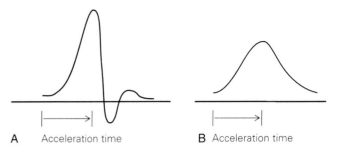

FIGURE 19–5. A normal common femoral artery tracing with a normal acceleration time (A), and an abnormal common femoral artery tracing with an abnormal acceleration time (B).

or less than 133 ms suggests the absence of significant aortoiliac disease. False-positive results can occur with technical errors, e.g., a Doppler angle ≥70°, which may dampen the Doppler signal qualities, and in the presence of poor cardiac output since the Doppler flow signal will be attenuated with the waveform detecting slow upstroke, rounded peak, and slow downslope.

Limitations of the Analog Wave Tracing Analysis

The Doppler waveforms may be affected by (1) ambient temperature; (2) uncompensated congestive heart failure resulting in dampened waveforms following exercise; (3) an inability to distinguish stenosis from occlusion; (4) an inability to precisely localize the occlusion; (5) and an inability to be applied on patients with casts or extensive bandages that cannot be removed. It is technologist-dependent, and the result can vary with the Doppler angle used.

Segmental Doppler Pressures

After completion of the examination and analysis of the arterial analogue tracings, the second component of the Doppler examination is started, i.e., determinations of the segmental systolic limb pressures. Doppler segmental pressures have the same capabilities of analog wave tracing, i.e., to help in identifying the presence and severity of arterial occlusive disease, to provide an objective baseline to follow the progression of peripheral vascular disease of the lower extremity and/or the postoperative course, and to somewhat evaluate the treatment plan. The results of this testing are usually combined with the Doppler velocity waveform analysis. The patient preparation and positioning are similar to those of the Doppler velocity waveform analysis.

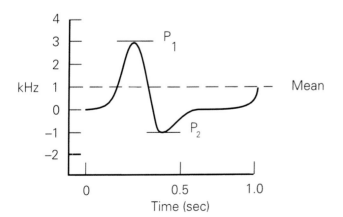

FIGURE 19–4. The method for calculating the pulsatility index.

Technique for Segmental Doppler Pressures

The brachial artery Doppler systolic pressures are measured in each arm. Cuffs of appropriate size (bladder dimension 12 × 40 cm) are placed on each arm. The brachial artery is palpated in the antecubital fossa, and a small amount of acoustic gel is applied to the skin over the artery. The arterial signal is found using the Doppler probe, and then the cuff is inflated until the signal disappears (20–30 mm Hg beyond the last audible Doppler signal). The cuff is slowly deflated until the arterial signal is again audible, at which time the pressure is recorded. Unlike the standard stethoscope, as the cuff is further deflated, the velocity signal will not disappear, so the diastolic pressure cannot be determined.

Four 12 × 40 cm pneumatic cuffs are applied at various levels on each leg: as high on the thigh as possible, just above the knee, just below the knee, and above the ankle (Figure 19–6A). The examiner then listens to the posterior tibial and the dorsalis pedis arterial signals (Figure 19–6B). The posterior tibial artery is found just posterior to the medial malleolus, and the dorsalis pedis artery is

found on the dorsum of the foot. Occasionally, the peroneal (lateral tarsal) artery is examined (found just anterior to the lateral malleolus). Of these vessels the one with the strongest Doppler signal is chosen for the ankle pressure. If none of the vessels can be located with the ultrasound probe, the popliteal artery signal is identified in the popliteal fossa. High-thigh, above-knee, below-knee, and ankle pressure readings are taken. An automatic cuff inflator may be used to save time.

Several important facts concerning cuff characteristics should be noted. It is most important that the pneumatic bladder of the cuff completely encircle the limb. The bladder of the cuff should be placed over the artery. This is especially important when the bladder does not encircle the limb. Just as bladder length affects the pressure determination, bladder width must also be related to the limb diameter. For the most accurate measurement of blood pressure, the width of the pneumatic cuff should be 20% greater than the diameter of the limb.[3] For all practical purposes, this means that larger arms require wider cuffs. When a cuff is too narrow relative to the limb diameter, an erroneously high pressure (30–90 mm Hg greater than arm pressure) results.

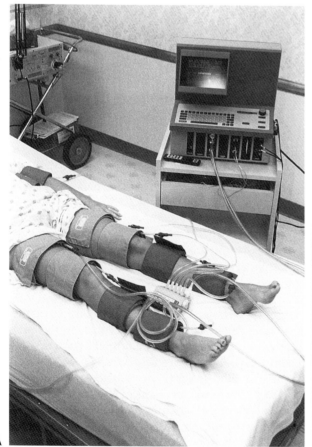

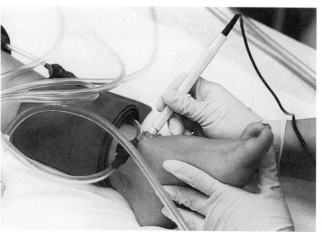

FIGURE 19–6. (A) Technique for measuring the segmental Doppler pressures using the four cuff method. (B) The application of the Doppler probe on the dorsalis pedis artery.

A

B

The four cuffs used in this test to determine the segmental pressures at different levels of the lower limb are all the same width (12×40 cm), making the pressures at the widest part of the limb (high thigh) erroneously high. Some laboratories use a large (19×40 cm) thigh cuff to satisfy the recommended width/girth relationship and thereby give a more accurate thigh pressure. However, the cuff is so wide that only one can be placed on the thigh. The three-cuff technique utilizes one large cuff placed as high as possible on the thigh. With this technique, a more accurate thigh pressure is obtained (a thigh pressure that is very similar to the higher brachial pressure).

Segmental Doppler pressures of the lower extremity are obtained bilaterally at the following sites and in this order using a hand-held or machine sphygmomanometer with automatic display: ankle pressure (using the posterior tibial artery and dorsalis pedis artery); below-knee pressure (calf pressure), using the best signal of the posterior tibial artery or the dorsalis pedis artery; above-knee pressure (same as below-knee pressure, although the popliteal artery can be used if the ankle Doppler signals are difficult to obtain); and high-thigh pressure (the same as above-knee pressure). If a pressure measurement needs to be repeated, the cuff should be fully deflated for about 1 min prior to repeat inflation.

Barnes[4] used a narrower cuff (12×40 cm) for measuring the proximal and distal thigh pressures and accepted the artificially high values obtained. This technique allows an approximation of the common femoral (inflow) artery pressure by the proximal cuff and the superficial femoral artery pressure by the above-knee cuff. When only one large cuff is used on the thigh, the single thigh pressure measured does not differentiate aortoiliac from superficial femoral artery occlusive disease. For convenience, the aeroid manometer is used rather than the mercury manometer. The aeroid manometer has the advantage of being portable, inexpensive, easily exchanged from cuff to cuff, and an accurate pressure registering system.

For the analog wave recording technique, diastolic pressure is taken as the pressure at which there is continuous forward flow during diastole. But this point of return of continuous forward flow in diastole would be difficult to determine in the vasoconstricted or high-resistant limb, because the tracing would be constantly crossing to zero during the period of net flow reversal. The problem is overcome by purposely inducing a state of reactive hyperemia in the vasoconstricted limb. This hyperemia is a state of vasodilation.

Interpretations

After determination of the segmental systolic limb pressures, analysis of the various segment pressures is done. Normally, the proximal thigh pressure should be 20–

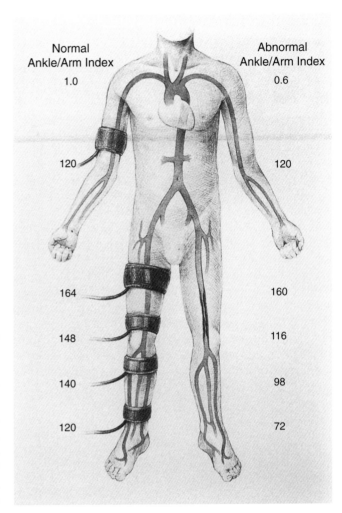

FIGURE 19–7. Segmental systolic limb pressures of a patient with severe stenosis of the left superficial femoral artery.

30 mm Hg higher than that of the arm, and the pressure gradient between adjacent levels of measurement in the leg should be no greater than 20–30 mm Hg. A low proximal thigh pressure signifies aortoiliac or common femoral occlusive disease. An abnormal gradient between the proximal thigh and the above- or below-knee cuff is indicative of superficial femoral or popliteal artery occlusive disease. An abnormal gradient between the below-knee and ankle cuffs indicates tibioperoneal disease. Figure 19–7 shows a patient with occlusion of the left superficial femoral artery as indicated by the pressure differential between the high-thigh and above-knee readings (160–116 mm Hg, respectively). A horizontal difference of 20–30 mm Hg or more suggests significant disease at or above the level of the leg with the lower pressure. Figure 19–8 shows a patient with significant stenosis or occlusion at the aortoiliac level as indicated by low high thigh pressures bilaterally.

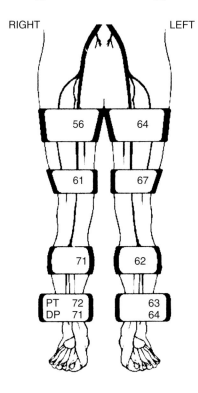

109	BRACHIAL	107
Indexes		
0.51	U.THIGH	0.59
0.56	L.THIGH	0.61
0.65	CALF	0.57
0.66	ANKLE-PT	0.58
0.65	ANKLE-DP	0.59

(*) Indexes use highest
brachial pressure

FIGURE 19–8. A patient with significant stenosis or occlusion at the aortoiliac level as indicated by low high-thigh pressures bilaterally.

Thigh Pressure Indexes

Thigh pressure/higher brachial pressures are normally greater than 1.2, while 0.8–1.2 suggests aortoiliac occlusive disease, and less than 0.8 indicates that proximal occlusion is likely. With the three-cuff technique, the large, single thigh cuff segmental pressure is normally similar to the brachial pressure.

Ankle-Brachial Index

Another component of the arterial lower extremity Doppler examination is the calculation of the ankle-brachial index (ABI). From the ankle and brachial sys-

tolic pressures, a ratio is obtained that is helpful in determining the presence and magnitude of occlusive disease. Since normal lower limbs have ankle pressures equal to or greater than their ipsilateral arm pressures (recorded in a supine position), a ratio of 1.0 or greater is taken as normal. However, mild to moderate atherosclerotic disease may not affect resting ankle pressures significantly, so all persons having an ABI of 1.0 or greater will probably benefit from stress testing, e.g., treadmill exercise as described in detail later.

It is generally agreed upon that an ABI of 0.9–1.0 signifies normalcy or minimal arterial occlusive disease, an ABI of 0.5–0.9 signifies a claudication level, less than 0.5 signifies the presence of ischemic rest pain or severe arterial occlusive disease, and less than 0.3 is compatible with trophic changes of the lower extremity. Some believe that an absolute ankle pressure of less than 50 mm Hg, rather than an ABI of 0.5, is better at predicting symptoms at rest. It has also been suggested that an ABI of equal to or more than 0.5 represents single segment involvement and that lower values are more indicative of multilevel disease.[5]

Technique for Toe Doppler Systolic Pressure

The digital study is often done in combination with a physiological lower extremity arterial test, usually a segmental Doppler pressure with or without Doppler waveform analysis. An appropriately sized cuff, the width of which should be at least 1.2 times that of the toe, is applied to the base of the toe (s). Two 2.5-cm cuffs are usually used for fingers and a 2.5- to 3-cm cuff for the great toe. The digital pulse can be examined using the usual Doppler probe, and a similar technique is applied to measure the Doppler toe pressure.

Normal toe pressures vary from 60% to 80% of the ankle pressures. Values significantly less than this signify digital arterial occlusive disease. The exception to this criteria is when the ankle pressure is artificially high (arterial calcinosis), in which case the toe pressure may be much lower than 80% of the ankle pressure in the absence of digital artery disease. It is generally believed that there is little difference between the toe pressures in diabetics and nondiabetics, which makes toe pressure determination very helpful in patients with very artificially high segmental Doppler pressures at the ankle level.[14]

Limitations and Sources of Error in Doppler Segmental Pressure Determination

1. *Media sclerosis:* This may cause falsely elevated Doppler pressures in those patients with calcified vessels, e.g., patients with diabetes or end-stage renal disease. Toursarkissian et al.[14] reported the results of a

retrospective review of 101 diabetic patients without aortoiliac disease to analyze the ability of various noninvasive tests to predict the level of >50% significant stenosis of intrainguinal arterial disease. Patients were studied with ABI, toe brachial indices (TBI), segmental pulse volume recording (pulse volume recording), segmental pressures, segmental Doppler waveforms, and arteriography. The results were classified as normal, disease at the femoropopliteal level, infrapopliteal level, or both levels (multilevel), or noninterpretable. Their findings showed that as a single test, the Doppler waveform appears to have the best angiographic correlation, although the summed diagnosis of combined Doppler waveform and pulse volume recording data was superior in distinguishing multilevel disease from isolated tibial disease. It was also concluded that segmental Doppler pressures were of limited value in patients with diabetes mellitus, even in multimodality testing.

2. *Hypertension:* When the systemic pressure is elevated, the absolute poststenotic values are also erroneously high. Since there is no linear relationship between the change in the systemic pressure and the peripheral pressure, the measurement should always be repeated after the systemic pressure has normalized.

3. In patients with multilevel occlusive disease it is difficult to interpret segmental pressures.

4. *Measurement of pressure postexercise:* Two examiners should carry out the examination simultaneously after physical exertion to evaluate both extremities, otherwise an adequate rest period between the measurement of the right and left sides is needed. The lower extremity that has the lower resting pressure should be measured first, because the recovery time, postexercise, is otherwise too long in pathological cases.

5. *Edema:* In solid edema, especially lipedema, adequate arterial compression may fail, causing erroneously high pressure values.

6. Patients with uncompensated congestive heart failure may show decreased ankle-brachial indexes after exercise.

7. This test cannot distinguish between stenosis and occlusion, and cannot precisely localize the area of occlusion, although it can identify a general location. Similarly, it cannot distinguish between common femoral artery disease and proximal external iliac artery disease.

8. *Resting period:* An adequate resting period of 10–20 min before measurements are taken must be observed. Where there are poorly compensated flow obstructions, the resting period should be longer, in order to avoid measuring erroneously low pressure values.

9. *Deflation errors:* Releasing the cuff pressure too quickly (above 5 mm Hg per second) causes erroneously low values. Therefore, a deflation velocity of around 2 mm Hg per second should be maintained.

10. *Arm–leg measurement intervals:* The time difference between Doppler pressure measurements should not be too long. Intraindividual systemic blood pressure fluctuations can occur and affect the results.

11. *Subclavian stenosis or occlusion:* The systolic blood pressure values measured in this situation are erroneously low; this may give a false impression of normal circulation of the lower extremities.

12. *Flow velocity in the arteries measured:* If the flow velocity in the arteries that are being measured is too low (less than 6 cm/s), it is not possible to receive a Doppler signal. This phenomenon usually occurs at pressures below 30 mm Hg.

13. *Effect of the girth of the limb:* When the girth of the limb is large in relation to the width of the cuff, the pressure in the cuff may not be transmitted completely to the vessels in the central part of the limb, and the measured pressures may be erroneously exaggerated. Such high false pressures are commonly encountered in the measurement at the level of the thigh.

14. *Effect of vasomotor tone changes:* Changes in the vasomotor tone may affect the arterial pressures. When the blood flow is increased during peripheral vasodilation induced by exercise, heat, or reactive hyperemia, more pressure energy is used in causing flow through stenotic lesions, small distal vessels, and collaterals; therefore distal pressure is reduced. Conversely, when the patient is cool, or when the flow is lower at rest, the pressure tends to be higher. These considerations will explain the normal pressures measured at rest in limbs with mild stenotic lesions and why ankle and digital pressures may be altered significantly by changes in the vasomotor tone. The high tone of the smooth muscle in the wall of the smaller distal vessels of the limbs may result in an artificial reduction of the measured systolic pressure.[15,16]

15. *Stenosis or occlusion in parallel vessels:* When several parallel vessels of comparable size are under the cuff, the measurement will usually reflect the pressure in the artery with the highest pressure and will not detect stenotic or occlusive lesions in the other vessel. Therefore, these measurements will not detect isolated disease in the internal iliac, profunda femoris, tibial, peroneal, ulnar, or individual digital arteries, or interruption of one of the palmer or plantar arches.

Clinical Studies and Results

An analysis of 150 patients (300 limbs) who had both arterial lower extremity Doppler studies (segmental Doppler pressures and analogue wave analysis) and arteriograms was done. Each limb was studied in four arterial segments: 300 iliofemoral, 300 femoral,

TABLE 19–2. Correlation of arterial leg Doppler (ALD) studies and arteriograms in detecting normal arterial segments.

Segment	Normal by ALD	Normal by arteriogram	True-negative	False-negative
Iliofemoral	201	192	96%	4%
Femoral	222	211	95%	5%
Poplitea	187	176	94%	6%
Trifurcation	183	179	98%	2%
Total	793	758	96%	4%

TABLE 19–4. Correlation of arterial leg Doppler (ALD) studies and arteriograms.

Segment	Total segments studied by ALD	Findings confirmed by arteriogram	Accuracy
Iliofemoral	300	282	93%
Femoral	300	280	95%
Popliteal	282	262	94%
Trifurcation	275	262	94%
Total	1157	1086	94%

282 popliteal, and 275 trifurcation segments. Eighteen popliteal and 25 trifurcation segments were excluded for lack of angiographic visualization (not enough dye).

The results are tabulated in Tables 19–2 through 19–4. In the 1157 segments studied, 793 were found to be normal, of which 758 were confirmed by the arteriogram (96% true-negative and 4% false-negative results). The other 35 segments, which were normal by arterial lower extremity Doppler, were found to have mild to moderate atherosclerotic disease. Of the 364 segments interpreted as abnormal by arterial lower extremity Doppler, 328 were confirmed by the arteriogram (90% true-positive and 10% false-positive results). In the other 36 segments, the arteriogram was normal or showed mild disease. Thus, in a total of 1157 segments studied, the findings in 1086 were confirmed by the arteriogram (94% correlation).[17,18]

Selective Use of Segmental Doppler Pressures and Color Duplex Imaging in the Localization of Arterial Occlusive Disease of the Lower Extremity

With the recent advances in noninvasive vascular technology, color duplex imaging (CDI) has become popular in the diagnosis and localization of aortoiliac and femoropopliteal occlusive disease with a very good correlation to angiography.[19–22] However, because of

TABLE 19–3. Correlation of arterial leg Doppler (ALD) studies and arteriograms in detecting abnormal arterial segments.

Segment	Abromal by ALD	Abromal by arteriogram	True-positive	False-positive
Iliofemoral	99	90	90%	10%
Femoral	78	69	88%	12%
Popliteal	95	86	93%	7%
Trifurcation	92	83	90%	10%
Total	364	328	90%	10%

the cost and time involved in performing a CDI of the lower extremity, many vascular laboratories still rely on segmental Doppler pressures to localize arterial occlusive disease, while others still combine both modalities.

In a previously published study,[23] we compared the abilities of segmental Doppler pressures and CDI to accurately categorize the severity of disease. We analyzed 134 patients (268 limbs) who underwent all three tests: segmental Doppler pressures, CDI, and arteriograms. Segmental Doppler pressures and CDI results were examined to determine their accuracy in localizing high grade (>50%) stenosis at three levels: aortoiliac-common femoral artery (Level I), superficial femoral artery (Level II), and popliteal artery (Level III).

The sensitivity, specificity, positive and negative predictive values, and overall accuracy for segmental Doppler pressures and CDI were as follows: Level I— 63%, 88%, 81%, 75%, and 77%; 93% 99%, 98%, 95%, and 96%, respectively ($p < 0.01$); Level II—51%, 99%, 99%, 57%, and 70%; 94%, 98%, 99%, 92%, and 96%, respectively ($p < 0.01$); Level III—55%, 92%, 60%, 90%, and 85%; 78%, 100%, 97%, 95%, and 95%, respectively ($p < 0.01$). There was exact agreement between the CDI and arteriogram in regards to the severity of disease in 88% of the limbs (1170 segments). The presence of superficial femoral artery disease in patients with Level I disease or aortoiliac-common femoral artery disease in patients with Level II disease did not significantly alter the ability of segmental Doppler pressures to localize the disease. The presence of diabetes significantly affected the accuracy of segmental Doppler pressures in localizing superficial femoral and popliteal artery stenosis. An analysis of the ability of segmental Doppler pressure to detect any segment as abnormal, as confirmed by arteriogram, revealed a sensitivity of 88%, specificity of 82%, positive predictive value of 96%, negative predictive value of 60%, and overall accuracy of 87%. We concluded that CDI was superior to segmental Doppler pressures in localizing arterial stenosis at all levels. However, since segmental Doppler pressure is cheaper, it can be used initially if no surgical or endovascular intervention is planned.

Summary

Doppler ultrasound has the advantage of being inexpensive, noninvasive, and easy to perform. Moreover, it can provide valuable information on the functional impairment caused by vascular lesions, a parameter that its invasive cohort, arteriography, cannot do. These characteristics make the ultrasonic technique an ideal test for the serial evaluation of disease progression and for postoperative follow-up study of reconstructive procedures.

Feigelson et al.[24] used the segmental Doppler pressure ratios and flow velocities by Doppler ultrasound to define cases of large vessel peripheral arterial disease. They noted that overall measurement of the posterior tibial flow showed the highest sensitivity, specificity, positive predictive value, negative predictive value, and overall accuracy. In addition, an absent or nonrecordable posterior tibial peak forward flow occurred in 96% of all limbs with isolated posterior tibial disease or an ankle ratio of equal to or less than 0.8 considered in parallel yielded a test with a sensitivity of 89%, specificity of 99%, positive predictive value of 90%, negative predictive value of 99%, and overall accuracy of 98%. They concluded that the majority of large vessel peripheral arterial disease cases can be detected with a single measurement using a hand-held Doppler flowmeter employed at the ankle.

Like most noninvasive vascular tests, the arterial leg Doppler examination has certain limitations. These include falsely high segmental pressure readings in areas with calcified arteries, artificially elevated high-thigh pressure in very large or obese patients, difficulty in interpretation of segmental pressures in patients with multilevel occlusive disease, difficulty in distinguishing occlusive disease in the aortoiliac segment and common femoral artery, interpretive problems for high-thigh pressures in patients with isolated hemodynamically significant superficial femoral and deep femoral occlusive disease, and false-negative results in patients with mild vascular occlusive disease who have normal resting segmental systolic pressures.

In patients with diabetes mellitus or chronic renal failure, the vessels may be heavily calcified, leading to factiously high segmental limb pressures. Since the digital arteries are seldom calcified, an accurate toe pressure can usually be measured in spite of an artificially high pressure proximally. Also, the analogue wave tracing might be abnormal and, thus, helpful in these patients.

Another difficulty in interpreting segmental pressures occurs in patients with multilevel occlusive disease. In these patients, the proximal lesion might mask distal disease, e.g., if both severe aortoiliac occlusive disease and femoral popliteal stenosis are present, the high-thigh pressure is low. The gradient between the high-thigh and the above-knee cuffs might be quite small, thus masking the disease present between these levels. Also giving a low high-thigh pressure is the combination of isolated, hemodynamically significant, superficial femoral and profunda femoris occlusive lesions.

These problems in the interpretation of high-thigh pressure may be solved in one of several ways. A normal femoral pulse and the absence of an iliac bruit suggest a more distal arterial disease as the cause of the low high-thigh pressure. The common femoral artery pressure may also be obtained noninvasively using an inguinal compression device. This pneumatic device presses the artery against the superior pubic ramus, thus allowing the pressure to be measured as the compression is slowly released. The return of the arterial Doppler signal distal to the groin establishes the endpoint. Despite the presence of a normal iliac segment, monophasic waveforms may occasionally be seen in the common femoral artery when there is a combination of superficial femoral artery occlusion and severe deep femoral artery stenosis.

Other methods, which may help in differentiating aortoiliac occlusive disease from disease of the common femoral artery and/or disease of the superficial femoral artery and deep femoral artery, are the determination of the pulsatility index[13] and the inverse damping factor. The amplitude of the Doppler waveform depends on the angle between the ultrasound probe and the axis of blood flow. As the angle of the probe is changed toward zero degrees, the amplitude of the wave increases, although the shape remains unchanged. Velocity can be calculated only if the probe vessel angle can be measured accurately. Unfortunately, this is usually not possible in humans with any reasonable degree of accuracy. Gosling and King[25] have suggested that the pulsatility index is useful and independent of the probe vessel angle in this regard. Several other researchers have found that it is useful for quantifying the Doppler waveform.[26,27]

As previously discussed, the segmental systolic limb pressure alone is somewhat limited in certain patients in localizing vascular occlusive disease. A combination of segmental limb pressure and analog tracing or color duplex imaging is helpful in determining the level of the vascular occlusion. Recently, Gale et al.[28] quantified improvements in accuracy compared with arteriography when ankle pressures alone (ABI) or segmental blood pressures were added to velocity waveforms obtained by Doppler ultrasound. They concluded that ABIs significantly improved Doppler waveform accuracy at all levels. Compared with ABI, the addition of segmental pressure to waveform data failed to improve accuracy.

The Value of Stress Testing in the Diagnosis of Peripheral Arterial Disease

A majority of lower limb arterial studies use Doppler ultrasound to measure the resting ankle pressure. While indicative of the presence and relative magnitude of peripheral arterial occlusive disease, the resting ankle pressure does not always correlate well with the degree of exercise limitation.

The most common complaint of patients with chronic arterial occlusion is intermittent claudication, yet functional disability among patients varies. One patient with a resting ankle pressure of 90 mm Hg may be able to walk two or three blocks before claudicating, while another with a similar ankle pressure may be forced to stop after walking only a block or less. The best functional test of the physiologic impairment associated with arterial occlusive disease is the measurement of the magnitude and duration of fall in ankle pressure following a constant load of exercise. Various methods of producing this constant stress have been used to evaluate the functional disability of patients with claudication, e.g., treadmill exercise, reactive hyperemia, and isolated leg exercises.[25–34] The two most commonly used methods are treadmill exercise and reactive hyperemia.

Treadmill Exercise

Patients with advanced arterial ischemia can be adequately evaluated by simply measuring the resting ankle pressure. However, an early lesion might not lower the resting ankle pressure enough to be detected by the usual methods. For example, a patient with typical claudication has normal or borderline resting ankle pressure. More accurate evaluation can be obtained by increasing the flow through exercise and exertion, thereby accentuating the hemodynamic affect of the stenosis.

Exercise testing can also isolate a patient's primary limitation when the patient complains of a combination of symptoms such as claudication and shortness of breath. If the symptoms are due to pulmonary disability, arterial reconstruction will not be of benefit. Further, exercise testing is useful in distinguishing true claudication from pseudoclaudication caused by neurologic or musculoskeletal conditions or venous insufficiency. It can also weed out suspected malingerers.

Treadmill exercise is preferred over reactive hyperemia because it produces physiological stress that reproduces the patient's ischemic symptoms. However, treadmill testing has the following limitations and/or contraindications: hypertension, shortness of breath, cardiac problems, stroke, or difficulty in walking.

Technique

The resting arm and ankle Doppler pressure are initially recorded with the patient in the supine position. The posterior tibial and dorsalis pedis systolic pressures are taken, and the highest reading is used as the ankle pressure. The ABI is then calculated. The treadmill exercise is done at 2 mph on a 12% grade for 5 min or less, if not tolerated by the patient because of claudication. The ankle and arm pressures are recorded immediately following the test and every minute thereafter for up to 20 min until the pressure returns to the preexercise level.

Electrocardiographic monitoring during the treadmill test is controversial. However, the majority of researchers agree that ECG monitoring is essential for patients who are more than 50 years of age or who have symptoms of heart disease, e.g., angina, myocardial infarction, congestive heart failure, and cardiac arrhythmias. Carroll et al. found that 11% of their patients had to stop the exercise because of ECG changes—5% excessive heart rate, 5% premature ventricular contractions, and 1% ST segment depression.[32]

Normally, an increase in the pressure is noted after exercise in healthy individuals and a drop in the pressure is noted in patients with peripheral vascular disease.

Interpretation

The time it takes for recovery, the symptoms that are experienced during exercise, and the pressure changes, if any, from pre- to postexercise status form the basis for interpretation of this test. Doppler ankle pressures that drop to low or unrecordable levels immediately following treadmill exercise and increase to resting level in 2–5 min suggest occlusion at a single level. Meanwhile, when ankle pressures remain reduced or unrecordable for up to 12 min, multilevel occlusions are usually present. Patients with severe or advanced peripheral vascular disease, e.g., with ischemic rest pain, may have unrecordable postexercise Doppler ankle pressure for 15–20 min.

Clinical Studies

From a cohort of 1000 arterial Doppler studies performed on 1000 patients (2000 limbs) at the Charleston Division of West Virginia University Medical Center, Charleston, West Virginia, 280 patients (560 limbs) who had resting arterial lower extremity Doppler (ALD) studies and arteriograms were selected. One hundred and twenty-four of these limbs had resting and exercise lower extremity Doppler studies and arteriograms. The Doppler technique described previously was used to measure the resting ankle pressure and the exercise ankle pressure and to calculate the ABI.

To facilitate the correlation, the findings on the arteriograms were classified as normal, mild (<30% stenosis), moderate (30–60% stenosis), severe (>60% stenosis), or occluded. The 124 limbs studied included 46 limbs with occluded arteries, 23 limbs with severe stenoses, 10 limbs with moderate disease, 11 limbs with mild disease, and 34 normal limbs.

The majority of normal limbs or limbs with mild disease had a resting ABI of 0.90 or greater. However, a significant number of patients with severe disease (11 out of 23) or with occluded arteries (8 out of 46) also had a resting index of 0.90 or above. After the treadmill test, most of the severely diseased limbs had a significant drop in the ABI.

After treadmill exercise, all patients with normal limbs had an exercise index above 0.90, signifying excellent correlation between the tests. In comparing patient symptoms to the exercise index, none of the patients with rest pain had an index greater than 0.59. However, 80 limbs out of 101 with claudication had an index greater than 0.59. Ninety-one percent of patients with resting pain had an exercise index less than 0.50 (21 out of 23), and 92% of patients with claudication had an exercise index greater than 0.50% (93 out of 101).

Test of Functional Capacity

The best functional evaluation of physiologic impairment associated with arterial occlusive disease is the measurement of the magnitude and duration of fall in the ankle pressure following the constant load treadmill exercise test. Table 19–5 presents the readings in a patient with resting right ankle pressure of 180 mm Hg and left ankle pressure of 130 mm Hg. After exercising on the treadmill for 5 min, the right ankle pressure remained above 180 mm Hg, while the left ankle pressure dropped to 50 mm Hg. It took 20 min for the left pressure to return to 130 mm Hg, indicating severely compromising arterial disease.

TABLE 19–5. Segmental pressure readings (mm Hg) and ankle-brachial index after exercise in a patient with severe peripheral vascular occlusive disease of the left leg.

Postexercise (min)	Right ankle (normal)	Left ankle (abnormal)	Arm
1	186	50	180
2	186	58	180
4	180	60	176
6	180	70	170
10	166	78	160
15	170	90	162
20	170	130	162
Ankle-brachial index	(186/180) 1.03	(50/180) 0.27	

Although the ankle pressure response provides physiologic information about the severity of peripheral arterial occlusive disease, it does not pinpoint the location of the arterial obstruction. Strandness and Bell noted that the location of disease had an effect on the magnitude of the pressure drop and the time required for the pressure to return to baseline.[30] Pressure drops following exercise indicate that the obstruction involves the arteries supplying the gastrocnemius and soleus muscles. A large portion of the blood supply to these muscles is derived from the sural arteries, which originate from the popliteal artery; hence, a drop in the ankle pressure following exercise signifies an obstruction of the upper popliteal or superficial femoral arteries or a more proximal vessel. When the obstruction is confined to vessels below the knee, exercise seldom causes claudication or a significant drop in ankle pressure; in fact, the pressure may even rise.

In general, the more proximal the occlusive disease, the more effect it has on the ankle pressure response to exercise. For example, an isolated aortoiliac lesion usually has more functional significance than a lesion confined to the superficial femoral artery. This phenomenon occurs because the more proximal arteries supply a greater muscle mass than do the distal arteries. Consequently, there is more severe and prolonged deviation of blood away from the ankle to the proximal muscle mass.

In patients who have aortoiliac obstruction combined with more distal limb arterial disease, a question of the severity of the aorotiliac disease is frequently raised. If the amplitude of the femoral pulses either at rest or following exercise is reduced, the disease may contribute significantly to the leg symptoms and require correction. However, moderate aortoiliac disease may not significantly affect pulses or high-thigh pressures. Such patients may be candidates for the segmental, reactive hyperemia test.

However, if a low high-thigh pressure is noted on the preexercise examination, the contribution by aortoiliac disease to the total limb ischemia may be evaluated by determining the high-thigh and ankle pressure responses following exercise. Normally, the high-thigh pressure will increase after exertion, but aortoiliac disease may diminish it. The relative drop in high-thigh and ankle pressures provides indices by which the contributions of aortoiliac and more distal arterial obstruction may be assessed.

The capacity for walking itself is not a particularly important indicator, mainly because it is not reproducible.[31] Motivation, pain tolerance, and accompanying symptoms may all affect its duration. It correlates poorly with estimated walk intolerance and with objective hemodynamic measurements. Of more importance is the observation of other symptoms that precede claudication. If a patient stops exercising due to shortness of breath, angina, or hip pain before claudication develops, the ankle pressure response may be small and of little help in isolating lower limb arterial insufficiency.

In conclusion, the three factors evaluated during treadmill exercise testing have to be taken into consideration in determining the severity of the vascular occlusive disease, i.e., the duration of exercise, the maximum drop in the ankle index, and the recovery time (the time required for return to baseline pressures).

Reactive Hyperemia

For some patients, treadmill exercise is not applicable (amputees or persons with musculoskeletal problems) or practical (patients with cardiopulmonary disease or severe claudication), because they cannot perform for a sufficient length of time. In such cases, reactive hyperemia may be used to increase blood flow in the extremities.

To increase blood flow, a thigh cuff is inflated above the systolic pressure (20–30 mm Hg above the brachial pressure) for 3–7 min to produce local circulatory arrest, resulting in hypoxia and local vasodilation. After release of the compression, ankle pressures are taken at 15, 20, or 30 s intervals for 3–6 min, or until the measurements return to reocclusion level. In normal limbs, the ankle pressures immediately decrease to about 80% of the preocclusion levels, but readily rise, reaching 90% levels within 30–60 s. It should be noted that ankle systolic pressures in a normal limb do not decrease after treadmill exercise, whereas a transient pressure decrease in the range of 15–35% does occur at the ankle of normal limbs after reactive hyperemia. In limbs with obstructive arterial occlusive disease, the decrease in pressure coincides well with that seen following exercise, but recovery to resting levels is much faster.[33] The magnitude of the pressure drop depends upon the anatomical extent of the disease process and the degree of functional impairment. Although recovery times are also correlated with the severity of the disease (from less than 1 min to more than 3 min), the correlation is not as good as that given by the maximal depression of the ankle pressure induced by exercise. Patients who have single level disease generally experience less than a 50% drop in the Doppler ankle pressure, whereas patients with multilevel arterial occlusive disease experience a pressure drop of greater than 50%.

To its benefit, the hyperemic stress test is less time-consuming than the treadmill exercise test, and it can be done in the patient's room, using simple inexpensive equipment. Since the duration of calf occlusion can be prescribed and walking time cannot, the stress may be more centralized than that of exercise testing. It is also less dependent upon patient motivation. The major disadvantage of the test is that it cannot duplicate the maximum exercise load of the treadmill, which is the most effective method in detecting small changes. It fails to elicit the patient's symptoms, and it does not identify any cardiopulmonary disability that might actually be more limiting than the arterial insufficiency. The test is also uncomfortable and thigh compression may be hazardous in limbs with femoral popliteal grafts. Finally, rapid pressure measurements are required to get reproducible results.

Other methods of stress testing have been described in the literature. Isolated leg exercises provide a simple form of stress testing for patients who cannot walk satisfactorily on the treadmill because of cardiac, pulmonary, or orthopedic reasons. In the test's simplest form, the patient flexes and extends the ankles repeatedly. Some investigators have used ankle exercise performed against a fixed load, accomplished by having the patient repeatedly rise up and down on the toes.

References

1. Satomura S. Study of flow patterns in peripheral arteries by ultrasonics. J Acoust Soc Jpn 1959;15:151–153.
2. Strandness DE Jr, McCutcheon EP, Rushmer RF. Application of transcutaneous Doppler flow meter in evaluation of occlusive arterial disease. Surg Gynecol Obstet 1966;122:1039–1045.
3. Kirkendall WM, Burton AC, Epstein FH, et al. Recommendation for human blood pressure determinations by sphygmomanometers: Report of sub-committee of the postgraduate education committee, American Heart Association. Circulation 1967;36:980–988.
4. Barnes RW. Noninvasive diagnostic techniques and peripheral vascular disease. Am Heart J 1979;97:241–258.
5. Holland T. Utilizing the ankle brachial index in clinical practice. Ostomy Wound Manage 2002;48:38–40.
6. Adam DJ, Naik J, Hartshorne T, Bello M, London NJ. The diagnosis and management of 689 chronic leg ulcers in a single-visit assessment clinic. Eur J Vasc Endovasc Surg 2003;25:462–468.
7. Carser DG. Do we need to reappraise our method of interpreting the ankle brachial pressure index? J Wound Care 2001;10:59–62.
8. Yao JST, Bergan JJ. Predictability of vascular reactivity to sympathetic ablation. Arch Surg 1973;106:676–680.
9. AbuRahma AF, Robinson PA. Clinical parameters for predicting response to lumbar sympathectomy with severe lower limb ischemia. J Cardiovasc Surg 1990;31:101–106.
10. Barnes RW, Shanik GD, Slaymaker EE. An index of healing of below knee amputation: Leg blood pressure by Doppler ultrasound. Surgery 1976;79:13–20.
11. Sumner DS, Strandness DE Jr. An abnormal finger pulse associated with cold sensitivity. Ann Surg 1972;175:294–298.
12. Barnes RW. Noninvasive assessment of arteriovenous fistula. Angiology 1978;29:691–704.
13. Johnson KW, Maruzzo BC, Kassam M, et al. Methods for obtaining processing and quantifying Doppler blood flow

velocity waveforms. In: Yao JST, Nicolaides AN (eds). *Basic Investigation in Vascular Disease.* London: Churchill Livingstone, Inc., 1981.

14. Toursarkissian B, Mejia A, Smilanich RP, Schoolfield J, Shireman PK, Sykes MT. Noninvasive localization of infrainguinal arterial occlusive disease in diabetics. Ann Vasc Surg 2001;15:73–78.

15. Sawka AM, Carter SA. The effect of temperature on digital systolic pressures in the lower limb in arterial disease. Circulation 1992;85:1097–1101.

16. Carter SA, Tate RB. The effect of body heating and cooling on the ankle and toe systolic pressures in arterial disease. J Vasc Surg 1992;16:148–153.

17. AbuRahma AF, Diethrich EB, Reiling M. Doppler testing in peripheral vascular occlusive disease. Surg Gynecol Obstet 1980;150:26–28.

18. AbuRahma AF, Diethrich EB. Doppler ultrasound in evaluating the localization and severity of peripheral vascular occlusive disease. South Med J 1979;72:1425–1428.

19. Hatsukami TS, Primozich JF, Zierler RE. Color Doppler imaging of infrainguinal arterial occlusive disease. J Vasc Surg 1992;16:527–533.

20. Moneta GL, Yeager RA, Lee RW. Noninvasive localization of arterial occlusive disease: A comparison of segmental Doppler pressures and arterial duplex mapping. J Vasc Surg 1993;17:578–582.

21. Collier P, Wilcox G, Brooks D. Improved patient selection for angioplasty utilizing color Doppler imaging. Am J Surg 1990;160:171–173.

22. Cossman DV, Ellison JE, Wagner WH, *et al.* Comparison of contrast arteriography to arterial mapping with color-flow duplex imaging in the lower extremities. J Vasc Surg 1989;10:522–529.

23. AbuRahma AF, Khan S, Robinson PA. Selective use of segmental Doppler pressures and color duplex imaging in the localization of arterial occlusive disease of the lower extremity. Surgery 1995;118:496–503.

24. Feigelson HS, Criqui MH, Fronek A. Screening for peripheral arterial disease: The sensitivity, specificity, and predictive value of noninvasive tests in a defined population. Am J Epidemiol 1994;140:526–534.

25. Gosling RG, King DH. Continuous wave ultrasound as an alternative and compliment to x-rays in vascular examination. In: Rebeman RS (ed). *Cardiovascular Applications of Ultrasound.* Amsterdam: North Holland Publishers, 1974.

26. Harris PL, Taylor LA, Cave FD, *et al.* The relationship between Doppler ultrasound assessment and angiography in occlusive arterial disease of the lower limbs. Surg Gynecol Obstet 1974;138:911–914.

27. Johnson KW, Cobbold RSC, Kassam M, *et al.* Real time frequency analysis of peripheral arterial Doppler signals. In: Diethrich EB (ed). *Noninvasive Cardiovascular Diagnosis.* Littleton, MA: PSG Publishing, 1980.

28. Gale SS, Scissons RP, Salles-Cunha SX, *et al.* Lower extremity arterial evaluation: Are segmental arterial blood pressures worthwhile? J Vasc Surg 1998;27:831–839.

29. AbuRahma AF. Correlation of the resting and exercise Doppler ankle arm index to the symptomatology and to the angiographic findings. In: Diethrich EB (eds). *Noninvasive Assessment of the Cardiovascular System,* pp. 287–290. Littleton, MA: John Wright-PSG, Inc., 1982,

30. Strandness DE Jr, Bell JW. An evaluation of the hemodynamic response of the claudicating extremity to exercise. Surg Gynecol Obstet 1964;119:1237–1242.

31. Quriel K, McDowell AE, Metz CE, *et al.* Critical evaluation of stress testing in the diagnosis of peripheral vascular disease. Surgery 1982;91:686–693.

32. Carroll RM, Rose HB, Vyden J, *et al.* Cardiac arrhythmias associated with treadmill claudication testing. Surgery 1978;83:284–287.

33. Baker JD, Daix D. Variability of Doppler ankle pressures with arterial occlusive disease: An evaluation of ankle index and brachial ankle gradient. Surgery 1981;89:134–137.

34. Halperin JI. Evaluation of patients with peripheral vascular disease. Thromb Res 2002;106:V303–311.

20
Pulse Volume Recording in the Diagnosis of Peripheral Vascular Disease

Jeffrey K. Raines and Jose I. Almeida

Introduction

The pulse volume recorder (PVR) was introduced by Raines almost 35 years ago in a thesis based on graduate work conducted at the Massachusetts Institute of Technology (MIT), Harvard Medical School and Massachusetts General Hospital.[1] The work was sponsored by the National Institutes of Health. The work built on earlier pioneering efforts by investigators such as T. Winsor[2] and E. Strandness.[3] The research took advantage of major recent advances in electronics, specifically in the area of pressure transducer design. However, the driving force was the increasing ability of the vascular surgeon to reconstruct peripheral arteries and the associated need to perform accurate diagnostic studies preoperatively and in follow-up.

In 1972 Raines, along with R. Darling, B. Brener, and W. Austen, presented the first clinical paper on the PVR at the Annual Meeting of the Society of Vascular Surgery; this was later published in *Surgery*.[4] Earlier that year (in April 1972) this same group of investigators established the first clinically oriented vascular laboratory at the Massachusetts General Hospital. A similar laboratory was established at about the same time at Northwestern's Medical School by Yao and Bergan. Founding these laboratories included obtaining codes for reimbursement from Medicare and other third party insurance carriers. Three years later the early experience of this laboratory was presented at the 1975 Annual Meeting of the Society for Vascular Surgery and again published in *Surgery*.[5] At that time studies within the vascular laboratory were expanding to include functional evaluation of venous disorders and extracranial arterial occlusive disease. At this point many other centers had developed vascular laboratories and began publishing their results.

The early PVR was available in either a box or cart model. The first units also included a built-in continuous-wave Doppler in two frequencies (9 MHz and 5 MHz). Within 5 years of its introduction the PVR became an extremely popular device and was widely used throughout the world. In vascular laboratories its frequency of use was second only to the continuous-wave Doppler systems.

Guidelines for establishing vascular laboratories were published along with accuracy studies comparing noninvasive functional studies with angiography and clinical outcome in the areas of peripheral arterial occlusion,[6-8] deep venous thrombosis,[9-11] and extracranial arterial occlusive disease.[12-14]

In 1978, W. Glenn introduced B-mode ultrasound. The first clinical studies using this technique were performed in the Vascular Laboratory of the Miami Heart Institute, which was directed at that time by Raines, who a number of years earlier introduced the PVR.[15] Within several years B-mode ultrasound was producing images of peripheral arterial and venous vessels that were very useful clinically and augmented information obtained from functional studies. With B-mode ultrasound as a basis, ultrasound engineers developed duplex scanning, color duplex scanning, power duplex imaging, and more recently improved imaging with internal computer enhancement, storage, and image transfer.

Clearly technology in the field of noninvasive medical imaging as applied to peripheral vascular disease has been explosive and has made significant clinical contributions. Despite this, functional studies remain an integral component in the investigation of most forms of peripheral vascular disorders, and functional technology has also kept pace. In the remainder of this chapter a description of how the PVR has been improved over nearly 35 years will be given. This will be followed by descriptions of how the PVR may be used most effectively in today's modern vascular laboratory.

Before closing the introduction it is instructive to note two important items. First, peripheral vascular disease of the elderly and in the United States the elderly is now the fastest growing segment of the population. The Census Bureau estimates this trend is expected to continue to the year 2030.[16] This is compounded by the fact that in the United States over the past 20 years mortality from coronary artery disease has been decreasing. This means that more survivors who would have died of coronary artery disease live to present to the vascular laboratory with peripheral vascular disease.

Second, while there will be increasing pressure to provide services for peripheral vascular disease, medical providers will be asked to do so at less cost. This means more accurate less costly outpatient diagnostic studies coupled with effective, less costly therapy. This is both a challenge and an opportunity for manufacturers of equipment and providers of care in peripheral vascular disease.

Pulse Volume Recorder—2005

As described in the original PVR development work at MIT,[1] to maintain proper system calibration when a PVR cuff is placed on an extremity, the system and operator must inflate the cuff to a known cuff pressure (i.e., 65 mmHg thigh/calf/ankle) and also know the amount of injected atmospheric air necessary to produce the cuff pressure. If the volume of injected air does not meet an

established criterion (i.e., $75 \pm 10\,cm^3$, calf/ankle; $400 \pm 75\,cm^3$, thigh) the operator must reapply the cuff. Whereas a number of manufacturers market PVR-like devices, some do not include this important calibration. These manufacturers have suggested to operators that after cuff application it is necessary to inflate the cuff *only* to the recommended pressure. This assumes each cuff is applied to the same tension despite variation in limb size; we have found results can vary significantly based on operator application and technique. There are manufacturers who provide a good *external* calibration as described above. These systems provide reproducible PVR data that almost eliminate operator application and technique errors. In our laboratory, working with industry, we have developed a computer-controlled *internal* calibration system that is very accurate and completely eliminates cuff reapplication at any level (Figure 20–1).

The ability to record and store data is most important to document testing for both reimbursement and certification purposes. The new PVR systems include patient interface ports (i.e., for PVR cuffs and Doppler probes), color monitor, keyboard, and color printer. Studies may be performed in a dedicated laboratory or at the patient's bedside. It should be acknowledged that when earlier systems were making the transition from non-PC-based to PC-based units, the PC units were slow,

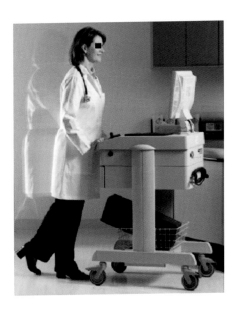

A

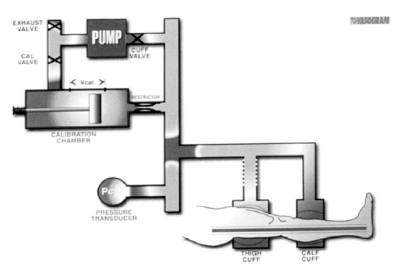

B

FIGURE 20–1. (A) Picture of a prototype *internally* calibrated pulse volume recorder (PVR). This system is controlled by a computer. The operator interfaces with the unit via Keyboard, Joystick, and Monitor. The system also has a dedicated Printer and Modem for report generation. (B) This schematic illustrates how *internal* calibration is accomplished. During the early

phase of diastole, the piston in the calibration chamber rapidly increases the system volume by a known amount. The resultant instantaneous pressure reduction is measured along with the pressure differential from tracing foot to peak. This allows the total volume change to be calculated in near real-time.

difficult for even experienced operators to use, and inflexible. With time, technician input, and fast processors this has changed and the new systems are both rapid and flexible.

In our view the major advantages of current systems over earlier PVR systems are accuracy of calibration, clarity and rapid development of data reporting, and rapid storage and transmission.

The primary purpose of performing any level of vascular laboratory testing is to provide the referring physician with information that will improve patient management. If a rapid, accurate, complete, and understandable report is not generated this is not possible. New PVR systems provide a protocol-like format for general testing, compile the data in a logical sequence, and provide guidelines for interpretation.

We compared the time taken to perform a lower extremity arterial study using a standard PVR with a PC-based PVR. Evaluation time was divided into three components: (1) time to obtain and record demographics, clinical history, and pulse and bruit grading; (2) time to perform 10 PVR arterial tracings and six segmental limb pressures; and (3) time to prepare a final report excluding interpretation. In obtaining background information for the standard PVR, the technician recorded the data on a preprinted form that became part of the final report. The technician entered background information for the PC-based PVR directly into the system via a keyboard. Testing was performed using standard protocols for each system and included PVR tracings at the thigh, calf, ankle, metatarsal (TM), and first digital levels bilaterally and limb systolic pressures bilaterally by Doppler technique at the thigh, calf, and ankle levels. Using the standard PVR, the technician had to cut three cardiac cycles from the PVR strip charts and using tape affix them to the final report. For the PC-based system the technician electronically selects cycles for reporting and printing. This latter area is where the PC-based system is clearly faster (Table 20–1).

PVR vascular technicians not familiar with the PC-based systems require approximately 3 h of formal training to perform the testing and an additional 10 h of use to obtain the skills to perform the testing at the same degree of speed and confidence obtained by experienced workers.

Indications and Guidelines for Functional Lower Extremity Arterial Studies

Diagnostic technique and therapeutic methods for peripheral vascular disease have changed significantly since the development of the PVR. However, the questions posed to the vascular laboratory by referring physicians have not changed. These include the following:

1. Is resting ischemia present?
2. Is current perfusion adequate for lesion healing?
3. Will a particular amputation site heal properly?
4. Is vascular claudication present?

Further, for all of the above questions there is an associated interest in describing as accurately as possible the anatomic location of hemodynamically significant lesions. However, it should be carefully noted that while these are the important questions in over 90% of patients referred to a vascular laboratory for lower extremity occlusion, these questions *cannot* be answered by knowing the anatomy. These are purely questions of function. Later we will discuss questions primarily of anatomy.

Before proceeding, it is helpful to describe the patient population presenting to our vascular laboratory. We have carefully reviewed our patient demographics and when possible have compared our figures with those of other vascular laboratories; in most cases the numbers have been very similar. The average age of our patients is 67 years. Two-thirds are male. Over 75% are current or past cigarette smokers. Approximately 40% have a history of hypertension and 25% are diabetic. Approximately 20% have elevated blood lipids and 20–25% are obese by routine criteria. In our series one-third have had a previous myocardial infarction and one-tenth (9%) have a history of previous cerebrovascular accident.

TABLE 20–1. Time taken to perform lower extremity arterial study using a standard pulse volume recorder (PVR) and a PC-based PVR.

Component	Standard PVR (min)	PC-based PVR (min)
Background	11	11
Testing	18	20
Report	10	4
Total ($n = 10$)	39	35

Is Resting Ischemia Present?

Patients with rest pain as their *initial* presentation may be either diabetic or nondiabetic; however, nondiabetics are more frequent in this category as will be described. Their description of pain will also almost exclusively be limited to the forefoot. The pain will develop at rest and will transiently be relieved by dangling the foot. This temporarily decreases the local peripheral resistance, increasing local blood flow. Although ischemia pain may present more proximally, more proximal resting pain in the absence of forefoot pain is often not of vascular origin. Since ischemia is a clear indication for surgical reconstruction, its diagnosis must be made with accuracy.

In making this judgment the following four parameters, in the limb of interest, must be obtained carefully with a PVR at the correct pneumatic gain settings:

PVR amplitude and contour at the ankle level.
PVR amplitude and contour at the TM level.
PVR amplitude and contour at the first digit or most symptomatic digit.
Ankle pressure.

If the ankle pressure is <40mm Hg in the nondiabetic patient or <60mm Hg in the diabetic patient *resting ischemia may be present*. The difference in criteria is based on the fact that diabetics often have medial calcinosis that artificially elevates distal pressures. It should also be stated that in 10–15% of diabetic cases distal pressures cannot be measured at all, due to medial calcinosis; in these cases PVR recordings are the only measurements available.

The diagnosis is secured on the basis of the amplitude of the PVR tracings. If a digit of interest has a flatline PVR amplitude, ischemia is very probable. The probability is further increased if the TM and ankle PVR tracings are also flatline or near flatline. It is not hemodynamically possible to have a flatline tracing proximal to a nonflatline tracing. If this occurs, the operator should look for a technical error in the testing. In the ischemic setting all tracings should be markedly blunted with no reflected wave present in diastole.

It is possible to have transient borderline ischemia with digital amplitudes as high as 2mm; however, this is rare.

Is Current Perfusion Adequate for Lesion Healing?

Ischemic arterial lesions are almost always present at the digit or near digit levels. More proximal foot lesions (i.e., TM level or heel) are most often secondary to a degree of ischemia *and* chronic trauma (pressure ulceration). In this class of patients the initial presenters include a higher percentage of diabetics than in the rest pain group. This is due to the clinically recognized fact that diabetic patients are more prone to develop traumatic lesions due to neuropathic loss of sensation and combined large and small vessel involvement.[5]

TABLE 20–2. Guidelines for determining whether current perfusion is adequate for healing.

	Nondiabetic	Diabetic
Ankle pressure (mm Hg)	≥60	≥70
Pulse volume recorder amplitude in digit of interest (mm)	≥1	≥2

As in the rest pain case, in making this judgment the following four parameters in the limb of interest must be obtained carefully with a PVR at the correct pneumatic gain settings:

PVR amplitude and contour at the ankle level.
PVR amplitude and contour at the TM level.
PVR amplitude and contour at the first digit or most symptomatic digit.

Ankle Pressure

Hemodynamics indicates that local perfusion is a function of mean arterial pressure (MAP), mean venous pressure (MVP), and size and number of perfusion vessels. We use systolic pressure as a surrogate for MAP; MVP in a supine subject is near 0mm Hg and PVR amplitude can be shown to be an adequate surrogate for size and number of perfusing vessels. Table 20–2 is a helpful guideline in determining whether a lesion will heal with the current level of perfusion in the absence of infection, chronic trauma, and microvessel diabetic disease. These stipulations are significant and require a degree of clinical judgment.

Will a Particular Amputation Site Heal Primarily?

There is a sizable group of patients with advanced arteriosclerotic peripheral vascular disease in whom arterial reconstruction is not possible and who come to amputation. Significant morbidity and mortality rates are present in these patients, particularly in those in whom a more distal amputation fails and who require a second procedure. Measurements in a vascular laboratory with a PVR are helpful in reducing this complication by predicting which amputation site is most likely to heal primarily.

There are four major lower extremity amputations that can be addressed by these measurements. The functional noninvasive measurements necessary for determining amputation site healing potential are a function of the

TABLE 20–3. Guidelines for amputation site healing (applicable to diabetic and nondiabetic patients).

Site	Thigh	Calf	Ankle	TM	Digital
Above-knee (AK)	≥2 mm ≥50 mm Hg	NA	NA	NA	NA
Below-knee (BK)	NA	≥1 mm ≥50 mm Hg	NA	NA	NA
TM	NA	NA	≥40 mm Hg	≥1 mm	NA
Digital	NA	NA	≥50 mm Hg	≥1 mm	≥1 mm

site. Table 20–3 gives guidelines for amputation site healing that are applicable to the diabetic and nondiabetic patient.

Is Vascular Claudication Present?

Patients in the age range associated with peripheral vascular disease often present with lower extremity pain on exertion. It is important to distinguish symptoms due to neurologic or orthopedic processes from those produced by vascular insufficiency. In fact, both entities may coexist. With vascular insufficiency it is also important to determine accurately the patient's degree of disability and to establish a quantitative baseline with which the results of medical or surgical treatment can be compared.

In our experience the presence of vascular claudication and its associated degree of disability cannot accurately be determined from history/physical examination *or hemodynamic measurements taken at rest.* We have therefore evaluated various methods of stressing vascular patients and have determined that a small treadmill operating at a fixed grade of 10% at either 1.5 mph (2.4 km/h) or 2.25 mph (3.6 km/h)—choice of speed being a function of the subject's ability—is the most physiologic and is tolerated by the largest percentage of vascular patients. Following resting studies, we determine on the treadmill what we call maximum walking time (MWT). MWT is the point at which the patient experiences a rapid increase in symptoms. This develops between the initial onset of pain and the point at which the patient can no longer continue. This point has consistently been reproducible. We have *not* found that following PVR amplitudes and/or limb pressures beyond the immediate postexercise measurement are helpful in making the diagnosis more secure.

The guideline we use to establish vascular claudication is a postexercise ankle pressure of <70 mm Hg and an ankle PVR amplitude of <5 mm. Note that this criterion represents significant hemodynamic alteration and that it is therefore possible to have significant anatomic disease that does not produce symptoms even with exertion.

Due to the fact that many investigators use the ankle/arm (ankle/brachial) index as a guideline it deserves mention.[17] We have found the ankle/arm index is helpful in determining the degree of arterial occlusion from the aortic root to the ankle, but it is of far less value than absolute values in criteria associated with resting and exertional vascular insufficiency.

Location of Arterial Obstruction in the Lower Extremities

As mentioned in the beginning of this section, the major questions to be addressed in the vascular laboratory are functional. However, with attention to detail, hemodynamic studies can also localize the major levels of arterial obstruction. The following guidelines are helpful in the anatomical localization of arterial lesions in the lower extremity.

Pulse Volume Recorder Reflected Wave

The contour of a PVR tracing is closely associated with the intraarterial pressure contour. If at rest the reflected wave is absent, this implies the peripheral resistance distal to the point at which the tracing was taken has been reduced. Reduction in peripheral resistance is most often caused by proximal arterial obstruction.

Of course, reduced peripheral resistance and loss of PVR reflected wave are expected following exercise (Figure 20–2).

Pulse Volume Recorder Amplitude

The greater the PVR amplitude, the greater the local pulsatile component of total flow rate (Qp). Generally, Qp tracks total flow. Further, PVR amplitude is a function of local pulse pressure and pulse pressure is reduced with arterial occlusion proximal to the point at which the tracing is taken. Therefore, the more reduced the PVR amplitude the greater the proximal obstruction and the poorer the local perfusion.

PULSE VOLUME RECORDINGS*

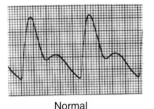 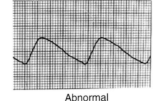

Normal   Abnormal

*Ankle Level
Cuff Pressure – 65 mm Hg
Cuff Volume – 75 cc

FIGURE 20–2. Normal PVR tracings illustrate rapid rise and fall during systole and the presence of a clear reflected wave in early diastole. When proximal arterial obstruction is present, PVR amplitude (foot to peak) is reduced and the reflected wave is absent.

Pulse Volume Recorder Amplitude Relationships

When PVR tracings are properly calibrated, with an open superficial femoral artery, the PVR calf amplitude is always increased when compared with the thigh and ankle amplitudes. If this is not the case a superficial femoral artery occlusion should be expected. If the PVR tracing at the thigh level is normal with an open aortoiliac system, and the calf PVR tracing amplitude does not augment, an occlusion at the level of Hunter's canal should be suspected.

If the contours of the thigh, calf, and ankle tracings are abnormal (i.e., loss of reflected wave, amplitude reduction) but the calf amplitude is augmented compared with the thigh, this suggests aortoiliac disease with an open superficial femoral/popliteal system.

Whenever there is an abrupt change in PVR amplitude and contour from a proximal measurement to the next segment (i.e., calf to ankle; ankle to TM; TM to digit) occlusion between the two levels should be suspected.

Postexercise Measurements

Exercise testing is very helpful in both localizing arterial lesions and determining exercise-related symptoms such as claudication. This has been mentioned previously. Aortoiliac disease produces symptoms in the calf, thigh, and finally in the buttock if exercise is continued. Superficial femoral artery occlusions produce symptoms at the calf level and do not rise to the buttock level. Further, significant aortoiliac disease always produces flatline ankle PVR amplitudes after exercise.

Superficial femoral artery occlusions reduce postexercise ankle PVR amplitude, but a flatline tracing is rarely seen without proximal involvement.

Segmental Systolic Limb Pressures

Segmental systolic limb pressures should always be taken bilaterally at the thigh, calf, and ankle levels and compared with the highest brachial pressure. In a normal arterial system the distal systolic pressures should be slightly higher than the brachial value. When there is a reduction of >20 mm Hg between segments, arterial obstruction between segments should be suspected.

It is important to note that often PVR results and systolic limb pressures are supportive. However, since they are derived from different hemodynamic principles they may differ. It is a good rule of thumb to consider PVR findings more representative of local perfusion and systolic limb pressures more representative of the degree of native vessel occlusion.

Role of Lower Extremity Arterial Imaging

Clearly over the past 30 years the ability to image accurately vessels in the lower extremities and measure local velocities with ultrasound has improved dramatically. What has not changed is the *inability* of ultrasound to address the functional questions of ischemia, perfusion, amputation site healing, and the presence of vascular claudication. For this reason the importance of functional hemodynamic measures should not be lost as our abilities to image continues to improve. Having said that, there are several areas in which lower extremity arterial ultrasound is crucial.

Imaging Improves Anatomic Localization

In the best of hands the localization criteria described above have an overall accuracy in multilevel disease of 90%. By definition, the ability to directly image obstruction at the aortoiliac and superficial femoral/popliteal systems can improve this accuracy and should be used in cases of multilevel disease and/or where anatomic considerations are of major importance.

Graft Surveillance

Vascular grafts placed in lower extremities may occlude acutely or fail over an extended period of time. It is known that grafts in which corrections are made before total occlusions develop have a greater overall patency.

Minor changes in graft diameter (area) secondary to an obstructive process may not produce significant hemodynamic changes, but may be identified by abnormalities in graft appearance. This is most often true at anastomotic sites.

Aneurysmal Disease

Functional studies in only selected situations are helpful in identifying femoral or popliteal aneurysms and are never able to measure the size of an aneurysm. In contrast, ultrasound can be used very effectively to identify, measure, and follow femoral and popliteal aneurysms.

Indications and Guidelines for Functional Lower Extremity Venous Studies

In the previous section we stated that the average age of patients presenting to a vascular laboratory for lower extremity arterial disease is 67 years, with 75% being male. For venous disease the age is two decades younger and the majority of patients are female.

In the era of the modern vascular laboratory, lower extremity hemodynamic measurements were first made in the arterial system and expanded to the venous system. For many years, the major question posed to vascular laboratories in the area of venous disease by referring physicians has been: is deep venous thrombosis (DVT) present? The second most frequently asked question has been: is venous vascular insufficiency present? It should be acknowledged that duplex ultrasound has replaced other hemodynamic measurements in most modern vascular laboratories. Ultrasound has become the "gold standard" in the diagnosis of extremity DVT and in determining superficial venous system incompetence. The role of the PVR in these settings has been reduced to situations in which detailed knowledge of deep venous resistance is required. This use is described below.

Is Deep Venous Thrombosis Present?

In 1975 Raines produced a monograph entitled *Application of the Pulse Volume Recorder for Noninvasive Diagnosis of Deep Vein Thrombosis.*[18] This work suggested the measurement of two parameters described as maximum venous outflow (MVO) and segmental venous capacitance (SVC). This investigation was performed at the Massachusetts General Hospital and involved developing a scoring system for DVT using MVO, SVC, venous respiratory waves, and Doppler ultrasound at the femoral and popliteal venous levels. The noninvasive measurements were compared with venography. The details of this work have been published many times and will not be repeated here. The work was also duplicated by many investigators and published extensively.[9–11] Some published studies using this technique have reported a sensitivity as high as 96% with a specificity of 90%.[11] In the author's hands for DVT excluding minor nonextending calf thrombi, the sensitivity has been 95% with an 85% specificity when compared with venography.[19]

The modern PVR completely automates the measures of MVO and SVC. Further, the system allows the determination of venous respiratory waves and venous velocity measurements. These data are input to the system and a color report is generated; this report includes the scoring system described above. This information is obtained in less that 30 min with the patient supine on an examining table. This functional method is extremely useful in making a rapid and safe assessment of DVT and is also helpful in determining the degree of hemodynamic venous obstruction present, which correlates with degree of expected valvular damage.

DVT can lead to acute death. For that reason alone, the diagnosis cannot be taken lightly. We have described accurate functional diagnostic studies. However, today all subjects suspected of having DVT should undergo a vascular laboratory examination that includes venous imaging. The vascular technologist should look for deep venous obstruction in the veins of the lower extremities. In the early stages of DVT this is often characterized by noncompressibility of the venous structures.

Is Venous Valvular Insufficiency Present?

The major hemodynamic culprit in venous valvular insufficiency is venous ambulatory hypertension. In the senior author's laboratory, before the development of photoplethysmography, measurements of venous ambulatory hypertension were taken using a needle in a subject's foot connected to a fluid column. Many PVR systems now include an easy-to-use photoplethysmograph that quickly allows the determination of venous valvular insufficiency at the deep and superficial levels. Details have been published and will not be repeated here.[19]

Functional Studies of the Upper Extremities

Upper Extremity Arterial Studies

Assessment of the upper extremity arterial system can be performed with the PVR. PVR and limb pressures may be obtained in the upper arm, forearm, and digital levels. These measurements give a clear indication as to the location and degree of compromise associated with the upper extremity. Atherosclerosis in the upper extremities in comparison with the lower extremities is relatively rare. However, obstruction due to catheter injury and trauma are common. Vasospastic disease also generates patients for this investigation.

Miscellaneous Studies

The PVR can perform abbreviated protocols for a number of miscellaneous studies. These include upper extremity measurements for thoracic outlet syndrome and vasospastic studies for Raynaud's disease or scleroderma. In the lower extremity, miscellaneous studies may be performed for popliteal entrapment syndrome and arteriovenous and venovenous malformations. PVR and Doppler measurements are also used in the evaluation of male impotence.

References

1. Raines JK. Diagnosis and analysis of arteriosclerosis in the lower limbs from the arterial pressure pulse. Ph.D. thesis, Massachusetts Institute of Technology, Cambridge, 1972.
2. Winsor T, Hyman C. *A Primer of Peripheral Vascular Disease.* Philadelphia: Lea & Febiger, 1965.
3. Strandness DE Jr. *Peripheral Arterial Disease.* Boston: Little Brown, 1969.
4. Darling RC, Raines JK, Brener BJ, Austen WG. Quantitative segmental pulse volume recorder: A clinical tool. Surgery 1972;72:873–887.
5. Raines JR, Darling RC, Buth J, Brewster DC, Austen WG. Vascular laboratory criteria for the management of peripheral vascular disease of the lower extremities. Surgery 1976;79:21–29.
6. Rutherford RB, Lowenstein DH, Klein MF. Combining segmental systolic pressures and plethysmography to diagnose arterial occlusive disease of the legs. Am J Sur 1979;138:211–218.
7. Raines J, Larsen PB. Practical guidelines for establishing a clinical vascular laboratory. Cardiovasc Dis Bull Texas Heart Inst 1979;6:93–123.
8. Barringer M, Poole GV, Shircliffe AC, Meredith JW, Hightower F, Plonk GW. The diagnosis of aortoiliac disease. Ann Surg 1983;197:204–209.
9. Sufian S. Noninvasive vascular laboratory diagnosis of deep venous thrombosis. Am Surg 1981;47:254–258.
10. van Rijn ABB, Heller I, Van Zijl J. Segmental air plethysmography in the diagnosis of deep vein thrombosis. Surgery 1987;165:488–490.
11. Naidich JB, Feinberg AW, Karp-Harman H, Karmel MI, Tyma CG, Stein HL. Contrast venography: Reassessment of its role. Radiology 1988;168:97–100.
12. Raines J, Schlaen H, Brewster DC, Abbott WM, Darling RC. Experience with a non-invasive evaluation for cerebral vascular disease. Angiology 1979;30:600–609.
13. Kempczinski RF. A combined approach to the non-invasive diagnosis of carotid artery occlusive disease. Surgery 1979;85:689–694.
14. Berkowitz HD. Diagnostic accuracy of ocular pneumoplethysmography attachment for pulse volume recorder. Arch Surg 1980;115:190–193.
15. Hashway T, Raines JK. Real-time ultrasonic imaging of the peripheral arteries: Technique, normal anatomy and pathology. Cardiovasc Dis 1980;7:257–264.
16. United States Population Projections. Bureau of the Census 1993;23–178.
17. Yao ST, Hobbs JT, Irvine WT. Ankle systolic pressure measurements in arterial disease affecting the extremities. Br J Surg 1969;56:677.
18. Raines JK. Application of the pulse volume recorder for non-invasive diagnosis of deep venous thrombosis [monograph]. Life Sciences, 1975.
19. Abramowitz HB, Queral LA, Finn WR, et al. The use of photoplethysmography in the assessment of venous insufficiency: A comparison to venous pressure measurements. Surgery 1979;86:434.

21
Duplex Scanning for Lower Extremity Arterial Disease

Paul A. Armstrong and Dennis F. Bandyk

Introduction

An accurate diagnosis of lower extremity peripheral artery disease (PAD) can usually be established based on the clinical history, vascular examination including pulse palpation, and Doppler survey of the femoral and pedal arteries. With the development of symptomatic PAD, i.e., disabling claudication, critical limb ischemia (ischemic rest pain, tissue loss), or peripheral aneurysmal disease, more detailed vascular testing is necessary for disease management. Peripheral arterial testing is best performed in an accredited facility by certified technical personnel and physicians experienced in test interpretation. Measurement of limb blood pressure in conjunction with duplex mapping of the arterial tree should be performed to assess disease location and severity. Duplex ultrasound scanning provides hemodynamic and anatomic information at no risk to the patient and ensures an accurate diagnosis.[1-4] Based on disease location and morphology, a decision to proceed with endovascular or surgical intervention is possible.[5-9] Other vascular imaging modalities [contrast arteriography, computed tomography (CT) angiography, magnetic resonance angiography (MRA)] do not provide hemodynamic information essential for the evaluation of symptomatic PAD, and formulating an individualized treatment plan.

The versatility of duplex testing allows its use in all phases of disease management, including diagnosis, intraprocedural assessment, and surveillance for residual or recurrent stenosis. Often, the improvement in PAD symptoms can often be accomplished using less invasive endovascular techniques making duplex detection of appropriate lesions important. When duplex ultrasound is used in conjunction with Doppler-derived pressure measurements, i.e., ankle-brachial index (ABI), the need for a catheter-based diagnostic contrast angiogram can be obviated.[9-13] A high-quality peripheral duplex scan is diagnostic in the majority of PAD patients, and provides sufficient information to recommend and proceed with either endovascular or surgical intervention (Table 21–1). Other arterial lesions important in patient care can also be addressed such as concomitant extracranial carotid stenosis, associated aneurysmal disease, and the presence of an adequate lower limb (saphenous, femoral-popliteal) or arm (cephalic, basilica) vein for arterial bypass grafting.

Preintervention Arterial Testing

The extent of peripheral arterial testing should be individualized based on patient symptoms, signs of limb ischemia, and other physical findings (swelling, ulceration, gangrene, pulsatile masses). The presence and severity of lower limb occlusive disease should be evaluated by performing segmental pressure measurements in combination with Doppler or plethysmographic (pulse volume) waveform analysis (Figure 21–1). Measurement of toe systolic pressure is especially helpful in the evaluation of diabetic patients in whom calcified, incompressible tibial vessels may produce erroneously high (>1.3) ABI in the presence of significant occlusive disease. Patients with atypical exertion leg pain and an abnormal ABI (<0.90) should undergo exercise treadmill testing with assessment of ankle systolic pressure reduction in response to walking to verify or exclude vascular claudication. Other indications for peripheral arterial testing, including absent pulses, disabling claudication, ulceration, gangrene, or rest pain, should prompt a color duplex examination to characterize disease location, morphology (atherosclerosis, aneurysm), severity, and extent. Duplex testing can also identify other relevant concomitant vascular conditions (renal artery stenosis, abdominal or peripheral aneurysm, venous thrombosis).

Duplex scanning is used to detect and classify disease (occlusive, aneurysmal) in the aortoiliac, femoropopliteal, and popliteal-tibial arterial segments.[2-4,10-13] Multilevel disease is commonplace and should be expected when

TABLE 21–1. Interventional options based on color duplex scan findings.

Duplex diagnosis	Endovascular	Surgery
Aortoiliac lesions		
Focal stenosis	Stent	Endarterectomy
Diffuse disease	Stent	Aortofemoral bypass
	Subintimal angioplasty	Femorofemoral bypass
Infrainguinal lesions		
Femoropopliteal segment		
Common femoral	—	Endarterectomy
Profunda femoris		Patch angioplasty
Superficial femoral	Balloon angioplasty	Endarterectomy
	(cryoplasty balloon)	Patch angioplasty
	(cutting balloon)	Interposition graft
	Atherectomy	Bypass reconstruction
Popliteal aneurysm	Stent-graft	Exclusion with bypass
		Interposition grafting
Pseudoaneurysm		
Iatrogenic	Ultrasound-guided thrombin injection	Surgical repair
Graft	Covered stent	Interposition graft
Arteriovenous fistula	Embolization	Surgical repair
Vein graft stenosis	Balloon angioplasty	Surgical revision

scanning patients with critical limb ischemia. Accepted clinical applications for duplex scanning include the following:

- The evaluation of symptomatic patients with abnormal (<0.9) ABIs to identify occlusive lesions amenable to endovascular intervention, e.g., percutaneous transluminal angioplasty (PTA), or surgical bypass.

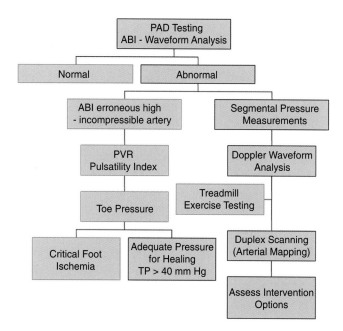

FIGURE 21–1. Vascular laboratory evaluation of peripheral artery disease by ankle-brachial index (ABI), Doppler waveform analysis, pulse volume recordings (PVR), digit pressures, exercise testing, and duplex arterial mapping to assess intervention options.

- The assessment of femoral artery catheterization sites for pseudoaneurysm.
- The exclusion of occult inflow (aortoiliac) disease in patients requiring lower limb femoral-distal bypass grafting.
- The evaluation of the hemodynamics of specific diseased arterial segments visualized on diagnostic arteriography when clinical significance is ambiguous.
- The provision of arterial imaging to avoid angiographic contrast exposure in patients with renal insufficiency.
- The identification of peripheral lesions causing atheroembolism, i.e., blue toe syndrome.
- The evaluation of vascular (arterial, venous) injury following blunt and penetrating limb trauma.
- The surveillance of arterial bypass grafts or reconstructions, endovascular angioplasty, or dialysis access for stenosis, caused by myointimal hyperplasia, fibrosis, or atherosclerosis.

The accuracy of duplex scanning is sufficient to permit arterial mapping analogous to contrast arteriography in body regions accessible to diagnostic ultrasound imaging. Classification of lesion severity is based on the same physical principles that apply to the duplex evaluation of cerebrovascular, renal, and mesenteric circulations. Compared to arteriography, the "gold standard" for peripheral arterial imaging, duplex scanning has a diagnostic accuracy of >80% for the detection of a >50% diameter reducing stenoses or occlusion (Table 21–2).[1,2,4,7–9] Diagnostic accuracy decreases when multilevel disease is present. In the absence of multilevel disease, diagnostic accuracy exceeds 90% for the detection of high-grade stenosis or occlusion involving iliac, femoral, popliteal, or tibial arterial segments. In more than 50% of patients with symptomatic PAD, duplex scanning will identify disease

TABLE 21–2. Diagnostic accuracy (sensitivity/specificity) of color duplex ultrasonography compared with contrast arteriography or magnetic resonance angiography for hemodynamically significant lesions.[a]

Author	IA	CFA	DFA	SFA	Pop	Tib
Cossman et al.[1,b]	81/98	70/97	71/95	97/92	78/97	50/8
Moneta et al.[2,b]	89/99	76/99	83/97	87/98	67/99	90/2
Allard et al.[4,b]	84/97	36/98	44/97	92/96	37/92	—
Kohler et al.[6,b]	89/90	67/98	67/81	84/93	73/97	—

	Aortoiliac	Femoropopliteal	Tibial
Hingorani et al.[16,c]	81/84	75/90	43/65

[a]IA, iliac artery; CFA, common femoral artery; DFA, deep femoris artery; SFA, superficial femoral artery; Pop, popliteal artery; Tib, tibial arteries.
[b]Contrast angiography.
[c]Magnetic resonance angiography.

amenable to endovascular therapy.[9,13] Duplex imaging to plan infrainguinal bypass procedures for occlusive disease has also been studied in prospective trials with results compared to contrast angiography. Patient outcomes (limb salvage, graft patency) were similar indicating that the clinical accuracy of duplex testing to select appropriate inflow-outflow anastomotic sites for lower limb arterial bypass was equivalent to angiography.[10,11]

Whether an arterial lesion is suitable for endovascular repair depends on specific anatomic characteristics. Duplex findings of TransAtlantic Intersociety Consensus (TASC) category A or B lesions indicate endovascular intervention is the preferred treatment (Table 21–3).[11] Technical success rates in excess of 95% can be achieved with clinical results similar to surgical reconstruction. Category C lesions (>4 cm length calcified stenosis, mul-

tilevel disease, 5–10 cm length chronic occlusions) may also be amenable to endovascular repair depending on the experience of the vascular surgeon. Endovascular treatment of category 4 (diffuse stenosis, >10 cm occlusions) lesions is not associated with outcomes comparable to "open" surgical repair or bypass grafting.[11] In applying duplex scanning to patient evaluation, the intent is to characterize the extent and severity of occlusive disease to permit a clinical decision regarding intervention options.

Color Duplex Peripheral Arterial Examination

Patient examination should be conducted in a warm (75–77°F) room to avoid vasoconstriction. A time of 30–45 min should be allotted for testing, and the patient informed not to smoke (>1 h) or eat (overnight fasting, >4 h) prior to testing. Imaging in the morning is recommended to minimize the presence of intestinal gas that obscures imaging of the infrarenal aorta and iliac arteries. Abdominal imaging is performed using a 3–5 MHz phased array transducer beginning at the level of the renal arteries. From the groin (femoral artery) to the ankle (tibial arteries), a 5–7 MHz linear array transducer should be used. Multiple scanning windows (anterior, flank, umbilical, posterior) may be required to achieve adequate arterial insonation/imaging of the aorta, iliac, and infrainguinal arteries due to obesity (vessels >15 cm deep), bowel gas, large limbs, edema, surgical wounds, ulcers, joint contractures, small vessels, and vessel calcification. Scanning should proceed sequentially from proximal to distal with recording of centerstream pulsed Doppler velocity

TABLE 21–3. TACS (TransAtlantic Intersociety Consensus) classification of lower limb arterial occlusive lesions suitable for percutaneous transluminal angioplasty (PTA).[19,20]

Category	Site of arterial lesion[a]	
	Aortoiliac	Femoropopliteal
A	<3 cm focal stenosis	<3 cm focal stenosis or occlusion
B	Single stenosis 3–10 cm	3–5 cm single stenosis or occlusion
	Unilateral CIA occlusion	Heavily calcified lesions ≤3 cm
	Two stenosis <5 cm	Lesions with tibial occlusion
		Multiple lesions <3 cm
C	Unilateral EIA occlusion not involving CFA	Single stenosis or occlusion >5 cm
	Unilateral EIA stenosis extending into CFA	Multiple lesions 3–5 cm
	Bilateral stenosis 5–10 stenosis	Multiple lesions >5 cm
	Bilateral CIA occlusion	Complete CFA or SFA and popliteal or proximal tibial vessel occlusion
D	Iliac stenosis associated with aortic or iliac aneurysm	
	Diffuse stenosis >10 cm of CIA, EIA, CFA	
	Unilateral occlusion CIA and EIA	
	Bilateral EIA occlusion	

[a]CIA, common iliac artery; EIA, external iliac artery; CFA, common femoral artery; SFA, superficial femoral artery.

TABLE 21–4. Mean arterial diameter and peak systolic flow velocity (PSV) measured by duplex scanning patients with normal ankle-brachial indices (ABI).[7]

Artery	Diameter ± SD[a] (cm)	Velocity ± SD (cm/s)
Infrarenal aorta	2.0 ± 0.3	65 ± 15
Common iliac	1.6 ± 2	95 ± 20
External iliac	0.79 ± 0.13	119 ± 22
Common femoral	0.82 ± 0.14	114 ± 25
Proximal superficial femoral	0.60 ± 0.12	91 ± 14
Distal superficial femoral	0.54 ± 0.11	94 ± 14
Popliteal	0.52 ± 0.11	69 ± 14
Tibial		55 ± 10

[a]SD, standard deviation.

TABLE 21–5. Most common locations of lower limb atherosclerosis, or stenosis after infrainguinal bypass grafting.

Arterial segment	Site of occlusive disease
Aortoiliac	Distal aorta, proximal-mid common iliac artery, proximal external iliac artery
Femoropopliteal	Common femoral artery, superficial femoral artery at the adductor, i.e., "Hunter" canal, origins of superficial and deep femoral artery
Tibial	Tibioperoneal trunk
Vein bypass	Proximal graft segment after reversed saphenous vein bypass, distal graft segment after nonreversed or *in situ* vein bypass grafting, graft–graft anastomosis
Prosthetic bypass	Distal anastomotic region

spectra in a segmental (iliac, femoral, popliteal, distal tibial) manner. Normal values of arterial diameter and peak systolic velocity (PSV) for lower limb arterial segments are shown in Table 21–4.[6,7] Infrarenal aorta diameter is documented as the technologist moves from the renal to iliac arteries. Aorta wall-to-wall diameter should be measured in both transverse and sagittal scan planes. Real-time color and power Doppler imaging facilitates location of stenosis by identifying lumen narrowing, plaque formation, color-map aliasing (turbulent flow), presence of color flow jet, and tissue bruits (Figure 21–2). At sites of stenosis, changes in PSV and spectral content are assessed by moving the "sample volume" of pulsed Doppler through the area of narrowing. To classify stenosis severity, velocity spectra are recorded at a 60° Doppler angle relative to the artery wall for calculation of peak-systolic and end-diastolic velocity. Identification of vessel branching, exit and reentry collaterals, vessel occlusion, aneurysmal change, and atherosclerotic plaque is an important component of arterial imaging. Occlusive lesions tend to develop at specific arterial sites (Table 21–5). These segments should be examined in detail when proximal-to-distal changes in PSV or spectral broadening are identified. Limitations of duplex imaging include obesity (vessels >15 cm deep to skin), bowel gas, edema, surgical incisions, ulcers, joint contracture, and arterial wall calcification producing acoustic shadowing.

Recording pulsed Doppler velocity spectra from tibial arteries at the ankle is recommended to correlate PSV and waveform pulsatility with measured ABI values (Figure 21–3). Correlation is necessary when calcified

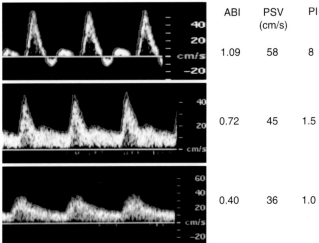

ABI	PSV (cm/s)	PI
1.09	58	8
0.72	45	1.5
0.40	36	1.0

FIGURE 21–3. Duplex scan of mid-thigh superficial femoral artery stenosis in a patient with calf claudication. At rest, a triphasic waveform was recorded proximal and at a focal stenosis with a PSV of 441 cm/s (criteria indicating a >50% diameter reducing stenosis). Treadmill exercise (12% grade at 1.5 mph) resulting in a decrease in ankle pressure from 132 mm Hg at rest (ABI = 0.8) to 50 mm Hg after walking for 2 min. The patient underwent percutaneous transluminal balloon angioplasty of the lesion with restoration of normal limb hemodynamics (ABI > 1.0).

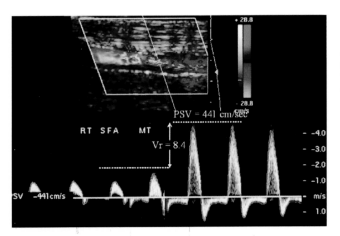

FIGURE 21–2. Iatrogenic common femoral artery pseudoaneurysm with narrow stalk amenable to duplex guided thrombin injection. Velocity spectra recording from the stalk demonstrates characteristic to-and-fro arterial flow.

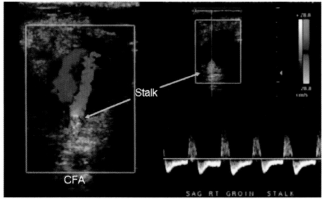

FIGURE 21–4. Pulsed Doppler velocity spectra recorded form the posterior tibial artery at the ankle. Note changes in the velocity spectral waveform (triphasic to monophasic), decrease in peak systolic velocity (PSV), and pulsatility index (normal: >4) with decrease in ankle-brachial index (ABI) from normal (>0.95), to the levels seen in claudicants (ABI: 0.5–0.09), and with critical limb ischemia (ABI < 0.5).

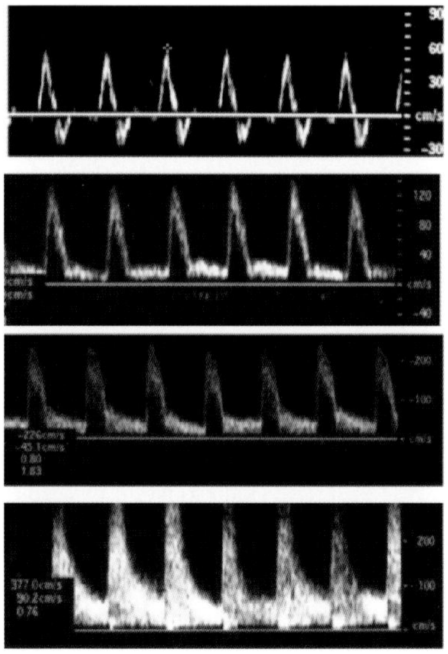

A Normal, no stenosis

B PSV < 150 cm/sec

C PSV 200–300 cm/sec

D PSV > 300 cm/sec

FIGURE 21–5. Lower extremity duplex spectral waveforms typical of normal (A) 1–19% diameter reduction, (B) 20–49% diameter reduction, (C) 50–75% diameter reduction, and (D) >75% diameter reduction stenosis as classified in Table 21–6.

tibial arteries are imaged, when patients are diabetic, or incompressibility is suggested by an ABI value > 1.3. Segmental pulsed Doppler spectra should be recorded from arterial segments (common femoral, popliteal, tibial) without severe (>50%) stenosis as this allows diagnosis of multilevel disease by comparison of pulsatility index, acceleration time, and waveform damping (pulsus tardus) between adjacent arterial segments.

Duplex testing is the recommended diagnostic modality to evaluate the arterial catheterization sites for pseudoaneurysm. Ultrasound imaging can distinguish between a hematoma with no flow and color Doppler characteristics of a pseudoaneurysm (Figure 21–4). The finding of a stalk indicates suitable anatomy for ultrasound-guided thrombin injection.

Duplex Criteria for Grading Arterial Stenosis

A number of duplex-derived velocity criteria to grade stenosis severity have been validated by comparison with contrast arteriography.[1–3,6] Use of PSV, end-diastolic velocity (EDV), and the velocity ratio (Vr) of PSV proximal to and at the site of maximum stenosis, in conjunction with the velocity spectral waveform distal to the stenosis, is recommended to categorize first- and second-order (tandem) stenoses. Assessment of the common femoral waveform is an accurate predictor of normal inflow (aortoiliac segment) if its configuration is tri- or multiphasic. If the superficial femoral artery is occluded,

a monophasic common femoral waveform may be present, but the acceleration time is <130 ms when no pressure-reducing iliac lesion is present. Symptoms of mild claudication (ABI >0.8) may be associated with a tibial artery triphasic Doppler waveform at rest, but with exercise treadmill testing, the ankle pressures decrease and a monophasic, damped waveform develops distal to the occlusive lesion.

Stenosis severity based on PSV and Vr values recorded at the lesion is useful in grading mild (<50%), moderate (50–75%), and severe (>75% or occlusion) peripheral stenosis (Figure 21–5 and Table 21–6).[6,7,13] Lesions with a velocity spectra indicating a >75% stenosis are typically associated with a >20 mm Hg reduction in systolic pressure (Figure 21–6). Duplex criteria that reliably predict a hemodynamically significant stenosis, i.e., associated with resting peripheral pressure and flow reduction include the following:

- Loss of triphasic waveform configuration at stenosis
- Damping or reduction in the pulsatility index in the distal artery velocity waveform.
- PSV >250–300 cm/s.
- EDV >0.
- Vr >3 across the stenosis.

By using a modified Bernoulli equation, an estimation of the systolic pressure gradient across a stenosis can be obtained, where

$$\text{Systolic pressure gradient (mm Hg)} = 4 \times (\text{PSV}_{\text{at the stenosis}} - \text{PSV}_{\text{proximal to the stenosis}})^2$$

TABLE 21–6. University of South Florida duplex criteria for lower limb arterial occlusive disease.[6,13,a]

Percent stenosis (%)	Peak systolic velocity (cm/s)	End diastolic velocity (cm/s)	Velocity ratio	Distal arterial waveform
Normal, (1–19%)	<150	<40	<1.5	Triphasic
20–49%	150–200	<40	1.5–2.0	Triphasic
50–75%	200–300	<90	2.0–3.9	Poststenotic turbulence distal to stenosis, monophasic distal waveform
>75%	>300	>90	>4.0	Damped distal waveform and low PSV[b]
Occlusion	Absent flow by color Doppler/pulsed Doppler spectral analysis; length of occlusion estimated by scan distance between exit and reentry collateral arteries			

[a]Adapted from University of Washington Criteria.
[b]PSV, peak systolic velocity.

Example:

Common iliac stenosis: $PSV_{stenosis} = 3.5\,m/s$;
$$PSV_{proximal} = 0.5\,m/s$$

$$\Delta P = 4 \times (3.5 - 0.5)^2$$

$$\Delta P = 36\,mm\,Hg$$

As stenosis severity increases, distal arterial pulsatility and flow velocity decrease, EDV in the stenosis increases, and flows in the inflow artery decrease. The flow pattern in the arterial segment proximal to high-grade (>75%) stenosis or occlusion depends on the extent of collateral development. In the setting of acute limb ischemia, a high resistance (no flow in diastole) flow pattern should be identified. Velocity criteria thresholds for grading >50% and >70% iliac artery stenosis and validated diagnostic accuracy compared to biplane, contrast arteriography are shown in Table 21–7.[8,12,13] High-grade (>70%) iliac artery stenosis was associated with an EDV >40cm/s and Vr >5 across the stenosis; the positive predictive value is 65%.

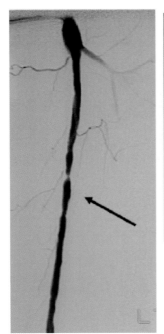
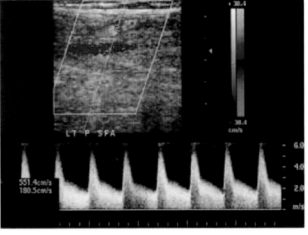

PSV 551 cm/sec, Vr 12
EDV 180 cm/sec
ABI = 0.65

FIGURE 21–6. Duplex scan and corresponding arteriogram of a >75% superficial femoral artery stenosis (arrow) with increased peak systolic velocity (PSV), velocity ratio (Vr), and end-diastolic velocity (EDV) and turbulent spectra characteristic of a pressure reducing lesion accounted for the abnormal ankle-brachial index (ABI) of 0.68 measured at rest.

TABLE 21–7. Diagnostic accuracy of color duplex ultrasonography criteria in detection of the occlusive disease involving aortoiliac segment compared with arteriography.[5,14]

Duplex criteria predictive[a]	Positive predictive value (%)	Negative predictive value (%)
50–70% DR stenosis		
Vr > 2.8	86	84
PSV > 200 cm/s	68	91
>70% DR stenosis		
Vr > 5.0	65	91
EDV > 40 cm/s	64	92

[a]DR, diameter reduction; Vr, peak systolic velocity ratio across the stenosis; PSV, peak systolic velocity; EDV, end diastolic velocity.

Occlusion of an arterial segment is identified by absence of color Doppler flow in the lumen, a preocclusive thump (staccato waveform), dampening of distal waveforms, and the presence of exit collateral vessels. Real-time Doppler imaging can be used to estimate the length (± 4 cm) of vessel occlusion based on flow in the lumen and imaging the distance between the exit and reentry collaterals.[1] The diagnostic accuracy of duplex scanning in grading stenosis severity decreases distal to an occlusion. The presence of proximal >75% stenosis or occlusion reduces duplex accuracy in the femoropopliteal segment approximately 10%. The grading of second-order stenosis relies on high-resolution imaging using power Doppler and modification of the velocity criteria for stenosis grading. A velocity ratio >2.5 combined with significant lumen narrowing demonstrated by B-mode/power Doppler imaging indicates a >50% diameter reduction stenosis.[4] The reduced sensitivity of color Doppler mapping to accurately identify >50% stenosis in low-flow conditions, e.g., limbs with critical limb ischemia, limits is application as the sole vascular imaging study prior to intervention. In these circumstances, MR or CT angiography is required for disease management.

Endovascular and Surgical Intervention Based on Duplex Scanning

The application of duplex arterial mapping as a sole diagnostic modality to proceed with, or for monitoring arterial interventions continues to expand.[1–7,14–17] This approach is recommended in patients at increased risk for developing contrast-induced renal failure, with a contrast allergy, or when arterial access for a catheter-based diagnostic study is limited. Newer duplex ultrasound systems provide enhanced resolution and other imaging features (power Doppler, B-flow) important for arterial mapping studies and accurate disease detection. Vascular

surgeons have also acquired confidence by performing duplex-guided therapeutic interventions, including thrombin injection of femoral artery pseudoaneurysms, angioplasty of peripheral and carotid stenoses, placement of vena cava filters, and closure of saphenous vein using radiofrequency or laser energy.

In the treatment of lower limb occlusive disease, duplex testing can reliably distinguish between single and multilevel (aortoiliac, femoropopliteal, popliteal-tibial) segment involvement. Single segment disease, characterized by focal (<5 cm) stenosis or occlusion, is typically associated with claudication symptoms of varying disability. Medical therapy consisting of risk factor PAD modification, a walking exercise program, and drug therapy (cilostazole) should be initiated. Vascular laboratory surveillance at 6-month intervals is recommended for treatment response and disease progression. If claudication symptoms are disabling and medical therapy has failed, duplex testing can identify limbs with lesions amenable to PTA.

Clinical features of an occlusive lesion suitable for endovascular intervention include a duplex-detected focal stenosis or short segment (<5 cm) occlusion and recent (<3 months) onset of limb ischemia. Endovascular treatment of TASC A and B lesions is associated with high (>95%) technical success rates and acceptable clinical outcomes when postprocedure duplex surveillance is performed.[17–20] Endovascular repair of TASC C and D is less durable with outcomes inferior to surgical endarterectomy and/or bypass. Both endovascular and "open" surgical interventions are prone to the development of myointimal restenosis and thus duplex surveillance has an important role in monitoring functional patency and detection of "correctable" occlusive lesions. The application of intraluminal stent-grafts to treat lower limb occlusive and aneurysmal disease has further expanded the use of duplex scanning to identify lesions with appropriate anatomy for this type of endovascular repair.

Patients with multilevel occlusive disease may require a combined endovascular-surgical approach for disease management. Duplex arterial mapping can be used to identify common femoral disease, best treated by open repair, and iliac or superficial femoral artery (SFA) lesions amenable to endovascular therapy. The use of duplex testing to design an arterial intervention procedure is well accepted by the patients who, by nature, favor using less invasive procedures when possible. Duplex-guided surgical bypass and peripheral aneurysm repair are associated with outcomes similar to evaluations using contrast angiography.[9–11,15,19,20] Patient evaluation using duplex arterial mapping has the potential to reduce patient care costs by reducing the need for diagnostic arteriography, and facilitate the use of endovascular therapies.

Duplex-Monitored Endovascular Procedures

Early failure after endovascular procedures, defined as an initial technical failure or technical success without clinical improvement 1 month after treatment, has been correlated with the presence of a residual duplex-detected stenosis. Factors such as elastic recoil, plaque dissection, and spasm are reported as factors contributing to early PTA failure rates ranging from 9% to 47%.[14,15] Even in limbs with improved ABI following PTA, abnormal hemodynamics at the angioplasty site have a negative influence on durability. Mewissen et al.[14] demonstrated that PTA sites with duplex-detected residual stenosis are predictive of clinical failure. By life-table analysis, a >50% PTA site stenosis (PSV >180 cm/s, Vr >2) was associated with a 15% 1-year clinical success compared to 84% stenosis-free patency when <50% was verified by duplex scanning, $p < 0.01$. Other reports indicated that completion arteriography following PTA can mask a hemodynamic stenosis in up to 25% of procedures. These observations provide the rationale for duplex monitoring of angioplasty procedures. Some vascular groups have championed the use of intravascular ultrasound, which provides unique anatomic information at the PTA compared to arteriography. Given the versatility and accuracy of duplex ultrasound, we prefer this diagnostic modality for evaluating the outcome of endovascular interventions.

The evaluation algorithm for peripheral angioplasty using PTA-site arteriography and duplex ultrasound is shown in Figure 21–7. The goal of duplex-monitored angioplasty is to terminate the procedure when duplex testing has confirmed normal PTA site hemodynamics. Pre-PTA velocity spectra typically indicate high-grade, pressure-reducing stenosis with PSV >300 cm/s and end-diastolic velocity >40 cm/s. A successful PTA should have

TABLE 21–8. University of South Florida experience with duplex-monitored percutaneous transluminal balloon angioplasty (PTA) of femoropopliteal or infrainguinal vein graft stenosis.

PTA site	Number of sites	Treatment altered[a]	Early failure	Late failure
Femoropopliteal segment	32	8	0	3
Vein grafts	54	15	1	6[b]

[a]Larger balloon ($n = 15$); longer inflation time ($n = 5$); stent placement ($n = 3$).
[b]80 stenosis-free patency at 2 years.

a PSV less than 180 cm/s and/or a Vr across the treated stenotic segment less than 2. Duplex assessment is performed after the PTA site arteriogram confirms <20% residual stenosis. If a residual stenosis is identified by duplex scanning, reintervention using a larger balloon, prolonged balloon inflation, atherectomy, or stent deployment is performed. Duplex testing is repeated to verify normal PTA site hemodynamics. If a lesion is judged to be maximally dilated, i.e., in treating a vein graft stenosis, duplex scanning demonstrates persistent stenosis, careful surveillance or operative intervention (PSV exceeds 250 cm/s) is recommended depending on the severity of the residual stenosis. A duplex-detected stenosis at the angioplasty site has in our experience been correlated with early failure by progression to stenosis with similar hemodynamics of the primary lesion, or to occlusion. Approximately 20% of infrainguinal PTAs were found to have residual stenosis by intraprocedural duplex assessment (Table 21–8). Reintervention resulted in normal PTA site hemodynamics in 82 of the 86 angioplasty procedures. Subsequent duplex surveillance demonstrated an 80% stenosis-free patency, and reintervention for recurrent stenosis was performed at six sites.

Duplex Surveillance following Intervention

Late failure following endovascular or surgical interventions can be caused by myointimal hyperplasia or atherosclerotic disease progression. Identification of a "failing" arterial reconstruction allows intervention prior to thrombosis thereby extending functional patency. In general, a repeat PTA is associated with an outcome similar to the primary procedure. Lower limb arterial repairs should be assessed by duplex scanning and measurement of ABI within 1–2 weeks of the procedure. If normal repair site hemodynamics are recorded, subsequent surveillance is performed 3 months later and then at 6-month intervals. If the postprocedure duplex identifies a 50–75% stenosis but the ABI has appropriately

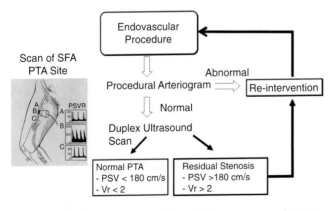

FIGURE 21–7. Evaluation algorithm of infrainguinal endovascular angioplasty procedures using arteriography and duplex ultrasound.

increased, a repeat scan in 3–4 weeks should be performed to assess for improvement or deterioration in the repair site hemodynamics. A progressive stenosis with PSV >300 cm/s, Vr >3.5 should be subjected to repeat angiographic imaging and consideration for angioplasty or surgical repair based on anatomic characteristics of the arterial segment.

Conclusion

Duplex scanning has demonstrated an established and continually expanding role in the management of PAD. While duplex arterial mapping is not a replacement for arteriography or other vascular imaging modalities, its routine use in patient evaluation allows rapid, safe assessment of a wide spectrum of lower limb vascular conditions. The diagnostic accuracy of lower limb duplex scanning is similar to contrast arteriography, and superior to MRA, for defining arterial anatomy in patients undergoing revascularization. In this emerging era of endovascular therapy, duplex arterial testing is ideally suited to identify lesions appropriate for PTA, and then at the time of the procedure to be used to monitor technical adequacy. Normalization of lower limb or arterial repair hemodynamics is an important treatment principle and should be a goal of intervention since a stenosis-free repair predicts long-term clinical success. As clinical experience with peripheral arterial duplex is gleaned, clinicians acquire confidence in its accuracy and are willing to proceed with intervention based solely on duplex findings.

References

1. Cossman DV, Ellison JE, Wagner WH, *et al.* Comparison of contrast arteriography to arterial mapping with color-flow duplex imaging in the lower extremities. J Vasc Surg 1989; 10:522–529.
2. Moneta GL, Yeager RA, Antonovic R, *et al.* Accuracy of lower extremity arterial duplex mapping. J Vasc Surg 1992;15:275–284.
3. Kerr, TM, Bandyk DF. Color duplex imaging or peripheral arterial disease before angioplasty or surgical intervention. In: Bernstien EF (ed). *Vascular Diagnosis,* 4th ed., pp. 527–533. St. Louis: CV Mosby, 1993.
4. Allard L, Cloutier G, Durand LG, *et al.* Limitations of ultrasonic duplex scanning for diagnosing lower limb arterial stenosis in the presence of adjacent segment disease. J Vasc Surg 1994;19:650–657.
5. de Smet AA, Ermers EJ, Kitslaar PJ. Duplex velocity characteristics of aortoiliac stenoses. J Vasc Surg 1996;23: 628–636.
6. Kohler TR, Zierler G, Strandness DE, *et al.* Duplex scanning for diagnosis of aortoiliac and femoropopliteal disease: A prospective study. Circulation 1987;76:1074–1080.
7. Jager KA, Risketts HJ Strandness DE Jr. Duplex scanning for the evaluation of lower limb arterial disease. In: Bernstien EF (ed). *Noninvasive Diagnostic Techniques in Vascular Disease,* pp. 619–631. St. Louis: CV Mosby, 1985.
8. Whelan JF, *et al.* Color flow Doppler ultrasound comparison with peripheral arteriography for the investigation of peripheral arterial disease. J Clin Ultrasound 1992;20: 369–374.
9. Ligush J Jr, Reavis SW, Preisser JS, *et al.* Duplex ultrasound scanning defines operative strategies for patients with limb threatening ischemia. J Vasc Surg 1998;28:482–491.
10. Grassbaugh JA, Nelson PR, Ruicidlo EM, *et al.* Blinded comparison of preoperative duplex ultrasound scanning and contrast arteriography for planning revascularization at the level of the tibia. J Vasc Surg 2003;37: 1186–1190.
11. Standards of Practice Committee of the Society of Cardiovascular and Interventional Radiology. Guidelines for percutaneous angioplasty. Radiology 1990;177:619.
12. Edwards JM, Coldwell DM, Goldman ML, *et al.* The role of duplex scanning in the selection of patients for transluminal angioplasty. J Vasc Surg 1991;13:69–74.
13. Langsfeld, M, *et al.* The use of deep duplex scanning to predict significant aortoiliac stenosis. J Vasc Surg 1988;7: 395–399.
14. Merwissen MW, Kenney EV, Bandyk DF, *et al.* The role of duplex scanning versus angioplasty in predicting outcome after balloon angioplasty in the femoropopliteal artery. J Vasc Surg 1992;15:960–966.
15. Spijkrboer AM, Nass PC, de Valois JC, *et al.* Evaluation of femoropopliteal arteries with duplex ultrasound after angioplasty. Can we predict results at one year? Eur J Vasc Surg 1996;12:418–423.
16. Hingorani A, Markevich N, Sreedhar K, *et al.* Magnetic resonance angiography versus duplex arteriography in patients undergoing lower extremity revascularization: Which is the best replacement for contrast arteriography? J Vasc Surg 2004;39:717–722.
17. Surowiec SM, Davies MG, Shirley WE, *et al.* Percutaneous angioplasty and stenting of the superficial femoral artery. J Vasc Surg 2005;41:269–278.
18. Timaran CH, Prault TL, Stevens SL, *et al.* Iliac artery stenting versus surgical reconstruction for TASC (Trans-Atlantic Inter-Society Consensus) type B and type C iliac lesions. J Vasc Surg 2003;38:272–278.
19. Tielbeek AV, Rietjens E, Buth J, *et al.* The value of duplex surveillance after endovascular intervention for femoropopliteal obstructive disease. Eur J Vasc Surg 1996;12:145–150.
20. Avino AJ, Bandyk DF, Gonsalves AJ, *et al.* Surgical and endovascular intervention for infrainguinal vein graft stenosis. J Vasc Surg 1999;29:60–71.

22
Duplex Surveillance of Infrainguinal Bypass Grafts

Patrick A. Stone and Dennis F. Bandyk

Introduction

Vascular laboratory surveillance using duplex ultrasound is recommended after infrainguinal bypass grafting as it benefits patient outcome by improving graft patency.[1,2] Ideally, duplex testing should begin in the operating room to survey the graft and anastomotic sites for stenosis and to document augmented flow in the runoff arteries and foot. Color duplex imaging is more sensitive than arteriography for intraoperative assessment and detects unrecognized graft abnormalities in 5–10% of reconstructions, permitting immediate correction.[3] The application of duplex graft surveillance has been shown to reduce the incidence of both early (<30 days) and late bypass failure.[1,2,4] Infrainguinal arterial bypasses, constructed of either autologous vein or a prosthetic graft, are prone to develop intrinsic stenotic lesions, which when progressive to cause thrombosis if graft flow is reduced below the "thrombotic threshold velocity."[5–9] Myointimal hyperplasia producing lumen reduction is the most common etiology for graft stenosis, but its temporal occurrence and site(s) of development differ between vein and prosthetic grafts. The occurrence of vein graft stenosis is highest in the 6 months following the procedure, and decreases thereafter. Myointimal stenosis is most common at vein valve and anastomotic sites, and has anatomic features of a smooth, typically focal (<2 cm) stricture. This acquired lesion has been implicated in nearly 80% of vein bypass failures, with other graft failures caused by technical errors, intrinsic graft lesions, or hypercoagulable states.[1,2,6,10] Following prosthetic grafting, intragraft abnormalities are rare (<10% of all stenoses) with graft stenosis developing most commonly at the distal anastomosis and the adjacent runoff artery. The failure rate of prosthetic grafts (10–15%/year) is higher than autologous vein grafts (2–5%/year) and has been attributed to differences in "thrombotic threshold velocity," myointimal hyperplasia development, and atherosclerotic disease progression.[8,9]

The patterns of infrainguinal graft failure mandate using color duplex ultrasound for effective surveillance. Clinical assessment for symptoms or signs of limb ischemia, even when combined with measurements of segmental limb pressures, lack the diagnostic sensitivity to detect a developing graft stenosis. Less than 50% of patients found to have a >70% diameter reducing graft stenosis admit to symptoms of claudication or recognized changes in limb perfusion. Duplex surveillance is used to detect changes in graft flow, identify sites of intrinsic graft lesions or developing stenosis, and grade lesion severity. Serial testing permits timely revision of hemodynamically significant lesions that if unrepaired would result in graft thrombosis. The criteria for intervention of an identified "failing graft" are based on duplex-measured peak systolic flow velocity and/or reduction of ankle-brachial index (ABI) compared to initial postoperative levels. The efficacy of surveillance has been demonstrated in prospective clinical trials by a 15–30% improvement in long-term graft patency rates: higher for autologous vein than for prosthetic bypass grafts.[2,7,11–13] Multiple investigators have observed graft failure rates of approximately 25% in stenotic bypass grafts with a policy of no intervention. Idu et al. reported a 10% graft occlusion rate when a duplex-detected stenosis of >70% was repaired, compared to a 100% graft failure rate when the lesions were untreated.[13] Infrainguinal prosthetic graft patency is also improved by duplex surveillance. Calligaro et al. demonstrated duplex scanning was more sensitive (81%) than ABI with clinical evaluation (24%) with 50% of correctable stenosis found at anastomotic sites.[9]

The goal of graft surveillance is to avert failure by the detection and elective correction of graft abnormalities (technical errors, intrinsic graft lesions, myointimal hyperplasia, and graft aneurysm). Surveillance should be initiated prior to discharge from the hospital and continue indefinitely, with the majority of patients requiring 6 month or yearly evaluation after the first year. It has been estimated that a duplex surveillance program is cost-effective if limb loss can be prevented in 2% of enrolled patients.

Mechanisms and Hemodynamics of Graft Failure

The interpretation of duplex surveillance studies requires an understanding of the mechanisms of graft failure, arterial bypass graft hemodynamics, and the physiology of graft stenosis. Graft failure occurs by one of three mechanisms: occlusion by thrombosis, hemodynamic failure, or structural failure (aneurysmal degeneration or infection).[1,6,13–16] Graft thrombosis is most frequent during the perioperative (operating room to hospital discharge) period, with a reported incidence of 3–8%. Thereafter, the rate of graft failure is approximately 1% per month during the first year and then decreases to <5%/year. The attrition of patency is highly dependent on application of graft surveillance, patient compliance, and the success of graft revision procedures.

Early (<30 days) graft failure is the result of technical errors in bypass construction (anastomotic stricture, retained vein valves, unrecognized intrinsic graft lesions, tunneling errors, graft kinking), a hypercoagulable condition, or inadequate runoff to maintain graft flow above the "thrombotic threshold velocity."[12] Recognition of technical errors and abnormal graft hemodynamics caused by poor runoff is best accomplished by duplex assessment at operation.[17] Graft thrombosis despite a "normal" intraoperative duplex scan as a rule indicates the presence of a hypercoagulable state.

Graft failure beyond 30 days can result from infection, structural degeneration of the conduit, or graft stenosis caused by intrinsic vein disease or myointimal hyperplasia. The incidence of graft stenosis varies with graft type ranging from 12% following *in situ* saphenous vein bypass grafting to 44% for arm vein bypasses.[1,10,18] The temporal occurrence of graft stenosis follows a "bell-shaped" curve with the highest prevalence at 6 months following the procedure. Infection producing graft failure is rare (<1%) with autologous venous conduits, but 3–5% with prosthetic graft usage.

Beyond 2 years, atherosclerosis progression of the inflow/outflow arteries and venous aneurysm *development* account for the majority of late graft failures.[18] Atherosclerotic disease progression is related to effective control of the patient's risk factors, i.e., tobacco use, diabetes, hypertension, and hyperlipidemia. Inflow and outflow occlusive disease are suspected when duplex testing indicates reduction in graft blood flow velocity but no graft abnormality is identified. Aneurysm-related or thromboembolic graft failure should be suspected with graft thrombosis despite a prior duplex showing no stenotic lesions and normal graft flow. Aneurysmal degeneration is infrequent and tends to occur in arm vein conduits and in patients with aortic/popliteal aneurysmal disease. The presence of mural thrombus in a vein or prosthetic conduit is abnormal and indicates the graft is at increased risk for thrombosis.

Arterial Bypass Hemodynamics

Factors that influence duplex-measured flow velocity and spectral waveforms of graft blood flow include conduit diameter, status of inflow/outflow arteries, severity of preoperative ischemia, and cardiac hemodynamics. The range of peak systolic velocities (PSV) recorded from infrainguinal vein bypasses varies but the mean graft flow velocity (GFV) recorder from three or four sites along the graft length ranges from 50 to 80cm/s (Table 22–1 and Figure 22–1).[19–21] The PSV in nonstenotic vein grafts of >3mm diameter should be over 40cm/s and the graft spectra waveform should demonstrate low outflow resistance, i.e., antegrade flow throughout the pulse wave cycle. Flow velocity varies with graft diameter and type (Figure 22–2). Belkin *et al.* reported graft PSV was lower in inframalleolar (pedal) grafts (59 ± 4cm/s) compared to tibial (77 ± 6cm/s) and popliteal (71 ± 8cm/s) vein bypasses.[21] A low graft PSV can be measured in large (>6mm) diameter vein conduits, i.e., basilic vein, and in grafts with disadvantaged runoff (pedal bypass, isolated popliteal/tibial artery segments). If the graft PSV is <40cm/s in a conduit <6mm in diameter, a careful search for inflow or outflow arterial lesions should be conducted. The combination of low PSV and absent diastolic flow indicate high outflow resistance and indicates a bypass at increased risk for thrombosis. A low PSV is abnormal but does not predict graft failure in all cases. When identified at operation it

TABLE 22–1. Peak systolic velocity measured by duplex ultrasound from mid- or distal segments of femoropopliteal and femorotibial saphenous vein and PTFE[a] bypass grafts.[19–21]

Graft type	No.	Peak systolic velocity (cm/s) (mean ± SD)
In situ saphenous vein		
Femoropopliteal	65	76 ± 12
Femorotibial	95	72 ± 16
Femoral-pedal	25	52 ± 12
Reversed saphenous vein		
Femoropopliteal	20	80 ± 16
Femorotibial	12	69 ± 14
Cephalic/basilic arm vein		
Femoropopliteal/tibial	68	63 ± 12
PTFE, 6mm diameter		
Femoropopliteal	20	80 ± 16
Femorotibial	12	69 ± 14
PTFE, 5mm diameter		
Femorotibial	5	77 ± 11

[a]PTFE, polytetrafluoroethylene.

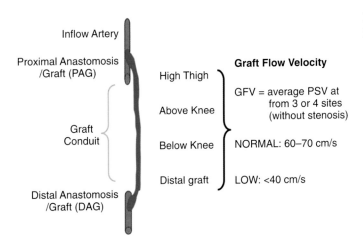

FIGURE 22–1. Schematic depicting the recording sites used for the calculation of mean graft flow velocity.

provides the rationale for the perioperative administration of anticoagulation (heparin, warfarin) regimens, or altering the primary procedure by adding a sequential bypass to a second outflow artery or construction of a distal arteriovenous fistula, procedures intended to increase graft flow velocity.

A graft flow pattern of low outflow resistance is prognostic of successful bypass grafting. A bypass graft performed for critical limb ischemia should demonstrate this "hyperemic" flow pattern in the distal graft segment and runoff artery. Within days to weeks, the hyperemia of revascularization abates and the Doppler waveform changes to a triphasic pattern with normalization of the ABI (Figure 22–2). Failure of the graft flow to convert from a biphasic to triphasic spectral waveform has been associated with reduced graft patency. Taylor *et al.* reported that 54 (86%) of 63 grafts with persistent biphasic waveforms more than 3 months after operation developed a graft stenosis or subsequently occluded.[5] Bypass grafts to the peroneal artery or an isolated popliteal arterial segment may not develop a triphasic flow pattern if limb pressure (ABI) does not become normal (<0.85). In

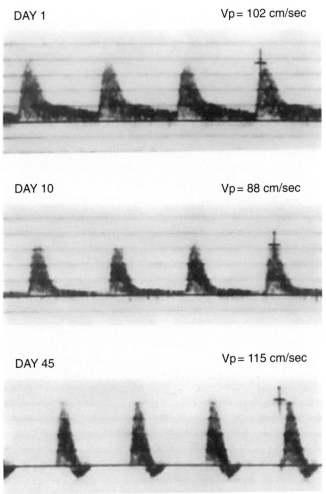

FIGURE 22–3. Velocity spectra recorded from the distal segment of a femoral-peroneal *in situ* saphenous vein bypass at 1, 10, and 45 days. A low-resistance spectral waveform (flow throughout the pulse cycle) is normal and expected after bypass grafting for critical ischemia. Flow resistance increased with time as evidenced by the decrease in diastolic flow. No significant change in peak systolic velocity (Vp) occurred and the development of a triphasic spectral waveform at day 45 indicates normal bypass graft hemodynamics and distal limb perfusion (ABI > 0.9).

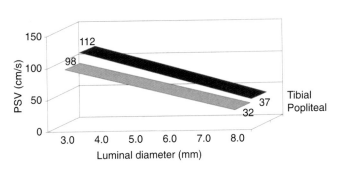

FIGURE 22–2. Duplex ultrasound measured peak systolic flow velocity (PSV) for tibial and popliteal grafts showing relationship with lumen diameter.

4-months after bypass grafting

7-months after bypass grafting

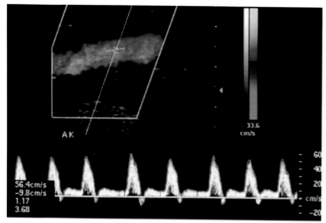
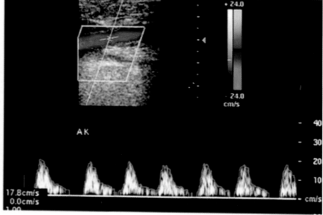

FIGURE 22–4. Duplex-recorded velocity spectra recorded from the above-knee segment of a femoropopliteal vein bypass demonstrating change in waveform configuration (triphasic to biphasic) and reduction in peak systolic velocity (PSV) from 56 to 18 cm/s caused by the development of a distal anastomotic graft stenosis.

patients with dialysis-dependent end-stage renal disease and severely calcified tibial arteries, a low flow (PSV in the range of 30–45 cm/s) bypass with minimal or no diastolic flow can occur due to diseased runoff and associated high outflow resistance.

Following changes in graft PSV is important in detecting "failing" bypass grafts. Development of a low (<40 cm/s) PSV or a decrease in PSV of >30 cm/s compared to a prior study indicates a significant change in graft flow and a search for a graft stenosis should be initiated (Figure 22–3). The duplex features of a >70%, pressure-reducing stenosis included lumen reduction with color Doppler aliasing, PSV increase to >300 cm/s with spectral broadening, and a PSV ratio (at stenosis compared to proximal to stenosis) >3.5. (Figures 22–4 and 22–5). The increase in diastole flow velocity is due to flow limitation during systole requiring flow throughout the pulse cycle to supply adequate volume flow to the distal limb. If

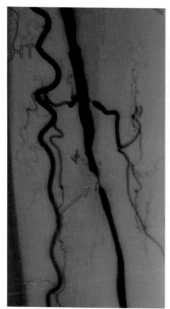
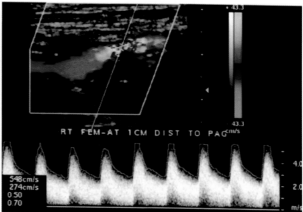

PSV = 548 cm/s; Vr = 12
Vend-diastole = 274 cm/s
ABI = 0.69

FIGURE 22–5. Angiogram and duplex ultrasound scan of a >75% diameter reducing stenosis of the proximal segment of a superficial femoral artery to anterior tibial artery vein bypass. Peak systolic velocity (PSV) is 548 cm/s, velocity ratio is 12, end-diastolic velocity is 274 cm/s, and ABI is 0.69 decreased from the initial postoperative value of 0.95.

duplex scanning of the bypass does not identify a stenosis, graft imaging by contrast arteriography or computed tomography (CT) angiography is recommended. Elevated PSV (>150 cm/s) in the graft conduit or anastomosis is abnormal and may be caused by small graft caliber or a stenosis. Graft PSV in the range of 120–160 cm/s can be measured along the entire course of small (3 mm diameter or less) vein conduits. More frequent (every 4–6 weeks) surveillance of these "high"-velocity grafts is recommended because of their propensity to develop long-segment strictures. When a progressive increase in PSV to >300 cm/s is identified, replacement of the stricture with an interposition vein bypass should be performed.

The development of graft stenosis and impending graft occlusion can be recognized from the graft spectral waveform. A low-velocity, biphasic waveform is the most common configuration associated with an acquired graft stenosis (Figure 22–3). An abnormal graft waveform of this type is recorded from 50% of grafts with stenosis; the ABI had decreased to 0.4–0.7 and mean graft velocity (MGV) has decreased by 20–30 cm/s. The reduction in waveform pulsatility and return of diastolic flow indicate arteriolar dilation in response to a pressure-reducing lesion. Other types of abnormal graft waveforms include a monophasic waveform with low (<45 cm/s) PSV seen in one-third of graft stenosis with an ABI in the range of 0.7–0.9, and a staccato graft waveform seen in approximately 6% of abnormal grafts and always associated with a high-grade outflow stenosis. This staccato flow pattern indicates a to-and-fro blood flow within a compliant venous conduit, extremely low graft flow, and impending graft thrombosis. Grafts with this flow feature are difficult to evaluate using contrast arteriography and the condition has been referred to as a graft "pseudoocclusion." The combination of graft PSV measurements, color duplex imaging for anatomic lesions, and ABIs analyzed sequentially during the postoperative period provides a comprehensive characterization of graft and limb hemodynamics. The objective data provided by duplex testing allow detection of graft stenosis, the progression of lesions, and identification of grafts at increased risk for thrombosis.

Intraoperative Duplex Scanning

Assessment of infrainguinal bypass grafts at operation for technical adequacy can be performed using continuous-wave (CW) Doppler flow analysis, arteriography, angioscopy and CW Doppler after flow is restored, or color duplex ultrasonography.[22–24] Color duplex ultrasound is the preferred methods because it provides both anatomic and hemodynamic assessment of graft function and limb perfusion. When used at operation, approximately 15% of procedures have an unrecognized abnor-

mality with velocity spectra of a stenosis identified. Repair of these problems and documentation of normal graft hemodynamics are associated with a low (<1%) incidence of graft thrombosis. In a series of 626 consecutive infrainguinal vein bypasses, duplex scanning prompted revision of 104 lesions in 96 bypass grafts, which included 82 vein/anastomotic stenoses, 17 vein segments with platelet thrombus, and 5 low-flow grafts. The revision rate was highest ($p < 0.01$) for alternative vein bypass grafts (27%) compared with the other grafting methods (reversed vein bypass grafts, 10%; nonreversed translocated, 13%; in situ, 16%). A normal intraoperative scan on initial imaging ($n = 464$ scans) or after revision ($n = 67$ scans) is associated with a 30-day thrombosis rate of 0.2% and a revision rate of 0.8% for duplex-detected stenosis (PSV > 300 cm/s). By comparison, 20 (21%) of 95 bypass grafts with a residual ($n = 29$ grafts) or unrepaired duplex stenosis ($n = 53$ grafts) or low flow ($n = 13$ grafts) had a corrective procedure for graft thrombosis ($n = 8$) or stenosis ($n = 12$); $p < 0.001$. Correction of residual graft defects and rescanning to document no residual stenosis reduced the incidence of graft problems identified on postoperative duplex surveillance.

The algorithm for intraoperative duplex ultrasound assessment of an infrainguinal vein bypass involves imaging the entire arterial reconstruction and classification of findings into one of four categories (Figure 22–6 and Table 22–2). Scanning is performed after completion of the bypass graft and patency is verified by clinical inspection and pulse palpation. A 10–15 MHz linear array transducer, placed in a sterile plastic sleeve containing acoustic gel, is used to scan exposed vessels and grafts segments beneath the skin. Imaging of the vein graft, anastomoses, and adjacent native arteries is performed in a longitudinal plane along the vessels, beginning at the

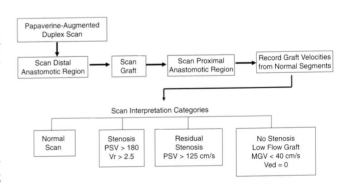

FIGURE 22–6. Algorithm for intraoperative duplex scanning of an infrainguinal vein bypass. Following duplex assessment, the study is classified into one of four categories: normal, stenosis identified, residual stenosis identified, or no stenosis identified but hemodynamic assessment of graft flow demonstrates low [peak systolic velocity (PSV) < 40 cm/s] velocity and high resistance (no flow in diastole, Ved = 0).

TABLE 22–2. Interpretation of intraoperative duplex ultrasound studies of infrainguinal vein bypasses and suggested perioperative management.

Duplex scan category	Graft flow velocity (cm/s)	Peripheral vascular resistance	Interpretation and perioperative management
Normal	>40	Low	No stenosis identified and graft PSV[a] is normal; administer with dextran-40 (25 ml/h, 500 ml) and oral aspirin (325 mg/day)
Stenosis PSV > 180 cm/s Vr > 2.5	<40	Low	Correct lesion and rescan graft, if no residual stenosis is identified but graft PSV is low <40 cm/s—administer heparin anticoagulation (weight-based) or low-molecular-weight heparin (1 mg/kg sc bid), dextran-40 (25 ml/h), and oral aspirin (325 mg/day)
Residual stenosis PSV < 180 cm/s Vr < 2.5	>40	Low	Rescan after 10 min to confirm no progression; administer low-molecular-weight heparin (1 mg/kg sc bid), dextran-40 (25 ml/h), and oral aspirin (325 mg/day)
Low flow, no graft stenosis	<40	High	Consider an adjunctive procedure to increase graft flow (distal arteriovenous fistula, jump/sequential graft to another outflow artery); if not possible treat as low flow graft with an antithrombotic regimen of heparin anticoagulation, dextran-40, and aspirin (325 mg/day)

[a]PSV, peak systolic velocity.

distal graft anastomotic segment and then proceeding proximal to include the entire venous conduit and the inflow artery-proximal anastomosis graft segment. Papaverine-HCl (30–60 mg) is injected into the distal vein bypass via a 27-gauge needle to augment flow thereby increasing the diagnostic sensitivity for stenosis detection. Graft PSV is measured (60° or less Doppler angle) at the proximal and distal anastomosis, at selected sites along the graft length (high-thigh, HT; above-knee, AK; below-knee, BK; and distal graft), and from inflow and outflow arteries. Following *in situ* saphenous bypass, imaging for patent side branches is performed and the absence of a side-branch flow is confirmed by the presence of a staccato waveform with distal graft occlusion.

Vein conduit stenosis is the most frequent abnormality found with intraoperative duplex scanning, and other abnormalities, in decreasing frequency, include anastomotic stenosis, platelet thrombus, and low graft flow as a result of outflow disease. Immediate repair is indicated for vein valve/anastomotic sites with PSV >180 cm/s and a velocity ratio (Vr = PSV at lesion/PSV proximal) of >2.5 (Figure 22–7). Velocity spectra of a high-grade stenosis (PSV > 300 cm/s) at the site of the imaging graft abnormality may represent formation of platelet thrombus. This graft segment should be replaced and a thrombolytic agent infused downstream to lyse thrombus embolized to the distal graft and runoff arteries. In vein grafts of normal (3–5 mm) caliber, a low PSV was measured in only 13 of the 626 grafts, of which 6 were to blind

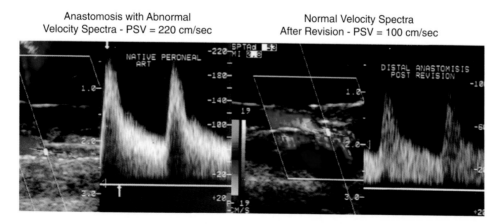

FIGURE 22–7. Intraoperative color duplex scan of a residual stenosis at the distal anastomosis of a femoral-peroneal saphenous vein bypass (left). Following revision by vein patch angioplasty, repeat scanning shows normal velocity spectra [peak systolic velocity (PSV) < 150 cm/s].

segments. Five of the 13 grafts failed within 90 days. Rzucidlo *et al.*[26] also reported a high rate of early graft thrombosis when duplex scanning demonstrated no or low (<8 cm/s) flow in diastole in the distal graft. When a high-resistance, low graft flow is identified, a careful search for a technical error should be performed, and if none is identified, perioperative heparinization or a procedure to increase graft flow (sequential bypass, distal arteriovenous fistula) should be considered.

Postoperative Graft Surveillance

Duplex ultrasound is used to confirm graft patency, identify stenotic lesions, assess their risk for producing graft thrombosis, and, if not repaired, monitor stenosis progression. Testing should include a clinical evaluation for symptoms or signs of limb ischemia, measurement of ABI, and color duplex imaging of the entire bypass graft including anastomosis and inflow/outflow arteries. A "predischarge" scan is recommended to confirm normal functional patency, identify the presence of technical problems and the progression of a residual stenosis detected at operation, and provide baseline graft flow velocities. Upon discharge, patients should be counseled and their primary care physician notified regarding the importance and necessity of graft surveillance. Graft failure has been associated with lack of a surveillance examination within 3 months of the procedure.[27] At each graft surveillance study, patients should also be queried regarding current use of tobacco products and whether they are taking antiplatelet medications. Modifying these two factors associated with graft failure can improve long-term patency.

Testing Intervals

Factors affecting the frequency of surveillance include the type of bypass and results of the predischarge duplex scan (Figure 22–7). Grafts at higher risk include those with residual stenosis, those modified during surgery, and those with low graft velocities. If the predischarge scan is normal, the first outpatient graft surveillance is performed 1 month after discharge. At this time, complete graft imaging should be possible, and if no abnormalities are identified the next surveillance study is scheduled for 3 months later, and every 6 months thereafter if normal surveillance studies are obtained. Bypasses with low-flow, residual graft lesions or constructed of arm veins should be evaluated every 3 months for the first year.

Threshold Velocity Criteria for Graft Revision

Repair of duplex-detected graft stenosis with a PSV > 300 cm/s and Vr > 3.5 is recommended, especially

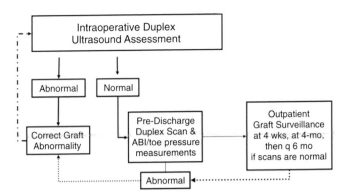

FIGURE 22–8. Duplex surveillance protocol beginning at operation with rescanning prior to discharge and in the outpatient clinic at regular intervals.

if the lesions have demonstrated progression on serial examinations and MGV has decreased to <45 cm/s.[28] Duplex imaging should demonstrate an anatomic stenosis on power Doppler and other features of lesion should be characterized including stenosis length, site (graft vs. anastomosis vs. native artery), and the diameter of the graft proximal to the lesion (Figure 22–8). Similar threshold velocity criteria have been published by other vascular groups:

- PSV > 300 cm/s, Vr > 4.0: Mills *et al.*[29]
- PSV > 300 cm/s, Vr > 3.0: Sladen *et al.*[30]
- PSV > 250 cm/s, Vr > 3.4: Papanicolauo *et al.*[31]
- PEDV > 20 cm/s: Buth *et al.*[32]
- Vr > 3.0: Bell *et al.*[33]

The risk of graft thrombosis is predicted by using the combination of high- and low-velocity duplex criteria discussed above, and the ABI values (Tables 22–3 and 22–4). In the highest risk group (Category I), the development of a pressure-reducing stenosis (PSV > 300 cm/s) has produced low flow velocity (GFV < 45 cm/s) in the graft, which if it decreases below the "thrombotic threshold velocity" will result in graft thrombosis. Prompt repair of Category I lesions is recommended, while Category II lesions (PSV > 300 cm/s, GFV > 45 cm/s) can be scheduled for elective repair within 1–2 weeks. A Category III stenosis (PSV of 150–300 cm/s, Vr < 3.5) is not pressure or flow reducing in the resting limb. Serial scans at 4–6 week intervals are recommended to determine hemodynamic (Figures 22–9 and 22–10) progression or regression of these lesions. Among graft stenosis detected within the first 3 months of surgery, regression of the lesion occurs in 30–35% of cases, while 40–45% remain stable. Approximately 50% of these "index" graft lesions progress to high-grade (PSV > 300 cm/s, Vr > 3.5) stenosis. In general, serial (4–6 week intervals) duplex scans will determine if a lesion will progress and become "graft threatening"

TABLE 22–3. Risk stratification for graft thrombosis based on surveillance data.[a]

Category[b]	High-velocity criteria		Low-velocity criteria		ΔABI
I (highest risk)	PSV > 300 cm/s or Vr > 3.5	and	GFV < 45 cm/s	or	>0.15
II (high risk)	PSV > 300 cm/s or Vr > 3.5	and	GFV > 45 cm/s	and	<0.15
III (intermediate risk)	180 < PSV > 300 cm/s or Vr > 2.0	and	GFV > 45 cm/s	and	<0.15
IV (low risk)	PSV < 180 cm/s and Vr < 2.0	and	GFV > 45 cm/s	and	<0.15

[a]PSV, duplex-derived peak systolic velocity at site of flow disturbance; GFV, graft flow velocity (global or distal); Vr, PSV ratio at maximum stenosis compared to proximal graft segment without disease; ABI, Doppler-derived ankle-brachial systolic pressure index.
[b]Category I: prompt repair of lesion is recommended—patients are hospitalized and anticoagulated prior to repair. Category II: lesions are repaired electively (within 2 weeks). Category III: lesions are observed with serial duplex examination at 4–6 week intervals and repaired if they progress. Category IV: lesions are at low risk for producing graft thrombosis—follow-up every 6 months; few (<3%/year) failures observed in this group.

TABLE 22–4. Potential of a graft lesion to cause graft thrombosis.

High-grade stenosis producing low graft flow	High
Graft entrapment	High
Flow-limiting graft stenosis	Moderate
Graft—anastomotic site aneurysm with mural thrombus	Moderate
Nonflow limiting graft stenosis (PSV < 300 cm/s)[a]	Low
Residual arteriovenous fistula after *in situ* vein bypass	Low

[a]PSV, peak systolic velocity.

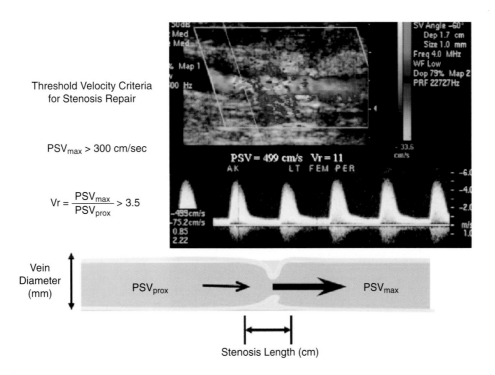

FIGURE 22–9. Duplex characterization of a graft stenosis, including velocity criteria for stenosis repair, vein diameter, and stenosis length.

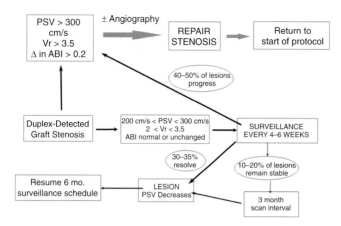

FIGURE 22–10. Algorithm for the surveillance and management of duplex-detected graft stenosis based on peak systolic velocity (PSV), velocity ratio (Vr), and ankle-brachial index (ABI) measurements.

within 4–6 months of identification.[8,9] In a natural history study of intermediate graft stenosis, Mills et al.[22] found that 63% of lesions progressed, 22% resolved, 10% remained unchanged, and one graft (2%) thrombosed despite more frequent surveillance.

No stenosis is identified in the majority (approximately 80%) of bypass grafts studied with ultrasound, i.e., Category IV scans. For these patients, surveillance at 6-month intervals is generally recommended. For Category IV grafts with a GFV < 45 cm/s, a diligent search should be conducted for additional inflow or outflow occlusive lesions. If none is detected, oral anticoagulation (sodium warfarin) is prescribed to maintain the prothrombin time at an INR of 1.6–2.2, as well as aspirin (81 mg/day).

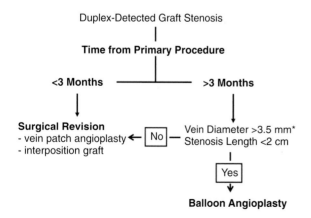

FIGURE 22–11. Treatment algorithm for duplex-detected stenosis based on appearance time (less than or more than 3 months) from operation and anatomic characteristics (vessel diameter, stenosis length). *Stenosis in a graft outflow artery >2 mm in diameter can be considered for endovascular intervention.

This anticoagulation regimen is also prescribed following femorodistal prosthetic bypass grafting when a GFV of <60 cm/s is measured in the graft by duplex scanning prior to discharge. The rationale for oral anticoagulation is based on the concept of the "thrombotic threshold velocity," which is higher in prosthetic than in vein arterial bypass grafts.

Infrainguinal bypasses constructed with arm (basilic, cephalic) veins require vigilant surveillance because of an observed 42% revision rate for stenosis. Of note, 82% of all spliced arm vein grafts required revision within 1 year of operation compared to 28% of basilic vein grafts (p < 0.01). With duplex surveillance and repair of duplex-detected stenosis, a graft patency of 91% at 3 years was achieved. A surveillance program is extremely important in this patient group since failure of the alternative vein bypass would require either a redo prosthetic revascularization, a procedure with poor long-term success, or amputation.[31]

Duplex Criteria for Endovascular Repair of Graft Stenosis

Methods for repair of graft stenosis include open surgical revision using path angioplasty, interposition grafting or jump, and endovascular repair using balloon angioplasty. Duplex testing can be used to select lesions appropriate for balloon angioplasty based on criteria that include severity of stenosis, lesion length, conduit diameter, and appearance time from bypass procedure:

Stenosis severity: PSV > 300 cm/s, Vr > 3.5
Stenosis length: ≤2 cm
Conduit diameter: ≥3.5 cm
Appearance time: >3 months from bypass grafting.

Over a 6-year period, 118 (22%) of 525 infrainguinal vein bypasses monitored by duplex ultrasound underwent revision for stenosis. One-half of the lesions met the criteria for endovascular intervention. Stenosis-free patency at 2 years was identical for surgical (63%) and endovascular (63%) interventions. However, the stenosis-free patency varied with timing and type of procedure. The endovascular treatment of a focal (<2 cm) vein graft stenosis >3 months from the initial procedure was associated with an 89% 1-year stenosis- free patency.[34] Following either surgical or endovascular repair, surveillance is similar to that performed after the primary procedures with an initial scan with 1 week to verify no residual stenosis at the repair site. Outcome of balloon angioplasty for graft stenosis is varied in the literature (Figure 22–11). Alexander et al.[35] used balloon angioplasty to treat 101 cases of vein graft stenosis with failure rates of 35% at 6 months and 54% at 1 year. Graft angioplasty was associated with an 8% complication rate. Kasirajan et al.[36] evaluated angioplasty using a "cutting" balloon in 19 patients.

During a mean follow-up of 11 months, one (5%) angioplasty site developed stenosis, and no surgical conversions were required.

While the majority of graft stenosis develop during the first postoperative year, Erickson et al.[37] emphasized the need for indefinite bypass surveillance in a study of 556 bypasses followed up to 13 years. Approximately 20% of the graft abnormalities developed after 2 years. The majority (63%) of the graft defects involved the conduit or the anastomoses. These findings support the continued annual evaluation of infrainguinal bypass for the development of stenosis and for disease progression or aneurysmal changes in the venous conduit.

Conclusion

Routine duplex ultrasound surveillance of lower limb vein and prosthetic bypass grafts is recommended. Optimum results are obtained when duplex surveillance is initiated in the operating room or prior to discharge. Since the majority of graft abnormalities identified occur in asymptomatic patients, criteria for intervention should be based on duplex-measured velocity spectra. High-grade lesions that produce low graft flow have the greatest potential to produce graft thrombosis and should be repaired promptly. Duplex findings can also be used to select either percutaneous balloon angioplasty or open surgical repair. The likelihood of graft revision varies with the vein bypass type, and is increased when a graft defect is identified on a "predischarge" or early (<6-week) duplex scan. With time, the incidence of vein graft stenosis decreases, but because of atherosclerotic disease progression in native arteries and aneurysm formation in the vein conduit, life-long surveillance (yearly after 3 years) is recommended.

References

1. Bandyk DF, Schmitt DD, Seabrook GR, et al. Monitoring functional patency of in situ saphenous vein bypasses: The impact of a surveillance protocol and elective revision. J Vasc Surg 1989;11:280–294.
2. Moody AP, Gould DA, Harris PL. Vein graft surveillance improves patency in femoropopliteal bypass. Eur J Vasc Surg 1990;4:117–120.
3. Bandyk DF, Mills JL, Gahtan V, et al. Intraoperative duplex scanning of arterial reconstructions: fFate of repaired and unrepaired defects. J Vasc Surg 1994;20:426–433.
4. Bandyk DF, Johnson BL, Gupta AK, Esses GE. Nature and management of duplex abnormalities encountered during infrainguinal vein bypass grafting. J Vasc Surg 1996;24:430–436.
5. Taylor PR, Wolfe HN, Yyrrell MR, et al. Graft stenosis: Justification for 1-year surveillance. Br J Surg 1990;77:1125–1128.
6. Mills JL, Harris EJ, Taylor LM, et al. The importance of routine surveillance of distal bypass grafts with duplex scanning: A study of 379 reversed vein grafts. J Vasc Surg 1990;12:379–389.
7. Lundell A, Linblad B, Bergqvist D, Hansen F. Femoropopliteal graft patency is improved by an intensive surveillance program: A prospective randomized study. J Vasc Surg 1995;21:26–34.
8. Lawlike NJ, Hanel KC, Hunt J, et al. Duplex scan surveillance of infrainguinal prosthetic bypass grafts. J Vasc Surg 1994;20:637–641.
9. Calligaro KD, Musser DJ, Chen AY, et al. Duplex ultrasonography to diagnose failing arterial prosthetic grafts. Surgery 199;120:455–459.
10. Gupta AK, Bandyk DF, Cheanvechai D, Johnson BL. Natural history of infrainguinal vein graft stenosis relative to bypass grafting technique. J Vasc Surg 1997;25:211–225.
11. Mills JL, Bandyk DF, Gahtan V, Esses GE. The origin of infrainguinal vein graft stenosis: A prospective study based on duplex surveillance. J Vasc Surg 1995;21:16–25.
12. Giannoukas AD, Adrouulakis AE, Labropoulos N, Wolfe JHN. The role of surveillance after infrainguinal bypass grafting. Eur J Vasc Endovasc Surg 1996;11:279–289.
13. Idu MM, Blankenstein JD, de Gier P, Truyen E, Buth J. Impact of a color-flow duplex surveillance program on infrainguinal vein graft patency: A five-year experience. J Vasc Surg 1993;17:42–53.
14. Bandyk DF, Bergamini TM, Towne JB, et al. Durability of vein graft revision: The outcome of secondary procedures. J Vasc Surg 1991;13:200–210.
15. Donaldson MC, Mannick JA, Whittemore AD. Causes of primary graft failure after in situ saphenous vein bypass grafting. J Vasc Surg 1991;13:137–149.
16. Bergamini TM, Towne JB, Bandyk DF, et al. Experience with in situ saphenous vein bypass during 1981 to 1989: Determinant factors of long-term patency. J Vasc Surg 1991;13:97–106.
17. Johnson BL, Bandyk DF, Back MR, Avino AJ, Roth SM. Intraoperative duplex monitoring of infrainguinal vein bypass procedures. J Vasc Surg 2000;31:678–690.
18. Armstrong PA, Bandyk DF, Wilson JS, Shames ML, Johnson BL, Back MR. Optimizing infrainguinal arm vein bypass patency with duplex ultrasound surveillance and endovascular therapy. J Vasc Surg 2004;40:724–731.
19. Bandyk DF, Kaebnick HW, Bergamini TM, et al. Hemodynamics of in situ saphenous vein arterial bypass. Arch Surg 1988;123:477–482.
20. Bandyk DF, Seabrook GR, Moldenhauer P, et al. Hemodynamics of vein graft stenosis. J Vasc Surg 1988;8:688–695.
21. Belkin M, Mackey WC, Maclaughlin R, et al. The variation in vein graft flow velocity with luminal diameter and outflow level. J Vasc Surg 1992;15:991–999.
22. Mills JL, Fujitani RM, Taylor SM. The contribution of routine intraoperative completion arteriography to early graft patency. Am J Surg 1992;164:506–511.
23. Miller Maracaccio EJ, Tannerbaum GE, et al. Comparison of angioscopy and angiography for monitoring infrain-

guinal bypass grafts: Result of a prospective randomized trial. J Vasc Surg 1993;17:382–398.

24. Rzucidlo EM, Walsh DB, Powell RJ, Zwolak RM, Fillinger MF, Schermerhorn ML, Cronenwett JL. Prediction of early graft failure with intraoperative completion duplex ultrasound scan. J Vasc Surg 2002;36:975–981.

25. Giswold ME, Landry GJ, Sexton GJ, Yeager RA, Edwards JM, Taylor LM, Moneta GL. Modifiable patient factors associated with reverse vein graft occlusion in the era of duplex scan surveillance. J Vasc Surg 2003;37:47–53.

26. Gahtan V, Payne LP, Roper LD, et al. Duplex criteria for predicting progression of vein graft lesions. J Vasc Tech 1995;19:211–215.

27. Westerband A, Mills JL, Kistler S, et al. Prospective validation of threshold criteria for intervention in infrainguinal vein grafts undergoing duplex surveillance. Ann Vasc Surg 1997;11:44–48.

28. Caps T, Cantwell-Gab, K, Bergelin RO, Strandness DE. Vein graft lesions: Time of onset and rate of progression. J Vasc Surg 1995;22:466–475.

29. Mills et al. Mills JL, Wixon CL, James DC, Devine J, Westerband A, Hughes JU. The natural history of intermediate and critical vein graft stenosis: Recommendations for continued surveillance or repair. J Vasc Surg 2001;33:273–280.

30. Sladen JG, Reid JDS, Cooperberg PL, et al. Color flow duplex screening of infrainguinal grafts combining low and high-velocity criteria. Am J Surg 1989;158:107–112.

31. Papanicoloauo G, Zierler RE, Beach RW, et al. Hemodynamic parameters of failing infrainguinal bypass grafts. Am J Surg 1995;169:238–244.

32. Buth J, Disselhoff B, Sommeling C, et al. Color flow duplex criteria for grading stenosis in infrainguinal vein grafts. J Vasc Surg 1991;14:729–738.

33. Bell P, et al. At what PSV ratio value should grafts be revised. Eur J Vasc Endovasc Surg 1998;15:258–261.

34. Avino AJ, Bandyk DF, Gonsalves AJ, Johnson BL, Black TJ, Zwiebel BR, Rahaim MJ, Cantor A. Surgical and endovascular intervention for infrainguinal vein graft stenosis. J Vasc Surg 1999;29:60–71.

35. Alexander JQ, Katz SG. The efficacy of percutaneous transluminal angioplasty in the treatment of infrainguinal vein bypass graft stenosis. Arch Surg 2003;138:510–513.

36. Kasirajan K, Schneider PA. Early outcome of "cutting" balloon angioplasty for infrainguinal vein graft stenosis. J Vasc Surg 2004;39:702–708.

37. Erickson CA, Towne JB, Seabrook GR, et al. Ongoing vascular laboratory surveillance is essential to maximize long term in situ saphenous vein bypass patency. J Vasc Surg 1996;23:18–27.

23
Rationale and Benefits of Surveillance After Prosthetic Infrainguinal Bypass Grafts

Stephen Kolakowski, Jr., Keith D. Calligaro, Sandy McAffe-Benett, Kevin J. Doerr, Kathy Mueller, and Matthew J. Dougherty

Introduction

Infrainguinal revascularization with autogenous conduit remains the gold standard of care for the treatment of critical lower extremity ischemia when bypass is required. One of the major factors diminishing long-term patency of these grafts is the development of stenosis of the graft or inflow and outflow arteries. Twenty to forty percent of all infrainguinal bypass grafts will develop stenosis due to different factors.[1] It is critical to identify these lesions while grafts are patent, as treatment with minor procedures will maintain patency, while treatment after thrombosis is significantly more morbid and less successful. Clinical examination looking for signs and symptoms of limb ischemia, including pulse evaluation and with measurement of ankle systolic pressure, can usually identify only the very high grade stenoses or occlusions. Over the past two decades there has been increasing evidence to support postoperative surveillance of arterial bypass grafts to improve long-term patency. The use of duplex ultrasound (DU) surveillance for infrainguinal vein grafts has become widely accepted.[2] We have suggested that DU is also applicable for prosthetic bypass grafts.[3]

Natural History

Primary patency of a graft is defined as uninterrupted patency without need for further procedures to maintain patency. Any surgical or percutaneous procedure performed on a patent graft, its anastomosis, or inflow and outflow vessels, serves as an endpoint to primary patency, but maintains "assisted primary patency." When a graft thromboses, "secondary" patency can be achieved by restoring patency to the graft.[4] As noted, the outcome of procedures performed to prevent graft thrombosis is better than that of procedures to restore patency of an occluded graft.[5]

In a large prospective randomized multicenter study, Veith and co-workers compared patency rates of infrainguinal bypasses using autologous vein grafts with those of prosthetic [polytetrafluoroethylene (PTFE)] grafts.[6] For infrainguinal bypasses to the above-knee popliteal artery, primary patency at 48 months was 76% for vein grafts and 54% for PTFE grafts, a difference that was not statistically different. For bypasses to the infrapopliteal arteries, primary patency rates at 48 months were 49% for vein grafts and 12% for PTFE grafts, respectively. This study performed prior to routine duplex surveillance gives a picture of the natural history of these revascularization efforts, since graft failure was recorded when graft thrombosis occurred or when any secondary intervention became necessary to treat graft thrombosis.

Prospective observational studies with the use of DU have demonstrated that 20–30% of infrainguinal vein bypasses develop discrete stenoses during the first postoperative year.[7] These lesions are usually the result of myointimal hyperplasia. If these lesions are not corrected, they have been associated with 80% of all graft failures within 3–5 years of the original procedure.

The natural history of bypass grafts with documented DU abnormalities when left untreated is unclear. Approximately 100 total grafts with varying DU abnormalities in one series were followed without revision.[8] Idu and co-workers reported high occlusion rates in a small group of bypass grafts both autogenous and prosthetic with 50% diameter-reducing stenoses on arteriography if left unrevised. In a subsequent prospective randomized study, superior patency rates were found in grafts that were revised based on DU abnormalities.[8,9] However, only 18 grafts were treated in this series. Mattos and co-workers followed 38 grafts with DU abnormalities and found similarly inferior patency rates in failing grafts that were left unrevised when compared with failing grafts that were revised.[10] We followed 46 failing arterial bypass grafts over a median of 10 months that were not treated for a variety of reasons (difficult anatomy, patient reluctance, etc.)[11] Only five (10.9%) showed progression of abnormal findings. Only 3 of the 46 failing grafts (6.5%) occluded during the follow-up period.

Clearly intervening for a failing graft is more beneficial than for failed grafts. In a retrospective series of 213 patients from the Mayo Clinic who underwent graft revision of pedal bypasses, 2 year patency rates in failing vs. failed grafts were reported to be 58% and 36%, respectively.[12] These data are supported by Wixon and co-workers who demonstrated that revision of a duplex-identified stenosis was significantly less costly over a 1-year period than revision after graft thrombosis ($17,688 vs. $45,252, respectively).[13]

Duplex Ultrasonography

Prior to the routine use of DU, clinical parameters, such as return of ischemic symptoms, and reduction in ankle-brachial indices and pulse volume recordings were used to detect failing grafts. These modalities lack sufficient sensitivity to detect some stenoses and some become abnormal only after graft occlusion. Two European studies relying on clinical symptoms to diagnose greater than 50% reduction in graft diameter missed 62–89% of duplex-defined lesions.[14,15] Even by adding the measurement of ankle-brachial indices, only 46% of grafts with greater than 50% stenoses were diagnosed.[16] In contrast, duplex ultrasonography detected 100% of grafts with the same diameter reduction.[15] Contrary to prior thought, the value of ankle-brachial index appears to be limited in predicting graft failure.[16,17]

In 1985 Bandyk and co-workers published one of the earliest reports about the use of DU-derived blood flow velocity measurements to define graft stenosis that might predict graft failure.[18] The two most important predictors in this series were low peak systolic velocities (<45 cm/s) throughout the graft and the absence of diastolic forward flow, indicating high outflow resistance. The authors also noted that all grafts experienced some degree of increased outflow resistance in the early postoperative period, as evidenced by a generalized drop in peak systolic velocities during follow-up studies. These results were later confirmed by Mills and co-workers on a much larger patient cohort.[19] Once again, a peak systolic velocity of 45 cm/s was suggested as the threshold to predict early graft failure. If the peak systolic velocity was higher than 45 cm/s in this series, the chance for graft failure was 2.1% compared with a 12.6% graft failure rate if the peak systolic velocities were routinely less than 45 cm/s. Only 29% of failing grafts, as diagnosed by DU, showed a reduction in ankle-brachial index measurement greater than 0.15, clearly indicating the higher sensitivity of DU surveillance.

These studies were performed using DU sampling at three positions: proximal anastomosis, mid graft, and distal anastomosis. This method may miss focal stenoses within the body of the graft, or in inflow and outflow vessels. The current technique in most reliable noninvasive vascular laboratories includes sampling the graft with segmental peak systolic velocity measurements along its entire length. In our noninvasive laboratory, velocities are measured every 10 cm along the graft, along with measurements at both anastomosis, and proximal and distal to the anatomy. It appears that the benefit of DU surveillance is most apparent in the highest risk autogenous grafts.

A recent retrospective review by Armstrong and co-workers found a statistically significant benefit of DU surveillance in optimizing the patency of infrainguinal grafts constructed with an arm vein.[20] They found the combination of DU and endovascular therapy achieved an excellent assisted graft patency rate (91%) and limb salvage rate (97%) at 3 years. These statistics are impressive considering half of the bypass required a graft intervention and one-third required surgical revision.

Surveillance programs for infrainguinal vein grafts have been well supported.[21] It would follow that given that prosthetic grafts do have a higher propensity to fail, DU surveillance might be correspondingly more valuable. However, the surveillance of infrainguinal prosthetic grafts has received mixed reviews.[8,22–28] A prospective randomized study by Lundell and co-workers demonstrated a 25% improvement in infrainguinal vein bypass patency at 3 years (78% vs. 53%) with DU surveillance, but no significant benefit was appreciated with PTFE or PTFE-vein composite graft patency.[29] However, the number of prosthetic infrapopliteal arterial grafts was very small, which may limit he statistical value of the analysis.

We and others have observed significant benefits for surveillance programs for prosthetic grafts.[3,5,30,31] Many feel that prosthetic graft failure often occurs without the harbinger of a discrete stenosis developing. The nature of the lesions that can cause prosthetic graft failure is similar to that of autologous vein grafts. They tend to be located primarily at an anastomosis, in adjacent inflow or outflow arteries, or much less commonly within the body of the graft.

As has been demonstrated for vein grafts, patency rates of thrombosed prosthetic grafts undergoing revision are inferior to assisted primary patency rates for failing prosthetic grafts.[5] Sullivan and co-workers demonstrated that thrombolysis for occluded vein grafts had significantly better long-term patency than for prosthetic grafts (69.3% vs. 28.6% at 30 months), which supports aggressive surveillance of prosthetic grafts.[32]

Prosthetic grafts are much more sensitive to low-flow states and resulting thrombosis than autologous vein grafts. When reviewing DU surveillance data on 89 infrainguinal prosthetic bypass grafts at our institution, we found that the sensitivity of abnormal DU findings that correctly diagnosed a failing graft was 88% for femorotibial bypasses but only 57% for femoropopliteal bypasses.[3] The positive predictive value (correct abnormal studies/total abnormal studies) was 95% for femorotibial grafts and 65% for femoropopliteal grafts. Therefore we concluded that DU surveillance is indicated and worthwhile for prosthetic femorotibial grafts, while its utility for prosthetic femoropopliteal grafts remains unproven.

Several studies have shown that DU surveillance is cost effective when compared with performing graft revisions based on clinical indications alone.[13,33] Wixon and co-workers concluded that the 1-year and 5-year costs of DU surveillance ($7,742 vs. $12,194, respectively) were markedly less than performing graft revisions based on clinical indications alone ($10,842 vs. $16,352, respectively).[13] They also found that patent grafts revised after DU detected stenoses had an improved 1-year patency (93% vs. 57%), were associated with fewer amputations (2% vs. 33%) and less frequent multiple graft revisions, and generated fewer expenses 1 year after revision compared to grafts revised after they occluded.

In our protocol, both vein and prosthetic bypass grafts are routinely evaluated by duplex sonography in the early post discharge period.[11] Thereafter, the graft is followed every three months for the first year after bypass operation, every six months for the second year, and annually thereafter if no problems are found. A 4.0–7.5 MHz probe is utilized with color map imaging. It is essential that the examiner is aware of the origin of the graft and its course. Due to their more superficial location, in situ vein grafts are much easier to follow than anatomically tunneled grafts. The entire graft is scanned beginning at the inflow artery, crossing the proximal anastomosis, moving along the body of the graft every 10 cm, and beyond the distal anastomosis. Peak systolic and diastolic velocities are recorded at these sites. Color flow is used to identify areas of turbulence, which are also sampled. Significant focal increase in flow velocities is more precisely investigated with measurements performed proximal and distal to the focus. At the distal anastomosis the Doppler angle must be carefully adjusted, due to the relatively steep angle of the graft. If consistently low peak systolic velocities are detected throughout the graft, a more detailed examination of the inflow and outflow vessels is necessary. These findings, however, could be consistent with normal flow through a relatively large diameter graft.

TABLE 23–1. Criteria to identify failing arterial bypass grafts at Pennsylvania Hospital.

Monophasic signal throughout the graft
Uniform peak systolic velocities <45 cm/s
Any focal peak systolic velocity >300 cm/s
Peak systolic velocity ratio between two adjacent segments >3.5

Abnormal Findings

There is no firm consensus on strict criteria for defining stenosis with duplex ultrasonography or on what degree of abnormality mandates revision.[10,34–36] The published literature has focused on low peak systolic flow velocities (PSFV)[17,18,21] and focal increases in peak systolic flow velocities with reference to adjacent areas.[8,9,30,37–39] A combination of these two parameters has also been recommended.[40] A consensus appears to be evolving away from low flow velocity criteria toward use of a PSFV ratio of 3–4. The criteria used at our institution to determine failing grafts are illustrated in Table 23–1.

Indications for Interventions

The optimal threshold of intervention for arterial bypass grafts is still controversial. Most authorities would agree that impending failure of a graft is suggested by the following:

1. Lack of diastolic forward flow throughout the graft as evidenced by monophasic Doppler signals.
2. Decreased peak systolic velocities less than 45 cm/s throughout the graft.
3. Focal elevations of peak systolic velocities greater than 250–350 cm/s.
4. Elevated peak systolic velocity ratios between two adjacent segments, suggested by abnormal elevated ratios, range between 3.5 and 4.0.[8,10,41–46]

Gupta and co-workers recommended peak systolic velocity ratios greater than 3.4 and focal peak systolic velocities greater than 300 cm/s.[44] Similar values were also suggested by Mills et al.[19]

Bandyk created a graft surveillance risk stratification model to predict graft thrombosis as illustrated in Table 23–2.[33] Patients with Category I lesions were hospitalized, anticoagulated, and promptly treated. Patients with Category II lesions were repaired electively within 2 weeks. Category III lesions were closely observed with serial duplex examinations and repaired if the lesions progressed in severity. Category IV lesions at the lowest risk were safely observed. Westerband and co-workers were able to support these criteria with a prospective study and demonstrate all grafts at risk for thrombosis.[45]

TABLE 23–2. Risk stratification for graft thrombosis based on surveillance data.[a]

Category	High-velocity criteria		Low-velocity criteria		ΔABI
I (highest risk)	PSV > 300 cm/s or Vr > 3.5	and	GFV < 45 cm/s	or	>0.15
II (high risk)	PSV > 300 cm/s or Vr > 3.5	and	GFV > 45 cm/s	and	<0.15
III (intermediate risk)	180 < PSV > 300 cm/s or Vr > 2.0	and	GFV > 45 cm/s	and	<0.15
IV (low risk)	PSV < 180 cm/s or Vr < 2.0	and	GFV > 45 cm/s	and	<0.15

[a]PSV, duplex-derived peak systolic velocity; Vr, velocity ratio of stenosis to more proximal graft segment of same caliber; GFV, graft flow velocity; ABI, Doppler-derived ankle-brachial index.

An interesting finding in Bandyk's series was that of lesion regression when a Category III (intermediate graft stenosis (PSV 150–300 cm/s, Vr < 3.5) lesion is discovered in the first 3 months after surgery; it may regress (30–35%), remain stable, or progress to a high-grade stenosis (40–50%).[33] Given the variable biological behavior, it is critical to perform serial duplex studies at 4–6 week intervals for Category III abnormalities. These lesions will usually stabilize or progress within 4–6 months.[10,44]

As suggested by the previous study from our group, abnormal duplex findings do not always mandate further therapy.[1,47] This is especially true if the abnormal finding is moderate PSV ratio elevation near the proximal anastomosis. We speculate that the hemodynamics at vessel bifurcations, which occurs at the typical end-to-side proximal anastomosis, is not strictly comparable to flow dynamics within the graft because of size discrepancies between the graft and native artery. Possibly this turbulence and the resulting abnormalities in peak systolic velocity ratios at the proximal anastomosis are less predictive of graft thrombosis than the same abnormalities at other locations.

Recommendation of Lifelong Surveillance

Clearly duplex surveillance of infrainguinal bypass grafts is beneficial, but how long does the surveillance program need to continue? Most reviews have shown a definite benefit up to 2 years based on the fact that 70–80% of all graft abnormalities develop and require revision during this time period. Erickson and co-workers recommend that surveillance continue indefinitely for autogenous bypass grafts.[48] They reported that 18% of the initial interventions for a duplex-detected lesion occurred after the initial 24-month period. Sixty-three percent of theses defects occurred at an anastomosis. Although the incidence of vein graft stenosis developing decreases over time, atherosclerotic changes continue in native arteries. Another important finding to look for in older vein grafts is aneurysmal degeneration of the vein. Vein dilation is usually focal and can be associated with mural thrombus, which may warrant segmental graft revision. We support the concept of lifelong vein graft surveillance, which also gives the vascular surgeon the opportunity to monitor development of atherosclerosis in other vascular beds.

Summary

Duplex ultrasonography is the method of choice for the surveillance of infrainguinal bypass grafts. Every noninvasive vascular laboratory should continuously correlate its interpretations with arteriographic findings and clinical outcomes. Any focal peak systolic velocity >300 cm/s or a peak systolic velocity ratio >3.5 between two adjacent segments is generally accepted as a strong indicator for a focal stenosis that may threaten graft patency. Low peak systolic velocities throughout the graft (<45 cm/s), as well as lack of diastolic forward flow as evidenced by loss of biphasic Doppler signals throughout the graft, may also indicate inflow or outflow problems and warrant further investigation. Arteriography and appropriate endovascular or open surgical revision of failing grafts should be judiciously implemented by the vascular surgeon to improve long-term patency and limb salvage rates.

References

1. Ryan SV, Dougherty MJ, Chang M, Lombardi J, Raviola C, Calligaro K. Abnormal duplex findings at the proximal anastomosis of infrainguinal bypass grafts: Does revision enhance patency? Ann Vasc Surg 2001;15:98–103.
2. Lundell A, Lindblad B Bergqvist D, Hansen F. Femoro-popliteal-crural graft patency is improved by an intensive surveillance program: A prospective randomized study J Vasc Surg 1995;21:26–33.
3. Calligaro KD, Doerr K, McAffee-Bennett S, Krug R, Raviola CA, Dougherty MJ. Should duplex ultrasonography be performed for surveillance of femoropopliteal and femorotibial arterial prosthetic bypasses? Ann Vasc Surg 2001;15:520–524.
4. Rutherford RB, Baker JD, Ernst C, Johnston KW, Porter JM, Ahn S, Jones DN. Recommended standards for reports

dealing with lower extremity ischemia: Revised version. J Vasc Surg 1997;26:517.

5. Sanchez LA, Suggs WD, Veith FJ, et al. Is surveillance to detect failing polytetrafluoroethylene bypasses worthwhile? Am J Surg 1993;18:981–990.

6. Veith FJ, Gupta SK, Ascer E, et al. Six-year prospective multicenter randomized comparison of autologous saphenous vein and expanded polytetrafluoroethylene grafts in infrainguinal arterial reconstructions. J Vasc Surg 1986;3:104–114.

7. Mills JL, Harris EJ, Taylor LM, Beckett Wc. The origin of infrainguinal vein graft stenosis: A prospective study based duplex surveillance. J Vasc Surg 1995;21:16–25.

8. Idu MM, Blankenstein JD, de Gier P, et al. Impact of color-flow duplex surveillance program on infrainguinal vein graft patency: A five-year experience. J Vasc Surg 1993;17:42–53.

9. Lundell A, Linblad B, Bergqvist D, et al. Femoropopliteal-crural graft patency is improved by an intensive surveillance program: A prospective randomized study. J Vasc Surg 1995;21:26–34.

10. Mattos MA, van Bemmelen PS, Hodgson KJ, et al. Does correction of stenoses identified with color duplex scanning improve infrainguinal graft patency? J Vasc Surg 1993:17:54–66.

11. Dougherty MJ, Calligaro KD, Delaurentis DA. The natural history of "failing" arterial bypass grafts in a duplex surveillance protocol. Ann Vasc Surg 1998;12:255–259.

12. Rhodes JM, Gloviczki P, Bower TC, Panneton JM, Canton LG, Toomey BJ. The benefits of secondary interventions in patients with failing or failed pedal bypass grafts. Am J Surg 1999;178:151–155.

13. Wixon CL, Mills JL, Westerband A, Hughes JD, Ihnat DM. An economic appraisal of lower extremity bypass graft maintenance. J Vasc Surg 2000;32:1–12.

14. Moody P, Gould DA, Harris PL. Vein graft surveillance improves patency in femoropopliteal bypass. Eur J Vasc Surg 1990;4:117–121.

15. Disselhoff B, Bluth J, Jakimowicz J. Early detection of stenosis of femoral-distal grafts: A surveillance study using color-duplex scanning. Eur J Vasc Surg 1989;3:43–48.

16. Barnes RW, Thompson BW, MacDonald CM, et al. Serial noninvasive studies do not herald postoperative failure of femoropopliteal or femorotibial bypass grafts. Ann Surg 1989;210:486–492.

17. Berkowitz J, Hobbs C, Roberts B, et al. Value of routine vascular laboratory studies to identify vein graft stenoses. Surgery 1981;90:971–979.

18. Bandyk DF, Cato RF, Towne JB. A low flow velocity predicts failure of femoropopliteal and femorotibial bypass grafts. Surgery 1985;98:799–809.

19. Mills JL, Harris EJ, Taylor LM Jr, et al. The importance of routine surveillance of distal bypass grafts with duplex scanning: A study of 379 reversed vein grafts. J Vasc Surg 1990;12:379–386; discussion 387–389.

20. Armstrong PA, Bandyk DF, Wilson JS, Shames ML, Johnson BL, Back MR. Optimizing infrainguinal arm vein bypass patency with duplex ultrasound surveillance and endovascular therapy. J Vasc Surg 2004;40:724–730; discussion 730–731.

21. Bandyk DF, Schmitt DD, Seabrook GR, et al. Monitoring functional patency of in situ saphenous vein bypasses: The impact of a surveillance protocol and elective revision. J Vasc Surg 1989;9:284–296.

22. Strandness DE, Andros G, Bake D, et al. Vascular laboratory utilization and payment report of the Ad Hoc Committee of the Western Vascular Society. J Vasc Surg 1992;16:163–168.

23. Lalak NJ, Hanel KC, Junt J, et al. Duplex scan surveillance of infrainguinal prosthetic bypass grafts. J Vasc Surg 1994;20:637–641.

24. Providers' News. April 1, 1993. Medicare Services, Louisiana.

25. Baker JD. The vascular laboratory: Regulations and other challenges. J Vasc Surg 1994;19:901–904.

26. TASC Working Group. Management of peripheral arterial disease. J Vasc Surg 2000;31:S1–S296.

27. Hobollah JJ, Nassal MM, Ryan SM, et al. Is color duplex surveillance of infrainguinal polytetrafluoroethylene grafts worthwhile? Am J Surg 1997;174:131–135.

28. Fasih T, Rudol G, Ashour H, Mudawi A, Bhattacharya V. Surveillance versus nonsurveillance for femoro-popliteal bypass grafts. Angiology 2004;55(3):251–256.

29. Lundell A, Lindblad B, Bergqvist D, Hansen F. Femoropopliteal-crural graft patency is improved by an intensive surveillance program: A prospective randomized study. J Vasc Surg 1995;21:26–33.

30. Calligaro KD, Musser DJ, Chen AY, et al. Duplex ultrasonography to diagnose arterial prosthetic grafts. Surgery 1996;120:455–459.

31. Sanchez LA, Gupta SK, Veith FJ, et al. A ten-year experience with one hundred fifty failing or threatened vein polytetrafluoroethylene arterial bypass grafts. J Vasc Surg 1991;14:729–738.

32. Sullivan KL, Gardiner GA Jr, Kandarpa K, Bonn J, Shapiro MJ, Carabasi RA, Smullens S, Levin DC. Efficacy of thrombolysis in infrainguinal bypass grafts. Circulation. 1991;83(2 Suppl):I99–105.

33. Bandyk DF. Infrainguinal vein bypass graft surveillance: How to do it, when to intervene, and is it cost-effective?. J Am Coll Surg 2002;194(1 Suppl):S40–52.

34. Nyamekye I, Sommerville K, Raphael M, Adiseshiah M, Bishop C. Non-invasive assessment of arterial stenoses in angioplasty surveillance: A comparison with angiography. Eur J Vasc Endovasc Surg 1996;12:471–481.

35. Buth J, Disselhoff B, Sommeling C, et al. Color-flow duplex criteria for grading stenosis in infrainguinal vein grafts. J Vasc Surg 1991;14:716–728.

36. Grigg MJ, Nicolaides AN, Wolfe JHN. Detection and grading of femorodistal vein graft stenoses: Duplex velocity measurements compared with angiography. J Vasc Surg 1988;8:661–666.

37. Bergamini TM, George SM, Massey HT, et al. Intensive surveillance of femoropopliteal-tibial autogenous vein bypasses improves long-term graft patency and limb salvage. Ann Surg 1995;221:507–516.

38. Gahtan V, Payne LP, Roper LD, et al. Duplex criteria for predicting progression of vein graft lesions: Which stenoses can be followed? J Vasc Tech 1995;19:211–215.

39. Belkin M, Schwartz LB, Donaldson MC, *et al.* Hemodynamic impact of vein graft stenoses and their prediction in the vascular laboratory. J Vasc Surg 1997;25:1016–1022.

40. Sladen JG, Reid JDS, Cooperberg PL, *et al.* Color-flow duplex screening of infrainguinal grafts combining low and high velocity criteria. Am J Surg 1989;158:107–112.

41. Bandyk DF, Johnson BL, Gupta AK, *et al.* Nature and management of duplex abnormalities encountered during infrainguinal vein bypass grafting. J Vasc Surg 1996;24:430–438.

42. Caps MT, Cantwell-Gab K, Bergelin RO, *et al.* Vein graft lesions: Time of onset and rate of progression. J Vasc Surg 1995;22:466–474.

43. Chalmers RT, Hoballah JJ, Kresowik TF, *et al.* The impact of color duplex surveillance on the outcome of lower limb bypass with segments of arm veins. J Vasc Surg 1994;19:279–286.

44. Gupta AK, Bandyk DF, Cheanvechai D, *et al.* Natural history of infrainguinal vein graft stenosis relative to bypass grafting technique. J Vasc Surg 1997;25:211–220.

45. Westerband A, Mills JL, Kistler S, *et al.* Prospective validation of threshold criteria for intervention in infrainguinal vein grafts undergoing duplex surveillance. Ann Vasc Surg 1997;11:44–48.

46. Idu MM, Buth J, Hop WC, *et al.* Vein graft surveillance: Is graft revision without angiography justified and what criteria should be used? J Vasc Surg 1998;27:399–411.

47. Dougherty MJ, Calligaro KD, DeLaurentis DA. Revision of failing lower extremity bypass grafts. Am J Surg 1998;178:126–130.

48. Erickson CA, Towne JB, Seabrook GR, Freischlag JA, Cambria RA. Ongoing vascular laboratory surveillance is essential to maximize long-term in situ saphenous vein bypass patency. J Vasc Surg 1996;23:18–26.

24

Rationale and Benefits of Surveillance After Percutaneous Transluminal Angioplasty and Stenting of Iliac and Femoral Arteries

Evan C. Lipsitz and George L. Berdejo

Introduction

Duplex surveillance of lower extremity bypass grafts significantly improves both primary assisted and secondary patency rates.[1,2] In this setting duplex ultrasound provides objective, hemodynamic data, and can provide detailed anatomic information both in terms of degree of stenosis as well as plaque characteristics and morphology. It can also be cost-effective.[3] The goal of any surveillance protocol is to reduce procedural failures by detecting disease progression within the treated segment and allow for reintervention before a failure is realized. Such a protocol will ideally be cost-effective based on the assumption that the cost of reintervention is less than the cost of treating a failure of that procedure, which is likely to require a more complex intervention with potentially greater morbidity.

Although reporting standards are well-established for the surveillance of lower extremity bypass grafts there are currently no such standards for surveillance after lower extremity angioplasty. Therefore, duplex surveillance protocols following angioplasty of the iliac and femoral arteries have largely been based on the concepts and results derived from duplex surveillance of lower extremity bypass grafts.

Rationale

All interventions are finite. Although angioplasty has less patency than bypass grafting, it is a less invasive option for lower extremity revascularization. If symptoms resolve a successful angioplasty may postpone or ultimately preclude the need for the more invasive intervention. A surveillance protocol, with appropriate reintervention when needed, can therefore extend the patency of angioplasty sites and delay or prevent the need for a more invasive bypass procedure. Different vascular beds have different rates of restenosis following angioplasty. In general, the larger the artery is, the lower the restenosis rate. One year patency rates following iliac artery angioplasty for stenoses range from 67% to 92%, whereas patency rates for occlusions range from 59% to 94%. Primary patency rates for angioplasty of femoropopliteal lesions at 1 year range from 47% to 86%.[4] Other considerations such as clinical indication (claudication vs. limb salvage), lesion length, location within the vessel, degree of calcification, eccentricity of the lesion, the presence and extent of inflow and outflow disease, and overall medical condition will also affect restenosis rates. Finally, female sex and renal insufficiency in the presence of critical ischemia are associated with deceased patency rates in patients undergoing iliac angioplasty and stenting.[5]

As is the case for bypass procedures, failure following interventional procedures may occur early or late. There are also similar causes of failure at each stage. Although somewhat simplified, early failures (<30 days) following angioplasty and/or stenting are usually due to technical failures secondary to the presence of residual or newly created defects, or to a thrombogenic state. These technical failures may be due to incomplete angioplasty, recoil of the vessel, or the presence of a residual flow limiting lesion. Midterm failures (30 days–18 months) are generally due to the development of intimal hyperplasia while late failures (>18 months) are frequently due to progression of the underlying atherosclerotic disease process.

To justify any surveillance protocol, it is necessary to show that primary assisted and/or secondary patency rates exceed primary patency rates to a degree that justifies the surveillance (Figure 24–1).[6] In addition, the justification for such a protocol depends on the ability of the method to detect treated sites at risk (positive predictive value), the implications of failure of the procedure, and the durability of potential secondary interventions that may be performed.

Duplex ultrasound has been used increasingly in both the preprocedural planning and intraprocedural performance of lower extremity angioplasty.[7] Advantages of this approach include reduced radiation exposure to the

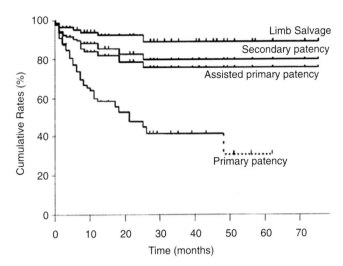

FIGURE 24–1. Increased assisted primary patency, secondary patency, and limb salvage rates above primary patency rates with duplex surveillance. (Adapted from Kudo T, Chandra FA, Ahn SS. The effectiveness of percutaneous transluminal angioplasty for the treatment of critical limb ischemia: A 10-year experience. J Vasc Surg 2005;41:423–35. With permission.)

patient and staff, as well as reduced risk of contrast toxicity, especially renal effects. Occasionally, duplex ultrasound may identify lesions not identified by conventional arteriography, such as the presence of intimal flaps (Figure 24–2).[8] Another major advantage is the ability to obtain a baseline evaluation at the completion of the procedure, which may then be used for comparison during follow-up surveillance examinations. One study found that the detection of a residual stenosis on duplex did not correlate with angiographic appearance, but predicted clinical failure.[9]

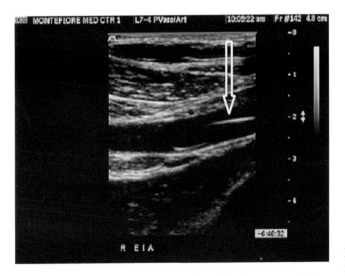

FIGURE 24–2. External Iliac artery dissection (open arrow). The dissection was not evident on angiography and was repaired under duplex guidance.

Outcome Measures

The ultimate utility and outcomes of a duplex surveillance protocol will depend on the definitions used to define success. In other words, how are outcomes defined in restorative as opposed to reconstructive procedures? The difference between a widely patent and an occluded segment is straightforward, but the degree of stenosis, as determined by peak systolic velocity (PSV) or other measures, may not be as obvious. This is largely because these determinations are being made in a vessel that is still diseased, despite the angioplasty that was performed. By extrapolating from the reporting standards adopted for the surveillance of lower extremity bypasses the following comparisons can be made.

To assess the optimal value of PSV for surveillance, i.e., that providing the greatest sensitivity and specificity, receiver operating characteristic (ROC) curve analysis can be performed. This analysis plots sensitivity and specificity against a range of PSV values. Such an analysis was performed for iliac interventions.[10] In this study a threshold PSV of 300 cm/s as determined by the need to reoperate was most optimal for the detection of technical failure, having the highest accuracy (81%) and specificity (90%), although the sensitivity was relatively low (58%) (Figure 24–3).

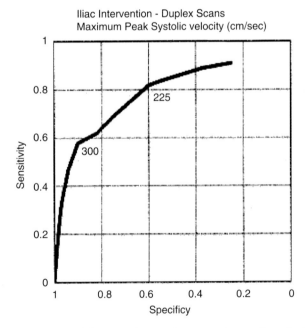

FIGURE 24–3. ROC curves for maximum peak systolic velocity following iliac intervention. (From Myers KA, Wood SR, Lee V. Vascular ultrasound surveillance after endovascular intervention for occlusive iliac artery disease. Cardiovasc Surg 2001;9:448–54. With permission.)

The criteria chosen to define technical success and patency will impact on technical success rates, patency rates, reintervention rates, and the number of reported failures. This fact underscores the need for evaluation of both hemodynamic and clinical results when evaluating a procedure. For example, subintimal angioplasty, which has been used in the treatment of long-segment lower extremity arterial occlusions in patients with severe lower extremity ischemia, has relatively low reported patency rates but high limb salvage rates, from which it derives much of its support, especially for use in high-risk patients.[11]

In most cases anatomic success of angioplasty is defined as residual luminal stenosis of less than 30% compared to normal diameter as determined by angiography or other accepted imaging techniques.[12] Anatomic failure is defined as restenosis of 50% or greater compared to the normal diameter by angiographic or other imaging assessment.[12]

Reporting standards for bypass procedures state that criteria used to determine a failing graft include a PSV above a certain level (e.g., 150 cm/s) or a PSV greater than that of an adjacent "normal" segment (e.g., at least 2.5 times).[13] End diastolic velocity also increases with greater degrees of stenosis. Failure on the basis of decreased graft flow velocity (e.g., below 45 cm/s) has also been predicted in femoropopliteal vein grafts. Absolute flow velocities may not be applicable to tibial or prosthetic bypass grafts. However, relative decreases in flow velocities on serial examinations are suggestive of problems in both bypass and angioplasty procedures.

Primary patency is defined as uninterrupted patency of the treated vessel without any interventional or open procedures that maintain or restore patency. Assisted primary patency is uninterrupted patency of the treated vessel with a secondary intervention, e.g., reballoon angioplasty designed to preserve patency in the setting of restenosis. As noted above, because the effects of angioplasty are not limited to the segment in which the balloon is inflated or where the stent is placed these definitions should include the entire artery(ies), or treated vessel(s) and not just the treated segment. Secondary patency is defined as patency of a vessel after an intervention, e.g., thrombolysis was undertaken to restore patency following occlusion of the vessel. For the purposes of lower extremity angioplasty, the difference between primary and assisted primary patency is the most important in assessing the benefits of a surveillance protocol since this difference is where most of the benefit will be realized. Reinterventions designed to restore patency (secondary patency) may not be required immediately upon the time of failure. For example, if an angioplasty performed for a gangrenous lesion that has healed goes on to fail but the patient remains asymptomatic, i.e., the lesion remains healed, no further intervention is required at that time.

Surveillance of Angioplasty with and Without Stents

The question can be raised as to whether there should be any difference in the indications for surveillance in patients undergoing angioplasty versus those undergoing angioplasty with stenting? We believe that protocols for the surveillance of angioplasty alone should not differ from those designed to follow angioplasty with stenting. Although many studies show no difference in restenosis rates, justifying surveillance in both cases, these may represent different cohorts of patients, with stented patients having more severe disease. There are some special concerns regarding stents. The presence of a stent may make visualization of the flow lumen somewhat difficult due to shadowing. Stents also decrease the compliance of the artery and may lead to velocities that are falsely elevated relative to the predicted degree of stenosis.

Surveillance of Angioplasty Versus Bypass Procedures

Although angioplasty is a "minimally invasive" procedure, it is nonetheless still an invasive procedure. While it differs in many ways from bypass procedures both these differences and its invasive nature need to be taken into account when considering a surveillance protocol. Angioplasty is a "restorative procedure," defined as "one in which the obstructing element (often clot or plaque) is removed or displaced from the lumen of an arterial or venous segment, allowing flow through the lumen to be restored to normal or near normal without direct reconstruction."[13] By its nature, it involves "controlled trauma" to a given narrowed area of the affected vessel. During dilatation of the vessel the plaque is split and the media is stretched. These events hopefully have the net effect of increasing the luminal diameter and the total cross-sectional area of the artery in question. There are, however, several negative effects resulting from angioplasty including the presence of irregularly fractured plaque, damage to the media that occurs from stretching, and desquamation of endothelium. There is also the potential for embolization and the creation of intimal flaps. In addition, longitudinal dissection planes are created and plaque fracture can extend a good distance proximal and/or distal to the actual angioplasty site. Because of these negative effects the already diseased vessel may be at increased risk of restenosis or occlusion along an even greater length than was encompassed by the original lesion. Thus, the entire arterial segment may be considered somewhat vulnerable and must be closely followed.

There are several new technologies that seek to improve upon the results of traditional angioplasty by reducing some of the negative effects indicated above. The evaluation of these technologies will be dependent on the performance of adequate duplex ultrasound surveillance protocols. One such device is the cutting balloon, which contains multiple longitudinally arranged circumferential microtomes, designed to cut the plaque before it ruptures and allow for a more uniform dilatation of the vessel with less plaque fracture and dissection. Another device is the cryoplasty balloon, which freezes the plaque prior to dilatation. In this case the plaque develops microfractures, again allowing for a more uniform dilatation without large plaque fracture or dissection. Another proposed advantage of the latter system is the prevention of intimal hyperplasia by inhibitory effects on the proliferation of vascular smooth muscle cells.

Bypass is a "reconstructive procedure," defined as "an open procedure that is performed to remove, replace, or bypass an obstructive or aneurysmal lesion involving the vessel wall and restore pulsatile flow beyond the involved segment."[13] In bypass procedures the inflow and outflow sites are chosen specifically such that anastomoses are constructed to the most normal area of the vessels possible. There should be minimal or no disease above the inflow site and minimal or no disease below the outflow site (the occluded segment as well as any diseased or otherwise unfavorable segments are excluded). However, with angioplasty only the most diseased segments of the artery are treated and the remaining, less diseased segments, left untreated, may still impact on the overall outcome of the procedure and its durability. Thus, bypass graft surveillance begins (ideally) with a relatively disease-free inflow, conduit (vein or prosthetic), and outflow vessel. In the case of surveillance following angioplasty there may be a patent, but nonetheless extensively diseased vessel in which quantitative and qualitative assessments are more difficult. This is especially true considering the variety of endoluminal procedures that are now being performed including traditional angioplasty, which dilates the native true lumen, subintimal angioplasty, which creates and dilates a new lumen, and atherectomy, in which plaque causing stenosis or occlusion is mechanically debulked. These considerations argue for close monitoring of the *entire* vessel following angioplasty.

A bypass graft that develops intimal hyperplasia or other lesions within the graft, as well as the progression of proximal or distal disease, can produce signs and symptoms of hemodynamic deterioration in patients without producing concomitant thrombosis of the bypass graft. This condition is referred to as a "failing graft" because, if not corrected, graft thrombosis will almost certainly occur.[14] The importance of this failing graft concept lies in the fact that many difficult lower extremity revascularizations can be salvaged for long periods by relatively simple interventions if the lesion responsible can be detected and treated before graft thrombosis occurs. The patency of a graft (or angioplasty site) is greater when treated prior to thrombosis than when treated after thrombosis occurs. Additionally, if recanalization is not possible, the secondary reconstruction may be difficult or impossible.

Because the entire artery is generally diseased, the reference diameter by which the degree of stenosis is judged may be smaller than that of the true, undiseased "normal" vessel diameter and as such lead to an underestimation of the actual degree of stenosis.

Alternative Surveillance Methods

Other surveillance methods have been considered and evaluated but none has proven to have the same utility as duplex scanning.[15–17] Physical examination, while simple, inexpensive, and readily available, is also unreliable in terms of predicting failures and is generally useful only once failure has occurred or in rare cases where failure is imminent. Resting ankle-brachial indices (ABIs) are less time consuming to perform than are duplex studies but are also subject to significant interobserver variability. In addition, the ABI is affected by the presence of both proximal and distal occlusive disease. While a decrease in ABI is indicative of some compromise in circulation, these decreases in ABI may therefore be due to the progression or development of lesions either within the treated segment, proximal to the treated segment, distal to the treated segment, or any combination thereof. Finally, ABIs are not reliable in patients with diabetes, end-stage renal disease, and/or heavy vascular calcifications. For these reasons resting ABIs are not considered to be an adequate method for long-term follow-up of patients undergoing angioplasty. Postexercise ABIs have also been found to be highly variable and have many of the same shortcomings as those described for resting ABIs. Other indirect measures, such as assessment of the common femoral artery waveform following iliac angioplasty, may be of benefit but are generally combined with other indirect measures for surveillance. Lastly, angiography, considered the current gold standard for the evaluation of lower extremity occlusive disease, is both invasive and costly and, as such, is not suitable for use as a surveillance tool.

Surveillance Duplex Protocol

Currently we utilize the following duplex surveillance protocol. Patients are scanned preprocedurally, within 1 month postprocedurally, every 3 months for the first year, every 6 months for the next year, and yearly thereafter.

If a patient requires a reintervention the protocol is restarted beginning from the time of the most recent reintervention. The protocol may also be adjusted to allow for increased frequency of screening if a stenosis of moderate severity is detected and the patient remains asymptomatic. The importance of follow up and the purpose of the surveillance protocol must be communicated to the patient as noncompliance may be a significant issue. This is especially true in patients who are asymptomatic or in those having limited mobility.

We and others also utilize a standardized scanning protocol for the surveillance of patients who have undergone angioplasty. Duplex Doppler with a 60°angle of insonation is employed. The entire treated segment is evaluated in addition to one complete vessel above and one complete vessel below the treated vessel. The maximum PSV is calculated at predetermined, standardized points within the vessel(s) examined. The PSV at the site of suspected stenosis is the most consistent measurement available and therefore minimizes interobserver variability. Other secondary criteria that can be used to evaluate restenosis include the PSV ratio at the stenosis (calculated by dividing the peak velocity at the stenosis by the velocity at a normal segment proximal to it), the end diastolic velocity, and evaluation of spectral waveforms.

The examination is performed using a high-resolution duplex scanner that provides color flow capability. The equipment selected must allow enough penetration to permit adequate insonation of the deep structures in the abdomen and pelvis with color flow sensitivity that allows the detection of slow flow velocities, all at reasonable frame rates. A low-frequency (2.5–4MHz) sector or curved array transducer is necessary to visualize these deep structures; often, however, a variety of differently configured (linear) and higher frequency (7–4MHz) transducers are needed to accomplish a complete iliofemoropopliteal study.

For iliac interventions, Doppler color-flow imaging is performed from the distal aorta, along the treated and native iliac segments, and through the common, proximal profunda, and superficial femoral arteries. Spectral velocity waveforms are sampled from the center-line of flow at multiple sites along the aortoiliofemoral segment. Spectral waveforms and measured PSVs within angioplastied and/or stented iliac segments are compared to velocities in adjacent native iliac artery segments. For femoropopliteal interventions, Doppler color-flow imaging is performed from the common femoral artery with evaluation of the waveform, along the treated and native femoropopliteal segments, and through the origin of the anterior tibial artery and tibioperoneal trunk. Spectral velocity waveforms are sampled from the center-line of flow at multiple sites along the femoropopliteal segment. Spectral waveforms and meas-

ured PSV within angioplastied and/or stented femoropopliteal segments are compared to velocities in adjacent native femoropopliteal artery segments.

We recommend that the first postprocedural scan be performed within 1–2 weeks following the procedure to obtain an adequate baseline study and to assess for any otherwise undetected residual stenosis. The PSV at the treated site and elsewhere in the vessel should be <200cm/s and the PSV ratio should be <2.

The reason to scan not only the treated segment but the entire vessel as well as one vessel above and below is because failure of the procedure can and does occur within any of these segments. In their series Meyers et al. found that restenosis in relation to a stent occurred above the stent in 11% of cases, within the stent in 56% of cases, and in the artery below the stent in 33% of cases (Figure 24–4).[10] Vroegindeweij et al. evaluated 62 femoropopliteal recannalizations with a 3 year patency of 44%.[18] They found that the majority of restenoses occurred within the first year following the procedure and that restenosis occurred within the distal one-half of the treated segment in 16 of 21 patients with recurrent stenosis.

The importance of residual stenosis is highlighted in a study from Kinney et al. In this study 77 balloon-dilated arterial segments were scanned using duplex ultrasound within 1 week of a technically successful angioplasty. Moderate (defined as 20–49% diameter reduction) or severe (defined as greater than 50% diameter reduction) residual stenosis was identified in 49 (63%) of the treated arterial segments. In segments with a greater than 50%

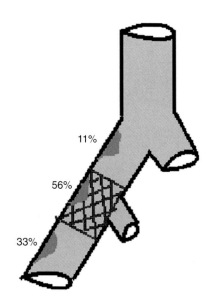

FIGURE 24–4. Distribution of restenoses following iliac angioplasty and stenting.

diameter reduction, further restenosis and late clinical failure were significantly more likely (11% success rate at 1 year) than in segments where the degree of residual stenosis was less than 50% diameter reduction (80% success rate at 2 years), including patients with critical ischemia, poor runoff, or diabetes mellitus.[19]

The vascular system is dynamic in nature and there are instances where regression of residual stenosis may be seen on serial duplex examinations. Spijkerboer *et al.* analyzed a series of 70 limbs in 61 patients undergoing iliac angioplasty.[20] In their series, 15 residual stenoses (as characterized by a PSV ratio >2.5) were identified on early postprocedural duplex. Of these 15 residual stenoses, 6 resolved by the 3-month duplex and 4 of these 6 remained improved at 1 year. Of the 9 that had not improved at the time of the month duplex one ultimately improved by 1 year. Back *et al.* reported a series of 84 iliac angioplasties undergoing surveillance, and identified 2 residual stenoses that regressed by the 3-month duplex.[21] This is not to suggest that high-grade residual stenoses be left untreated or that the presence of residual stenosis is not a predictor of failure, but rather to note that with remodeling and other less well understood factors improvement that obviates the need for reintervention can occur.

Plaque Morphology

Although there are many factors that predict technical success and durability of angioplasty within the arterial system the degree of stenosis is the parameter that has been most widely utilized. Other factors such as the degree of calcification, plaque ulceration, intraplaque hemorrhage, and other morphologic characteristics are also important but are not routinely analyzed. While not a formal part of most duplex surveillance protocols at present, evaluation of plaque morphology is an area of active investigation for the preprocedural and postprocedural evaluation of plaques in all vascular beds.[22,23] Such investigations may ultimately lead to a delineation of characteristics that can define which plaques are most amenable to angioplasty and/or stenting and which plaques will yield the most durable results. The use of B-mode imaging allows the observer to measure the plaque thickness and characteristics at all areas of the circumference of the vessel. The maximum and minimum luminal diameters can also be evaluated by this method. A method has been developed for evaluating the actual plaque morphology.[23] The process involves using computer image standardization of grayscale images. All digitized images (including those obtained by ultrasound) are made of pixels, the smallest units of information. All pixels in a grayscale image can be assigned a value from 0 (black) to 256 (white). The grayscale median represents the median value of all pixels within a given area of inter-

est. An image is taken and the values for blood and adventitia are normalized to 0–5 and 185–195, respectively. The image is then rescanned with these normalized values in place (to allow standardization across different scans) and a grayscale median (GSM) is calculated for the plaque. Echolucent plaques are plaques defined as having a GSM less than 25. They appear black on B-mode imaging and have a higher content of lipids and cholesterol. As such, they are more prone to rupture and embolization and in patients with carotid artery disease are more frequently seen in symptomatic patients. Conversely, echogenic plaques have a GSM greater than 25 and appear white on B-mode imaging. They contain larger amounts of fibrous tissue and calcium and are thereby less prone to rupture and embolization. In patients with carotid artery disease, these types of plaques are more commonly seen in asymptomatic patients.

The effect of GSM on lower limb angioplasty has been investigated by Ramaswami and colleagues.[22] They evaluated the value of ultrasonic plaque characteristics for identifying patients at "high risk" for restenosis following angioplasty. Thirty-one iliac or femoropopliteal stenoses were followed with serial duplex at 1 day, every week for 8 weeks, at 3 months, 6 months, and 1 year. Total plaque thickness, minimal luminal diameter, and PSV ratios were recorded. The authors found a significantly greater reduction in plaque thickness when the GSM was less than 25 (3.3 ± 1.8 mm) than when it was more than 25 (1.8 ± 1.6 mm). Using a 2-fold increase in the PSV ratio as the criterion for restenosis, the overall restenosis rate was 41% at 1 year. For lesions with a GSM of less than 25, restenosis occurred in 11% of cases, while in lesions with a GSM of more than 25, restenosis occurred in 78% of cases. This difference was highly significant (Figure 24–5). The

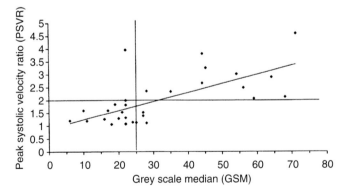

FIGURE 24–5. Relationship between grayscale median (GSM) and peak systolic velocity ratio following angioplasty. There is an increased restenosis rate with increasing GSM value for plaque. (From Ramaswami G, Tegos T, Nicolaides AN, *et al.* Ultrasonic plaque character and outcome after lower limb angioplasty. J Vasc Surg 1999;29:110–21. With permission.)

authors concluded that plaque echodensity can be used to evaluate stenoses prior to angioplasty to predict initial success and to identify a subgroup of plaques that has an increased likelihood of restenosis.

Other Factors

There may be as yet unrealized medical/physiologic factors that affect the durability of angioplasty and/or stenting in the iliac and femoral arteries. The use of statins has recently been shown to improve patency in lower extremity bypass grafts and there is reason to expect the same may be true for lower extremity angioplasty procedures.[24] In addition, stent technology continues to improve and both drug-eluting and covered stent technologies are currently undergoing evaluation. To date, convincing long-term results for these devices have not been presented. Determination of improved results due to both medical and mechanical developments will depend on the presence of reliable and consistent surveillance procedures that will take on a heightened importance in the assessment of these adjuncts.

Conclusion

Duplex ultrasound surveillance of iliac and femoral angioplasty and/or stenting provides essential hemodynamic information. Arterial duplex can provide useful anatomic information both pre- and postprocedurally, and is increasingly being used intraprocedurally. The implementation of such a surveillance protocol requires standardization for both the timing and technical performance of scans. A surveillance protocol can improve long-term patency of angioplasty sites and potentially delay or eliminate the need for additional, more invasive therapies.

References

1. Lundell AN, Lindblad B, Bergqvist D, *et al.* Femoropopliteal-crural graft patency is improved by an intensive surveillance program: A prospective, randomized study. J Vasc Surg 1995;21:26–34.
2. Fasih T, Rudol G, Ashour H, *et al.* Surveillance versus non-surveillance for femoro-popliteal bypass grafts. Angiology 2004;55:251–6.
3. Idu MM, Buth J, Cuypers P, *et al.* Economising vein-graft surveillance programs. Eur J Vasc Endovasc Surg 1998;15:432–38.
4. Dormandy JA, Rutherford RB. Management of peripheral arterial disease (PAD). TASC Working Group. Trans-Atlantic Inter-Society Concensus (TASC). J Vasc Surg 2000;31:S1–S296.
5. Timaran CH, Stevens SL, Freeman MB, Goldman MH. Predictors for adverse outcome after iliac angioplasty and stenting for limb-threatening ischemia. J Vasc Surg 2002;36:507–13.
6. Kudo T, Chandra FA, Ahn SS. The effectiveness of percutaneous transluminal angioplasty for the treatment of critical limb ischemia: A 10-year experience. J Vasc Surg 2005;41:423–35.
7. Wain RA, Berdejo G, Delvalle W, *et al.* Can duplex scan arterial mapping replace contrast arteriography as the test of choice before infrainguinal revascularization? J Vasc Surg 1999;29:100–9.
8. Cruz J, Lipsitz EC, Berdejo GL. Diagnosis and ultrasound-guided repair of an iliac artery dissection. JVU 2004;28:96–100.
9. Mewissen MW, Kinney EV, Bandyk DF, *et al.* The role of duplex scanning versus angiography in predicting outcome after balloon angioplasty in the femoropopliteal artery. J Vasc Surg 1992;15:860–66.
10. Myers KA, Wood SR, Lee V. Vascular ultrasound surveillance after endovascular intervention for occlusive iliac artery disease. Cardiovasc Surg 2001;9:448–54.
11. Lipsitz EC, Veith FJ, Ohki T. The value of subintimal angioplasty in the management of critical lower extremity ischemia: Failure is not always associated with a rethreatened limb. J Cardiovasc Surg (Torino) 2004;45:231–37.
12. Ahn SS, Rutherford RB, Becker GJ, *et al.* Reporting standards for lower extremity arterial endovascular procedures. Society for Vascular Surgery/International Society for Cardiovascular Surgery. J Vasc Surg 1993;17:1103–7.
13. Rutherford RB, Baker JD, Ernst C, *et al.* Recommended standards for reports dealing with lower extremity ischemia: revised version. J Vasc Surg 1997;26(3):517–38. Erratum in J Vasc Surg 2001;33:805.
14. Lipsitz EC, Veith FJ. Femoral-popliteal-tibial occlusive disease. In: Moore W (ed). *Vascular Surgery: A Comprehensive Review*, 6th ed, pp. 523–547. Philadelphia, PA: WB Saunders Company, 2002.
15. Fisher CM, Burnett A, Makeham V, *et al.* Variation in measurement of ankle-brachial pressure index in routine clinical practice. J Vasc Surg 1996;24:871–75.
16. Bray AE, Liu WG, Lewis WA, *et al.* Strecker stents in the femoropopliteal arteries: Value of duplex ultrasonography in restenosis assessment. J Endovasc Surg 1995;2:150–60.
17. Nyamekye I, Sommerville K, Raphael M, *et al.* Non-invasive assessment of arterial stenoses in angioplasty surveillance: A comparison with angiography. Eur J Vasc Endovasc Surg 1996;12:471–81.
18. Vroegindeweij D, Tielbeek AV, Buth J, Vos LD, van den Bosch HC. Patterns of recurrent disease after recanalization of femoropopliteal artery occlusions. Cardiovasc Intervent Radiol 1997;20:257–62.
19. Kinney EV, Bandyk DF, Mewissen MW, *et al.* Monitoring functional patency of percutaneous transluminal angioplasty. Arch Surg 1991;126:743–7.
20. Spijkerboer AM, Nass PC, de Valois JC, *et al.* Iliac artery stenoses after percutaneous transluminal angioplasty:

Follow-up with duplex ultrasonography. J Vasc Surg 1996; 23:691–7.

21. Back MR, Novotney M, Roth SM, et al. Utility of duplex surveillance following iliac artery angioplasty and primary stenting. J Endovasc Ther 2001;8:629–37.

22. Ramaswami G, Tegos T, Nicolaides AN, et al. Ultrasonic plaque character and outcome after lower limb angioplasty. J Vasc Surg 1999;29:110–21.

23. Elatrozoy T, Nicolaides A Tegos T, et al. The effect of B-mode ultrasonic image standardisation on the echodensity of symptomatic and asymptomatic carotid bifurcation plaques. Int Angiol 1998;17:179–86.

24. Abbruzzese TA, Havens J, Belkin M, et al. Statin therapy is associated with improved patency of autogenous infrainguinal bypass grafts. J Vasc Surg 2004;39:1178–85.

25
Duplex Ultrasound in the Diagnosis and Treatment of Femoral Pseudoaneurysms

Patrick A. Stone

The use of percutaneous methods for coronary interventions continues to grow, with more than 500,000 coronary interventions performed annually in the United States.[1] In concert, the frequency of postcatheterization false aneurysms continues to rise. Larger sheath sizes as well as more advanced anticoagulation regimens during and following percutaneous procedures have resulted in larger arterial defects with decreased ability to obtain hemostasis at the puncture site. Attempts at addressing this problem with closure devices and/or mechanical compression devices have failed to show clinical superiority to focal manual pressure. With the mounting push for less invasive treatment of cardiovascular and peripheral vascular disease, the vascular surgeon will frequently be faced with a "swollen" groin following these percutaneous procedures.

During the past three decades, the diagnosis and treatment algorithm for this iatrogenic problem has undergone multiple changes. As in other areas of arterial and venous pathology, the diagnosis of false aneurysms has become a minimally invasive procedure. Like carotid disease, once requiring arteriography prior to intervention, evaluation for iatrogenic pseudoaneurysms (IPA) today almost exclusively begins and ends with arterial duplex. Until the early 1990s, open surgical repair was the first-line, and really only, therapy widely offered for IPA.

Beginning in the late 1980s and through the mid 1990s, several centers reported results of observation and duplex follow-up for small pseudoaneurysms. In 1991, Fellmeth introduced ultrasound-guided compression (UGC), which was met with great enthusiasm. This minimally invasive option spared many patients an open surgical repair. However, the UGC technique had many limitations: long procedure times, treatment pain, and very mixed success in patients currently treated with anticoagulation.

The shortcomings of compression therapy were surmounted with the introduction of duplex-guided thrombin injection (DGTI), first described in 1986, whereby a small amount of thrombin is injected directly into the pseudoaneurysm sac with the assistance of ultrasound. DGTI treatment is less painful, faster, and more successful than UGC. Diagnosis and treatment of IPA in the twenty-first century are handled almost exclusively by duplex technology. With groin-related false aneurysms accounting for the majority of those encountered in practice, the focus of this chapter will be on postcatheterization femoral pseudoaneurysms and their contemporary management.

Definition and Incidence

Pseudoaneurysms result when a disruption in one or more layers of the arterial wall occurs. Should an arterial puncture site not seal, subsequent arterial bleeding into the soft tissue can result in hematoma formation. Occasionally, the hematoma maintains a soft liquid central region while developing a firm outer pseudocapsule that permits blood to freely circulate from the injured vessel, thereby forming a pseudoaneurysm. Since a femoral arterial approach offers the interventionalist a wide variety of diagnostic and treatment options, it is no surprise that IPA most commonly occurs with percutaneous intervention for cardiac and peripheral vascular disease. Other risk factors for development of pseudoaneurysms have been identified such as the use of anticoagulation either at the time of arterial cannulation or in the immediate postprocedure period, increased age, female gender, concomitant venous puncture, and large sheath/catheter size[2] (Table 25–1). Naturally, attention to technical factors remains an important part of a successful arterial access procedure. For example, double arterial entry during access can result in the development of arterial bleeding in the posterior arterial wall or inaccuracy in arterial entry can inadvertently puncture the superficial or deep femoral arteries. Puncture above the inguinal ligament into the external iliac artery can also result in

TABLE 25–1. Risk factors for iatrogenic pseudoaneurysms.

Increasing sheath size
Cannulation of artery other than common femoral artery
Calcified artery
Increased body mass index
Concurrent anticoagulation
Combined arterial and venous puncture
Failure to provide appropriate postoperative compression

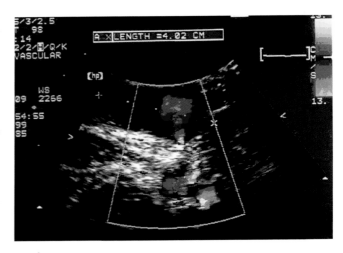

FIGURE 25–1. Characteristics of duplex imaging.

an arterial laceration creating a risk of retroperitoneal bleeding.

The incidence of IPA ranges widely from 0.05% up to 9%. This wide range results from variations in methods used to assess IPAs. In a prospective study of over 500 patients with routine evaluation with duplex, regardless of symptomatology, an incidence of 7.7% was reported.[3] This figure is substantially larger than that seen in clinical practice, in that generally only symptomatic patients are assessed. According to The Society of Cardiovascular and Interventional Radiology, an acceptable rate of IPA and/or arteriovenous fistula should be ≤0.2%.[4]

Diagnosis

Clinical suspicion for IPA should follow any percutaneous intervention resulting in a swollen groin or soft tissue hematoma. Hard signs of continued bleeding include pulsatile bleeding at the access site or expanding hematoma. The presence of a femoral bruit or thrill may also indicate an IPA, however, their absence does not exclude IPA. Most commonly, IPA is associated with a somewhat painful, nonbleeding access site and associated hematoma of varying size. Unfortunately, physical examination alone is notoriously inaccurate in identifying IPA. Angiography was the definitive mode of diagnosis until Mitchell et al. reported successful diagnosis by color duplex ultrasound in 1987.[5] Arterial duplex evaluation has emerged as the gold standard for diagnosis should a patient have concern for IPA, as duplex scanning is associated with nearly 100% diagnostic accuracy.

Generally, to diagnose an IPA, a 5- to 7-mHz probe in a longitudinal orientation is used with vessel sampling and velocity measurements to identify IPA neck and confirm flow. Changing orientation to the transverse plane allows diagnostic confirmation, size measurement, and evaluation for thrombus. Duplex evaluation should include views of the inflow distal external iliac, common femoral, deep femoral, and proximal superficial femoral arteries. Visualization of the common femoral vein is particularly important to exclude the presence of an associated arteriovenous fistula. Evaluation of IPA anatomic features should include sac size, sac shape, neck diameter, and neck length. The sac size of the false aneurysm should be measured in largest squared centimeters, which is one of the most important parameters for determining treatment options. However, the length and width of the neck are equally important to record in that a larger neck width often directly correlates with larger arterial defects that are generally more refractory to treatment with minimally invasive techniques. Multilobed IPA(s) likewise may be more difficult to treat. In our previous series up to 20% of IPA(s) were multilobed. Finally, the presence of native artery or IPA thrombus should be confirmed.

Typical characteristics noted on duplex imaging include a swirling of color flow in a mass distinct from the underlying artery, color flow signal through a tract leading to a sac, and to-and-fro Doppler waveform in the pseudoaneurysm neck (Figure 25–1).

Treatment Options

Observation

Several small studies have reported successful closure in more than 50% of pseudoaneurysms by observation alone. However, these studies were not able to identify variables that could accurately predict which IPA(s) could be safely observed. In a prospective study evaluating the natural history of femoral vascular complications following coronary catheterization, Kresowik et al. had vascular surgery fellows evaluate all puncture sites with physical examination prior to patient discharge. This series observed seven femoral pseudoaneurysms that were less than 3.5 cm over a 4-week period with no complications and 100% thromboses within 4 weeks.[2] In a series of similar size, Kent et al. reported 9 of 16 iatrogenic IPA(s) thrombosed with observation. Larger IPA(s) and those associated with anticoagulation use required repair more frequently.[6]

Toursarkissian et al.[7] reported one of the largest series using duplex surveillance of observed IPA(s). This series also had strict inclusion criteria for observation of the IPA(s): a maximum sac size less than 3 cm, nonexpanding, an association with severe pain, or in patients on anticoagulation. Additionally, patients who could not comply with a scheduled follow-up regimen underwent surgical repair and were excluded. Eighty-two IPA(s) were followed at 2-, 4-, 8-, and 12-week intervals. A spontaneous thrombosis rate was observed in 89% of the group with no adverse events or circulatory complications occurring. The mean time for spontaneous closure was 23 days, with a mean 2.6 duplex examinations per patient required.[7]

Unfortunately, adoption of an observation policy for all IPA(s) is not without concern. Problems with patient follow-up tend to develop and the cost accrued with a mean of 2.6 duplex examinations per patient approaches $750–1,000 in patient charges. Additionally, as many patients require chronic antiplatelet therapy for which newer generation medications are now used, the thrombosis rate may not be as predictable.

Ultrasound-Guided Compression

In 1991, Fellmeth et al. described a nonoperative technique for thromboses of IPA and arteriovenous fistula. With an overall success rate of 93%, this alternative to open repair was welcomed.[8] Following this initial report, the use of UGC became the first-line treatment of choice for those who were hemodynamically stable and without associated infection or skin necrosis. This technique includes the use of a linear or curvilinear probe (5 or 7 MHz) to compress the IPA and arrest IPA blood flow. Real time, duplex, and color Doppler are used to identify the neck of the pseudoaneurysm. Manual compression is subsequently applied to the neck via the transducer, which allows flow through the native artery while preventing flow into the aneurysm sac. Flow is continuously studied during the compression. Pressure is maintained for 10-min intervals, at the end of which pressure is slowly released and flows into the pseudoaneurysm assessed. This is continued until thrombosis, operator fatigue, or patient discomfort occurs. Success with this treatment modality generally ranges from 60 to 90%.[9–11] Despite this acceptable success rate, compression times in excess of 1 h can be required and multiple compression sessions are needed to treat at least 10% of IPA(s).

Factors associated with failed compression have been evaluated in multiple previous publications. Ongoing anticoagulation has been shown in many series to significantly reduce successful compression, as reported by Coley et al. and Eisenburg et al.[10,12] They describe failure rates of 38% and 70%, respectively, in anticoagulated patients, whereas failure rates in the groups without concurrent anticoagulation were 5% and 26%. In addition, 75% of those in Coley's series ultimately had their anticoagulation stopped and underwent repeat UGC with successful thrombosis. Several other series have shown similar results. In contrast, Dean et al. found a 73% success rate of UGC in 77 patients with uninterrupted anticoagulation, with seven patients requiring multiple compressions (12.5%) to induce sustained thrombosis. The only factor found in this study influencing success of UGC was the size of the pseudoaneurysm.[13]

Pseudoaneurysm size has been shown by most series to have a trend toward significance. In addition to Dean, Coley and Eisenburg also showed increased success with compression in those with smaller pseudoaneurysms. Coley et al. achieved a 100% success rate in those less than 2 cm with only a 67% success in those between 4 and 6 cm. Although it seems intuitive that a shorter tract length and larger neck diameter would have less success with compression, this has not been widely reported. Diprete and Cronan did report a short tract length (<5 mm) had unfavorable compression outcomes, however, this study was limited by a sample size of only 12 patients.[14]

Complications following UGC can include arterial or venous thrombosis. Case reports of aneurysm rupture have also been reported following UGC. In the series by Eisenberg et al., the six complications that occurred included acute enlargement or rupture requiring emergent surgery. In general, complications with UGC are infrequent. Successful thrombosis occurs at an acceptable rate, but limitations including lengthy procedure times, local patient discomfort, and newer methods have surpassed this treatment as the first line treatment of iatrogenic pseudoaneurysms.

Ultrasound-Guided Thrombin Injection

In 1986, Cope and Zeit described a technique of ultrasound-guided percutaneous injection of bovine thrombin into a pseudoaneurysm sac with successful thrombosis.[15]

Although an appealing method for handling IPA, rapid acceptance of this technique was slow to develop, taking over a decade. In 2002, Friedman et al. reported a review of over 400 patients with a success rate of 99% for UGTI and success rates have been compared to that of ultrasound-guided compression in multiple studies in the literature (Table 25–2).

Thrombin is an active form of factor II (prothrombin). It transforms inactive fibrinogen to its active form—fibrin. Fibrin subsequently contributes to thrombus formation. As a result of a limited blood flow in the pseudoaneurysm sac, thrombin can propagate thrombus that would often be cleared in sites of normal blood flow,

TABLE 25–2. Ultrasound guided compression (UGC) vs. ultrasound guided thrombin injection (UGTI).

Reference	N (UGC)/(UGTI)	Success (UGC)/(UGTI)
Weinmann et al.[16]	30/33	87%/100%
Gorge et al.[17,a]	36/30	17%/93%
Taylor et al.[18]	40/29	63%/93%
Stone et al.[19]	47/27	57%/96%
Paulson et al.[20]	281/26	74%/96%
Khoury et al.[21]	189/131	75%/96%
Lonn et al.[22,b]	15/15	40%/100%

[a]Prospective—all patients initially UGC; UGTI if failed compression.
[b]Prospective randomized trial.

which limits this mechanism by natural thrombolytic systems.

The procedure can be performed at bedside or in the vascular laboratory. Some clinicians use local nesthetic, however, with experience single punctures can be achieved. A 1-ml syringe and spinal needle (20–22 gauge) is used to administer the bovine thrombin (100–1000 units/ml). Using B-mode imaging, the needle tip is visualized and directed into the IPA sac (Figure 25–2). The clinician should take care to keep the needle tip just inside the capsule and as far from the IPA neck as technically possible. This minimizes the chance of forcing thrombus or thrombin into the neck and native circulation. Injection is preformed into the sac under duplex visualization at 0.1-ml increments until successful obliteration of flow is achieved. After successful thrombosis, the native circulation is reassessed including the distal tibial circulation and compared to preprocedural studies. Following successful thrombosis, bed rest is recommended typically for a period of 4–8h.

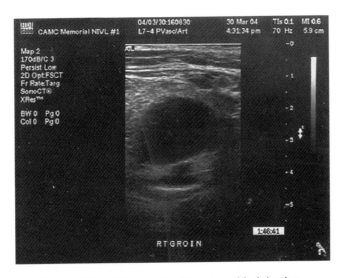

FIGURE 25–2. Utrasound guided thrombin injection.

Complications following thrombin injection are reported infrequently. In over 80 PSAs treated at our institution over a 3-year period, there have been no instances of infected pseudoaneurysm postinjection. The most feared complications are arterial thrombosis and distal embolization, but we have not seen any instances of arterial or venous thrombosis at our institutions. Distal embolization has occurred in less than 1% of the reviewed literature, with some authors noting improved circulation spontaneously. Others have been successfully treated with intraarterial thrombolytic therapy or surgical thrombectomy. Limited evidence suggests that distal embolization is associated with short and wide pseudoaneurysm necks.

Other complications seen only in case reports include allergic reactions to bovine thrombin with severity ranging from generalized urticaria to anaphylaxis. Infection after injection has also been reported occasionally, and one case of rupture was identified in a complete literature review.

Experience from Our Institution

As a high volume cardiac and peripheral intervention center, we have extensive experience with pseudoaneurysms. We reported our early results of duplex-guided thrombin injection versus ultrasound-guided compression. With success in only 57% of those with compression therapy as opposed to 97% with duplex-guided thrombin injection, the use of compression therapy has mostly stopped. Further experience was presented at the Society of Vascular Ultrasound Annual Meeting in June of 2004. Ninety-seven percent of patients ($n = 82$) with iatrogenic pseudoaneurysms, of which 12 were complex, were successfully treated with UGTI. Additionally, in that cohort we reported a mean number of ultrasounds per patient of slightly more than three. These included diagnostic, treatment, and follow-up examinations. Upon evaluation of this routine, we found only 5% of the follow-up ultrasounds could be deemed clinically significant. Two pseudoaneurysms recurred after successful thrombosis and two new pseudoaneurysms were found that had not been previously detected, both of which were less than 2.5cm. With such a low yield from follow-up duplex examinations, we recommended follow-up ultrasound only in symptomatic patients. We also considered our recurrence rate with that of over 600 iatrogenic pseudoaneurysms in the available literature, and determined a 3.2% recurrence rate after successful duplex-guided thrombin injection (Table 25–3).

As a result of these excellent technical success rates, low recurrence rates, and overall patient acceptance and applicability, most vascular specialists now consider duplex-guided thrombin injection as the initial

TABLE 25–3. Literature review of PSA recurrences.

Reference	Number of successful DGTI	Recurrence at follow-up
Liau et al.[23]	5	0 (24h)
Kang et al.[24]	20	0 (1–4 days)
Lennox et al.[25]	30	0 (1 day and 3 weeks)
Brophy et al.[26]	15	0 (1 week)
Sackett et al.[27]	29	0 (24h)
Pezzullo et al.[28]	23	1 (24h)
Paulsen et al.[20]	23	0 (24h)
Tamim et al.[29]	10	0 (1 and 3 weeks)
La Perna et al.[30]	66	3 (24h)
Calton et al.[31]	52	2 (24h)
Sheiman et al.[32]	50	0 (within 10 days)
Olson et al.[33]	17/15	1 (24h)/1 (1 week)
Friedman et al.[34]	40	0 (24h)/1 (1 week)
Khoury et al.[21]	126	9 (1–30 days)
Chattar-Cora et al.[35]	39	0 (24h)
Stone et al. (unpublished)	80	2
Total	**625**	**20[b]**

[a]PSA, pseudoaneurysms; DGTI, duplex-guided thrombin injection.
[b]Overall recurrence rate of 3.2%.

treatment of choice as compared to other options for IPA management.

Surgical Intervention

Under some circumstances, surgical repair remains the best treatment strategy to address IPA. Patients presenting with hemodynamic instability and soft tissue infection and those requiring immediate coronary artery bypass grafting should all have surgical repair. In addition, those patients with failed minimally invasive techniques should undergo surgical repair (Figure 25–3).

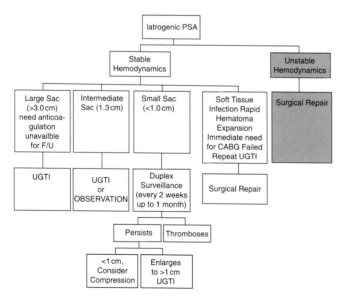

FIGURE 25–3. Algorithm for surgical intervention.

Conclusion

Increasing demand for minimally invasive treatments will undoubtedly be accompanied by associated complications such as IPA. Fortunately, a minimally invasive treatment solution is available and exhibits a high technical success and satisfaction rate for treatment of IPA. Duplex imaging has now arisen to uniquely facilitate both the diagnostic acumen and interventional success displacing routine observation, manual compression, and surgical repair in most instances.

References

1. Koreny M, Riedmuller E, Nikfardjam M, Siostrzonek P, Mullner M. Arterial puncture closing devices compared with standard manual compression after cardiac catheterization: Systemic review and meta-analysis. JAMA 2004; 291(3):3507.
2. Kresowik TF, Khoury MD, Miller BV, et al. A prospective study of the incidence and natural history of femoral vascular complications after percutaneous transluminal coronary angioplasty. J Vasc Surg 1991;13:328–36
3. Katzenschlager R, Ugurluoglu A, Ahmade A, et al. Incidence of pseudoaneurysm after diagnostic and therapeutic angiography. Radiology 1995;195:463–66.
4. Standards of Practice Committee of the Society of Cardiovascular and Interventional Radiology. Standard for diagnostic arteriography in adults. J Vasc Interv Radiol 1993; 4:385.
5. Mitchell DG, Needleman L, Bezzi M, Goldberg B, Kurtz AB, Penneli RG, Rifkin MD, Vialaro M, Balatrowich OH. Femoral artery pseudoaneurysm: Diagnosis with conventional duplex and color Doppler US. Radiology 1987;165: 687–90.
6. Kent KC, McArdle CR, Kennedy B, Baim DS, Anninos E, Skillman JJ. A prospective study of the clinical outcome of femoral pseudoaneurysms and arteriovenous fistulas induced by arterial puncture. J Vasc Surg 1993;17:125–33.
7. Toursarkissian B, Allen BT, Petrinec D, Thompson RW, Rubin BG, Reilly JM, Anderson CB, Flye MW, Sicard GA. Spontaneous closure of selected iatrogenic pseudoaneurysms and arteriovenous fistulae. J Vasc Surg 1997;25: 803–9.
8. Fellmeth BD, Roberts AC, Bookstein JJ, Freishlag JA, Forsythe JR, Buckner NK. Postangiographic femoral artery injuries: Nonsurgical repair with ultrasound guided compression. Radiology 1991;178:671–5.
9. Cox GS, Young JR, Gray BR, Grubb MW, Hertzer NR. Ultrasound-guided compression repair of postcatheterization pseudoaneurysms: Results of treatment in one hundred cases. J Vasc Surg 1994;19(4):683–6.
10. Coley BD, Roberts AC, Fellmeth BD, Valji K, Bookstein JJ, Hye RJ. Postangiographic femoral artery pseudoaneurysms: Further experience with ultrasound guided repair. Radiology 1995;194(2):307–11.
11. Hood DB, Mattos MA, Douglass MG, Barkmeier LD, Hodgson KJ, Ramsey DE, et al. Determinants of success of

color-flow duplex guided compression of repair of femoral pseudoaneurysms. Surgery 1996;120(4):585–88.

12. Eisenburg L, Paulson EK, Kliewer MA, *et al.* Sonographically guided compression repair of pseudoaneurysms: Further experience from a single institution. AJR Am J Roentgenol 1999;173:1567–73.

13. Dean SM, Olin JW, Piedmonte M, Grubb M, Young JR. Ultrasound-guided compression closure of postcatheterization pseudoaneurysms during concurrent anticoagulation: A review of seventy-seven patients. J Vasc Surg 1996;23:28–35.

14. Diprete DA, Cronan JJ. Compression ultrasonography: Treatment for acute femoral artery pseudoaneurysms in selected cases. J Ultrasound Med 1992;11:489–92.

15. Cope C, Zeit R. Coagulation of aneurysms by direct percutaneous thrombin injection. AJR AM J Roentgenol 1986; 147:383–87.

16. Weinmann EE, Chayen D, Kobzantzev ZV, Zaretsky M, Bass A. Treatment of postcatheterization false aneurysms: Ultrasound-guided compression vs. ultrasound-guided thrombin injection. Eur J Endovasc Surg 2002;23:68–72.

17. Gorge G, Kunz T, Kirstein M. A prospective study on ultrasound-guided compression therapy of thrombin injection for treatment of iatrogenic false aneurysms in patients receiving full-dose anti-platelet therapy. Z Kardiol 2003;92(7):564–70.

18. Taylor BS, Rhee RY, Muluk S, Trachtenberg J, Walters D, Steed DL, Makaroun MS. Thrombin injection versus compression of femoral artery pseudoaneurysms. J Vasc Surg 1999;30:1052–9.

19. Stone P, Lohan J, Copeland SE, Hamrick RE Jr, Tiley EH, Flaherty SK. Iatrogenic Pseudoaneurysms: Comparison of treatment modalities, including duplex-guided thrombin injection. WV Med J 2003;99(6):230–32.

20. Paulson EK, Sheafor DH, Kliewer MA, Nelson RC, Eisenberg LB, Sebastin MW, Sketch MH Jr. Treatment of iatrogenic femoral arterial pseudoaneurysms: Comparison of US-guided thrombin injection with compression therapy. Radiology 2000;215(2):403–8.

21. Khoury M, Rebecca A, Greene K, Rama K, Colaiuta E, Flynn L, Berg R. Duplex scanning-guided thrombin injection for the treatment of iatrogenic pseudoaneurysms. J Vasc Surg 2002;35:517–21.

22. Lonn L, Olmarker A, Geterud K, Risberg B. Prospective randomized study comparing ultrasound-guided thrombin injection to compression in the treatment of femoral pseudoaneurysms. J Endovasc Ther 2004;11(5):570–6.

23. Liau CS, Ho FM, Chen MF, Lee YT. Treatment of iatrogenic femoral artery pseudoaneurysm with percutaneous thrombin injection. J Vasc Surg 1997;26(1):18.

24. Kang SS, Labropoulos N, Mansour MA, Baker WH. Percutaneous ultrasound guided thrombin injection: A new method for treating postcatheterization femoral pseudoaneurysms. J Vasc Surg 1998;27(6):1032–8.

25. Lennox AF, Delis KT, Szendro G, *et al.* Duplex-guided thrombin injection for iatrogenic femoral artery pseudoaneurysm is effective even in anticoagulated patients. Br J Surg 2000;87(6):796–801.

26. Brophy DP, Sheiman RG, Amatulle P, Akbari CM. Iatrogenic femoral pseudoaneurysms: Thrombin injection after failed US-guided compression. Radiology 2000;214(1):278–82.

27. Sackett WR, Taylor SM, Coffey CB, *et al.* Ultrasound-guided thrombin injection of iatrogenic femoral pseudoaneurysms: A prospective analysis. Am Surg 2000;66(10): 937–42.

28. Pezzullo JA, Dupuy DE, Cronan JJ. Percutaneous injection of thrombin for the treatment of pseudoaneurysms after catheterization: An alternative to sonographically guided compression. AJR Am J Roentgenol 2000;175(4):1035–40.

29. Tamim WZ, Arbid EJ, Andrews LS, Arous EJ. Percutaneous induced thrombosis of iatrogenic femoral pseudoaneurysms following catheterization. Ann Vasc Surg 2000; 14(3):254–59.

30. La Perna L, Olin JW, Goines D, *et al.* Ultrasound-guided thrombin injection for the treatment of postcatheterization pseudoaneurysms. Circulation 2000;102(19):2391–95.

31. Calton WC Jr, Franklin DP, Elmore JR, Han DC. Ultrasound-guided thrombin injection is a safe and durable treatment for femoral pseudoaneurysms. Vasc Surg 2001;35(5): 379–83.

32. Sheiman RG, Brophy DP. Treatment of iatrogenic femoral pseudoaneurysms with percutaneous thrombin injection: Experience in 54 patients. Radiology 2001;219(1):123–27.

33. Olsen DM, Rodriguez JA, Vranic M, *et al.* A prospective study of ultrasound-guided thrombin injection of femoral pseudoaneurysm: A trend toward minimal medication. J Vasc Surg 2002;36(4):779–82.

34. Friedman SG, Pellerito JS, Scher L, *et al.* Ultrasound-guided thrombin injection is the treatment of choice for femoral pseudoaneurysms. Arch Surg 2002;137(4):462–64.

35. Chattar-Cora D, Pucci E, Tulsyan N, *et al.* Ultrasound-guided thrombin injection of iatrogenic pseudoaneurysm at a community hospital. Ann Vasc Surg 2002;16(3):294–96.

26

Lower Extremity Arterial Mapping: Duplex Ultrasound as an Alternative to Arteriography Prior to Femoral and Popliteal Reconstruction

Enrico Ascher, Sergio X. Salles-Cunha, Natalie Marks, and
Anil Hingorani

Introduction

The objectives of this chapter are to (1) summarize specific goals of distinct vascular laboratory arterial examinations, (2) describe protocols for duplex ultrasound arterial mapping (DUAM), (3) describe philosophies of implementation of a preoperative arterial ultrasound mapping program, and (4) summarize advantages of DUAM over X-ray, contrast arteriography (XRA), magnetic resonance angiography (MRA), and computed tomographic arteriography (CTA). The following sections represent the experience acquired with over 1000 arterial procedures performed in the lower extremity based on preoperative and perioperative ultrasound imaging.[1-13]

The distinct goals of arterial examinations include (1) screening, (2) definitive diagnosis, (3) preoperative or preprocedural mapping, (4) intraoperative or perisurgical imaging, either during open or endovascular surgery, and (5) postoperative follow-up for procedure and/or patient evaluation. The protocols for arterial imaging can be complete and time consuming or short and very specific. High-level communication between sonographer and surgeon in charge of the patient is necessary to create imaging shortcuts.

The philosophies or steps of implementation of a peripheral arterial mapping program include (1) discussion of what is the primary objective to be accomplished by arterial mapping, (2) comparison of ultrasonographic and arteriographic findings for specific segments of the peripheral arterial tree, (3) evaluation of virtual decision making based on ultrasound examinations, (4) appraisal of real decision making, and (5) assessment of procedures based entirely on preoperative and perioperative ultrasound imaging.

Advantages of DUAM are primarily based on imaging of the arterial wall and hemodynamic data besides lower cost, portability, noninvasiveness, and freedom of malignancy risk. Concomitant mapping of veins to be used as arterial conduits is another advantage of the preoperative ultrasound assessment.

Arterial Examinations

This section summarizes details of specific arterial examinations according to their goals and objectives.[1-18] It fulfills the first two objectives of this chapter.

Screening

Peripheral arterial screening is commonly based on the measurement of ankle pressures. Systolic ankle pressures are compared to brachial pressures and the ankle-brachial systolic blood pressure ratio, or ankle-brachial index (ABI), is calculated. An ABI below 1 is abnormal and warrants a medical investigation of the cardiovascular system. An ABI below 0.5 suggests severe peripheral arterial disease and evaluation by a vascular surgeon. Contrary to popular belief, the lowest ABI should be employed as a screening criterion.[19] Relation of calf flow rate is stronger to the lowest than highest ABI.

Flow waveform analysis of the anterior and posterior tibial arteries at the ankle may replace ABI as a screening method, particularly in the diabetic patient with arterial incompressibility. Arterial incompressibility may be total or partial, resulting in nonmeasurable or falsely elevated ABI.[20] The toe-brachial index could also be used as a screening method in patients with incompressible tibial arteries.[21-23] Triphasic flow waveforms are normal. Monophasic waveforms suggest severe peripheral arterial occlusive disease. Detection and evaluation of tibial arteries waveforms are a first training step toward arterial mapping.

Definitive Diagnosis

Although pulse volume recording (PVR) and segmental pressure measurements have been used in the vascular laboratory, a protocol based on ABI and flow waveforms obtained at the common femoral, mid superficial femoral, popliteal, and distal tibial arteries is recommended from the perspective of arterial mapping. With this protocol, an expert interpreter can predict the levels of significant arterial obstruction with an accuracy greater than 80% when compared to X-ray arteriography.[24,25] Upper calf and thigh pressures may not present additional information once the ABI and waveforms are analyzed. From the arterial mapping learning point of view, the early experience can be acquired with a continuous-wave Doppler. The sooner the sonographer starts using a duplex scanner to obtain the waveforms, the better. The next training step would be to scan the femoropopliteal arteries while looking for the sites to collect the waveforms. With this approach, the sonographer is acquainted with arterial mapping of the ankle and from below the knee to the groin. Proper imaging at the adductor canal level requires specific training. Additional experience is needed for upper calf and aortoiliac arterial mapping.

Preoperative Mapping

DUAM of the lower extremities requires information about the procedure being considered based on clinical findings and definitive diagnosis. Clinical findings may dictate if treatment is limited to the aortoiliac segment or the femoropopliteal segment or if a distal bypass is being considered. The aortoiliac or femoropopliteal treatment may be a bypass or an endovascular procedure. The protocols for arterial mapping described below are subdivided into three segments: (1) aortoiliac, (2) femoropopliteal, and (3) infrapopliteal. They are complemented by venous mapping if an autogenous conduit is considered.

Aortoiliac Segment

A long protocol demands an attempt at a complete aortoiliac mapping from the renal arteries down to the groin. Imaging of the aortoiliac segment may be suspended (1) if the primary objective is infrainguinal revascularization, (2) if the waveform of the common femoral artery is clearly triphasic, and (3) if intraoperative pressure measurements are scheduled following the infrainguinal procedure.

The patients receive instructions to get ready for an abdominal ultrasound scan. They should not eat, chew gum, or smoke for about 10h prior to the examination, usually scheduled in the morning. Antigas medication is recommended if not contraindicated.

A low-frequency abdominal transducer is commonly used to image the aorta and its bifurcation. Imaging is performed in transverse, longitudinal, and oblique planes, pending aortic elongation and tortuosities. Aortic flow waveforms are obtained above and below the level of the renal arteries and proximal to the aortic bifurcation. Occlusion, aneurysms, conditions of the arterial wall, and degree of stenosis are assessed based on B-mode, color flow, or power Doppler imaging. Local increase in velocity may be employed to grade severe stenosis. If dilatation of a stenosis is considered, the test may be repeated after treadmill exercise.

The iliac arteries are also commonly imaged with a low-frequency abdominal transducer. Patient size may allow the use of a linear transducer, particularly during imaging of the external iliac artery. Images are obtained in transverse, longitudinal, and several oblique positions. Patient and transducer positioning are constantly changed to obtain appropriate images. Forceful pressure to bring the transducer closer to the iliac artery segment under scrutiny is common. Flow waveforms are obtained at the proximal and distal common iliac arteries and at various segments of the external iliac artery. Occlusion, aneurysms, stenosis, and conditions of the arterial wall are observed with B-mode, color flow, and power Doppler imaging. Aliasing and increased velocities are scrutinized at stenotic sites. Usually, a local doubling in peak systolic velocity represents a hemodynamic significant stenosis corresponding to a 50% diameter reduction. A local tripling in peak systolic velocity corresponds to a severe stenosis greater than 75% diameter reduction. A significant stenosis should result in a monophasic flow waveform distal to the stenotic site. Plaques in large iliac arteries, however, may not alter the triphasic characteristic of the common femoral waveform. Examination after treadmill exercise is recommended to evaluate such cases.[26]

Patency or obstruction of the iliac arteries and aorta are reevaluated during the treatment procedure. Intraarterial pressure measurements are performed from the groin and compared to brachial pressures. A decrease greater than 20 mm Hg indicates the presence of a hemodynamically significant stenosis. Pressure measurements are more sensitive to detection of a stenosis once iliac flow is increased after an infrainguinal procedure. The drop in pressure across a stenosis is proportional to the flow rate through the lesion. Pending intraarterial pressure evaluation, dilatation and perhaps stenting of the iliac artery may be considered in addition to infrainguinal reconstruction.

In summary, the long protocol requires imaging from the perirenal aorta to the groin in both extremities. The short protocol does not include aortoiliac mapping if the common femoral waveforms are clearly triphasic and intraarterial pressures are going to be measured during the treatment procedure.

Femoropopliteal Segment

DUAM is commonly performed with a high-frequency linear transducer. Imaging of the adductor canal may have to be performed with a low-frequency sector probe in the patient with a large thigh. A monophasic flow waveform in the popliteal artery is indicative of severe stenosis or segmental occlusion of the femoropopliteal segment. The scan of these arteries is performed in transverse and/or longitudinal sections to obtain B-mode, color flow, and/or power Doppler images. High persistence and low velocity scale improve detection of low flow in obstructed arteries. Many patients requiring treatment have segmental occlusion(s) of the femoropopliteal arteries.

Endovascular treatment of this segment requires complete mapping. Serial significant stenoses or occlusions can be present.

A short protocol can be established if the patient is a candidate for a distal bypass or even a femoropopliteal bypass. The arterial mapping continues from the common femoral to the site of most proximal occlusion or severe stenosis. The site of a proximal anastomosis is then selected within this patent segment. The scan is then restarted at the popliteal artery. This artery is scanned in its entirety to determine if it is a candidate for the site of the distal anastomosis (Figure 26–1).

Occlusions are confirmed by lack of color flow or Doppler waveforms performed in very low, high sensitive velocity scales. The first stenosis may be graded based on velocity measurements. Doubling or tripling at the stenotic locale indicates a hemodynamic significant or severe stenosis, usually equated to a 50% or 75% diameter reduction (Figure 26–2). The hemodynamic energy lost in the first stenosis precludes velocity grading of additional, distal, sequential stenoses. It may be possible to locate such stenoses based on aliasing at low, high sensitive color flow velocity scales. An apparent aliasing signal

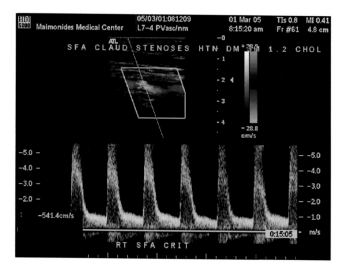

FIGURE 26–2. Significant increase in local velocity, corroborated by aliasing in color. Color flow bleeding beyond stenotic lumen or noncircular lumen requires additional imaging for a complete evaluation.

may be obtained. Otherwise, stenoses are perceived based on narrowing of the color flow channel (Figure 26–3). Branch analysis clarifies sites of collateral flow take-off prior to severe obstructions and/or collateral flow reentry distal to such obstructions.

In summary, a long femoropopliteal imaging protocol is required prior to an endovascular procedure. A short protocol from the common femoral down to the first occlusion/severe stenosis site is acceptable to select the location of the proximal anastomosis of a bypass graft. Imaging of the entire popliteal artery is recommended in both instances.

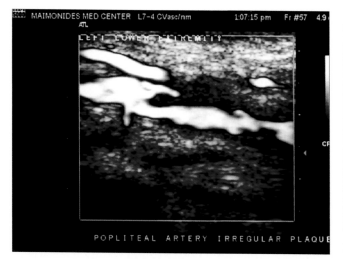

FIGURE 26–1. Longitudinal image of the popliteal artery showing irregular plaquing. Imaging must continue distally in search of a distal anastomotic site.

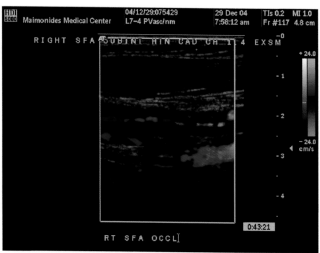

FIGURE 26–3. Preocclusive "string-sign" at the superficial femoral artery.

Infrapopliteal Arteries

Imaging of diseased infrapopliteal arteries demands appropriate patient preparation. The room and the patient must be warm. Creating conditions for vasodilation of the peripheral arteries helps detection of patent segments. Mapping may actually be easier in patients with inflammatory or infectious conditions due to the degree of vasodilation already present. Detection of patent, small segments is most difficult in extremities with severe rest pain and cold feet. Manual compression maneuvers may elicit blood movement in apparently occluded segments. Performing the scan with the leg dependent may actually help visualization of small arteries dilated by the hydrostatic pressure. Contrast ultrasound mapping is recommended prior to amputation based on lack of a distal target for a bypass graft.

DUAM is performed with high-frequency linear transducers. The posterior artery at the ankle is an easy start. Occlusion or patency is determined. If patent, the scan continues until the tibioperoneal trunk, if anatomically or ultrasonographically possible, or until a reentry branch distal to an occlusion. Edema, large legs, and occlusions make imaging difficult. Occlusions are documented by association with the posterior tibial veins (Figure 26–4). Large legs and edema may have to be scanned with a low-frequency sector probe.

On occasion color flow imaging of a patent distal posterior tibial artery is followed toward the posterior terminal branch of the peroneal artery into the peroneal artery. Once the proximal scan of the posterior tibial artery is completed, the scan continues distally through the common plantar artery and its bifurcation. The objectives of the distal scan are to find a potential plantar

target for a distal anastomosis or to evaluate the posterior tibial artery runoff in case the distal anastomosis is to be placed at the calf or ankle level. A short protocol may start at the ankle and stop at the most distal location of a stenosis or occlusion that needs to be bypassed. Wasting time imaging occluded or diseased arteries that are going to be bypassed is avoided.

The mapping of the anterior tibial artery follows a similar routine in the anterior compartment. First, the segment at the ankle is evaluated. The relation to the tibia and fibula is essential for identification of the anterior tibial artery. The learning of cross-sectional anatomy is extremely valuable. A monophasic waveform indicates proximal severe stenosis or occlusion. The scan toward the popliteal artery can be performed in transverse or longitudinal sections. Although a B-mode scan is potentially feasible, longitudinal color-flow or power Doppler imaging is most common and practical. A patent distal anterior tibial may be fed via the anterior terminal branch of the peroneal artery. The anterior tibial veins are smaller than the posterior tibial veins. Therefore, identification of potentially occluded segments must rely on other secondary information. For example, the arterial channel may appear irregular in sites where the flow is diverged via short collaterals. Long collaterals may also take over the task to deliver blood to patent distal segments. A sector probe may be needed to image the proximal part of the anterior tibial artery. From a posterior approach, the anterior tibial artery branches deeply from the popliteal artery. A common beginner's error is to identify a superficial, posterior branch of the popliteal artery as the anterior tibial artery instead of a geniculate branch or an artery toward the gastrocnemius muscle.

Once the proximal scan of the anterior tibial artery is completed, the scan continues distally through the dorsal pedal artery. It is necessary to pay attention to anatomic variants that include tarsal arteries or unusual endings of the anterior terminal branch of the peroneal artery. The dorsal pedal divides into the a deep plantar branch that communicates with the posterior circulation and a more superficial transmetatarsal artery that eventually feeds the digits. The objectives of the distal scan are to find a potential pedal target for a distal anastomosis at the dorsal pedal artery or to evaluate the anterior tibial artery runoff in case the distal anastomosis is to be placed at the calf or ankle level. A short protocol may start at the ankle and stop at the most distal location of a stenosis or occlusion that needs to be bypassed. Wasting time imaging occluded or diseased arteries that are going to be bypassed is avoided.

The peroneal artery is approached with a high-frequency probe at a posterolateral position. Learning cross section anatomy to identify the peroneal vessels in relation to the fibula is recommended. Longitudinal color-flow or power Doppler scanning is preferred to

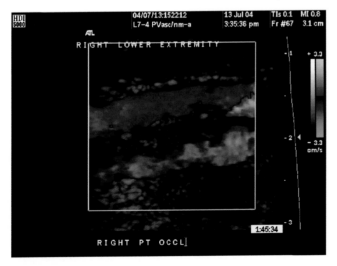

FIGURE 26–4. Imaging of the posterior tibial veins identify the occluded artery as the posterior tibial artery.

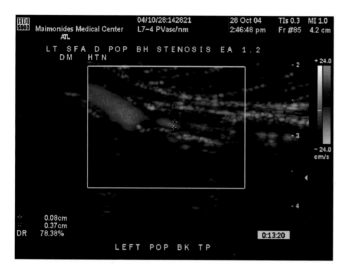

FIGURE 26–5. Severe narrowing of the tibioperoneal trunk, with an estimated stenosis greater than 75%.

transverse or B-mode imaging for practical reasons. If possible, a transverse scan is highly informative about other arteries, veins, and anatomic references. Completion of a peroneal artery scan is less likely than completion of a posterior tibial or anterior tibial artery scan. The problems are encountered in a large, edematous calf. The proximal peroneal artery and the tibioperoneal trunk are often difficult (Figure 26–5) and they may have to be studied with a low-frequency sector probe. Branching and collateral networks may create difficulties in identifying a patent peroneal artery. Bypasses have been extended to a branch of the peroneal artery initially identified as the peroneal artery on arteriography. Ultrasound has the advantage of identifying the peroneal veins adjacent to the peroneal artery. The anterior and posterior terminal branches of the peroneal artery may feed the distal posterior tibial and anterior tibial arteries. Therefore, posterior or anterior tibial ABIs may actually represent peroneal pressures. A short protocol may start at the ankle and stop at the most distal location of a stenosis or occlusion that needs to be bypassed. Wasting time imaging occluded or diseased arteries that are going to be bypassed is avoided.

The Anastomotic Site

Ultrasound B-mode imaging allows for detailed examination of the arterial walls. A thin, flexible, compressible arterial segment can be selected. A rigid, calcified wall can be avoided (Figure 26–6). Although calcification may be a hindrance for ultrasonic evaluation of some stenoses, a great advantage of ultrasound is to identify calcified wall segments and redirect the anastomotic site to a soft arterial segment. The surgeon may opt for a local

endarterectomy and patch over a stenotic site to provide blood flow not only distally but proximally also. Often the bypass graft provides enough pressure to dilate small arteries and collaterals that feed the muscles upstream.

A decision has to be made if the arterial wall is thickened. Initially, the tendency is to avoid a thickened wall as a site for a distal anastomosis. Close examination, however, has shown that vascular surgeons have approached thickened arteries and have performed anastomoses in arteries apparently normal by arteriography. Indeed, if needed, an anastomosis may even be performed over a calcified segment.[27] Nevertheless, ultrasound imaging can classify the segments into soft, thickened, or calcified.

Vein Mapping

Arterial mapping should either start or end with vein mapping, particularly if a distal bypass graft is being considered as treatment.[15] Anastomotic sites may be altered based on length of vein available for the bypass. Saphenous or arm vein mapping is performed with high-frequency transducers. Venous patency and conditions of the vein wall are evaluated. Diameters and length of vein available are measured. Location of the vein may be marked on the skin to facilitate the surgical procedure. Tributaries may be marked if an *in situ* bypass is being considered. A cephalic vein 2 mm in diameter often dilates to become a 4-mm bypass graft.[28] The arm veins dilate with placement of a tourniquet in the upper arm.

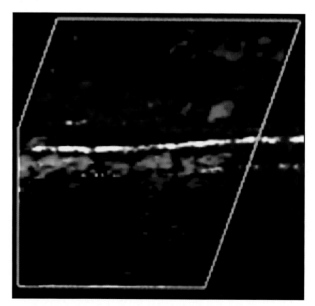

FIGURE 26–6. This arterial segment was not selected as a distal anastomotic site due to calcification as demonstrated by the shadows through the color flow signal.

Saphenous veins do not dilate as much. A dilation maneuver to determine if vein diameter can increase with temperature or hydrostatic pressure is recommended if the saphenous vein diameter is less than 4mm. The vein wall must be thin. Thickened walls suggest a previous event of venous thrombosis. Usually these vein segments are avoided. Valve sinuses can be disrupted. The ultrasound imaging shows various structures apparently floating in the vein valve sinus region. The potential for causing graft stenosis or occlusion exists if these segments are implanted.

In summary, veins are mapped in conjunction with the arteries to plan for arterial revascularization. The conditions of the venous wall, vein diameters, and length available are recorded.

Posttreatment Follow-up

Ultrasound or physiologic testing is recommended to follow patients (1) with mild peripheral arterial disease, (2) treated medically, (3) who had an endovascular procedure, or (4) who had open surgery, particularly a bypass graft.

Procedure Follow-up

Follow-up of bypass grafts in the postoperative period and at 3, 6, 9, 12, 18, and 24 months and yearly thereafter is recommended. Long protocols include evaluation of the bypass graft and proximal and distal arteries, particularly the bypass runoff arteries. A stenosis can be graded based on the B-mode/color flow imaging or on increased velocities. The scan must continue after one defect is found. The graft or arteries may have additional stenoses. A short protocol can be performed based on the measurements of volumetric blood flow rate in milliliters/minute. If a first ultrasound scan is normal, then flow rate can become a parameter to indicate the need for another complete scan. If flow rate decreases by 20–30% between tests, then a complete scan is indicated. Several details, however, must be followed during flow rate measurement. Only pulsatile flow must be considered. Diastolic flow is variable and adaptable to numerous conditions of vasodilation. It is recommended that measurements be performed in similar conditions of vasodilation as indicated by toe temperatures. Recommended toe temperature for such measurements is 28°C (26–30°C). Another indication for a full duplex ultrasound evaluation is if pulsatile flow rate falls below a minimum flow threshold value indicating poor perfusion: <50, 40, 30ml/min of pulsatile flow for bypass grafts to the popliteal, tibial, or paramalleolar level, respectively. Low flow states are not caused only by graft or peripheral arterial obstruction. A failing heart is often the cause of a low flow state. A low flow state with unobstructed peripheral conduits is an indicator of a poor heart condition with a high mortality rate within 1 year.

The natural history of endovascular procedures has yet to be determined for most of the procedures now performed. Follow-up, therefore, should be more stringent than that for bypass grafts. A full duplex ultrasound evaluation is recommended. Sites of wall thickening, neointimal proliferation, and stenoses are documented with imaging and velocity measurements. Stents have different compliance than arteries apparently causing increases in velocity. Criteria used to classify arteries as normal or stenosed still need to be adapted to stented conduits.

In summary, peripheral arterial procedures must be followed routinely and constantly at least for the first 12 months. Detection and treatment of stenoses provide better long-term patency rates than thrombectomy of an occluded bypass or than a secondary vascular reconstruction.[29]

Patient Follow-up

Patient follow-up includes testing the contralateral limb besides evaluation of an extremity treated with open or endovascular surgery. Eventually the contralateral limb will demand similar treatment. Patients treated medically are often tested annually in the vascular laboratory. Patients at risk of developing significant peripheral arterial occlusive disease should also be tested routinely. All these patients benefit from a vascular rehabilitation program designed to educate patients on risk factors, peripheral arterial disease, dieting, and exercise habits. Indeed, patient conditioning is suggested prior to surgical treatment to potentially minimize the operative morbidity.

Implementation

This section deals with the third objective of this chapter. It discusses several philosophies to prepare a team for DUAM as the sole preoperative imaging modality prior to open or endovascular surgery to treat the ischemic leg.

Fundamental Objective

Many have the misconception that the fundamental objective of DUAM is to replace X-ray contrast arteriography. Such a concept is fundamentally wrong. As an analogy, one of the problems with a nuclear power plant that had to be closed was that they were not monitoring the fundamental variable. A valve was being monitored as closed or opened. That is an indirect variable. The fundamental information needed was if there was flow or not through the valve. The valve could be closed and defective, allowing flow of unwanted material through the conduit.

The fundamental objective of DUAM is to permit safe and effective treatment. For a bypass, for example, if DUAM permits appropriate selection of the locations for the proximal and distal anastomoses, then agreement with arteriography becomes secondary.

An important point to consider is that several alternatives of treatment exist. A patient may go to different doctors and receive different proposals of treatment. Indeed, a study demonstrated that the same surgeon, receiving the same clinical and imaging information, may opt for different forms of treatment in almost one-third of the cases![30] More specifically, one service may have preference to perform a bypass to the peroneal artery while another service may use the anterior tibial artery as the preferred target. The fundamental concept is that DUAM becomes very effective if it is the target for the particular surgeon or team that is actually treating the patient. Constant and specific communications between the ultrasonographer and the surgical team is a major prerequisite for successful preoperative arterial mapping. This principle is also applicable to arteriography. If a clinical decision has been made to treat the aortoiliac segment, an infrainguinal arteriogram is unnecessary. In contrast, a beautiful arteriogram of the proximal arteries is unnecessary if the surgeon needs a detailed evaluation of the arteries of the leg and foot.[31]

In summary, the fundamental objective of DUAM is to provide information for effective treatment, not to mimic arteriography. The needs of the treatment team must be met. Continuous interaction between the vascular laboratory and the surgical team creates the basis to accomplish the fundamental objective of DUAM.

Learning Phase

The learning phase includes a gradual evolution from detection of flow waveforms with a continuous-wave Doppler to complete or limited imaging protocols to define the operative procedure. Progressively, this phase includes detection of flow waveforms at the common femoral, superficial femoral, and distal infrapopliteal arteries with a duplex ultrasound scanner. Segmental imaging and flow evaluation are accomplished. The next step is to image the entire femoropopliteal segment as waveforms are recorded during a segmental physiologic evaluation. Imaging of the aortoiliac segment and of infrapopliteal arteries then becomes the hardest step. As the training, skills, and confidence improve, then the steps described below represent alternatives to document the qualifications of the team.

Comparison with Arteriography

The initial training most likely includes comparison between DUAM and arteriography or, now, MRA.[6,9,10,13,15]

Several studies have compared accuracy, sensitivity, specificity, and predictive values of ultrasound mapping to arteriographic findings. Some have had better success in detecting obstructions in the aortoiliac segment and others in the femoropopliteal segment. Agreement in the comparison of infrapopliteal findings has been inferior to agreement in the comparison of findings in the most proximal segments. One error is to consider arteriography or MRA as reference standards. These techniques often fail to demonstrate arteries distal to occlusions or do not have enough anatomical landmarks for the necessary identification of the vessels visualized. Ultrasound is often incomplete in large, edematous segments with calcified arteries. Another drawback noted in several studies was the strict dependence on velocity measurements only. Increased velocities are inadequate for analysis of secondary, distal stenoses. All color-flow duplex-Doppler information must be considered. Apparently, documentation of a patent segment by any technique should be the standard. Nevertheless, segmental comparison with arteriography or MRA helps training of the ultrasonographer and improves confidence to determine if the ultrasound is informative, in agreement or not with other techniques.

Virtual Decision Making

Studies have compared surgical decisions based on ultrasound mapping with decisions based on arteriographic imaging.[13,32] Usually, such decisions were from different interpreters. Although this process is effective for training, it fails to consider that multiple alternatives for treatment are possible in many patients. Furthermore, interpersonal variability in surgical decision making must be taken into consideration.

A variant of virtual decision making that was successful at the Maimonides Medical Center was to analyze the decision made by one vascular surgeon based on the surgeon's own ultrasound scanning. A senior vascular surgeon accepted or rejected the surgical decision based on ultrasound while observing the corresponding arteriogram. This learning phase demonstrated that 15 cases were needed to educate the ultrasonographer and to perceive the preferences of the vascular surgeon. Another lesson was to recognize when the ultrasound examination was incomplete either due to anatomic or pathologic constraints or to lack of patient cooperation with the study. Patients in contracted positions, or constantly moving, for example, are not ideal for ultrasound mapping.

Actual Decision Making

Several variants at various levels are available for actual decision making:[13]

1. The patient may be scheduled for surgery based on the ultrasound mapping with the plan to perform an intraoperative, pretreatment, or prebypass arteriogram.
2. The treatment plan or the bypass may be actually carried out based on the preoperative ultrasound mapping and completion X-ray arteriography is performed at the end of the procedure.
3. The treatment plan is carried out based on ultrasound and a completion *ultrasound* arteriogram is performed at the end of the procedure.

Conditions to perform X-ray arteriography and to measure intraarterial pressures are highly desirable, even if the entire treatment is planned based on preoperative and perioperative ultrasound imaging. Such techniques become prominent if treatment of an iliac artery follows infrainguinal revascularization.

Disadvantages of Ultrasonography

Ultrasound (US) has several limitations as mentioned below. Some frequently mentioned disadvantages, however, may be dogmatic, while others can be reinterpreted as potential advantages.

1. US requires contact with the skin. Certain patients have profound wounds that preclude appropriate placement of the US probe to conduct a high-quality examination.
2. US often requires patient collaboration. Although possible to perform an US examination in a sedated patient, a preoperative examination is most commonly performed with the patient awake. High-quality US is almost impossible in patients with major contractures.
3. US is "operator dependent." This is a common saying that should be considered extremely dogmatic. It is true that US is operator dependent. As if the other technologies were not operator dependent! Skill is required not only to perform an arteriogram, for example, but detailed knowledge is essential for the selection of the proper arteriographic, MR, and CT sequences. Tridimensional reconstruction also requires special training and specific knowledge. In conclusion, all technologies employed for peripheral arterial imaging are "operator dependent."
4. US is inadequate in large patients and in edematous segments. The list of conditions that preclude a high-quality US examination may be comparable or even smaller than the lists that preclude a high-quality arteriogram, MR, or CT.
5. US fails to categorize stenosis in the presence of calcified walls or plaques. This disadvantage of US can be used advantageously during DUAM. A significant stenosis or even occlusion may not be properly diagnosed in calcified arterial segments. However, this information is valuable in the selection of an anastomotic site, the primary goal of DUAM.
6. US has a small field of view. The other techniques can be presented as images that are readily understood and quickly assimilated. In contrast, many small US images need to be interpreted. This problem may be circumvented with drawings that describe the US findings. Extended or panoramic images address this issue to a certain extent. Computer reconstruction of a large image using cropping, rotation, and collage of small pictures is not too different than selecting two-dimensional MR images of a tridimensional data set.

Advantages of Ultrasound Mapping

DUAM has multiple advantages over arteriography, MRA, and CTA:

1. DUAM is a noninvasive technique. Not even MRA can claim the degree of noninvasiveness associated with US. MRA requires injection of a contrast agent via a venous catheter. The magnetic field can dislodge body implants and affect the behavior of cardiac pacemakers. Indeed, at the Maimonides Medical Center, the contraindications to the performance of MRA reach double digits. The morbidity associated with X-ray, contrast arteriography is well known. Hematomas, pseudoaneurysms, and even fistulas have been created by needle puncture and catheter placement. Allergic reaction to contrast and renal morbidity are serious contraindications to arteriography, especially if the patient is a diabetic in renal failure. The latest claim against X-ray technology is that it is carcinogenic. In particular, the use of CT must be restricted significantly.
2. DUAM is portable. Arterial mapping can be performed in the vascular laboratory, in the emergency room, in the patient's room, in the operating room, in the recovery room, or almost everywhere. Access to the other technologies is limited.
3. DUAM shows the arterial wall and the obstructive plaque. Arteriography is strictly a luminogram, showing only flow. MRI and CT could, theoretically, show the arterial wall and the obstructive material. Their resolution at present, however, is inferior to that of US B-mode characterization.
4. DUAM provides hemodynamic data. Although theoretically possible with MRA, none of the other techniques presently available provides velocity and volumetric flow rate data. Hemodynamic data detected with US improves evaluation of the cardiovascular conditions including the peripheral runoff.
5. DUAM detects low flow in any direction. Arteriography often fails to detect flow distal to an obstruction.[33,34]

MRA often fails to detect flow in directions not predicted by the algorithm employed. CTA often fails to demonstrate flow in small arteries. In contrast, US is capable not only of detecting low flow but also of demonstrating blood movement in arteries without apparent flow.

6. DUAM provides information in all three dimensions. X-Ray arteriography fails to describe properly stenoses that cause noncircular lumens. One single projection is inadequate in many applications. Two, even three projections or rotational arteriography cause an overload of contrast and radiation. MRA can be tridimensional, but in practice, only the longitudinal lumen is described in multiple projections. The contrast and radiation doses to obtain images of small infrapopliteal vessels with CTA are large and often fail to provide needed information. US allows for examination in all directions, creating images in transverse, longitudinal, and oblique planes.

7. DUAM provides anatomic information. US can identify the major arteries in the leg and even foot by observation of concomitant veins and other adjacent anatomical structures. CT and MRI could perform the same task if algorithms to detect both arteries and veins are developed. MRA and X-ray arteriography may provide misleading information related to the actual vessel being visualized. The interpretation of collaterals, for example, can be erroneous with luminograms.

8. DUAM is "fast." Depending on how time is measured, a 1-h DUAM procedure can be considered fast compared to the other techniques. MRA can be time consuming. CTA and even MR need expert reconstruction that may not be available until the data are analyzed overseas, for example. If the time spent by the patient in the recovery room after X-ray arteriography is included, then this technique must be considered slower than ultrasonography.

9. DUAM is inexpensive. However, reimbursement for preoperative arterial mapping that replaces other, more expensive technologies must increase to make the US testing viable. Hospitals and physicians will continue to use X-ray arteriography, MRA, and even CTA if reimbursement for DUAM is not competitive and if they have to continue subsidizing the DUAM procedure.

Conclusions

Duplex ultrasound arterial mapping provides information leading to effective treatment of the lower extremity. Personnel training, open mindedness, and increased reimbursement could make DUAM a preferred option for most cases in a service geared toward patient and personnel safety and simplicity of diagnosis, perioperative imaging, and follow-up.

References

1. Ascher E, Mazzariol F, Hingorani A, Salles-Cunha SX, Gade P. The use of duplex ultrasound arterial mapping as an alternative to conventional arteriography for primary and secondary infrapopliteal bypasses. Am J Surg 1999;178:162–5.
2. Mazzarriol F, Ascher E, Salles-Cunha SX, Gade P, Hingorani A. Values and limitations of duplex ultrasonography as the sole imaging method of preoperative evaluation for popliteal and infrapopliteal bypasses. Ann Vasc Surg 1999;13:1–10.
3. Mazzariol F, Ascher E, Hingorani A, Gunduz Y, Yorkovich W, Salles-Cunha SX. Lower-extremity revascularization without preoperative contrast arteriography in 185 cases: Lessons learned with duplex ultrasound arterial mapping. Eur J Vasc Endovasc Surg 2000;19:509–15.
4. Ascher E, Hingorani A, Markevich N, Costa T, Kallakury S, Khanimoy Y. Lower extremity revascularization without preoperative contrast arteriography: Experience with duplex ultrasound arterial mapping in 485 cases. Ann Vasc Surg 2002;16:108–14.
5. Hingorani A, Ascher E. Dyeless vascular surgery. Cardiovasc Surg 2003;11:12–8.
6. Soule N, Hingorani A, Ascher E, Kallakuri S, Yorkovich W, Markevich N, et al. Comparison of magnetic resonance angiography (MRA) and duplex ultrasound arterial mapping (DUAM) prior to infrainguinal arterial reconstruction. Eur J Vasc Endovasc Surg 2003;25:139–46.
7. Ascher E, Markevich N, Schutzer RW, Kallakuri S, Jacob T, Hingorani A. Small popliteal artery aneurysms: Are they clinically significant? J Vasc Surg 2003;37:755–60.
8. Ascher E, Hingorani A, Markevich N, Schutzer RW, Kallakuri S. Acute lower limb ischemia: The value of duplex ultrasound arterial mapping (DUAM) as the sole preoperative imaging technique. Ann Vasc Surg 2003;17:284–9.
9. Hingorani A, Ascher E, Markevich N, Kallakuri S, Hou A, Schutzer RW, Yorkovich W. Magnetic resonance angiography versus duplex arteriography in patients undergoing lower extremity revascularization: Which is the best replacement for contrast arteriography? J Vasc Surg 2004;39:717–22.
10. Hingorani A, Ascher E, Markevich N, Kallakuri S, Schutzer RW, Yorkovich W, Jacob T. A comparison of magnetic resonance angiography, contrast arteriography and duplex arteriography for patients undergoing lower extremity revascularization. Ann Vasc Surg 2004;18:294–301.
11. Ascher E, Hingorani A, Markevich N, Yorkovich W, Schutzer RW, How A, et al. Role of duplex arteriography as the sole preoperative imaging modality prior to lower extremity revascularization surgery in diabetic and renal patients. Ann Vasc Surg 2004;18:433–9.
12. Ascher E, Markevich N, Schutzer RW, Kallakuri S, How A, Nahata S, et al. Duplex arteriography prior to femoral-popliteal reconstruction in claudicants: A proposal for a new shortened protocol. Ann Vasc Surg 2004;18:544–51.
13. Ascher E, Salles-Cunha SX, Hingorani A, Markevich N. Duplex ultrasound arterial mapping before infrainguinal revascularization. In: Mansour MA, Labropoulos N (eds). Vascular Diagnosis. Philadelphia: Elsevier Saunders, 2005.

14. Salles-Cunha S, Andros G. *Atlas of Duplex Ultrasonography: Essential Images of the Peripheral Vascular System.* Pasadena, CA: Appleton and Davis, Publ., 1988.

15. Salles-Cunha SX, Andros G. Preoperative duplex scanning prior to infrainguinal revascularization. Surg Clin North Am 1990;70:41–59.

16. Beebe HG, Salles-Cunha SX. Rational use of the vascular diagnostic laboratory. In: Zelenock GB (guest ed). *Problems in General Surgery*, pp. 527–541. Philadelphia: J.B. Lippincott Company, 1994.

17. Beebe HG, Salles-Cunha SX. Vascular laboratory testing for arterial disease. In: Greenfield LJ, Mulholland MW, Oldham KT, Zelenock GB, Lillimoe KD (eds). *Surgery: Scientific Principles and Practice*, 3rd ed., pp. 1604–1613. Philadelphia: Lippincott Williams & Wilkins, 2001.

18. Salles-Cunha SX, Wakefield TW. Vascular diagnostics with special emphasis on ultrasound. In: Mulholland MW, Lillemoe KD, Doherty G, *et al.* (eds). *Greenfield's Surgery: Scientific Principles and Practice,* 4th ed. Philadelphia: Lippincott Williams & Wilkins, 2006.

19. Salles-Cunha S, Andros G, Harris R, Dulawa L, Oblath R, Schneider P. Poster. Infrapopliteal hemodynamics in patients with different anterior and posterior tibial artery pressures. Program of the 6th San Diego Symposium on Vascular Diagnosis, San Diego, CA, February 15–21, 1992, p. 31.

20. Salles-Cunha SX, Vincent DG, Towne JB, Bernhard VM. Noninvasive ankle blood pressure measurements by oscillometry. Texas Heart Inst J 1982;9:349–57.

21. Vincent DG, Salles-Cunha SX, Bernhard VM, Towne JB. Noninvasive assessment of toe systolic pressures with special reference to diabetes mellitus. J Cardiovasc Surg 1983;24:22–8.

22. Vollrath KD, Salles-Cunha SX, Vincent DG, Towne JB, Bernhard VM. Noninvasive measurement of toe systolic pressures. Bruit 1980;4:27–30.

23. Sondgeroth TR, Salles-Cunha SX, Vollrath KD, Towne JB. Variability of toe pressure measurements. Bruit 1982;6:14–6.

24. Gale SS, Scissons RP, Salles-Cunha SX, Dosick SM, Whalen RC, Pigott JP, Beebe HG. Lower extremity arterial evaluation: Are segmental arterial blood pressures worthwhile? J Vasc Surg 1998;27:831–9.

25. AbuRahma AF, Khan S, Robinson PA. Selective use of segmental Doppler pressures and color duplex imaging in the localization of arterial occlusive disease of the lower extremity. Surgery 1995;118:496–503.

26. Coffi SB, Ubbink DT, Zwiers I, van Gurp JA, Legemate DA. Improved assessment of the hemodynamic significance of borderline iliac stenosis with use of hyperemic duplex scanning. J Vasc Surg 2002;36:575–80.

27. Ascer E, Veith FJ, Flores SA. Infrapopliteal bypasses to heavily calcified rock-like arteries. Management and results. Am J Surg 1986;152:220–3.

28. Salles-Cunha SX, Andros G, Harris RW, Dulawa LB, Oblath RW. Preoperative, noninvasive assessment of arm veins to be used as bypass grafts in the lower extremities. J Vasc Surg 1986;3:813–6.

29. Bandyk D, Bergamini TM, Towne JB, Schmitt DD, Seabrook GR. Durability of vein graft revision: The outcome of secondary procedures. J Vasc Surg 1991;13:200–8.

30. Kohler TR, Andros G, Porter JM, Clowes A, Goldstone J, Johansen K, *et al.* Can duplex scanning replace arteriography of lower extremity arterial disease? Ann Vasc Surg 1990;4:280–7.

31. Schneider PA, Ogawa DY. Is routine preoperative aortoiliac arteriography necessary in the treatment of lower extremity ischemia? J Vasc Surg 1998;28:28–34.

32. Wain RA, Berdejo GL, Delvalle WN. Can duplex scan arterial mapping replace contrast arteriography as the test of choice before infrainguinal revascularization? J Vasc Surg 1999;29:100–7.

33. Salles-Cunha SX, Engelhorn C, Miranda F Jr, Burihan E, Lourenco MA, Engelhorn AL, Cassou MF. Distal revascularization: Comparison of incomplete images of infrapopliteal arteries in severely ischemic lower extremities. J Vasc Bras 2003;2(Suppl 1):S34.

34. Engelhorn CA. Comparison of expanded field-of-view ultrasound imaging and arteriography in the diagnosis of infrainguinal arterial obstructions. Doctoral dissertation. Universidade Federal de Sao Paulo, Escola Paulista de Medicina, 2001.

27
Preoperative Saphenous Vein Mapping

Benjamin B. Chang, Ann Marie Kupinski, R. Clement Darling III, Philip S.K. Paty,
Paul B. Kreienberg, Sean P. Roddy, Kathleen J. Ozsvath, Manish Mehta, and Dhiraj M. Shah

The successful performance of any arterial bypass procedure starts with, ideally, the surgeon being armed with the maximal amount of information about the patient. This is commonly thought of as a history, physical examination, arteriography, and any preoperative testing for medical clearance. Most surgeons would not willingly abandon some effort to image both the inflow and outflow arteries, whether by conventional angiography, ultrasound, magnetic resonance arteriography, computerized tomography, or other more arcane techniques. However, these same surgeons often pay little attention to the greatest portion of their bypass, the vein itself.

That this is so is probably because the saphenous vein was most frequently encountered by surgeons during vein stripping, and certainly preoperative anatomic definition of the saphenous vein was not performed. In addition, it has taken the surgical community time to regard veins as more than passive tubes awaiting use as an arterial bypass. As the importance of the physiologic importance of the live autogenous vein became revealed to the surgical community, methods were progressively developed to preserve the live vein. In this context, it became increasingly apparent that minimizing intraoperative injury to the vein conduit was desirable. In addition, because of the frequent anatomic variations seen in any of the cutaneous veins used for arterial bypass, improved preoperative knowledge of the vein allowed surgeons to select the most satisfactory veins available while avoiding those that were too small or otherwise diseased while minimizing the incisions and dissections required to make this choice. This last point cannot be overemphasized as wound complications from vein harvest sites are a frequent and troublesome complication of arterial bypass surgeries.

The overall goal of this chapter is to supply the clinician or technologist with the specific knowledge necessary to perform preoperative vein mapping while, hopefully, convincing him or her of its utility and ultimate logic. Like many technologic advances, the need for vein mapping may seem obscure, especially to surgeons who have performed these surgeries for decades without this knowledge. But like personal computers, post-it notes, and remote controls, vein mapping, once used, makes the life of the operator so much easier that it soon becomes indispensable.

Preoperative Imaging with Venography

At Albany Medical Center, preoperative vein imaging evolved hand in hand with the reintroduction of the *in situ* bypass technique.[1] While the initial cases were done by incising the skin overlying the saphenous vein and incising the valves with the modified Mills valvulotome ("open" technique), further evolution of the instrumentation led to the development of the Leather and then other valvulotomes, which are passed blindly up the vein from a below-knee incision to the groin incision ("closed" technique). The use of a closed technique, although attractive in terms of decreasing operative dissection and operative time, is very sensitive to variations in saphenous vein anatomy, as the surgeon does not directly expose and thereby examine the entire vein or veins available, making the selection of the best available vein more problematic. In addition, certain branching patterns, when unrecognized, are frequently points of injury to the bypass when a closed technique is used.

For these reasons, the saphenous vein was for several years imaged with contrast venography. The results of these studies were summarized in part by Shah *et al.*[2] The methods reported in that paper are still effective and useful in some selected cases. The saphenous vein is punctured in the foot, ideally in one of the many prominent sidebranches covering the medial aspect of the foot. The use of a tourniquet is helpful for the puncture, but should be removed subsequently. Contrast medium is injected into the saphenous vein. Importantly, the vein is then flushed with heparinized saline after the venogram is completed to minimize the chance of contrast-induced thrombosis.

Alternatively, the same information may be gained intraoperatively at the beginning of the bypass procedure. An incision is made over the saphenous vein, usually just below the knee. Once the vein is thought to be identified, it is cannulated through an opened side-branch with a 22-gauge plastic angiocath (sheath only) and a single film is taken of the thigh after 10–12 ml of contrast is instilled into the vein. This has the advantage of not requiring the delay and inconvenience of preoperative venography, but is less likely to give the surgeon the complete picture of the vein.

Although these venographic techniques were used in several hundred bypass procedures, they are both invasive. In addition, venography gives relatively little information in regard to vein wall thickness, calcification, and other aspects of vein quality that are more apparent with ultrasonographic techniques. Venography is also not a practical method of imaging multiple limbs in the same patient at the same time.

There are some circumstances in which these methods are still of use. First, when first starting to perform duplex vein mapping, accuracy may be monitored by performing venograms. This is especially important when the imager encounters variations that he or she has not seen previously and helps shorten the learning period for the imager. Second, there are individuals in whom the vein anatomy is sufficiently complicated and/or difficult to image with duplex due to patient anatomy (extreme obesity) or inability to cooperate in whom an intraoperative venographic study would be useful. Third, emergency cases done late at night when duplex may not be available may benefit from on-table venography instead.

Ultrasound Imaging of the Saphenous Vein

After duplex ultrasound became available at our institution, its potential advantages over contrast venography were readily apparent. After a period of time trying to develop a technique and method of duplex imaging, this new technology became the method of choice for venous imaging in 1985 and has continued with a few minor modifications until the present day.[3,4]

The noninvasive nature of ultrasound is its most attractive feature. This is most significant in patients who have contrast sensitivity who may require imaging of more than one vein at a time. This is most common in redo cases with imaging of the contralateral greater saphenous vein, bilateral lesser saphenous veins, residual ipsilateral greater saphenous vein, and arm veins. This allows the surgeon to pick and choose among several conduit options in order to complete the reconstruction in the most efficient manner possible with the fewest incisions.

There is a wealth of other information that ultrasound can deliver that has proven to be of use for the surgeon. It has become apparent that the "quality" of the vein affects vein performance as an arterial conduit. While this has been long understood to include vein diameter, quality also reflects other aspects of vein morphology such as the presence of recanalization, sclerotic areas, and thick vein walls.[5,6] This information allows the operator to avoid the use of suboptimal veins whenever possible and to thereby help maximize bypass patency.

Method of Imaging

The equipment necessary for adequate saphenous and other cutaneous vein mapping is that commonly available and employed in vascular imaging studies of most kinds. A 10- to 12-MHz transducer is what is generally employed. Lower MHz probes are occasionally useful to image deeper veins in extremely obese individuals, but lack the resolution necessary for delineating the important details seen with the higher MHz probes. A 4.5-MHz pulsed Doppler is also occasionally employed primarily to check for vein patency. Color is rarely, if ever, necessary and may in some circumstances obfuscate important details. The reason that color flow is usually not helpful is that the unaugmented flow rates in these cutaneous veins provides only sporadic color filling of the vessel, which is of little use in outlining their course. The transmit power (decibels) of the transducer probe is generally turned down as this delivers a cleaner, clearer image by minimizing backscatter. Focal zones should be adjusted to maximize the near-field resolution (Figure 27–1).

Because the course of the vein is drawn upon the skin with indelible marker and then stain, the unprotected probe head may become permanently stained, especially through the relatively porous probe membrane. To avoid this, the probe is covered with a plastic sandwich bag containing ultrasound gel.

Preparation of the examination area or room is of vital importance for successful mapping. The room should be well heated to minimize peripheral venoconstriction. In a similar fashion, the patient should remain clothed and covered, exposing only the necessary limb. Sometimes keeping the exposed foot covered is also useful. Finally, the room is generally kept dark in order to assist with visualization of the ultrasound image on the display.

Positioning for imaging of the greater saphenous vein usually requires the stretcher to be placed in reverse Trendelenburg with the knee slightly flexed and the hip externally rotated. Standing the patient is usually not necessary for the majority of cases and is certainly not well tolerated by many in this patient group. Occasionally, the

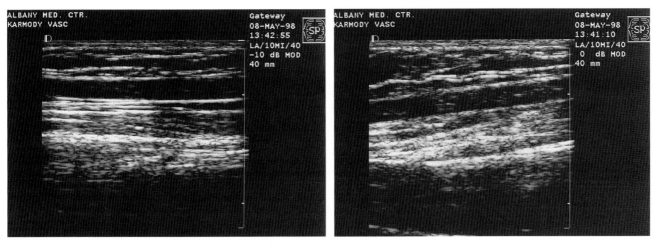

FIGURE 27–1. (A) Ultrasound power low. (B) Ultrasound power high.

patient may be stood at the end of the procedure to check the vein size under maximal pressure. In the past, tourniquets were employed in an effort to maximally dilate these veins but this has proven to be poorly tolerated by the patients and has therefore been abandoned.

Imaging of the saphenous vein can be started at either one of three logical sites: the ankle, the knee, or the groin. Generally, the groin is favored as the saphenofemoral junction can usually be positively identified with its characteristic relationship to the common femoral vein and artery ("Mickey Mouse," Figure 27–2). In very obese patients, however, this may be difficult to image even with the lower frequency transducers. Beginning imaging at the knee may avoid some of the above problems, but it is much easier to follow the wrong vein or to miss double systems.

The scanning technique is very different from that used with, say, carotid imaging. Because these veins are superficial and have very little internal pressure, they are exquisitely sensitive to external pressure such as from the probe itself. Therefore the weight of the probe and the examiner's hand should be supported by the fourth and fifth fingers offset from the course of the vein. The examiner can check his or her technique by examining the vein in cross section: it should be round, not elliptical (Figure 27–3).

Held in this way, the probe is applied at or near the groin in a transverse plane. Held in this plane, the probe may be moved in a medial-lateral direction until the vein is visualized. Generally, the vein runs slightly medial to the midline of the thigh at this point. The vein may be followed into the saphenofemoral junction to confirm its identity. The vein may be compressed to confirm patency. If this is in doubt, pulsed Doppler may be used in conjunction with manual compression of the distal leg.

Care should be taken to keep the probe as perpendicular to the skin as possible in order to help the surgeon make the incisions as directly over the vein as possible. This is entirely possible in most cases where the leg is normal, but can be unavoidably inaccurate if the skin is sagging or otherwise very redundant. Correct marking of the course of the vein on the skin requires some experience and constant feedback from the operating room findings.

Once the vein is identified in the transverse plane, the probe is slowly rotated 90° to insonate the vein in a sagittal plane. The position of the vein may then be marked at either end of the probe. We use a Sharpie King Size Permanent Marker with a chisel tip because it will mark through gel and it will stay wet when left uncapped. As the probe is moved distally, a new dot is made every inch

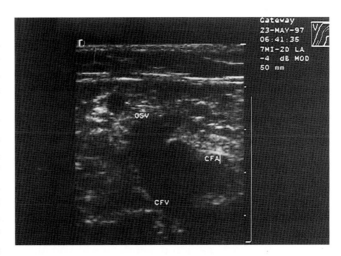

FIGURE 27–2. Mickey Mouse.

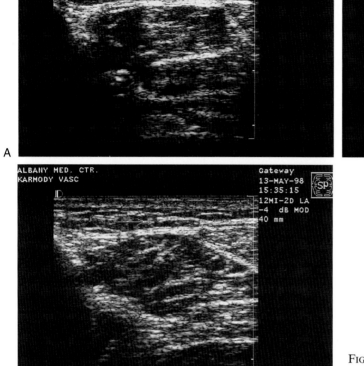

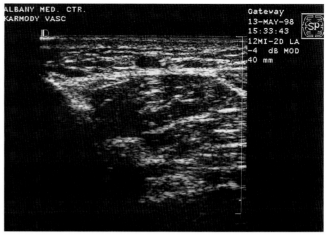

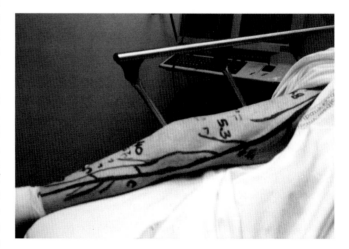

FIGURE 27–3. (A) Transverse vein image, no pressure, vein round. (B) Transverse vein image, mild pressure, vein elliptical. (C) Transverse vein image excess pressure, vein not visualized.

or so. After the remainder of the scan is completed, the dots are painted over with a continuous line. For this purpose, we use carbol fuchsin stain (originally obtained from the radiation oncology department) applied with a cotton-tip applicator. This provides the operator with a map of the underlying vein (Figure 27–4). This map should provide the operator with a detailed picture of the vein but it does not necessarily precisely indicate the best place for the operator to place the incisions; this requires some judgment from the surgeon in addition to the external map.

The size of the vein can also be measured. This is best done with the vein imaged in the transverse plane. Usually the vein size is determined in the groin, the distal thigh, and three equidistant points along the lower leg. Any marked changes in vein diameter along the course of the vein should also be marked. The limitations of these measurements should be stressed. Because they are obtained with the vein under venous pressure, they generally underestimate the diameter of the vein when the vein is connected to arterial pressure. In addition, these measurements are taken of the inside diameter of the vein, not the outside diameter. The surgeon should regard these measurements as the minimum size of the available vein. It is very important that the surgeon does not abandon the thought of using the vein without visually

FIGURE 27–4. Vein map.

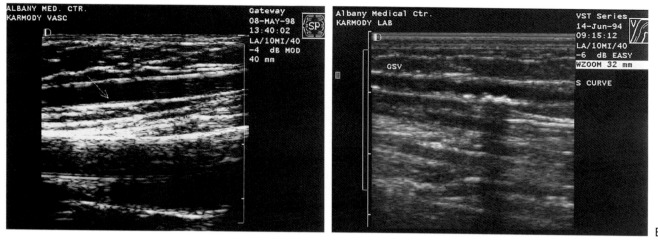

FIGURE 27–5. (A) Normal vein wall. (B) Thickened (?sclerotic) vein wall.

inspecting the vein at the time of operation. The vein by ultrasound may appear quite small and actually be quite acceptable upon arterialization. The vein size is roughly underestimated by a millimeter or more by ultrasonography under venous pressure.

As the probe is moved from the groin to the ankle, the vein is held in a sagittal plane. As marks are made on the skin, the probe is rotated to a transverse plane every 3–4 inches at which time the vein may be compressed to confirm patency and its diameter measured and recorded. Other data that should be generally noted include the relationship of the vein to the superficial and deep fascia and the relative depth of the vein in regards to the skin. It does help if the ultrasonographer has some direct experience with the relationship of the saphenous vein to the fascia. Knowing that the main vein usually runs below the superficial fascia, for instance, allows the imager to avoid tracking more superficial subdermal veins that may be as large or larger.[7] This is especially the case when the patient has large varicosities of the thigh where selecting the proper vein to track and follow is largely a matter of identifying the vein with the proper relationship to the fascial layers.

Other more subtle but no less important data that may be obtained include information about the vein wall. Normally, the intimal-medial complex appears as a thin, single, well-delineated reflection. With the probe in the sagittal plane, an abnormal appearance of the vein wall should be noted (Figure 27–5). This may be expressed in the report by describing the vein wall as being thickened (worrisome), calcified (worrisome but often usable), irregular (very worrisome, with possible recanalization), or sclerotic (almost certainly not usable). These notations are somewhat subjective and really describe a whole class of vein wall abnormalities but are of paramount importance to the surgeon as it allows for some preoperative planning to avoid using these diseased veins whenever possible.

Patients in this group may have variable amounts of peripheral edema. This complicates imaging considerably as the layers of edematous tissue may appear similar to a vein on ultrasound. This is the one condition in which use of color flow imaging is useful; distal compression will help define the vein from the surrounding fluid-filled tissue planes.

At this point, the entire vein should have been completed in the first pass from the groin to the ankle. There should be a line of black dots along the course of the vein. At this time, the vein is rescanned again, from the top down but with the probe held in the transverse plane. During this pass, major branches are noted and marked. This includes known named tributaries such as the medial and lateral accessory veins in the upper thigh as well as major perforators, which are seen as posterior or posteriolateral branches that then dive through the deep fascia to communicate with the deep venous system (Figure 27–6). Preoperative identification of these points will

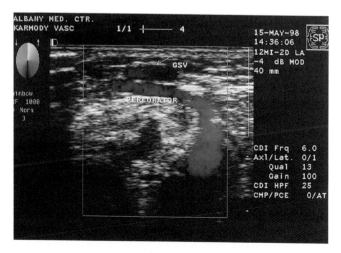

FIGURE 27–6. Perforator to deep system from saphenous vein.

allow the surgeon to gain access to the vein with a minimum amount of dissection and to ligate these perforators efficiently.

After the main branches are marked, the scan may be completed by connecting the dots with the carbol fuchsin stain, leaving the surgeon a cutaneous map upon which the operation may be planned. In addition, a form depicting the leg (or arm) in question is filled out. This form has a diagram of the mapped vein and notation for abnormalities, configuration, vein size, depth, and any other data felt to be useful to the operator. This entire procedure may take as little as 15 min with a single simple system, although longer periods of time are required for more complicated cases.[8]

Saphenous Vein Variants

During imaging, many branches of the vein may be encountered. Some of these branches will prove, upon imaging, to be long parallel venous systems.[9] While most operators regard the greater saphenous vein as a single tube running up the medial aspect of the leg, this has proven to be the case in only 55% of the several thousand limbs now scanned. Familiarity with these variations is important for both the ultrasonographer and the surgeon.

For most purposes, the variations in saphenous vein anatomy may be classified into two groups: above the knee and below the knee. The most common single configuration of the thigh saphenous vein is what is termed a single medial dominant vein, seen in about 60% of cases. This is the "typical" configuration in which the vein is a single trunk running medially along the thigh and deep to the superficial fascia. In addition, it curves away from the patient's midline (concave outward).

In the other 40% of cases, important variations exist in the thigh. The thigh saphenous vein may have a single lateral dominant system in 8% of cases (Figure 27–7). In this setting, the thigh vein runs more laterally than usual and is superficial to the superficial fascia. In addition, it has many more, smaller branches, is more thin walled, and curves toward the patient's midline (concave inward). The lateral system arises as the lateral accessory vein, usually the first and largest lateral branch just distal to the saphenofemoral junction. Although a single lateral dominant system can be used for bypass, closed *in situ* techniques should be employed more cautiously due to its thin wall and profusion of branches.

The saphenous vein may have both medial and lateral systems running along the entire thigh that remain relatively separate from each other even below the knee.[10] These double systems may have a larger medial (medial dominant double system) or lateral (lateral dominant double system) branch, or both systems may be relatively

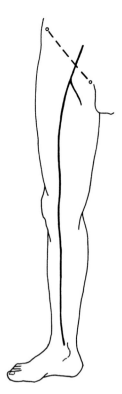

FIGURE 27–7. Single lateral dominant system 8%.

equal in caliber (Figure 27–8). This pattern occurs in about 8% of cases. It is vitally important for the ultrasonographer to pick up this variant and to give the surgeon some idea which vein is better so that the surgeon can place the incisions over the appropriate place. In addition, the surgeon can use the ultrasound information to avoid wasting time chasing the less satisfactory vein.

The saphenous vein may have a closed loop in the thigh portion in about 7% of cases (Figure 27–9). This type of vein tends to be a poor candidate for closed *in situ* bypass valvular disruption, as there is no assurance the surgeon has been able to instrument the larger of the branches of the loop, and the start and finish of the loop are points especially prone to injury from intraluminal instrumentation.

In about 16% of cases, the saphenous vein divides in the distal two-thirds of the thigh (Figure 27–10). Both branches run parallel into the lower leg. If not identified by mapping, the surgeon can easily isolate the wrong (smaller) system at the knee. Furthermore, the point of division of the vein is likewise prone to injury from blind intraluminal instrumentation.

In 1–2% of cases, the saphenous vein anatomy is sufficiently complicated, usually reflecting multiple loops and parallel systems, as to be difficult to characterize ultrasonographically. The surgeon should be

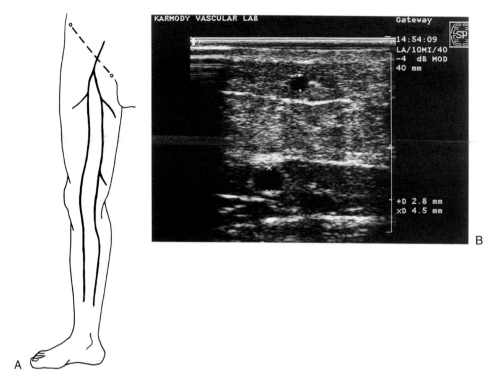

FIGURE 27–8. (A) Superficial lateral and deeper medial systems. (B) Components of a double system 8%.

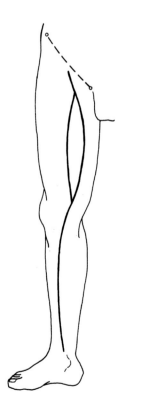

FIGURE 27–9. Closed loop in thigh 7%.

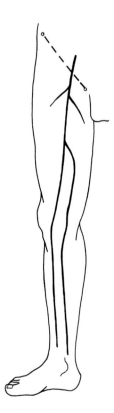

FIGURE 27–10. Branching of saphenous vein in distal thigh.

notified of this. Careful exploration and the use of intra-operative venography (see above) are called for in these cases. These are rarely pleasurable and often tedious experiences.

Calf Saphenous Vein Anatomy

The saphenous vein commonly divides at or just below the knee joint into an anterior and posterior system. The common situation, seen in 58% of cases, has the anterior branch being the dominant system and the posterior remaining clearly a tributary (Figure 27–11). The anterior system is generally deeper, thicker walled, and has fewer branches than the posterior system. It can be seen to lie between the deep and superficial fascia and to travel with the saphenous nerve.

The posterior system is the single dominant system in about 7% of cases (Figure 27–12). This vein runs in a sub-cutaneous plane, is thinner walled, and has many small branches. This vein is generally harder to work with but delivers good results when the dominant system. Incisions for this variant tend to be more posterior in the calf and less deep than the usual situation.

The saphenous vein has both complete anterior and posterior systems in about 35% of cases. The systems divide at the knee and rejoin at the junction of the upper two-thirds and lower one-third of the lower leg. In this situation, the anterior system is dominant in most (85%)

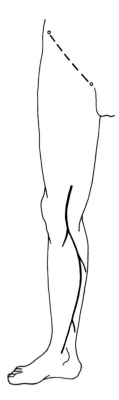

FIGURE 27–12. Single posterior dominant 7%.

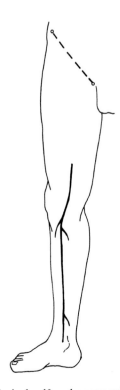

FIGURE 27–11. Typical calf saphenous vein anatomy 58%.

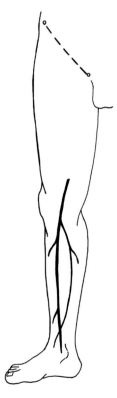

FIGURE 27–13. Double calf system 35% (anterior dominant 85%).

cases and posterior dominant in 15% of this subgroup (Figure 27–13).

In less than 1% of the time the veins are tripled or otherwise too complex for accurate imaging by ultrasound.

Proper Use of Mapping Data

Like any test, there are limitations in the data the study purports to deliver. First, like any ultrasound data, mapping is highly dependent upon a close working relationship between the technologist and surgeon. The technologist needs to become familiar with the anatomic variants of the saphenous vein and the details of vein anatomy that affect the bypass procedure. The surgeon, in turn, must close the loop by informing the ultrasonographer in a noncontentious manner if the map was accurate or if the data provided were not accurate.

Mapping is very good at defining the presence or absence of vein. It is good at defining the minimum size of the vein. Conversely, it does not do a good job of defining the size of the vein under arterial pressure. Thus in good hands, if the surgeon is told that there is no vein, this is probably true. If the surgeon is told that the vein is present but small, the vein should be examined in the operating room to decide if it is usable.

The map drawn upon the skin can be fairly accurate, but less so in obese patients. It can serve as a guide in the placement of the first two (proximal and distal) incisions over the vein, but the vein should then be identified before the incisions are connected. The map does not obviate the need for surgical judgment in regard to this point.

Venous anatomic variants are very well delineated with good mapping. This requires considerable training for both parties and mistakes will be made early on.

Branches and perforators are moderately well identified. Valves are not well imaged.

Irregularities of the vein wall, when identified, are very accurately identified with ultrasonography. Many of these findings are somewhat subtle at first and require experience. The lack of identified irregularities on the mapping is no guarantee that the vein quality is good.

References

1. Leather RP, Shah MD, Karmody AM. Infrapopliteal arterial bypass for limb salvage: Increased patency and utilization of the saphenous vein used in-situ. Surgery 1981;90:1000–1008.
2. Shah DM, Chang BB, Leopold PW, Corson JD, Leather RP, Karmody AM. The anatomy of the greater saphenous venous system. J Vasc Surg 1986;3:273–283.
3. Leopold PW, Shandall AA, Kupinski AM, Chang BB, et al. The role of B-mode venous mapping in infrainguinal arterial bypasses. Br J Surg 1989;76:305–307.
4. Darling RC III, Kupinski AM. Preoperative evaluation of veins. In: Leather RP (ed). Seminars in Vascular Surgery, Vol. 6, pp. 193–196. Philadelphia: Saunders, 1993.
5. Marin ML, Veith FJ, Panetta TF, et al. Saphenous vein biopsy: A predictor of vein graft failure. J Vasc Surg 1993;18:407–414.
6. Marin ML, Gordon RE, Veith FJ, et al. Human greater saphenous vein: Histologic and ultrastructural variation. Cardiovasc Surg 1994; 2(1):56–62.
7. Ricci S, Georgiev M. Ultrasound anatomy of the superficial veins of the lower limb. J Vasc Tech 2002;26:183–199.
8. Kupinski AM. Ultrasound mapping of the superficial venous system. Vasc US Today 2002;7:25–44.
9. Kupinski AM, Evans SM, Khan AM, et al. Ultrasonic characterization of the saphenous vein. Cardiovasc Surg 1993;1:513–517.
10. Caggiati A, Bergan JJ, Gloviczki P, Janter G, Wendell-Smith CP, Partsch H. Nomenclature of the veins of the lower limb: An international interdisciplinary consensus statement. J Vasc Surg 2002;36:416–422.

28
Noninvasive Diagnosis of Upper Extremity Vascular Disease

Jocelyn A. Segall and Gregory L. Moneta

Introduction

Symptomatic arterial disease of the upper extremity is uncommon and accounts for approximately 5% of all cases of extremity ischemia. Unlike the lower extremity, where atherosclerosis is by far the most common disorder, ischemia in the upper extremity may be caused by a variety of systemic diseases. The diagnosis of upper extremity arterial disease is often complex and requires a complete history and physical examination, laboratory screening, and noninvasive and possibly invasive examination of the arteries of the upper extremity. In contrast to lower extremity ischemia, surgical intervention is rarely required in patients with upper extremity ischemia and the diagnosis of upper extremity ischemia can often be sufficiently accomplished using only noninvasive diagnostic tests. We have had a long-standing interest in upper extremity ischemia at the Oregon Health & Science University and over the past 30 years have evaluated over 1500 patients. Our noninvasive testing includes segmental arm pressures, digital pressures and arterial waveforms using photoplethysmography (PPG), and testing for cold-induced vasospasm. Duplex evaluation plays a minor role, and arteriography is rarely employed. The noninvasive tests, in combination with the history and physical examination, generally give all the necessary information to secure the diagnosis and guide the treatment for upper extremity ischemia. In this chapter, we will review the disease processes that result in upper extremity ischemia and our diagnostic approach to patients presenting with it.

Presentation

Most clinical syndromes involving upper extremity ischemia include Raynaud's syndrome as one of the major clinical manifestations. This condition is characterized by episodic attacks of digital artery vasospasm in response to cold exposure or emotional stimuli. The vasospasm causes closure of the small arteries of the distal parts of the extremities. Classic attacks consist of intense pallor of the distal extremities followed by cyanosis and rubor upon rewarming with full recovery not occurring until 15–45 min after the inciting stimulus is removed (Figure 28–1). Some patients, however, develop only pallor or cyanosis during attacks and it is now clear that the classic tricolor attacks do not occur in all patients. In addition, a number of patients have been recognized who complain of cold hands without digital color changes. These patients have abnormal findings on noninvasive examinations identical to patients with classic digital color changes, thus suggesting that digital color change may not be essential for diagnosis.

Patients with Raynaud's syndrome have traditionally been divided into two groups, as described by Allen and Brown in 1932.[1] The term Raynaud's disease was used to describe a benign idiopathic form of intermittent digital ischemia occurring in the absence of associated diseases, while the term Raynaud's phenomenon was used to describe a similar symptom complex occurring in association with one or more of a variety of systemic diseases. This classification is not based on the underlying cause of the symptoms, and it is well recognized that associated diseases may not be diagnosed at the time of initial presentation but may develop years later. Therefore, using this classification scheme, patients may make the transition between disease and phenomenon sometime after their initial presentation. Thus we believe there is no need to attempt to separate Raynaud's disease from Raynaud's phenomenon and refer to the condition as Raynaud's syndrome.

Episodic digital ischemia is not limited to primary vasospasm and may be seen in association with other diseases involving the small vessels of the hands, as well as in large artery disease due to embolization from an upstream lesion or occlusion of the major arteries sup-

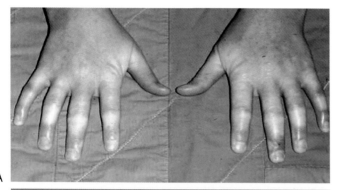

A

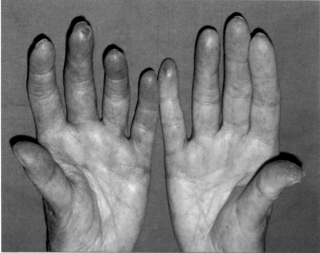

B

FIGURE 28–1. Raynaud's syndrome.

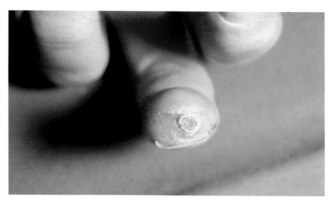

FIGURE 28–2. Digital ulcer.

plying the arm or hand. A small group of patients present with intermittent ischemia overlying symptoms of chronic ischemia. These patients may have chronic limb pain or severe pain with minimal arm exertion. Such patients are likely to have digital ulcers or fingertip gangrene at the time of presentation (Figure 28–2). They also report episodic worsening of digital ischemia consistent with Raynaud's syndrome.

A useful classification scheme for both the diagnosis and treatment of upper extremity ischemia is to divide patients into those with large artery disease and those with small artery disease. Patients are then further divided into those with vasospasm and those with arterial obstruction. We have found this classification scheme to be helpful in categorizing patients and predicting their long-term outcome.

Pathophysiology

The etiologies associated with small and large artery occlusive disease are quite distinct, although the underlying pathophysiology of Raynaud's syndrome attacks is the same. It is important to note, however, that small

artery occlusive disease in the upper extremity accounts for 90–95% of patients presenting with upper extremity ischemia. Only 5–10% of patients will have large vessel disease. Upper extremity ischemia resulting from small artery disease may be as mild as intermittent cold sensitivity of the fingertips, or may be severe enough to result in gangrene of the fingertips.

The variety of diseases resulting in small artery disease is wider than those seen in large artery disease (Tables 28–1 and 28–2). In contrast to large artery diseases, in which symptoms are caused predominantly by arterial obstruction, small artery diseases often result in symptoms that are caused by vasospasm of the palmar and digital arteries and arterioles. In clinical practice, the most common cause of upper extremity ischemia, which results from small vessel disease, is idiopathic vasospasm. It is well established that in cool, damp climates 6–20% of the population, particularly young females, will report symptoms of Raynaud's syndrome if questioned.[2]

Patients with vasospastic Raynaud's syndrome do not have significant proximal arterial, palmar, and/or digital artery obstruction and accordingly have normal digital

TABLE 28–1. Causes of small artery disease in the upper extremity.

Idiopathic vasospasm
Connective tissue disease
  Scleroderma
  Rheumatoid arthritis
  Sjögren's syndrome
  Systemic lupus erythematosus
  Mixed connective tissue disease
Undifferentiated connective tissue disease
Hypercoagulable states
Neoplasm
Hypersensitivity angiitis
Frostbite
Emboli
Buerger's disease
Chemical exposure
Vibration injury

TABLE 28–2. Causes of large artery disease in the upper extremity.

Atherosclerosis
Aneurysmal disease
Giant cell arteritis
Takayasu's arteritis
Radiation arteritis
Cardiac emboli
Trauma
Fibromuscular dysplasia
Arterial thoracic outlet syndrome

artery pressure at room temperature. A markedly increased force of cold-induced arterial spasm causes arterial closure in these patients. Patients with obstructive Raynaud's syndrome have a significant obstruction of the arteries between the heart and the distal phalanx. To experience a Raynaud's attack, the patient must have sufficiently severe arterial obstruction to cause a significant reduction in resting digital artery pressure. This condition requires obstruction of both arteries of a single digit. In such patients, a normal vasoconstrictive response to cold is sufficient to overcome the diminished intraluminal distending pressure and cause arterial closure. This theory predicts that all patients with hand arterial obstruction sufficient to cause resting digital hypotension will experience cold-induced Raynaud's attacks.[3] In our experience this appears to be true. Figure 28–3 demonstrates the relationship between finger pressure and finger temperature for normal patients and for those patients with vasospastic and obstructive Raynaud's syndrome.

A major focus in the search for the abnormalities in Raynaud's syndrome pathophysiology has been on alter-

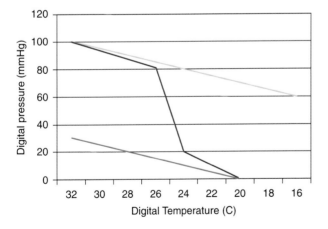

FIGURE 28–3. The relationship between digital blood pressure and digital temperature is illustrated in a diagrammatic fashion for normal (red), patients with vasospastic Raynaud's syndrome (yellow), and patients with obstructive Raynaud's syndrome (green).

ations in peripheral adrenoceptor activity. Increased finger blood flow was noted in patients following α-adrenergic blockade with drugs such as reserpine. Oral and intraarterial or intravenous reserpine was the cornerstone of medical management of Raynaud's syndrome for many years.

α_2-Adrenoreceptors appear to play an important role in the production of the symptoms of Raynaud's syndrome, as they are involved in the regulation of digital vascular tone.[4] Receptor levels in circulating cells appear to mirror tissue levels. Due to the difficulty in obtaining digital arteries from human subjects, levels of platelet α-adrenoceptors have been measured as a surrogate. An increased level of platelet α_2-adrenoceptors in patients with Raynaud's syndrome has been demonstrated.[5,6] Increased finger blood flow during body cooling was noted in human controls treated with the α_2-adrenergic antagonist yohimbine. The α_1-adrenergic antagonist prazosin had only a mild effect.[7] α_2-Adrenoceptors are believed to be necessary for the production of vasospastic attacks in idiopathic Raynaud's syndrome.[8] Possible mechanisms of α_2-adrenergic-induced Raynaud's syndrome include an elevation in the number of α_2-receptor sites, receptor hypersensitivity, and alterations in the number of receptors exposed at any one time. Additionally, increased vasoconstrictive responses to serotonin and angiotensin II have been demonstrated in Raynaud's patients with an increase of tyrosine phosphorylation upon cooling. This effect was reversed with protein tyrosine kinase inhibitors.[9]

The possible roles of the vasoactive peptides endothelin-1, a potent vasoconstrictor, and calcitonin gene-related peptide (CGRP), a vasodilator, have also been investigated. Elevated endothelin-1 levels have been found in Raynaud's syndrome patients.[10] Depletion of endogenous CGRP may also contribute to Raynaud's syndrome. Increased skin blood flow in response to CGRP infusion has been demonstrated in patients with Raynaud's syndrome compared with controls.[11] Additionally, investigations into the role of nitric oxide (NO) have been and are continuing to be performed. It is believed that with endothelial damage, NO is underproduced. Furthermore, estrogens are thought to have some control in vasodilation, especially in small artery circulation, via an NO pathway.[12] The deficiency of NO, in combination with circulating inhibitors of NO, may have a substantial role in the disease process.[13]

Platelet activation has also been implicated in the pathophysiology of Raynaud's syndrome and vibration has been recognized as a cause of platelet activation. This fact has been demonstrated by the increase in circulating levels of thromboxane and α-thromboglobulin, both of which are released by platelets. Thromboxane is a well-known potent vasoconstrictor and platelet aggregator and its actions, especially with cooling, are increased in patients with Raynaud's syndrome. Additionally, serotonin is released from platelets and may contribute to the complex pathway that causes symptoms in Raynaud's patients.[14]

Small Artery Diseases

The most frequently associated disease process seen in patients presenting with upper extremity ischemia is connective tissue disease. Of the various connective tissue diseases, scleroderma is the most common in patients presenting with Raynaud's syndrome (Figure 28–4) The incidence of connective tissue disease in patients with upper extremity ischemia varies widely in the literature from 16% to 80%.[2] The reason for this variation includes the fact that tertiary referral centers see patients with the most severe ischemia, which likely includes a disproportionate number of patients with connective tissue diseases. It is important to realize that while most patients with connective tissue disease will have Raynaud's syndrome, most patients with Raynaud's syndrome do not have a connective tissue disease. In our patient population, 21% of patients had a connective tissue disease at their initial presentation, with an additional 5.9% developing some type of connective tissue disease during long-term follow-up.[15]

Patients with connective tissue disease may have either obstructive or vasospastic Raynaud's syndrome, and may progress from vasospasm to obstruction over time. Patients with connective tissue disease are more likely to have obstructive Raynaud's syndrome at the time of initial presentation and are more likely to develop obstruction over time. The obstructive process appears to result from a vasculitis that is common to the connective tissue disease.

A variety of hypercoagulable states including cryoglobulins, protein C and protein S deficiencies, and antiphospholipid antibodies have been associated with the development of upper extremity ischemia and digital and palmar artery occlusion. Patients with cancer, likely through a hematologic abnormality, have also presented with digital and palmar artery occlusive disease.[16,17] We see several patients a year who present with the acute onset of upper extremity ischemia with widespread obstruction of the digital and palmar arteries in whom we are not able to find a cause of the obstruction. We have used the term "hypersensitivity angiitis" to describe the process in these patients and postulate that they have formed antibodies as a result of some environmental or infectious exposure. These antibodies then precipitate in the digital arteries resulting in obstruction.

Cold injuries such as frostbite and prolonged immersion lead to upper extremity ischemia. The mechanism in this type of injury includes digital artery obstruction, which is seen in frostbite, and nerve damage resulting in vasospasm, which occurs with both frostbite and immersion injuries.

Buerger's disease, also known as thromboangiitis obliterans, is a clinical syndrome characterized by the occurrence of segmental thrombotic occlusions of small- and medium-sized arteries in the upper and lower extremities accompanied by a prominent arterial wall inflammatory cell infiltrate.[18] Affected patients are predominantly young male smokers (mean age 34 years) who usually present with distal limb ischemia frequently accompanied by localized digital gangrene[19] (Figure 28–5).

About 10% of patients with Buerger's disease have isolated upper extremity involvement, and 30–40% have upper and lower extremity involvement. Central to the diagnosis of Buerger's disease is the onset of symptoms before age 45 years, a uniform exposure to tobacco, and the absence of arterial lesions proximal to the knee or elbow.[19] In the upper extremity, the lunar or radial artery is frequently occluded, and extensive digital and palmar arterial occlusion is uniformly present. The etiology of Buerger's disease remains unknown. Although a strong association with tobacco use has been clinically recognized, a causal relationship has not been conclusively demonstrated.[20]

Occupational causes of small vessel disease include vibration, toxin exposure, and perhaps long-term cold exposure. The most common toxin reported to cause upper extremity ischemia is polyvinylchloride, which is no longer widely used. There have been several studies that have looked at employees exposed to long-term cold, particularly in the food packaging industries.[21,22] There does appear to be an increase in Raynaud's

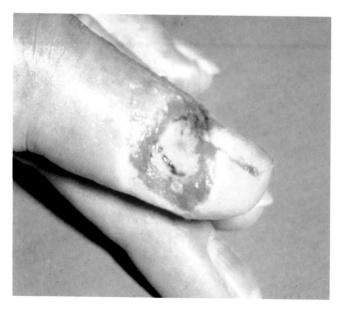

Figure 28–4. Scleroderma.

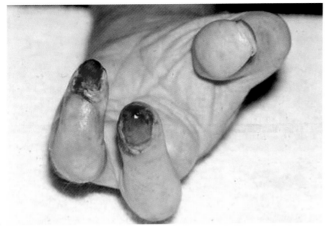

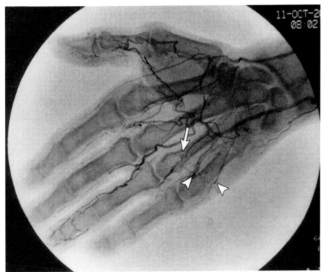

FIGURE 28–5. Buerger's disease. (A) Minor finger amputations. (B) Segmental thrombotic occlusion of small and medium arteries in the upper and lower extremities of young smokers.

symptoms with long-term cold exposure, but a cause and effect link has not been established.

Use of vibrating tools has long been known to cause upper extremity ischemia, starting with the first reports from stonecutters in the early 1900s. Long-term use of tools that vibrate at certain frequencies first causes vasospasm both with the exposure to cold and vibration, and later leads to palmar and digital artery obstruction. As new industries have arisen over the years and vibrating mechanical tools have been invented to make the work easier, new waves of patients with "vibration white finger" have appeared.[2] A prime example of this is in the timber industry. The earliest chain saws were little more than a motor attached to a blade and caused widespread damage to the hands of those using them. The newer antivibration saws have been carefully designed to isolate the damaging frequencies from the user's hands.

Large Artery Diseases

The causes of large artery disease in the upper extremity are similar to those seen in the lower extremity but the proportional distribution of diseases is different. The most common cause of larger artery disease in the upper extremity is atherosclerosis. However, atherosclerosis is responsible for only a small proportion of disease, in contrast to the lower extremities where atherosclerosis is by far the most frequent cause. A large variety of other conditions may also affect the arteries of the upper extremity proximal to the wrist (Table 28–2).

Although a small proportion of disease, atherosclerosis in the upper extremity is the most frequently seen cause of large artery upper extremity ischemia, particularly in older males (Figure 28–6). The disease may be at the origin of the great vessels or more distally in the axillary or brachial arteries. Atherosclerosis may present with chronic ischemia of the limb or as intermittent ischemia due to embolic events. Aneurysms of the brachiocephalic, subclavian, and axillary arteries may result in upper extremity ischemia through thrombosis or by showering emboli, which occlude the distal circulation. Treatment of occlusive or aneurysmal disease consists of thrombolysis, angioplasty and/or stenting, or bypass of the lesion with resection or isolation of the aneurysm if present.

Giant cell arteritis and Takayasu's arteritis are autoimmune disorders involving the arteries of the head, neck, and arms and are characterized by long segment stenoses, occlusion, or aneurysms of the affected arteries.[23] Giant cell arteritis is most commonly seen in elderly white females. These patients often have systemic symptoms such as polymyalgia rheumatica, malaise, headache, and an elevated sedimentation rate.[24] Takayasu's arteritis frequently presents in young Asian females. Fever, myalgias, and anorexia are common. It is important to identify these disease processes correctly since surgery is contraindicated in the active phase and steroid therapy is essential.

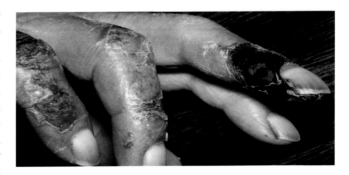

FIGURE 28–6. Atherosclerosis.

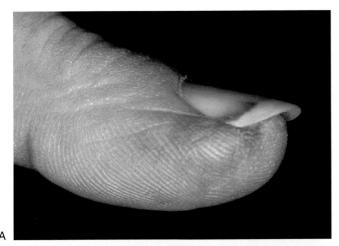

A

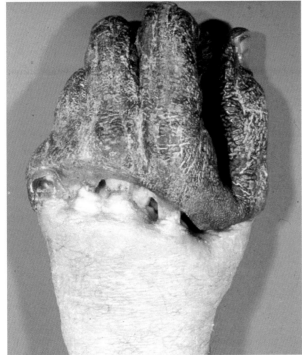

B

FIGURE 28–7. Embolization.

Radiation arteritis is known to involve the subclavian and axillary arteries and has led to critical limb ischemia in a small group of patients.[25] Treatment of these patients may be difficult because of the radiation injury to the surrounding tissue, but bypass with veins is often technically possible.

Ten to twenty percent of cardiac emboli lodge in the upper extremity. Emboli may also originate in diseased upper extremity arteries or a heavily diseased and calcified aortic arch, but approximately 70% of upper extremity emboli originate in the heart.[26] The severity of symptoms a patient has depends in part on the acuteness of the episode and the location of the embolus (Figure 28–7). Emboli lodging proximal to the origin of the pro-

funda brachii artery usually result in severe extremity ischemia because of the paucity of collaterals. Emboli lodging distal to the profunda brachii do not usually cause limb-threatening ischemia but may result in disabling chronic symptoms of ischemia with arm use. For these reasons surgical embolectomy is the recommended treatment for emboli. The operative mortality of repair is high, approximately 10%, and is due to underlying diseases. Occasionally, particularly in the acute setting, thrombolytic therapy may be effective in treating the embolus.

Traumatic injuries to the upper extremity arteries may be of a blunt or penetrating nature. Angiographic misadventures, particularly those seen with brachial artery catheterization, are another traumatic etiology. Most traumatic arterial injuries present acutely with little doubt as to the etiology. One exception to this is among patients with occupations in which the hand is used as a hammer to align or force objects. These patients, often carpenters, mill workers, or machinists, may develop chronic traumatic aneurysms of the ulnar artery at the wrist. This so-called hypothenar hammer syndrome may cause ischemia by thrombosis of the ulnar artery, embolization to the digital arteries from the aneurysm, or a combination of the two (Figure 28–8).

Extremely rare causes of large artery upper extremity ischemia include fibromuscular dysplasia with occlusion or aneurysm formation, and true arterial thoracic outlet syndrome, which may cause subclavian artery aneurysms or occlusions.[27,28] Buerger's disease, as described previously, may also cause large artery disease.

Noninvasive Diagnostic Techniques

Segmental Arm Pressures

Blood pressure using a 10-cm pneumatic cuff is measured above the elbow, below the elbow, and above the wrist while insonating the radial or ulnar artery at the wrist using continuous wave Doppler. Waveforms can also be recorded at the different levels. Abnormal waveforms or pressures will help diagnose arterial disease proximal to the wrist (Figure 28–9).

Digital Pressure and Plethysmography

Digital pressure and plethysmography have proven to be extremely useful in the diagnosis of upper extremity arterial disease. Either PPG or strain gauge plethysmography can be used to measure digital blood pressure and to obtain pulse waveforms. We prefer PPG because the equipment is easier to use and more durable. The photo cell is attached to the fingertip pulp with double-sided tape or small strain gauges are placed around the finger-

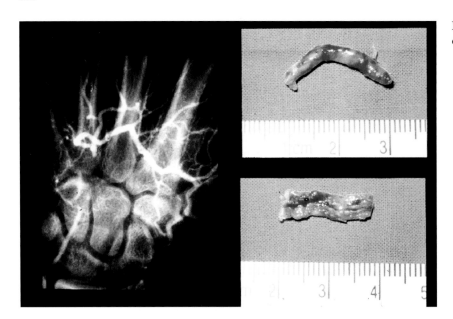

FIGURE 28–8. Hypothenar Hammer syndrome (ulnar artery aneurysm).

tip. One-inch (2.5-cm) blood pressure cuffs are placed around the proximal phalanx (Figure 28–10). Waveforms are recorded at rest, and then the cuff is inflated to measure blood pressure, which is indicated by the cessation of pulsatile blood flow. It is extremely important to measure and record finger temperature before performing this test. If the finger temperature is less than 28–30°C then false-positive results may be obtained secondary to cold-induced vasospasm. We recommend hand and/or whole body warming in patients with low finger temperatures, and require the technologist to record the finger temperature on the test form. Digital blood pressure is normally within 20–30 mm Hg of brachial pressure. This corresponds to a ratio of finger systolic pressure to brachial systolic pressure of greater than 0.80. Waveforms are normal if the upstroke time is less than 0.2 s. The absolute height of the waveform is not important since the test is qualitative, not quantitative. Diagrammatic

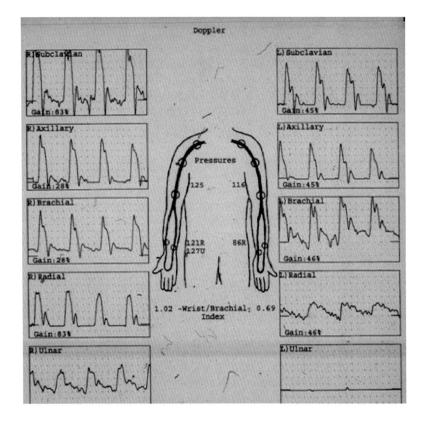

FIGURE 28–9. Segmental pressures and waveforms.

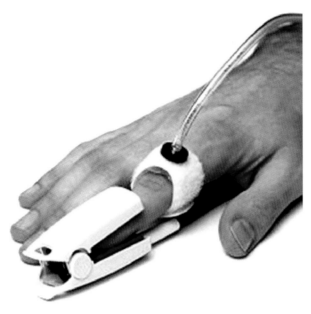

FIGURE 28–10. Digital artery waveforms/pressures.

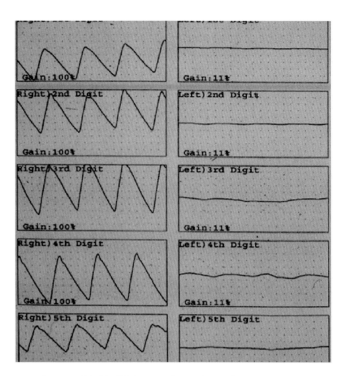

FIGURE 28–12. PPG waveforms in unilateral disease.

representations of PPG waveforms are shown in Figures 28–11 and 28–12. It is important to remember that there are occasional patients with very distal digital artery occlusive disease who will have normal finger pressures measured since the digital cuff is around the proximal phalanx.

Cold Challenge Testing

The simplest cold intolerance test is to measure the digital temperature recovery time after immersion of the hand in ice water for a short time period. This test is uncomfortable and poorly tolerated by patients. Using a thermister probe to measure finger temperatures, the patient's hand is immersed in a container of ice water for 30–60 seconds. After the hand is dried, the fingertip pulp temperatures are measured every 5 minutes for 45 minutes, or until the temperature returns to preimmersion levels. The preimmersion digital temperature must be above 30°C and therefore hand and body warming may be required prior to immersion. When cold sensitivity testing is performed the hands are immersed in ice water. Normal individuals will have a recovery time to preimmersion levels of less than 10 minutes. This test is very sensitive for detecting cold-induced vasospasm but is quite nonspecific, with approximately 50% of patients with a positive test having no clinical symptoms of cold sensitivity.[29]

A better test for cold sensitivity is the digital hypothermic challenge test as described by Nielsen and Lassen[30] (Figure 28–13). This test involves placing a finger cuff around the proximal phalanx on the test finger and perfusing the cuff with progressively cooler fluid. The pressure in the test finger is then compared with that in a reference finger that is not cooled. This test has become our preferred test for cold-induced vasospasm. The Nielsen test is interpreted as positive for abnormal cold-induced vasospasm if the test finger pressure is reduced by more than 17% compared with the reference finger (Figure 28–14). Other tests for cold-induced vasospasm include thermal entrainment, digital laser Doppler response to cold, thermography, venous occlusion plethysmography, and digital artery caliber measurement, but these test are not widely accepted or used.[31–33]

Upper Extremity Duplex Scanning

Duplex scanning of the upper extremity is carried out in a manner similar to arterial examination elsewhere in the body. The arteries are relatively superficial and fairly constant in location. Even digital arteries can be visualized in some patients by careful examination. Digital arterial lesions may be associated with more proximal disease, and therefore all arteries from the subclavian artery to the digital and palmar arteries should be imaged, even if

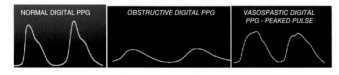

NORMAL DIGITAL PPG	OBSTRUCTIVE DIGITAL PPG	VASOSPASTIC DIGITAL PPG - PEAKED PULSE

FIGURE 28–11. Diagrammatic representation of normal, obstructive, and vasospastic digital PPG waveforms.

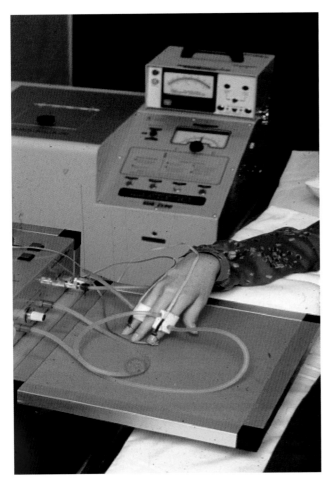

FIGURE 28–13. Digital hypothermic challenge test.

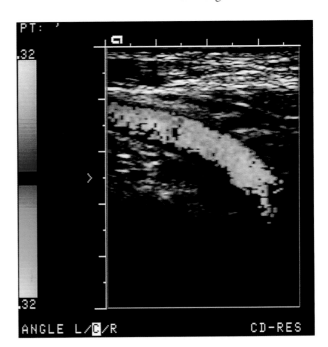

FIGURE 28–15. Duplex image of the origin of the right subclavian artery demonstrating a normal color flow image.

the suspected lesion is at one extreme of the upper extremity.

For examination of the origin of the subclavian artery a 3- or 5-MHz probe generally gives the best images (Figure 28–15). The remaining upper extremity arteries are superficial and are best scanned with a higher-frequency probe such as a 7.5- or 10-MHz probe. Either a sector or linear scan head may be used, but in either case a standoff or mound of acoustical gel is helpful to visualize the vessel clearly and to assess the flow pattern within it. Color duplex scanners facilitate identification of the vessels (Figure 28–16), and tortuosity of the upper

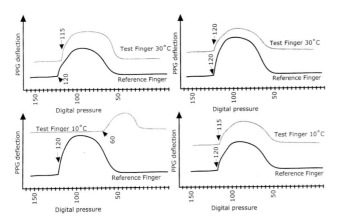

FIGURE 28–14. Diagrammatic representation of the digital hypothermic challenge test, showing an abnormal (left column) and normal examination (right column). During the abnormal examination the digital blood pressure in the test finger, which is normal at rest, drops to approximately 50% of the pressure in the reference finger at 10°C. In the normal examination there is a minimal pressure drop in the test finger with local cooling.

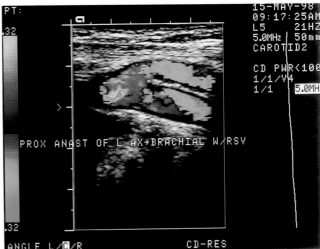

FIGURE 28–16. Duplex image of a patent origin of a left axillary brachial vein graft.

TABLE 28-3. Techniques for visualizing upper extremity arteries.

Artery	Probe	Approaches	Acoustical standoff
Subclavian	2–5 MHz	Supraclavicular Infraclavicular Sternal notch	No
Axillary	7–10 MHz	Anterior Axillary	Occasionally helpful
Brachial	7–10 MHz	Anterior	Yes
Radial	7–10 MHz	Anterior	Yes
Ulnar	7–10 MHz	Anterior	Yes

extremity arteries may be more easily seen with color-flow imaging. Table 28–3 summarizes the techniques used to visualize each upper extremity artery by duplex scanning.

The interpretation of duplex findings in the upper extremity is similar to the interpretation of B-mode images and Doppler signals gathered in other arterial systems.[34] Stenoses will result in high-velocity jets, post-stenotic turbulence, and dampened distal waveforms. At present there are no specific frequency or velocity criteria with which to gauge the severity of stenoses in the upper extremity, as there are for carotid or lower extremity arteries.

Normal waveforms in the upper extremity arteries are usually triphasic. With cooling of the limb, the amplitude of the velocity waveform decreases dramatically, but the triphasic pattern persists. Heating of the limb results in decreased hemodynamic resistance and monophasic signal with flow throughout diastole. The diagnosis of arterial occlusion is made by imaging the artery and using the Doppler to show that there is no flow within the lumen. Although the use of color may aid in the performance of the examination, the important diagnostic information resides in the Doppler spectra.

Diagnosis

The evaluation of the patient presenting with upper extremity ischemia begins with a detailed history and physical examination. In addition to the standard questions regarding the onset, severity, and timing of symptoms, the patient should be questioned specifically for symptoms of connective tissue disease including arthralgias, dysphagia, skin tightening, xerophthalmia, or xerostomia. An occupational history determining exposure to toxic substances is important. Historical information should be sought regarding exposure to trauma or frostbite, drug history, and a history of malignancy. Symptoms

in the lower extremity should also be sought. Patients, especially those who present with sudden onset of digital ischemia, should be questioned about coagulation abnormalities and a history of previous thromboembolic episodes.

On physical examination, the digits should be carefully inspected for the presence of ulcers and hyperkeratotic areas suggesting healed ulcers. The hands and fingers should also be examined for telangectasias, skin thinning, tightening, or sclerodactyly, which may suggest an associated autoimmune disease. Signs and symptoms of nerve compression syndrome should also be sought since carpal tunnel syndrome is seen in about 15% of Raynaud's patients.[1] A thorough pulse examination of all extremities should be performed with attention to the strength and quality of pulses as well as the presence of aneurysms or bruits. Four limb blood pressures should be obtained and carefully charted. It should be noted that the physical examination is frequently completely normal in patients with Raynaud's syndrome.

The extent of laboratory evaluation will vary somewhat depending on the findings of the history and physical examination. Our current basic evaluation includes a complete blood count, erythrocyte sedimentation rate, chemistry panel, rheumatoid factor, antinuclear antibody to aid in the diagnosis of any associated autoimmune disease, and hand radiographs for calcinosis or tuft resorption in patients with suspected systemic disease. Additional information such as serum protein electrophoresis and antibodies to a variety of nuclear antigens may subsequently be obtained as indicated. An upper extremity nerve conduction test should be considered if there is any clinical suspicion of carpal tunnel syndrome. We further evaluate patients with sudden onset of hand ischemia and no evidence of autoimmune disease for hypercoagulable states. Our current hypercoagulable screen consists of prothrombin time/partial thromboplastin time (PT/PTT), antithrombin III, protein C, protein S, lipoprotein (a) levels, homocysteine levels, as well as screening for antiphospholipid antibodies, anticardiolipin antibodies, hereditary resistance to activated protein C (Factor V Leiden), prothrombin gene mutation (G20210A), and dilute viper venom test (DVVT).

Vascular laboratory testing consists initially of segmental arm pressures, finger pressures and PPG waveforms, and cold challenge testing. Segmental pressures are carried out at the wrist, below the elbow, and above the elbow. There is normally no change in blood pressure at each level, and the pressures should be equal to systemic pressure. Abnormal waveforms and decreased pressures at the above-elbow cuff site indicate axillary, subclavian, or brachiocephalic arterial occlusive disease. Similarly, abnormalities at the below-elbow and above-wrist sites indicate brachial and proximal ulnar/radial arterial occlusive disease, respectively.

Digital blood pressures and waveforms are obtained. It is very important to ensure that the hands are not cold when measuring finger pressures and waveforms to avoid false-positive results. Normal digital artery pressure is within 20–30 mm Hg of brachial pressure with a finger-brachial ratio of >0.80. A normal digital PPG artery waveform will have a rapid upstroke (less than 0.2s) and may or may not have a dicrotic notch. It is important to remember that finger PPG waveforms are not quantitative, as the height of the waveform is dependent on the gain setting, not blood flow. Patients with vasospasm will often have an abnormally shaped waveform termed a "peaked pulse," which is thought to represent abnormal elasticity and rebound of the palmar and digital vessels. Obstructive waveforms have a slow upstroke (greater than 0.2s) and generally a more rounded peak (Figure 28–11). We have found that PPG is as accurate as arteriography in assessing patients with hand ischemia.[35]

To confirm the diagnosis of vasospasm in response to cold exposure we prefer to use the digital hypothermic challenge (Nielsen) test, as the ice water immersion test is not well tolerated. Patients with vasospastic and obstructive Raynaud's syndrome will have digital pressure drops of greater than 17% with cooling compared with a test finger, which is not cooled.

The combination of upper extremity pulses, digital pressures, and waveforms will allow the differentiation of large artery disease from small artery disease. Dampened digital waveforms with diminished digital pressures will lead to a diagnosis of occlusive small vessel disease when the proximal arm pressures are normal. Normal digital waveforms and a positive digital hypothermic challenge test will clearly distinguish vasospastic from obstructive disease. Raynaud's syndrome can be confidently diagnosed from the history and these studies. Other diseases such as scleroderma, Buerger's disease, hypersensitivity angiitis, and hypercoagulable states can also be differentiated and diagnosed with this approach in association with judicious laboratory blood testing.

Patients with abnormal arterial pressures at the wrist and above can be considered to have large artery disease and require further evaluation. Duplex scanning is proving useful in evaluating patients in whom there is no evidence of a systemic disease process that may be responsible for the obstructive ischemic symptoms. For those patients with unilateral symptoms who may have a surgically correctable lesion such as a subclavian artery aneurysm or stenosis, duplex scanning has been the most useful.[36] The duplex evaluation of aneurysms is based upon the B-mode image appearance, with the most important feature being the size of the enlarged artery. Presence or absence of flow within the aneurysm can be determined by the Doppler component. Duplex scanning may be of use in patients with suspected embolization to identify proximal aneurysms, but the evaluation should also include echocardiography to look for mural thrombi and valvular lesions. While duplex scanning alone cannot be used to make the diagnosis of Takayasu's arteritis, it is a helpful adjunct in following the progression or regression of arterial involvement in response to treatment.[37]

We rarely use arteriography in the upper extremity, even in patients with tissue loss. We have realized that the vascular laboratory can provide almost all the diagnostic information we require. We reserve arteriography for those patients with significant hand ischemia in whom no underlying disease process can be detected with noninvasive testing, particularly if the symptoms are unilateral. When arteriography is performed it is important to study both upper extremities because the presence of bilateral small artery occlusive disease is an indication that there is a systemic process involved. We find that magnified cut film views of the hands provide greater detail than digital subtraction techniques. We continue to obtain arteriograms on all patients requiring surgical correction of arterial lesions.

Treatment and Outcome

The primary treatment of upper extremity ischemia is cold avoidance. We further recommend cessation of tobacco use if present, and a reduction of caffeine if intake is heavy. Since most of the patients we see have vasospastic Raynaud's syndrome and are moderately symptomatic, these therapeutic recommendations are generally sufficient. Patients with more severe symptoms are treated with a variety of vasodilators. Our first line drug is extended-release nifedipine (30 mg at bedtime).[38] While this causes a reduction in the severity of vasospastic episodes, it is rarely curative and is associated with frequent side effects, the most common of which is headache. Other drugs that appear to be effective include captopril, losartan, guanethidine, prazosin, and sustained-release transdermal glyceryl trinitrate patches and slidenafil.[39–41] Selective serotonin reuptake inhibitors (SSRIs) have been studied recently as well and may be helpful in the treatment of Raynaud's syndrome.[42] Behavioral modification with biofeedback has helped many patients, and acupuncture has even proved beneficial in one small study.[43,44] We empirically treat patients with digital ulcers with pentoxifylline until their ulcers have resolved. The digital ulcers are treated with local care and judicious use of antibiotics for cellulitis. Distal phalangeal amputation is occasionally required for either pain control or protruding bone. These amputations heal slowly but there is often dramatic pain relief.

Patients with no evidence of large or small artery obstruction and no laboratory abnormalities can be considered to have idiopathic Raynaud's syndrome and have an excellent long-term prognosis with a low probability of developing either a connective tissue disease or ischemic ulcers.[15] Patients with positive serologic tests or other laboratory abnormalities clearly are at increased risk of having or developing an associated disease process, which may or may not require further evaluation and treatment. If these patients have no evidence of obstructive disease they have an intermediate prognosis along with those patients who have obstruction but no evidence of an associated disease. The patients with obstruction and an associated disease are the group that fare the worst over the long term and are most likely to have or develop digital ulcers.[15] Approximately 50% of patients who present with digital ulcers will have recurrent ulcers.[16,35]

In the few patients with large artery disease, surgical bypass or repair is frequently indicated.[28] Unfortunately, patient recovery may be limited since many large artery diseases are associated with distal emboli, which cannot be retrieved at the time of surgical repair. This leaves the patient with normal circulation to the wrist but with symptoms due to residual small artery occlusive disease.

We have not found any improvement in ulcer healing with sympathectomy as compared with local wound care and have not performed upper extremity sympathectomy for upper extremity ischemia in over a decade. Periarterial digital sympathectomy has been recommended as a more direct approach.[45] While we have several patients who have had satisfactory results from this procedure, there are no convincing data concerning its efficacy. We have tried arteriovenous reversal in a limited number of difficult cases but have not noted any significant clinical improvement and have abandoned this procedure.[46]

Conclusions

Upper extremity ischemia is an unusual clinical entity. Using a careful history and physical examination, detailed noninvasive vascular laboratory testing (segmental pressures, PPG, cold challenge test), and serologic tests, determining the cause is possible in nearly every patient. Duplex scanning appears to offer some additional information in selected cases. If the diagnosis cannot be established by noninvasive testing or if therapeutic intervention is planned, arteriography remains an important diagnostic test for upper extremity vascular disease. The primary treatment of upper extremity ischemia remains cold avoidance, with the addition of pharmacologic treatment for a limited number of patients. The long-term outcome for the majority of patients who present with Raynaud's syndrome appears quite good with a low risk of developing a connective tissue disease or tissue loss.

References

1. Allen E, Brown G. Raynaud's disease: A critical review of minimal requisites for diagnosis. Am J Med Sci 1932;83:187–200.
2. Edwards JM. Basic data concerning Raynaud's syndrome. Ann Vasc Surg 1994;8:509–513.
3. Hirai M. Cold sensitivity of the hand in arterial occlusive disease. Surgery 1979;85:140–146.
4. Freedman RR, Moten M, Migaly P, Mayes M. Cold-induced potentiation of α2-adrenergic vasoconstriction in primary Raynaud's disease. Arthritis Rheum 1993;36:685–690.
5. Graafsma SJ, Wollersheim H, Droste HT, et al. Adrenoceptors on blood cells from patients with primary Raynaud's phenomenon. J Vasc Med Biol 1990;2:101–106.
6. Edwards JM, Phinney ES, Taylor LM Jr, et al. Alpha$_2$-adrenergic receptor levels in obstructive and spastic Raynaud's syndrome. J Vasc Surg 1987;5:38–45.
7. Coffman JD, Cohen RA. Alpha$_2$-adrenergic and 5-HT2 receptor hypersensitivity in Raynaud's phenomenon. J Vasc Med Biol 1990;2:101–106.
8. Freedman RR, Baer RP, Mayes MD. Blockade of vasospastic attacks by alpha$_2$-adrenergic but not alpha$_1$-adrenergic antagonists in idiopathic Raynaud's disease. Circulation 1995;92:1448–1451.
9. Furspan PB, Chatterjee S, Freedman RR. Increased tyrosine phosphorylation mediates the cooling-induced contraction and increased vascular reactivity of Raynaud's disease. Arthritis Rheum 2004;50:1578–1585.
10. Zamora MR, O'Brien RF, Rutherford RB, et al. Serum endothelin-1 concentrations and cold provocation in primary Raynaud's phenomenon. Lancet 1990;336;1144–1147.
11. Shawket S, Dickerson C, Hazleman B, et al. Selective suprasensitivity to calcitonin-gene-related peptide in the hands in Raynaud's phenomenon. Lancet 1989;II:1354–1357.
12. Generini S, Seibold JR, Matucci-Cerinic M. Estrogens and neuropeptides in Raynaud's phenomenon. Rheum Dis Clin North Am 2005;31:177–186.
13. Rajagopalan S, Pfenninger D, Kehrer C, et al. Increased asymmetric dimethylarginine and endothelin 1 levels in secondary Raynaud's phenomenon. Implications for vascular dysfunction and progression of disease. Arthritis Rheum 2003;48:1992–2000.
14. Herrick AL. Pathogenesis of Raynaud's phenomenon. Rheumatology 2005;44:587–596.
15. Landry GJ, Edwards JM, McLafferty RB, et al. Long-term outcome of Raynaud's syndrome in a prospectively analyzed patient cohort. J Vasc Surg 1996;23:76–85.
16. Taylor LM Jr, Hauty MG, Edwards JM, Porter JM. Digital ischemia as a manifestation of malignancy. Ann Surg 1987;206:62–71.
17. Paw P, Dharan SM, Sackier JM. Digital ischemia and occult malignancy. Int J Colorectal Dis 1996;11:196–197.
18. Buerger L. Thromboangiitis obliterans: A study of the vascular lesions leading to presenile spontaneous gangrene. Am J Med Sci 1908;136:567–580.
19. Mills JL, Porter JM. Buerger's disease: A review and update. Semin Vasc Surg 1993;6:14–23.

20. Papa M, Bass A, Adar R. Autoimmune mechanisms in thromboangiitis obliterans (Buerger's disease): The role of the tobacco antigen and the major histocompatibility complex. Surgery 1992;111:527–531.

21. Mackiewicz Z, Piskorz A. Raynaud's phenomenon following long-term repeated action of great differences of temperature. J Cardiovasc Surg 1977;18:151–154.

22. Kaminski M, Bourgine M, Zins M, et al. Risk factors for Raynaud's phenomenon among workers in poultry slaughterhouses and canning factories. Int J Epidemiol 1997;26:371–380.

23. Sharma S, Rajani M, Talwar KK. Angiographic morphology in nonspecific aortoarteritis (Takayasu's arteritis): A study of 126 patients from North India. Cardiovasc Intervent Radiol 1992;15:160–165.

24. Pountain G, Hazelman B. Polymyalgia rheumatica and giant cell arteritis. BMJ 1995;310:1057–1059.

25. McCallion WA, Barros S. Management of critical upper extremity ischemia long after irradiation injury of the subclavian and axillary arteries. Br J Surg 1991;78:1136–1138.

26. Abbott WM, Maloney RD, McCabe CC, et al. Arterial embolism: A 44 year perspective. Am J Surg 1982;143:460.

27. McCready PA, Pairolero PC, Hollier LH, et al. Fibromuscular dysplasia of the right subclavian artery. Arch Surg 1982;117:1243–1245.

28. Nehler MR, Taylor LM Jr, Moneta GM, et al. Upper extremity ischemia from subclavian artery aneurysm caused by bony abnormalities of the thoracic outlet. Arch Surg 1997;132:527–532.

29. Porter JM, Snider, RL, Bardana EJ, et al. The diagnosis and treatment of Raynaud's phenomenon. Surgery 1975;77:11–23.

30. Nielsen SL, Lassen NA. Measurement of digital blood pressure after local cooling. J Appl Phys: Respir Environ Exerc Phys 1977;43:907–910.

31. Lafferty K, de Trafford JC, Roberts VC, Cotton LT. Raynaud's phenomenon and thermal entrainment: An objective test. BMJ Clin Res 1983;286:90–92.

32. Singh S, de Trafford JC, Baskerville PA, et al. Digital artery caliber measurement: A new technique of assessing Raynaud's phenomenon. Eur J Vasc Surg 1991;5:199–205.

33. Lutolf O, Chen D, Zehnder T, Mahler F. Influence of local finger cooling on laser Doppler flux and nailfold capillary blood flow velocity in normal subjects and in patients with Raynaud's phenomenon. Microvasc Res 1993;46:374–382.

34. Strandness DE. Peripheral Arterial System. Duplex Scanning in Vascular Disorders. New York: Raven Press, 1993.

35. McLafferty RB, Edwards JM, Talyor LM Jr, et al. Diagnosis and long-term clinical outcome in patients presenting with hand ischemia. J Vasc Surg 1995;22:361–369.

36. Grosveld WJ, Lawson JA, Eikelboom BC, et al. Clinical and hemodynamic significance of innominate artery lesions evaluated by ultrasonography and digital angiography. Stroke 1988;19:958–962.

37. Reed AJ, Fincher RME, Nichols FT. Case report: Takayasu's arteritis in a middle-aged Caucasian woman: Clinical course correlated with duplex ultrasonography and angiography. Am J Med Sci 1989;298:324–327.

38. Corbin DO, Wood DA, Macintyre CC, Housley E. A randomized double blind cross-over trial of nifedipine in the treatment of primary Raynaud's phenomenon. Eur Heart J 1986;7:165–170.

39. Teh LS, Manning J, Moore T, et al. Sustained-release transdermal glyceryl trinitrate patches as a treatment for primary and secondary Raynaud's phenomenon. Br J Rheum 1995;34:636–641.

40. Pancera P, Sansone S, Secchi S, et al. The effects of thromboxane A_2 inhibition (picotamide) and angiotensin II receptor blockade (losartan) in primary Raynaud's phenomenon. J Intern Med 1997;242:373–376.

41. Anderson ME, Moore TL, Hollis S, et al. Digital vascular response to topical glyceryl trinitrate, as measured by laser Doppler imaging, in primary Raynaud's phenomenon and systemic sclerosis. Rheumatology 2002;41:324–328.

42. Coleiro B, Marshall SE, Denton CP, et al. Treatment of Raynaud's phenomenon with the selective serotonin reuptake inhibitor fluoxetine. Rheumatology 2001;40:1038–1043.

43. Rose GD, Carlson JG. The behavioral treatment of Raynaud's disease: A review. Biofeedback Self Regul 1987;12:257–272.

44. Appiah R, Hiller S, Caspary L, et al. Treatment of primary Raynaud's syndrome with traditional Chinese acupuncture. J Intern Med 1997;241:119–124.

45. el-Gammal TA, Blair WF. Digital periarterial sympathectomy for ischaemic digital pain and ulcers. J Hand Surg 1991;16:382–385.

46. King TA, Marks J, Berrettoni BA, Seitz WH. Arteriovenous reversal for limb salvage in unreconstructible upper extremity arterial occlusive disease. J Vasc Surg 1993;17:924–932.

29
Ultrasound Imaging of Upper Extremity Arteries: Clinical Applications

Sergio X. Salles-Cunha

Introduction

The objectives of this chapter are to review applications and describe protocols of duplex ultrasound arterial mapping (DUAM) of the upper extremities. A literature search revealed multiple arterial applications of duplex ultrasound in the upper extremity. Situations in which ultrasound may replace arteriography or other techniques actually employed are also mentioned. The examples cited expand the role of the noninvasive vascular laboratory to many medical specialties, including vascular surgery, vascular medicine, radiology, neurology, nephrology, orthopedics, plastic surgery, emergency medicine, trauma, and physiology.

Applications

Although the incidence of severe ischemia is low in the upper compared to the lower extremity,[1] a variety of pathological arterial conditions have been investigated with duplex ultrasound.

Acute and Chronic Obstructions

The large and small arteries feeding the upper extremity may be imaged with DUAM pending the patient's body habitus and availability of high-grade, high- and low-frequency transducers and ultrasound scanners. Examples of applications include detection of acute embolization of the axillary, subclavian, and/or brachial arteries, severe stenosis of the innominate artery, occlusion of the brachial artery (Figure 29–1), and obstruction of digital arteries.[2–4] Ultrasound has high sensitivity for the detection of occlusive disease at nine different levels of the arterial circulation.[5] It is a common technique to follow treatment, including endovascular procedures of large arteries, and digital transplantation.[6–8]

Subclavian Steal Syndrome

Occlusion or severe stenosis of the subclavian artery is commonly detected by differences in arm pressure measurements or observation of reverse flow in the vertebral artery (Figure 29–2). DUAM corroborates the diagnosis by direct imaging and detection of monophasic or abnormal waveforms distal to the obstruction.

Trauma

Ultrasound can be as effective as arteriography in detecting arterial wall injuries caused by trauma.[9] Occlusion, pseudoaneurysms (Figure 29–3), fistulas, wall injuries, and intimal flaps can be properly identified in the subclavian, axillary, brachial, and forearm arteries. Vasospasm without injury can also be evaluated.

Vasculitis

Inflammation of blood vessels can cause thromboangiitis obliterans or Buerger's disease. Arteries of the hands and feet are particularly affected, becoming constricted or severely obstructed. The large arteries and the arteries of the hand and fingers, all the way to the nail level, can be insonated.[10] Takayasu's arteritis can be recognized by the arterial wall characteristics and narrowed lumen as imaged by B-mode ultrasound (Figure 29–4). Alterations in shape, as imaged by color flow ultrasound and velocity waveforms, have been detected in patients with secondary Raynaud's phenomenon.[11] Drug treatment can be monitored and controlled by DUAM.[12] The ultrasound evaluation helps define the location and amount of drug delivered.

Aneurysms of Subclavian/Axillary Arteries

Distal embolization may originate from mural thrombus located at the proximal arteries (Figure 29–5). Saccular

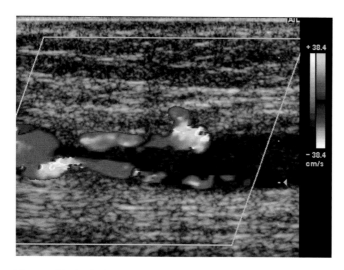

FIGURE 29–1. Color duplex image: Pseudoaneurysm with long neck and to and fro color in sac.

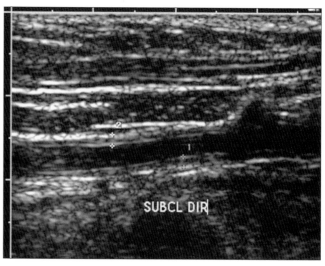

FIGURE 29–4. Arterial wall thickening extending to the subclavian artery in a patient diagnosed with Takayasu's arteritis. Manual measurements of wall thickness were 1.2 mm in the near wall and 1.3 mm in the far wall.

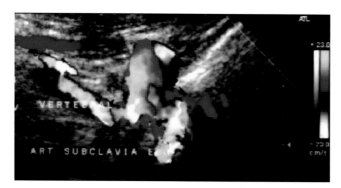

FIGURE 29–2. B mode image: Tip of needle in center of pseudoaneurysm sac. Note thrombus forming in inferior aspect of sac.

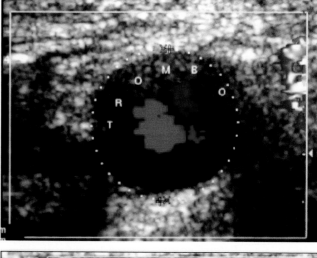

A

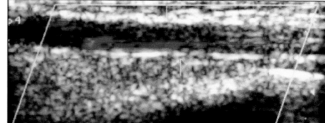

B

FIGURE 29–3. Current treatment algorithm for postcatheterization pseudoaneurysms.

FIGURE 29–5. Partially thrombosed aneurysm of the axillary artery (A) causing thrombosis of the radial artery (B). (Courtesy of Fanilda Barros, M.D., Angiolab Vitoria, ES, Brazil.)

aneurysms of the subclavian or axillary arteries can be diagnosed with ultrasound. The treatment can be via open surgery or endovascular.[13] Pending the location and access of the aneurysm, DUAM could be employed for guidance for puncture or even implantation during the endovascular procedure.

Stump of an Occluded Axillofemoral Bypass

The rare, acute embolic consequences of axillofemoral bypass occlusion were diagnosed with DUAM. The ultrasound technique complements arteriography, magnetic resonance, and transesophageal echography in determining the source and consequences of the embolic episode.[2]

Thoracic Outlet Syndrome

Thoracic Outlet Syndrome (TOS) affects nerves, veins, and arteries. Congenital or posttraumatic pseudarthrosis, hypertrophic callus, arterial restriction by a screw in a clavicular plate, bone tumors, and Paget's disease usually demonstrate arterial lesions that are symptomatic during postural changes. An embolic stenosis of the subclavian artery followed by poststenotic dilatation is a common finding.[14]

Radial Artery Mapping for Coronary Bypass

Arterial mapping has been increasingly accepted prior to harvesting the radial artery for coronary bypasses. Radial artery diameter and reactivity can be assessed.

The radial artery has several favorable features as a coronary graft, including a caliber similar to that of the coronary arteries, adequate length for complete coronary revascularization, and adequate wall thickness and resistance. Presently, several cardiovascular surgeons request that the vascular laboratories perform preoperative noninvasive mapping of the forearm vessels prior to radial artery harvesting to assess the suitability of the radial artery for graft replacement and to avoid ischemic complications to the hand.

Harvesting the radial artery may occasionally lead to ischemic complications of the hand (particularly the thumb and the index finger), which could be deprived of blood flow in patients with anatomical variations that do not allow adequate collateral flow across the palm. The incidence of this complication is generally low.[15,16] There are several contraindications to using the radial artery as a graft conduit, including ischemic symptoms in the upper extremity, history of arterial trauma, and Raynaud's syndrome. The use of the radial artery in the dominant arm is generally avoided, but this contraindication seems to be less important when adequate noninvasive evaluation confirms that it is appropriate. The two major objectives

of this evaluation are (1) to ensure that the radial artery is free of disease and is of appropriate size, and (2) to eliminate the possibility of postharvest ischemia of the hand.

The contribution of increased ulnar flow (Figure 29–6) in the absence of radial artery flow has been assessed by digital pressures and other signs of increased collateral circulation. The value of increased ulnar velocities during radial artery compression remains a controversial issue.[17] Examination of the digits includes the contribution of other arteries besides the ulnar.

The anatomic feature that permits radial artery harvesting without ischemic complications is the presence of collateral anastomosis across the palm between the radial and ulnar arteries, in the form of several arches. The most significant collateral pathway is the superficial palmar arch, which typically originates from the ulnar artery and

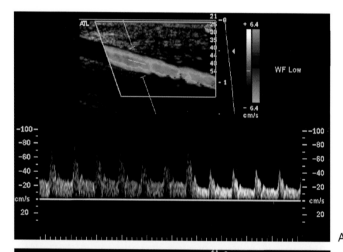

A

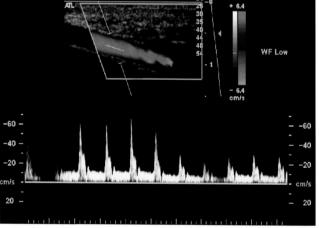

B

FIGURE 29–6. Increased blood flow velocities through the ulnar artery during compression of the radial artery. Variations in velocity with this maneuver, such as the increase in ulnar artery velocities with radial compression and the corresponding decrease after release of compression, depend on the degree of vasodilatation (A) or vasoconstriction (B) of the hand and digits. Incorporation of testing response to radial compression in worst-case condition with a constricted hand is suggested.

provides the majority of arterial supply to the digits. The dorsal and deep palmar arches usually originate from the radial artery and are generally smaller than the superficial palmar arch and its branches. Overall, if the superficial palmar arch is intact, collateral flow to the radial aspect of the hand should be adequate, if the radial artery is harvested. However, there are several anatomic variations that may lead to hand ischemia with radial artery harvesting, e.g., incomplete superficial palmar arch, radial artery dominance of the superficial palmar arch, and absence or malformation of the ulnar artery. These variations have been reported to vary from 6% to 34%.[18]

Several methods were advocated to evaluate the capability of the ulnar artery to provide adequate perfusion to the hand in the event of radial artery harvesting. These include the clinical modified Allen test, digital blood pressure measurement,[19] segmental pressure measurement,[20] laser Doppler flowmetry,[19] pulse oximetry,[21] flow measurement with photoplethysmography,[21] and modified Allen test with Doppler ultrasound.[15,18,22] In the clinical modified Allen test, the hand is deprived of perfusion by clinching the fist and compressing the ulnar and radial arteries until the hand is exsanguinated, and is then observed for return of color upon release of the ulnar artery. This test is believed to be subjective and unreliable with a significant number of false-negative and false-positive results.[23] The measurement of digital systolic blood pressure is objective, and although a pressure drop of more than 40 mm Hg has been proposed as an indicator of hand ischemia, the choice of this value is somewhat arbitrary and needs validation. The measurement of oxygen saturation in the digits with radial artery compression is also objective, but substantial variations in perfusion do not always result in changes in saturation.[16,21]

A Doppler ultrasound version of the clinical Allen test has been used in several studies, mostly using continuous-wave Doppler ultrasound and some with color Doppler ultrasound.[15,18,22] This examination involves Doppler interrogation of the radial portion of the superficial palmar arch before and after radial artery compression, and assessment for the presence and/or reversal of flow as an indicator of an intact arch providing adequate collateral flow.[15,18,22] In three previously reported studies,[15,18,22] using the modified ultrasound Allen test with continuous-wave Doppler, in the follow-up of patients who underwent radial artery harvesting, none of the 113 patients who had negative studies (i.e., intact palmar arches) had signs of hand ischemia. Zimmerman et al.[24] examined 358 patients who underwent coronary artery bypass graft replacement, who were evaluated using modified ultrasound Allen test, and reported 53 radial arteries were harvested with no single case of hand ischemia. They began their examination with a modified ultrasound Allen test. If this test indicated that the arch

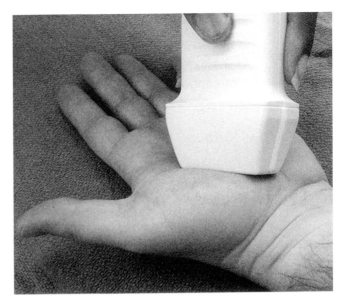

FIGURE 29–7. Transducer positioning for insonation of the superficial palmar branch of the radial artery in the crease at the base of the thumb. (Reprinted from Zimmerman P, Chin E, Laifer-Narin S, et al. Radial artery mapping for coronary artery bypass graft placement. Radiology 2001;220:299–302. With permission from the Radiological Society of North America.)

was not intact, the examination was ended. If collateral flow through the ulnar artery was demonstrated, they proceeded to evaluate the radial and ulnar arteries for any evidence of obstructive disease or atherosclerosis.

The ultrasound Allen test utilizes a 7- to 10-MHz linear transducer that is placed in the crease of the proximal palm at the base of the thumb (Figure 29–7). The superficial palmar arch of the radial artery can be identified coursing anteriorly at this location. The approximate place of this vessel can generally be found by drawing a line along the longitudinal axis of the center of the index finger to the point of its intersection with the crease at the base of the thumb or the thenar eminence. Flow in this artery is normally directed toward the transducer and into the superficial palmar arch. The direction of flow in this artery can be easily determined by using color Doppler ultrasound. Color Doppler ultrasound is generally used to locate the artery and spectral imaging to evaluate and document the change in flow direction. While the superficial palmar arch is insonated, the radial artery is compressed at the wrist, and the ultrasonographer watches for a reversal of flow, implying that the arch is complete, or lack of flow, implying that the arch is incomplete (Figure 29–8). Reversal of flow implies that the radial artery may be harvested with safety. Complete lack of flow in this artery with compression essentially precludes the use of the ipsilateral radial artery.

Although there are no specific velocity criteria to grade stenoses in the upper extremity arteries, the application

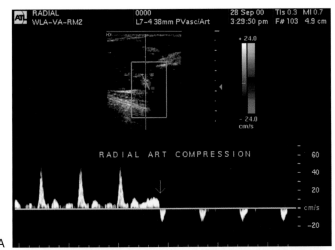

A

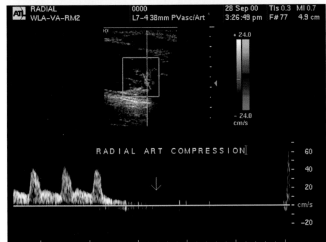

B

FIGURE 29–8. Color (inset box) and spectral Doppler ultrasound images of the superficial palmar branch of the radial artery (red area in inset box) in a healthy volunteer demonstrate blood flow toward the transducer before radial artery compression (left of arrow.) (A) In one hand, flow reverses after radial artery compression (right of arrow), indicating a continuous palmar arch. (B) In the contralateral hand, flow does not reverse after radial artery compression (right of arrow), indicating an incomplete arch. (Reprinted from Zimmerman P, Chin E, Laifer-Narin S, *et al.* Radial artery mapping for coronary artery bypass graft placement. Radiology 2001;220:299–302. With permission from the Radiological Society of North America.)

of velocity criteria on other vessels may apply. These include a focal increase in peak systolic velocity, post-stenotic turbulence, and dampening of the waveform distal to the lesion.

Radial Forearm Flap

Mapping of the upper extremity arteries is recommended for appropriate decision making in selecting a radial flap for plastic surgery.[25] Preexisting vascular disease as detected by echography eliminates donor vessels, reduces the risk of hand ischemia, and reduces failure of free flaps. Excision of the radial artery during harvesting of the forearm flap significantly alters the flow patterns of the distal upper extremity.[26] Compensatory increased flow rates were noted in the anterior and posterior interosseous and ulnar arteries. Mapping the ulnar artery alone is, therefore, an insufficient evaluation if the radial artery is being harvested. The contributions of the interosseous arteries must be taken into consideration.

Arterial Mapping Prior to Constructing a Dialysis Fistula

Patients now are less likely to have suitable arteries and veins for autogenous fistulas in classical locations.[27,28] Stenosis of forearm arteries is a common finding altering fistula configuration. DUAM is usually performed to determine patency and adequate inflow to the brachial (Figure 29–1), radial, and ulnar arteries.[29] The examination is particularly recommended if the patient has had prior revascularization or arterial catheters implanted. An integrated approach that includes preoperative ultrasound improves utilization and outcome of primary forearm fistulas.[30,31] Ultrasound examinations can also document improvement in arterial and venous diameters and in flow-mediated dilatation following prefistula exercise training.[32]

Steal Syndrome

Digital ischemia associated with a dialysis access may be caused by (1) elevated flow through the fistula, (2) stenosis of an inflow artery, and (3) disease of the palmar arch.[33] Measurement of blood flow rate through the inflow artery, access and outflow vein(s), imaging of inflow arteries, and evaluation of high-resistance flow in the ulnar and radial arteries are evaluated to determine actual causes of the steal syndrome.

Arteriovenous Malformations

DUAM complements diagnosis of high-flow arteriovenous malformations,[34] could be employed during embolotherapy, and helps access the results of treatment.

Hypothenar Hammer Syndrome

This condition reduces blood flow to the fingers and is caused by workers such as carpenters repeatedly using the palm of the hand, the hypothenar eminence in particular, as a hammer to deal with various objects. These actions damage blood vessels, specially the ulnar artery. A traumatic aneurysm of the ulnar artery, for example, can thrombose and cause digital embolization. DUAM complements history and clinical diagnosis, and could be used to monitor thrombolytic therapy.

Microsurgical Operations

Plastic reconstructions of the hand and digits often require appropriate monitoring of brachial, radial, ulnar, and digital inflow. Due to vasospasm, blockade of the brachial plexus may be performed to increase flow.[35] Preoperative mapping, evaluation of brachial plexus blockade, perioperative evaluation, and postoperative follow-up of plastic reconstruction of the upper extremity can be accomplished with DUAM. Digital arteries may be followed all the way to below the nail bed (Figure 29–9).

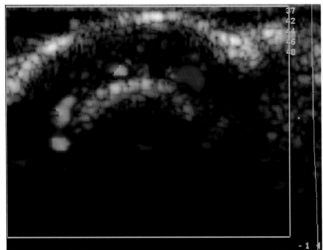

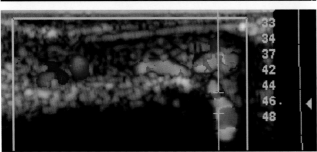

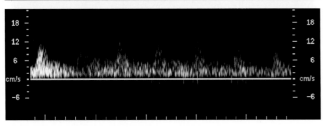

FIGURE 29–9. Small arteries detected beneath the nail in the tip of the finger in transverse (A) and longitudinal (B) imaging with corresponding blood flow rate waveforms (C).

Sympathetic Activity

Measurements of artery diameter, velocities, and resistive indices permit objective evaluation of sympathetic tone and stellate ganglion blockade.[36]

Tumor Detection

The vascularity and size of digital glomus tumors have been evaluated preoperatively to facilitate excision.[37]

Adventitial Cystic Disease

Very few cases of adventitial cystic disease have been reported.[38] Lesions in the popliteal fossa, external iliac, axillary, distal brachial, radial, and ulnar arteries as well as in the proximal saphenous vein at the ankle have been described. Anatomic images of a lobulated arterial wall and flow disturbances are detected in conjunction with this pathology.

Brachial Artery Reactivity

Duplex imaging and/or M-mode imaging have been employed to detect flow-mediated dilatation (FMD) or brachial artery reactivity in response to postocclusive reactive hyperemia. Such measurements have been used to evaluate endothelium function and drug influence on the arterial walls.[39]

Carpal Tunnel

Changes in radial and ulnar diameters and respective blood flow rates have quantitated the effectiveness of carpal tunnel release.[40]

Summary

DUAM can be employed for definitive diagnosis, preoperative mapping, periprocedural imaging, and patient follow-up in a variety of medical conditions. Intraoperative ultrasound guidance is a hot topic for development in the near future.

Protocols

This section briefly describes basic protocols for duplex ultrasound imaging of the arteries of the upper extremities.

Patient Positioning

The examination is usually performed with the patient supine and the arm alongside the body. In this position, the arteries of the forearm and hand can be easily assessed. The proximal large arteries, the subclavian and axillary, can also be imaged in this position. Imaging of the arteries in the arm often requires lateral extension and rotation to provide space between the body and the medial aspect of the arm.

Patient positioning is changed to accomplish the objectives of specific tests. For thoracic outlet syndrome, for example, the head and the arm are rotated and forcefully moved in an attempt to cause arterial blockage. The baseball pitcher's position while preparing to throw the ball is particularly useful. Positioning, however, should try to mimic conditions that cause symptoms according to the patient's complaints. Patient's position is also adapted to examination with immersion of the hand in cold or warm water. Immersion of a hand in water with ice is contraindicated. We recommend that the hand be immersed in tap water and ice be placed in the water until the patient cannot tolerate the discomfort any more. A warning is warranted about changes in pressure caused by raising or lowering of the hands above or below heart levels. Pressure in the vessels of the hand decreases or increases with changes in hydrostatic pressure. Such positioning must be taken into consideration during pressure measurements or interpretation of the DUAM results.

Worst-Case Conditions

It is recommended that some examinations be performed in worst-case conditions also. For example, if the radial artery is to be excised, the remaining collateral flow must be enough to feed the hand comfortably in conditions of severe vasoconstriction. The patient should be tested in a cold environment, with cold hands and perhaps a colder than usual central body temperature. This philosophy can be expanded to other situations such as plastic implantations, arteriovenous fistulas for dialysis, and evaluation of bypass grafts. Potential for success or failure can be demonstrated. Testing in worst-case conditions does not preclude examination in normal conditions.

Best-Case Conditions

Arterial imaging improves if physiological and technical parameters are optimized. Arteries dilate and blood flow rates increase with heat. The patient then should be mapped while warm, in a warm environment and after maneuvers to promote vasodilatation such as exercise and immersing the hand in warm water.

Several technical factors facilitate imaging of small or diseased arteries:

- High-frequency transducers improve resolution.
- Low scale applied to color flow and duplex Doppler increases sensitivity.

- Some instruments have special algorithms for detection of low velocity or low volume.
- Proper steering improves color flow and duplex Doppler signals.
- Increased persistence augments perception of color flow.

Large Proximal Arteries

Sector probes with a small footprint are often needed to image the proximal arteries as we approach the aortic arch (Figure 29–2). A small footprint, or size of the ultrasound probe also facilitates imaging of the arteries around the clavicle. As patient size and anatomy vary, the rules for imaging the large arteries change. Forcing the shoulders forward or backward and head positioning away from the area of interest may improve imaging.

Brachial Artery

Most brachial arteries are easily imaged with a linear transducer in the 5–10 MHz range. Problems may surface in the presence of anomalous anatomy such as a high brachial bifurcation (Figure 29–10), and dilated interosseous arteries mimicking the radial or ulnar arteries segmentally.

Forearm Arteries

Forearm arteries can be imaged with the same transducer used to examine the brachial artery. This transducer is commonly needed to evaluate the interosseous arteries and to visualize radial and ulnar arteries with meandering superficial and deep tunnels. Otherwise, a transducer with high frequencies above 10 MHz can be used to improve resolution and visualization of small superficial arteries.

An expanded field of view of the radial artery facilitates transfer of information. It requires training and it may take time if the artery is diseased or has an irregular course.

Hand and Digit Arteries

High-frequency high-resolution transducers are recommended for improved imaging. Probes in the 10–20 MHz range are now commonly available for most scanners. Small probes facilitate the approach to digital arteries. Large probes improve the overall visualization of the complex anatomy of the palm arch.

Summary

Two or three ultrasound probes may be needed to evaluate the arteries of the upper extremity from the

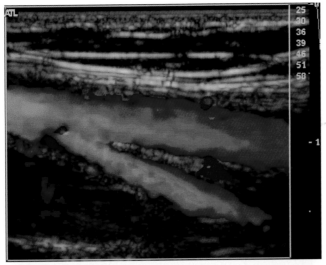

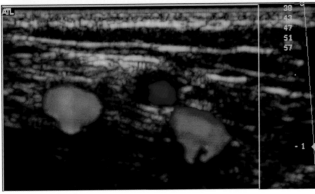

FIGURE 29–10. High brachial artery bifurcation at the upper arm (A.) Identification of the radial and ulnar arteries was accomplished only after continuous scanning to the distal forearm. The presence of a large interosseus artery above and below the elbow complicated identification of the arteries (B).

subclavian to the nail bed. Protocols must adapt to the objectives of the test, using normal, best, or worst-case conditions and performing examinations before, during, and after provocative maneuvers.

References

1. Harris RW, Andros G, Dulawa LB, Oblath RW, Salles-Cunha SX, Apyan R. Large vessel arterial occlusive disease in the symptomatic upper extremity. Arch Surg 1984;119: 1277–82.
2. Kallakuri S, Ascher E, Hingorani A, Markevich N, Schutzer R, Hou A, Yorkovich W, Jacob T. Endovascular management of axillofemoral bypass graft stump syndrome. J Vasc Surg 2003;38:833–5.
3. Zeller T, Frank U, Burgelin K, Sinn L, Horn B, Schwarzwalder U, Roskamm H, Neumann FJ. Treatment of acute embolic occlusions of the subclavian and axillary arteries using a rotational thrombectomy device. Vasa 2003;32:111–6.
4. Langholz J, Ladleif M, Blank B, Heidrich H, Behrendt C. Color coded duplex sonography in ischemic finger artery disease—a comparison with hand arteriography. Vasa 1997;26:85–90.
5. Tola M, Yurdakul M, Okten S, Ozdemir E, Cumhur T. Diagnosis of arterial occlusive disease of the upper extremities: Comparison of color duplex sonography and angiography. J Clin Ultrasound 2003;31:407–11.
6. Korner M, Baumgartner I, Do DD, Mahler F, Schroth G. PTA of the subclavian and innominate arteries: Long-term results. Vasa 1999;28:117–22.
7. Schmidt DM, McClinton MA. Microvascular anastomoses in replanted fingers: Do they stay open? Microsurgery 1990;11:251–4.
8. Walter J, Hofmann WJ, Ugurluoglu A, Magometschnigg H. False aneurysm after balloon dilation of a calcified innominate artery stenosis. J Endovasc Ther 2003;10:825–8.
9. Kuzniec S, Kauffman P, Molnar LJ, Aun R, Puech-Leao P. Diagnosis of limbs and neck arterial trauma using duplex ultrasonography. Cardiovasc Surg 1998;6:358–66.
10. Pokrovskii AV, Kuntsevich GI, Dan VN, Chupin AV, Kalinin AA, Alekperov RT, Makhmudova LS. Diagnosis of occlusive lesions of upper extremity arteries in patients with thromboangiitis obliterans. Angiol Sosud Khir 2003;9: 86–94.
11. Steins A, Hahn M, Volkert B, Duda S, Schott U, Junger M. Color duplex ultrasound of the finger arteries. An alternative to angiography? Hautarzt 1998;49:646–50.
12. Noel B, Panizzon RG. Use of duplex ultrasonography in the treatment of thromboangiitis obliterans with iloprost. Dermatology 2004;208:238–40.
13. Danzi GB, Sesana M, Bellosta R, Capuano C, Baglini R, Sarcina A. Endovascular treatment of a symptomatic aneurysm of the left subclavian artery. It Heart J 2005;6: 77–9.
14. Garnier D, Chevalier J, Ducasse E, Modine T, Espagne P, Puppinck P. Arterial complications of thoracic outlet syndrome and pseudarthrosis of the clavicle: Three patients. J Mal Vasc 2003;28:79–84.
15. Serricchio M, Gaudino M, Tondi P, et al. Hemodynamic and functional consequences of radial artery removal for coronary artery bypass grafting. Am J Cardiol 1999;84:1353–56.
16. Nunoo-Mensah J. An unexpected complication after harvesting of the radial artery for coronary artery bypass grafting. Ann Thorac Surg 1998;66:929–31.
17. Sullivan VV, Higgenbotham C, Shanley CJ, Fowler J, Lampman RM, Whitehouse WM Jr, Wolk SW. Can ulnar artery velocity changes be used as a preoperative screening tool for radial artery grafting in coronary artery bypass? Ann Vasc Surg 2003;17:253–9.
18. Starnes SL, Walk SW, Lampman RM, et al. Noninvasive evaluation of hand circulation before radial artery harvest for coronary artery bypass grafting. J Thorac Cardiovasc Surg 1999;117:261–66.
19. Levinsohn DG, Gordon L, Sessler DI. The Allen's test: Analysis of four methods. J Hand Surg Am 1991;16:279–82.
20. Winkler J, Lohr J, Rizwan HB, et al. Evaluation of the radial artery for use in coronary artery bypass grafting. J Vasc Technol 1998;22:23–9.

21. Fuhrman TM, Pippin WD, Talmage LA, Reilley TE. Evaluation of collateral circulation of the hand. J Clin Monit 1992;8:28–32.

22. Pola P, Serricchio M, Flore R, Manasse E, Favuzzi A, Posati GF. Safe removal of the radial artery for myocardial revascularization: Doppler study to prevent ischemic complication to the hand. J Thorac Cardiovasc Surg 1996;112:737–44.

23. Grenhow DE. Incorrect performance of Allen's test: Ulnar artery flow erroneously presumed inadequate. Anesthesiology 1972;37:356–57.

24. Zimmerman P, Chin E, Laifer-Narin S, Ragavendra N, Grant EG. Radial artery mapping for coronary artery bypass graft placement. Radiology 2001;220:299–302.

25. Thomson PJ, Musgrove BT. Preoperative vascular assessment: An aid to radial forearm surgery. Br J Oral Maxillofac Surg 1997;35:419–23.

26. Ciria-Llorens G, Gomez-Cia T, Talegon-Melendez A. Analysis of flow changes in forearm arteries after raising the radial forearm flap: A prospective study using color duplex imaging. Br J Plast Surg 1999;52:440–4.

27. Malovrh M. The role of sonography in the planning of arteriovenous fistulas for hemodialysis. Semin Dial 2003;16: 299–303.

28. Malovrh M. Native arteriovenous fistula: Preoperative evaluation. Am J Kidney Dis 2002;39:1218–25.

29. Huber TS, Ozaki CK, Flynn TC, Lee WA, Berceli SA, Hirneise CM, Carlton LM, Carter JW, Ross EA, Seeger JM. Prospective validation of an algorithm to maximize native arteriovenous fistulae for chronic hemodialysis access. J Vasc Surg 2002;36:452–9.

30. Silva MB Jr, Simonian GT, Hobson RW 2nd. Increasing use of autogenous fistulas: Selection of dialysis access sites by duplex scanning and transposition of forearm veins. Semin Vasc Surg 2000;13:44–8.

31. Shemesh D, Zigelman C, Olsha O, Alberton J, Shapira J, Abramowitz H. Primary forearm arteriovenous fistula for hemodialysis access—an integrated approach to improve outcomes. Cardiovasc Surg 2003;11:35–41.

32. Russ RR, Ponikvar R, Kenda RB, Buturovic-Ponikvar J. Effect of local physical training on the forearm arteries and veins in patients with end-stage renal disease. Blood Purif 2003;21:389–94.

33. Malik J, Slavikova M, Maskova J. Dialysis access-associated steal syndrome: The role of ultrasonography. J Nephrol 2003;16:903–7.

34. Tan KT, Simons ME, Rajan DK, Terbrugge K. Peripheral high-flow arteriovenous vascular malformations: A single-center experience. J Vasc Interv Radiol 2004;15:1071–80.

35. Kurt E, Ozturk S, Isik S, Zor F. Continuous brachial plexus blockade for digital replantations and toe-to-hand transfers. Ann Plast Surg 2005;54:24–7.

36. Celiktas M, Birbicer H, Aikimbaev K, Ozbek H, Akgul E, Binokay F. Utility of color duplex sonography in the assessment of efficacy of the stellate ganglion blockade. Acta Radiol 2003;44:494–7.

37. Chen SH, Chen YL, Cheng MH, Yeow KM, Chen HC, Wei FC. The use of ultrasonography in preoperative localization of digital glomus tumors. Plast Reconstr Surg 2003;112: 115–9.

38. Elster EA, Hewlett S, DeRienzo DP, Donovan S, Georgia J, Yavorski CC. Adventitial cystic disease of the axillary artery. Ann Vasc Surg 2002;16:134–7.

39. Malik J, Melenovsky V, Wichterle D, Haas T, Simek J, Ceska R, Hradec J. Both fenofibrate and atorvastatin improve vascular reactivity in combined hyperlipidaemia (fenofibrate versus atorvastatin trial—FAT). Cardiovasc Res 2002;54: 191–2.

40. Schuind F, Nguyen T, Vancabeke M, Wautrecht JC. Modifications of arterial blood flow to the hand after carpal tunnel release. Acta Orthop Belg 1998;64:296–300.

30
Protocol and Technique of Dialysis Ultrasound Surveillance

Niten Singh, Cameron M. Akbari, and Anton N. Sidawy

Introduction

Surgery for access for hemodialysis (HD) is the most commonly performed vascular surgical operation in the United States, predominantly due to a steady rise in the incidence and prevalence of end-stage renal disease (ESRD). Despite a concomitant increase in the mean age of these patients and more coexisting morbidities, advances in the management of renal failure and dialysis have resulted in longer survival among patients on HD. However, the "Achilles heel" for these patients remains access, with poor patency rates resulting in multiple interventions for thrombosis and maintenance, and, in many patients, the eventual need for life-long catheter placement. Access failure is the second leading cause of hospitalization among patients with ESRD, and the annual cost of access maintenance is estimated to be $1 billion in the United States.[1]

Multiple studies have confirmed the improved patency rate and lower infection rates for native arteriovenous fistulas compared to prosthetic arteriovenous grafts. Although approximately 60–90% of nonautogenous grafts are functional at 1 year, the patency falls to 40–60% at 3 years.[2] Despite inferior patency rates, however, prosthetic grafts continue to be more common than native fistulas in the United States, accounting for 65% of all access procedures. In contrast, data from Canada and Europe demonstrate greater use of autogenous fistulas in those countries, with prosthetic grafts accounting for less than 35% in Canada and 10% in Europe.[3]

In an effort to promote more standardized practice patterns and greater success with autogenous access placement, the National Kidney Foundation produced the Dialysis Outcome Quality Initiative (DOQI).[4] The guidelines recommend that more than 50% of all access grafts be autogenous; furthermore, to decrease thrombosis rates, guideline 10 (Table 30–1) provides information on surveillance and monitoring of dialysis access. Based on the current data, routine surveillance of dialysis access appears warranted, but the best method of surveillance has yet to be devised. Ultrasound appears to be an attractive tool for monitoring dialysis access based on its noninvasive nature and its success with lower extremity bypass surveillance, but it has not gained popularity as evidenced by its ranking as the last acceptable method of arteriovenous (AV) access surveillance in guideline 10 of DOQI.

Non-Ultrasound-Based Methods of Surveillance

Physical Examination

The DOQI guidelines recommend weekly physical examination of dialysis access. This includes palpation of the access for a thrill over the arterial and venous anastomosis as well as the mid portion of the access.[4] The access site should be auscultated for an audible bruit and inspected for evidence of hematomas and pseudoaneurysms over the length of the access and in relation to the puncture sites. It should also be monitored for signs of possible infection along the access.

Venous Pressures

Elevation in the venous pressure on the dialysis machine can signify a significant stenosis at the venous anastomosis or outflow. Both static venous pressure (SVP) and dynamic venous pressure (DVP) can be measured. The SVP is measured with no dialyzer flow and varies among patients. The DVP is measured when the dialyzer flow rate is kept constant; pressures greater than 125 mm Hg signify venous outflow stenosis.[5]

Access Recirculation

This refers to already dialyzed blood returned through the venous needle that reenters the extracorporeal circuit

TABLE 30–1. Guideline 10 from NKF/DOQI.

Definition of terms

Monitoring—This term refers to the examination and evaluation of the vascular access by means of physical examination to detect physical signs that would suggest the presence of pathology.

Surveillance—This term refers to periodic evaluation of the vascular access by means of tests that may involve special instrumentation, for which an abnormal test result suggests the presence of pathology.

Diagnostic testing—This term refers to testing that is prompted by some abnormality or other medical indication and that is undertaken to diagnose the presence of pathology.

Monitoring dialysis arteriovenous (AV) grafts

Physical examination of an access graft should be performed weekly and should include, but not be limited to, inspection and palpation for pulse and thrill at the arterial, mid, and venous sections of the graft. (Opinion)

   A. Intraaccess flow (Evidence)
   B. Static venous dialysis pressure (Evidence)

Acceptable

   C. Dynamic venous pressures (Evidence)

Other studies or information that can be useful in detecting AV graft stenosis:

   D. Measurement of access recirculation using urea concentration (Evidence)
   E. Measurement of recirculation using dilution techniques (nonurea-based) (Evidence)
   F. Unexplained decreases in the measured amount of hemodialysis delivered (URR, Kt/V) (Evidence)
   G. Physical findings of persistent swelling of the arm, clotting of the graft, prolonged bleeding after needle withdrawal, or altered characteristics of pulse or thrill in a graft (Evidence/Opinion)
   H. Elevated negative arterial prepump pressures that prevent increasing to acceptable blood flow (Evidence/Opinion)
   I. Doppler ultrasound (Evidence/Opinion)

via the arterial needle. The blood urea nitrogen (BUN) concentration ratio between the arterial line, venous line, and systemic values is used to calculate this parameter. Normal recirculation is less than 10% with greater values indicating an outflow stenosis.[5]

Ultrasound and Dialysis Access Creation and Surveillance

Preoperative Planning

Ultrasound may be incorporated into preoperative planning, particularly for autogenous access placement. Duplex ultrasound (DU) has been used for preoperative planning in dialysis access, and studies have shown a proven benefit of ultrasound in predicting success in patients who have undergone a preoperative ultrasound.[6] Robbin et al. noted an increase in autogenous AV access creation from 32% to 58% after a preoperative DU program was started.[7] With preoperative ultrasonography, Silva et al. were also able to demonstrate an increase in autogenous access placement from 14% to 63% and a decrease in failure of the autogenous access from 38% to 8.3%. In that study, veins greater than 2.5 mm were required for autogenous access placement and greater than 4 mm for nonautogenous placement.[8] Using the criteria of a 2-mm vein at the wrist and greater than 3 mm in the upper arm, Ascher et al. reported a similar increase in autogenous access placement with preoperative DU.[9]

Most preoperative ultrasound procedures can be performed in an office/vascular laboratory setting. The forearm venous network is superficial and easily imaged (Figure 30–1). The superficial veins can be visualized both longitudinally as well as in cross section. If these veins are compressible and greater than 2.5 mm, then an autogenous access can likely be performed. Mendes et al. studied the cephalic vein preoperatively with DU to determine whether a minimal cephalic vein size in the forearm could predict successful wrist autogenous access. He noted that patients with a cephalic vein size of 2.0 mm or less were less likely to have a successful wrist autogenous access than if the cephalic vein was greater than 2.0 mm.[10] If the patient's history suggests previous central venous lines or arm swelling, the deep veins such as the axillary and distal subclavian can also be interrogated. The bony clavicle limits accurate assessment at the mid to proximal subclavian level. Color flow DU may also be used to assess the arterial inflow. Starting at the wrist the radial artery can be identified and followed proximally to the brachial artery. Using color flow in the longitudinal view occlusive arterial disease can be identified. Unobstructed arterial inflow of 2.0 mm has been used as a predictor of success.[11,12]

Ultrasound Monitoring and Surveillance of Dialysis Access

DU has been studied for monitoring dialysis access and has been noted to correlate well with the degree of stenosis. The accuracy has been reported to be as high as 90% when confirmed by contrast studies of the accesss.[13,14] An estimation of a greater than 50% diameter reduction in stenosis is a peak systolic velocity (PSV) of greater than 400 cm/s, end-diastolic velocity (EDV) of greater than 250 cm/s, and residual lumen of less than 2 mm diameter.[5] Additionally, almost all protocols also utilize flow rates within the access, which are calculated from acquired measurements of diameter, area, and flow velocity (Figure 30–2). Doppler ultrasound-derived direct vascular access blood flow determination is simple and noninvasive, and may be used within a serial surveillance protocol (see below). In addition, DU can interrogate the entire length of the access including the anastomosis (Figure 30–3).

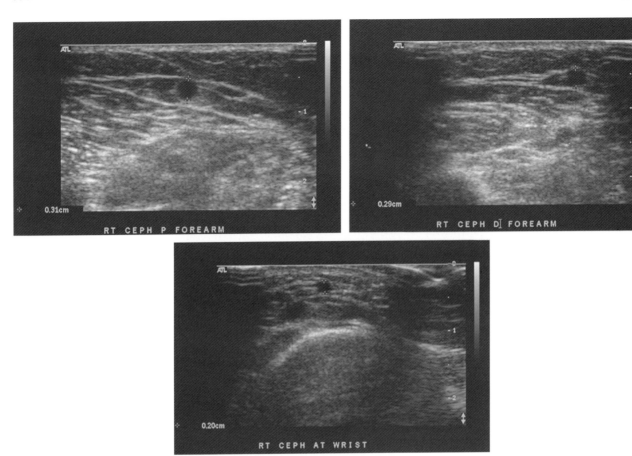

FIGURE 30–1. Preoperative ultrasound images of the cephalic vein at the proximal and distal forearm and at the wrist, obtained prior to planned radiocephalic fistula creation.

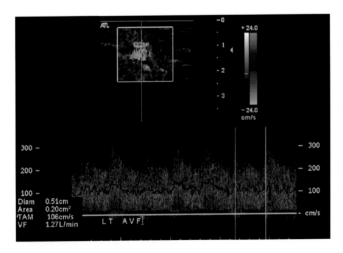

FIGURE 30–2. Duplex images of a well-functioning autogenous brachial-basilic fistula (basilic vein transposition), with Doppler-derived flow rates of 1270 ml/min.

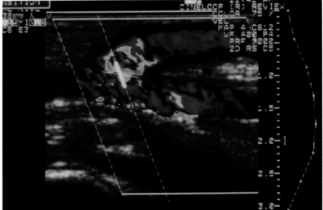

FIGURE 30–3. Duplex ultrasound study clearly showing the arteriovenous anastomosis of an autogenous access.

The results of the impact of DU on patency and secondary interventions vary widely. Sands et al. studied 55 patients with polytetrafluoroethylene (PTFE) grafts and randomized the patients to DU followed by angioplasty if a greater than 50% stenosis was identified and a control group in which no angioplasty was performed. He noted that in the intervention group the thrombosis rate was 19 per 100 patient-years versus 126 per 100 patient-years in the control group. There was a clear advantage of the ultrasound group in regards to complications related to the dialysis access.[15] Detecting stenosis without access malfunction may not be useful, however, as a prospective study by Lumsden et al. found that stenosis detection alone was not predictive of access failure. This group studied patients with PTFE grafts and used color flow duplex to detect patients with a greater than 50% diameter reduction. They then randomized these patients to

observation or balloon angioplasty, and noted no significant difference in 6-month and 12-month patency rates among the two groups. They concluded that a "blanket" approach to angioplasty for all stenoses greater than 50% does not prolong graft patency and cannot be supported.[16]

Advantages of DU include its noninvasiveness, and, as opposed to contrast studies, the fact that it can render more anatomic information regarding extraluminal pathology such as fluid collections, hematomas, and pseudoaneuyrsms while still characterizing luminal stenoses. Indeed, in Europe, DU is the standard of care for evaluation of AV access dysfunction and some believe it should be included in an integrated program of vascular access management.[17] On an individual basis, DU evaluation should be correlated with the clinical examination of the access to plan treatment (Figure 30–4).

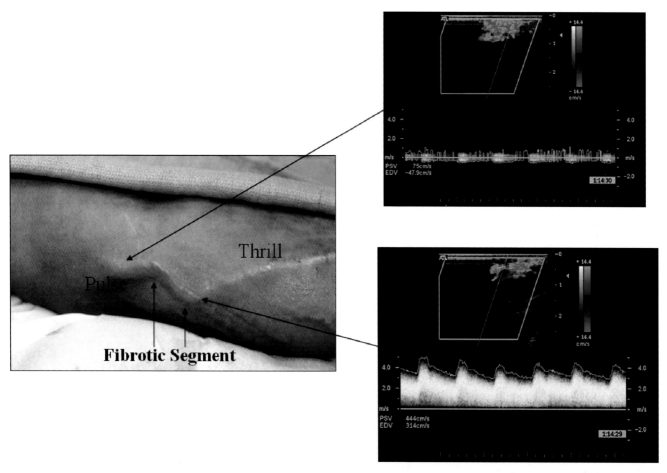

FIGURE 30–4. The correlation that is necessary between the clinical evaluation of the access and the findings on Duplex ultrasound (DU). This recently placed forearm basilic vein transposition to the radial artery was found to have poor flow on hemodialysis. Physical examination of the access revealed a fibrotic segment that was easily palpable; proximal to this segment the access was pulsatile and distal to it a very faint thrill was felt. DU study showed a peak systolic velocity (PSV) of 75 cm/s in the pulsatile area and a PSV of 444 cm/s and an end diastolic velocity of 314 cm/s in the fibrotic area indicating a significant stenosis. No other abnormality was detected along the length of the vein or at the anastomosis. This stenosis was easily repaired with a vein patch angioplasty.

The main disadvantage of DU relates to operator dependency. Standardization must be performed in each laboratory to minimize potential sources of variance such as cross-sectional areas of the vessels and an adequate duplex angle, and the skills of an experienced vascular technologist are integral to its success.[18] Another source of variance is the variability of individual ultrasound machines. Winker et al. compared five different ultrasound machines and noted a wide range of underestimation and overestimation of flow volume, due to different algorithms used to compute the velocity of access blood flow.[19]

Vascular Access Blood Flow

Measurement of access blood flow (Qa) has been shown to identify access stenosis. A low Qa or a decrease in Qa from one study to another is associated with an increased risk of access thrombosis.[20] Monitoring of Qa requires additional technology, expertise, and time. The technique involves indicator dilution technology, whereby the ultrasound velocity through blood is the indicator and dilution is provided by a bolus of normal saline. The Transonic Hemodialysis Monitor (HD01; Transonic Systems Inc.) and dual flow/dilution sensors are used for the process.[21] Ultrasound transducers are placed on the arterial and venous dialysis tubing and the lines are reversed so that the arterial line is downstream of the venous line within the access conduit. The circuit flow is fixed and rapid injection of saline into the venous line dilutes the red cell mass in blood flowing through the access and results in alterations of the Doppler-derived waveform recorded by the arterial line transducer.[5] Table 30–2 outlines the DOQI recommendations for access blood flow measurement.[4]

Several studies have shown that Qa is the surveillance method of choice to detect stenosis before thrombosis. Grafts with a Qa < 600 ml/min have a higher rate of thrombosis than grafts with a Qa > 600 ml/min.[22] Smits

TABLE 30–2. Access flow surveillance from the NKF/DOQI.

Access flow measured by ultrasound dilution, conductance dilution, thermal dilution, Doppler or other technique should be performed monthly

The assessment of flow should be performed during the first 1.5 h of the treatment to eliminate error caused by decreases in cardiac output related to ultrafiltration

The mean value of three separate determinations performed at a single treatment should be considered the access flow

Arteriovenous (AV) graft and AV fistula

Access flow less than 600 ml/min; the patient should be referred for a fistulogram

Access flow less than 1000 ml/min that has decreased by more than 25% over 4 months; the patient should be referred for a fistulogram

et al. compared static and dynamic venous pressure (SVP and DVP, respectively) monitoring to Qa alone, Qa plus DVP, and Qa plus SVP. Venous pressures were performed weekly and Qa every 8 weeks; it was concluded that SVP alone, Qa alone, or a combination of Qa and SVP reduced the thrombosis rate below 0.5 per patient-year.[23] Another study found the addition of Qa to standard surveillance increases the detection of stenosis as indicated by the number of angioplasties in their treatment group. However, there was no difference in time to thrombosis or overall graft survival.[20] Studies have shown that Qa monitoring accurately detects stenosis but interventions with "prophylactic" endovascular angioplasty do not improve graft survival.

The use of access flow rates correlates well with the presence of significant stenosis, with some series reporting greater than 90% positive predictive value. However, prophylactic intervention (i.e., angioplasty) does not necessarily improve graft survival after detection of these stenoses by Qa monitoring.[24] The NKF/DOQI guideline suggests that Qa should return to baseline, but there is no clear recommendation as to when to repeat Qa after an intervention.

Other Uses of Ultrasound in Dialysis Access Surveillance

Other uses of ultrasound in dialysis access monitoring include the potential use of intravascular ultrasound (IVUS). Arbab-Zadeh et al. investigated the assessment of dialysis access with IVUS and compared it to angiography of the access. They noted that IVUS detected more lesions than conventional angiography.[25] Further studies will be needed to prove whether these results are reproducible.

More recently, a new ultrasound instrument using vector Doppler and embedded machine intelligence has been developed to measure access flow rates by nonvascular specialists. The advantage of this technique is that it can be performed with the patient off the dialysis machine. This new technology has yet to be studied on a large population but is promising in that it can eliminate the need for a vascular technologist to perform the study.[26]

Ultrasound Surveillance Protocol

To date, no randomized prospective studies have established the optimal surveillance protocol. Bowser and Bandyk have instituted a surveillance program that involves preoperative DU to maximize autogenous access creation. Postoperatively, B-mode ultrasound with calculation of volume flow rates is performed. Any abnormality noted is corrected. Routine duplex surveillance of the access is subsequently performed every 3 months.[5]

Based on extensive experience with infrainguinal bypass graft surveillance, DU surveillance of access grafts appears intuitively attractive and would appear to offer similar advantages of extending patency. However, in contradistinction to extremity bypass grafts, routine surveillance of dialysis access has not been accepted by the Center for Medicare and Medicaid services (CMS) as a reimbursable procedure except in specific circumstances. Reimbursement is allowed for DU surveillance of the access when certain abnormalities are noted, carefully documented in the records, and furnished for reimbursement. Examples of these clinical indications include (1) elevated DVP over 200 mm Hg, (2) access recirculation of 12% or higher, (3) an otherwise unexplained urea reduction ratio of less than 60%, and (4) the presence of an access water hammer pulse. Even with these indications CMS would allow reimbursement for either DU or contrast study of the access. In rare occasions, when adequate justification is provided, CMS may allow payment for both (CMS Program Memo #AB-01–129, September 15, 2001).

In summary, several recent studies have indicated that Duplex ultrasonography has made the most impact in the preoperative planning process with consequent increased numbers of autogenous access creation. These changing practice patterns, from prosthetic grafts to autogenous fistulas, are consistent with current DOQI guidelines aimed at prolonging access patency and minimizing short- and long-term complications of hemodialysis access.[27,28] With further studies, refinements in technology, and changes in reimbursement, ultrasonography may play an even greater role, either primarily or as an adjunct, in prolonging the lifespan of dialysis access.

References

1. United States Renal Data System. The economic cost of ESRD, vascular access procedures, and Medicare spending for alternative modalities of treatment. Am J Kidney Dis 1997;30:S160–S177.
2. Schwab S, Harrington J, Singh A, Rohrer R, Shohaib S, Perrone R, Meyer K, Beasley D. Vascular access for hemodialysis. Kidney Int 1999;55:2078–2090.
3. Dixon BS, Novak L, Fangman J. Hemodialysis vascular access survival: Upper-arm native arteriovenous fistula. Am J Kidney Dis 2002;39:92–101.
4. NKF-K/DOQI clinical practical guidelines for vascular access: Update 2000. Am J Kidney Dis 2001;29:223–229.
5. Bowser AN, Bandyk DF. Surveillance program for hemodialysis access. In: Pearce WH, Matsumura J, Yao JST (eds). Trends in Vascular Surgery, pp. 371–383. Chicago: Precept, 2002.
6. Koskoy C, Kuzu A, Erden I. Predictive value of color Doppler ultrasonography in detecting failure of vascular access grafts. Br J Surg 1995;82:50–52.
7. Robbin ML, Gallichio MH, Deierhoi MH, Young CJ, Weber TM, Allon M, et al. US vascular mapping before hemodialysis placement. Radiology 2000;217:83–88.
8. Silva MB Jr, Hobson RW 2nd, Pappas PJ, Jamil Z, Araki CT, Goldberg MC, Gwertzman G, Padberg FT Jr. A strategy for increasing the use of autogenous hemodialysis access procedures: impact of preoperative noninvasive evaluation. J Vasc Surg 1998;27:302–308.
9. Ascher E, Gade P, Hingorani A, Mazzariol F, Gunduz Y, Fodera M, Yorkovich W. Changes in the practice of angioaccess surgery: Impact of the dialysis outcome and quality initiative recommendations. J Vasc Surg 2000;31:84–92.
10. Mendes RR, Farber MA, Marston WA, Dinwiddie LC, Keagy BA, Burnham SJ. Prediction of wrist arteriovenous fistula maturation with preoperative vein mapping with ultrasonography. J Vasc Surg 2002;36:460–463.
11. Parmley MC, Broughan TA, Jennings WC. Vascular ultrasonography prior to dialysis access surgery. Am J Surg 2002;184:568–572.
12. Malovrh M. The role of sonography in the planning of arteriovenous fistulas for hemodialysis. Semin Dialysis 2003;16:299–303.
13. Tordoir JH, de Bruin HG, Hoeneveld H, Eikelboom BC, Kitslaar PJ. Duplex ultrasound scanning in the assessment of arteriovenous fistulas created for hemodialysis access: comparison with digital subtraction angiography. J Vasc Surg 1989;10:122–128.
14. Dousset V, Grenier N, Douws C, Senuita P, Sassouste G, Ada L, Potaux L. Hemodialysis grafts: Color Doppler flow imaging correlated with digital subtraction angiography and functional status. Radiology 1991;181:89–94.
15. Sands J, Gandy D, Finn M, et al. Ultrasound—angioplasty program decreases thrombosis rate and cost of PTFE graft maintenance. J Am Soc Nephrol 1997;8:171.
16. Lumsden AB, MacDonald MJ, Kikeri D, Cotsonis GA, Harker LA, Martin LG. Prophylactic balloon angioplasty fails to prolong the patency of expanded polytetrafluoroethylene arteriovenous grafts: Results of a prospective randomized study. J Vasc Surg 1997;26:382–392.
17. Sands J. The role of color flow Doppler ultrasound in dialysis access. Semin Nephrol 2002;22:195–201.
18. Sands JJ. Doppler ultrasound and hemodialysis access management. In: Gray R, Sands JJ (eds). Dialysis Access: A Multidiscipline Approach, pp. 133–136. Philadelphia: Lippincott, Williams & Wilkins, 2002.
19. Winkler AJ, Wu J, Case T, Ricci MA. An experimental study of the accuracy of volume flow measurements using commercial ultrasound systems. J Vasc Technol 1995;19:175–180.
20. Moist LM, Churchill DN, House AA, Millward SF, Elliot JE, Kribs SW, et al. Regular monitoring of access flow compared with monitoring of venous pressure fails to improve graft survival. J Am Soc Nephrol 2003;14:2645–2653.
21. Tonelli M, Jhangri GS, Hirsch DJ, Marryatt J, Mossop P, Wile C, Jindal KK. Best threshold for diagnosis of stenosis or thrombosis within six months of access flow measurement in arteriovenous fistulae. J Am Soc Nephrol 2003;14:3264–3269.

22. Rehman SU, Pupim LB, Shyr Y, Hakim R, Ikzler TA. Intra-dialytic serial vascular access flow measurements. Am J Kidney Dis 1999;34:471–477.

23. Smits JH, van der Linden J, Hagen EC, Modderkolk-Cammeraat EC, Feith GW, Koomans HA, Blankestijn PJ. Graft flow as a predictor of thrombosis in hemodialysis grafts. Kidney Int 2001;59:1551–1558.

24. McCarley P, Wingard RL, Shyr Y, Pettus W, Hakim RM, Ikizler TA. Vascular access blood flow monitoring reduces access morbidity and costs. Kidney Int 2001;60:1164–1172.

25. Arbab-Zadeh A, Mehta RL, Ziegler TW, Oglevie SB, Mullaney S, Mahmud E, et al. Hemodialysis access assessment with intravascular ultrasound. Am J Kidney Dis 2002;39: 813–823.

26. Vilkomerson D, Chilipka T, Nazarov A. Kuhlman M, Levin NW. Non-specialist ultrasound measuring of access flow: New technology. Blood Purif 2004;22:78–83.

27. Schuman E, Standage BA, Ragsdale JW, Heinl P. Achieving vascular access success in the quality outcome era. Am J Surg 2004;187:585–589.

28. Huber TS, Ozaki CK, Flynn TC, Lee WA, Berceli SA, Hirniese CM, et al. Prospective validation of an algorithm to maximize native arteriovenous fistulae for chronic hemodialysis access. J Vasc Surg 2002;36:452–459.

31
Noninvasive Evaluation for Congenital Arteriovenous Fistulas and Malformation

Robert B. Rutherford

Introduction

This chapter addresses the application of noninvasive vascular diagnostic laboratory (VDL) tests in diagnosing vascular anomalies containing arteriovenous fistulas (AVFs). These developmental defects can take several forms, diffuse microfistulas, groups of macrofistulas that involve major artery distributions, and more mature maturational defects, which tend to involve a single artery. Together these lesions are categorized by the Hamburg classification[1] as predominantly AVFs, and constitute just over one-third of all vascular anomalies.[2] AVFs can also be present in more complex mixed anomalies, e.g., in those that are predominantly venous. The VDL can provide much useful clinical decision-making information regarding peripheral AVFs. The diagnostic methods described here are all aimed at detecting AVFs and can even be used, albeit with some differences, in diagnosing acquired AVFs, those due to iatrogenic and other penetrating trauma.

The instrumentation employed is basically the same used in diagnosing peripheral arterial occlusive disease: segmental limb pressures and plethysmography, velocity waveform analysis, and duplex scanning.[3] A number of considerations govern how these diagnostic methods can be applied in diagnosing AVFs. First, a basic understanding of the hemodynamic characteristics of arteriovenous fistulas is needed to perform and properly interpret these tests. Second, the diagnostic capabilities and limitations of the different tests described must be understood in applying them. "Physiologic" VDL tests simply gauge the pressure, volume, or velocity changes associated with peripheral AVFs but do not visualize the AVFs, as duplex ultrasound imaging can do. Most of these tests are qualitative and not quantitative, and most can be applied only to peripheral or extremity AVFs and arteriovenous malformations (AVMs). Third, congenital and acquired AVFs differ from each other significantly in terms of their anatomic localization. Congenital AVFs are rarely iso-lated lesions; they more commonly are in clusters within major arterial distributions, but may be even more diffuse in location. As a result they can be localized to a particular limb segment only by so-called physiologic tests and even visualization by Doppler ultrasonography may not completely encompass them. Fourth, the diagnostic goals may vary considerably in different clinical settings and this significantly affects the application of the tests. The simplest diagnostic goal may be to determine the presence or absence of an AVF, but beyond the presence of an AVF, which may be clinically obvious, it is the relative magnitude of its peripheral hemodynamic effects that needs to be gauged, or the overall effect on the peripheral circulation, for example, the presence of a distal steal and the severity of the associated ischemia.

The main focus of this chapter will be on diagnostic approaches that are available in most VDLs. The basic diagnostic methods and the instrumentation behind each of these diagnostic methods will be covered elsewhere in this book, and will not be described at length. Rather their utility in this setting will be discussed, in terms of the instrumentation used, the interpretation or analysis of the test results, and appropriate clinical applications as well as diagnostic limitations.

Clinical Evaluation

Those utilizing the VDL tests to be described should have some basic knowledge about clinical diagnosis, by history and physical examination, for diagnostic testing is an adjunct superimposed on these. Most clinically significant AVMs will present well before adult life because a vascular "birthmark," localized skin color change, overlying varicose veins or other prominent blood vessels, or occasionally a distinct vascular mass or tumor or enlargement of the limb (swelling, increase in the length or girth) has gained the attention of a parent or child. Changes in limb dimension are unusual in the absence of significant AVFs, and minor differences may be overlooked. Characteristically, these occur as the result of long-standing AVFs present during the growth period, but they are also reported to occur with pure venous anomalies, in the absence of AVFs. Whether or not this relates to failure to detect occult microfistulous AVFs in venous anomalies described earlier before noninvasive tests (NITs) were employed is debatable, but it is true that such fistulas are often missed by angiography.[4]

Most "birthmarks" represent either true hemangiomatous lesions or cutaneous capillary or superficial venous malformations, the latter also still being referred to as "cavernous malformations." Differentiating between these is extremely important in early childhood and usually can be done on clinical grounds given their time of appearance and their growth or lack of growth with time. Juvenile hemangiomas are true tumors with a rapid endothelial turnover, which undergo rapid early growth then involute, usually between 2 and 8 years of age, whereas true malformations are present at birth and maintain the same size relative to the growing child.

Localized warmth and vascular-based color changes, compressibility of vascular masses, the presence of a thrill or bruit, and inequalities in the dimensions of the limb should all be noted, but it must be remembered that true hemangiomas, during their rapid growth phase, are hypervascular or high flow lesions and this will be reflected by their appearance and associated physical signs. Finally, the triad of birthmark, varicose veins, and limb enlargement is well known, and usually sought, but a limb presenting with these may or not may not harbor major AVFs. The presence of AVFs has been the basis for the traditional distinction between the Parkes Weber and Klippel-Trenaunay syndromes, the former being associated with AVFs and the latter not. Furthermore, these physical findings are inconsistent even in the presence of AVFs. In Sziylagyi's classic study of 82 cases of congenital AVMs, the classic triad was present in only 57%.[4]

Diagnostic Studies for Congenital Arteriovenous Fistulas or Arteriovenous Malformations

The vascular diagnostic techniques described below can be valuable in determining the presence or absence of AVFs in this setting, in patients presenting with atypical (location, age of onset) varicose veins and/or a birthmark, with or without limb enlargement.[5] Depending on their location and localization, the same simple physiologic tests used in diagnosing peripheral arterial occlusive disease can be employed in diagnosing AVFs or AVMs, and can do it quickly and inexpensively, avoiding the need for angiography, which is particularly important since many of the presenting patients are young children. Although

qualitative in nature, the degree of abnormality observed in these tests in association with congenital AVFs gives the clinician a rough impression of their relative magnitude. Increasingly, the current workhorse of the VDL, the duplex scan, has found useful application in evaluating AVFs.

Characteristic Hemodynamic Changes Associated with Arteriovenous Fistulas: Diagnostic Implications

AVFs can be considered a "short-circuit" between the high-pressure arterial and the low-pressure venous systems. If the AVFs present in vascular anomalies are hemodynamically significant enough, they will result in an arterial pressure drop, a significant diversion of flow into the venous system rather than through the microcirculation, increased pulsatility (a volume change), and an increase in velocity, often with turbulence. The *mean* arterial blood pressure distal to an AVF is always reduced to some degree. This is the result of blood being shunted away from the distal arterial tree into the low-resistance pathway offered by the arteriovenous communication. The reduction in mean pressure is greatest when the fistula is large and the arterial collaterals are small. On the other hand, when the fistula is small and the collaterals are large, there may be little or no perceptible pressure effects away from the fistula itself. AVMs, being made up of a number of relatively smaller AVFs, may, in combination, have the same hemodynamic effects as a single large AVF. Thus, the magnitude of the pressure drop across an AVM, or the limb segment containing them, can provide a fair assessment of its hemodynamic significance. If the pressure drop and flow diversion are severe enough, there may be distal ischemia, which can be measured by standard VDL tests. If overall fistula flow is great enough, there will be associated venous hypertension. This is not readily measured noninvasively but increased flow velocity in the major draining vein, compared to its normal contralateral counterpart, can be assessed. An AVF or AVM can produce significant pressure swings, locally perceived as increased pulsatility, which are reflected in associated volume changes in the involved limb segment, and these can be detected plethysmographically. Finally AVFs are associated with significant velocity changes that are greatest closest to the AVF. To appreciate the basic nature of these velocity changes, and how best to detect them, it is first necessary to understand that a pattern of low flow and high resistance characterizes the *normal resting* extremity circulation. This is in contrast to the high flow and low resistance pattern associated with exercise. The velocity patterns associated with peripheral AVFs are similar to those associated with exercise, and readily distinguished from those observed in the normal resting limb by studying arterial velocity in the VDL. Thus, by understanding the characteristic underlying hemodynamic changes associated with AVFs, congenital lesions containing them can be detected and their severity assessed by studying the arterial pressure, volume, and velocity changes they produce, using VDL tests designed to gauge these same hemodynamic parameters.

Diagnostic Tests: Descriptions and Applications

The focus of this section will be on diagnostic approaches available in most VDLs that can be applied to the diagnosis of peripheral AVFs, whether they be single, or multiple, as characteristic of AVMs. The noninvasive "physiologic" tests that are employed are the same as those used for many decades in the diagnosis of peripheral arterial occlusive disease. More recently duplex scanning has greatly supplemented these. The basic diagnostic methods and the instrumentation behind these tests have been covered earlier in this book (Chapters 17–19) and will not be described at length here, but their utility in this setting will be discussed, as will their interpretation, appropriate clinical applications, and limitations. It should be emphasized that while the pressure, flow volume, and velocity changes associated with AVFs located in an extremity can be readily assessed in the VDL, particularly with noninvasive physiologic tests, this *requires that the findings be compared to those of the normal contralateral extremity.*

Segmental Limb Pressures

Segmental limb pressure measurements are a standard technique described in greater detail earlier in this book (Chapter 19). Noninvasive methods of measuring systolic blood pressure are reasonably accurate and reproducible and are painless, rapid, and simple in application. Briefly, a pneumatic cuff is placed around the limb segment at the required site and inflated to above systolic pressure. As the cuff is deflated, the *systolic* pressure at which blood flow returns distal to the cuff is noted on an aneroid or mercury manometer. Return of flow can be detected with a Doppler flowmeter placed over a distal artery (or a mercury-in-Silastic strain gauge, or a photoplethysmograph or pulse volume recorder cuff placed distally). In the upper extremity, pressure measurements can be made at the upper arm, forearm, wrist, or finger levels; in the lower extremity, pressure measurements can be made at the high or low thigh, and the calf, ankle, foot, or toe. Although ankle pressures are primarily used in studying occlusive disease, multiple segmental cuffs are used to detect and localize AVFs, particularly AVMs. Impor-

tantly, cuffs should be applied bilaterally to allow comparison with the normal contralateral limb.

A hemodynamically significant AVF will reduce *mean* pressure in the limb or at least in the arterial tree close to the fistula. But it must be remembered that these cuffs measure *systolic* pressure, and even though mean pressure is reduced in the arterial tree when approaching an AVM, the pressure swings between systolic and diastolic pressure (i.e., the pulse pressure) are *increased*, so that systolic pressure is likely to be elevated *proximal to a fistula*. The *systolic* pressure can be detected as being elevated only by comparison with that of the opposite limb at the same level.[5] It will also be elevated if the pressure cuff has been placed directly over the site of the AVM or its afferent branches. Compared to the contralateral extremity, cuffs at or above a hemodynamically significant fistula or group of fistulas (AVM) will usually record a higher systolic pressure, but those below the fistula will record a normal or lower systolic pressure, depending on the magnitude of the fistula, with major fistulas being associated with a detectable degree of distal steal. Such pressure differences between equivalent limb segments or levels, greater than measurement variability, indicate a significant AVM.

Segmental Plethysmography

Segmental plethysmography is also a standard technology described earlier in this text (Chapter 20), in which cuffs of precise dimensions are applied at various levels/locations along an extremity, much as for measuring segmental limb pressures. Air-filled cuffs are normally used. The contour of the resulting tracing is generally assessed in terms of magnitude and shape. When the pulse-sensing device is placed over the fistula or just proximal to it, the pulse volume may actually be increased.[5,6] This is commonly seen in a limb with significant congenital AVFs, the increased pulsations being quite diagnostic (Figure 31–1). Although the pulse contour may be normal (or nearly so) in a limb *distal* to an AVF or AVM, it is frequently reduced, particularly in the presence of a steal (Figure 31–2).[7] As in the case of segmental limb pressure measurements, the reduction in pulse volume distally depends on the size of the fistula and the adequacy of the collateral vessels. Therefore, very much as described for segmental limb pressures above, plethysmography tracings are increased in magnitude above or at the level of an AVF, or group of AVFs, and, depending on the degree of distal steal, the tracings below the fistula will be reduced, or, at best, normal in magnitude. A study of the tracings compared with the contralateral extremity will not only detect an AVF but allow its segmental location or level to the identified.

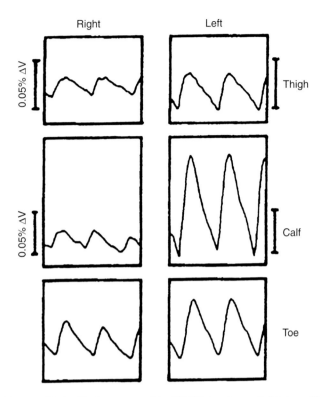

FIGURE 31–1. Plethysmographic (PVR) tracings at thigh, calf, and toe levels in a 4-year-old girl with multiple congenital AV fistulas involving the entire left leg. [From Rutherford RB (ed). *Vascular Surgery*, 5th ed. W.B. Saunders, 2000.]

Velocity Waveform Analysis

Velocity tracings can be recorded over any extremity artery by a Doppler probe connected to the DC recorder and strip chart, or by the velocity readout of a Duplex scan. However, this is increasingly being done by the latter technique because it offers other valuable information in this setting (see below) and the strip chart recording of velocity waveforms generated by a Doppler probe is uncommonly done today as a separate test. Nevertheless, the characteristic findings will be described here. In evaluating for AVFs, the velocity is recorded over the major proximal inflow artery, e.g., femoral or axillary. The reason for selecting this location, rather than directly over the suspected fistula(s), will become apparent later, in describing Duplex scan findings. A high-velocity flow pattern in an artery leading to the area of suspicion is good evidence that the artery is serving as the inflow for AVFs.[7,8] For many if not most clinical purposes, a qualitative estimate of flow velocity and the contour of the analog velocity tracings or "waveforms" obtained in this manner with a directional Doppler velocity detector provides sufficient information for clinical diagnosis, and the magnitude of the changes provides some indication of the size of the fistula(s).

To recognize a tracing diagnostic of AVFs, it is necessary to realize that the velocity tracings of a *resting* normal extremity is characterized by end-systolic reversal following peak systolic flow, followed by low flow in early diastole and negligible flow in late diastole. Such a low-flow, high-resistance pattern is most pronounced in the lower extremity. In the upper extremity there may be little end-systolic reversal. In contrast, a high-flow low-resistance arterial velocity pattern is seen in a number of high-flow visceral arteries (e.g., the renal, carotid, celiac arteries), but in the extremities, such high-flow patterns are seen after exercise and, importantly, in association with AVFs. In these settings peak systolic velocity may be quite high but more diagnostic is the *continuous flow throughout diastole and that the dip in the tracing between systole and diastole does not approach the zero velocity baseline*, let alone show an end-systolic reversal, as it does in the normal resting extremity. The characteristic arterial pattern associated with AVFs, shown in Figure 31–3, thus consists of an *elimination of end-systolic reversal and a marked increase in diastolic velocity, which "elevates" the entire tracing above the zero-velocity baseline*. The degree of elevation in end-diastolic velocity correlates directly with the flow increase caused by the AVF.[5,6] By using these characteristic Doppler velocity signals as a guide, it is possible to detect and localize congenital arteriovenous communications that otherwise might escape detection.[9,10] Peripheral AVFs constituting 5% of extremity flow or more can be readily detected by these means. This test is more sensitive than segmental pressures and plethysmography.

Although these changes are diagnostic enough that comparison with the other extremity would not seem necessary, this comparison still holds value, to rule out hyperemia and similar velocity signals there. Hyperdynamic flow is associated with conditions such as beriberi or

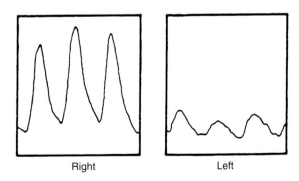

FIGURE 31–2. Toe plethysmographic tracings from a patient with a congenital AVM involving the left calf. The reduced PVRs reflect a distal steal from this, but not to critical ischemic levels for some pulsatility remains. The left ankle pressure was 55 mm Hg. [From Rutherford RB (ed). *Vascular Surgery*, 5th ed. W.B. Saunders, 2000.]

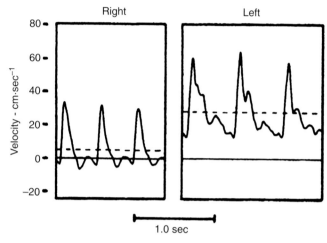

FIGURE 31–3. Velocity tracing from the femoral arteries in a 4-year-old girl with a large AVM involving the left thigh. Note that the tracing on the left, compared to the normal right tracing, has a higher peak and mean (dashed line) systolic velocity, and there is no end systolic reversal. Rather, there is high flow continuing throughout diastole, as a result of which the tracing does not drop back to the zero baseline at the end of diastole, but is elevated well above the zero baseline. [From Rutherford RB (ed). *Vascular Surgery*, 5th ed. W.B. Saunders, 2000.]

thyrotoxicosis, but since it is generalized it would affect all extremities. False positives can occur unilaterally in other hyperemic settings, e.g., inflammation associated with superficial thrombophlebitis, lymphangitis, bacterial infection, and thermal or mechanical trauma. Other causes of hyperemia isolated to an individual vessel or limb (e.g., exercise or reactive hyperemia following a period of ischemia) are transient. Externally applied heat, local infection (e.g., cellulitis or abscess), or sympathetic blockade can also increase flow velocity and give this pattern, but none of these should create any significant confusion in the usual patient referred to the VDL for evaluation of congenital AVFs.

Evaluation for Congenital Arteriovenous Fistulas Using These Three Physiologic Tests in Combination

These three tests are usually done in combination for they reinforce each other, and they share the advantages that they are inexpensive, quickly applied, and require only basic operator or interpretive skill. The instrumentation is simple and used on an everyday basis in most VDLs. On the other hand, these tests give qualitative rather than quantitative information and can be applied only to AVFs located in the extremity proper (i.e., at or below the highest cuff or point of Doppler probe interrogation). It should be noted that in children appropriately smaller cuffs are required. These tests may not detect diffuse congenital microfistulas or overall fistula

flow constituting less than 5% of total extremity flow. Single limb studies may not be diagnostic unless compared with a normal contralateral extremity. Nevertheless, in combination, these tests can be very useful in screening for congenital AVFs in the extremities of patients presenting with suggestive signs (e.g., a vascular "birthmark," atypical varicose veins, limb enlargement), and for detecting, roughly localizing, and assessing the relative magnitude of such congenital lesions.. With anatomically localized lesions, these tests, with or without duplex scanning (see below), suffice for most clinical decision making.

Duplex Scanning

The basic Duplex scanner combines an ultrasound image with a focused directional Doppler probe. In modern instruments the velocity signal is color coded so that red represents arterial flow and blue represents venous flow (going in opposite directions). The velocity signal is also displayed on the screen as needed for specific applications.

Because the duplex scanner provides velocity information, it can serve as a means of performing velocity waveform analysis, as described above, the pattern serving as a simple yet sensitive means of diagnosing an AVF. Because of the other additional information obtainable from duplex scanning, it has mostly replaced using a simple Doppler probe connected to a DC recorder and strip chart for this purpose. High peak mean velocity readings recorded over the main inflow artery of the involved extremity, compared with those at the same location of the contralateral normal extremity, will confirm the presence of an AVF in that limb. The characteristic pattern of the velocity tracing, already described in detail above, will distinguish this high-velocity reading from the more focused high-velocity reading observed in association with an arterial stenosis.

The software of some of today's duplex scanners also allows a rough estimation of volume flow, with diameter measurements being used to estimate cross-sectional area and the velocity signals and the angle of incidence of the probe allowing the Doppler equation to be applied [Flow = velocity (frequency shift) × cosine theta (angle of incidence of the ultrasound beam) × cross-sectional area, divided by C (velocity of sound in tissue, a constant]. However, a significant problem in using the Duplex scan to obtain accurate velocity or flow measurements *directly over* an AVF is the presence of turbulence, multidirectional flows, and aliasing. On the other hand, flashes of yellow representing turbulent fistula flow will be seen, and along with higher than normal velocities these are diagnostic of an AVF. So the diagnosis is readily made, but quantification is not possible at the fistula site.

Congenital AVFs are more complex, but their high-flow patterns are readily recognized and the nature and extent of the more localized superficial lesions can be well delineated. This in itself can be diagnostic, and is particularly useful when applied to mass lesions, which often present with a network of varicosities near the surface of the skin. Higher than normal flows in these veins will betray an underlying AVM. The diagnostic dilemma, that these varicosities may either be part of a venous malformation or be associated with an underlying arteriovenous malformation, can thus be resolved by this approach. The problem of not being able to *directly* measure fistula flow can be addressed by comparing velocity readings obtained proximally over the major inflow artery of the involved limb with those from the contralateral normal extremity recorded at the same level. The latter approach is recommended when quantitative measurements of fistula flow are desired. Subtracting the contralateral normal limb flow from that of the involved limb will provide a fairly reliable estimate of AV shunt flow as long as the interrogation sites and monitoring techniques are the same for both limbs.

Duplex scanners offer the advantage that they are in everyday use in today's VDLs for many other applications, so the necessary instrumentation and the operator skills are there. The duplex scan is rather versatile in evaluating AVFs, used to interrogate either a penetrating wound or groin hematoma following a catheterization procedure or the limb of a young patient suspected of harboring congenital AVFs. It may directly visualize and interrogate AVFs as well as provide velocity evidence of their existence, e.g., high flow in the artery leading to suspected AVFs. On the other hand, in some congenital anomalies, where multiple AVFs may not be spread out over a larger area, the duplex scanner may be as useful, not being able to directly visualize all the fistulas, and in larger mass lesions it may not be able to assess the full anatomic extent of an AVM. Like the previously described "physiologic" tests it can be applied to extremity lesions but not to central lesions, e.g., in the trunk or pelvis. Much of its application is qualitative not quantitative, although flow estimates are possible using the technique described. So, it can detect and generally localize AVMs and guide or monitor thrombotic or embolic therapy in those congenital lesions that are relatively superficially located and reasonably well localized.

Competing and Complementary Diagnostic Studies

Arteriography

Arteriography was the gold standard in the past, before noninvasive tests and imaging became available. Unfortunately, many if not most primary care physicians presented with such patients today perpetuate this primary reliance on angiography due to lack of awareness of the value of noninvasive tests and imaging. This misguided "AGA" (always get an angiogram) approach is particularly unfortunate because angiography is required only *if* the need for therapeutic intervention for congenital AVFs has been determined *and* will be undertaken soon, in which case it can be obtained at the same time as embolotherapy. The presence or absence of congenital AVFs, and their relative severity, can be determined by noninvasive methods in most cases, allowing management decisions to be made on the basis of these tests alone, without angiography. Furthermore, arteriography may fail to demonstrate the fistula or fistulas either because they are too small or because the flow is too rapid. In addition, arteriography is invasive, associated with certain risks (contrast allergy, idiosyncratic reaction, renal toxicity), expensive, uncomfortable, and a major consideration in infants and young children is that it risks injury to their smaller arteries and requires either general anesthesia or heavy sedation and analgesia, usually requiring admission.

However, while this addiction to contrast angiography deserves opposition, there are a number of noninvasive or miniinvasive imaging approaches that have emerged in recent years that deserve mention here in that they offer significant additional perspectives over what can be achieved by the VDL diagnostic methods described, particularly in the evaluation of congenital AVFs. These diagnostic modalities include radionuclide quantification of AV shunting, computed tomography (CT) and magnetic resonance imaging (MRI). Additional discussion of these is included here to provide the reader with sufficient knowledge of their capabilities and clinical applications, as additional diagnostic options that must be considered in this setting. On the other hand, these new imaging methods are considerably more expensive and time consuming than VDL testing, so that if the additional perspective they offer is not required for decision making, their use may be inappropriate or at least delayed until later, an advantage in dealing with children.

Radionuclide Arteriovenous Shunt Quantification

Radionuclide-labeled albumen microspheres can be used to diagnose and *quantitate* arteriovenous shunting. The basic principle behind the study is simple: radionuclide-labeled albumen microspheres too large to pass through capillaries are injected into the inflow artery proximal to the suspected AVM. Those passing through arteriovenous communications are trapped in the next vascular bed, in the lung, and may be quantified by counting the increased radioactivity of the lungs with a gamma camera, or a discrete sample of it, by maintaining a rectilinear scintillation scanner in a fixed position over a limited pulmonary field.[6,11] The fraction of microspheres reaching the lungs is determined by comparing these counts with the lung counts following another injection of microspheres introduced into *any* peripheral vein, 100% of which should lodge in the lungs. The agent commonly used consists of a suspension of 35-μm human albumin microspheres labeled with technetium-99m (similar to that commonly used in lung scans), but other radionuclide labels have been used.

The study is minimally invasive, relatively simple to perform, causes little discomfort, and carries a negligible risk. It quantifies the degree of AV shunting, something none of the other tests can do. Because shunt flow can be quantified, the results have prognostic value.[5,6] It is possible to better estimate the hemodynamic significance of an AVM and thus be better able to predict the need for intervention. Serial measurements can also be used to gauge the success of interventions designed to eliminate or control AVMs. Radionuclide-labeled microspheres are most useful for studying patients with suspected congenital AVFs.[2,6] In patients with diffuse or extensive congenital vascular malformations presenting with a vascular "birthmark," varicose veins, and/or limb overgrowth, it may be difficult to distinguish clinically between patients with multiple AVFs (so called Parkes Weber syndrome), some so small they cannot be visualized arteriographically, and those with the same triad but with predominantly venous malformations (e.g., Klippel-Trenaunay syndrome). The labeled microsphere study solves this dilemma. Importantly, the success of surgical or endovascular interventions in eliminating or controlling AVMs can be adequately gauged by pre- and postintervention studies. Finally, serial measurements will indicate whether the fistula is following a stable or a progressive course and whether previously dormant arteriovenous communications have begun to open up or "grow."

Although naturally occurring "physiologic" arteriovenous shunts are present in normal human extremities, less than 3% of the total blood flow (and usually much less) is diverted through these communications, so they normally do not produce an interpretive error.[11] However, measurements made during anesthesia are not accurate because anesthesia, both general and regional, significantly increases shunting through these naturally occurring arteriovenous communications. The examiner must also be aware that the percentage of blood shunted through arteriovenous communications can be quite significant, in the range of 20–40%, in the limbs of patients soon after sympathetic denervation, and in patients with cirrhosis, or hypertrophic pulmonary osteopathy.[12] Finally, this study shares the limitation of the physiologic studies previously described in that it does not ordinarily localize the lesion. However, several injections can be made at key locations in the arterial tree at the time of arteriography, if a gamma camera is present, and these can be quantified against a later venous injection, to give localizing information.

Magnetic Resonance Imaging and Computed Tomgraphy Scanning

The previously described VDL studies cannot properly assess the anatomic extent of large or deep vascular malformations, and even angiographic studies tend to underestimate their full anatomic extent. CT will usually demonstrate the location and extent of the lesion and even the involvement of specific muscle groups and bone.[13,14] Offsetting these desirable features of CT are the need for contrast, the lack of an optimum protocol for its administration, and the practical limitation of having to use multiple transverse images to reconstruct the anatomy of the lesion. Three-dimensional reconstruction of CTA data overcomes some of these limitations, but subtracting away muscle, skin, and bone, as performed in most vascular applications, prevents the true anatomic extent of AVMs from being accurately determined.

MRI possesses a number of distinct advantages over CT in evaluating vascular malformations. There is no need for contrast, the anatomic extent is more clearly demonstrated, longitudinal as well as transverse sections may be obtained, and the flow patterns in the congenital malformation can be characterized. As a result, MRI has become the pivotal diagnostic study in the evaluation of most vascular malformations presenting with mass lesions.

Overall Diagnostic Strategy and Clinical Correlation

Although venous malformations are more common than arteriovenous malformations (roughly one-half vs. one-third of all vascular anomalies), determining whether or not a vascular anomaly or malformation contains AVFs is the usual starting point, even in presumed venous lesions, and particularly in presumed Klippel-Trenaunay syndrome. The VDL can provide much useful information in this regard, using segmental limb pressures and plethysmography, velocity wave form analysis, and duplex scanning, and most vascular malformations containing AVFs can be evaluated adequately enough with these basic VDL tests for clinical decision making. A radionuclide-labeled microsphere shunt study can be added if it is important to quantify the AV shunting, and MRI is used in mass lesions to determine their anatomic extent, particularly the involvement of adjacent muscle, bone, and nerves, which in turn determines resectability of mass lesions. It also demonstrates the lesion's flow characteristics (e.g., distinguishing venous from arteriovenous malformations).

After utilizing the above diagnostic tests, *without the use of angiography*, it should be possible to categorize the lesion as one of the following: a localized AVF, an extensive malformation with macrofistulous AVFs (an AVM) fed by specific named vessels, diffusely scattered microfistulous AVFs (which may or may not be associated with venous malformations), venous angiomas (an extratruncular venous malformation consisting of multiple venous lakes), a congenital defect of the deep veins, or an arterial anomaly. In most cases duplex scanning will aid in sorting these out if the noninvasive "physiologic" tests are not definitive. Angiography is rarely used initially, being saved to guide interventions once they have been deemed necessary. The need for intervention is limited to the more localized AV malformations, which may be resectable (less than 10%), to larger AVMs composed of macro-AVFs, which can be controlled best by modern embolotherapy and some venous or lymphatic mass lesions. Diffuse micro-AVFs and extensive or diffuse venous malformations usually require no treatment other than conservative management of the associated venous hypertension (e.g., by elastic stockings and intermittent elevation). Thus the noninvasive studies featured in today's VDL, and described above, can and should play a pivotal role in the diagnosis of AVMs, and in determining whether AVFs are significant components of other congenital vascular anomalies.

References

1. Belov S. Anatomopathological classification of congenital vascular defects. Semin Vasc Surg 1993;6:219–224.
2. Tasnadi G. Epidemiology and etiology of congenital vascular malformations. Semin Vasc Surg 1993;6:200–203.
3. Rutherford RB, Fleming PW, Mcleod FD. Vascular diagnostic methods for evaluating patients with arteriovenous fistulas. In: Diethrich EB (ed). *Noninvasive Cardiovascular Diagnosis: Current Concepts*, pp. 189–203. Baltimore: University Park Press, 1978.
4. Szilagyi DE, Smith RF, Elliott JP, et al. Congenital arteriovenous anomalies of the limbs. Arch Surg 1976;111:423.
5. Rutherford RB. Congenital vascular malformations of the extremities. In: Moore WS (ed). *Vascular Surgery: A Comprehensive Review*, 5th ed. Philadelphia: W.B. Saunders, 2000.
6. Rutherford RB. Noninvasive testing in the diagnosis and assessment of arteriovenous fistula. In: Bernstein EF (ed). *Noninvasive Diagnostic Techniques in Vascular Disease*, pp. 430–442. St. Louis: C.V. Mosby, 1982.
7. Brener BJ, Brief DK, Alpert J, et al. The effect of vascular access procedures on digital hemodynamics. In: Diethrich EB (ed). *Noninvasive Cardiovascular Diagnosis: Current Concepts*, pp. 189–203. Baltimore: University Park Press, 1978.
8. Barnes RW. Noninvasive assessment of arteriovenous fistula. Angiology 1978;29:691.
9. Bingham HG, Lichti EL. The Doppler as an aid in predicting the behavior of congenital cutaneous hemangioma. Plast Reconstr Surg 1971;47:580.
10. Pisko-Dubienski ZA, Baird RJ, Bayliss CE, et al. Identification and successful treatment of congenital microfistulas with the aid of directional Doppler. Surgery 1975;78:564.
11. Rhodes BA, Rutherford RB, Lopez-Majano V, et al. Arteriovenous shunt measurement in extremities. J Nucl Med 1972;13:357.
12. Rutherford RB. Clinical applications of a method of quantitating arteriovenous shunting in extremities. In: *Vascular Surgery*, 1st ed., pp. 781–783. Philadelphia: WB Saunders, 1977.
13. Rauch RF, Silverman PM, Korobkin M, et al. Computed tomography of benign angiomatous lesions of the extremities. J Comput Assist Tomogr 1984;8:1143.
14. Pearce WH, Rutherford RB, Whitehill TA, Davis K. Nuclear magnetic resonance imaging: Its diagnostic value in patients with congenital vascular malformations of the limbs. J Vasc Surg 1988;8:64.

32
Clinical Implications of the Vascular Laboratory in the Diagnosis of Peripheral Arterial Disease

Ali F. AbuRahma

The rightful place of the vascular laboratory and its various tools in the evaluation of the patient with peripheral vascular disease is ever changing. Our expanding understanding of the pathophysiology, clinical manifestations, and natural history of peripheral vascular disorders[1-3] must constantly be coupled with an appreciation of current diagnostic and therapeutic tools (magnetic resonance angiography, operating room angiography, radiographic suite angiography, and angioplasty/stenting). This section will provide an entry point into clinical problem solving by considering the areas of screening, assessment prior to and immediately after intervention, surveillance (long-term, usually after intervention), and certain special areas of the peripheral arterial system.

Screening: "Does Peripheral Arterial Disease Exist?"

The most practical, well-studied method is resting ankle-brachial index (ABI).[4] Values in the range of 0.85–0.90 are usually chosen to signify a positive result. Attention to operator training is important for valid results.[5] Post-exercise or reactive hyperemia studies are not usually performed for screening purposes. An individual with a positive test is at increased risk for all cardiovascular events (cardiac, cerebral, or extremity).

Assessment of Location and Severity of Peripheral Vascular Disease

The primary use of noninvasive tests in patients with lower extremity vascular problems is to obtain objective, quantitative determinations instead of the subjective categories resulting from the physical examination. Measurements permit reproducibility among different examiners as well as from one time to another. Both Doppler ultrasound (continuous-wave) and the pulse volume recorder (PVR) have proved useful in defining the severity and the location of arterial occlusive disease.[6-11] However, the application of duplex ultrasonography over the past 20 years has been more helpful in localizing and grading the severity of peripheral vascular disease.[12]

In the patient presenting with lower extremity pain on exercise, it is most important to distinguish symptoms due to neurologic or orthopedic diseases from those produced by vascular insufficiency. In fact, both entities may coexist. If a true claudication is present, it is also important to accurately determine the patient's degree of disability and to establish a quantitative baseline with which the effect of medical or surgical therapy can be compared.

In the initial evaluation for the presence or absence of true claudication, the arterial leg Doppler study, using the segmental pressure determination with the analog wave tracing or PVRs, should be used, preferably measured after treadmill exercise. The simplest, most reliable means of confirming peripheral vascular occlusive disease of the lower extremity is measurement of the ankle systolic pressure and the calculation of the ABI. As described in Chapter 19, the normal resting ABI is generally around 1.0. In patients whose resting values are borderline, stress testing should be induced by treadmill exercise or reactive hyperemia. Although normal patients may transiently lower their ankle systolic pressure 15–20 mm Hg, those with even mild occlusive disease usually show a prolonged pressure decrease in excess of 50 mm Hg. In persons who become symptomatic during treadmill exercise, but whose ankle pressure remains normal, a nonvascular cause for their pain should be evaluated. Although an abnormal response to exercise confirms the presence of hemodynamically significant arterial disease, it does not exclude the possibility of coexistent neurospinal compression. The magnitude of the pressure drop should parallel the severity and location of the patient's symptoms. The ABI has also been helpful in determining the severity of vascular occlusive disease as described in previous chapters.

Raines et al.[8] classified the PVRs into five categories, which, when combined with pressure data, were helpful in defining various clinical states of ischemia, e.g., claudication, rest pain, or foot necrotic lesions.

Anatomic localization of hemodynamically significant peripheral vascular lesions by noninvasive testing is another important contribution to patient management. It is important to note that laboratory findings and physical findings must be combined to localize a lesion accurately. One parameter (physiologic testing) is generally not sufficient. The case of combined disease (aortoiliac and femoropopliteal-tibial) is by far the most challenging. In 5–10% of patients with combined disease, noninvasive analysis, while defining the hemodynamics, cannot accurately localize the main contributing lesion. In these cases, an invasive femoral artery pressure study may be indicated. Localization of the disease is of critical importance; e.g., in the patient who has thigh and buttock pain secondary to a neurospinal compression and a well-collateralized, asymptomatic superficial femoral artery occlusion, both resting and postexercise ABIs may be appropriately abnormal. Yet, if the postexercise thigh pressure and the PVRs are normal, a nonvascular cause for the patient's symptoms is suggested. Furthermore, since angiography is notoriously inaccurate in assessing the functional significance of iliac artery stenosis, some physiologic measurement of arterial inflow is essential before a distal bypass is constructed.

As described previously, the combination of the segmental Doppler pressures and the analog wave tracings could be helpful in the localization of peripheral vascular occlusive disease. However, determination of segmental pressure has certain limitations in patients with multilevel occlusive disease. In these patients, the proximal lesion might mask the distal disease; e.g., if both severe aortoiliac occlusive disease and femoral popliteal stenosis are present, the high-thigh pressure is low. The gradient between the high-thigh and the above-knee cuffs might be quite small, thus masking the disease present between these levels. Also giving a low high-thigh pressure is the combination of isolated, hemodynamically significant, superficial femoral and profunda femoral occlusive lesions. These problems in the interpretation of the pressure may be solved in one of several ways. A normal femoral pulse and the absence of an iliac bruit suggest a more distal arterial disease as the cause of the low high-thigh pressure. The common femoral artery pressure may also be obtained noninvasively using an inguinal compression device. This pneumatic device presses the artery against the superior pubic ramus, thus allowing the pressure to be measured as the compression is slowly released. The return of the arterial Doppler signal distal to the groin establishes the endpoint. Despite the presence of a normal iliac segment, monophasic waveforms may occasionally be seen in the common femoral artery when there is a combination of superficial femoral artery occlusion and severe deep femoral artery stenosis.

Other physiologic methods, which might help in differentiating aortoiliac occlusive disease from disease of the common femoral artery and/or disease of the superficial femoral artery and deep femoral artery, are the determination of the pulsatility index (PI) and the inverse damping factor. These were described in Chapter 19. Hemodynamically significant aortoiliac stenosis is unlikely if the femoral artery PI is greater than 6.0 at rest, whereas significant disease is probable if the PI is less than 5.0. When the value is between 5.0 and 6.0, the aortoiliac segment may be normal or abnormal, and further assessment is required by Doppler recording or direct pressure measurement after exercise or reactive hyperemia. Superficial femoral artery occlusion or severe stenosis is usually present if the inverse femoral popliteal damping factor is less than 0.9. A value between 0.9 and 1.1 may be normal or abnormal. When the inverse tibial damping factor is less than 1.0, significant tibial arterial occlusive disease is present.

Another hemodynamic method of determining the location of peripheral vascular occlusive disease relies on the amplitude of the calf pulse volume recording. With the use of a single large thigh cuff for lower extremity PVRs, the amplitude of the calf PVR is constantly increased relative to that of the thigh when the superficial femoral artery is patent. This finding is an artifact due to the relative volumes of the thigh and calf cuffs. Since the thigh cuff contains five to seven times more air than the calf cuff, segmental pulse volume changes that occur with each cardiac cycle result in relatively smaller pressure changes within the thigh cuff and, hence, relatively smaller thigh PVRs. Despite its basis in cuff artifact, calf augmentation is a reliable indicator of superficial femoral artery patency. If the amplitude of the calf PVR is equal to or only slightly greater than that of the thigh (less than 25%), and if there is an obvious deterioration in the contour of the waveform, superficial femoral artery stenosis or a short, well-collateralized occlusion should be suspected. For augmentation to occur, the superficial femoral artery must be patent to the origin of the sural artery in the midpopliteal region. When augmentation is noticed, but there is a 20 mm Hg or greater decrease in the segmental pressure from the thigh to the calf, distal popliteal or proximal tibial artery occlusions are usually found.[13]

Recently, duplex ultrasonography has been used more frequently for localizing and grading the severity of peripheral vascular disease with accuracies of greater than 90%.[1,2,12,14] The first step prior to vascular intervention is segmental pressure determination, which is often followed by Doppler duplex mapping of the involved arteries.

If intervention is deferred, identified lesions can be followed to detect changes. If surgical intervention is chosen, an operating room angiogram with or without magnetic resonance angiography may provide a cost-effective solution, bypassing the need for formal preoperation angiography. If angioplastic intervention appears to be warranted, it is prudent to do it concurrently with the diagnostic study. A reasonable idea of lesion location and severity will help to make these practical decisions, along with the availability of ever improving operating room radiology apparatus.

Koelemay et al.[14] evaluated the value of duplex scanning in allowing selective use of arteriography in the management of patients with severe lower leg arterial disease. Management was based on duplex scanning and intraarterial subtraction angiography was performed only when indicated. A total of 125 limbs in 114 patients were evaluated (74% of which were for rest pain or tissue loss). In 97 (78%) of limbs, management was based on duplex scanning only. It compromised conservative treatment [number = 33, 0% after intraarterial digital subtraction angiography (DSA)], PTA (number = 25, 16% intraarterial DSA), femoropopliteal bypass graft (number = 29, 17% intraarterial DSA), femorotibial bypass graft (number = 29, 62% intraarterial DSA), and other surgical procedures (number = 8, 4% intraarterial DSA). Overall, the 30-day mortality rate was 4%, and the 2-year survival rate was 83%. The 2-year primary and secondary patency and limb salvage rates were 75%, 93%, and 93% after femoropopliteal bypass operations, respectively.

The 1-year primary and secondary patency and limb salvage rates were 35%, 73%, and 74%, respectively, after a femorocrural bypass operation. There was no difference in patient characteristics, indications for a specific treatment, and immediate and intermediate term outcome between the study and reference population. They concluded that management of patients with severe lower leg ischemia could be based on duplex scanning in most patients without a negative effect on clinical outcome, whether early or at 2-year follow-up.

Prognosis and Medical Therapeutic Implications

Several noninvasive vascular tests, particularly the Doppler ankle pressures, have been applied to the study of the progression of peripheral vascular occlusive disease.[15–19]

Wilson et al., in a study of nondiabetic patients with claudication who were followed for 5 years, reported that symptomatic improvement was likely without surgery when the ABI exceeded 0.60, but was unlikely when the ABI was less than 0.50.[17] In patients with severe ischemia, Paaske and Tonnesen found that 82% of those with a toe pressure index (toe pressure divided by brachial pressure) of less than 0.07 underwent a major amputation within 2 years and 27% died.[18] These results indicate that toe pressures provide important information that can be helpful in making clinical decisions about the management of individual patients on a more rational basis.

Development of peripheral vascular occlusive disease in the second limb in patients with unilateral occlusive disease process is frequent.[16] Some of these patients show objective improvement during the first year after the onset of symptoms, and then there are no significant changes in many others over periods of several years.[15] It has also been reported that patients with disease affecting the femoral and popliteal arterial segments showed a more variable clinical course than did those with localized superficial femoral artery disease,[15] and limbs with poor runoff that eventually required amputation had significantly lower ABIs than those with poor runoff that did not require amputation.[15] Serial Doppler pressure measurements often showed deterioration without obvious clinical changes, suggesting that intervention in such cases might improve limb salvage.[15]

The American Heart Association recognized that Doppler pressure measurements provide a sensitive index of arterial obstruction and can be performed repeatedly.[20] The brachial-ankle pressure difference was noted to correlate significantly with various risk factors of atherosclerosis, e.g., smoking, hyperlipidemia, and hypertension.[21] Several researchers noted that such measurements could also be used to quantitate the severity of the arterial sclerotic process and to evaluate the relationship to the factors that influence its progression. Ankle pressure measurements were used to estimate prevalence of peripheral arteriosclerotic disease and were applied to the study of the prevalence of atherosclerosis in patients with diabetes mellitus.[22–24]

Recently, McLafferty et al.[25] reported that the ABI is relatively insensitive in identifying the progression of lower extremity arterial occlusive disease as demonstrated by the use of imaging studies. They studied patients with prior suprainguinal or infrainguinal lower extremity revascularization. Progression of lower extremity arterial occlusive disease in native arteries was determined by comparing a preoperative (baseline) arteriogram with late follow-up arteriography or duplex scanning. Progression of lower extremity arterial occlusive disease was defined as a decrease in the ABI of 0.15 or greater, and progression by imaging studies was defined as an increase in one category of stenosis. They concluded that in studies of natural history or therapy for atherosclerosis, imaging studies should be used in preference to the ABI to evaluate progression of lower extremity arterial occlusive disease more accurately.[25]

Measurement of Doppler pressures can also be used to guide and evaluate medical therapy. Vasodilators have been noted to decrease digital blood pressure distal to occlusion and are probably not indicated, particularly in the presence of severe ischemia.[26] Meanwhile, clofibrate resulted in a significant improvement in the response of ankle pressure to exercise in patients with intermittent claudication and a high plasma fibrinogen level.[27] Quick and Cotton,[28] in a study of patients with intermittent claudication, noted that cessation of smoking was followed by significant improvement in the walking distance, resting Doppler ankle pressure, and ankle pressures after exercise, whereas patients who continued to smoke showed no significant changes. Segmental pressure measurements have also been helpful in the management of patients with arterial obstruction secondary to ergotism that may regress spontaneously,[29] and to assist in the treatment of severe ischemia with drug-induced systemic hypertension by monitoring distal systolic pressure.[26]

Perioperative Evaluation

Direct examination with the Doppler detector or duplex imaging has been applied preoperatively to determine whether there is a flow in the distal vessels, which may help to plan distal bypass operations in the calf.

Ascher et al. reported previously on the efficacy of duplex arteriography as the sole imaging technique (without contrast angiography) in the management of patients with chronic and acute lower limb ischemia.[30,31] A reliable assessment of inflow and outflow arteries could be made with duplex ultrasonography, even in very low flow situations.[31] Duplex arteriography is also an effective method for preoperative diagnosis of a thrombosed popliteal artery aneurysm and for identifying the available outflow vessels for urgent revascularization. Duplex arteriography identifies the inflow, patent distal runoff vessels, and the presence of a suitable saphenous vein for revascularization.

Although routine intraoperative arteriography might detect intraoperative accident or inadequate vascular reconstruction, it is cumbersome and occasionally may be misleading since it provides visualization in only one plane. Noninvasive intraoperative physiologic monitoring provides an immediate, quantitative assessment of the success or failure of arterial surgery. Doppler ankle systolic pressures can be measured intraoperatively or immediately after surgery. Depending on the nature of the arterial reconstruction and extent of uncorrected distal disease, the postoperative change in the ABI will vary. However, if the ABI has not risen to 50% of preoperative levels within 1 h after declamping, the graft should be systematically checked for technical problems, and an intraoperative or immediate postoperative angiogram should be considered.[32]

Segmental plethysmography or duplex imaging for intraoperative monitoring might be more practical than Doppler ultrasound because of the difficulty in preventing movement of the Doppler probe during operation. Also, some patients with multilevel disease arrive in the recovery room after successful aortofemoral bypass so vasoconstricted that no Doppler signal can be detected in the lower legs. In the recovery room, serial determination of the ABI or the PVRs provide objective evidence of the graft function. Since pulses are palpable in only 25% of patients, and their feet frequently remain cold and pale for several hours following surgery,[33] such objective measurements provide nursing personnel with valuable parameters to monitor continued function of the vascular reconstruction.

Selection of the Arterial Reconstructive Procedure

Choice of Treatment Based on Duplex Scanning

Based on duplex findings, patients found to have unilateral focal stenosis or short <5 cm occlusions of recent onset (less than 3 months) involving the common iliac or superficial femoral arteries should be considered for PTA (balloon angioplasty/stent with or without catheter-directed thrombolysis). The arterial lesion should be verified by angiography and if a category 1 or 2 lesion, based on the Society of Cardiovascular and Interventional Radiology guidelines,[34] is confirmed, endovascular intervention is performed. Such treatment results in high (>95%) technical success and can yield clinical results similar to those following surgical intervention. When duplex scanning indicates features of category 3 or 4 lesions (>4 cm length calcified stenosis, multilevel disease, 5–10 cm length chronic occlusions) use of PTA is possible, but to date endovascular treatment does not yield long-term patency comparable to bypass grafting, especially in treatment of arterial occlusion. PTA of these lesions should be considered only for patients with critical ischemia who are deemed a surgical risk, or patients with unfavorable anatomy for bypass grafts, or in the absence of a suitable autologous vein for use as a bypass conduit.

Most patients with critical limb ischemia have multilevel occlusive disease and require additional vascular imaging studies (contrast arteriography, magnetic resonance angiography) beyond that afforded by duplex scanning. Duplex scanning can be used to determine whether iliac angioplasty is feasible for patients with combined aortoiliac and infrainguinal disease.[35,36] The surgeon can then decide whether to proceed with a staged iliac PTA followed by distal bypass or perform a simultaneous inflow/outflow revascularization. For patients with unilateral or contralateral absence of femoral pulses and long-segment arterial occlusion by duplex imaging, proceeding with aortofemoral, femorofemoral, or axillofemoral bypass grafting without arteriography is appropriate. In treatment of infrainguinal disease, surgical intervention (endarterectomy, bypass grafting) without arteriography is possible in selected patients with single segment occlusive or aneurysmal disease. Femoral endarterectomy with or without profundaplasty, femoropopliteal bypass grafting, and repair of femoral or popliteal aneurysms can be performed based on duplex scan findings. If imaging of the distal vessels is not optimal, intraoperative arteriography can be performed to exclude downstream lesions. Patients with arteriomegaly and diffuse atherosclerosis with multiple tibial artery involvement should undergo preoperative arteriography prior to bypass grafting.

Aortofemoral Popliteal Reconstruction

Garrett et al. suggested that if the ABI does not increase by 0.1 or more immediately following aortofemoral bypass, concomitant distal bypass should be considered.[37] However, other authors have noted that the immediate index was the same or actually lower than the preoperative value in some of their patients with multilevel disease who subsequently improved significantly over the next 4–6 h,[38] thus seriously challenging the validity of this observation. Studies by Dean et al. indicate that 90% of femoral popliteal grafts inserted in limbs with an ABI of less than 0.20 failed in the early postoperative period.[39] This merely reflects the adverse effect of high runoff resistance of graft patency. Nevertheless, a few patients with an ABI less than 0.20 will obtain satisfactory results. A successful outcome can be expected in limbs with a preoperative ABI of greater than 0.50.[40]

Others reported the importance of the pressure measurements in the assessment of patients prior to vascular surgery or angioplasty, in the immediate and long-term follow-up after the procedures, and in the objective evaluation of the results.[41,42]

Profundaplasty

The segmental systolic pressure determination can also be helpful in determining whether profundaplasty is successful or not. When performed for limb salvage, profundaplasty as an isolated procedure is effective in 33–86% of cases.[43] For a profundaplasty to be successful, the profunda femoris artery must be severely stenotic, and the profunda-popliteal collateral bed must be well developed. If the collateral resistance is too high, profundaplasty will reduce the total limb resistance by an insufficient amount, and the distal portions of the limb will remain ischemic. To predict the outcome of profundaplasty, Boren et al. developed an index of collateral arterial resistance across the popliteal segment.[43] This index is calculated by dividing the gradient across the knee (above-knee pressure minus below-knee pressure) by the above-knee pressure. When the index was less than 0.25, successful results were obtained in 67% of cases; but when the index was greater than 0.50, there were no successful results.

Lumbar Sympathectomy

Sympathectomy does not relieve claudication and is performed only as a means of improving the skin blood flow in ischemic areas. Although pressure measurement does not directly indicate the magnitude of the local blood flow, the level is correlated with the ability of the peripheral arteries to dilate. The arterioles tend to be maximally dilated in ischemic tissues. When the perfusion pressure is quite low, this dilatation is necessary to maintain adequate tissue nutrition. Sympathectomy might also be questionable in patients with diabetes mellitus in which a significant number of patients had autosympathectomy; hence, the objective evidence of sympathetic activity in the terminal vascular bed is important.

During deep inspiration, an individual with normal sympathetic activity has a prompt decrease in digital pulse volume.[44] This can be documented using a mercury-in-Silastic strain gauge or the PVR. Another important point is whether the resistance vessels in the affected extremity are capable of further vasodilation. This can be answered by demonstrating a doubling of the resting digital pulse volume following the reactive hyperemia test (a 5-min period of ischemia induced by inflating a proximal pneumatic cuff above the systolic pressure) or by direct warming of the extremity. In normal extremities, the pulse volume after induced reactive hyperemia is several times that of the resting pulse, thus reflecting the ability of the peripheral arterioles to dilate further. This effect can be demonstrated even in the presence of proximal arterial occlusive disease.

Yao and Bergan,[45] in a study of patients with ischemic rest pain and pregangrenous changes of the foot who were not candidates for reconstructive surgery and who underwent lumbar sympathectomy, reported that 96% of limbs with an ABI below 0.21 failed to benefit from lumbar sympathectomy and required amputation. All limbs with an ABI greater than 0.35 had a satisfactory response. More recently, Walker and Johnston[46] observed that sympathectomy was unlikely to be successful in an ischemic limb with associated neuropathy, regardless of the level of the ankle pressure. In the absence of neuropathy, a successful outcome was likely in limbs with rest pain or digital gangrene, provided that the ankle pressure exceeded 30 mm Hg. Their analysis suggested that a favorable response might be expected in about 50% of limbs with more severe ischemia (forefoot or heel gangrene) when the ankle pressure was greater than 60 mm Hg. Using these criteria, their accuracy in predicting failure was 78%, and in predicting success was 93%.

Recently, in a prospective study of 85 lumbar sympathectomies for inoperable peripheral vascular disease, we analyzed the correlation between lumbar sympathectomy, ABI, popliteal-brachial index, and the clinical presentation. These patients were also studied to determine if predicted clinical criteria, single or combined, could be defined for selection of patients who might benefit from lumbar sympathectomy. Good results were obtained if at 6 months after surgery pain at rest was absent, ischemic ulcers had healed, and there were no major amputations. In this study, 77% of all limbs with a preoperative ABI ≥ 0.3 had a good outcome in contrast to a 94% failure for an index of <0.3 ($p < 0.001$). Sixty-nine percent of all limbs with a popliteal-brachial index ≥ 0.7 had a good outcome vs. 52% if the index was <0.7 ($p = 0.199$). Patients with rest pain, simple leg ulcers, and toe gangrene had a good outcome if the ABI was ≥ 0.3 and if the postoperative ABI increased by ≥ 0.1. The popliteal-brachial index and diabetic status had no prognostic value.[47]

Tiutiunnik[48] studied the microcirculation state in lower extremities using laser Doppler flowmetry in 37 patients with obliterating atherosclerosis before and after lumbar sympathectomy performance. It was established that laser Doppler flowmetry may be applied for estimation of the microcirculation bed function state and prognosis of the lumbar sympathectomy results.[48]

In general, patients with an ABI of greater than 0.25% have a favorable response to lumbar sympathectomy. However, patients with indices even higher than that might fail to respond and eventually might require amputation, thus demonstrating that other factors such as infection, neuropathy, and patency of the pedal vessels might adversely affect the outcome.

Postoperative Follow-up

The vascular laboratory has also been helpful in detecting impending graft failure.[49,50] Stenoses may develop in the femoropopliteal or femorotibial graft without producing any symptoms or alteration in the pulses of the graft or at the periphery. These silent stenoses, which often evolve into total occlusion, can be detected if the ankle pressure is followed closely in the months and years after operation. Close observation is particularly impor-

tant during the first year, since about 75% of such events occur within this period. A previously stable ABI that drops by 0.20 or more suggests the need for arteriographic investigation.[32] As a rule, operative correction is easy and the ankle pressure often returns to normal levels.

Calligaro et al.[51] conducted a study of the role of ultrasonography in the surveillance of femoropopliteal and femorotibial arterial prosthetic bypasses. In this study, 89 infrainguinal grafts in 66 patients were entered into a postoperative prosthetic graft surveillance protocol, which included clinical evaluation, segmental pressures, pulse volume recordings, and duplex ultrasounds performed every 3 months. Patients with follow-up of less than 3 months were excluded, unless the graft thrombosed. An abnormal duplex ultrasound considered predictive of graft failure included (1) peak systolic velocity (PSV) >300 cm/s at inflow or outflow arteries, in the graft or at an anastomosis (unless an adjunctive arteriovenous fistula had been performed); (2) adjacent PSV ratio >3.0; (3) uniform PSVs < 45 cm/s; or (4) monophasic signals throughout the graft. Duplex ultrasound was considered to have correctly diagnosed a failing graft if a stenosis >75% of the luminal diameter of the graft, at an anastomosis, or in an inflow/outflow artery was confirmed by operative or arteriographic findings or if the graft thrombosed after an abnormal duplex ultrasound, but before intervention. Their results support the routine use of duplex ultrasound as a part of a graft surveillance protocol for femorotibial, but not femoropopliteal, prosthetic grafts.

Over the past decade, duplex ultrasound has been frequently used for postoperative graft surveillance, described in detail in Chapters 22 and 23.

If one waits for a significant change in ABI or segmental pressures, the golden opportunity to correct a stent or graft while still patent may be lost. Waiting for thrombosis and then doing a secondary procedure carries a reduced chance for long-term success.

Healing Response

Ischemic Skin Lesions

Skin ulcers of the lower extremities may be arterial, venous stasis, neuropathic (e.g., diabetic), or occasionally related to other systemic causes. Raines et al.[8] suggested that healing of ischemic ulcers was likely in nondiabetic patients at an ankle pressure >65 mm Hg, and in diabetic patients if the ankle pressure was >90 mm Hg. Healing was unlikely if the ankle pressure was <55 mm Hg in nondiabetic patients and <80 mm Hg in diabetic patients. They also emphasized the importance of the forefoot or digital plethysmography, stating that if a pulsatile, metatarsal PVR was present, the probability of healing was 90%. Carter reported that all limbs with ischemic ulcers required amputation when the ankle pressure was <55 mm Hg.[52] With pressures >55 mm Hg, 92% of the lesions in nondiabetics healed. In diabetics, 33% healed with an ankle pressure in the 55–70 mm Hg range. He also found that foot lesions usually healed if the toe pressure was >30 mm Hg in nondiabetics or 55 mm Hg in diabetics. Ramsey et al.[53] reported that toe pressures had more prognostic value than ankle pressures. Lesions failed to heal in 92% of limbs with an ankle pressure <80 mm Hg, but they also failed to heal in 45% of limbs with higher ankle pressures. When the toe pressure was <30 mm Hg, the failure rate was 95%; but when the toe pressure was >30 mm Hg, only 14% did not heal.

These figures can help the vascular surgeon decide what therapy to use in patients with ulceration, e.g., revascularization, amputation, or conservative therapy. For example, continuing to dress and debride an ulcer on the foot of a patient with diabetes and a toe pressure of 20 mm Hg or an ankle pressure of 45 mm Hg is probably a futile exercise; but this same regimen is likely to be valuable when the toe pressure is >30 mm Hg. These figures also serve to point out the beneficial effects that a relatively small increase in ankle pressure can have in regard to skin healing. If, for example, an iliac reconstruction or profundaplasty raises the ankle pressure only 20 mm Hg, from 50 to 70 mm Hg, or the toe pressure from 20 to 35 mm Hg, the chance of healing an ischemic lesion may be greatly enhanced, despite the persistence of severe femoropopliteal or below-knee lesions.

Amputation Sites

The selection of amputation site can make the difference between a bed or wheelchair existence versus successful prosthetic rehabilitation. A successful amputation must remove all necrotic or infected tissue, and it must be possible to fit the amputation stump with a functional and easily applied prosthesis with a good blood supply at the level of the proposed amputation to allow primary healing. This, particularly, is very critical when it comes to a mid-thigh amputation versus a below knee amputation, which deprives the patient of the opportunity for subsequent ambulation under most circumstances, even though the amputation might heal without difficulty if an above knee amputation is done. On the other hand, if a distal amputation site, e.g., a below knee, is selected and the blood supply is inadequate, this will necessitate further surgery with higher morbidity and mortality. A below knee amputation as opposed to above knee amputation has several advantages including making it easier to ambulate, a consideration that is extremely important in older patients. In most series, older patients who undergo unilateral below knee amputation show a >90%

success rate of rehabilitation to ambulation in contrast to only 30% for patients with above knee amputations.

The presence of pulses in the affected lower extremity, or nonobjective assessment of skin temperature based on clinical judgment, or clinical judgment alone, does not yield information with consistent enough correlation to amputation healing to serve as a sound basis for clinical decision making. Robbs and Ray[54] retrospectively analyzed the results of healing in 214 patients who underwent lower limb amputation in which the amputation level was determined by such objective criteria. They reported a failure rate of 9% for above knee amputation in contrast to 25% for below knee amputation. They concluded that skin flap viability could not be predicted by the extent of the ischemic lesion in relation to the ankle joint, the popliteal pulse status, or angiographic findings. van Den Broek et al.[55] challenged these findings in recent reports in which 53 patients undergoing amputations of the lower limb were evaluated in terms of clinical criteria, PVR, Doppler pressures, photoplethysmographic skin perfusion pressures, and angiography. They reported that although not as reliable as photoplethysmographic skin perfusion pressures, angiographic findings correlated significantly with the success of healing.

Various noninvasive methods were described to assess the level of amputation sites. These included Doppler ankle and calf systolic blood pressure measurements with or without PVR,[56–60] xenon-133 skin blood flow studies,[61–63] digital or transmetatarsal photoplethysmographic pressures,[64] transcutaneous oxygen determination,[65–69] skin fluorescence after the intravenous infusion of fluorescent dye,[70–72] laser Doppler skin blood flow,[73] skin temperature evaluation,[74] pertechnetate skin blood pressure studies,[75,76] and photoelectrically measured skin color changes.[77]

Skin temperature, laser Doppler, and xenon-133 skin clearance were described in a previous chapter (Chapter 18). Transcutaneous oxygen pressure will be described in detail in a later chapter.

Skin Fluorescence

Skin fluorescence holds significant promise as a minimally invasive test. Initial studies measured skin fluorescence with a Wood's ultraviolet light after the intravenous injection of fluorescene. This technique is somewhat more invasive than the Doppler ankle systolic pressure measurement or PVR, however, it is less complicated and less invasive than xenon-133 skin blood flow or pertechnetate skin perfusion measurement. New fluorometers that can provide objective numerical readings quickly without the need for a Wood lamp have enhanced the value of this technique. Silverman et al.[78] reported on the use of fiberoptic fluorometry for selecting digital, transmetatarsal, below knee, and above knee amputation levels. In 86 cases with cellulitis at the site of amputation, preoperative fluorometry clearly distinguished between healing and nonhealing sites. The amputation healed in all but one patient whose dye fluorescene index was >42. This technique maintained its high accuracy even in patients with diabetes mellitus. These authors pointed out that dye fluorescene index values between 38 and 42 constitute a transitional zone in which the precision of fluorometric determination is unclear. Fluorometry has an advantage over other techniques such as laser Doppler perfusion and transcutaneous oximetry in assessment of patients with multiple sites on the same limb.

Doppler Systolic Pressure Determinations in Amputation Sites

Raines et al.[8] reported that primary healing of below-knee amputation was likely if the calf pressure was above 65 mm Hg or the ankle pressure was above 30 mm Hg. Healing was unlikely if the calf pressure was <65 mm Hg or the ankle pressure was <30 mm Hg. Transmetatarsal amputation will generally heal primarily if any detectable amplitude is present at the transmetatarsal level. Toe amputation has a very good prognosis for healing if an amplitude is measurable at the digit base. Others reported that in patients with a calf systolic pressure of 50–75 mm Hg, primary healing of below-knee amputations can be expected in 88–100%.[79] However, in another study Barnes et al. concluded that there was no significant difference in the mean blood pressure between the groups with healed and failed amputations, regardless of the level of pressure measurement, and observed healing in 90% of below-knee amputations in extremities with unobtainable pressure at the below-knee or ankle levels.[57]

Verta et al.[58] reported that there was little chance that toe amputations would heal if the ankle pressure was <35 mm Hg. However, Nicholas et al.[59] noted failure of 60% of forefoot amputations when the ankle pressure was <75 mm Hg. Thus, a low ankle pressure appears to be an ominous sign. High ankle pressure, on the other hand, does not signify a favorable prognosis, since this high pressure could be secondary to arterial calcification and might not reflect the presence of pedal or digital arterial obstruction. Consequently, failure of toe amputations or transmetatarsal amputation is not unusual, even when the ankle pressure exceeds 100 mm Hg.[57,80]

In general, a calf pressure >40 mm Hg or an ankle pressure above 30 mm Hg provides reasonable assurance that the below-knee amputation will heal, but lower values should not deter the surgeon from attempting an amputation at this level if other signs are favorable.

Apelquist et al.[56] reported on the value of systolic ankle and toe pressure measurements in predicting healing in patients with diabetic foot ulcers and presented data for both patients who underwent amputation and those who did not. Primary healing was achieved in 85% of patients with a toe pressure of >44 mm Hg, whereas 63% of patients with toe pressures of <45 mm Hg experienced healing without amputation. In contrast, below-knee amputations with ankle pressures in excess of 80 mm Hg were associated with healing, and 20 of 21 of these patients who underwent amputation had toe pressures in excess of 50 mm Hg. They concluded that different Doppler pressure levels have to be used to predict primary healing for diabetic ulcers compared to healing after minor amputation.

Compression Syndromes

Vascular laboratory testing can be helpful in thoracic outlet syndrome[81–83] and popliteal artery entrapment.[84,85]

Thoracic Outlet Syndrome

Thoracic outlet syndrome occurs when there is a compression of the neurovascular bundle by shoulder structures that may include the cervical rib, costoclavicular space, or scalene muscle. The symptoms of this syndrome generally include numbness or tingling of the arm and pain or aching of the shoulder and forearm. Exercise and upward arm positions can increase the symptoms.[81] It should be noted that around 25% of the population have asymptomatic compression.

Most authorities believe that the pain associated with thoracic outlet syndrome is neurogenic, secondary to nerve compression at the lowest trunk of the brachial plexus by the first rib or occasionally a cervical rib. The subclavian artery or vein is occasionally compressed, and this might be associated with arterial ischemia of the upper extremity or symptoms and signs of axillary subclavian vein thrombosis.

Various noninvasive techniques can be used in the diagnosis of thoracic outlet syndrome, which may include plethysmographic techniques and/or Doppler waveform analyses to detect vascular changes. The photoplethysmograph (PPG) is attached to the index finger, or the continuous wave Doppler is used to monitor the radial artery, or a brachial cuff is applied to monitor plethymographic pulse volume waveforms. Resting waveforms are obtained, and then the patient's arm is placed in various positions as the pulsations are monitored at each position. The following technique is applied for the application of PVR in patients with thoracic outlet syndrome.

The patient is first asked to sit erect on the side of an examining table. A PVR monitoring cuff is placed on the upper arm and is inflated to 65 mm Hg. Recordings are taken in the following positions: (1) erect, with hands in lap; (2) erect, with arm at a 90° angle in the same plane as the torso; (3) erect, with arm at a 120° angle in the same plane as the torso; (4) erect, with arm at a 90° angle in the same plane as the torso, with the shoulders in extended military-type brace; (5) the same position as in (4), but with head turned sharply toward the monitored arm; and (6) the same position as in (4), but with the head turned sharply away from the monitored arm.

In general, PVR amplitude increases as the arm is elevated. Arterial compression is present if the PVR amplitude goes flat in any of the above positions. However, many asymptomatic patients (around 25%) may have a positive test in some of the positions outlined. Since the syndrome is often bilateral, the other arm should always be studied.

Duplex imaging with or without color can also be used to aid in the diagnosis of thoracic outlet syndrome where both axillary subclavian arteries or veins can be imaged at resting and at various maneuvers as described above. Wadhwani et al.[83] studied color Doppler sonographic findings in five clinically suspected cases of thoracic outlet syndrome. The subclavian artery and vein were studied in varying degrees of abduction to assess the severity of the syndrome. Significant changes, including increased velocities, preocclusion, and occlusion in the subclavian artery in varying degrees of abduction, were noted in four of five cases. Blunted flow in the axillary artery (four patients) and a rebound increase in velocities on release of abduction were noted in three patients. These changes suggested that significant narrowing was causing symptoms. They concluded that color Doppler sonography is a noninvasive, effective method compared with digital subtraction angiography in the diagnosis of thoracic outlet syndrome.

Gillard et al.[82] evaluated the diagnostic usefulness of provocative tests, Doppler ultrasonography, electrophysiological investigations, and helical computed tomography (CT) angiography in thoracic outlet syndrome. They prospectively evaluated 48 patients with clinical suspicion of thoracic outlet syndrome. Standardized provocative tests such as an eletromyogram and somatosensory evoked responses, a Doppler ultrasonogram, and a helical CT arterial and/or venous angiogram with dynamic maneuvers were done on each patient. The final diagnosis was established by excluding all other causes based on all available data. The agreement between the results of each investigation and the final diagnosis was evaluated. Provocative tests had mean sensitivity and specificity values of 72% and 53%, respectively, with better values for the Adson test [positive predictive value (PPV), 85%], the hyperabduction test (PPV, 92%), and the Wright test. Using several tests in combination improved specificity. Doppler ultrasonography visualized vascular parietal abnormalities and confirmed the diagnosis in patients with at least five positive provocative tests. Electrophysiologic studies were useful mainly for the differ-

ential diagnosis in detecting concomitant abnormalities. It was concluded that although helical CT angiography provided accurate information on the locations and mechanism of vascular compression, the usefulness of this investigation for establishing the diagnosis of thoracic outlet syndrome and for obtaining pretherapeutic information remains unclear.

Popliteal Artery Entrapment Syndrome

Ischemic pain with exercise (running, not walking) may occur because of intermittent compression of the popliteal artery by the medial head of the gastrocnemius muscle.[84] In such cases, the popliteal artery passes medial to or through the fibers of the medial head of the gastrocnemius muscle, which may have an anomalous origin on the femur either cephalad or lateral to its normal position on the posterior surface of the medial femoral condyle. This will cause episodic and functional occlusion of the popliteal artery that occurs with each active plantar flexion. The syndrome may be characterized by a history of unilateral intermittent claudication in young men and the laboratory findings of diminution of ankle PVRs with sustained plantar flexion and/or passive dorsiflexion of the foot or abnormal Doppler pulse waves with decreased ankle systolic pressure.[84] The demonstration of the medial deviation of the popliteal artery on arteriogram will confirm it. Popliteal artery entrapment syndrome can also be induced during reconstruction of femoral popliteal bypass, and this can also be detected by using PVR. Duplex ultrasound can also be helpful in the diagnosis of this syndrome.[85]

Penile Circulation

Impotence can be psychogenic, neuorogenic, hormonal, vascular, or drug related. Diabetes mellitus is often a factor in both neurogenic and vasculogenic impotence. Doppler penile pressure studies are helpful in identifying a possible vascular cause.[86] Similarly, plethysmography has been used effectively to quantitate penile blood flow.[87]

A pneumatic cuff measuring 2.5 cm in width (2.5 × 12.5 cm or 2.5 × 9 cm) is applied to the base of the penis. A return of blood flow when the cuff is deflated can be detected by a mercury strain-gauge plethysmograph, a photoplethysmograph applied to the anterolateral aspect of the shaft, or a Doppler flow probe (Figure 32–1). Although some investigators have positioned the probe over the dorsal penile arteries, others have emphasized the importance of detecting flow in the cavernosal artery. Because the penile blood supply is paired, an obstruction may occasionally be limited to only one side. It has been recommended that the pressures be measured on both sides of the penis.[88] In normal individuals under 40 years of age, the penile-brachial index (penile pressure divided

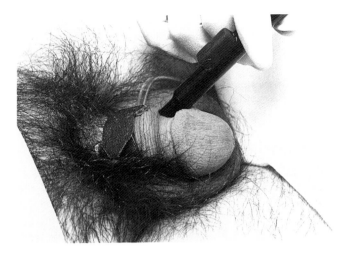

FIGURE 32–1. Method for measuring the penile Doppler pressures using a Doppler flow probe on the dorsal penile artery.

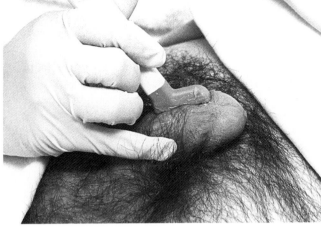

FIGURE 32–2. Position of the scan head (duplex ultrasound) for examination of the cavernous artery. Note the scan head is positioned on the ventral aspect of the penis.

by the brachial systolic pressure) was found to be 0.99 ± 1.15.[86]

Patients over the age of 40 years without symptoms of impotence tend to have lower indices. Penile-brachial indices >0.75–0.8 are considered compatible with normal erectile function; an index of <0.60 is diagnostic of vasculogenic impotence.[86,89]

Knowledge of the penile pressure can be used to guide the surgeon in planning the operative approach to aneurysmal or obstructive occlusive disease of the aortoiliac segment. Maintenance of blood flow to the internal iliac artery will preserve potency and restoration of flow to this artery and will often improve penile pressure and erectile function.

Imaging Techniques for Penile Circulation

Duplex imagings can be used to assess penile circulation as follows. The cavernous arteries are measured bilaterally in an A/P transverse orientation. Color Doppler imaging is also a sensitive means of detecting cavernous artery blood flow, thus permitting more rapid identification of these vessels (Figures 32–2 and 32–3).[90] The examiner measures the PSVs in the dorsal and cavernous arteries bilaterally (Figures 32–4 and 32–5). This is followed by injections of specific medications, e.g., papaverine and/or prostaglandin by the urologist utilizing the lateral aspect of the proximal shaft of the penis (Figure 32–6). Repeat velocity measurements are obtained postinjection. These can be measured at 1 or 2 min after injection; multiple measurements may be obtained at various increments for up to 6 min after the injection. PSV and end-diastolic velocity measurements are obtained from the proximal cavernous arteries before full erection is achieved. This may require taking several measurements to obtain the highest velocity recording. The deep dorsal vein flow velocity is also measured from

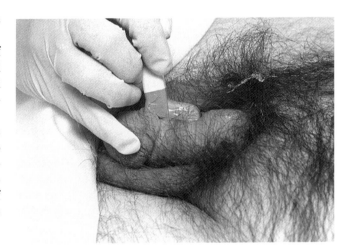

FIGURE 32–3. Position of the scan head to show the dorsal penile artery. Note the position of the scan head on the dorsal aspect of the penis.

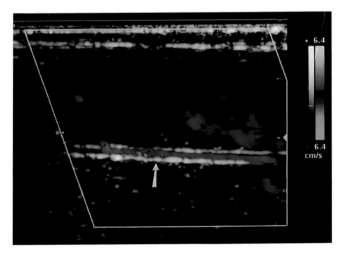

FIGURE 32–4. A color duplex image of the cavernous artery. Note the color flow as indicated by the arrow.

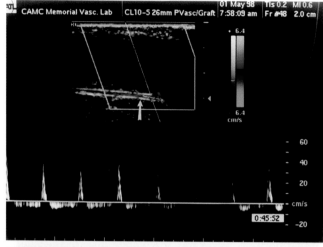

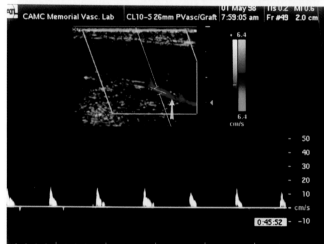

FIGURE 32–5. (A) A color duplex image of the cavernous artery (see arrow). The Doppler flow velocity spectrum with a peak systolic velocity of approximately 40 cm/s is shown at the bottom of the figure. (B) A color duplex image of the cavernous artery (see arrow). The Doppler flow velocity spectrum with a peak systolic velocity of approximately 15 cm/s is shown at the bottom of the figure.

a dorsal approach, with light probe pressure. The dimensions of the cavernous arteries are also measured in the A/P and transverse views during systole. The examiner should observe the time elapsed since injection and document when velocities are recorded.

It has been noted that PSVs generally increase after injection: a normal velocity is equal to or greater than 30 cm/s, 25–29 cm/s is a marginal value, and <25 cm/s is considered an abnormal velocity. To be noted, since the time when the highest PSV is reached after injection varies among individuals, it is imperative to obtain serial measurements. These velocities may occur 5, 10, 15, or 20 min after injection, with a nearly equal distribution. Postinjection, the deep dorsal venous flow velocity should not increase with the following criteria to be followed: normal—<3 cm/s, moderate increase—10 to 20 cm/s, and

markedly increased—>20 cm/s. It has been suggested that an increase to >4 cm/s may indicate a venous leak, which could contribute to the erectile dysfunction. The diameter of the cavernous arteries normally increases (dilates) after injection.

Measurement of PSVs in the cavernousal arteries after intracavernousal injection currently appears to be the best ultrasound approach for evaluating patients with suspected arteriogenic impotence.[90–92]

Several other studies recently reported on the value of color duplex ultrasonography in the diagnosis of vasculogenic erectile dysfunction.[93–96]

Roy et al.[95] conducted a study to evaluate the role of duplex sonography for flaccid penis and the potential role in the evaluation of impotence. Their goal was to assess the potential value of PSV measurements on the flaccid penis in the diagnosis of arteriogenic impotence. Forty-four men underwent duplex Doppler sonography with peak systolic measurements before and after intracavernous injection of prostaglandin E(1). Three different cutoff values for lowest normal PSV before injection—5, 10, and 15 cm/s—were tested. Thirteen patients had arteriogenic insufficiency based on postintracavernous injection duplex sonography and clinical response. Results for different cutoff PSV values of 5, 10, and 15 cm/s in diagnosing arteriogenic impotence were, respectively: sensitivity 29%, 96%, and 100%; specificity 100%, 92%, and 23%; negative predictive value 80%, 92%, and 100%; positive predictive value 100%, 81%, and 41%; and overall accuracy 79%, 93%, and 44%. In the flaccid state, there was a significant difference in mean PSV between the "normal" group (12.6 ± 0.9 cm/s) and the arteriogenic impotence group (7.7 ± 1.1 cm/s). Twenty-nine patients with a bilateral PSV of 10 cm/s or less before intracavernous injection had a normal clinical response. They

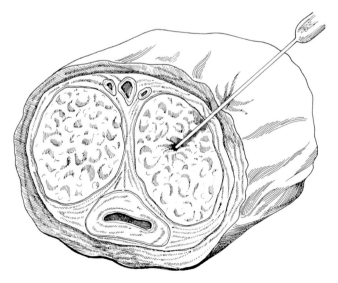

FIGURE 32–6. An illustration of the structure of the penis with the position of the needle used for injection of vasodilators.

concluded that a cutoff PSV value of 10 cm/s in the flaccid state had the best accuracy in predicting arterial insufficiency. Duplex Doppler sonography is proposed as the initial test to evaluate the penile arterial supply and to determine whether patients are good candidates for therapy with intracavernous injection.

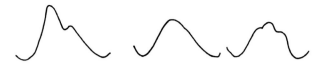

FIGURE 32–7. Digit pulse contours. From left to right: normal contour, obstructive contour, peaked contour.

Upper Extremity Ischemia and Vasospastic Diseases

Upper extremity ischemia is relatively infrequent and can be caused by atherosclerosis, vasospasm, emboli, and trauma, which might be caused by diagnostic arterial catheterization. The segmental pressures and Doppler flow or PVRs can be measured at the level of the upper arm, forearm, and wrist, as well as in one or more digits to aid in diagnosing and localizing the obstructing lesion. Doppler ultrasound can accurately assess the patency of the palmar arch, which should be considered in all patients suspected of having intrinsic small vessel disease of the hand, or prior to cannulation of either the radial or the ulnar arteries. After catheterization, pressure data can be used to determine whether an accident has occurred. With spasm, the blood pressure drops only moderately and recovers rapidly.

Sumner and Strandness[97] described the characteristic peaked pulse seen in the digit volume pulse contours of patients with cold sensitivity secondary to collagen vascular disease or other forms of intrinsic digital artery disease. This is in contrast to patients with pure vasospasm where the contour is normal in configuration, but of decreased amplitude. Figure 32–7 shows three typical digit pulse contours obtained with a mercury-in-Silastic plethysmograph. The normal pulse contour has a sharp systolic upswing that rises rapidly to a peak, and then drops off rapidly toward the baseline. The downslope of this curve is bowed toward the baseline and usually contains a prominent dicrotic notch midway between the peak and baseline. In contrast, the pulse found distal to an arterial obstruction is considerably more rounded as seen in the obstructive contour. The upswing is delayed, the downslope is bowed away from the baseline, and there is no dicrotic notch. In several cases of arterial obstruction, no pulse is perceptible. The peaked pulse has a somewhat more delayed upswing than the normal pulse. Near the peak there is an anacrotic notch. On the downslope, a dicrotic notch is present that is less prominent and located closer to the peak than normally seen.

At room temperature, digital perfusion may be normal in persons with early vasospastic disease. To examine these patients, baseline PVRs of all digits are obtained. The hands are then immersed in iced water for 3 min, or as long as tolerated. Serial digital PVRs are measured as rewarming occurs. If they fail to return to baseline levels within 5 min, a pathologic degree of vasospasm is likely. Measuring digit or toe pressure might also be helpful in distinguishing between primary vasospastic Raynaud's disease and obstructive organic disease or Raynaud's syndrome. In the primary disease the digital pressure is almost normal, but in the obstructive disease the digital pressure is markedly decreased. It should be noted that the toe pressure is normally a few millimeters of mercury less than the arm pressure and the finger pressure is a few millimeters higher than the arm pressure in young adults, but almost equal to the arm pressure in old patients. After the hands are immersed in iced water, the digital pressure in a normal individual will drop very slightly, but will return to normal very rapidly. In patients with primary vasospastic disease, the digital pressure will drop more significantly and might take a few minutes or more to come back. The digital pressure in organic obstructive disease will drop very dramatically (from 60 to 0 mm Hg) and will take longer to return to normal. Further details of upper extremity vascular evaluation will be described in another chapter.

Arteriovenous Malformations

Arteriovenous malformations (AVMs) or fistulas can be congenital or acquired (e.g., traumatic). They consist of an abnormal connection between a high-pressure arterial system and a low-pressure venous system, causing marked hemodynamic and anatomic changes. AVMs may involve proximal and distal arteries and veins as well as collateral arteries and veins. Its diameter and length predict the resistance it offers. If the fistula is proximal in its location (close to the heart), the potential for cardiac complications, primarily cardiac failure, increases. This is in contrast to peripheral fistulas, which are less likely to cause congestive heart failure, but more likely to cause limb ischemia. Generally, flow in the artery proximal to the fistula is greatly increased, especially during diastole, because the fistula markedly reduces resistance, and this is in contrast to what is seen in a normal artery. The proximal venous flow is also increased and becomes more pulsatile in character. The blood pressure distal to the fistula is somewhat reduced. The direction of the blood flow, on the other hand, is normal if the fistula resistance exceeds that of the distal vascular bed. If the fistula is chronic and large, arterial blood flow may be retrograde. A long-standing chronic fistula tends to elevate venous pressure, and blood flow is retrograde in the distal vein, which is associated with an incompetent valve.

Diagnosis of AVM may be evident on physical examination by (1) the presence of a characteristic bruit, (2) the presence of secondary varicosities and cutaneous changes of chronic venous insufficiency, (3) the obliteration of the thrill producing bradycardiac response, or (4) the association of a birthmark and limb overgrowth in patients with congenital AVM. However, such combinations are often lacking. Szilagyin et al.[98] reported in one of the largest series of AVMs that the classic triad of birthmark, varicosities, and limb enlargement was present in only 30% of patients, with various other combinations of signs present in 38% and 32% of those presenting with only a single physical finding. Various noninvasive diagnostic tests have been used for the diagnosis of extremity AV fistula including (1) Doppler segmental limb systolic pressure determination, (2) segmental limb plethysmography or PVRs, and (3) analysis of arterial velocity waveforms.

The reduced peripheral resistance associated with AVM decreases the mean arterial pressure proximally, but increases the pulse pressure.[99] Accordingly, proximal to the malformation, segmental systolic pressures are usually increased compared with the contralateral normal extremity. Beyond the malformation, they are normal, except in the case of stealing from distal arterial flow, when they may be decreased. The decreased peripheral resistance eliminates the reverse flow, which is seen in the normal Doppler analog wave tracing and increases the forward flow, particularly during diastole. Consequently, the end-diastolic velocity waveforms are elevated above the zero baseline in direct proportion to the decrease in peripheral resistance. However, this pattern can be seen in cases of reactive hyperemia, after vasodilator drugs, in warming of the extremity, in inflammation, and after sympathectomy. In the absence of these conditions, it is diagnostic of AVM.

The PVR can also be helpful in the diagnosis of these malformations. The AVM increases the segmental limb volume changes normally produced by pulsatile arterial flow and can be detected with the PVR. The PVRs proximal to the fistula are uniformly increased. The anacrotic slope and peak are sharper with loss of the dicrotic wave. Distal to the fistula, the PVRs are often entirely normal. The same principles can be applied in evaluating patients with angioaccess for kidney failure, premature atypical varicose veins, unequal limb growth, or hemangiomas of the extremity.

Labeled microsphere methods can be used to estimate the AV shunt flow of an extremity. The percentage of total extremity flow that passes through AVMs may be meas-

ured by comparing the relative levels of pulmonary radioactivity following an arterial, and then a peripheral venous injection of a radionuclide-labeled human albumin microsphere.[99] These methods may be used to confirm or exclude the diagnosis of AVM, particularly if the results of the noninvasive vascular tests are equivocal. They also provide a quantitative estimate of the AV shunt flow, which may be helpful in determining its prognosis and the need for any therapeutic interventions.

Patients with congenital AVM may also present primarily as venous pathology, e.g., varicose veins. Some of these may harbor AVM and have secondary venous insufficiency, whereas others may have a venous anomaly, but no AVM (e.g., Klippel-Trenaunay or Parks-Weber syndrome). These can be investigated by various venous noninvasive studies that will be described later. Various venous abnormalities can be detected, including deep venous valvular insufficiency, which can be diagnosed by simple Doppler ultrasound or venous duplex imaging or PPG.

In spite of the role of various noninvasive vascular tests described earlier, other testing may be necessary in many patients with AVM of the extremities to achieve sufficient information on which to base major clinical decisions. Magnetic resonance imaging, which is preferable to contrasted enhanced CT, might be necessary in evaluating congenital vascular malformation.[100] Magnetic resonance imaging gives a better definition of the anatomic extent and the feasibility of surgical resection than CT and allows multiplanar views (Figure 32–8). This subject is described in more detail in Chapter 31.

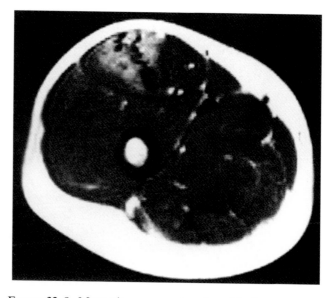

FIGURE 32–8. Magnetic resonance imaging of the lower extremity showing a vascular mass with high flow changes in the anterior medial compartment of the thigh region (involving the vastus medialis muscle) as noted in the upper portion of this transverse view.

Hemodialysis Access Graft Imaging

Duplex scanning of hemodialysis access grafts documents abnormalities and abnormal velocity or volume flow measurements commonly associated with a graft malfunction. Imaging of these grafts is indicated in the following circumstances: elevated venous pressure, difficult needle placement, loss of graft thrill, swelling around the graft site, perigraft mass, recirculation, abnormal laboratory values, and underdeveloped Cimino fistula.

Technique

No specific preparation is required prior to the examination. The patient may sit or lie in the supine position and clothing may need to be removed, depending on the location of the access graft. The extremity is inspected for raised or flattened areas of edema, or discoloration of the hand or digits. The presence of a pulse is abnormal and the presence of a palpable thrill is a normal finding. Brachial pressures should be obtained and should be equal bilaterally. A five to ten MHz linear transducer can be used and the graft should be examined in both transverse and longitudinal scan planes. Both the inflow artery, the entire length of the graft, and the outflow veins should be imaged. Velocities or volume flow measurements must be done at the anastomotic sites, mid-graft, puncture sites, and sites of obvious lumen reduction. If color flow imaging is available, observe the image for frequency increases, turbulence, and flow channel changes. The following can be some of the limitations of this technique: excessive swelling, infection, anatomic variations, uncooperative patients, and visualization of the graft less than 48 h after placement. The technician or examiner should be familiar with the type of hemodialysis access graft to facilitate mapping. Figure 32–9 is an example of these grafts.

Interpretations

As indicated earlier, the following should be identified and documented as to location, extent, and type: aneurysmal changes (including pseudoaneurysms), puncture sites for hematomas or leaks, thrombus, and perigraft fluid collection.

PSVs vary according to the graft type and normally can be quite elevated. Presently, there are no standardized velocity criteria for hemodialysis access grafts. It is generally recommended to have follow-up studies, which will provide specific comparisons to previous studies. A low PSV obtained throughout the graft could suggest an arterial inflow dysfunction. It is generally believed that the venous anastomosis and outflow veins are the most common sites of stenosis in these grafts, which can be caused by an increased arterial pressure introduced through the vein and/or intima hyperplasia. Occasionally, steal syndrome can be observed whereby the distal arterial blood flow is reversed into the venous circulation of the lower systems. This can be manifested by pain on exertion of the affected extremity as well as pallor and coolness of the skin distal to the shunt.

Table 32–1 summarizes a generally agreed upon interpretation criteria that is adapted from an Advanced Technology Laboratory manual.

Volume Flow Criteria

Low blood flow volume through a hemodialysis graft can be predictive of graft failure. A noninvasively derived

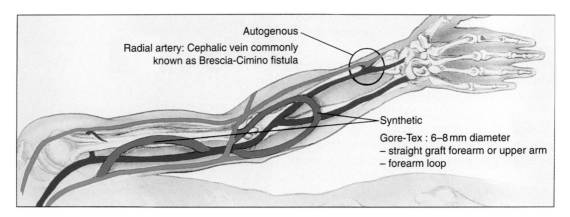

FIGURE 32–9. Illustration showing various AV grafts. As noted in this figure, these grafts can be autogenous (radial artery to cephalic vein) or synthetic (Gore-Tex graft between the brachial artery and the antecubital vein or between the brachial artery and the distal axillary or proximal brachial veins).

TABLE 32–1. Dialysis access graft imaging: interpretation criteria.

Classification	Velocity (cm/s)		Image characteristics
Normal	Mid graft >150 cm/s	Anastomotic sites >300 cm/s	No visible narrowing. Distended outflow veins. Aneurysms, puncture sites, perigraft fluid may be visible
Moderate stenosis	Mid graft 100–150 cm/s	Anastomotic sites >300 cm/s at stenosis	Decrease in lumen diameter. Echogenic narrowing. Wall abnormalities
Severe stenosis	Mid graft <100 cm/s		Intraluminal echogenicity. <2 mm lumen. >50% diameter reduction. Marked velocity acceleration. Marked reduction in lumen diameter with color Doppler
Inflow stenosis	Inflow anastomosis site >300 cm/s with turbulence. Monophasic spectra with graft compression	Mid graft <100 cm/s. No velocity acceleration at outflow anastomosis	Intraluminal echogenicity. <2 mm lumen at velocity acceleration
Outflow stenosis	Inflow anastomosis site <300 cm/s (decreases as distal stenosis progresses). Mid graft <100 cm/s	Focal velocity acceleration (could be mild, outflow, or distal vein). >300 cm/s	Intraluminal echogenicity. <2 mm lumen velocity acceleration. Prominent collateral veins around outflow
Occlusion	No Doppler signal		Intraluminal echogenicity. Graft walls appear collapsed. Occluded vein may not be visible

value of <450 ml/min has been associated with graft stenosis or dysfunction and impending failure, and some investigators use this finding as additional diagnostic criteria. However, it is to be noted that determination of the flow volume through a graft can produce variable results due to variations in technique and instrumentation as well as fundamental limitations of Doppler for this procedure.

Interpretation Pitfalls

This includes the following: low systemic pressure, poor Doppler angle, central venous stenosis or occlusion, well-collateralized occlusion, velocity acceleration without lumen reduction, and degree of stenosis is not absolute in predicting access failure.[101,102] This subject will be covered in more depth in a later chapter.

Arterial Aneurysms

An arterial aneurysm is generally defined as an abnormal dilatation of an artery of equal to or more than one and a half of the normal adjacent arterial segments. These aneurysms can be true aneurysms, which is defined as a dilatation of all layers of the arterial wall, differentiating it from a pseudoaneurysm, which does not contain arterial wall layers, but rather is a pulsating hematoma completely separate from the artery except for the communicating neck or channel through which the blood travels to reach it. The false or pseudoaneurysm is usually secondary to an injury that produces a hole in the arterial wall that permits the blood to escape under pressure, generating a false aneurysm. Once the hematoma is formed, and if confined by the surrounding structures and if there is continuous blood flowing from the artery to this region, a false aneurysm is created that is covered by a fibrous capsule. These are usually secondary to arterial catheterization as seen after a cardiac catheterization or peripheral arterial interventions, particularly if a larger sheath is used.

A dissecting aneurysm occurs when a small tear of the intima allows the blood to form a cavity between the two walls, a new lumen (false lumen) is formed, and blood may flow through this lumen as well as through the original true lumen to supply branch arteries. This condition is usually secondary to weakening of the media of the

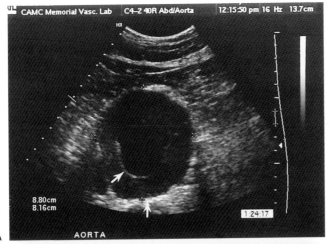

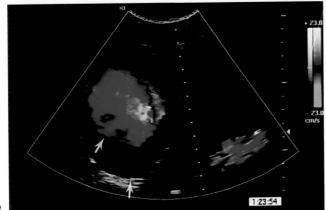

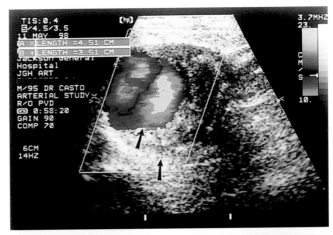

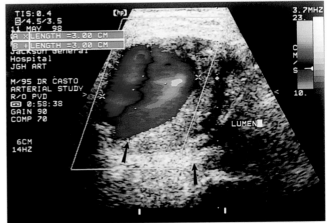

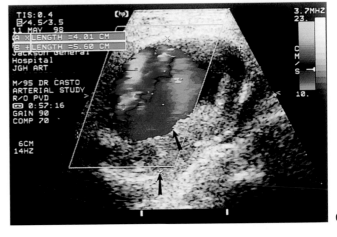

FIGURE 32–10. (A) A duplex ultrasound image of an abdominal aortic aneurysm measuring 8.8 cm in AP diameter and 8.16 cm in transverse diameter. Note the presence of thrombus between the inside and outside arrows. (B) A color duplex ultrasound image of the same abdominal aortic aneurysm showing the lumen as noted in color and the thrombus as indicated by arrows.

artery and the development of an intimal tear through which the blood then leaks into the media. Arterial dissection is most often seen or noted in the thoracic aorta, which may not be secondary to atherosclerosis.

The most common location of arterial aneurysms is the infrarenal abdominal aorta (Figure 32–10), but they can occur in nearly any artery of the body. Peripheral arterial aneurysms are commonly seen in the femoral and popliteal artery regions. These peripheral aneurysms can be bilateral (over 50%), as seen in Figures 32–11 and 32–12.

The causes of aneurysms are unknown, but may include atherosclerosis, poor arterial nutrition, congenital defects, infection, and iatrogenic injury. Aneurysms are usually fusiform, i.e., diffuse circumferential dilatation of the arterial segment, but can be saccular. The major complications of arterial aneurysms include rupture and

FIGURE 32–11. (A) A color duplex ultrasound image showing a right common femoral artery aneurysm in transverse view that measures around 4.51 cm in transverse diameter and 3.51 cm in AP diameter. Note the presence of thrombus between the outside wall as indicated by the outside arrow, and the inside lumen as indicated by the inside arrow. (B) A color duplex ultrasound image showing the same patient as in (A) with measurement of the inside lumen (3 cm in transverse diameter and 3 cm in AP diameter). Note the thrombus between the inside lumen and the outside wall (arrows). (C) A color duplex ultrasound image showing the same patient as in (A) with an aneurysm measuring 5.6 cm in length and 4.01 cm in AP diameter (longitudinal view).

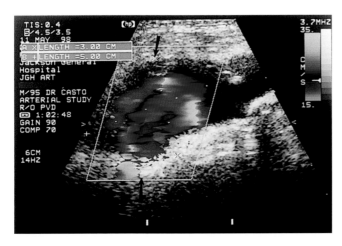

FIGURE 32–12. A color duplex ultrasound image of the same patient as in Figure 32–11A showing another aneurysm of the left common femoral artery that measures 5 cm in length and 3 cm in AP view.

distal embolizations. As noted in Figures 32–10, 32–11, and 32–12, these aneurysms have the propensity to form thrombotic material at the walls.

Abdominal aortic aneurysms are usually discovered incidentally in about 50% of patients, i.e., asymptomatic patients, 25% of patients present with symptoms that may vary from abdominal and/or back pain, and the remaining 25% of patients present with rupture with the classical triad of abdominal or back pain, pulsating mass, and hypotension. Peripheral arterial aneurysms can also be discovered incidentally as a pulsating mass, or can present with distal arterial embolization. The diagnosis is usually confirmed by B-mode ultrasonography or duplex ultrasound (Figures 32–10, 32–11, and 32–12). Other modalities used to confirm aneurysms include CT scanning and magnetic resonance imaging. This subject will be covered in more depth in a later chapter.

Endothelial Dysfunction

Long before atherosclerosis becomes clinically manifest, endothelial dysfunction is evident and can be demonstrated by changes in brachial artery size during reactive hyperemia. The fact that brachial artery dysfunction correlates with coronary artery dysfunction is an important discovery.[103]

References

1. Supplement to Circulation. Chronic critical leg ischemia. Circulation 1991;84:IV-1–IV-26.
2. Weitz JI, Byrne J, Clagett GP, et al. Diagnosis and treatment of chronic arterial insufficiency of the lower extremities: A critical review. Circulation 1996;94:3026–3049.
3. AbuRahma AF. Noninvasive assessment of critical leg ischemia. In: Bartolucci R, Battaglia L, D'Andrea V, De Antoni E (eds). Critical Lower Limb Ischemia—Principles and Practice, pp. 99–114. Rome: Nuova Editrice Grafica, 2002.
4. Feigelson HS, Criqui MH, Fronek A, et al. Screening for peripheral arterial disease: The sensitivity, specificity, and predictive value of noninvasive tests in a defined population. Am J Epidemiol 1994;140:526–534.
5. Ray SA, Srodon PD, Taylor RS, et al. Reliability of ankle:brachial pressure index measurement by junior doctors. Br J Surg 1994;81:188–190.
6. AbuRahma AF, Diethrich EB. The Doppler testing in peripheral vascular occlusive disease. Surg Gynecol Obstet 1980;150:26–28.
7. AbuRahma AF, Diethrich EB. The Doppler ultrasound in evaluating the localization and severity of peripheral vascular occlusive disease. South Med J 1979;72:1425–1428.
8. Raines JK, Darling RC, Buth J, et al. Vascular laboratory criteria for the management of peripheral vascular disease of the lower extremities. Surgery 1976;79:21–29.
9. Toursarkissian B, Mejia A, Smilanich RP, Schoolfield J, Shireman PK, Sykes MT. Noninvasive localization of infrainguinal arterial occlusive disease in diabetics. Ann Vasc Surg 2001;15:73–78.
10. Holland T. Utilizing the ankle brachial index in clinical practice. Ostomy Wound Manage 2002;48:38–40.
11. Adam DJ, Naik J, Hartshorne T, Bello M, London NJ. The diagnosis and management of 689 chronic leg ulcers in a single-visit assessment clinic. Eur J Vasc Endovasc Surg 2003;25:462–468.
12. AbuRahma AF, Khan S, Robinson PA. Selective use of segmental Doppler pressures and color duplex imaging in the localization of arterial occlusive disease of the lower extremity. Surgery 1995;118:496–503.
13. Kempczinski RF. Segmental volume plethysmography: The pulse volume recorder. In: Kempczinski RF, Yao JST (eds). Practical Noninvasive Vascular Diagnosis, pp. 105–117. Chicago: Year Book Medical Publishers, 1982.
14. Koelemay MJ, Legemate DA, de Vos H, van Gurp AJ, Balm R, Reekers JA, Jacobs MJ. Duplex scanning allows selective use of arteriography in the management of patients with severe lower leg arterial disease. J Vasc Surg 2001;34:661–667.
15. Lewis JD. Pressure measurements in the long-term follow-up of peripheral vascular disease. Proc R Soc Med 1974;67:443–444.
16. Strandness DE Jr, Stahler C. Arteriosclerosis obliterans. Manner and rate of progression. JAMA 1966;196:1–4.
17. Wilson SE, Schwartz I, Williams RA, et al. Occlusion of the superficial femoral artery: What happens without operation. Am J Surg 1980;140:112–118.
18. Paaske WP, Tonnesen KH. Prognostic significance of distal blood pressure measurements in patients with severe ischemia. Scand J Thorac Cardiovasc Surg 1980;14:105–108.
19. Nicoloff AD, Taylor LM Jr, Sexton GJ, Schuff RA, Edwards JM, Yeager RA, Landry GJ, Moneta GL, Porter JM. Hemocysteine and progression of atherosclerosis

study investigators. Relationship between site of initial symptoms and subsequent progression of disease in a prospective study of atherosclerosis progression in patients receiving long-term treatment for symptomatic peripheral arterial disease. J Vasc Surg 2002;35:38–46.

20. Prineas RJ, Harland WR, Janzon L, et al. Recommendations for use of noninvasive methods to detect atherosclerotic peripheral arterial disease—in population studies. Circulation 1982;65:1561A–1566A.

21. Janzon L, Bergentz SE, Ericsson BF, et al. The arm-ankle pressure gradient in relation to cardiovascular risk factors in intermittent claudication. Circulation 1981;63:1339–1341.

22. Beach KW, Brunzell JD, Strandness De Jr. Prevalence of severe arteriosclerosis obliterans in patients with diabetes mellitus. Arteriosclerosis 1982;2:275–280.

23. Criqui MH, Fronek A, Barrett-Connor E, et al. The prevalence of peripheral arterial disease in a defined population. Circulation 1985;71:510–515.

24. Hiatt WR, Marshall JA, Baxter J, et al. Diagnostic methods for peripheral arterial disease in the San Luis Valley diabetes study. J Clin Epidemiol 1990;43:597–606.

25. McLafferty RB, Moneta GL, Taylor LM, et al. Ability of ankle-brachial index to detect lower extremity atherosclerotic disease progression. Arch Surg 1997;132:836–841.

26. Gundersen J. Segmental measurements of systolic blood pressure in the extremities including the thumb and the great toe. Acta Chir Scand 1972;426:1–9.

27. Postlethwaite JC, Dormandy JA. Results of ankle systolic pressure measurements in patients with intermittent claudication being treated with clofibrate. Ann Surg 1975;181:799–802.

28. Quick CR, Cotton LT. The measured effect of stopping smoking on intermittent claudication. Br J Surg 1982;69:S24–S26.

29. Kempczinski RF, Buckley CJ, Darling RC. Vascular insufficiency secondary to ergotism. Surgery 1976;79:597–600.

30. Ascher E, Hingorani A, Markevich N, Costa T, Kallakuri S, Khanimoy Y. Lower extremity revascularization without preoperative contrast arteriography: Experience with duplex ultrasound arterial mapping in 485 cases. Ann Vasc Surg 2002;16:108–114.

31. Ascher E, Hingorani A, Markevich N, Schutzer R, Kallakuri S. Acute lower limb ischemia: The value of duplex ultrasound arterial mapping (DUAM) as the sole preoperative imaging technique. Ann Vasc Surg 2003;17:284–289.

32. O'Donnell TF, Cossman D, Callow AD. Noninvasive intraoperative monitoring: A prospective study comparing Doppler systolic occlusion pressure and segmental plethysmography. Am J Surg 1978;135:539–546.

33. Baird RN, Davies PW, Bird DR. Segmental air plethysmography during arterial reconstruction. Br J Surg 1979;66:718–722.

34. Standards of Practice Committee of the Society of Cardiovascular and Interventional Radiology. Guidelines for PTA. Radiology 1990;177:619.

35. van der Heijden FH, Legemate DA, van Leeuwen MS, Mali WP, Eikelboom BC. Value of duplex scanning in the selection of patients for percutaneous transluminal angioplasty. Eur J Vasc Surg 1993;7:71–76.

36. Whelan JF, Barry MH, Moir JD. Color flow Doppler ultrasonography: Comparison with peripheral arteriography for the investigation of peripheral vascular disease. J Clin Ultrasound 1992;20:369–374.

37. Garrett WV, Slaymaker EE, Heintz SE. Intraoperative prediction of symptomatic result of aortofemoral bypass from changes in ankle pressure index. Surgery 1977;82:504–509.

38. Brener BJ, Brief DK, Alpert J. Clinical usefulness of noninvasive arterial studies. Contemp Surg 1980;16:41–55.

39. Dean RH, Yao JST, Stanton PE, et al. Prognostic indicators in femoropopliteal reconstructions. Arch Surg 1975;110:1287–1293.

40. Corson JD, Johnson WC, LoGerfo FW, et al. Doppler ankle systolic blood pressure. Prognostic value in vein bypass grafts of the lower extremity. Arch Surg 1978;113:932–935.

41. Rutherford RB. Standards for evaluating results of interventional therapy for peripheral vascular disease. Circulation 1991;83:I-6–I-11.

42. Tooke JE. European consensus document on critical limb ischaemia. Vasc Med Rev 1990;1:85–89.

43. Boren CH, Towne JB, Bernhard VM, et al. Profunda-popliteal collateral index. A guide to successful profundaplasty. Arch Surg 1980;115:1366–1372.

44. Strandness DE Jr, Sumner DS. Hemodynamics for Surgeons, pp. 573–582. New York: Grune & Stratton, Inc., 1975.

45. Yao JST, Bergan JJ. Predictability of vascular reactivity to sympathetic ablation. Arch Surg 1973;107:676–680.

46. Walker PM, Johnston KW. Predicting the success of a sympathectomy: A prospective study using discriminant function and multiple regression analysis. Surgery 1980;87:216–221.

47. AbuRahma AF, Robinson P. Clinical parameters for predicting response to lumbar sympathectomy with severe lower limb ischemia. J Cardiovasc Surg 1990;31:101–106.

48. Tiutiunnik AA. The significance of laser Doppler flowmetry for the prognosis and outcome evaluation of lumbar sympathectomy in patients with obliterating vascular arteriosclerosis of lower extremities. Klin Khir 2003;3:49–51.

49. Berkowitz HD, Hobbs, CL, Roberts B, et al. Value of routine vascular laboratory studies to identify vein graft stenosis. Surgery 1981;90:971–979.

50. Bandyk DF, Schmitt DD, Seabrook GR, et al. Monitoring functional patency of in situ saphenous vein bypasses: The impact of a surveillance protocol and elective revision. J Vasc Surg 1989;286–296.

51. Calligaro K, Doerr K, McAffee-Bennett S, Krug R, Raviola CA, Dougherty MJ. Should duplex ultrasonography be performed for surveillance of femoropopliteal and femorotibial arterial prosthetic bypasses? Ann Vasc Surg 2001;15:520–524.

52. Carter SA. The relationship of distal systolic pressures to healing of skin lesions in the limbs with arterial occlusive disease with special reference to diabetes mellitus. Scand J Clin Lab Invest 1973;128(suppl 31):239–243.

53. Ramsey DE, Manke DA, Sumner DS. Toe blood pressure—valuable adjunct to ankle pressure measurement for assessing peripheral arterial disease. J Cardiovasc Surg 1983;24:43–48.

54. Robbs JV, Ray R. Clinical predictors of below-knee stump healing following amputation for ischemia. South Afr J Surg 1982;20:305–310.

55. van den Broek TA, Dwars BJ, Rauwerda JA, et al. A multivariate analysis of determinants of wound healing in patient after amputation for peripheral vascular disease. Eur J Vasc Surg 1990;4:291–295.

56. Apelqvist J, Castenfors J, Larsson J, et al. Prognostic value of systolic ankle and toe blood pressure levels in outcome of diabetic foot ulcer. Diabetes Care 1989;12:373–378.

57. Barnes RW, Thornhill B, Nix L. Prediction of amputation wound healing. Roles of Doppler ultrasound and digit photoplethysmography. Arch Surg 1981;116:80–83.

58. Verta MJ Jr, Gross WS, VanBellen B, et al. Forefoot perfusion pressure and minor amputation for gangrene. Surgery 1976;80:729–734.

59. Nicholas GG, Myers JL, DeMuth WE, Jr. The role of vascular laboratory criteria in the selection of patients for lower extremity amputation. Ann Surg 1982;195:469–473.

60. Baker WH, Barnes RW. Minor forefoot amputations in patients with low ankle pressure. Am J Surg 1977;133:331–332.

61. Cheng EY. Lower extremity amputation level: Selection using noninvasive hemodynamic methods of evaluation. Arch Phys Med Rehabil 1982;63:475–479.

62. Holloway GA Jr. Cutaneous blood flow responses to infection trauma measured by laser Doppler velocimetry. J Invest Dermatol 1980;74:1–4.

63. Malone JM, Anderson GG, Lalka SG, et al. Prospective comparison of noninvasive techniques for amputation level selection. Am J Surg 1987;154:179–184.

64. Schwartz JA, Schuler JJ, O'Conner RJ, et al. Predictive value of distal perfusion pressure in the healing of amputation of the digits and the forefoot. Surg Gynecol Obstet 1982;154:865–869.

65. Burgess EM, Matsen FA, Wyss CR, et al. Segmental transcutaneous measurements of PO2 in patients requiring below the knee amputations for peripheral vascular insufficiency. J Bone Joint Surg (Am) 1982;64:378–382.

66. Christensen KS, Klarke M. Transcutaneous oxygen measurement in peripheral occlusive disease: An indicator of wound healing in leg amputation. J Bone Joint Surg (Br) 1986;68:423–426.

67. Harward TR, Volny J, Golbranson F, et al. Oxygen inhalation induced transcutaneous PO2 changes as a predictor of amputation level. J Vasc Surg 1985;2:220–227.

68. Lee TQ, Barnett SL, Shanfield SL, et al. Potential application of photoplethysmography technique in evaluating microcirculatory status of STAMP patients: Preliminary report. J Rehabil Red Dev 1990;27:363–368.

69. Wyss CR, Harrington RM, Burgess EM, et al. Transcutaneous oxygen tension as a predictor of success after an amputation. J Bone Joint Surg (Am) 1988;70:203–207.

70. Graham BH, Walton RL, Elings VB, et al. Surface quantification of injection fluorescein as a predictor of flap viability. Plast Reconstr Surg 1983;71:826–833.

71. McFarland DC, Lawrence FF. Skin fluorescence: A method to predict amputation site healing. J Surg Res 1982;32:410–415.

72. Silverman DG, Roberts A, Reilly CA, et al. Fluorometric quantification of low-dose fluorescein delivery to predict amputation site healing. Surgery 1987;101:335–341.

73. Holloway GA Jr, Burgess EM. Preliminary experiences with laser Doppler velocimetry for the determination of amputation levels. Prosthet Orthot Int 1983;7:63–66.

74. Golbranson FL, Yu EC, Gelberman HH. The use of skin temperature determination in lower extremity amputation level selection. Foot Ankle 1982;3:170–172.

75. Dwars BJ, Rauwerda JA, van den Broek TA, et al. A modified scintigraphic technique for amputation level selection in diabetics. Eur J Nucl Med 1989;15:38–41.

76. Holstein P, Trep-Jensen J, Bagger H, et al. Skin perfusion pressure measured by isotope wash out in legs with arterial occlusive disease. Clin Physiol 1983;3:313–324.

77. Stockel M, Ovesen J, Brochner-Mortensen J, et al. Standardized photoelectric techniques as routine method for selection of amputation level. Acta Orthop Scand 1982;53:875–878.

78. Silverman DG, Rubin SM, Reilly CA, et al. Fluorometric prediction of successful amputation level in the ischemic limb. J Rehabil Res Dev 1985;22:23–28.

79. Barnes RW, Chanik GD, Slaymaker EE. An index of healing in below-knee amputation: Leg blood pressure by Doppler ultrasound. Surgery 1976;79:13–20.

80. Bone GE, Pomajzl MJ. Toe blood pressure by photoplethysmography: An index of healing in forefront amputation. Surgery 1981;89:569–574.

81. Dale WA, Lewis MR. Management of thoracic outlet syndrome. Ann Surg 1975;181:575–585.

82. Gillard J, Perez-Cousin M, Hachulla E, Remy J, Hurtevent JF, Vinckier L, Thevenon A, Duquesnoy B. Diagnosing thoracic outlet syndrome: Contribution of provocative tests, ultrasonography, electrophysiology, and helical computed tomography in 48 patients. Join Bone Spine 2001;68:416–424.

83. Wadhwani R, Chaubal N, Sukthankar R, Shroff M, Agarwala S. Color Doppler and duplex sonography in 5 patients with thoracic outlet syndrome. J Ultrasound Med 2001;20:795–801.

84. Darling RC, Buckley CJ, Abbott WM, et al. Intermittent claudication in young athletes: Popliteal artery entrapment syndrome. J Trauma 1974;14:543–552.

85. Abbas M. Calydon M, Ponosh S, Theophilus M, Angel D, Tripathi R, Prendergast F, Sieunarine K. Sonographic diagnosis in iatrogenic entrapment of a femoropopliteal bypass graft. J Ultrasound Med 2004;23:859–863.

86. Kempczinski RF. Role of the vascular diagnostic laboratory in the evaluation of male impotence. Am J Surg 1979;138:278–282.

87. Britt DB, Kemmerer WT, Robison JR. Penile blood flow determination by mercury strain gauge plethysmography. Invest Urol 1971;8:673–678.

88. Ramirez C, Box M, Gottesman L. Noninvasive vascular evaluation in male impotence. Technique. Bruit 1980;4: 14–19.

89. Nath RL, Menzoian JD, Kaplan KH, et al. The multidisciplinary approach to vasculogenic impotence. Surgery 1981;89:124–133.

90. Quam JP, King BF, James EM, et al. Duplex and color Doppler sonographic evaluation of vasculogenic impotence. AJR 1989;153:1141–1147.

91. Benson CB, Vickers MA. Sexual impotence caused by vascular disease: Diagnosis with duplex sonography. AJR 1989;153:1149–1153.

92. Paushter DM. Role of duplex sonography in the evaluation of sexual impotence. AJR 1989;153:1161–1163.

93. Aversa A, Caprio M, Spera G, Fabbri A. Non-invasive vascular imaging for erectile dysfunction. J Endocrinol Invest 2003;26:122–124.

94. Mancini M, Negri L, Maggi M, Nerva F, Forti G, Colpi GM. Doppler color ultrasonography in the diagnosis of erectile dysfunction of vascular origin. Arch Ital Urol Androl 2000;72:361–365.

95. Roy C, Saussine C, Tuchmann C, Castel E, Lang H, Jacqmin D. Duplex Doppler sonography of the flaccid penis: Potential role in the evaluation of impotence. J Clin Ultrasound 2000;28:290–294.

96. Altinkilic B, Hauck EW, Weidner W. Evaluation of penile perfusion by color-coded duplex sonography in the man-agement of erectile dysfunction. World J Urol 2004;22: 361–364.

97. Sumner DS, Strandness DE Jr. An abnormal finger pulse associated with cold sensitivity. Ann Surg 1972;175:294–298.

98. Szilagyi DE, Smith RF, Elliott JP, et al. Congenital arteriovenous anomalies of the limbs. Arch Surg 1976;111:423–429.

99. Rutherford E, Fleming PW, McLeod FD. Vascular diagnostic methods for evaluating patients with arteriovenous fistulas. In: Diethrich EB (ed). Noninvasive Cardiovascular Diagnosis, pp. 217–230. Baltimore: University Park Press, 1978.

100. Pearce WH, Rutherford RB, Whitehill TA, et al. Nuclear magnetic resonance imaging: Its diagnostic value in patients with congenital vascular malformations of the limbs. J Vasc Surg 1988;8:64–70.

101. Rittgers SE, Garcia-Valdez C, McCormick JT, et al. Non-invasive blood flow measurement in expanded polytetra-fluoroethylene grafts for hemodialysis access. J Vasc Surg 1986;3:635–642.

102. Tordoir JH, Hoeneveld H, Eikelboom BC, et al. The correlation between clinical and duplex ultrasound parameters and the development of complications in arteriovenous fistulas for hemodialysis. Eur J Vasc Surg 1990;4: 179–184.

103. Anderson TJ, Uehata A, Gerhard MD, et al. Close relation of endothelial function in the human coronary and peripheral circulations. J Am Coll Cardiol 1995;26:1235–1241.

Section V
Noninvasive Diagnosis of Venous Disorders of the Extremities

33
Overview of Venous Disorders

John J. Bergan

Anatomy

The term venous disorders implies that normal functioning is deranged. To understand the various venous disorders, it is necessary to start with an understanding of the normal anatomy (Table 33–1). The venous system of the lower extremities can be divided, for purposes of understanding, into three systems: the deep venous system, the superficial venous system, and the connecting veins, which are called perforating veins. The principal return of blood flow from the lower extremities is through the deep veins. In the calf, the deep veins are paired and named for the accompanying arteries. Therefore, the anterior tibial, posterior tibial, and peroneal artery are accompanied by their paired veins, which are interconnected. These join to form the popliteal vein, which may also be paired. As the popliteal vein ascends, it becomes the femoral vein.[1] Near the groin, this is joined by the deep femoral vein, which becomes the common femoral vein and then the external iliac vein proximal to the inguinal ligament. The superficial venous system of the lower extremities consists of two axial veins, the great and small saphenous veins, and many interconnecting tributaries, the communicating veins. The great saphenous vein begins on the dorsum of the foot and it ascends anterior to the medial malleolus at the ankle and anteromedial to the tibia. At the knee, the great saphenous vein is found in the medial aspect of the popliteal space. It then ascends in the anteromedial thigh to join the common femoral vein just below the inguinal ligament.

In 2001, an International Interdisciplinary Committee was designated by the Presidents of the International Union of Phlebology (IUP) and the International Federation of Anatomical Associations to update the official Terminologia Anatomica.[2] The Committee with the participation of Members of the Federative International Committee for Anatomical Nomenclature (FICAT) outlined a Consensus Document at a meeting held in Rome on the occasion of the 14th World Congress of the IUP. Terminological recommendations of the Committee were published[3] and these new, possibly unfamiliar terms are used throughout this chapter.

Throughout its course, the great saphenous vein is deep to the superficial fascia and superficial to the deep, muscular fascia. This enclosure is called the saphenous compartment.[4] It receives many tributaries, nearly all of which are superficial, to the superficial fascia. The small saphenous vein originates laterally from the dorsal venous arch of the foot and travels subcutaneously behind the lateral malleolus at the ankle. As it ascends in the calf, it enters deep to the deep fascia and ascends between the heads of the gastrocnemius muscle to join the popliteal vein behind the knee. There are many variations of the small saphenous vein connections to the popliteal vein in the popliteal fossa.

The third system of veins in the lower extremity is the perforating vein system. This connects the superficial to the deep venous system. These veins penetrate anatomic layers, which gives them the name perforating veins. Veins that interconnect on the same anatomic layer are called communicating veins. In the leg, and using the now disfavored eponyms, the principal perforating veins have been named for an English surgeon, Frank Cockett. The Cockett I perforating vein is approximately 6 cm, measured from the floor in the standing patient. The Cockett II perforating vein clusters at about 12 cm, and the Cockett III is at 18 cm. These, and the 24 cm perforating vein, may need to be identified as tibial perforating veins in limbs with severe chronic venous insufficiency as they become targets for the surgeon. These perforating veins connect the posterior arch circulation to the posterior tibial veins.

In the upper anteromedial calf, a perforating vein is found and in the distal thigh, there are perforating veins. Above these in the mid-thigh, the perforating veins are named for John Hunter (Figure 33–1).

TABLE 33–1. Important changes in nomenclature of lower extremity veins.

Old terminology	New terminology
Femoral vein	Common femoral vein
Superficial femoral vein	Femoral vein
Sural veins	Sural veins
	Soleal veins
	Gastrocnemius veins (medial and lateral)
Huntarian perforator	Mid thigh perforator
Cockett's perforators	Paratibial perforator
	Posterior tibial perforators
May's perforator	
Gastrocnemius point	Intergemellar perforator

TABLE 33–2. Venous disorders.

Acute
Superficial
Deep
Chronic
Primary venous insufficiency
   Telangiectasias
   Reticular veins
   Varicose veins
Secondary (Postthrombotic)
   Venous obstruction
   Venous reflux
Chronic venous insufficiency (CVI) (hyperpigmentation, edema, lipodermatosclerosis, cutaneous ulceration)

Venous Disorders

Terms used to describe the various manifestations of venous disorders lend confusion to the general topic. Some of these terms, such as phlegmasia cerulea dolens and superficial thrombophlebitis, are descriptive. Others memorialize largely dead physicians such as May-Thurner and Paget-von Schröetter. Order can be made out of apparent chaos by dividing venous disorders that are acute from those that are chronic. The acute disorders are largely thrombotic and may produce relatively severe manifestations (Table 33–2). For purposes of orientation, prognostication, and therapy, these can be divided into superficial and deep venous thrombosis. It is in the

chronic disorders, dominated by venous reflux through failed check valves, that disorientation reigns.

Primary Venous Insufficiency

The manifestations of simple primary venous insufficiency appear to be different from one another. However, reticular varicosities, telangiectasias, and major varicose veins are all elongated, dilated veins with incompetent valves. They respond to the same physical forces and acquired influences that cause the abnormality. Dilation and elongation are responses to abnormal forces. These responses are influenced by a hereditary predisposition, the effect of progesterone, which prevents smooth muscle contraction, weakness in the venous wall, and valvular abnormalities. Very little can be done to change either the

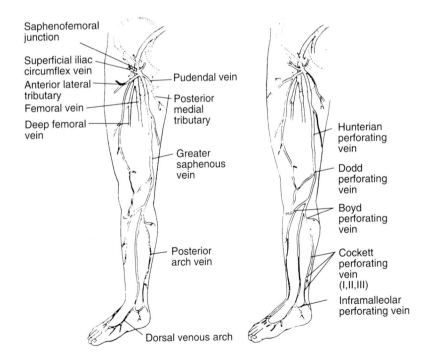

FIGURE 33–1. The main superficial veins and perforating veins. Note that the Cockett perforating veins are part of the posterior arch circulation and that important tributaries to the saphenous vein at the groin include the anterolateral and posteromedial tributaries, either of which may simulate a duplication of the saphenous circulation.

hereditary predisposition or the effect of progesterone on veins. However, investigations into venous wall abnormalities and valvular damage may eventually lead to an understanding of the problem, and, therefore, a solution by surgery or pharmacotherapy.

Scanning electron microscopy has shown varying degrees of thinning of the varicose venous wall. These areas of thinning coincide with areas of varicose dilation, and replacement of smooth muscle by collagen is also a characteristic of varicose veins.[5]

Our approach to this has been to assume that both the venous valve and the venous wall are affected by the elements that cause varicose veins. We and others have observed that in limbs with varicose veins, an absence of the subterminal valve at the saphenofemoral junction is common.[6] Further, perforation, splitting, and atrophy of saphenous venous valves have been seen both by angioscopy and by direct examination of surgical specimens.[7] Supporting the theory of weakness of the venous wall leading to valvular insufficiency is the observation that there is an increase in the vein wall space between the valve leaflets. This is the first and most commonly observed abnormality associated with valve reflux.[8,9] Realizing these facts, our investigations have led us to explore the possible role of leukocyte infiltration of venous valves and the venous wall as part of the cause of varicose veins. In our investigations of surgical specimens, leukocytes in great number have been observed in the venous valves and wall and monoclonal antibody staining has revealed their precise identification as monocytes.[10]

Chronic Venous Insufficiency

The discussion above refers to primary venous insufficiency. The clinical manifestations of severe chronic venous insufficiency (CVI) are somewhat different. Some time ago these were all classified as secondary or postthrombotic venous insufficiency. Later, it was realized that many limbs with severe skin changes had never experienced venous thrombosis—hence, the term chronic venous insufficiency. Among the earliest findings in CVI is hyperpigmentation. This has been found to be caused by red cell extravasation and hemosiderin deposition. This appears wherever inflammation has been manifest in the skin. That is, inflammation causes hyperpigmentation. The second manifestation of CVI is induration of the epidermis, dermis, and subcutaneous tissues. The term lipodermatosclerosis has been applied to this. This serves not only as a definition but as a description of the process. Investigations by histologic techniques and capillary microscopy have shown an apparent capillary proliferation. This is actually best explained by elongation of a single capillary loop rather than an increase in the number of capillaries. Such elongation does increase

the surface area of endothelium. Immunohistochemical investigations have revealed a pericapillary cuff that contains collagen IV, laminin, fibronectin, and tenascin in addition to fibrin. The endothelium of these capillaries expresses an increased amount of factor VIII-related antigen and adhesion molecules.[11] In particular, the intercellular adhesion molecule-I (ICAM-I) has been found. Endothelium expressing such adhesion molecules becomes a target for leukocytes, and a profound interstitial leukocyte infiltration has been identified in limbs of patients with venous ulcer.[12] These cells are further identified as macrophages and T-lymphocytes. Thus this can be thought of as a severe chronic inflammatory state (Figure 33–2).[9] Secondary venous insufficiency, or the true postphlebitic state, is caused by damage or destruction of venous conduits and their contained valves. The pathogenesis of the postthrombotic state is dominated by the phenomenon of reflux. Reflux in the postphlebitic limb is most important in the deep system. However, the superficial venous system is almost always involved and contributes by reflux to venous hypertension. Perforating veins that demonstrate outward flow, inward flow, or both inward and outward flow may transmit muscular compartment pressure outward or overload the deep venous system by directing refluxing blood inward into deep veins. In secondary venous insufficiency, a small fraction of the pathologic process is caused by residual venous occlusion. Venous occlusion is largely well compensated and not pathophysiologic. However, when it is of

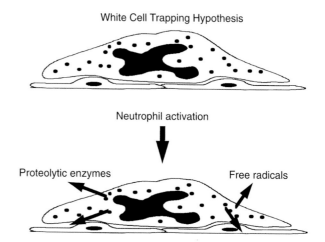

FIGURE 33–2. The causes of skin changes in chronic venous insufficiency are linked to white cell trapping. White cell endothelial interactions occur on the extended endothelial surface caused by precapillary venular elongation and dilation. White cells adhere under the influence of adhesion molecules and release proteolytic enzymes and free radicals as illustrated here. These, in turn, cause the tissue destruction that is manifested as the physical findings of chronic venous insufficiency. (Courtesy of Philip Coleridge Smith and the Middlesex Vascular Laboratory.)

importance physiologically, there is treatment available that can correct the observed abnormalities.

Acute Venous Disorders

As indicated above, acute venous disorders are entirely thrombotic. The differences in their manifestations are dictated by the venous bed that is affected. These cause syndromes to appear. Examples are superficial thrombophlebitis, acute deep venous thrombosis of the lower extremities, axillary subclavian venous thrombosis, and acute thrombosis of the portal venous system.

Superficial Thrombophlebitis

Superficial thrombophlebitis is a very commonly encountered pathologic entity. It may occur in nearly every patient who is hospitalized and certainly is dominant in patients receiving intravenous therapy. Its diagnosis is literally underneath the fingers of the examining hand as the cardinal signs of inflammation are nearly always present. These are calor, rubor, dolor, and tumor, which describe a linear, painful, erythematous swelling along the course of a superficial vein. The area is warm early on and cooler later. Similarly, it is tender early on and resolves into a cord-like structure later. The visible inflammation is usually aseptic, although it may occasionally be suppurative. The pathologic process does not require treatment by anticoagulation, corticosteroids, or antibiotics. It is best treated by limb elevation and elastic support, although some clinicians will advocate cooling with ice or warming with hotpacks. When the superficial thrombophlebitis is suppurative, it becomes a serious, potentially lethal complication that demands rapid intervention for removal of the affected vein. The most common pathogens are *Staphylococcus epidermidis*, *Staphylococcus aureus*, and *Pseudomonas*. Specialized forms of superficial thrombophlebitis include thrombophlebitis of varicose veins, migratory thrombophlebitis found in association with malignant tumor, and migratory thrombophlebitis associated with coagulopathies and/or Buerger disease. It is important to know that up to 20% of cases of superficial thrombophlebitis of the lower extremities are associated with deep venous thrombosis.

Acute Deep Venous Thrombosis

Risk factors in deep venous thrombosis are listed in Table 33–3. When thrombi develop in the deep venous system, the findings may include acute inflammation or an entirely bland pathologic process. While the thrombus does produce venous occlusion, such blockage may be partial or so well compensated that distal limb swelling does not occur. Therefore, diagnosis remains elusive except by imaging techniques. The findings of deep

TABLE 33–3. Risk factors for venous thromboembolism.

Age > 40 years
Obesity
Pelvic or multiple extremity trauma
Major abdominal surgery
Stroke/paraplegia
Congestive heart failure
Acute myocardial infarction
Malignancy
Oral contraceptives
Inflammatory bowel disease
Pregnancy

venous thrombosis will vary with the location of the thrombus as well as whether it occurs in isolated fashion or in multiple venous segments. It is the proximal iliofemoral veins that present the greatest risk for fatal pulmonary embolization, and it is the thrombi in distal or calf veins that present the least risk. In the past, it was thought that deep venous thrombosis inevitably caused chronic edema, hyperpigmentation, and other changes of CVI. Now it is well known that approximately one-third of thrombi will lyse quickly. In vein segments that experience total lysis within 3–5 days, valvular function is often maintained. Because of the risk for pulmonary embolization, urgent diagnosis is made by imaging techniques and treatment is given by immediate anticoagulation. Acute anticoagulation is achieved with heparin and chronic anticoagulation with warfarin. Thrombolytic therapy may be used in special clinical situations. Venous thrombectomy, long practiced on the European continent, has not found a sympathetic audience in North America and what little status it had has been largely replaced with aggressive catheter-directed thrombolysis.

Overview of Venous Disorders

Paget—von Schroeter Syndrome

While axillary subclavian venous thrombosis represents a small fraction of all cases of deep venous thrombosis, in fact it is an important clinical entity (Figure 33–3). In the past, it was thought to be benign and self-limiting, and conservative measures were advocated. More recently, it has been recognized that a considerable morbidity may occur and aggressive management is dominant in today's medical milieu. Similarly, in the past, spontaneous axillary subclavian venous thrombosis was referred to effort thrombosis and was associated with a variety of physical activities. Now, because of central lines and pacemaker wires, a more frequent cause is traumatic and iatrogenic. In fact, this element of axillary subclavian venous thrombosis is so common that it is believed that between one-third and two-thirds of patients with subclavian lines or

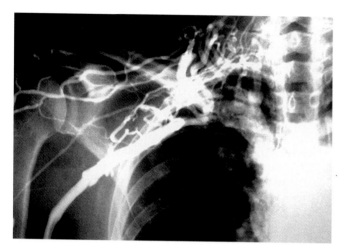

FIGURE 33–3. The pattern of occlusion in subclavian venous thrombosis. Note the profuse collateral circulation that has developed around the thrombus. The occlusion itself lies deep to the clavicular head just distal to the confluence of jugular and subclavian veins. Note the configuration of the valves in the axillary vein.

catheters develop deep venous thrombosis. Symptomatic patients with axillary subclavian venous thrombosis present with a swollen forearm, upper arm, and shoulder. A visible pattern of venous distention is present across the anterior aspect of the shoulder and chest wall. There may be venous distention of the antecubital veins as well as those in the hand. If a tender, palpable cord is present in the neck and/or axilla, this is due to a superficial thrombophlebitis accompanying the deep venous thrombosis. A bluish or cyanotic discoloration is commonly present in the hand and fingers, and an aching pain in the forearm exacerbated by exercise is also a common complaint. Some patients with upper extremity venous thrombosis will have abnormal clotting factors. The most important of these are listed in Table 33–4. While diagnosis of lower extremity deep venous thrombosis is dominated by imaging techniques and ultrasound, in fact, diagnosis of upper extremity venous thrombosis is dominated by catheter-directed phlebography because this can be followed by immediate infusion of lytic agents. This is done

TABLE 33–4. Abnormal clotting factors.

Antithrombin III deficiency
Protein C deficiency
Protein S deficiency
Activated protein C resistance
Factor V Leiden
Abnormal factor V cofactor activity
Dysfibrinogenemia
Hypoplasminoginemia
Hyperhomocysteinemia
Anticardiolipin antibody

to decrease the late sequelae of the venous occlusion. In the past, venous thrombectomy was done rarely, but now lytic therapy is applied frequently to spontaneous venous thrombosis. Secondary or catheter/pacemaker wire-induced venous thrombosis is allowed to undergo a normal developmental course.

Treatment after the acute event or after thrombolysis will vary from total thoracic outlet decompression by first rib resection and intraluminal stent placement to simple anticoagulation without intervention. Exact treatment will be prescribed according to the findings in each individual patient.

Thrombosis in the Portal Venous System

If thrombosis of the portal venous system is not recognized, the condition can be extremely serious and even fatal. However, modern methods of imaging have led to earlier diagnosis and therapy with anticoagulation, thus limiting the extent and seriousness of the condition. The symptoms are generally nonspecific but are entirely abdominal. They often follow a flu-like illness and the progression is slow with low-grade symptoms lasting more than 48 h in many cases. The most common symptoms are diffuse, nonspecific abdominal pain associated with a clinical appearance like a bowel obstruction with abdominal distention. The condition is primary when there are no associated conditions, but portal venous thrombosis also occurs in hypercoagulable states, cirrhosis, splenomegaly, abdominal malignancy, intraabdominal infection, pancreatitis, or even colon diverticular disease. Computed tomography (CT) scanning with contrast will reveal a portal vein with a hyperlucent wall and thrombus in the superior mesenteric vein. Bowel wall thickening, pneumatosis, or streaky mesentery may be present and are often late signs. Anticoagulation may halt the process but bowel necrosis will require resection.

Conclusions

This overview of venous disorders suggests dividing venous conditions into those that are acute and those that are chronic. The acute conditions are dominated by venous thrombosis, and these, in turn are classified according to the particular venous bed that is affected. Chronic venous disorders are dominated by venous reflux and can be divided into those that are primary and those that are secondary to thrombosis. In both instances, reflux is the dominating pathologic process, but specific individual chronic obstructive situations do arise and may call for direct venous reconstruction or venous intervention.

References

1. Bundens WP, Bergan JJ, Halasz NA, Murray J, Drehobl M. The superficial femoral vein: A potentially lethal misnomer. JAMA 1995;274:1296–1298.

2. Federative International Committee for Anatomical Terminology. *Terminologia Anatomica*. Stuttgart: George Thieme Verlag, 1998.

3. Caggiati A, Bergan JJ, Gloviczki P, Jantet G, Wendell-Smith CP, Partsch H; International Interdisciplinary Consensus Committee on Venous Anatomical Terminology. Nomenclature of the veins of the lower limbs: an international interdisciplinary consensus statement. J Vasc Surg 2002;36: 416–422.

4. Caggiati A. Fascial relationships of the long saphenous vein. Circulation 1999,100:2547–2549.

5. Mashiah A, Ross SS, Hod 1. The scanning electron microscope in the pathology of varicose veins. Isr J Med Sci 1991;27:202–206.

6. Travers JP, Brookes CE, Evans J, *et al.* Assessment of wall structure and composition of varicose veins with reference to collagen, elastin, and smooth muscle content. Eur J Vasc Endovasc Surg 1996;11:230–237.

7. Gradman WS, Segalowitz J, Grundfest W. Venoscopy in varicose vein surgery: Initial experience. Phlebology 1993;8: 145–150.

8. Van Cleef IF, Desvaux P, Hugentobler JP, *et al.* Endoscopie veineuse. J Mal Vasc 1991;16:184–187.

9. Van Cleef JF, Desvaux P, Hugentobler JP, *et al.* Etude endoscopique des reflux valvulaires sapheniens. J Mal Vasc 1992; 17:113–116.

10. Ono T, Bergan JJ, Schmid-Schönbein GW, Takase S. Monocyte infiltration into venous valves. J Vasc Surg 1998;27: 158–166.

11. Wilkinson LS, Bunker C, Edwards JC, Scurr JH, Coleridge Smith PD. Leukocytes: Their role in the etiopathogenesis of skin damage in venous disease. J Vasc Surg 1993;17:669–675.

12. Veraart JC, Verhaegh ME, Neumann HAM, Hulsmans RF, Arends JW. Adhesion molecule expression in venous leg ulcers. VASA 1993;22:213–218.

13. Herrick SE, Sloan P, McGurk M, Freak L, McCollum CN, Ferguson MW. Sequential changes in histologic pattern and extracellular matrix deposition during the healing of chronic venous ulcers. Am J Pathol 1992;141:1085–1095.

34
Overview: Plethysmographic Techniques in the Diagnosis of Venous Disease

M. Ashraf Mansour and David S. Sumner

Color-flow duplex scanning of the deep and superficial veins has largely replaced most other diagnostic testing. However, prior to the introduction of duplex scanning, plethysmography was the most widely used noninvasive method for the objective diagnosis of deep venous thrombosis (DVT). No other technique has been so thoroughly examined by so many distinguished investigators in the field. Its accuracy has been rigorously defined and documented by many carefully performed studies. Much valuable information concerning the prevalence, natural history, and clinical presentation of venous thrombosis has been acquired through the use of plethysmography.[1,2]

Nevertheless, plethysmography has a number of well-recognized limitations. It is insensitive to thrombi confined to the below-knee veins, profunda femoris vein, or internal iliac veins; may fail to detect nonocclusive thrombi, small clots, or clots in paired veins; provides little information concerning the distribution and extent of clots; and is limited in its ability to detect progression of disease or clot lysis.[3] These drawbacks were largely overcome by duplex imaging, which has now replaced plethysmography as the preferred method for detecting DVT in most vascular laboratories. Nonetheless, no text on noninvasive vascular diagnosis would be complete without a description of plethysmographic techniques for detecting DVT and venous reflux, if for no other reason than its historical importance. Furthermore, air plethysmography is now being used by some investigators to evaluate patients with chronic venous insufficiency (CVI) prior to intervention and for follow-up after surgical procedures.[4–6]

Plethysmographs

Plethysmography is a term derived from *Greek* and means to record (*graph* = write) an increase (*plethysmos* = increase). All plethysmographs measure the same thing, volume change. In the limbs, transient changes in volume are attributable to an increase or decrease in blood volume. Other tissues, bone, muscle, adipose tissue, and skin, have a relatively constant volume. Several of the various types of plethysmographs are adaptable to venous diagnostic studies. Air plethysmographs employ an air-filled cuff, which is proportional to the increase in limb volume. Mercury strain gauges use a fine Silastic tube filled with mercury or an indium-gallium alloy and are wrapped around the limb.[3] Changes in limb circumference produce a comparable change in the electrical resistance, which is proportional to relative volume change. Impedance plethysmographs consist of electrodes wrapped around the leg. An increase in blood volume decreases impedance and is amplified to reflect volume change. Thus, all methods measure changes in blood volume more or less indirectly.

Theory

Thrombi in the deep venous system increase venous outflow resistance and decrease venous compliance. These are the parameters that plethysmography measures as a means of detecting DVT. The increase in outflow resistance depends on whether the thrombi are totally or only partially occlusive, their length, the number of venous segments involved, and the location and extent of collateral development.[3] Clots located at bifurcation points or where collaterals originate or reenter the main venous tree are more likely to increase resistance than those in the midpoint of a long venous segment. Also clots in the profunda femoris or internal iliac veins, which are not part of the axial venous tree, have less effect on outflow resistance. Venous pressure distal to the site of thrombosis is elevated depending on the increase in outflow resistance. Since the volume of blood leaving the leg is ordinarily unchanged in the presence of a thrombus, the same volume of blood traversing an elevated

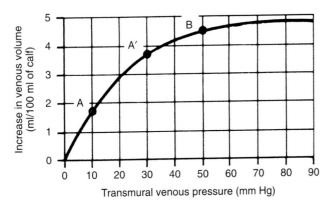

FIGURE 34–1. Calf venous pressure–volume curve. Pressure in the normal limb is low (A), but is elevated in the limb with acute deep venous thrombosis (A′). Inflating the thigh cuff to 50 mm Hg increases the volume of the normal limb by almost 3% (A to B); however, in the abnormal limb, the volume increase is less than 1% (A′ to B). [From Sumner DS: Diagnosis of deep vein thrombosis by strain-gauge plethysmography. In: Bernstein EF (ed). *Vascular Diagnosis.* St. Louis, MO: C.V. Mosby, 1993.]

resistance will result in an increase in venous pressure. If, however, clots are very extensive, involving both the deep and superficial systems, there may be a decrease in blood flow. This occurs in the condition known as phlegmasia cerulea dolens.

Thrombi may reduce apparent venous compliance in several ways. First, when venous pressure is already elevated, the volume of blood in veins peripheral to an obstruction is already increased, and further rise in venous pressure will result in less additional filling (Figure 34–1).[7] Second, venous walls become stiffer as they are distended by increased pressure. The third way is actually a reflection of the method used for measuring venous compliance. Compliance is usually measured as the volume change that occurs with a given rise in pressure divided by the baseline limb volume. If the veins are partially filled with thrombus, the degree to which they can expand by increasing their volume is limited since the residual capacity is limited. This might occur even when the venous elastic properties are unchanged. Since the potential for expansion is limited, the decreased volume change divided by the baseline volume makes the veins seem less compliant. Finally, another possible explanation for decreased compliance is that thrombi actually alter the elastic properties of venous walls, making them stiffer.

Venous Outflow Plethysmography

The volume sensor (air cuff, mercury strain gauge, or impedance electrodes) is placed around the calf or leg. An "occluding cuff" consisting of an air-filled bladder is wrapped around the thigh (Figures 34–2 and 34–3). When

this cuff is suddenly inflated to a pressure exceeding that in the underlying veins (usually about 50 mm Hg), venous outflow is prevented by the collapse of the veins.[8] Pressures of this level, which are well below diastolic arterial pressure, have little effect on the diameter of the underlying arteries. Since arterial inflow is not affected by cuff inflation, blood is trapped in the leg distal to the cuff until the venous pressure rises to equal that in the cuff. At this point, venous outflow resumes. When the veins are first occluded, the volume of blood in the calf rises in proportion to the rate of arterial inflow, gradually decreasing as the calf veins fill and their intraluminal pressure rises. Once venous pressure becomes equivalent to the cuff pressure, the calf volume ceases to increase and the recorded curve reaches a plateau (Figures 34–2 and 34–3).[9] The volume increase that occurs from baseline to the plateau is a measure of venous compliance.

Once a stable plateau is reached, the cuff is suddenly deflated, allowing the underlying thigh veins to expand. The blood trapped in the calf then rushes out, initially propelled by a pressure gradient equivalent to the 50 mm Hg developed during the time of occlusion. The initial rate of outflow, as reflected by the initial slope of the

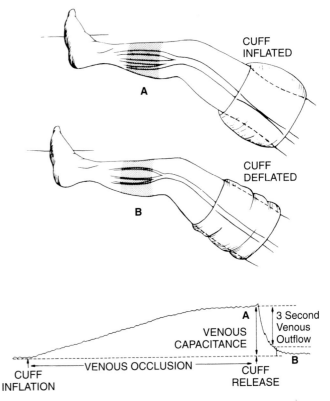

FIGURE 34–2. Venous outflow plethysmography. Above: correct positioning of the leg, cuff, and electrodes. Below: Typical normal tracing. [From Wheeler HB, Anderson FA Jr: Impedance plethysmography. In: Kempczinski RF, Yao JST (eds). *Practical Noninvasive Vascular Diagnosis.* Chicago: Year Book Medical Publishers, 1987. Permission requested.]

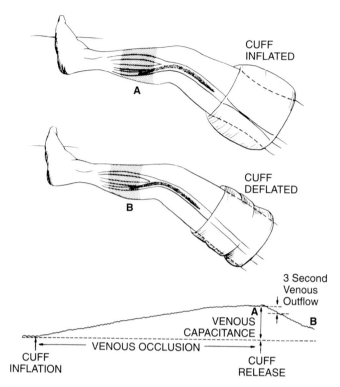

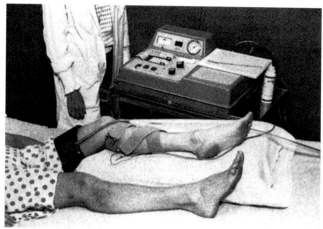

FIGURE 34–4. Impedance plethysmography (IPG): patient position.

FIGURE 34–3. Venous outflow plethysmography. Typical abnormal tracings. The 3-s outflow is markedly reduced with recent deep venous thrombosis. [From Wheeler HB, Anderson FA Jr: Diagnosis of DVT by impedance plethysmography. In: Bernstein EF (ed). *Vascular Diagnosis*. St. Louis, MO: C.V. Mosby, 1993. Permission requested.]

outflow curve, is inversely proportional to venous resistance. As blood leaves the calf, distal venous pressure falls, thus decreasing the pressure gradient and the rate of outflow. The outflow curve is, therefore, curvilinear, with the convexity facing the baseline (Figures 34–2 and 34–3). When the venous pressure again returns to the baseline level, the volume curve also returns to baseline.

Impedance Plethysmography

Technique

Examinations are performed with the patient supine. The leg being examined is elevated 20–30° to optimize venous drainage. This is accomplished by placing a pillow under the calf and heel (Figure 34–4). To ensure that the patient is relaxed and comfortable, the leg is allowed to rotate externally at the hip. The knee is flexed 10–20° to prevent compression of the popliteal vein. An 8-inch-wide pneumatic cuff is placed around the thigh and a set of two electrodes is wrapped around the calf. After the instrument has been electrically balanced and a stable baseline has been obtained, the thigh cuff is inflated to the manufacturer's specifications (about 50–70 cm H$_2$O). Pressure is

maintained until the tracing reaches a stable plateau; then the cuff is rapidly deflated and the tracing is allowed to return to baseline levels.[3]

The "rise" of the tracing from the baseline to the plateau measures venous capacitance, and the "fall" of the tracing from the peak value over a 3-s period measures venous outflow.[10] These measurements are plotted on a graph with the vertical axis representing the "fall" and the horizontal axis representing the "rise" (Figure 34–5). When the point described by these two parameters

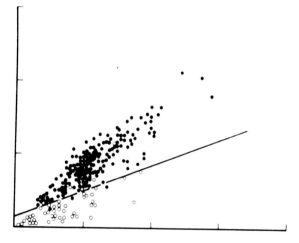

FIGURE 34–5. Impedance plethysmography (IPG) interpretation using the discriminant line method. Venographic findings: filled circles, no thrombus; open circles, proximal vein thrombus.

Impedance plethysmography results as a graph of 3-s venous outflow plotted as a function of venous capacitance (rise vs. fall). A diagonal line divides patients with normal venograms from those with recent proximal deep venous thrombosis. (Reproduced with permission from the American Heart Association. From: Hull R, van Aken WG, Hirsch J, *et al.* Impedance plethysmography: Using the occlusive cuff technique in the diagnosis of venous thrombosis. Circulation 1976; 53:696.)

lies above an experimentally determined discriminant line, the test is considered to be negative for DVT. Points below the line are indicative of DVT, provided they remain below the line after repeated testing. In other words, points above the line correspond to a high capacitance and high venous outflow, while points below the line represent an abnormally low compliance and venous outflow. To improve the accuracy of impedance plethysmography (IPG), a five-test sequence with occlusion times of 45, 45, 120, 45, 120 s, respectively, has been recommended by Hull et al.[11]

Sources of Error

In some patients with a previous DVT, venous collaterals are well developed. Therefore, occlusions in major deep veins may not be detected. Clots in tributary veins, such as the profunda femoris or internal iliac veins, do not impede venous outflow. Partially occluding clots or DVT in one of the paired crural veins may easily be missed. Contractions of the leg muscles in anxious patients who are unable to relax interferes with venous outflow. Also, false-positive results may be seen in patients with extrinsic compression from popliteal cysts or tumors, and in patients with an elevated central venous pressure, as in congestive heart failure.[3] Any other systemic conditions interfering with normal arterial inflow or venous outflow will lead to erroneous readings.

Limitations

To perform IPG, the patient must be able to cooperate. Anxiety, excessive muscle twitches, inability to lie flat because of respiratory problems, and severe edema are all conditions in which IPG cannot be performed. Also patients with leg bandages, casts, or skeletal traction cannot be studied because the electrodes and cuffs may not be applied. Some of these limitations do not interfere with the performance of duplex ultrasonography.

Accuracy

Venography is considered the "gold standard" for the diagnosis of DVT, although many would argue that color-flow scanning is superior to venography, particularly in the thigh and calf. In the early studies, IPG was compared to venography, but after the emergence of real time imaging modalities, it was compared to compression ultrasonography. Numerous investigators have examined the accuracy and fallibility of IPG and many refinements were proposed to improve its accuracy.[1,2,12,13] Despite these efforts, several investigators noted that the sensitivity of IPG was decreasing over time. In one report, this was explained by the fact that the patients being referred for testing had less severe symptoms and the patterns of DVT were changing.[14] Cogo et al. reviewed the

venograms performed in two different time periods separated by 8 years and found a change in the patient referral patterns and types of DVT.[15] They noted that patients were referred earlier after onset of symptoms, and that the prevalence of nonocclusive thrombi was higher and iliac DVT lower.

To improve the overall accuracy of IPG, the clinical probability of disease must be strongly considered. Wells et al. found that by multiple regression analysis, there were 9 variables from the patient's history and physical examination that improved the accuracy of IPG.[12] The identification of certain clinical conditions by history, such as cancer and paralysis, and by physical examination, such as local tenderness and swelling, improved the sensitivity of IPG. On the other hand, the use of IPG as a screening tool to detect DVT in asymptomatic patients proved unreliable in several studies.[1,2,16,17]

Direct comparison of serial IPG and serial compression ultrasonography has been performed.[18,19] Overall, duplex ultrasound had a higher sensitivity and specificity than IPG.[1] Both tests failed to detect discrete thrombi in asymptomatic patients, but IPG was worse than duplex ultrasound. IPG was especially unreliable in detecting calf thrombi and proximal DVT in asymptomatic patients. Repeated testing after a short interval (1–2 weeks) uncovered a small number of missed DVT. In one study, the conversion from a normal to abnormal IPG was 5.3% compared to a conversion rate of 1.4% for ultrasound.[13] It is generally acknowledged that if there is a reason for a high clinical suspicion of DVT in the face of negative IPG and duplex, a venogram should be obtained.[1–3]

Strain-Gauge Plethysmography

Technique

Strain-gauge plethysmography (SGP) involves the measurement of calf volume expansion in response to a standardized venous congesting pressure and the rate at which blood flows out of the leg after the pressure has been released. Mercury or indium-gallium strain-gauge instruments are highly accurate and sensitive in detecting volume changes in the calf. Patient positioning is identical to that in IPG. A rapidly deflating cuff measuring 22 × 71 cm is wrapped on the thigh.[20] Changes in calf volume are measured with a mercury-in-silicone strain gauge wrapped around the calf at its widest point (Figure 34–6). The length of the unstretched gauge should be 90% of the calf circumference. The gauge should be placed around the calf so as to ensure good contact but not with excessive pressure that might occlude the superficial veins. The cuff is inflated to 50–80 mm Hg for 2 min or until a stable plateau is reached when venous outflow equals the arterial inflow.[3]

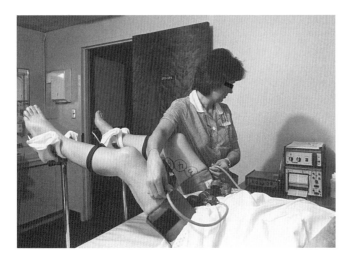

FIGURE 34–6. Strain-gauge plethysmography (SGP): patient position.

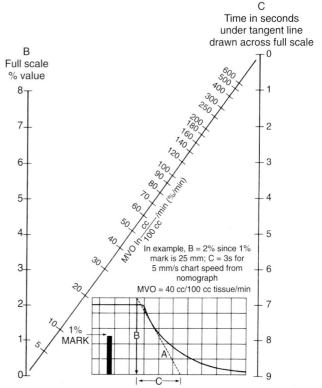

FIGURE 34–8. SGP: Nomograph for calculation of maximum venous outflow (MVO). [From AbuRahma AF. Strain-gauge plethysmography in diagnosis of deep vein thrombosis. In: AbuRahma AF, Diethrich EB (eds). *Current Noninvasive Vascular Diagnosis*. Littleton, MA: PSG Publishing Company, Inc., 1988. Permission requested.]

Calf volume expansion (also called venous volume or venous capacitance) is determined by comparing the rise of the curve from baseline with a 1% electrical calibration signal and is reported in terms of percent volume increase or as milliliters per 100 ml of calf volume. Calf volume expansion averages around 2–3% in normal limbs and is less than 2% in limbs with acute DVT (Figure 34–7).[21]

Measurement of maximum venous outflow (MVO) improves the sensitivity of SGP. To calculate the MVO, a tangent is drawn through the steepest part of the outflow curve after pressure in the cuff is released. MVO is expressed in milliliters per 100 ml of calf volume (Figure 34–8).[20] Cramer and colleagues devised a graph for plotting venous capacitance (VC) against venous outflow (VO) with a discriminant line specific for strain-gauge studies.[22] In a group of 45 patients, they found that the

VO/VC ratio was 100% sensitive and 92% specific in detecting DVT (Figure 34–9).

Sources of Error

There are several potential sources of error associated with measuring calf expansion. When the veins of the calf are not completely empty before the cuff is inflated, the response to a given congesting pressure will be reduced. This can be avoided by proper patient positioning ensuring complete emptying and collapse of the veins prior to cuff inflation. Also, if the veins have not undergone preliminary stretching, calf expansion may show incremental volumes with successive congesting pressures. To avoid this problem, two or three 45-s preparatory cuff inflations are done before the definitive measurements are taken. This will stretch the calf veins and reduce the effects of venous tone.[7] Finally, failure to use a standard congesting pressure or failure to adhere to the specifications of the thigh cuff will result in inconsistent measurements.[3,7,21] The thigh cuff must be of the recommended size and the pressure tubing must be at least 1 cm in internal diameter to allow rapid inflation and deflation.

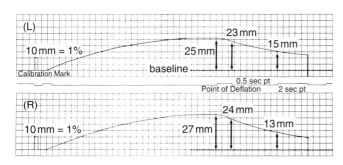

FIGURE 34–7. Strain-gauge plethysmography (SGP) diagram for the calculation of the venous outflow/venous capacitance (VO/VC) ratio. Note the response of the calf volume and venous pressure to inflation of a pneumatic cuff placed around the thigh. Although the venous pressure rises to equal the pressure in the thigh cuff in about 2 min, the calf volume continues to increase albeit at a much reduced rate.

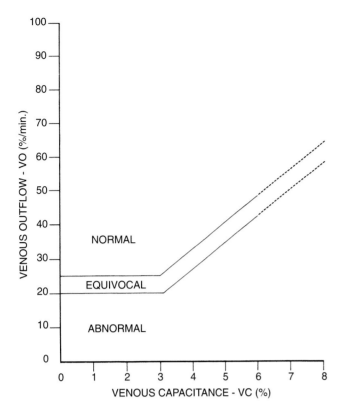

FIGURE 34–9. SGP: Venous outflow/venous capacitance (VO/VC ratio) discriminant line chart. [From AbuRahma AF. Strain-gauge plethysmography in diagnosis of deep vein thrombosis. In: AbuRahma AF, Diethrich EB (eds). *Current Noninvasive Vascular Diagnosis*. Littleton, MA: PSG Publishing Company, Inc., 1988.Permission requested.]

Acute venous thrombosis cannot be distinguished from other causes of increased venous resistance when the venous outflow method is used. Functional venous outflow obstruction, such as in a postphlebitic limb, extrinsic pressure from masses, tumors, or large hematomas will also give a false-positive result. Small nonocclusive thrombi will also escape detection.[7]

Limitations

SGP is subject to the same limitations previously described with IPG. An immobilized limb in a cast or bandage cannot be tested. Patients who are unable to cooperate also cannot be tested. The instruments must be calibrated and the correct cuffs and tubing must always be used.[7]

Accuracy

Barnes *et al.* and then AbuRahma and Osborne demonstrated that acute DVT can be detected with a high sensitivity, 91% and 96%, respectively, using the maximum

venous outflow method. They reported a specificity of 88% and 99%, respectively.[23,24] Warwick *et al.* used computerized SPG and reported a 100% sensitivity for detection of DVT above the popliteal confluence.[25]

Air Plethysmography

Technique

Raines *et al.* designed the air-filled plethysmograph, which is also known as the "pulse volume recorder."[26] It is used in much the same way as the strain-gauge plethysmograph. A single pneumatic cuff placed around the calf and inflated with $10\,cm^3$ of air serves as the volume sensor. An occlusion cuff is placed around the thigh and inflated to 50 mm Hg, then venous capacitance and MVO are measured (Figure 34–10). A venous score is calculated based on the 1-s outflow, the venous capacitance, a ratio of the venous capacitances of the two legs, the presence or absence of respiratory variations in limb volume, and Doppler ultrasonographic findings. A venous score of 4 or less excludes DVT, 5 to 7 is uncertain, and a score greater than 8 implies venous obstruction.[3,27,28] There has been wide variability in the accuracy of this technique in DVT detection and there have been no comparison studies with other noninvasive modalities in the same patients. Overall, it appears that APG is less accurate than either IPG or duplex ultrasonography in DVT detection.

Air plethysmography (APG) was found to be more useful in the evaluation of patients with CVI.[4–6] For this type of test, the air-filled cuff, usually 30–40 cm long, is placed on the leg. The patient initially lies supine with the leg elevated and the heel supported. The cuff is then inflated to a pressure of 6 mm Hg and a baseline volume is obtained with the patient supine and resting. The patient is then asked to stand using a rail or a walker, for support and balance, without transmitting weight to the

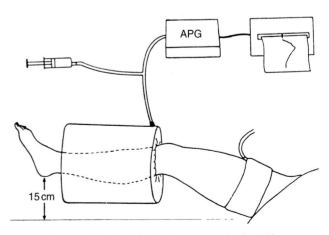

FIGURE 34–10. Air plethysmography (APG).

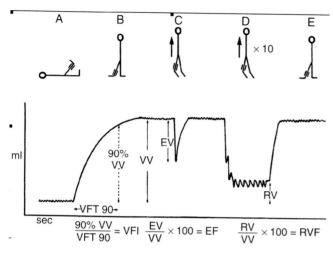

FIGURE 34–11. Diagrammatic representation of typical recording of volume changes during standard sequence of postural changes and exercise. The patient is in a supine position with the leg elevated 45° (A); patient standing with weight on the nonexamined leg (B); single tiptoe movement (C); 10 tiptoe movements (D); same as in (B)/(E). VV, functional venous volume; VFT, venous filling time; VFI, venous filling index; EV, ejected volume; RV, residual volume; EF, ejection fraction; RVF, residual volume fraction. [Reprinted from Marston WA[4] and Christopoulos DG, et al: Air plethysmography and the effect of elastic compression on venous hemodynamics of the leg. J Vasc Surg 1987;5:148–159. Copyright © 1987 with permission from The Society of Vascular Surgery.]

The patient is studied in the supine position with the bed tilted 10° with the foot down. Pneumatic cuffs designed to sense volume changes are placed around the thorax, the mid-thigh, the upper, middle, and lower calf, and the foot. The cuffs that are placed at the foot and lower calf also serve as compression devices. When the cuffs are used for sensing, they are inflated to 10 mm Hg. There are three operational modes. In the first mode, all cuffs on the thigh and leg serve as volume sensors while the foot cuff is inflated three times in rapid sequence up to 100 mm Hg. In the second, the mid-calf cuff is inflated three times to 50 mm Hg and the remaining cuffs are used to record volume changes. In the last mode, the ankle level cuff is inflated three times to 50 mm Hg while the remaining cuffs record volume changes. The study is read as normal if there are well-defined respiratory waves and no rise in the baseline of thigh, leg, and calf tracings during compression of the lower calf or foot (Figure 34–12). An abnormal study shows no respiratory waves and a rise in baseline of the limb tracings in response to foot and calf compression (Figure 34–13).[3,30,31]

Limitations

More than the other plethysmographic techniques, PRG is highly dependent on the skill of the technicians performing the test. The test cannot be performed in patients who have casts or bandages on the leg. Patients with abnormal breathing patterns, such as Cheyne-Stokes

limb being tested. The volume tracing shows a gradual increase until a plateau is reached. Then the patient performs one tip toe maneuver followed by rest, then a series of 10 consecutive tip toes. From the graph generated by these maneuvers, the venous volume (VV), venous filling index (VFI), ejection fraction (EF), and residual volume fraction (RVF) can be calculated (Figure 34–11: from Marston). A VFI < 2 ml/s is observed in normal limbs. Christoupoulos et al. found that an increasing VFI correlated well with worsening clinical symptoms in patients with CVI.[29] Criado et al. also found that an elevated VFI correlated well with increasing clinical severity of CVI.[5] More importantly, successful surgical intervention in patients with CVI lowered the VFI to a normal level.[6]

Phleborheography

Technique

Phleborheography (PRG) is another plethysmographic test, however, it is based on a different concept than venous occlusion plethysmography.[3] The test is designed to detect the effects of respiration and augmentation on venous outflow.

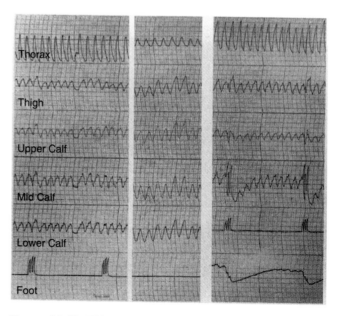

FIGURE 34–12. Phleborheography (PRG): normal tracing. Left: run A; center: respiratory mode; right: run B. Run A (foot compression) shows good respiratory waves; baseline remains level. Respiratory mode shows good waves after arterial pulses are filtered out. Run B (calf compression) shows good respiratory waves; baseline remains level.

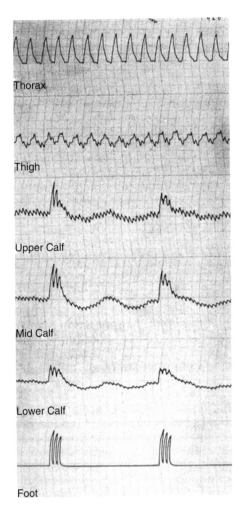

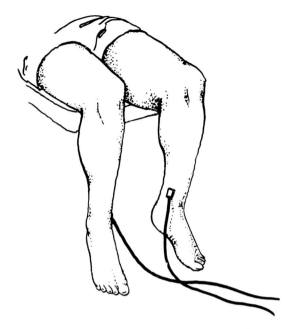

FIGURE 34–14. Photoplethysmography (PPG): patient positioning.

FIGURE 34–13. Phleborheography (PRG): acute popliteal thrombosis. Note the normal respiratory waves and level baseline in the thigh. In the calf, respiratory waves are absent and the baseline rises on foot and calf compressions, indicating deep vein obstruction at the popliteal level.

respiration, or patients on ventilators cannot be properly studied.[3,30,31]

Accuracy

PRG may fail to detect calf DVT for the same reasons that other plethysmographic techniques do. In a group of 60 patients with DVT confined to the calf, Cranley and Flanagan found a 25% false-negative rate. The overall accuracy in their hands was 94%, a rate slightly higher than in other reports.[30,31]

Photoplethysmography

Technique

Photoplethysmography (PPG) is an indirect method of measuring volume change occurring in the cutaneous

capillary network using a light (*photo*) source. PPG is mainly used to detect the presence of venous reflux (venous valvular incompetence). The test is performed by placing an infrared light source on the leg with an adjacent photoreceptor (sensor) to receive the backscattered light. This allows for the continuous recording on a strip chart of the signal intensity reflected from the cutaneous capillary network.

The patient is seated and the legs are allowed to hang freely (Figure 34–14). A baseline recording is obtained, then the patient performs five successive plantar flexion/extension maneuvers. The venous refill time with PPG measures the time it takes capillaries to empty and is dependent on the arterial inflow and efficiency of the venous outflow (Figure 34–15).[32,33] When reflux is identified by PPG, the placement of a tourniquet (or narrow occluding cuff inflated to 50 mm HG) alternately above and below the knee may help the investigator in localiz-

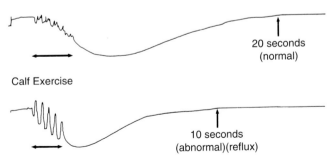

FIGURE 34–15. Venous reflux measured by photoplethysmography (PPG). Incompetent valves result in venous refilling time of less than 20s (below).

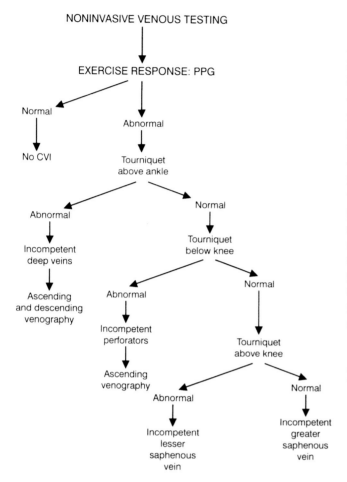

NONINVASIVE VENOUS TESTING

FIGURE 34–16. Protocol for evaluating patients with chronic venous insufficiency (CVI) using photoplethysmography (PPG).

ing the site of reflux (Figure 34–16).[33] Color-flow scanning can identify the sites of reflux more precisely and is currently the preferred method to evaluate patients with valvular incompetence and CVI.[34]

Limitations

There may be considerable variability in the measurements obtained from the same patient. Transducer position may also cause variations in measurements. PPG can detect reflux only in the superficial veins.[32]

Application of Plethysmography in the Modern Noninvasive Laboratory

Color-flow duplex scanning (CFS) has replaced plethysmographic testing in the modern noninvasive laboratory. However, in certain circumstances, IPG can play an important role, particularly in busy noninvasive laboratories with limited resources.[35] If cost cutting is a primary

concern, color-flow scanners can be used more efficiently to answer specific questions in patients with known or proven reflux, e.g., in the identification of incompetent perforators in a patient with recurrent venous stasis ulceration. On the other hand, the evaluation of a patient with leg swelling can be initiated with a less costly and relatively less time-consuming test such as IPG. Symptomatic patients with an abnormal IPG can be treated without any further diagnostic studies. In the past, symptomatic patients with a normal IPG were retested after 3–7 days. Wells *et al.* suggested a new algorithm based on the patient's clinical probability of having a DVT.[12] If the patient has a low pretest probability of harboring a DVT and a normal IPG, no further testing is required. On the other hand, patients with moderate or high pretest probability of having DVT and a normal IPG should be referred for a color-flow scan or venography. They felt that this algorithm was both cost efficient and safe, and in their hands would miss only six patients with isolated calf DVT from a total of 529 patients.[12]

References

1. Kearon C, Julian JA, Newman TE, Ginsberg JS. Noninvasive diagnosis of deep venous thrombosis. Ann Intern Med 1998;128:663–677.
2. Wheeler HB, Hirsch J, Wells P, Anderson FA. Diagnostic tests for deep vein thrombosis. Arch Intern Med 1994;154: 1921–1928.
3. Sumner DS. Diagnosis of deep venous thrombosis. In: Rutherford RB (ed). *Vascular Surgery,* pp. 1698–1743. Philadelphia: W.B. Saunders Company, 1995,
4. Marston WA. PPG, APG, Duplex: Which noninvasive tests are most appropriate for the management of patients with chronic venous insufficiency? Semin Vasc Surg 2002;15:13–20.
5. Criado E, Farber MA, Marston WA, *et al.* The role of air-plethysmography in the diagnosis of chronic venous insufficiency. J Vasc Surg 1998;27:660–670.
6. Owens LV, Farber MA, Young ML. The value of air plethysmography in predicting clinical outcome after surgical treatment of chronic venous insufficiency. J Vasc Surg 2000;32:961–968.
7. Sumner DS. Diagnosis of deep vein thrombosis by strain-gauge plethysmography. In: Bernstein EF (ed). *Vascular Diagnosis,* pp. 811–819. St. Louis, MO: C.V. Mosby, 1993.
8. Barnes RW, Collicott PE, Sumner DS, *et al.* Noninvasive quantitation of venous hemodynamics in postphlebitic syndrome. Arch Surg 1973;107:807.
9. Wheeler HB, Anderson FA Jr. Diagnosis of deep vein thrombosis by impedance plethysmography. In: Bernstein EF (ed). *Vascular Diagnosis,* pp. 820–829. St. Louis, MO: C.V. Mosby, 1993.
10. Hull R, van Aken WG, Hirsch J, *et al.* Impedance plethysmography: Using the occlusive cuff technique in the diagnosis of venous thrombosis. Circulation 1976;53:696.

11. Hull R, Taylor DW, Hirsch J, et al. Impedance plethysmography: The relationship between venous filling and sensitivity and specificity for proximal vein thrombosis. Circulation 1978;58:898.

12. Wells PS, Hirsch J, Anderson DR, et al. A simple clinical model for the diagnosis of deep vein thrombosis combined with impedance plethysmography: Potential for an improvement in the diagnostic process. J Intern Med 1998;243: 15–23.

13. Kearon C, Hirsch J. Factors influencing the reported sensitivity and specificity of impedance plethysmography for proximal deep vein thrombosis. Thromb Haemostas 1994; 72:652–658.

14. Ginsberg JS, Wells PS, Hirsch J, et al. Reevaluation of the sensitivity of impedance plethysmography for the detection of proximal deep vein thrombosis. Arch Intern Med 1994; 154:1930–1933.

15. Cogo A, Prandoni P, Villalta S, et al. Changing features of proximal deep vein thrombosis over time. Angiology 1994; 45:377–382.

16. Katz RT, McCullla MM. Impedance plethysmography as a screening procedure for asymptomatic deep venous thrombosis in a rehabilitation hospital. Arch Phys Med Rehabil 1995;76:833–839.

17. Agnelli G, Cosmi B, Radicchia S, et al. Features of thrombi and diagnostic accuracy of impedance plethysmography in symptomatic and asymptomatic deep vein thrombosis. Throm Haemostas 1993;70:266–269.

18. Heijboer H, Buller HR, Lensing AWA, et al. A comparison of real-time compression ultrasonography with impedance plethysmography for the diagnosis of deep vein thrombosis in symptomatic outpatients. N Engl J Med 1993;329: 1365–1369.

19. Wells PS, Hirsch J, Anderson FA, et al. Comparison of the accuracy of impedance plethysmography and compression ultrasonography in outpatients with clinically suspected deep vein thrombosis. Thromb Haemostas 1995;74:1423–1427.

20. AbuRahma AF. Strain-gauge plethysmography in diagnosis of deep vein thrombosis. In: AbuRahma AF, Diethrich EB (eds). Current Noninvasive Vascular Diagnosis, pp. 271–281. Littleton, MA: PSG Publishing Company, Inc., 1988.

21. Hokanson DE, Sumner DS, Strandness DE Jr. An electrically calibrated plethysmograph for direct measurement of limb blood flow. IEEE Trans Biomed Eng 1975;22:25.

22. Cramer M, Beach KW, Strandness DE Jr. The detection of proximal deep vein thrombosis by strain-gauge plethysmography through the use of an outflow-capacitance discriminant line. Bruit 1983;7:17.

23. Barnes RW, Collicott PE, Mozersky DJ, et al. Noninvasive quantitation of maximum venous outflow in acute thrombophlebitis. Surgery 1972;72:971.

24. AbuRahma AF, Osborne L. A combined study of the strain-gauge plethysmography and I–125 fibrinogen leg scan in the differentiation of deep vein thrombosis and postphlebitic syndrome. Am Surg 1984;50:585.

25. Warwick DJ, Thornton MJ, Freeman S, et al. Computerized strain-gauge plethysmography in the diagnosis of symptomatic and asymptomatic venous thombosis. Br J Radiol 1994;67:938–940.

26. Raines JK, Jaffrin MY, Rao S. A noninvasive pressure-pulse recorder: Development and rationale. Med Instrum 1973;7: 245.

27. Howe HR Jr, Hansen KJ, Plonk GW Jr. Expanded criteria for the diagnosis of deep venous thrombosis: Use of the pulse volume recorder and Doppler ultrasonography. Arch Surg 1984;119:1167.

28. Schroeder PJ, Dunn E. Mechanical plethysmography and Doppler ultrasound: Diagnosis of deep vein thrombosis. Arch Surg 1982;117:300.

29. Christopoulos D, Nicolaides AN, Szendro G: Venous reflux: Quantitation and correlation with clinical severity of chronic venous disease. Br J Surg 1988;75:352.

30. Cranley JJ. Diagnosis of deep venous thrombosis by plethysmography. In: Bernstein EF (ed). Vascular Diagnosis, pp. 801–810. St. Louis, MO: C.V. Mosby, 1993.

31. Cranley JJ, Flanagan LD. Phleborheograhy. In: AbuRahma AF, Diethrich EB (eds). Current Noninvasive Vascular Diagnosis, pp. 309–319. Littleton, MA: PSG Publishing Company, Inc., 1988.

32. Criado E. Laboratory evaluation of the patient with chronic venous insufficiency. In: Rutherford RB (ed). Vascular Surgery, pp. 1771–1785. Philadelphia: W.B. Saunders Company, 1995.

33. AbuRahma AF. Methods of noninvasive techniques in the diagnosis of venous disease. In: AbuRahma AF, Diethrich EB (eds). Current Noninvasive Vascular Diagnosis, pp. 263–269. Littleton, MA: PSG Publishing Company, Inc., 1988.

34. Labropoulos N, Giannoukas AD, Delis K, et al. Where does venous reflux start? J Vasc Surg 1997;26:736–742.

35. Hull RD, Feldstein W, Pineo GF, Raskob GE. Cost effectiveness of diagnosis of deep vein thrombosis in symptomatic patients. Thromb Haemostas 1995;74:189–196.

35
Venous Duplex Ultrasound of the Lower Extremity in the Diagnosis of Deep Venous Thrombosis

Bruce L. Mintz, Clifford T. Araki, Athena Kritharis, and Robert W. Hobson II

Duplex ultrasonography has dominated the clinical landscape for the diagnosis of acute deep venous thrombosis (DVT) since the early 1990s with utilization increasing in both the outpatient and inpatient milieu. Although this modality was initially flawed by high cost, cumbersome size, and low resolution, advancing technology has eliminated many of the early objections to the point where ultrasound has become the diagnostic test of choice. The recent advent of low cost, compact color duplex machines now enables even small laboratories and physician offices to play a larger clinical role in the diagnosis of and treatment for DVT.

Unfortunately, technological advances have not been matched by sufficient numbers of trained technologists with expertise in this clinical application and protocols vary among laboratories. Skilled ultrasonographers remain a requirement to achieve reproducible results of comparable accuracy but are not ubiquitous,[1] setting the need for standards of training and laboratory registry that could improve vascular laboratory findings.

We will review those factors that have shaped the diagnostic role that ultrasound plays in the diagnosis of DVT and discuss issues in protocol that influenced the perceptions from outside and within the vascular community.

Incidence and Risks of Deep Venous Thrombosis

DVT is a major U.S. health problem that affects 2.5 million people a year[2] and produces a lifetime risk for symptomatic DVT in one of every 20 persons.[3] While the risk to inpatients, postoperative patients, late trimester pregnancy females, and cancer patients is well known, the risk to outpatients is gaining recognition in previously healthy individuals, such as *coach class thrombosis in airline passenger flights* lasting longer than 12 h.[4]

Greater recognition leads to greater utilization and the availability of Duplex ultrasound has been associated with an increase in diagnosis for DVT. A survey of short-stay hospital discharges with a diagnosis of DVT documented a clinical practice trend over a 21-year period, from 1979 to 1999.[5] Discharges within the first decade of that period (1979–1989) remained relatively stable and then increased linearly from 1989 to 1999. The first decade also showed an increase in venography utilization that decreased sharply in the second decade from 1989 to 1996, to a low and stable baseline. Over the latter period, duplex ultrasound showed an inverse shift in utilization; it surpassed venography in 1989 and then supplanted it as the primary diagnostic modality for DVT. The large increase in duplex ultrasound utilization was also associated with the increase in DVT discharges, demonstrating the impact of ultrasound testing in changing clinical practice.

Although an increase in utilization may lead to overutilization, the increase in diagnosis has had a significant impact on patient care. Some form of symptomatic or asymptomatic pulmonary embolism (PE) is said to occur in the majority of patients with proximal DVT. The clinical consequence for an untreated DVT can be profound for the femoral, iliac, or caval DVT with a 42–51% incidence of PE.[6] Approximately 25% of patients with PE die and another 25% experience nonfatal recurrent DVT.[7]

Propagation and Resolution

Most DVT is said to arise from calf veins, where it can propagate into the proximal veins, resolve spontaneously, or produce residual defects.[8] Anticoagulation does not fully preclude propagation, which can be found in 19% of patients an average of 28 days after initial diagnosis.[9] Calf vein propagation to proximal DVT is estimated at 10–20%.[10–12] Complete resolution occurs in less than 40% of cases: 23% of patients in 11 months[9] or 38% within 6 months by venography.[13] The risk of recurrence has been estimated at 3% per year, but the risk increases above 10% per year with malignancy and a hypercoagulable state.[8]

Testing

Indications for lower extremity venous ultrasound testing in the diagnosis of DVT are quite varied and tend to be largely clinician dependent. The primary problem lies in the lack of adequate clinical signs and symptoms for DVT.[8,14] Because the clinical consequences of a missed DVT are extreme, clinicians will in many instances request testing even in the face of a low clinical suspicion. A clinical algorithm for predicting the probability for DVT proposed by Wells et al.[15] has gained popularity. By separating patients into high, moderate, and low pretest probability, based upon signs and symptoms, risk factors, and potential alternative diagnosis, the investigators were able to provide better patient stratification for duplex ultrasound testing. Meta-analysis demonstrated that the Wells clinical scoring was more predictable than individual clinical features but was not as valuable for the elderly and patients with a history of DVT or distal DVT.[14]

Equipment

Testing relies upon duplex ultrasound, since B-mode (brightness mode) ultrasound units are not sufficient for peripheral venous study. Along with duplex ultrasound, color-flow imaging aids the spectral Doppler flow assessment to determine vessel patency. A linear transducer, 5 MHz or greater, is used for the principal scanning. If the linear transducer does not provide the necessary imaging depth, a lower frequency sector transducer will often supplement the study.

Procedure

The protocol used in our laboratories is adapted from the one published by Talbot and Oliver.[16] We have found some modification necessary to fit our current application and the interpretation of results.

Patient Positioning

Patients are examined supine with the stretcher in a 45° reverse Trendelenburg position or semi-Fowler position for patient comfort. The patient's weight is shifted to the side of the examination with the hip externally rotated and the knee slightly flexed.

For popliteal and calf veins, the patient is examined in the same supine position as for the femoral vein segment: rolled into a lateral decubitus position, toward the examined leg, with the contralateral leg over and in front of the examined leg, in a prone position with knees flexed and ankles crossed, or laterally with the examined limb brought over and across the contralateral limb for visu-

alization of the popliteal vein and potentially better peroneal vein visualization.

Protocol

The study starts with an assessment of the common femoral vein (CFV) proximal to the saphenofemoral junction (SFJ) and then continues through tibioperoneal vein confluence to the posterior tibial, peroneal, gastrocnemius, and soleal veins within the deep system The study continues into the superficial system in the above-knee greater saphenous vein to the SFJ. The typical examination includes an evaluation of the contralateral limb as a bilateral study. At each stage, landmarks and the relationship of the vein(s) to the accompanying arteries are used to recognize the venous anatomy (Figure 35–1).

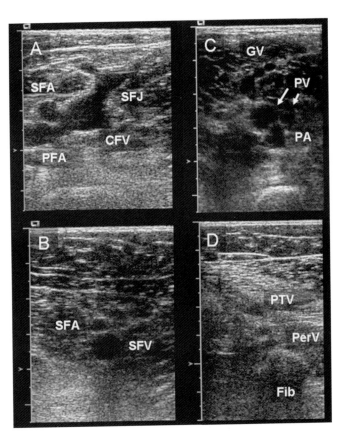

FIGURE 35–1. Normal cross-sectional appearance of the lower extremity veins. (A) The right common femoral vein (CFV) at the saphenofemoral junction (SFJ) lies medial to the superficial femoral artery (SFA) and profunda femoris artery (PFA). (B) Superficial femoral vein (SFV) is located deep to the superficial femoral artery (SFA). (C) Popliteal veins (PV) are found superficial to the popliteal artery (PA). The gastrocnemius veins (GV) project toward the PV in typical vein–artery–vein formation. (D) Peroneal veins (PerV) are imaged superficial to the fibula (Fib). The posterior tibial veins (PTV) approach the peroneal veins in the proximal calf.

FIGURE 35–2. Compression of the left common femoral vein (CFV) thrombus in serial images. Applying light pressure, the greater saphenous vein (GSV) compresses with minimal compression of the superficial femoral (SFA) and profunda femoris (PFA) arteries. Edema may blur the appearance of the deep vessels, while compression often increases visibility of veins and thrombus.

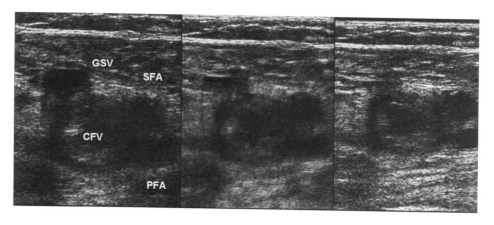

Testing is based upon the application of short, light excursion pressures that are just sufficient to cause full coaptation of the vein walls. Full wall apposition is consistent with vein patency. Intraluminal thrombus will prevent full vein closure (Figure 35–2) and light compressions should be applied to decrease the chance of thrombus embolization.

Spectral Doppler interrogation of the CFV is then used to demonstrate venous flow. The sample is taken with the vein imaged longitudinally. If phasic flow is not evident, the probe is steered to maximize the Doppler shift. Manual compressions are applied to demonstrate the characteristics of flow augmentation that can be elicited. Compression is applied at the abdominal, mid-thigh, and/or mid-calf levels. Flow characteristics are documented qualitatively, and no velocity calculations or velocity angle corrections are made.

Once flow is documented, the B-mode scan is continued on the medial aspect of the thigh through the length of the superficial femoral vein (SFV). Dual or duplicated SFV systems are documented when present along with the compressibility of each SFV limb. Manual vein compressions are applied every 3–4cm. Examination of the SFV and above knee popliteal vein (PV) ends from this approach when the knee is reached. Better visualization and vein apposition in the distal thigh often requires placing the contralateral hand under the limb to manually compress the thigh upward toward the probe.

The probe is then moved to the popliteal space to scan the PV from the posterior knee. The PV is imaged superficial to the popliteal artery, which is identified by its pulsation. Light serial compressions are applied to scan the above knee PV until the examined vessel overlaps the earlier examination of the SFV. Doppler flow is then documented in the above knee PV, with the vessel in long view to document spontaneity, phasicity, and augmentation.

The scan of the posterior calf to the confluence of the tibioperoneal trunk is made in B-mode with serial compressions. The gastrocnemius veins are evaluated to their confluence with the PV and the soleal sinusoids are imaged to their confluence with the tibioperoneal veins. The scan continues through the posterior calf to visualize the confluence of the posterior tibial vein (PTV) and peroneal veins as distally as possible when visualization is adequate.

The completion scan for the rest of the lower leg commences with the probe positioned at the medial aspect of the ankle. The PTVs are located between the medial malleolus and Achilles tendon. The probe is placed between the two, transverse to the vessel axis. Pulsations from the posterior tibial artery are used to identify the location of the vessels, while releasing compression allows two or three PTVs to expand around the artery. A series of light probe compressions is made from the ankle through the proximal calf, until an eventual overlap with the previous scan of the posterior calf. The scan track is repeated a second time to image the peroneal veins. The peroneal veins are first located in the distal calf, positioned several centimeters below the PTVs and just superficial to the fibula shadow. The peroneal veins may be larger than the PTVs but are less easily imaged. Frequently they can be completely evaluated by the same series of probe compressions.

Inclusion of the superficial veins varies by laboratory. Our laboratory typically evaluates the greater saphenous vein (GSV) trunk from the SFJ to the knee. The lesser saphenous vein (LSV) is evaluated as it approaches the PV as a standard part of the examination but is not normally evaluated along its superficial course unless symptoms suggest a superficial thrombophlebitis. Both the GSV and LSV are located between the deep and superficial fascial sheaths in the deep subcutaneous layer.

The anterior tibial veins (ATV) are not normally assessed unless signs or symptoms are focal to the paratibial location. When evaluated, the ATVs can be imaged with the leg rotated medially. The scan commences at the malleolar level at the flexure of the ankle. Light compressions with the probe are used to demonstrate the pulsation of the anterior tibial/dorsalis pedis artery. The

ATVs become visible on either side of the artery when compression is released. Scanning toward the knee, the ATVs are found cradled by the interosseous membrane, which connects tibia to fibula. Pulsations of the anterior tibial artery continually verify the location of the ATVs. Approaching the tibial plateau, vessels penetrate the interosseous fossa on their way toward the PV. Patency is confirmed by color flow imaging.

Venous Flow Characteristics

Doppler venous flow is used to extend the study beyond the directly imaged segments to provide indirect evidence of iliocaval vein patency from the CFV and SFV patency from the PV. Venous flow in the lower extremities is normally in phase with breathing (Figure 35–3). Obstruction in a more proximal vein (Figure 35–4) is expected to extinguish obviously phasic venous flow and possibly replace it with a continuous flow pattern.

The flow augmentation response with distal limb compression is used to support the findings of phasicity. Phasic venous flow should be accompanied by a good augmentation, which is an immediate acceleration of venous flow in response to compression that produces a high-velocity bolus ejection early in the compression. A period of quiescence follows once the venous reserve has been expressed (Figure 35–3). Poor augmentation is a sluggish flow response. Acceleration and deceleration are proportionate to the applied pressure, with low velocity amplitude. Augmentation maneuvers are ill-advised when a DVT has already been determined.

Doppler flow characteristics do not necessarily rule out a DVT. Phasic flow and qualitatively good augmentation can sometimes be observed upstream to an obstructed segment. On the other hand, continuous or absent venous flow is highly suggestive of a proximal thrombosis or extrinsic compression, or poor recanalization in post-thrombotic disease, particularly when it is associated with poor augmentation. When flow anomalies are encoun-

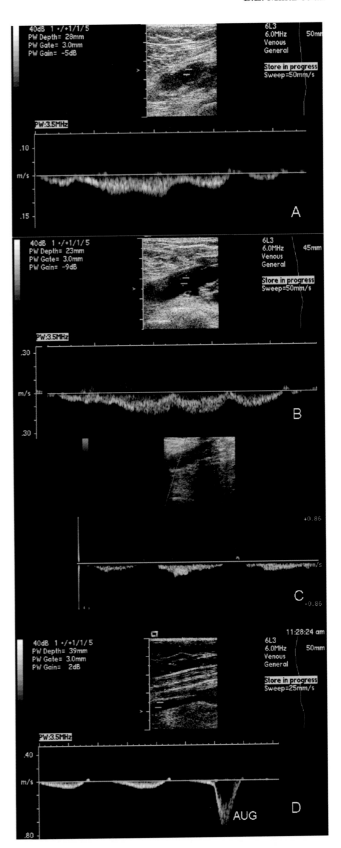

FIGURE 35–3. Normal lower extremity venous flow is strongly influenced by intraabdominal pressure, increasing during expiration and decreasing during inspiration (A). Secondary pulsations timed with right ventricular contraction may be present (B). Flow becomes pulsatile as central venous pressure increases and intraabdominal pressure becomes less influential (C). Congestive heart failure produces pulsatile venous flow (D), which may be observed in all insonated vessels. Venous valve closure in response to ventricular contraction occurs regularly as Dopplerable blips of flow reversals. Augmentation (AUG) in response to the manual compression of the distal limb is normally seen as the rapid ejection of a blood bolus from the limb segment. This should be followed by a quiescent phase that occurs after the venous reserve has been expressed.

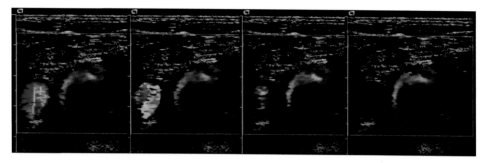

FIGURE 35–4. Near occlusive thrombosis of the common femoral vein revealed with color flow imaging. Serial images demonstrate the pulsation of the common femoral artery through one cardiac cycle. Continuous flow surrounds the thrombus throughout the cycle. Obstruction at this level is associated with the loss of venous flow phasicity in the distal limb. Continuous flow should be evident at the popliteal vein.

tered at the CFV, the iliocaval segments should be imaged, particularly if a filter has been placed and the signs are bilateral (Figure 35–5).

Acute Versus Chronic

Thrombus causes a vein to become noncompressible. Fresh thrombus produces a dilated, "spongily" compressible vein that softly deforms to light probe compression. It may be completely anechoic. Additional B-mode gain or dynamic range adjustments may demonstrate a thrombotic core composed of a hypoechoic homogeneous or laminating matrix that fills the vein lumen (Figure 35–2). Light compression of the tip of the thrombus may demonstrate a soft, loosely attached tail that "floats" within the surrounding venous flow. Fresh thrombus makes a soft, sticky contact with the vein wall when compressed. A partially compressible vein segment with a smooth surface that is poorly echogenic is typically considered to contain an acute non-occlusive thrombus.

Chronic, postthrombotic disease causes veins to become partially compressible. The remnants of the previous DVT, adherent to the wall, typically decrease the vein caliber. The wall becomes demonstrably irregular and often echogenic. The amount of residual material varies from patient to patient. In the extreme, postthrombotic disease may fully occlude a vein, causing it to become atrophic with a highly echogenic core. The well-aged, postthrombotic process, whether occlusive or partially occlusive, can often be recognized as chronic.

Between the extremes of the fresh thrombus and the echogenic postthrombotic disease, the age and risk of an intermediate thrombotic process are not simple to assess. A nonocclusive postthrombotic process is usually considered chronic, with patency verified by color flow. However, noncompressible anechoic and occlusive segments combined with irregular, partially compressible segments are difficult to assess, since they may be a mixture of acute thrombus overlying a chronic process. In other instances, the laboratory may consider a vein to contain a thrombotic process but will not attempt to characterize the acuteness of the disease, which may be best left to correlation with clinical findings and the duration of presenting symptoms.

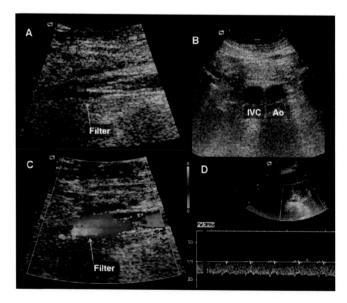

FIGURE 35–5. Ultrasound imaging of inferior vena caval (IVC) filter. Patent filter (A) is documented by color flow (C). Thrombosis produces IVC distention evident when compared to the aorta (Ao). Suprarenal involvement may be associated with continuous flow in the renal vein (D).

Interpretive and Performance Issues of the Duplex Scan

Accuracy

Accuracy of venous ultrasonography has been well documented. In general, ultrasound has a sensitivity and specificity in excess of 95% in the proximal deep veins for DVT when multiple vein segments are involved.[18] The utility of ultrasound is less definitive in other situations. Accuracy is known to decrease when thrombus is more localized, located in the calf, or associated with recurrent thrombosis.[18,19] While a greater than 90% sensitivity and specificity for isolated calf vein thrombosis has been published,[20–22] Wells et al.[15] found an 89% sensitivity for proximal DVT and 78% for all DVT, while the specificity for both proximal and all DVT was much higher (98%). The excellent diagnostic result has been associated with symptomatic limbs. In asymptomatic limbs, ultrasound has been noted to have a 54% sensitivity, 91% specificity, 83% positive predictive value, and 69% negative predictive value.[23] The lower sensitivity and high specificity are in line with how a duplex ultrasound examination is performed. Sonographers may miss a short segmental thrombus, a calf vein, iliac vein, or recurrent thrombus but when they identify a thrombus, the thrombus is most likely present.

The current situation has generated recommendations by other referring specialties that may not reflect current opinions within the vascular community. The American College of Emergency Physicians (ACEP)[19] in a clinical policy statement considered ultrasound to be unreliable for detecting calf vein, pelvic vein, or vena cava DVT and unable to distinguish acute from chronic DVT. Venography is considered essential for calf, recurrent DVT, and high-risk patients with negative ultrasound study. The ACEP considers the diagnostic utility of duplex ultrasound to decrease as the signs and symptoms for DVT become vague. The American College of Chest Physicians (ACCP) Consensus Guidelines recommend the treatment for calf DVT or, if anticoagulation is contraindicated, to monitor it with impedance plethysmography or duplex ultrasound serially.[17] The ACCP does consider a negative study by ultrasound to be associated with a low risk of clinically important PE.

The recognized deficiencies in these areas could be attributed to limitations in equipment, technical difficulties encountered by technologist inexperience, variability among laboratories in their inclusion of calf vein scanning, and the lack of standards. Ultrasound instrumentation once provided poor visualization of the small venous segments in the calf but advances in technology have dramatically improved and now allow more detailed visualization of iliac and calf veins. Statistical estimates of accuracy from 5 or more years ago are probably poor reflectors of today's technological climate.

While technology has improved, the ultrasonographer guides the study by what is gauged as normal or abnormal. Recognizing the role of lymph nodes (Figure 35–6), the appearance of Baker's cysts (Figure 35–7) and edema (Figure 35–8) will extend the examination to a more complete interpretation. In addition, identifying difficulties in

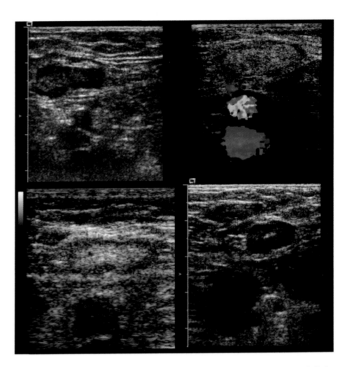

FIGURE 35–6. Inguinal lymph nodes are not normally visible when scanning the groin. Enlarged lymph nodes typically contain an echogenic core surrounded by a hypoechoic cortex. Found superficial to the common femoral artery and vein, they may be associated with the symptoms of tenderness and swelling that precipitated the request for a venous study.

the protocol described previously, such as poor visibility due to edema or inadequate vein compressions, may explain examination inaccuracies.

Technical difficulties are many. As noted above, sensitivity and specificity are greatest when multiple veins are incorporated in thrombus. Duplex scans become problematic when short segment or isolated distal thrombosis is involved. Within the protocol noted above, the more difficult areas encountered, which could affect accuracy, include the following:

1. Common femoral vein. Technologists do not always scan proximal to the SFJ. Isolated valve cusp or SFJ thrombus would not be imaged.
2. Deep femoral vein thrombosis, at the confluence with the CFV, may be missed. In some patients the deep femoral vein is a large vein that is almost continuous with the PV.
3. SFV assessment at the adductor canal is often difficult. Short cuts taken may allow inadequate vein compressions or a nonevaluated segment.
4. Edema caused by DVT may reduce visibility.
5. Venous flow assessments may be rushed to augmentation and spontaneous flow characteristics in phasicity not adequately examined.
6. The tibioperoneal trunk is often poorly visualized as the posterior calf projects away from the vessel.

FIGURE 35–7. Baker's cysts, when present, are located superficial to the popliteal vessels. Cysts contain an anechoic fluid-filled core and a brightly echogenic regular border. They are most often not completely spherical and may contain segments of irregular attachments. Color flow imaging will demonstrate Baker's cysts as avascular structures.

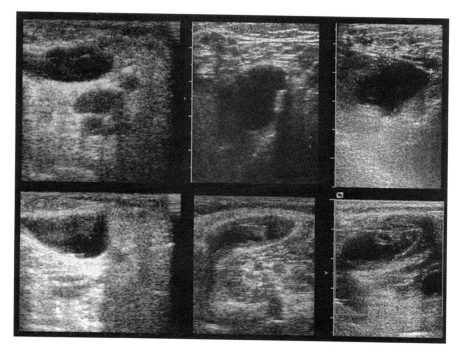

Adequate assessment is possible by applying slightly greater pressure to the scan.

7. PTV and peroneal confluence with the tibioperoneal trunk is similarly difficult to assess in patients with calf swelling.
8. Compression of the peroneal vein in its deep course may be difficult to assess, when the vein is surrounded by hypoechoic tissue.
9. Distinguishing chronic postthrombotic disease from acute thrombosis requires considerable experience.

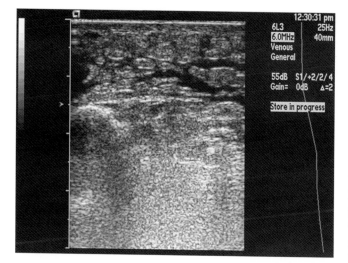

FIGURE 35–8. Edema, visible as irregular fractures in the subcutaneous interstitial space, is associated with a backup of lymphatic fluid. When present, it can be used to demarcate the region of swelling.

Even with experience, cases will be encountered that are poorly distinguishable.

These and other limitations to test accuracy can be corrected in individual laboratories with good quality assurance programs. Improving quality on a national scale requires greater standardization of laboratory practices, which are not currently uniform.[24] Two controversial examples of interlaboratory nonuniformity are the role of calf vein imaging and the use of unilateral instead of bilateral testing.

Calf Vein Imaging and Thrombosis

When a laboratory discovers an isolated calf vein thrombosis (Figure 35–9), patient outcome is seldom predictable. The clinical significance of below-knee thrombosis has long been the focus of considerable discussion. Clinicians vary in their concern for thrombi in the PTV, peroneal, gastrocnemius, and soleal veins.[25] Although reports in the literature have documented the potential for pulmonary embolus from calf thrombi, recommendations for clinical management have frequently been conservative, avoiding hospitalization and systemic heparinization. Most physicians (70%) would not treat symptomatic isolated calf vein thrombosis. Of those not treating, only 42% would use serial duplex scans to monitor propagation.[26] Yet, an isolated calf vein thrombosis is not inconsequential if most DVTs arise from calf veins and extend into the proximal veins at a 10–20% propagation rate.[8–12,27] The recommendation of the ACCP to treat or monitor calf vein DVT is increasingly being expressed.[27]

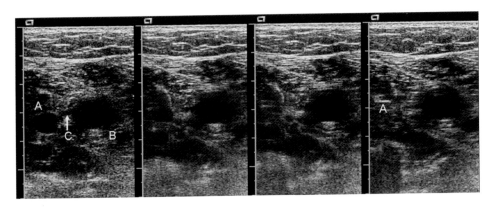

FIGURE 35–9. Compression of a soleal sinusoid pair (A and B). Probe compression collapses the patent vein (A). Thrombosis of vein (B) causes dilation and noncompressibility. The accompanying branch of the soleal artery (C) is situated between the venous pair.

The American College of Emergency Physicians[19] in a clinical policy statement considered ultrasound to be unreliable for detecting calf vein thrombosis. While this may reflect the accuracy statistics of a decade ago, the sensitivity and specificity for calf vein DVT should be continually improving with the advances in ultrasound technology. Those laboratories that still do not include calf vein imaging in their DVT protocol not only decrease test accuracies and compromise patient safety, but technologists in these laboratories are probably less capable of recognizing venous thrombosis outside the femoropopliteal segment.

Bilateral or Unilateral Testing

Medicare will reimburse bilateral or unilateral testing. Bilateral examinations have been standard since impedance plethysmographic testing was the noninvasive test modality of choice in the 1980s. Conversion to duplex ultrasound continued the tradition and is suggested by Intersocietal Commission for the Accreditation of Vascular Laboratories (ICAVL) accreditation. Many laboratories (75%) are now performing unilateral studies on patients who present with unilateral symptoms.[28] Unilateral testing recommendations do not, however, extend to inpatients[29] and probably should exclude patients with pregnancy, cancer, and recent discharge.

Some caution should be raised on the appropriateness of proceeding to unilateral scanning since this appears not to be accompanied by the development of clinical guidelines in the laboratories that perform unilateral testing.[28,30] Our laboratory routinely performs studies bilaterally. Both extremities may be fully evaluated but, at the very least, the asymptomatic limb will be evaluated from the CFV to the tibioperoneal trunk confluence. Our decision to perform bilateral testing is consistent with the logic of bilateral extracranial cerebrovascular testing in symptomatic patients, in a uniform belief that we better serve our patient population when we evaluate both extremities.

Summary

The role of duplex ultrasonography as the preferred test for the diagnosis of DVT is well established, and the ready availability of duplex ultrasound equipment has made it the preferred diagnostic examination for acute DVT in most healthcare facilities. Its low equipment cost, portability, and low complication rates due to its noninvasive approach make this technique particularly applicable for testing in either the ambulatory outpatient or the critically ill, intensive care patient.

Unfortunately the technical ease of its clinical application has not been so widely applied. Protocols vary among laboratories, and are in need of greater standarization. In addition, the availability of skilled ultrasonographers is important to achieving reproducible results, but the resource is far from ubiquitous.[1] As a result, limitations in uniformity and technical expertise have impacted the published accuracy data and the perceptions of the referring specialists.

Still, the acknowledged accuracy of ultrasound in the diagnosis of above-knee thrombi will allow it to maintain its premier role, as alternative imaging modalities gain presence. The results of prospective studies, including an evaluation of the technique's cost effectiveness, taking into account the decreasing expense of basic ultrasonographic equipment, will influence future application of duplex ultrasonography in clinical practice.

References

1. Zierler BK. Screening for acute DVT: optimal utilization of the vascular diagnostic laboratory. Semin Vasc Surg 2001;14:206–214.
2. Greenfield LJ. Venous thrombosis and pulmonary thromboembolism. In: Greenfield LJ, Mulholland M, Oldham KT, Zelenock GB, Lillemore KD (eds). Surgery: Scientific Principles and Practice, 2nd ed. Philadelphia: Lippincott-Raven Publishers, 1997.

3. Hull MB, Pineo GF. Prophylaxis of deep venous thrombosis and pulmonary embolism. Current recommendations. Med Clin North Am 1998;82:477–493.

4. Arfvidsson B, Eklof B, Kistner RL, et al. Risk factors for venous thromboembolism following prolonged air travel. Coach class thrombosis. Hematol Oncol Clin North Am 2000;14:391–400.

5. Stein PD, Hull RD, Ghali WA, et al. Tracking the uptake of evidence: Two decades of hospital practice trends for diagnosing deep vein thrombosis and pulmonary embolism. Arch Intern Med 2003;163:1213–1219.

6. Borst-Krafek B, Fink AM, Lipp C, Umek H, Kohn H, Steiner A. The proximal extent of pelvic vein thrombosis and its association with pulmonary embolism. J Vasc Surg 2003;37:518–522.

7. Barritt DW, Jordan SC. Anticoagulant drugs in the treatment of pulmonary embolism: A controlled study. Lancet 1960;1:1309–1312.

8. Kearon C. Natural history of venous thromboembolism Circulation 2003;107:I22–I30.

9. Ascher E, DePippo PS, Hingorani A, Yorkovich W, Salles-Cunha S. Does repeat duplex ultrasound for lower extremity deep vein thrombosis influence patient management? Vasc Endovasc Surg 2004;38:525–531.

10. Passman MA, Moneta GL, Taylor LM Jr, et al. Pulmonary embolism is associated with the combination of isolated calf vein thrombosis and respiratory symptoms. J Vasc Surg 1997;25:39–45.

11. Kazmers A, Groehn H, Meeker C. Acute calf vein thrombosis. Am Surg 1999;65:1124–1127.

12. Ohgi S, Tachibana M, Ikebuchi M, et al. Pulmonary embolism in patients with isolate soleal vein thrombosis. Angiology 1998;49:759–764.

13. Holmstrom M, Lindmarker P, Granqvist S, et al. A 6-month venographic follow-up in 164 patients with acute deep vein thrombosis. Thromb Haemost 1997;78:803–807.

14. Goodacre S, Sutton AJ, Sampson FC. Meta-analysis: The value of clinical assessment in the diagnosis of deep venous thrombosis. Ann Intern Med 2005;143:129–139.

15. Wells PS, Hirsh J, Anderson DR, et al. Accuracy of clinical assessment of deep-vein thrombosis. Lancet 1995;345:1326–1330.

16. Talbot SR, Oliver MA. Techniques of Venous Imaging. Pasadena, CA: Appleton Davies, 1992.

17. Hyers TM, Agnelli G, Hull RD, et al. Antithrombotic therapy for venous thromboembolic disease. Chest 2001;119:176S–193S.

18. Kearon C, Julian JA, Math M, et al. Noninvasive diagnosis of deep vein thrombosis. McMaster Diagnostic Imaging Practice Guidelines Initiative. Ann Intern Med 1998;128:663–677.

19. American College of Emergency Physicians (ACEP), Clinical Policies Committee and the Clinical Policies Subcommittee on Suspected Lower-Extremity Deep Venous Thrombosis. Clinical policy: Critical issues in the evaluation and management of adult patients presenting with suspected lower-extremity deep venous thrombosis. Ann Emerg Med 2003;42:124–135.

20. Rose SC, Zwiebel WJ, Nelson BD, et al. Symptomatic lower extremity deep venous thrombosis: Accuracy, limitations, and role. Radiology 1990;175: 639–644.

21. Bradley MJ, Spencer PA, Alexander L, et al. Colour flow mapping in the diagnosis of the calf deep vein thrombosis. Clin Radiol 1993;47:399–402.

22. Mattos MA, Londrey GL, Leutz DW, et al. Color-flow duplex scanning for the surveillance and diagnosis of acute deep venous thrombosis. J Vasc Surg 1992;15:366–375.

23. Borris LC. Comparison of real-time B-mode ultrasonography and bilateral ascending phlebography for detection of postoperative deep vein thrombosis following elective hip surgery. The Venous Thrombosis Group. Thromb Haemost 1989;61:363–365.

24. Zierler BK. Ultrasonography and diagnosis of venous thromboembolism. Circulation 2004;109:I9–I14.

25. O'Shaughnessy AM, Fitzgerald DE. The value of duplex ultrasound in the follow-up of acute calf vein thrombosis. Int Angiol 1997;16:142–146.

26. Zierler BK, Meissner MH, Cain K, Strandness DE. A survey of physicians' knowledge and management of venous thromboembolism. Vasc Endovasc Surg 2002;36:367–375.

27. Comerota AJ. Myths, mystique, and misconceptions of venous disease. J Vasc Surg 2001;34:765–773.

28. Blebea, J, Kihara TK, Neumyer MM, Blebea JS, Anderson KM, Atnip RG. A national survey of practice patterns in the noninvasive diagnosis of deep venous thrombosis. J Vasc Surg 1999;29:799–806.

29. Garcia ND, Morasch MD, Ebaugh JL, et al. Is bilateral ultrasound scanning of the legs necessary for patients with unilateral symptoms of deep vein thrombosis? J Vasc Surg 2001;34:792–797.

30. Hirsch AT, Zierler ER, Bendick PJ. Commentary re: A national survey of practice patterns in the noninvasive diagnosis of deep venous thrombosis. J Vasc Surg 1999;29:939–940.

36
Venous Imaging for Reflux Using Duplex Ultrasonography

Jeffrey L. Ballard, John J. Bergan, and Lisa Mekenas

Introduction

Surgical textbooks devote a great deal of space to clinical examination of the patient with varicose veins. Many of the clinical tests were described 100 years ago and carry the names of famous individuals interested in venous pathophysiology. Among these are the Trendelenburg test, the Schwartz test, the Perthes test, and the Mahorner and Ochsner modification of the Trendelenburg test.[1]

Evaluation of clinical findings with duplex ultrasound validation has shown that the above named clinical tests used in the examination of patients with primary varicose veins are inaccurate.[2] A comparison of preoperative evaluations using physical signs alone, physical findings combined with hand-held Doppler examination, and physical findings combined with duplex ultrasound validation has revealed that a traditional clinical examination alone can be improved by the use of hand-held Doppler ultrasonography. However, preoperative planning is best performed by incorporation of duplex ultrasound technology into the examination.[3]

Continuous-wave Doppler is certainly adequate for evaluation of greater saphenous vein incompetence but lesser saphenous incompetence must be validated by duplex ultrasonography as popliteal fossa anatomy is complex and requires high-resolution B-mode imaging for proper identification of pathologic processes.[4] Although phlebography has fallen into disuse, there is one study in which color-coded duplex sonography was compared to phlebography supplemented by varicography.[5] It was concluded that ascending venography was slightly superior to color-coded duplex sonography in detection of postphlebitic changes but there was good agreement between color-coded duplex sonography and descending phlebography in the grading of superficial and deep venous reflux. Similarly, there was agreement in evaluating greater and lesser saphenous vein reflux when phlebography and duplex scanning were compared. More

incompetent perforating veins were detected by ascending phlebography and varicography than by color-coded duplex sonography.[5]

Although duplex evaluation of varicose veins was first reported in 1986, routine use of duplex scanning prior to varicose vein surgery has not become an established practice.[6] In the mid-1990s, it was found that in the United States, 18% of noninvasive vascular laboratories did not use duplex ultrasound for vein mapping and another 37% did so only occasionally.[7] Citing lack of facilities and expense, some investigators have advocated using color-coded duplex sonography only for investigation of the popliteal fossa.[8,9] One group having adopted the procedure of routine stripping of the long saphenous vein in the thigh believes that this practice obviates the requirement for duplex scanning of the greater saphenous vein in such patients.[5,10]

We believe that duplex scanning for venous insufficiency is simple and cost effective. Color imaging facilitates the examination and evolved ultrasound methods have made standardization of the examination possible.[11] Duplex ultrasound precisely defines individual patient anatomy, and information is obtained that supplements the clinical impression. Measuring venous diameters allows for proper choice between radiofrequency or laser ablation and conventional stripping.[9]

Equipment

Precise information about venous reflux in the lower extremities can be obtained only by the use of proper equipment. The ability to detect blood flow rates as low as 6 cm/s is essential.[12,13] This is facilitated by a high-resolution duplex scanner that provides pulsed wave Doppler. Color Doppler is not absolutely necessary for evaluation of the deep and superficial venous systems. However, it is highly recommended for determining reflux in perforating veins and identifying small calf veins.

Transducers ranging from 5 MHz to 7.5 MHz are adequate regardless of body habitus. Additional materials needed for a complete examination include acoustic gel, towels, a walker, and a data collection sheet.

Clinical Examination

Subjective data regarding patient symptoms, clinical findings, previous venous history, and vascular procedures should be documented. These should be organized so that each limb studied can be classified according to the revised CEAP classification.[14] Clinical (C) class will be determined by the presence or absence of telangiectasias, dilated intradermal venules measuring 1 mm or less in size; reticular veins, nonpalpable, dilated subdermal venules less than 3 mm in diameter; varicose veins, palpable, dilated subcutaneous veins greater than 3 mm in diameter; edema; and severe skin changes including venous ulceration. Edema is usually observed in the lower calf and ankle area (gaiter area).[14,15] Also, hyperpigmentation, scars of previous ulceration or white cutaneous scars at the ankle area, termed atrophie blanche, may be encountered during physical examination. Atrophie blanche scars have a white porcelain appearance. These are thought by some to be a result of infarcted skin lesions.[15] Open ulceration, eczematoid dermatitis, and lipodermatosclerosis should be recorded and used to define the clinical class. These are all important physical findings that not only allow the clinical class to be pinpointed but also to assist in determining the extent of the reflux examination.

A history of previous deep venous thrombosis or pulmonary embolus will provide information for the etiology portion (E) of the CEAP classification.[14] A history of congenital arteriovenous malformation is also noteworthy. Lower extremity ulceration represents an advanced stage of chronic venous insufficiency.[15] While leg ulceration can also be arterial in origin, 75–95% are of venous etiology.[15] Arteriopathic ulcers are usually quite painful and have a punched-out, granulating base, whereas venous ulcers are less commonly painful and have a variable appearance. These ulcers are frequently accompanied by clear, yellow, or purulent exudate.[15] Important elements to document in addition to ulcer location are size, duration, number of recurrences, and previous treatment.

Ultrasound Examination

The protocol includes interrogation of specific points as listed in Table 36–1. The patient is examined in an upright position free of lower extremity clothing from the waist down except for nonconstricting underwear. The standing position is important in that it allows hydrostatic pressure from the column of venous blood to be applied to the valves. It also amplifies dilation of the venous system, which improves ultrasound imaging and enhances venous reflux detection.[16] Of particular importance is instruction to the patient to inform the ultrasonographer of any faint feelings, dizziness, or nausea. These symptoms seem to be associated with the overall atmosphere of the room and the presence of Doppler velocity signals. If a tendency to fainting because of vagovagal reflux is encountered, the examination may need to be modified with the patient in a semiupright but lying position.[17]

The full length of the axial venous system from ankle to groin is examined. The extremity is scanned with the probe in a transverse position which allows identification of specific named veins and their relationship to other limb structures. The veins are scanned by moving the probe up and down along their course. Double segments, sites of tributary confluence, and large perforating veins as well as their deep venous connections are identified. Varicose veins are often arranged in multiple parallel channels. It is a waste of time to follow reflux into all of the varicose clusters because these are obvious to the treating physician.

The miniaturized ultrasound unit (SonoSite Inc., Bothell, WA) has greatly enhanced the ease of scanning as the instrumentation is lightweight and easily movable. It is positioned close to the sonographer and the best resolution is obtained using the soft tissue setting. This setting gives the best edge definition to the vessels and soft tissues being scanned. Augmentation of flow (distal compression) should be done sharply, quickly, and aggressively and pressure applied to the calf to activate the gastrocnemius and soleus pump. The probe should be angled to provide a 60° or less insonation angle when using color or pulsed-wave Doppler.[11]

Examination should include both lower extremities initially. Posttreatment examinations may be targeted to a

TABLE 36–1. Interrogation points in the venous reflux examination.

Common femoral vein
Femoral vein
Upper third
Distal third
Popliteal vein
Gastrocnemius (sural) veins
Saphenofemoral junction[a]
Saphenous vein, above the knee
Saphenous vein, below the knee
Saphenopopliteal junction[b]
Mode of termination, lesser saphenous vein
Perforating veins, if indicated

[a] Diameter of the refluxing greater saphenous vein 2.5 cm distal to the junction.
[b] Distance from floor.

single extremity or a single area of an extremity. The search for perforating veins should be done in cases of severe chronic venous insufficiency with hyperpigmentation, lipodermatosclerosis, and healed or open ulcer, but the search for perforators in patients with venous insufficiency without skin changes at the ankle should be left up to the surgeon.

Terms in common use in addition to the greater saphenous vein and lesser saphenous vein are Cockett I, II, III perforating veins, 24-cm perforating vein, Boyd perforating vein, and intersaphenous communicating veins. There is a tendency not to use eponyms now and to follow the standard nomenclature as published in 2002.[18] Other veins can be referred to as unnamed. Perforating veins are defined as those veins that course from the subcutaneous tissue through deep fascia to anastomose with one of the named deep venous structures. Communicating veins are those that anastomose with one another within a single anatomic plane.

For the anterior examination, the patient faces the ultrasonographer with weight borne on the nonexamined lower extremity. The non-weight-bearing extremity is examined. The common femoral vein, saphenofemoral junction, and tributaries to the saphenofemoral junction can be examined with the Valsalva maneuver and with distal augmentation and release. The common femoral vein is examined first and then the greater saphenous vein junction. If reflux is present the diameter of the refluxing greater saphenous vein is noted for use in selecting the proper endovenous catheter during saphenous ablation. Tributaries to be searched for include the superficial epigastric, the circumflex iliac, the pudendal, the anterolateral tributary, as well as the posteromedial tributary. If reflux is present in any of these tributary veins, the reflux is followed peripherally and the extent noted.

The greater saphenous vein is identified by its relationship to the deep and superficial fascia that ensheathe it, anchoring it to the deep fascia and forming the saphenous compartment. This was first described by Thomson in 1979.[19] High-resolution B-mode ultrasound imaging of the superficial fascia in the transverse plane has shown this to be strongly ultrasound reflective, giving a characteristic image of the saphenous vein called the "saphenous eye."[20] The saphenous eye is a constant marker, clearly demonstrable in transverse sections of the medial aspect of the thigh. This differentiates the saphenous vein from varicose tributaries and other superficial veins (Figure 36–1). Casual examination of the thigh will often reveal an elongated, dilated vein that is considered to be the long saphenous vein. This is usually identified as an accessory saphenous vein by ultrasound scanning using the anatomic markers of the saphenous eye.[21,22]

Venous reflux can be elicited manually by squeezing calf muscles, by the Valsalva maneuver, or by pneumatic tourniquet release (Figure 36–2). In the study by Szendro

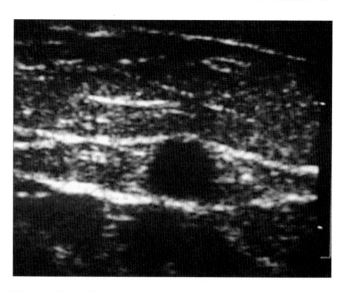

FIGURE 36–1. High-resolution B-mode ultrasound imaging of the superficial fascia in the transverse plane has shown this to be strongly ultrasound reflective, giving a characteristic image of the saphenous vein called the "saphenous eye."

et al., standing subjects were examined and manual compression of calf muscles followed by sudden release was used to assess reflux.[23] Normal healthy limbs had a duration of reflux of less than 0.5 s. Sarin's group, using manual calf compression in the standing position, showed duration of reflux in limbs with significant venous insufficiency to exceed 0.5 s in both the deep and the superficial veins.[24] The study by van Bemmelen et al. found similar duration of reflux in 95% of the limbs examined[16] and the study by Araki et al. found that there was no difference between pneumatic tourniquet release and manual compression and release.[25] As pneumatic tourniquet release is cumbersome and requires two vascular sonographers,

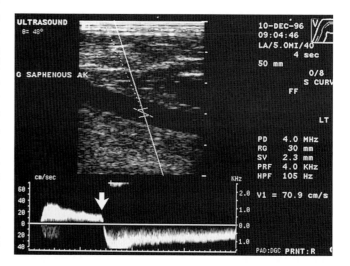

FIGURE 36–2. Doppler sample of the greater saphenous vein above the knee demonstrates venous reflux reflected by reversal of flow longer than 0.5 s. Arrow indicates rapid deflation.

the manual compression and release method has become very attractive. If saphenofemoral reflux exceeding 0.5 s in duration is present, the diameter of the saphenous vein is recorded 2.5 cm distal to the saphenofemoral junction. Present saphenous ablation technology with radiofrequency or laser energy is sometimes limited to saphenous veins <1.2 cm in diameter.

The examination continues distally along the greater saphenous vein, checking for reflux with distal augmentation. Reflux frequently ends in the region of the knee. The point at which reflux stops is noted in centimeters measured up from the floor. The femoral vein, formerly termed the superficial femoral vein, is checked for reflux and vein wall irregularities at the mid-thigh level.

The posterior examination is also done on the non-weight-bearing lower extremity and the examination begins at the saphenopopliteal junction with special attention being paid to reflux in the popliteal vein, the saphenopopliteal junction, and the gastrocnemius (sural) veins. Valsalva may be used to stimulate reflux as well as distal augmentation and release. Valsalva-induced reflux is halted by competent proximal valves. The lesser saphenous vein is followed from its retromalleolar position on the lateral aspect of the ankle proximally to the saphenopopliteal junction and augmentation maneuvers are used every few centimeters.

The termination of the lesser saphenous vein is noted and if the vein terminates proximally in the vein of Giacomini, the femoral vein, or otherwise, a specific check is made for a connection to the popliteal vein. If the lesser saphenous vein has pathologic reflux, measurement of the distance of the saphenopopliteal junction from the floor is recorded as this junction may be well above or below the skin crease in the popliteal fossa.

The search for incompetent perforating veins is done only in limbs with chronic venous insufficiency manifested by hyperpigmentation, atrophie blanche, woody edema, scars from healed ulceration, or open venous ulceration. Incompetent perforating veins in limbs without severe skin changes are associated with varicose veins and can be controlled by varicose phlebectomy.[26] Identification of perforating veins in the lower extremity can be difficult even for the experienced sonographer. However, a thorough understanding of surface anatomic landmarks can make this task less cumbersome.

In the calf, there are major groups of medial and lateral perforating veins. Five clusters of medial perforating veins are consistent in their location. These connect the posterior arch vein system with the posterior tibial veins. Using the heel pad as a reference point, these perforating veins are typically clustered 6, 12, 18, 24, and 28–32 cm above this reference point. The first three are still referred to as the Cockett I, II, and III perforating veins even though eponyms are discouraged.[18,27] The 24-cm perforator carries no special name but the highest antero-

medial perforating vein is called the Boyd perforator.[27] Localization of these medial perforators is important because they are responsible for nearly 40% of incompetent perforating veins.[28]

Lateral calf perforating veins are much more difficult to visualize with duplex ultrasound. In contrast to medial perforating veins, these perforating veins tend to vary in location.[27,28] In the proximal lateral aspect of the calf, there are two perforating veins that connect the lesser saphenous vein to the soleal or gastrocnemius vein(s).[27,28] In the distal lateral aspect of the calf there exist two perforating veins approximately 5 and 12 cm above the os calcis.[27,28] In the thigh the most commonly seen perforating vein connects the femoral vein to the greater saphenous vein at mid-thigh level.[27–29] This mid-thigh perforating vein is often referred to as the Hunterian perforator. There may also be perforators above or below this level. Therefore, careful scanning is essential.

Once a perforating vein is identified, manual compression can be used to determine reflux.[17,30] Manual compression is to be applied above and below the transducer.[17,29] The relationship of the pressure to the perforator will determine whether there is superficial-to-deep venous blood flow that is physiologically normal. Venous blood flow during pressure from above suggests perforator outflow and there should be an appropriate color change due to blood flow toward the transducer (Figures 36–3 and 36–4).

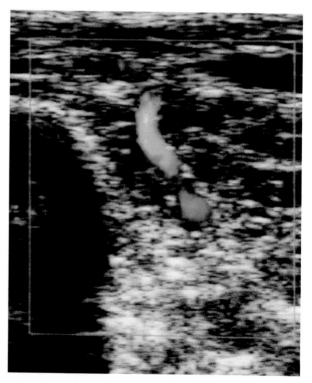

FIGURE 36–3. Color Doppler image demonstrating normal superficial to deep venous flow (away from transducer) of a medial perforating calf vein.

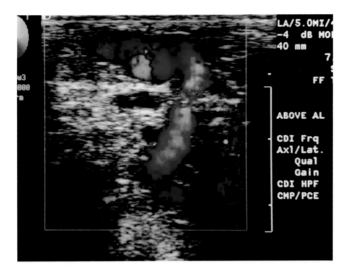

FIGURE 36–4. Color Doppler image demonstrating a dilated medial perforating calf vein with reversal of flow (toward the transducer) from the deep venous system to the superficial venous system.

Conclusions

Despite minor variations in imaging protocols, duplex ultrasonography provides accurate information about reflux in the superficial, deep, and perforating venous systems. These anatomic data are then used to plan therapy for patients with chronic venous insufficiency. Most authors agree that reversal of flow 0.5s or longer coincides with significant venous reflux.[13,17,29,31,32] In light of this definition, it is important for the sonographer not to confuse "transient" normal physiologic reflux with true venous reflux. In our experience, the standing patient position produces reversal of flow much longer than 0.5s when there is pathologic reflux. Shorter durations of reflux are considered to be normal.

Patients with telangiectasias/reticular varicosities and no superficial venous reflux are excellent candidates for sclerotherapy. Endovenous or sclerofoam ablation of greater or lesser saphenous vein reflux is appropriate in patients with superficial venous reflux and symptomatic varicose veins. Identification of perforating veins is indicated in those limbs with severe skin changes and evidence of healed or active ulceration. In this group, adjunctive perforator vein endovenous or sclerofoam ablation can frequently accelerate wound healing.[33]

References

1. Barrow DW. *The Clinical Management of Varicose Veins.* New York: P.B. Hoeber, 1948.
2. Kim J, Richard S, Kent PJ. Clinical examination of varicose veins: A validation study. Ann R Coll Surg Engl 2000; 82:171–175.
3. Singh S, Lees TA, Donlon M, Harris N, Beard JD. Improving the preoperative assessment of varicose veins. Br J Surg 1997;84:801–802.
4. Darke SG, Vetrivel S, Foy DMA, Smith S, Baker S. A comparison of duplex scanning and continuous-wave Doppler in the assessment of primary and uncomplicated varicose veins. Eur J Vasc Endovasc Surg 1997;14:457–461.
5. Baldt MM, Böhler K, Zontsich T, *et al.* Preoperative imaging of lower extremity varicose veins: Color-coded duplex sonography or venography? J Ultrasound Med 1996;15:143–154.
6. Sandager G, Williams LR, McCarthy WR, Flinn WR, Yao JST. Assessment of venous valve function by duplex scan. Bruit 1986;10:238–241.
7. Vascular technology in evolution: Results of the 1994 ARDMS task survey. J Vasc Technol 1995;19:127–145.
8. Darke SG. Preoperative duplex imaging is required before all operations for primary varicose veins. Br J Surg 1998; 85(11):1495–1497.
9. Meyer FJ, Taylor PR, Burnand KG. Preoperative duplex imaging is required before all operations for primary varicose veins. Br J Surg 1999; 86:569.
10. Phillips GWL, Paige J, Molan MP. A comparison of color duplex ultrasound with venography and varicography in the assessment of varicose veins. Clin Radiol 1995;50:20–25.
11. Rodriquez JH, Ballard JL, Rouse GA, De Lange M. Venous imaging for reflux. JDMS 1998;14:9–13.
12. Fronek HS. Noninvasive examination of the patient before sclerotherapy. In: Goldman MP (ed). *Sclerotherapy: Treatment of Varicose and Telangiectatic Leg Veins*, pp. 108–157. St. Louis, MO: Mosby, 1995.
13. Bays RA, Healy DA, Atnip RG, *et al.* Validation of air plethysmography, photoplethysmography, and duplex ultrasonography in the evaluation of severe venous stasis. J Vasc Surg 1994;20:721–727.
14. Eklof B, Rutherford RB, Bergan JJ, Carpentier PH, Gloviczki P, Kistner RL, Meissner MH, Moneta GL, Myers K, Padberg FT, Perrin M, Ruckley CV, Smith PC, Wakefield TW; American Venous Forum International Ad Hoc Committee for Revision of the CEAP Classification. Revision of the CEAP classification for chronic venous disorders: Consensus statement. J Vasc Surg 2004;40:1248–1252.
15. Goldman GP. Adverse sequelae and complications of venous hypertension. In: Goldman GP (ed). *Sclerotherapy: Treatment of Varicose and Telangiectatic Leg Veins*, pp. 32–85. St. Louis, MO: Mosby, 1995.
16. van Bemmelen PS, Bedford G, Beach K, Strandness DE. Quantitative segmental evaluation of venous valvular reflux with duplex ultrasound scanning. J Vasc Surg 1989;10: 425–431.
17. Masuda EM, Kistner RL, Eklof B. Prospective study of duplex scanning for venous reflux: Comparison of Valsalva and pneumatic cuff techniques in the reverse Trendelenburg and standing position. J Vasc Surg 1994;20:711–719.
18. Caggiati A, Bergan JJ, Gloviczki P, Jantet G, Wendell-Smith CP, Partsch H; International Interdisciplinary Consensus Committee on Venous Anatomical Terminology. Nomenclature of the veins of the lower limbs: An international interdisciplinary consensus statement. J Vasc Surg 2002;36: 416–422.

19. Thomson H. The surgical anatomy of the superficial and perforating veins of the lower limb. Ann R Coll Surg Engl 1979;61:198–203.

20. Zamboni P. *La Chirurgia Conservativa del Sistema Venoso Superficiale*, pp. 3–9. Faenza: Gruppo Editoriale Faenza Editrice, 1996.

21. Caggiati A. Fascial relationship of the long saphenous vein. Circulation 1999;100:2547–2549.

22. Caggiati A. The saphenous compartments. Surg Radiol Anat 1999;21:29–34.

23. Szendro G, Nicolaides AN, Zukowski AJ, *et al.* Duplex scanning in the assessment of deep venous incompetence. J Vasc Surg 1986;4:237–242.

24. Sarin S, Sommerville K, Farrah J, *et al.* Duplex ultrasonography for assessment of venous valvular function of the lower limb. Br J Surg 1994;81:1591–1595.

25. Araki CT, Back TL, Padberg FT Jr, *et al.* Refinements in the ultrasonic detection of popliteal vein reflux. J Vasc Surg 1993;18:742–748.

26. Bergan JJ. Varicose veins: Treatment by intervention including sclerotherapy. In: Rutherford RB (ed). *Vascular Surgery*, 6th ed., pp. 2251–2267. Philadelphia: W.B. Saunders Co., 2005.

27. Mozes G, Gloviczki P, Menawat S, *et al.* Surgical anatomy for endoscopic subfascial division of perforating veins. J Vasc Surg 1996;24:800–808.

28. O'Donnell TF. Surgical treatment of incompetent communicating veins: In: Bergan JJ, Kistner RL (eds). *Atlas of Venous Surgery*, pp. 111–118. Philadelphia: W.B. Saunders Co., 1992.

29. Polak JF. Chronic venous thrombosis and venous insufficiency. In Polak JF (ed). *Peripheral Vascular Sonography. A Practical Guide*, pp. 223–245. Baltimore: Williams & Wilkins, 1992.

30. Lees TA, Lambert D. Patterns of venous reflux in limbs with skin changes associated with chronic venous insufficiency. Br J Surg 1993;6:725–728.

31. Thibault PK, Warren LA. Recurrent varicose veins. J Dermatol Surg Oncol 1992;18:618–624.

32. Myers KA, Ziegenbein RW, Zeng GH, *et al.* Duplex ultrasonography scanning for chronic venous disease: Patterns of venous reflux. J Vasc Surg 1995;21:605–611.

33. Sparks SR, Ballard JL, Bergan JJ, Killeen JD. Early benefits of subfascial endoscopic perforator surgery (SEPS) in healing venous ulcers. Ann Vasc Surg 1997;11:367–373.

37
Duplex Ultrasound Use for Bedside Insertion of Inferior Vena Cava Filters

JimBob Faulk and Thomas C. Naslund

Introduction

Venous thromboembolic disease and subsequent pulmonary embolism are significant causes of morbidity and mortality in the United States affecting nearly 400,000 patients and causing approximately 200,000 deaths per year.[1-3] Anticoagulation has remained a standard of therapy for patients diagnosed with venous thromboembolism and pulmonary embolism. Vena cava interruption has emerged as an acceptable means of treating patients in whom anticoagulation is contraindicated or who fail anticoagulation with recurrent pulmonary embolism. Since its introduction in 1973, the Greenfield vena cava filter has become the filter to which all others are compared.[4] Due to a low complication rate, improved lower profile delivery systems, and the high degree of protection from pulmonary embolism, the indications for vena cava filters are being reevaluated.[5-7] This combined with more standardized methods of reporting and follow-up has resulted in a rapid growth in the number of filters placed in the past decade.[8,9]

Vena cava filters are now being routinely used in the trauma population where immobility, multiple long-bone fractures, traumatic brain injury, and spinal cord injury preclude the use of routine thromboembolic protective measures.[10-17] Additionally, the introduction of retrievable temporary filters has raised the question of their prophylactic use in perioperative patients who are morbidly obese or have other hypercoagulable conditions.[18]

Traditionally vena cava filters have been placed under fluoroscopic guidance with the aid of a contrast cavagram. This subjects the patient to ionizing radiation, intravenous contrast, and the inherent risk of transportation to the fluoroscopy suite. Some reports have shown intrahospital transport-related complication rates ranging from 5.9% to 15.5%.[19,20] With an increasing number of critically ill patients being evaluated for potential filter placement, placement at the bedside without transfer out of the intensive care unit (ICU) setting has become more desirable. Duplex-directed placement of a vena cava filter at the patient's bedside has been shown to be safe, cost-effective, and convenient.[10,17,21,22] Additionally, it avoids transfer of these critically ill patients from the ICU setting.

Indications

The absolute indications for vena cava filter placement have not changed for some time. They include a contraindication to anticoagulation, recurrent pulmonary emboli despite adequate anticoagulation, a significant complication developing while on anticoagulation, and an inability to undergo successful anticoagulation despite patient compliance.[23] The relative indications for filter placement have become somewhat of a moving target, and it is the expansion of this category that has led to the large increase in the number of vena cava filters being placed. With the improving safety profile of filter devices and the addition of removable filters, the use of filters for prophylaxis has grown considerably. It is outside the scope of this chapter to attempt to qualify this changing patient population.

Diagnostic Considerations

Patients in whom venous thromboembolism is suspected should undergo appropriate diagnostic tests as described elsewhere in this text. Patients with documented venous thromboembolism as well as those undergoing filter placements for prophylaxis should undergo a focused history and physical examination. Potential underlying hypercoagulable conditions should be elicited to avoid filter placement in patients with conditions such that the caval filter could serve as a nidus for clot propagation. Conversely, patients with an underlying bleeding diathesis deserve special attention as they are at increased risk for bleeding at the site of percutaneous insertion. A pertinent history of prior iliofemoral venous thromboembolism as well as operations involving any venous tributaries should be elicited. The physical examination should be aimed at identifying factors that will adversely affect filter placement. Bulky external fixators used to treat lower extremity and pelvic fractures can make access difficult but rarely impossible. Hematoma surrounding the site of planned percutaneous insertion can likewise make access difficult. Complex abdominal wounds, dressings, and orthotics overlying the right side of the abdomen can impair visualization with surface ultrasound.

Antecedent studies should be reviewed prior to proceeding. Many patients have undergone imaging of the abdomen and/or pelvis for other reasons during their hospitalization. Review of these images can often elicit important information regarding inferior vena cava diameter, renal vein location, the presence of venous anomalies, and the presence of iliac or caval thrombus. While these studies are not required prior to proceeding with bedside duplex-directed filter placement, they should certainly be reviewed if present. Additionally, it is ideal to withhold enteral nutrition for 6 h prior to the planned filter placement to help decrease obstructing bowel gas. While this is more of a convenience than a requirement, it does help decrease the incidence of failed ultrasound surface evaluation.

Technique

Positioning

Patients in the ICU setting provide ample space for positioning and locating the ultrasound machine. Smaller private patient rooms may require repositioning of the bed to allow adequate room for the physician and ultrasound. We have found it most convenient to position the ultrasound high on the patient's right side at shoulder level. The vascular technologist is then able to stand cephalad to the physician for a standard right femoral insertion. It is not necessary to shave the insertion site. The insertion field is prepped with betadiene or chlorhexidene. We have found it easiest to drape the insertion site with three sterile towels followed by a sterile drape for the lower half of the body. This leaves the abdomen free from obstruction for the vascular technologist (Figure 37–1).

Surface Ultrasound

Surface-directed ultrasound guidance (Ultramark 9/HDI, HDI 3000, and HDI 5000, Advanced Technology Laboratories, Bothell, WA) is performed by a registered

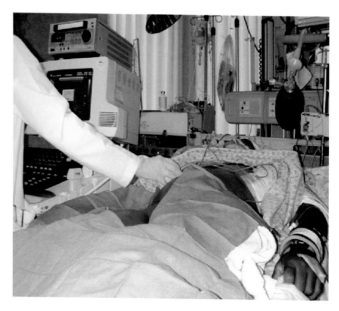

FIGURE 37–1. Typical patient and equipment positioning. Right groin prepped with betadiene and draped with three sterile towels and a sterile half sheet leaving the abdomen clear for ultrasound.

vascular technologist to verify visualization of the renal vein–inferior vena cava (IVC) junction (Figure 37–2). This is commonly obtained via an anterolateral transducer placement, but occasionally a more direct lateral transducer placement between the ribs will elicit better imaging when obstructing bowel gas is present. Identification of the right renal vein is crucial as this usually represents the lowest renal vein. Diameter measurements of the IVC are obtained in two dimensions. Additionally, patency of the proposed femoral cannulation site is evaluated as is the iliocaval junction. If the caval measurements exceed 28 mm in diameter (exclusion from Greenfield filter use), a Bird's Nest filter (Cook

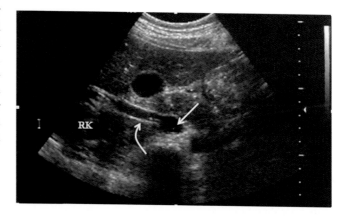

FIGURE 37–2. Suface ultrasound demonstrating the junction of the right renal vein (curved arrow) and the IVC (straight arrow). The right kidney (RK) is also seen.

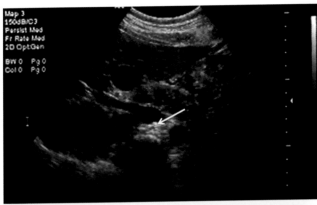

A

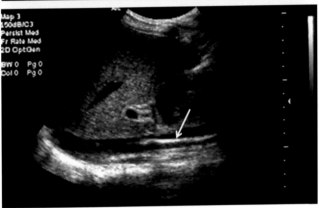

B

FIGURE 37-3. Surface ultrasound demonstrating guidewire (arrow) placement within the IVC in both transverse (A) and longitudinal (B) views.

Incorporated, Bloomington, IN) versus bilateral common iliac filter placement can be considered. If right iliofemoral vein thrombosis is identified or suspected, ultrasound evaluation of the left iliofemoral system is performed. Bilateral iliofemoral thrombosis or thrombus extending to the IVC bifurcation, large orthopedic external pelvic stabilization devices, or proximal injuries in the groins make femoral access difficult on occasion but rarely impossible. In the event of no femoral access, a transjugular route can be used. This often requires reversing the bed in smaller patient rooms, but it is feasible.

Filter Placement

The Medi-tech Stainless Steel Greenfield Vena Cava Filter (Boston Scientific Corporation, Watertown, MA) has been used most commonly. Percutaneous access is obtained using local anesthesia. A 0.035-inch superstiff guidewire is passed into the IVC with ultrasound scan guidance (Figure 37-3). After serial dilations over the guidewire, the 15 French introducer sheath for the Greenfield filter is inserted, which allows passage of

the 12 French preloaded filter introducer catheter. The positioning of the introducer catheter to the desired location is accomplished with visualization from surface ultrasound after removal of the guidewire (Figure 37-4). Removal of the guidewire improves visualization of the filter tip and simplifies accurate placement. The right renal vein–IVC junction is used as the anatomic land-

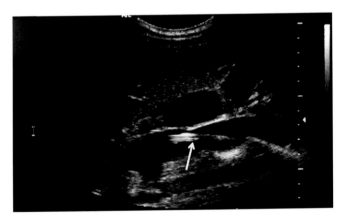

FIGURE 37-4. Surface ultrasound demonstrating placement of the introducer sheath (arrow) in the longitudinal view.

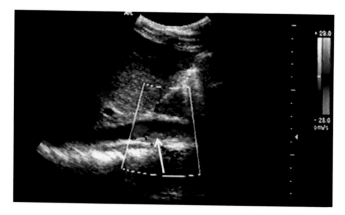

FIGURE 37–5. Duplex ultrasound in the longitudinal view demonstrating the right renal artery (arrow) passing behind the IVC.

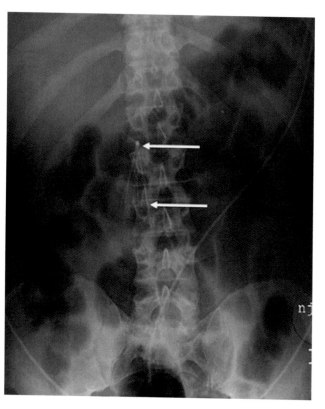

FIGURE 37–7. An abdominal radiograph following vena cava filter placement. The vena cava filter (arrows) is clearly seen with a vertical alignment and the tip located at the L1–L2 disc space.

mark for the identification of the proper location for filter placement. The right renal artery is also a useful landmark given its close association with the right renal vein and is best viewed in the longitudinal view (Figure 37–5). The filter and sheath are slowly withdrawn as a single unit while observing the renal vein–IVC confluence in the transverse view. The filter and sheath are withdrawn until the filter disappears from view. The sheath and filter are moved back and forth while observing with ultrasound to confirm placement. Once the filter tip is confirmed at the level of the right renal vein, deployment with duplex ultrasound guidance is accomplished. Postdeployment position is verified by surface ultrasound (Figure 37–6). Gentle manual pressure is used for hemostasis after the removal of the delivery apparatus. Postprocedure plain abdominal radiographs can be obtained for the confirmation of filter position (Figure 37–7).

Additional Considerations

The majority of patients in our series have received Meditech Greenfield Filters due to ease of visualization and encouraging long-term data. More recently the Günther Tulip Filter (Cook Incorporated, Bloomington, IN) has shown excellent ultrasound visualization should a removable filter be desired. With a slightly different delivery system, the Günther Tulip Filter can be placed with only minor alterations in the techniques described above.

Intravascular Ultrasound

In our initial series of patients, those with inadequate surface ultrasound underwent fluoroscopic filter placement, but more recently intravascular ultrasound (IVUS) placement has been used. It has now become exceedingly rare for any patient to require transport to the fluoroscopy suite for vena cava filter placement. The small numbers of patients who have inadequate surface ultrasound are now treated at the bedside using IVUS for successful visualization and placement with technical success in almost all patients. The use of IVUS is discussed in

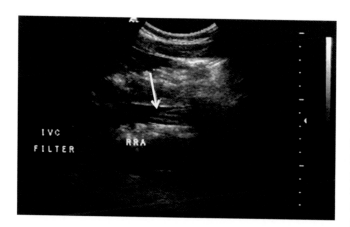

FIGURE 37–6. Surface ultrasound demonstrating the deployed IVC filter in the longitudinal view (arrow). The right renal artery can be seen cephalid to the filter tip.

greater depth elsewhere in this text. Additionally, techniques for IVUS-directed vena cava filter placement have been well described.[16,24–26]

Outcomes

From 1995 to 2003, we placed 486 bedside vena cava filters. Of these filters, 435 were placed using transabdominal duplex guidance and 51 were placed using IVUS. For all patients evaluated for duplex-directed vena cava filter placement, 13% of patients were found to be unsuitable for transabdominal duplex-directed filter placement. Of these patients 11% were felt to be unsuitable because of poor visualization usually due to obstructing bowel gas or body habitus. Less than 1% were judged to have vena cava diameters too large, and less than 1% had inferior vena cava thrombus precluding a transfemoral route of access. Complications occurred in fewer than 3% of patients. The complication most commonly encountered was filter misplacement in 2.4% of patients. This was treated with either additional filter placement or filter repositioning. There were no procedure-related deaths or septic complications.

Since the introduction of IVUS, our department has continued to gain experience with IVUS-directed filter placement. As a result, the majority of patients who have poor visualization with transabdominal surface ultrasound are still treated at the bedside using IVUS. Likewise, as our vascular technologists have gained expertise in vena cava visualization, the number of patients with poor visualization by surface ultrasound has decreased drastically. Improved experience with surface ultrasound combined with the introduction of IVUS has made trips to the interventional suite exceedingly rare thereby avoiding transport of nearly all critically ill patients undergoing vena cava filter placement. Including our early experience, the number of patients requiring fluoroscopic placement of IVC filters continues to fall and is currently 2.6% cumulative. A representative algorithm for vena cava filter placement is shown in Figure 37–8.

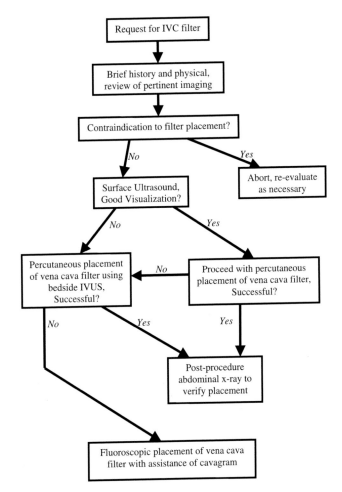

FIGURE 37–8. A proposed treatment algorithm for vena cava filter placement.

References

1. Bick R. Hereditary and acquired thrombophilia: Preface. Semin Thrombos Hemostas 1999;25:251–253.

2. Clagett G. Basic data related to venous thromboembolism. Ann Vasc Surg 1988;2:402–405.

3. Prevention of venous thrombosis and pulmonary embolism. NIH Consensus Development. J Am Med Assoc 1986(256);744–749.

4. Greenfield L, et al. A new intracaval filter permitting continued flow and resolution of emboli. Surgery 1973;73:599–606.

5. Jacobs D, Sing R. The role of vena caval filters in the management of venous thromboembolism. Am Surgeon 2003;69(8):634–642.

6. Duperier T, et al. Acute complication associated with Greenfield filter insertion in high-risk trauma patients. J Trauma 2003;54(3):545–549.

7. Simon M. Vena cava filters: Prevalent misconceptions. J Vasc Intervent Radiol 1999;10(8):1021–1024.

8. Stein P, Kayali F, Olson R. Twenty-one-year trends in the use of inferior vena cava filters. Arch Intern Med 2004;164:1541–1545.

9. Greenfield L, Rutherford R. Recommended reporting standards for vena caval filter placement and patient follow up. Vena caval filter consensus. J Vasc Intervent Radiol 1999;10(8):1013–1019.

10. Benjamin M, et al. Duplex ultrasound insertion of inferior vena cava filters in multitrauma patients. Am J Surg 1999;178(2):92–97.

11. Brasel K, Borgstrom D, Weigelt J. Cost-effective prevention of pulmonary embolus in high-risk trauma patients. J Trauma 1997;42(3):456–462.

12. Hoff W, et al. Early experience with retrievable inferior vena cava filters in high-risk trauma patients. J Am College Surg 2004;199(6):869–874.

13. Morris C, et al. Current trends in vena caval filtration with the introduction of a retrievable filter at a level I trauma center. J Trauma 2004;57(1):32–36.

14. Nunn C, et al. Cost-effective method for bedside insertion of vena caval filters in trauma patients. J Trauma 1997;43(5):752–758.

15. Quirke T, Ritota P, Swan K. Inferior vena caval filter use in U.S. trauma centers: A practitioner survey. J Trauma 1997;43(2):333–337.

16. Rosenthal D, et al. Role of prophylactic temporary inferior vena cava filters placed at the ICU bedside under intravascular ultrasound guidance in patients with multiple trauma. J Vasc Surg 2004;40(5):958–964.

17. Sato D, et al. Duplex directed caval filter insertion in multi-trauma and critically ill patients. Ann Vasc Surg 1999;13(4):365–371.

18. Sapala J, et al. Fatal pulmonary embolism after bariatric operations for morbid obesity: A 24-year retrospective analysis. Obesity Surg 2003;13(6):819–825.

19. Stearley H. Patients' outcomes: Intrahospital transportation and monitoring of critically ill patients by a specially trained ICU nursing staff. Am J Crit Care 1998;7:282–287.

20. Szem J, et al. High risk intrahospital transport of critically ill patients: Safety and outcome of the necessary "road trip." Crit Care Med 1995;23:1660–1666.

21. Conners M, et al. Duplex scan-directed placement of inferior vena cava filters: A five-year institutional experience. J Vasc Surg 2002;35:286–291.

22. Neuzil D, et al. Duplex directed vena cava filter placement: Report of initial experience. Surgery 1998;123(4):470–474.

23. Kinney T. Update on inferior vena cava filters. J Vasc Intervent Radiol 2003;14:425–440.

24. Garrett J, et al. Expanding options for bedside placement of inferior vena cava filters with intravascular ultrasound when transabdominal duplex ultrasound imaging is inadequate. Ann Vasc Surg 2004;18(3):329–334.

25. Wellons E, et al. Bedside intravascular ultrasound-guided vena cava filter placement. J Vasc Surg 2003;38(3):457–458.

26. Wellons E, et al. Real-time intravascular ultrasound-guided placement of a removable vena cava filter. J Trauma 2004;57(1):20–25.

38
Venous Stenting Using Intravascular Ultrasound

Peter Neglén

Venoplasty and stenting of the iliac vein now constitute the "method of choice" in the treatment of iliocaval chronic venous obstruction.[1–8] The importance of venous outflow obstruction in the pathophysiology of chronic venous disorders has been increasingly recognized, and it is apparent that reflux alone cannot explain the symptoms and signs in many patients. Although it is well known that the combination of reflux and obstruction creates the worst scenario, iliofemoral outflow obstruction alone may play a larger role in the pathophysiology of chronic venous disorders than previously thought. The iliac vein is the common outflow tract of the lower extremity and chronic obstruction of this segment appears to result in more severe symptoms than does lower segmental blockage. Distal obstructions appear to be better compensated by collateral formation than proximal lesions. Therefore, the iliocaval venous segment has become the most important target area for balloon dilation and stenting.

Since it is not known at what degree of obstruction the venous flow is restricted, no tests are presently available for the accurate diagnosis of hemodynamically significant venous outflow blockage.[9] Commonly used routine noninvasive tests such as outflow air or strain-gauge plethysmographic tests and duplex Doppler ultrasound may indicate an outflow obstruction, but a normal test does not exclude significant iliocaval blockage. Even invasive pressure tests, e.g., femoral exercise pressures, arm–foot venous pressure differential, and hyperemia-induced pressure increase, are not sufficiently accurate. Ultimately, the diagnosis of outflow obstruction must be made by morphologic investigations.

A single-plane transfemoral antegrade venogram is the routine morphologic investigation of the iliocaval outflow. This type of venogram in the anteroposterior plane is inferior to multiple oblique imaging, especially in the presence of iliac compression from external structures. These lesions compress the vein in different body planes and may therefore be visualized only in certain projections. Using arteriographic techniques including subtraction and power injection of contrast dye further increases the sensitivity (Figure 38–1). However, even multiplane venograms may underestimate the severity and extent of the obstructive lesion as compared to direct imaging by intravascular ultrasound (IVUS). This is currently superior to every other imaging technique in showing iliocaval venous outflow. Development of new magnetic resonance (MR) venography and spiral computed tomography (CT) techniques may replace invasive morphologic studies in the future. Although definition of a hemodynamically significant venous stenosis is lacking, a morphologic obstruction of more than 50% stenosis has arbitrarily been chosen to be significant and the treatment of choice is balloon venoplasty and stenting.

Venous outflow blockage will be found in patients with chronic venous disorders only if the treating physician is aware of its potential importance and suspects its presence. It is common to restrict venous work-up to duplex Doppler ultrasound of the lower extremity below the inguinal ligament for detection of reflux. This is insufficient to detect iliocaval outflow obstruction. A more aggressive approach toward diagnosis is warranted in selected patients. Ultrasound investigation should be complemented by morphologic studies such as multiplane transfemoral venograms or, preferably, IVUS. In our practice, IVUS is used generously in symptomatic patients with venographic findings of stenosis or visualization of collaterals as these can be considered as indicators of obstruction. Also, when plethysmographic or pressure tests are positive for obstruction, IVUS should be employed. Symptoms may range from painful swelling to severe lipodermatosclerosis or ulcer. Patients of special interest are those with symptoms (especially pain) out of proportion to detectable pathology or those with typical symptoms but no detectable lesions on standard tests, those with no improvement of symptoms after standard treatment, and those with previous deep vein thrombosis. The use of IVUS in these patients has the dual

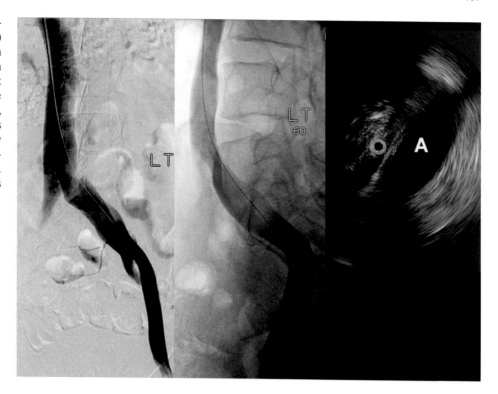

FIGURE 38–1. Transfemoral venogram in anteroposterior (AP) view (left) and with 60° rotation (middle). The right common iliac artery (A) makes a distinct corkscrew-like impression on the vein in the oblique projection, while only a slight translucency is seen on the AP view. The severity of the stenosis at the vessel crossing is better appreciated on IVUS. The black circle within the vein is the IVUS catheter (right).

purpose of accurately diagnosing the degree and nature of obstruction and aiding in appropriate treatment by placement of a stent.

The Intravascular Ultrasound Catheter Technique

IVUS was initially used to aid arterial endovascular interventions and was shown to be beneficial for complex procedures and diagnostic dilemmas.[10] Later IVUS was introduced to assist venous endovascular procedures. The IVUS catheters are disposable and designed in two configurations: rotating mirror catheter and multiple array transducers catheter. The rotating design type consists of an acoustic mirror and transducer assembly at the tip of the catheter. The mirror is rotated by a wire inside the catheter attached to a motor drive. The chamber in which the mirror rotates is filled with saline, taking care not to avoid introduction of air bubbles. The signal travels from the rotating mirror through the fluid-filled chamber to the transducer, producing a 360° cross-sectional image. An example of this design is the Sonicath Ultra imaging catheter used with the Galaxy imaging system (Boston Scientific Corporation, Natick, MA). The multiarray IVUS design incorporates an integrated circuit in the tip

of the catheter, has no movable parts and no chamber, and thus does not require any fluid injection. An example of this configuration is the Visions PV imaging catheter connected to the EndoSonics In-Vision Gold Imaging System (Volcano Therapeutics Inc., Rancho Cordova, CA).

Each individual catheter comes with a preset frequency. The depth of penetration is greater with lower frequency, while the resolution is greater with higher frequencies. For appropriate coverage of the entire lumen in the iliocaval system, a catheter of approximately 12.5 MHz will penetrate to a depth of 30 mm. The catheter does not always track in the center of the vessel at all vessel sites and obtain optimal visualization because of the curvature of the vessel. Often the catheter runs along the wall in an eccentric position. The resulting cross-cut lumen area is therefore not necessarily perpendicular to the longitudinal axis of the vessel (Figure 38–2). The oblique cross-cut area may be oblong and may not reflect the true lumen area. In the off-center position the ultrasound must penetrate the entire diameter of large venous capacitance vessels and with outside compression and oblique projection the longest diameter may even exceed 30 mm.

The IVUS catheter is always placed in the vein percutaneously. Ultrasound-guided cannulation of the femoral or popliteal vein is performed well below the

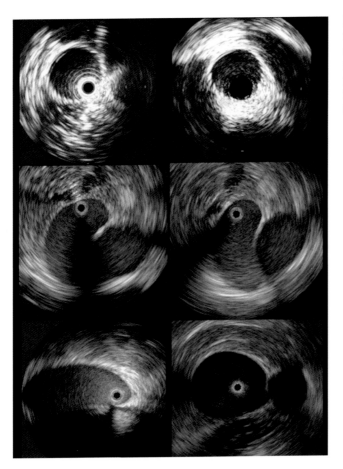

FIGURE 38–2. The bright echoes close to a multiarray catheter may be "ringed down" (top). The guidewire of a monorail type of catheter may create a wedge-formed acoustic shadow. By rotating the catheter the hidden areas can be visualized (middle). Rarely is the IVUS catheter tracking in the center of the vessel to register a true cross-cut area. An eccentric position of the IVUS may exaggerate the lumen (bottom).

suspected obstruction. A guidewire (usually 0.038 inch) is inserted and manipulated through the obstruction. A sheath (usually 9F) is placed percutaneously to facilitate repeated access. The IVUS catheter is threaded over the guidewire to assist the passage of the catheter within the venous lumen. The catheter rides either coaxially over the guidewire, which is placed in a central lumen along the catheter, or in a monorail fashion, where the catheter is attached only at the distal 1–2 cm of the tip. The coaxial placement of the guidewire improves tracking and prevents kinking and thus has an advantage in that aspect. A monorail-style catheter may be problematic when a tight stenosis or severe tortuosity of the vein is encountered. Advancing the catheter and the guidewire as one unit may sometimes facilitate passage. After advancing the IVUS catheter to a level above the area of interest, images are obtained during catheter withdrawal through the lumen. This allows a smooth and continuous image acquisition not always possible during insertion of the catheter. The images are seen in real time and may be stored digitally for later analysis by the built-in software of the ultrasound imaging system.

Bright echoes are produced close to the high frequency ultrasound tip, which is more noticeable with the multi-array IVUS catheter (Figure 38–2). This catheter allows digital subtraction of ringdown artifact, but in so doing limits the visualization close to the catheter. This maneuver is not necessary with the rotating mirror catheter. The guidewire in the monorail system often creates an acoustic shadow, hiding a wedge of the cross-cut area. This error is not seen with coaxial guidewires. By rotating the IVUS catheter the "shadowed" areas can be visualized (Figure 38–2).

The anatomic orientation of the visualized structures is often not accurate. The image is variably rotated. The only way to correctly orient the field during iliocaval imaging is to relate the image to the position of constant anatomic landmarks. The right renal artery most commonly crosses posterior to the IVC; the left common iliac artery crosses above the right common iliac vein, which is anterior to the dense bone; and the iliac artery is usually lateral and anterior to the iliac vein (Figure 38–3). The anatomic orientation, however, is not a major issue in diagnosis of venous obstruction or venous stenting.

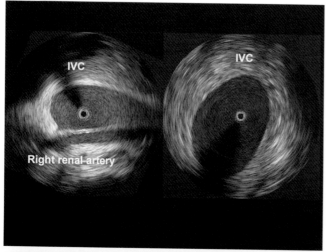

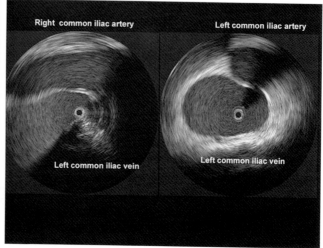

A

B

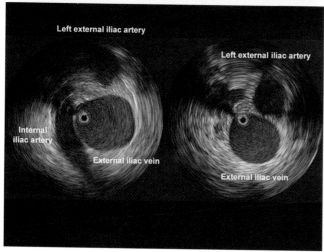

C

FIGURE 38–3. (A) Constant anatomic landmarks allow a correct rotation of the IVUS catheter. The right renal artery usually transverses posterior to the IVC (left). The aorta along the normal below-renal IVC is not seen with this magnification (right). The black circle within the vein is the IVUS catheter. (B) The right iliac artery crosses anterior to the left iliac vein, sometimes creating varying degrees of compression (left). The left and right common iliac artery follow the vein in an antero-lateral position (right). The black circle within the vein is the IVUS catheter. (C) The internal iliac artery crosses over the iliac vein medially as it leaves the common iliac artery and dives down into the pelvis following the internal iliac vein (left). The external iliac artery continues distally in the anterolateral position to the vein (right). The black circle within the vein is the IVUS catheter.

Diagnostic Venous Intravascular Ultrasound

Using the built-in software program, the actual cross-cut lumen area can be calculated by planimetry and the length of different diameters measured (Figure 38–4). Regardless of its shape and varying diameters in different projections, the true stenosis can be delineated and compared to the nonobstructed proximal or distal vein lumen. Several studies have shown that IVUS is superior in detection of the extent and morphologic degree of stenosis as compared to single-plane venography.[1,11–13] On average the transfemoral venogram significantly under-estimates the degree of stenosis by 30%. The venogram has been actually considered "normal" in 25% of limbs despite the fact that IVUS showed >50% obstruction.[2] In a similar population of limbs, the stenosis was less than 50% in 42% of venograms but in only 10% of the IVUS. On the other hand, the venous stenosis was greater than 70% in 32% of venograms, but twice as often with IVUS.

Using the IVUS result as the standard, the venogram had a poor sensitivity (45%) and a negative predictive value of 49% in detecting an obstruction of greater than 70%.[11]

The lack of correlation of the extent of venous lesion on venography and findings on IVUS is striking. More often than not, the extent of stenosis both in thrombotic and nonthrombotic obstruction is greater on IVUS. This is of great importance for placement of stents. The true extent and severity of in-stent restenosis can be assessed only by IVUS.

Finer intraluminal lesions are difficult to visualize with venography. The injected contrast dye may hide such lesions. Delicate intraluminal details, such as webs, frozen valves, and trabeculations, can be detected by ultrasound, but they are rarely seen on venography (Figure 38–5).[14] Despite the high resolution of IVUS, it is inferior to angioscopy in identifying the thin valve leaflets. IVUS failed to detect 76% of valve stations identified by angioscopy.[13]

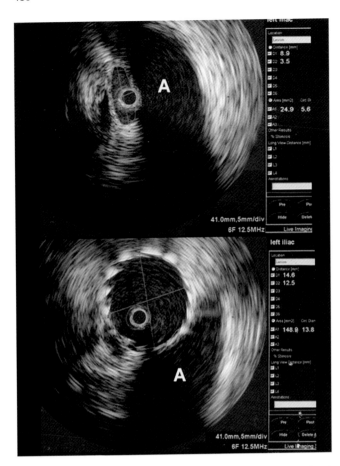

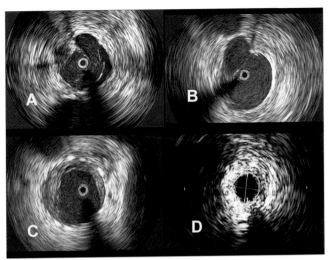

FIGURE 38–5. Images obtained by venous intravascular ultrasound (IVUS). (A) Trabeculation with multiple lumina; (B) intraluminal septa; (C) in-stent restenosis precisely identifying the stent, neointimal hyperplasia, and remaining lumen; (D) compression of the IVC by a circumferentially growing liver cancer. The black circle inside the vein represents the inserted IVUS catheter.

FIGURE 38–4. Measurement of the cross-cut area before (top) and after (below) venous stenting. The measurements are displayed at the right aspect of the screen. The area increased from 24.9 mm² to 148.9 mm² with the dilation. The longest and shortest diameters are given in addition to the calculated diameter as if the measured area represented a circle. The adjacent artery is marked with an A. The black circle within the vein is the IVUS catheter.

The IVUS can detect varying degrees of echogenicity in intraluminal masses, the vessel wall, and the surrounding tissue. Increased echogenicity of the vessel wall may indicate increased fibrosis and wall thickness often seen in postthrombotic veins. Varying echogenicity of intraluminal thrombi may correlate with the age of the thrombus. Fresh thrombus appears more transluscent than old and is surrounded by inflammatory edema (Figure 38–6). This may allow age determination of different parts of an extensive deep vein thrombus. Compliance of the venous wall is reflected by phasic movement during respiration. Lack of respiratory variations of the vein wall indicates less compliance with a stiffer wall. None of these observations is possible with venography. In contrast, collateral formation is poorly shown by IVUS. Only axial collateral formation in close proximity to the native vein can be detected by IVUS. Venograms may occasionally fail to distinguish these from the main vein.[14]

Arterial obstruction is usually due to thickening of the wall with plaque formation. Only rarely does outside compression play a major role. In the venous system, outside compression mainly by arterial structures appears to play a major role even in limbs with post-

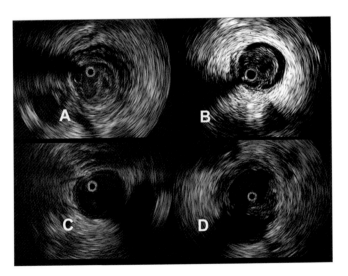

FIGURE 38–6. (A) Relatively acute DVT with partial obstruction of the lumen and surrounding inflammatory edema; (B) an older, well-defined thrombus adherent to the vessel wall, which is fibrosed with increased echogenicity; (C) complete clearance of a thrombus after lysis, but edema of the vessel wall (double-contour) remains; (D) partial lysis of a thrombus after lysis, but the vessel is more than 50% patent. The black circle inside the vein represents the inserted IVUS catheter.

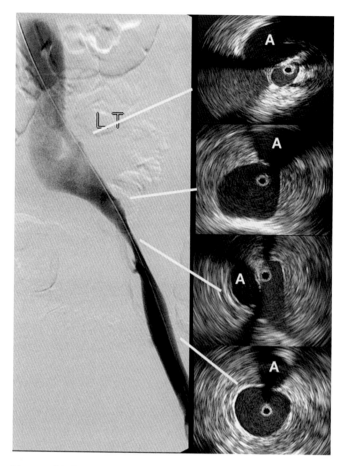

FIGURE 38–7. IVUS images and corresponding transfemoral venogram show a complex nonthrombotic obstruction due to an iliac compression syndrome. The common iliac vein is compressed in the frontal plane with a formation of septum clearly shown by IVUS. The external iliac vein is compressed in the sagittal plane by the internal iliac artery. The adjacent artery is marked with an A. The black circle within the vein is the IVUS catheter.

thrombotic obstruction. The relationship between the left iliac vein compression by the right iliac artery and deep venous thrombosis (DVT) of the left lower extremity is well known.[15] Typically, a stenosis of the left proximal common iliac vein is caused by compression by the right common iliac artery with secondary band or web formation (Figure 38–7).[16] Approximately 30% of the limbs with compression disease, however, have been shown to have stenosis beyond the common iliac vein.[2] Although this lesion is classically described as occurring in the left iliac vein in younger females, it is not an uncommon finding in males, in elderly patients, and in the outflow of the right limb.[17] On venogram such a compression may be indirectly suggested by showing a widening of the iliac vein, a "thinning" of the contrast dye resulting in a translucence of the area, and the presence of transpelvic collaterals, sometimes despite a normal appearance of the iliofemoral vein (Figure 38–8). With IVUS the com-

pressed vein can be clearly delineated between the overriding artery and the posterior bone structure.[8,18] This compression results in an hourglass deformity of the vein of varying degrees with frequently observed secondary intraluminal lesions such as web formation. IVUS investigation in 16 limbs with iliac compression syndrome showed that the iliac vein compression extended distally, involving the external iliac or common femoral veins in 68% (11/16). A filling defect representing thrombi was identified in 25% (4/16) and synechia in the compressed vein lumen was seen in 44% (7/16). These additional findings on IVUS led to modification of the intervention in 50% of limbs.[12]

Intravascular Ultrasound Assistance during Stenting

As indicated above, the IVUS is an invaluable diagnostic tool, but it is also vital for correct placement of stents.[11,12] First, the appropriate diameter of the stent is determined by using IVUS. The lumen dimensions below and above an obstruction can be defined. In stenosis close to the IVC, the prestenotic dimensions of the vein are usually used. The intrinsic software of the ultrasound machine calculates the greatest and least diameters. It also calculates a diameter as though the lumen area was circular. It is important to oversize the average stent diameter by at least 2–3 mm. Excessive oversizing is rarely a problem in venous obstruction as compared to arterial obstruction. The risk of rupture with hemorrhage is minimal in the low-pressure venous system. In our experience of more than 1000 venous stent procedures no clinical rupture has occurred although completely occluded veins have been dilated to 12–16 mm diameter. Dissection of the vascular wall does not develop in the vein because of a wall structure and disease process different from those found in the artery. The venous wall is more homogeneous with postinflammatory fibrosis as compared to the arteriosclerotic wall with heterogeneous plaque formation and with varying calcification. On the other hand, undersizing a venous stent is often a problem. Insertion of a stent with too small a diameter will not allow satisfactory fixation to the venous wall and may result in an immediate proximal migration. This will necessitate percutaneous stent recovery from the IVC or right atrium, which may be a laborious undertaking.

After determining the stent diameter, the proximal and distal disease-free endpoints of the area to be stented are determined by IVUS. When treating a stenosis close to the confluence of the iliac veins and the IVC with a Wallstent, it is important to place the top of the stent well into the inferior vena cava (IVC). The braided nature of that stent may otherwise allow retrograde migration (squeezing) of the stent when the proximal end is placed too near

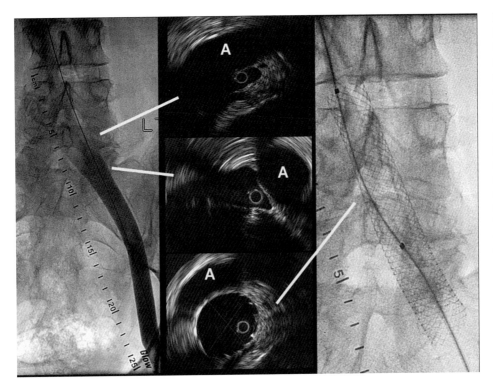

FIGURE 38–8. AP view of a transfemoral antegrade venogram, which appears normal with no obvious stenosis or collateral formation (left). IVUS of the same vein at different levels shows severe proximal common iliac vein (CIV) stenosis due to compression by the crossing iliac artery and partial obstruction of the mid-CIV (top and middle, center). A stent was inserted (right) and the final result is shown by IVUS (bottom, center). The adjacent artery is marked with an A. The black circle within the vein is the IVUS catheter.

the stenosis.[1] The diseased vein segment is frequently more extensive in reality than appreciated by venography. Therefore, the accurate extent of the diseased venous segment is determined by measuring the length of withdrawal of the IVUS catheter from proximal to distal landing points. IVUS is essential in recanalization of occluded iliofemoral veins. The recoil is frequently complete and short of performing a contralateral transfemoral venogram, IVUS is the only way to determine the stenting endpoints adequately. It is vital to cover the entire obstruction as outlined by the IVUS to avoid early restenosis and occlusion and ensure a sufficient venous inflow to maintain patency.

The guidewire is kept in place throughout the stenting procedure. The IVUS is repeated after stent placement and dilation of the stent (Figure 38–8). The degree of recoil and the apposition to the venous wall can be visualized and repeat dilation or additional stenting can be performed as necessary.

The use of IVUS decreases considerably the use of contrast during the stenting procedure. If there are absolute or relative contraindications to the use of contrast dye, the procedure can be performed completely without venography, using only IVUS in combination with fluoroscopy.

The IVUS is a valuable adjunct to surgical thrombectomy or thrombolysis of iliofemoral DVT. Remaining thrombus attached to the wall, the age of the thrombus, postlytic edema of the venous wall, and possible external compression may be identified (Figure 38–6). This may

assist in determining the duration of lytic treatment and any adjuvant stent placement.

The role of IVUS in the diagnosis of morphologic venous outflow obstruction may in the future be replaced by noninvasive studies such as MR venography or spiral CT of later generations. However, the additional information obtained by using IVUS as an adjuvant tool at the stenting procedure (accurate degree and extent of obstruction and finding of previously nonrevealed lesions) is most valuable and will be difficult to replace. Presently, the IVUS is vital for adequate stenting of venous obstruction. The future aim is to develop appropriate, preferably noninvasive, hemodynamic tests to assess outflow obstruction. At that time only patients with known hemodynamically significant obstruction will undergo IVUS-assisted venous stenting.

References

1. Neglén P, Raju S. Balloon dilation and stenting of chronic iliac vein obstruction: Technical aspects and early clinical outcome. J Endovasc Ther 2000;7:79–91.
2. Neglén P, Berry MA, Raju S. Endovascular surgery in the treatment of chronic primary and post-thrombotic iliac vein obstruction. Eur J Vasc Endovasc Surg 2000;20:560–71.
3. Raju S, Owen S Jr, Neglén P. The clinical impact of iliac venous stents in the management of chronic venous insufficiency. J Vasc Surg 2002;35:8–15.
4. Raju S, McAllister S, Neglén P. Recanalization of totally occluded iliac and adjacent venous segments. J Vasc Surg 2002;36:903–11.

5. Juhan C, Hartung O, Alimi Y, Barthelemy P, Valerio N, Portier F. Treatment of nonmalignant obstructive iliocaval lesions by stent placement: Mid-term results. Ann Vasc Surg 2001;15:227–32.

6. Nazarian GK, Austin WR, Wegryn SA, et al. Venous recanalization by metallic stents after failure of balloon angioplasty or surgery: Four-year experience. Cardiovasc Intervent Radiol 1996;19:227–33.

7. Blättler W, Blättler IK. Relief of obstructive pelvic venous symptoms with endoluminal stenting. J Vasc Surg 1999;29:484–8.

8. Hurst DR, Forauer AR, Bloom JR, Greenfield LJ, Wakefield TW, Williams DM. Diagnosis and endovascular treatment of iliocaval compression syndrome. J Vasc Surg 2001;34:106–13.

9. Neglén P, Raju S. Proximal lower extremity chronic venous outflow obstruction: Recognition and treatment. Semin Vasc Surg 2002;15:57–64.

10. Nishanian G, Kopchok GE, Donayre CE, White RA. The impact of intravascular ultrasound (IVUS) on endovascular interventions. Semin Vasc Surg 1999;12:285–99.

11. Neglén P, Raju S. Intravascular ultrasound scan evaluation of the obstructed vein. J Vasc Surg 2002;35:694–700.

12. Forauer AR, Gemmete JJ, Dasika NL, Cho KJ, Williams DM. Intravascular ultrasound in the diagnosis and treatment of iliac vein compression (May-Thurner) syndrome. J Vasc Intervent Radiol 2002;13:523–7.

13. Satokawa H, Hoshino S, Iwaya F, Igari T, Midorikawa H, Ogawa T. Intravascular imaging methods for venous disorders. Int J Angiol 2000;9:117–21.

14. Neglén P, Raju S. In-stent recurrent stenosis in stents placed in the lower extremity venous outflow tract. J Vasc Surg 2004;39:181–7.

15. Cockett FB, Thomas ML, Negus D. Iliac vein compression. Its relation to iliofemoral thrombosis and the post-thrombotic syndrome. Br Med J 1967;2:14–9.

16. Negus D, Fletcher EW, Cockett FB, Thomas ML. Compression and band formation at the mouth of the left common iliac vein. Br J Surg 1968;55:369–74.

17. Raju S, Neglén P. Laser, "closure", stents and other new technology in the treatment of venous disease. J Miss State Med Assoc 2004;45:290–7.

18. Ahmed HK, Hagspiel KD. Intravascular ultrasonographic findings in May-Thurner syndrome (iliac vein compression syndrome). J Ultrasound Med 2001;20:251–6.

39
Ultrasound Guidance for Venous Therapy: VNUS, Endovenous Laser Treatments, and Foam

John J. Bergan and Luigi Pascarella

Introduction

Duplex ultrasound sonography (US) represents the best choice in the evaluation of venous reflux in lower limbs.[1] This test is noninvasive, generally acceptable to the patient, and inexpensive.[2] It provides direct imaging, localization, and extent of venous reflux with a surprisingly high sensitivity (95%) and specificity (100%).[3] Duplex US findings have also been confirmed with angioscopic observations of incompetent vein valves in advanced chronic venous insufficiency (CVI).[4] As demonstrated by Yamaki, high peak reflux velocities (>30cm/s), reflux duration greater than 3s, and an enlarged valve annulus measured by duplex US at the saphenofemoral junction (SFJ) are closely related to angioscopically deformed and incompetent terminal valves (Type III and Type IV valves of Hoshino).[4]

Preoperative Assessment

The examination should always begin with a complete medical history. Data concerning family and personal venous history, symptoms, clinical findings, and previous venous treatments are collected. Comorbidities, allergies, and pharmacologic history must be documented.[2] The body mass index (BMI) is calculated from the patient's height and weight and should be recorded.

The patient should be examined in a standing position to demonstrate patterns of telangiectasias and reticular and varicose veins.[5] Cold light transillumination of the skin (vein light) may be used to identify reticular veins, while a hand-held Doppler device can verify the presence of reflux in some superficial veins as a screening examination.[5] Thus the three levels of pathologic veins are evaluated. Telangiectasias in the skin are visually inspected, reticular veins are transilluminated with the vein light, and varicosities and the saphenous veins with US.

Clinical data should be integrated into the CEAP classification.[6,7]

Equipment

The US duplex scanner should be able to detect blood flow rates as low as 6cm/s.[2] This can be done by dedicated high-resolution vascular scanners with color and/or power-Doppler functions as well as the pulsed-wave Doppler. Linear transducers in the range of 4–7MHz are used.[5,8] The inferior vena cava, pelvic veins, and deep veins of the limbs in obese patients may be imaged with 3-MHz transducers.[1] Linear hockey-stick transducers in the range of 5–12MHz can provide detailed imaging of smaller veins and perforating veins.

With the advances in technology, duplex scanners have become smaller, more transportable, and more operator friendly.[5] Miniaturized devices feature transducers designed with advanced architecture that allow a single probe to image across a greater range of depths within an application and across applications.[5] The transducer for peripheral vascular examinations operates from 10 to 5MHz and provides resolution from the skin surface to 7cm in depth.[5] The technology incorporates power Doppler sonography, tissue harmonic imaging, and direct connectivity to a personal computer.[5] Their overall performance is comparable to the more traditional and much larger US equipment.[5]

Venous Reflux Examination and Venous Mapping

A detailed duplex US study of the normal and pathologic venous anatomy (reflux) is essential. A clear graphic notation (mapping) of significant vein diameters, anomalous anatomy, superficial venous aneurysms, perforating

FIGURE 39–1. This data entry form outlines the saphenous veins and the relevant deep veins. Refluxing veins are added in heavy black lines. Location of perforating veins and aneurysms can be added and distance from the floor indicated. Diameters of perforating veins at the fascial level should also be noted.

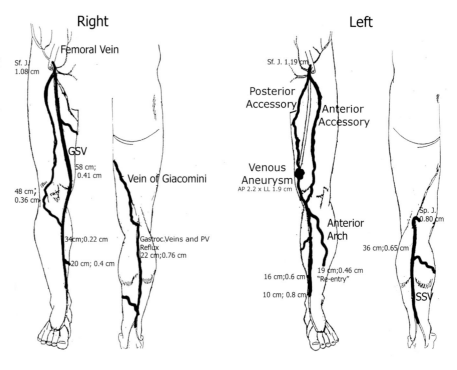

veins, and the presence and extent of reflux should always be recorded during the examination (Figure 39–1).[2,5]

The US examination is conducted with the patient standing.[9] This position has been found to maximally dilate leg veins and challenge vein valves. Sensitivity and specificity in detecting reflux are increased in examinations performed with the patient standing rather than when the patient is supine.[8,9] Supine examinations for reflux are unacceptable.

The veins are scanned by moving the probe vertically up and down along their course. Duplicated segments, sites of tributary confluence, and large perforating veins, and their deep venous connections are identified. Their location measured in centimeters from the floor provides a therapeutic guide. Measurements from the medial malleolus are not as precise. Transverse, in addition to longitudinal scans combined with continuous scanning are performed in order to provide a clear mapping of the venous system. Patency is usually assessed by compression of the vein with the transducer.[8] Reflux is detected by flow augmentation maneuvers such as distal compression and release of the thigh and calf or the Valsalva maneuver for only the SFJ.[8] Automated rapid inflation/deflation cuffs are cumbersome but may be used for this purpose and offer the advantage of a standardized stimulus.[10–12] Reflux greater than 500 ms is considered pathologic.[9,13]

The diameters of the SFJ and femoral vein are recorded for use in judgment for radiofrequency (RF) VNUS closure and endovenous laser treatments (EVLT).[14–16] Important information is also offered by the diameters of the great saphenous vein (GSV) at mid thigh and distal thigh. RF ablation is commonly applied to treat veins from 2 to 12 mm in diameter.[16] The supragenicular, infragenicular, or immediate subgenicular GSV is often the access point for its laser or RF ablation.[16,17] Therefore the depth of the GSV in these regions provides additional data to be recorded.

Accessory veins by definition run parallel to the GSV in the thigh[18] (Figure 39–1). It is imperative to map their course accurately and to note their eventual communication with the GSV (Figure 39–1). They are easily confused with the GSV, especially during continuous longitudinal scanning when the saphenous vein appears to leave the saphenous compartment.[18]

The GSV is then scanned in the leg and the thigh so that tributaries to the GSV should be noted (Figure 39–1).

The diameter of the popliteal vein and the small saphenous vein (SSV) is recorded as well as diameters of the SSV along its course in the leg. Intersaphenous veins should also be identified and the variability in SSV termination carefully recorded.

The venous reflux examination also includes the mapping of exit and reentry perforating veins (PV).[19] PV reflux is detected as outward flow duration greater than 350ms on the release phase of a flow augmentation maneuver (distal compression has higher sensitivity in detecting PVs reflux).[1] PVs should be accurately located in their different locations in the leg. Their position should be measured as distance (centimeters) from the floor in the extended limb.[18,20]

Ultrasound Monitoring during Endovenous Laser Treatments and VNUS Closure of the Great Saphenous Vein and Small Saphenous Vein

A thermic coagulation is caused by the application of electromagnetic energy to the endothelial surface of targeted veins.[16,21,22] It has been suggested that the coagulation process is related to the intravascular vaporization of blood (steam) with intimal denudation and collagen fiber contraction. Vein wall thickening and rapid reorganization of the vessel to form a fibrotic cord follow.[21,22] Occlusion is usually visualized within 10–20s from the laser or RF energy application.[22] These techniques have been proven to be safe and effective.[23] Percutaneous introduction of the laser or RF catheter has made formerly extremely invasive therapy (SFJ ligation and GSV stripping) more acceptable to the patient in terms of posttreatment pain, number of cutaneous incisions, and postprocedural disability.[15,16]

Before the procedure, it is always necessary to rescan the patient for better identification of the venous segment to cannulate. In this preparatory phase some anatomic landmarks have to be clearly recognizable:

1. Femoral vein
2. SFJ
3. Saphenous compartment
4. GSV
5. Small saphenous junctional anatomy.

Introduction of the introducer sheath is performed percutaneously using the Seldinger technique. The supragenicular saphenous vein is usually the access point of choice (Figure 39–2).[17] The intraluminal position of the sheath is ascertained by aspiration of nonpulsatile venous blood. The sheathed laser fiber or a 6 or 8F VNUS catheter is advanced to a point just distal to the entrance of the epigastric vein.[17] The position of the laser fiber is confirmed by direct visualization of the red aiming beam and that of the VNUS catheter by ultrasound[16] (Figures 39–3 and 39–4).

The catheter or sheath appears as a hyperechoic line in the GSV lumen.[14,15] Its placement must be precisely at the SFJ 1cm distal to the epigastric vein (Figure 39–4).[16]

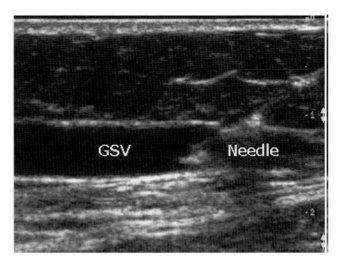

FIGURE 39–2. The great saphenous vein (GSV) is cannulated using the Seldinger technique. The puncturing needle is echogenic and can be easily visualized. (Adapted from Pichot O. *Atlas of Ultrasound Images.* Copyright VNUS Closure.)

Administration of the tumescent anesthesia into the saphenous compartment is monitored by US.[17] The vein is seen as "floating" in an anechogenic sea of the anesthetic solution (Figure 39–5). It is always wise to recheck the catheter position at the SFJ prior to the application of the energy (Figure 39–6).[22]

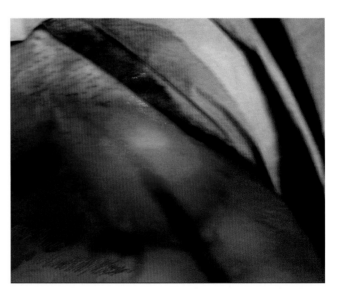

FIGURE 39–3. The laser catheter is advanced proximally toward the SFJ. The position of the laser fiber is confirmed by direct visualization of the red aiming beam through the skin. [Adapted from Navarro L, Min RJ, Bone C. Endovenous laser: A new minimally invasive method of treatment for varicose veins: Preliminary observations using an 810 nm diode laser. Dermatol Surg 2001;27(2):117.]

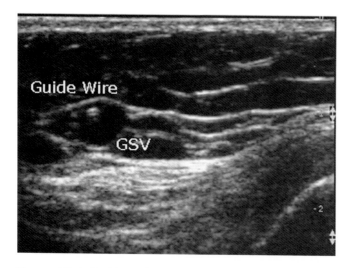

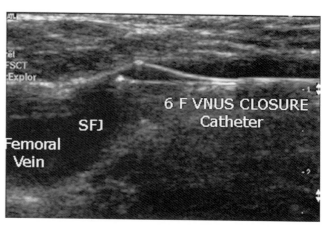

FIGURE 39–4. Position of the guidewire and radiofrequency catheter is monitored by ultrasound visualization. GSV, great saphenous vein. (Adapted from Pichot O. *Atlas of Ultrasound Images.* Copyright VNUS Closure.)

FIGURE 39–6. The ablation starts at the SFJ and proceeds in a distal direction.

It is always wise to recheck the catheter position at the SFJ prior to the application of the energy. (Adapted from Pichot O. *Atlas of Ultrasound Images.* Copyright VNUS Closure.)

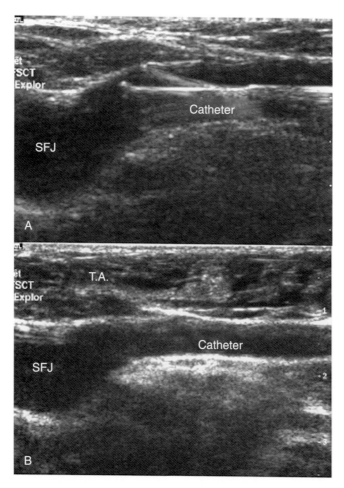

FIGURE 39–5. (A, B) Administration of the tumescent anesthesia into the saphenous compartment is monitored by ultrasound. SFJ, saphenofemoral junction; TA, tumescent anesthesia.

(Adapted from Pichot O. *Atlas of Ultrasound Images.* Copyright VNUS Closure.)

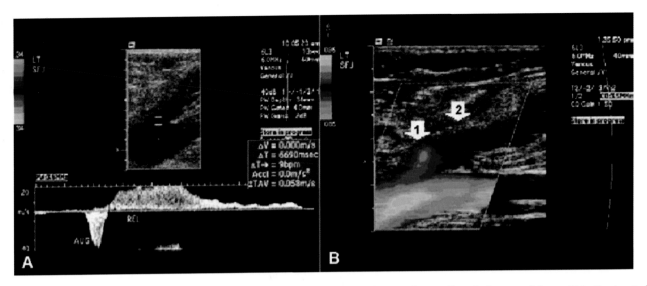

FIGURE 39–7. Duplex examinations (longitudinal views) of the great saphenous vein (GSV) at the saphenofemoral junction (SFJ). (A) Pretreatment scan demonstrated an incompetent SFJ after augmentation. (B) Intraoperative color duplex interrogation showed successful occlusion of the GSV with a patent, 3-mm proximal stump (arrow 1) and absence of flow within the treated segment (arrow 2). [Adapted from Puggioni A, Kalra M, Carmo M, Mozes G, Gloviczki P. Endovenous laser therapy and radiofrequency ablation of the great saphenous vein: Analysis of early efficacy and complications. J Vasc Surg 2005;42(3):488–93.]

The ablation starts at the SFJ and proceeds in a distal direction.[16] Successful obliteration is confirmed by contraction of the saphenous vein to a residual diameter of <2 mm.[16] Patency of the common femoral artery and vein is confirmed by US (Figure 39–7). A thrombus may be seen as a hyperechogenic core in the vessel (Figure 39–7B).[15,24]

Early posttreatment duplex scanning should be performed. Evidence of a protruding thrombus from the saphenous vein into the femoral vein should be looked for (Figure 39–8).[24] Evidence of a noncompressible GSV with thickened walls and absence of flow on color US analysis are signs of successful obliteration (Figure 39–9).[9]

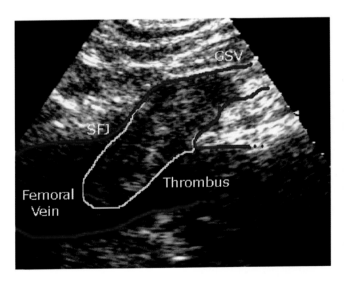

FIGURE 39–8. Early posttreatment duplex scanning should be performed. Evidence of a protruding thrombus from the saphenous vein into the femoral vein should be looked for. GSV, great saphenous vein; SFJ, saphenofemoral junction. (Adapted from Pichot O. *Atlas of Ultrasound Images.* Copyright VNUS Closure.)

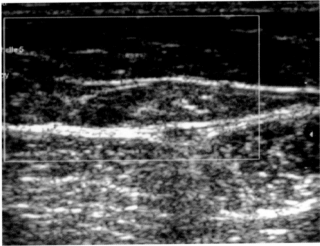

FIGURE 39–9. Evidence of a noncompressible GSV with thickened walls and absence of flow on color ultrasound analysis are signs of successful obliteration. (Adapted from Pichot O. *Atlas of Ultrasound Images.* Copyright VNUS Closure.)

Ultrasound Monitoring during Sclerofoam Ablation of Varicose Veins

Advent of foam sclerotherapy has added a new tool for the treatment of CVI. Sclerosant agents provoke endothelial damage by several mechanisms.[25] They change either the surface tension of the plasma membrane (detergents) and/ or the intravascular pH and osmolarity. The final result is a chemical fibrosis of the treated vessel.[25]

Sclerosing foams (SF) are mixtures of gas with a liquid solution with surfactant properties. In 1993, Cabrera proposed the use of SF, made of sodium tetradecylsulfate or polidocanol, in the treatment of varicose veins.[26] One of the intrinsic limits of liquid sclerosants in the treatment of varicose veins is dilution by the bloodstream with reduction of their efficacy.[27] Also, they are rapidly cleared by the moving bloodstream. Sclerosing foams do not mix with blood and instead remain in the vessel continuing to strip the endothelium.[27] This persistence of the agent in the vessel causes increased contact time with the intimal surface. Foam preparation is remarkably simple.[27] The Tessari's three-way stopcock method is the most commonly used.[27,28]

As in electromagnetic ablation, the treatment starts with clear US mapping. Varicose veins can be accessed by the placement of a 25-gauge butterfly needle or the GSV or the SSV can be directly cannulated with an angiocath, an echogenic Cook needle, or a 25-gauge butterfly.[27,29,30] Most descriptions of the technique explain direct US-guided access to the saphenous vein.[27,31] In contrast, we achieve a satisfactory and rapid obliteration of the GSV and SSV by cannulating a peripheral varicosity.[30] Although the saphenous vein cannot be cannulated with a catheter by way of a varicosity because of its angle of connection, there is no such obstacle to the flow of foam.

Foam functions as an efficient US contrast medium because of its air content. Its injection can be easily monitored. Its US appearance is that of a solid hyperechogenic core with an acoustic shadow projected in the tissue below (Figure 39–10).

Foam is introduced into a varix or the saphenous vein with the patient supine. As the foam reaches the SFJ as monitored by US, compression of the SFJ or the saphenopopliteal junction (SPJ) is effected in order to reduce flowing of foam into the systemic circulation.

Vasoconstriction and vasospasm can be induced by intermittent compression of the vein by the US transducer and by elevating the limb. This minimizes the blood content of the saphenous vein and its connected varices. Foam will be seen by US to flow distally in the elevated limb. It flows selectively through incompetent valves and is effectively blocked by competent valves. These maneu-

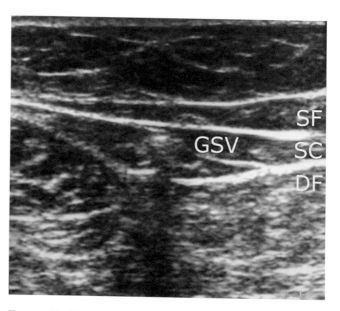

FIGURE 39–10. Foam functions as an efficient ultrasound contrast medium because of its air content. Its injection can be easily monitored. Its US appearance is that of a solid hyperechogenic core with an acoustic shadow projected in the tissue below. GSV, great saphenous vein.

vers have the effect of prolonging the action of the foamed sclerosant on the intima, improving the efficacy of the entire treatment. The femoral, popliteal, and deep veins of the leg are scanned throughout the entire procedure. Foam particles are washed out of deep veins such as the gastrocnemius or tibial veins by flexion–extension maneuvers of the foot. Quick movements of dorsiflexion of the foot completely clear the deep veins. Despite much concern about the problem, major thrombotic events in the femoral and popliteal veins have rarely been described with use of sclerofoam. In a study of over 1200 sclerotherapy sessions over half of which involved foam only a single femoral vein thrombus was encountered.[32]

Thromboses of the gastrocnemius, tibial, and peroneal veins have been reported only occasionally.[30,33] Intraarterial injections can also occur in monitoring the foam treatment of severe CVI (CEAP 4, 5, and 6).[30,33] US has confirmed the presence of a tangled network of varicose veins of small caliber, reticular varices, and incompetent perforating veins under lipodermatosclerotic plaques and under venous ulcers (Figure 39–11).[30] US monitoring is used to confirm the fact that these vessels are filled with foam during the therapeutic maneuvers. US guidance is also used in the treatment of incompetent perforating veins by direct cannulation and controlled injection of the SF under direct visual control.[27] More often superficial peripheral veins can be directly injected with obliteration of the inciting perforator and the network of the incompetent veins.

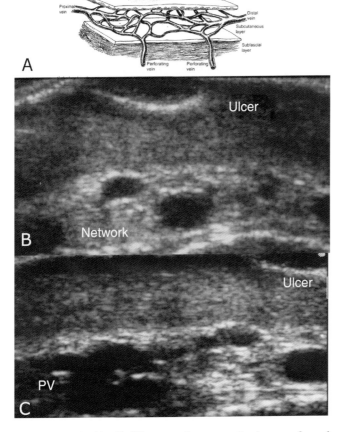

A

B

C

FIGURE 39–11. (A–C) Ultrasound sonography has confirmed the presence of a tangled network of varicose veins of small caliber, reticular varices, and incompetent perforating veins (PV) under lipodermatosclerotic plaques and under venous ulcers.

Discussion

Compression therapy and surgery have been the cornerstone of CVI treatment for years and they are still useful. New minimally invasive techniques such as RF ablation of saphenous veins, EVLT, and GSV and SSV ablation with sclerofoam of superficial varicose veins have been demonstrated to be safe, effective, and more acceptable to the patient.[16] The contribution of US in general and duplex technology in particular has given reliability to the diagnosis of CVI and has enhanced the development of these minimally invasive therapies. Intraprocedural and postprocedural US duplex ultrasound monitoring offers the best control of the entire procedure with early prevention of complications (thrombosis of deep veins) and eventual minimalization of failure.

Conclusion

Duplex US is essential in every phase of CVI patient care. Experience, critical thinking, uniform testing, and insight in the pathology are necessary to achieve satisfactory results.

References

1. Labropoulos N, Leon LR Jr. Duplex evaluation of venous insufficiency. Semin Vasc Surg 2005;18(1):5–9.
2. Ballard J, Bergan J, Delange M. Venous imaging for reflux using duplex ultrasonography. In: AbuRahma AF, Bergan JJ (eds). *Noninvasive Vascular Diagnosis*, 1st ed., pp. 339–334. London: Springer-Verlag, 2000.
3. Depalma RG, Kowallek DL, Barcia TC, Cafferata HT. Target selection for surgical intervention in severe chronic venous insufficiency: Comparison of duplex scanning and phlebography. J Vasc Surg 2000;32(5):913–20.
4. Yamaki T, Sasaki K, Nozaki M. Preoperative duplex-derived parameters and angioscopic evidence of valvular incompetence associated with superficial venous insufficiency. J Endovasc Ther 2002;9(2):229–33.
5. Mekenas L, Bergan J. Venous reflux examination: Technique using miniaturized ultrasound scanning. J Vasc Technol 2002;2(26):139–46.
6. Kistner RL, Eklof B, Masuda EM. Diagnosis of chronic venous disease of the lower extremities: The "CEAP" classification. Mayo Clin Proc 1996;71(4):338–45.
7. Eklof B, Rutherford RB, Bergan JJ, Carpentier PH, Gloviczki P, Kistner RL, Meissner MH, Moneta GL, Myers K, Padberg FT, Perrin M, Ruckley CV, Smith PC, Wakefield TW. Revision of the CEAP classification for chronic venous disorders: Consensus statement. J Vasc Surg 2004;40(6): 1248–52.
8. Lynch TG, Dalsing MC, Ouriel K, Ricotta JJ, Wakefield TW. Developments in diagnosis and classification of venous disorders: Non-invasive diagnosis. Cardiovasc Surg 1999;7(2): 160–78.
9. Labropoulos N, Tiongson J, Pryor L, Tassiopoulos AK, Kang SS, Ashraf Mansour M, Baker WH. Definition of venous reflux in lower-extremity veins. J Vasc Surg 2003;38(4): 793–8.
10. Masuda EM, Kistner RL, Eklof B. Prospective study of duplex scanning for venous reflux: Comparison of Valsalva and pneumatic cuff techniques in the reverse Trendelenburg and standing positions. J Vasc Surg 1994;20(5):711–20.
11. Marke A, Meissner MH, Manzo RA, Bergelin RO, Strandness DE Jr. A comparison of the cuff deflation method with Valsalva's maneuver and limb compression in detecting venous valvular reflux. Arch Surg 1994;129(7):701–5.
12. Delis KT, et al. Enhancing venous outflow in the lower limb with intermittent pneumatic compression. A comparative haemodynamic analysis on the effect of foot vs. calf vs. foot and calf compression. Eur J Vasc Endovasc Surg 2000;19(3): 250–60.
13. Vasdekis SN, Clarke GH, Nicolaides AN. Quantification of venous reflux by means of duplex scanning. J Vasc Surg 1989;10(6):670–7.

14. Pichot O, *et al.* Role of duplex imaging in endovenous obliteration for primary venous insufficiency. J Endovasc Ther 2000;7(6):451–9.

15. Min RJ, Khilnani N, Zimmet SE. Endovenous laser treatment of saphenous vein reflux: Long-term results. J Vasc Intervent Radiol 2003;14(8):991–6.

16. Sadick NS. Advances in the treatment of varicose veins: Ambulatory phlebectomy, foam sclerotherapy, endovascular laser, and radiofrequency closure. Dermatol Clin 2005; 23(3):443–55.

17. Puggioni A, Kalra M, Carmo M, Mozes G, Gloviczki P. Endovenous laser therapy and radiofrequency ablation of the great saphenous vein: Analysis of early efficacy and complications. J Vasc Surg 2005;42(3):488–93.

18. Caggiati A, Bergan JJ, Gloviczki P, Jantet G, Wendell-Smith CP, Partsch H. Nomenclature of the veins of the lower limbs: An international interdisciplinary consensus statement. J Vasc Surg 2002;36(2):416–22.

19. Delis KT, *et al.* In situ hemodynamics of perforating veins in chronic venous insufficiency. J Vasc Surg 2001;33(4): 773–82.

20. Caggiati A, Bergan JJ, Gloviczki P, Eklof B, Allegra C, Partsch H. Nomenclature of the veins of the lower limb: Extensions, refinements, and clinical application. J Vasc Surg 2005;41(4):719–24.

21. Weiss RA. Comparison of endovenous radiofrequency versus 810 nm diode laser occlusion of large veins in an animal model. Dermatol Surg 2002;28(1):56–61.

22. Weiss RA, Weiss MA. Controlled radiofrequency endovenous occlusion using a unique radiofrequency catheter under duplex guidance to eliminate saphenous varicose vein reflux: A 2-year follow-up. Dermatol Surg 2002;28(1): 38–42.

23. Morrison N. Saphenous ablation: What are the choices, laser or RF energy. Semin Vasc Surg 2005;18(1):15–8.

24. Pichot O, *et al.* Duplex ultrasound scan findings two years after great saphenous vein radiofrequency endovenous obliteration. J Vasc Surg 2004;39(1):189–95.

25. Goldman M. Mechanisms of action of sclerotherapy. In: *Sclerotherapy: Treatment of Varicose and Telangiectatic Leg Veins*, 2nd ed., pp. 244–279. St. Louis, MO: Mosby, 1995.

26. Cabrera J. Dr J. Cabrera is the creator of the patented polidocanol microfoam. Dermatol Surg 2004;30(12 Pt 2): p. 1605; author reply 1606.

27. Coleridge Smith P. Saphenous ablation: Sclerosant or sclerofoam? Semin Vasc Surg 2005;18(1):19–24.

28. Tessari L, Cavezzi A, Frullini A. Preliminary experience with a new sclerosing foam in the treatment of varicose veins. Dermatol Surg 2001;27(1):58–60.

29. Cabrera J, *et al.* Ultrasound-guided injection of polidocanol microfoam in the management of venous leg ulcers. Arch Dermatol 2004;140(6):667–73.

30. Bergan JJ, Pascarella L. Severe chronic venous insufficiency: Primary treatment with sclerofoam. Semin Vasc Surg 2005;18(1):49–56.

31. Guex JJ. Foam sclerotherapy: An overview of use for primary venous insufficiency. Semin Vasc Surg 2005;18(1): 25–9.

32. Guex JJ, Allaert FA, Gillet JL, Chleir F. Immediate and midterm complications of sclerotherapy: Report of a prospective multicenter registry of 12,173 sclerotherapy sessions. Dermatol Surg 2005;31(2):123–8; discussion 128.

33. Bergan JJ, Weiss RA, Goldman MP. Extensive tissue necrosis following high-concentration sclerotherapy for varicose veins. Dermatol Surg 2000;26(6):535–41; discussion 541–2.

40
Clinical Implications of the Vascular Laboratory in the Diagnosis of Venous Disorders

John J. Bergan

Introduction

After nearly 50 years of rapid advances in vascular surgery and after 25 years of progress in developing noninvasive vascular investigations the venous system remains enigmatic. Its pathophysiology is a fruitful area of clinical investigation because the component elements of venous dysfunction are incompletely understood. Investigations into venous dysfunction are continuing and research studies and individual patient examinations are being refined. Prospective, randomized studies are appearing in print and meta-analyses are being published.

Clinical examination of the dysfunctional venous system in the vascular laboratory has experienced a transition from indirect examinations such as photoplethysmography and impedance plethysmography to direct imaging and interrogation by means of duplex ultrasound imaging.

As indicated in Chapter 33, the overview of venous disorders, it is wise to separate those conditions that afflict patients into the two categories of acute and chronic. Acute problems deal with venous thrombosis. This may occur in the deep venous system and be quite serious, or in the superficial venous system and remain trivial (Table 40-1). A number of acute syndromes relate to particular venous beds that are afflicted by thrombosis.

Chronic venous disorders may range from trivial telangiectasias to serious and disabling intractable lower extremity venous ulceration. Nearly all these conditions have to do with venous reflux. The application of venous testing to these conditions is the subject of this chapter.

Obstruction

Venous obstruction is almost always the result of venous thrombosis. Less frequently, extrinsic compression may lead to total obstruction, such as on the subclavian vein or left common iliac vein. Patients with one or more elements of the Virchow triad (stasis, hypercoagulability, or vein wall abnormalities) are susceptible to thrombosis.[1] The clinical presentation can be totally asymptomatic or may progress to flagrant phlegmasia cerulea dolens and venous gangrene. The magnitude of symptoms and findings depends to some extent on the location and number of venous segments affected by thrombus.

Superficial Thrombophlebitis

Phlebitis in a superficial vein is readily diagnosed clinically. Varicose veins in the lower extremity and intravenous therapy in the upper extremity predispose a patient to phlebitis. Physical diagnosis of superficial thrombophlebitis can be made by detecting an erythematous streaking in the distribution of superficial veins. Tenderness is present and the extent of thrombosis is identified by a palpable cord. Thus, the diagnosis can be made by physical examination, but accurate estimation of the proximal extent of the disease process or deep venous penetration depends upon objective testing in the vascular laboratory.

Duplex ultrasonography is a reliable technique for evaluation of superficial venous thrombosis just as it is for deep venous thrombosis (DVT). The examination provides objective evidence of the diagnosis and a clear definition of its extent. This is particularly important in thrombosis of the great saphenous vein because surgeons believe that intervention is necessary to treat ascending thrombophlebitis of the saphenous vein in the upper third of the thigh.[2] Surgical treatment has fallen into disuse. Instead, low-molecular-weight heparin and other anticoagulants are given in situations in which it is believed that superficial thrombophlebitis is becoming dangerous.

Although the initial diagnosis can be made clinically, it is now known that approximately 20% of patients with

TABLE 40-1. Venous disorders.

Acute venous thrombosis
Deep venous thrombosis
    Proximal—iliofemoral
    Distal—popliteal, calf vein
Subclavian-axillary
Jugular
Cavernous sinus
Sagittal sinus
Mesenteric

Chronic venous dysfunction
Telangiectasias
Reticular varicosities
Varicose veins
Chronic obstruction and reflux
Deep venous reflux
Perforating vein dysfunction

superficial phlebitis will also have an associated occult DVT (Table 40-2).[3-7] Further, in approximately one-third of those with only initial superficial phlebitis the thrombus will eventually extend to the deep system via the saphenofemoral junction or perforating veins. Phlebitis of the great saphenous vein above the knee is particularly susceptible to progression to DVT. Therefore, it is prudent to perform a duplex examination for DVT[8] and, in selected cases, a follow-up examination in patients with suspected or proven ascending superficial phlebitis.

Evaluation of the lower extremity venous system for DVT has revealed thrombosis of the great saphenous vein in approximately 1% of limbs.[9] Thus, examination of the saphenofemoral junction should be a part of the examination of the lower extremity venous system when DVT is suspected.

Varicose Phlebitis

A special case of superficial thrombophlebitis is found in patients with lower extremity varicose veins. Before the advent of duplex testing, it was thought that superficial thrombophlebitis in varicose veins was isolated and not associated with DVT. However, recent experience suggests that superficial thrombophlebitis in varicose veins is not a benign condition. Clinical experience has identified particular factors that influence superficial thrombophlebitis in varicose veins. External trauma, a tight stocking band at the proximal calf, and an insect bite all can initiate varicose phlebitis. Sclerotherapy is another risk factor. Treatment of large varicose veins by injection is frequently followed by venous inflammation, but it is believed that this inflammation does not progress to thrombosis and that DVT and pulmonary embolism are rare. Guex observed three DVT patients in over 1200 patients treated by him. With his careful studies even Guex states that the overall incidence is unknown.[10]

Surgical procedures can be followed by spontaneous thrombosis in varicose veins and specific surgical procedures used in treatment of varicose veins may be followed by DVT in 0.2–0.4% of patients.

Diagnostic testing may be associated with superficial thrombophlebitis affecting varicose veins. Phlebography is particularly risky, but duplex scanning is not a risk factor. Because superficial thrombophlebitis may be associated with DVT, it is suggested that scanning of the deep and superficial veins of both limbs should be done in patients with superficial thrombophlebitis affecting varicose veins.

Deep Venous Thrombosis

DVT of the lower limbs is very common. An estimated 5 million cases occur in the United States yearly[11]. In addition to the acute problem, DVT can lead to death from pulmonary embolism or significant morbidity from the postphlebitic syndrome. Unlike superficial phlebitis, where the diagnosis is literally under the examining finger, the accuracy of clinical diagnosis of DVT is unreliable (Table 40-3). Clinical diagnosis of DVT has demonstrated accuracy only ranging from 50% to 70% in both retrospective and prospective studies.[12] Thus, if DVT is part of a differential diagnosis, an objective test must be done to confirm or refute the diagnosis. In addition,

TABLE 40-2. Incidence of occult deep venous thrombosis associated with superficial thrombophlebitis.

Year	Reference	Method	Incidence
1993	Jorgensen et al.[3]	Duplex scanning	23%
1991	Prountjos et al.[4]	Venogram	20%
1991	Lutter et al.[5]	Duplex scanning	28%
1990	Skillman et al.[6]	IPG[a] and venogram	12%
1986	Bergqvist et al.[7]	Venogram	44%,[b] 3%[c]

[a]IPG, impedance plethysmography.
[b]Patients without varicose veins.
[c]Patients with varicose veins.

TABLE 40-3. Sensitivity and specificity of clinical findings of deep venous thrombosis.[a]

Finding	Sensitivity	Specificity
Calf pain	60–85%	15–22%
Calf tenderness	50–75%	25–50%
Ankle edema	30–40%	15–25%
Leg/ankle swelling	35–50%	10–70%
Redness	5–15%	80–90%
Superficial vein dilation	25–30%	30–80%
Homan sign	15–40%	50–80%

[a]Modified from leClerc JR. *Venus Thromboembolic Disease*. London: Lea & Febiger, 1991, Table 13.2.

because up to two-thirds of DVTs are clinically silent, screening of high-risk patients may be justified even though it may not be cost effective.[14–17] Duplex scanning is now used to diagnose lower extremity DVT in most vascular laboratories and ultrasound departments. Perhaps it is redundant to state that duplex ultrasound with compression is now the standard test for DVT. However, a number of techniques have been used in the past but are seldom employed in clinical medicine today. Among these are contrast phlebography, isotope phlebography, and impedance plethysmography. Diagnostic modalities in use in vascular laboratories can be assessed in three ways. The first is determination of the sensitivity and specificity of the test versus an accepted gold standard; another is observation of clinical outcome analysis after a positive or negative test; and third there is determination of reproducibility.

When duplex ultrasound was compared with contrast phlebography, it was admitted that contrast phlebography might not detect all DVT but, as a valid test, it did exclude clinically significant DVT. This was proven by outcome analyses. However, interobserver variation of approximately 10% in interpretation of contrast phlebograms has been documented. This tends to invalidate the examination.

Radionuclide scans are used in the diagnosis of a pulmonary embolism. Therefore, there has been interest in imaging of the veins with isotopes. Difficulties with study methodology have led to questions about the accuracy and utility of radionuclide phlebography.[18]

Because no technique is as widely acceptable as ultrasound, this has become entirely dominant and it is accepted now that sensitivities of 83–100% and specificities of 86–100% are accurate descriptions of the method. Even in the late 1990s there remained some controversy about the place of impedance plethysmography. The late Professor Kenneth Moser stated that "we believe that the optimal diagnostic approach to a patient with suspected venous thrombosis is impedance plethysmography, followed by the selective use of compression ultrasonography, venography, or both." However, there has been gradual change toward early referral of patients with suspected venous thrombosis to the diagnostic laboratory. Therefore, there is a higher likelihood of nonocclusive proximal thrombi. While these can be imaged with duplex ultrasonography, impedance plethysmography is much less sensitive.

Ultrasonography is preferable to impedance plethysmography and has been compared in a direct, randomized comparison.[19] Up to 15–30% of limbs with venous thrombosis have persistent abnormal results on impedance plethysmography for up to 6 months. This presents difficulties when symptoms recur. Compression ultrasonography can be used in such patients with recurrent symptoms and can quantify the new thrombus mass.

Venous Disorders of the Extremities

Although physiologic testing [mercury in silastic strain gauge plethysmography (MSG) and impedance plethysmography (IPG)] dominated older methods of diagnosis of DVT in the past, imaging studies have emerged and are now dominant. Duplex ultrasound is only one such method of deep venous imaging. Contrast phlebography is another. It is available in most clinics and is highly sensitive and specific. It produces a direct image of the thrombus and its extent. It is invasive, objectionable to patients, and not portable. Ultrasonography removes those objections, is relatively inexpensive, but is highly operator dependent. It is less sensitive in calf vein thrombosis and differentiation of acute from chronic changes with duplex ultrasonography can be difficult. Magnetic resonance imaging may be useful in specific circumstances. It images pelvic veins as well as calf veins but it is an expensive technique, somewhat operator dependent, and may not be available in all clinics.[20]

Traditional teaching, largely derived from autopsy studies, holds that most lower extremity venous thrombosis begins in soleal sinuses or calf veins. However, duplex scanning has cast doubt on the universality of this concept. Primary iliac venous thrombosis (described below) is an important exception to the old dogma. Although two-thirds of DVT in the calf will lyse spontaneously, the remainder may propagate into the popliteal vein or embolize directly to the lungs. Such emboli are small and often silent. There is controversy over how to manage patients with isolated below-knee DVT. Some disagreement comes from the fact that a single small thrombus in one paired vein is different from multiple tibial venous occlusions or total obliteration of all crural veins. Some experts recommend anticoagulation at the time of diagnosis just as for above-knee DVT.[21,22] Others advocate careful follow-up examinations until the DVT lyses or extends to the popliteal vein.[23] Some vascular laboratories completely eliminate examination of the calf veins. Despite the management controversy, such thrombi should be looked for and, if found, should not be ignored. Unfortunately, accuracy of a duplex study for below-knee DVT is inferior to that for above-knee occlusion.

Iliac Vein Thrombosis

Isolated iliac vein thrombosis is said to be rare. One report using phlebography found none in 164 consecutive patients.[24] Another study using duplex scanning in 833 patients found only one isolated iliac (common iliac) thrombosis in 209 patients with DVT,[25] while another study of 237 patients found DVT in 56 and isolated iliac DVT in three.[26] These studies included all patients referred to a vascular laboratory with suspicion of DVT and those referred for postoperative surveillance after orthopedic surgery. However, it is known that pregnancy and pelvic abnormalities such as cancer, trauma, and recent surgery can also predispose to iliac thrombosis.[27] The true incidence of isolated pelvic DVT in these subgroups is not known as duplex diagnosis of iliac thrombosis is often difficult and accuracy has not been established.

The noninvasive laboratory has been particularly useful in defining the natural history of DVT. Serial studies have shown that at 3 months and 6 months of follow-up following DVT, between 55% and 75% of initially occlusive thrombi were recanalized. [28,29] Thrombus resolution occurs faster and more completely in situations of popliteal or calf thrombi. Long-term observations have suggested a very low incidence of postthrombotic syndrome sequelae (hyperpigmentation, lipodermatosclerosis, venous ulcer) in patients in whom anticoagulants and compression therapy have been used. Follow-up studies have indicated a high mortality (14%) and rate of recurrence (24%) in patients with DVT.

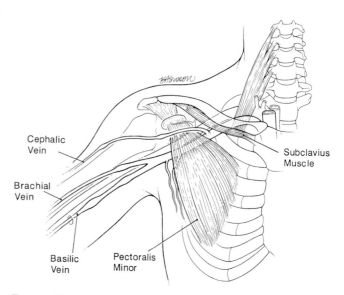

FIGURE 40–2. The structures that will be visualized in imaging the thoracic outlet. Note that the subclavian vein lies anterior to the scalenus anticus muscle and that muscle separates the subclavian vein from the subclavian artery. The cephalic vein is seen entering the subclavian vein and the brachial and basilica veins are illustrated.

Subclavian Axillary Venous Thrombosis

Another special circumstance in the general category of DVT is subclavian axillary vein thrombosis. The descriptive terms primary, spontaneous, idiopathic, effort, and traumatic have all been used to describe this condition (Figure 40–1). It is recognized that strenuous upper body activity as well as resting arm position are predisposing factors, as are anatomic abnormalities that produce venous compression in the thoracic outlet (Figure 40–2). Local intravascular conditions, including chemical irritation from intravenous fluids or traumatic catheterization as well as pacemaker wires, all induce occlusion of the subclavian axillary axis.

In contrast to the lower extremity, in which duplex Doppler ultrasonography is dominant, invasive phlebography is widely used in subclavian axillary venous thrombosis. Nevertheless, duplex ultrasonography remains useful. It is safe, reliable, and may be repeated. Unfortunately, duplex ultrasonography has its limitations because of acoustic shadowing from the clavicle. This reveals a blind spot exactly in the area that may be the nidus for thrombosis. Furthermore, the presence of large collateral vessels can make interpretation of the scan difficult. It is generally accepted that a positive Doppler ultrasound scan is definitive but a negative scan may call for mandatory phlebography.[30]

While radiologic catheterization of the thrombosed axillary subclavian vein is traumatic and invasive, the technique does allow fragmentation of the thrombus and installation of local lytic agents. Lytic agent treatment of spontaneous axillary subclavian venous thrombosis has been shown to be more efficient and efficacious than anticoagulant treatment[31,32] and, while it is expensive, its prevention of disability is believed to be worth the additional cost.

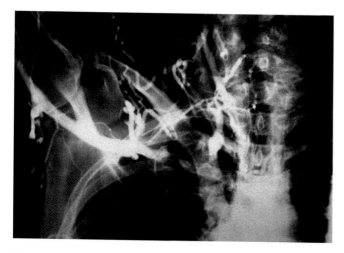

FIGURE 40–1. Axillary phlebogram with the arm in a provocative hyperabducted position. Note the apparent occlusion of the axillary vein beneath the clavicle and also the profuse network of collateral veins that has developed to counteract the physiologic effects of the subclavian venous obstruction. Also note the competent valves in veins in the axilla that prevent retrograde flow of contrast medium.

Duplex examination of the upper extremity is done by the vascular technologist to visualize the veins and determine their function. Commonly, patients are referred because of arm pain, swelling, and inflammation. Occasionally, the indication for the upper extremity study is a pulmonary embolus.

While there are no contraindications to the procedure, it may be difficult to perform if the patient is confused or uncooperative. Other limitations of the procedure are grossly obese patients or those with massively swollen upper extremities.

The investigation is done with ultrasound technology with pulsed Doppler capability. A generous supply of aquasonic gel and towels is necessary. The examination can be done on the examining table or at the bedside but a VHS, professional-grade videotape should also be on hand. A history should be obtained from the patient or family members and this should focus on the acute problem. The procedure should be explained to the patient and there should be time for the patient to ask questions. Best images are obtained with a 5–7.5 MHz phased-array probe. The patient should be placed in a comfortable position with the head up and the arm positioned outward to prevent costoclavicular occlusion of the subclavian vein.

The best images should be obtained by adjusting the grayscale and samples should be obtained at a 60° angle to the vein. The volume control should be adjusted to make the sound comfortable. Testing should include a longitudinal as well as a transverse view of the structures. The examination should start with the subclavian vein located just beneath the clavicle. The vein should be examined both above and below the clavicle and then the examination should proceed distally along the axillary vein followed by examination of the brachial vein. The cephalic vein should be located and followed along the medial aspect of the upper forearm. The basilic vein should be located in the upper portion of the arm medial to the cephalic vein. In all of the named veins, it is necessary to obtain a Doppler signal and augment flow looking for signs of distention of the vessel walls.

Primary Venous Insufficiency

An enormous variety of testing modalities have been employed in the evaluation of patients and limbs with primary venous insufficiency. As a result of this, it is necessary to make some broad generalizations about their use in present-day vascular laboratories.

Primary venous insufficiency includes telangiectasias or spider web veins, reticular flat blue-green varicosities, and varicose veins as a single entity. However, the use of diagnostic testing is different for each of these entities. Clinical examination is always used in evaluating limbs

TALBE 40–4. New clinical classification of venous disease.[a]

Class 0	No visible or palpable signs of venous disease
Class 1	Telangiectasias or reticular veins
Class 2	Varicose veins
Class 3	Edema
Class 4	Skin changes (pigmentation, eczema, lipodermatosclerosis)
Class 5	Skin changes with healed ulcer
Class 6	Skin changes with active ulceration

[a]Modified from Porter JM, Moneta GI. International Consensus Committee on Chronic Venous Disease. Reporting standards in venous disease: An update. J Vasc Surg 1995;21:635–645.

with primary venous insufficiency and each clinician is quite confident of his or her diagnostic abilities. Yet, objective testing of the clinician against the vascular laboratory shows that the vascular laboratory is much more accurate.[33] An attempt has been made to classify conditions of venous dysfunction (Table 40–4). Using this classification in reporting may clarify the condition that is being studied.

Most clinicians believe that patients with primary varicose veins can be adequately assessed by clinical examination aided by hand-held Doppler ultrasound. Most would agree that patients with only telangiectasias can be assessed clinically without recourse to other noninvasive methods. However, when ultrasound is added to the clinical examination for telangiectasias, a number of reflux sites and perforating veins can be identified that would otherwise be invisible.

Varicose veins require use of Doppler testing before planning therapy. Axial reflux in saphenous veins will dictate the need for surgical intervention. Absence of such reflux allows treatment by sclerotherapy.

A generalization can be made about physiologic testing. The majority of these techniques, including strain-gauge plethysmography, photoplethysmography, foot volumetry, and isotope plethysmography, provide an overall function of the calf muscle pump. This is similar to the direct measurement of foot vein pressure and there is a close correlation between venous pressure and venous volume testing. Many investigators add the obstruction of superficial veins by a vein-occluding tourniquet as a routine part of the investigation. However, others have challenged this concept and have shown that the application of a tourniquet is notoriously inaccurate. It should be added that the vascular laboratory can help immeasurably in determining whether visible varicose veins are the cause of a patient's symptoms.

Interested physicians have come to rely on standing duplex scanning in the assessment of venous reflux.[34] Gradually, in institutions interested in treating venous disorders, such reflux testing has become routine. Experienced clinicians believe that the duplex examination adds to their assessment of the patient and frequently refutes their clinical impressions. Of particular importance is the detection of the nonsaphenous origin of reflux in the femoral area. In such situations, the saphenous vein may be spared during surgical removal of refluxing veins.

While the territory of the greater saphenous vein is responsible for varicose veins in the vast majority of patients with primary venous insufficiency, in fact, the saphenofemoral junction is found to be competent in 30% of limbs.[35] When this is true, attention can be directed to the varicosities themselves and not to the junction; thus portions of the saphenous vein are preserved.

Doubt has been raised about the actual involvement of the saphenous vein in varicosities and, because of specific findings on ultrasound evaluation,[36] the answer is not yet final. Involvement of the lesser saphenous vein in varicose vein disease occurs in 15–20% of limbs.

Of particular importance to the vascular laboratory is the evaluation of limbs with recurrent varicose veins. Studies have shown that duplex scanning is an important adjunct to management of recurrent varicose veins.[37] It defines the pathways of incompetence and shows that the saphenofemoral junction and retained long saphenous vein are the key to the treatment of recurrent varicosities.[38,39]

Chronic Venous Insufficiency

DVT may permanently damage the affected vein segment. The thrombotic obstruction may recanalize and restore normal flow or the recanalization may produce an irregular surface that impedes flow. This leads to the opening of venous collaterals around the obstruction. Such collaterals are usually so extensive that physiologic tests of venous function are unable to detect the anatomic obstruction. Furthermore, intrinsic damage by thrombus to the venous valves produces shortening, thickening, and scarring that absolutely preclude normal functioning. Thus, the postthrombotic venous segment can be expected to reflux and may also obstruct. In addition to reflux through the damaged venous valves, the collateral vessels formed around the obstruction will dilate, their valves will fail, and this adds to the reflux.

Reflux, or flow away from the heart, does not occur in every venous segment subjected to thrombosis. Nevertheless, a sufficient number will be affected. The interested physician expects venous dysfunction after every episode of DVT.

In severe chronic venous insufficiency, lower extremity skin changes of hyperpigmentation, induration, and ulceration occur. The induration is commonly referred to as lipodermatosclerosis. In the past, such skin changes were referred to as postthrombotic, and the limb con-

taining these changes was referred to as the postthrombotic or postphlebitic limb. Gradually, it became known that the stigmata of the postthrombotic limb also appears in limbs without any episode of previous DVT. Now, the terms postphlebitic and postthrombotic are relatively obsolete and have been replaced by the term chronic venous insufficiency (CVI). This is important because the terms postphlebitic and postthrombotic have a connotation of hopelessness or inevitability. Very little can be done with a partially obstructed, valveless venous segment. In contrast, the term CVI connotes the possibility of surgical repair. If the refluxing segments can be removed or repaired, the severe condition of CVI may be ameliorated. It is testing in the noninvasive laboratory that will identify the venous segments that are dysfunctioning and will define for the clinician the procedures that will benefit the patient. Thus, the noninvasive evaluation of a limb with venous dysfunction will allow proper prescription of treatment. Examinations relevant to this are those that identify reflux, those that indicate obstruction, and those that localize perforating vein outflow.

Reflux

While most acute venous problems are concerned with obstruction by thrombosis, most chronic venous problems are caused by reflux. Reflux is defined as the retrograde flow of blood in veins of the lower extremity caused by absent or incompetent valves. The result is venous hypertension, which is attributable to one of three possible mechanisms: (1) The column of blood is not interrupted by functioning valves between the right atrium and the veins of the lower extremities. This allows full pressure of gravitational, hydrostatic forces to be exerted on the vein walls. (2) The calf muscle pump mechanism becomes ineffective. Ejection of blood from the limb by muscular compression of deep veins is inadequate and residual venous volume is increased. (3) Perforating veins, including calf perforators and the saphenofemoral or saphenopopliteal junctions, fail to function, allowing venous blood to flow outward and distally rather than inward and proximally. This failure of check valves in calf perforating veins allows high pressures (up to 250 mm Hg) generated by muscular contraction to be transmitted directly to the unsupported superficial veins. The resultant venous hypertension causes symptoms of heaviness, aching, and fatigue as well as findings of edema and dilated veins (varicosities and telangiectasias). In some limbs, venous hypertension is associated with skin pigmentation, lipodermatosclerosis, and/or ulceration. In such situations, axial and/or perforating vein reflux is common and is associated with the cutaneous changes.

Uncomplicated venous reflux is common. By age 20 years, 20% of the population may have some reflux, although they may not have varicosities.[40] The valves of varicose veins are always incompetent. Following DVT, valve damage is common and reflux can be detected in approximately half the veins that were thrombosed.[41]

Although it is easy to define reflux and appreciate its importance, as yet there is no universally accepted standard of diagnosis. Various tests may be invasive or noninvasive. Of the invasive tests, ambulatory venous pressure was an historic "gold standard." However, this test is a global measure of limb reflux. Pressures obtained in various categories of severity of venous stasis may be identical.

Pressures obtained do not aid in planning therapy nor do they correlate closely with stages of venous insufficiency. Descending phlebography is often used clinically to confirm and grade venous reflux, but this is occasionally inaccurate because of seepage of relatively high-density radiographic contrast media through competent valves.

The vascular laboratory has made a monumental contribution to the understanding of CVI.[41] Because of the influence of the noninvasive laboratory, it is known that the severe skin changes of CVI are not always due to post-thrombotic deep venous reflux. Recent studies show that extensive deep venous reflux is actually not dominant in CVI and superficial venous reflux is frequently present in limbs with the complications of severe CVI. In particular, the finding of a high prevalence of superficial venous incompetence in such limbs leads to more aggressive surgical management and even cure of the condition.[42]

While surgeons have been encouraged to correct superficial reflux in treatment of severe CVI, others are influenced by teaching that excision of secondary varicosities following DVT is contraindicated. It has been feared that stripping of the saphenous vein and its varices in the presence of deep venous obstruction would lead to worsening of the obstructive condition. This might even cause catastrophic venous congestion, jeopardizing the viability of the entire limb. Many surgeons, even today, believe that confirmation of deep venous patency is essential to the preoperative investigation before stripping of the saphenous vein. This is the basis for performing phlebography or duplex ultrasonography to determine patency prior to saphenectomy. However, more recent studies have shown that even in conditions of severe venous obstruction, the results of saphenectomy are very good in limbs with severe CVI.[43] Saphenectomy may, in fact, be strongly indicated in patients with true postthrombotic syndrome who still have a mixture of venous obstruction and venous reflux. The procedure of saphenectomy is well tolerated and is without adverse sequelae in the true postthrombotic limb. Removing the reflux parameters improves limb functioning and cutaneous abnormalities without jeopardizing the limb in any way.[43]

Perforating Veins and Chronic Venous Insufficiency

Because of increased emphasis on bidirectional flow in perforating veins and the relationship of perforating veins to the severe changes of CVI, the vascular laboratory has been increasingly employed to detect these vessels. Conventional wisdom holds that deep venous insufficiency is an important part of severe CVI and that outflow through perforating veins may be related to the skin changes.[44] Duplex imaging of perforating veins appears to be more effective than phlebography in detecting outward flow through the perforators.[45] However, both positive and negative findings have occurred when duplex evaluation was compared with direct surgical assessment.[46] Surgeons interested in treating severe CVI agree that a duplex examination is of value and that if a perforating vein is found on duplex, it probably will be found at surgery. However, surgeons will acknowledge that approximately 20% of existing perforating veins found at surgery are not seen by duplex examination. Other methods of detecting perforating veins include fluorescein testing as well as radionuclide scanning.[47,48] Thermography is another method that has been attempted.[49]

Duplex reflux study is recommended for all limbs with severe CVI. A search for perforating veins on the medial and lateral aspects of the limb should always be added to this examination. Even though limbs with severe CVI have a large component of superficial reflux as a cause of the cutaneous stigmata, the perforating veins are usually associated with the areas of lipodermatosclerosis or ulceration. These may be the target of surgical intervention. Therefore, perforating veins should be identified, located, and measured from the sole of the heel to guide surgeons and aid their discovery at the time of operation. Today, most operations for severe CVI consist of correction of all the superficial venous reflux as well as interruption of the perforating veins.

Pulmonary Embolism

About 90% of pulmonary emboli arise from DVT of the lower extremities and pelvis; the rest originate from the upper extremities, heart, or pulmonary arteries. While in most patients with established pulmonary embolism, diagnosis of DVT may be confirmed by noninvasive testing or venography, only about 30% will present with clinical manifestations of venous thrombosis. In the appropriate clinical setting, suspicion usually is aroused by the sudden onset of chest pain, dyspnea, hemoptysis, and low PO_2. These findings, however, have almost no predictive value. Tachycardia, tachypnea, and low PCO_2 are perhaps slightly more indicative of pulmonary embolism. Electrocardiographic tracings may be suggestive, but are not diagnostic; their main value is in ruling out myocardial infarction. Unfortunately, there are no reliable typical chest film findings that are diagnostic of pulmonary embolism. The information provided by the chest film, electrocardiogram (ECG), and blood gases is nevertheless helpful in the differential diagnosis, in assessing the general condition of the patient, and in determining the extent of pathophysiologic changes secondary to embolism. With the availability of pulmonary perfusion and ventilation scanning as well as pulmonary angiography, it is possible to diagnose pulmonary embolism with great accuracy.

The patient thought to have pulmonary embolism should have a preliminary chest film, an ECG, blood gas determinations, and noninvasive venous testing of the lower extremities (duplex ultrasound). These tests are to be followed by perfusion and ventilation lung scanning. If the clinical setting is appropriate, the patient may be started on heparin sodium while these tests are being done. If the scan is normal, pulmonary embolism may be safely excluded, heparinization discontinued, and the search for other pathologic changes made. If the perfusion scan shows defects and the ventilation scan is normal, or if both scans are abnormal and mismatched, pulmonary embolism is a highly probably diagnosis, and the patient should be treated for it. If both scans are abnormal and the defects are matched, the findings are suggestive, but not diagnostic of pulmonary embolism. However, if, in addition to these findings, the noninvasive venous testing of the lower extremities is positive for DVT, the diagnosis of pulmonary embolism is highly probable, and the patient should be treated for it. If noninvasive studies of the lower extremities are negative for DVT, it is necessary to proceed with pulmonary angiography, which, if positive, confirms the diagnosis of pulmonary embolism. If the pulmonary angiogram is negative, however, then pulmonary embolism is ruled out.

References

1. Virchow R. Die Cellularpathologic. In: Ihrer Begrundung auf Physiologische und Pathologische Gewebelehere. Berlin: A. Hirschewald, 1858.
2. Kock HJ, Krause U, Albrecht KH, et al. Die Crossektomie bei aszendierender oberflächlicher Thrombophiebitis der Beinvenen. Zentralb Chir 1997;122:795–200.
3. Jorgensen JO, Hanel KC, Morgan AM, Hunt JM. The incidence of deep venous thrombosis in patients with superficial thrombophlebitis of the lower limbs. J Vasc Surg 1993;18:70–73.
4. Prountijos P, Bastounis E, Hadjinikolaou L, Felekuras E, Balas P. Superficial venous thrombosis of the lower extremities coexisting with deep venous thrombosis. Int Angiol 1991;10:63–65.
5. Gillet JL, Allaert FA, Perrin M. Superficial thrombophlebitis in non varicose veins of the lower limbs. A prospective analysis in 42 patients. J Mal Vasc. 2004;29:263–272.
6. Skillman JJ, Kent KC, Porter DH, Kim D. Simultaneous occurrence of superficial and deep thrombophlebitis in the lower extremity. J Vasc Surg 1990;11:818–824.
7. Bergqvist D, Jaroszewski H. Deep vein thrombosis in patients with superficial thrombophlebitis of the leg. BMJ 1986;292:658–659.
8. Chengelis DL, Bendick PJ, Glover JL, Brown OW, Ranval TJ. Progression of superficial venous thrombosis to deep venous thrombosis. J Vasc Surg 1996;24:745–749.
9. Leon L, Giannoukas AD, Dodd D, Chan P, Labropoulos N. Clinical significance of superficial vein thrombosis. Eur J Vasc Endovasc Surg 2005;29:10–17.
10. Guex JJ. Thrombotic complications of varicose veins: A literature review of the role of superficial venous thrombosis. Dermatol Surg 1996;22:378–382.
11. Moser KK. Pulmonary embolism. In: Murray J, Nadel J (eds). Respiratory Medicine, 2nd ed., p. 653. Philadelphia: W.B. Saunders, 1994.
12. Sover ER, Brammer HM, Rowedder AM. Thrombosis of the proximal greater saphenous vein: ultrasonographic diagnosis and clinical significance. J Ultrasound Med 1997; 16:113–116.
13. Haeger K. Problems of acute deep venous thrombosis: The interpretation of signs and symptoms. Angiology 1969;20: 219–223.
14. Browse NL, Burnand KG, Lea Thomas M. Diseases of the Veins: Pathology, Diagnosis, and Treatment, p. 478. London: Edward Arnold, 1988.
15. Salzman EW. Venous thrombosis made easy. N Engl J Med 1986;314:847–848.
16. Mattos MA, Londrey GL, Leutz DW, et al. Color-flow duplex scanning for the surveillance and diagnosis of acute deep venous thrombosis. J Vasc Surg 1992;15:366–376.
17. Hillner BE, Philbrick JT, Becker DM. Optimal management of suspected lower extremity deep vein thrombosis. Arch Intern Med 1992;152:165–175.
18. Kilpatrick TK, Gibson RN, Lichtenstein M, Neerhut P, Andrews J, Hopper J. A comparative study of radionuclide venography and contrast venography in the diagnosis of deep venous thrombosis. Aust NZ J Med 1993;23:641–645.
19. Heijboer H, Büller HR, Lensing AWA, Turpie AGG, Colly LP, Wouter ten Cate J. A comparison of real-time compression ultrasonography with impedance plethysmography for the diagnosis of deep vein thrombosis in symptomatic outpatients. N Engl J Med 1993;329: 1365–1369.
20. Barloon TJ, Bergus GR, Seabold JE. Diagnostic imaging of lower limb deep venous thrombosis. Am Family Physician 1997;56:791–801.
21. Rotert EM, Basarich JR, Nashelsky J. Treatment of calf deep venous thrombosis. Am Fam Physician 2005;71: 2157–2158.
22. Lohr JM, James Ky, Deshmukh RM, Hasselfeld KA. Calf vein thrombi are not a benign finding. Am J Surg 1995;170: 86–90.

23. Solis MM, Ranval TJ, Nix ML, *et al.* Is anticoagulation indicated for asymptomatic postoperative calf vein thrombosis? J Vasc Surg 1992;16:414–419.

24. Rose SC, Zwiebel WJ, Miller FJ. Distribution of acute lower extremity deep venous thrombosis in symptomatic and asymptomatic patients: Imaging implications. J Ultrasound Med 1994;13:243–250.

25. Markel A, Manzo RA, Bergelin RO, Strandness DE Jr. Pattern and distribution of thrombi in acute venous thrombosis. Arch Surg 1992;127:305–309.

26. Sarpa MS, Messina LM, Smith M, Chang L, Greenfield U. Reliability of venous duplex scanning to image the iliac veins and to diagnose iliac vein thrombosis in patients suspected of having acute deep venous thrombosis. J Vasc Technol 1991;15:299–302.

27. Duddy MJ, McHugo JM. Duplex ultrasound of the common femoral vein in pregnancy and puerperium. Br J Radiol 1991;64:785–791.

28. Uindhagen A, Bergqvist D, Hallböök T, Efsing HO. Venous function five to eight years after clinically suspected deep venous thrombosis. Acta Med Scand 1985;2l7:389–395.

29. Lindner DJ, Edwards JM, Phinney ES, Taylor UM Jr, Porter JM. Long-term hemodynamic and clinical sequelae of lower extremity deep venous thrombosis. J Vasc Surg 1986;4:436–442.

30. Molina JE, Hunter DW, Dietz CA Jr. Occlusion of subclavian-innominate veins: The increasing problem of receiving improper care. Minn Med 2004;87:38–40.

31. AbuRahma AF, Short YS, White III JF, Boland JP. Treatment alternatives for axillary-subclavian thrombosis: Long-term followup. Cardiovasc Surg 1996;4:783–787.

32. AbuRahma AF, Sadler D, Stuart P, Khan MZ, Boland JP. Conventional versus thrombolytic therapy in spontaneous (effort) axillary subclavian venous thrombosis. Am J Surg 1991;161:459–465.

33. Szendro G, Nicolaides AN, Zukowski AJ, *et al.* Duplex scanning in the assessment of deep venous incompetence. J Vasc Surg 1986;4:237–242.

34. Guex JJ, Hiltbrand B, Bayon JM, Henri F, Allaert FA, Perrin M. Anatomical patterns in varicose vein disease. Phlebology 1995;10:1094–1097.

35. Zamboni P, Cappelli M, Marcellino MG, Murgia AP, Pisano L, Fabi P. Does a varicose saphenous vein exist? Phlebology 1997;12:74–77.

36. Canonico S, Campitiello F, Lauletta V, Pacifico F, Sciaudone G. Diagnostic and surgical approaches to recurrent varicose veins of lower limbs. Panminerva Med l997;39:287–290.

37. Blomgren L, Johansson G, Bergqvist D. Randomized clinical trial of routine preoperative duplex imaging before varicose vein surgery. Br J Surg 2005;92:688–694.

38. Tong Y, Royle J. Recurrent varicose veins following high ligation of long saphenous vein: A duplex ultrasound study. Cardiovasc Surg 1995;3:485–487.

39. Stucker M, Reich S, Robak-Pawelczyk B, Moll C, Rudolph T, Altmeyer PJ, Weindorf NG, Hirche H, Gambichler T, Schultz-Ehrenburg U. Changes in venous refilling time from childhood to adulthood in subjects with apparently normal veins. J Vasc Surg 2005;41:296–302.

40. van Ramshorst B, van Bemmelen PS, Hoeneveld H, Eikelboom BC. The development of valvular incompetence after deep vein thrombosis: A followup study with duplex scanning. J Vasc Surg 1994;20:1059–1066.

41. Myers KA, Ziegenbein RW, Zeng GH, Matthews PG. Duplex ultrasonography scanning for chronic venous disease: Patterns of venous reflux. J Vasc Surg l995;21:605–612.

42. Shami SK, Sarin S, Cheatle TR, Scurr JH, Coleridge Smith PD. Venous ulcers and the superficial venous system. J Vasc Surg 1993;17:487–490.

43. Raju S, Easterwood U, Fountain T, *et al.* Saphenectomy in the presence of chronic venous obstruction. Surgery 1998;123:637–644.

44. Welch HJ, Young CM, Semegran AB, Lafrati MD, Mackey WC, O'Donnell TF Jr. Duplex assessment of venous reflux and chronic venous insufficiency: The significance of deep venous reflux. J Vasc Surg 1996;24:755–762.

45. Hanrahan UM, Araki CT, Fischer JB, *et al.* Evaluation of the perforating veins of the lower extremity using high-resolution duplex imaging. J Cardiovasc Surg 1991;32:87–97.

46. Engelhorn C, Picheth F, Castro N Jr, Dabul JN, Cunha SXS. Color flow localization of insufficient communicating or perforating veins prior to surgical ligation. J Vasc Technol 1993;17:251–253.

47. Rulli F, Muzi M, Sanguigni V, Giordano A, Zanella E. Diagnostic accuracy of radionuclide venography in the assessment of incompetent perforating veins of the legs. Vasc Surg 1996;30:489–493.

48. Lofqvist J, Jansson I, Thomsen M, Elfström J. Evaluation of the fluorescein test in the diagnosis of incompetent perforating veins. VASA 1983;12:46–50.

49. Patil KD, Williams JR, Williams KU. Thermographic localization of incompetent perforating veins in the leg. BMJ 1970;1:195–197.

Section VI
Deep Abdominal Doppler

41
Deep Doppler in the Liver Vasculature

Peter N. Burns, Heidi Patriquin, and Michel Lafortune

Introduction

The widespread availability of duplex Doppler instruments that combine high-quality ultrasound imaging with spectral and color pulsed Doppler at ultrasonic frequencies suitable for abdominal scanning has brought several exciting new areas of clinical diagnosis into view. These include the assessment of blood flow in the vasculature of the liver and splanchnic veins in a variety of pathologic conditions. It has become apparent that there are numerous circumstances in which the addition of information related to blood flow can complement the role of conventional abdominal ultrasound imaging.[1,2] The Doppler sonographer of the abdomen must therefore be capable of interpreting the Doppler spectrum under a relatively wide range of hemodynamic circumstances: it is perhaps because of the varied objectives of the Doppler technique in the abdomen that there are so few firm guidelines for its use. A critical appreciation of the basic principles and limitations of the Doppler method applied to the splanchnic circulation is an essential prerequisite for its successful clinical use.

Instrumentation

The basic instrument for the deep Doppler examination is the duplex scanner.[3] As in peripheral vascular work, the ultrasound image serves as a guide for the location of the Doppler sample volume. In contrast to peripheral vascular applications, however, Doppler signals in the abdomen are frequently elicited from vessels that are tortuous, far from the transducer, and difficult to visualize throughout their entire course with grayscale sonography. The image must be relied upon to demonstrate the appropriate anatomic area for the positioning of the Doppler sample volume or the color region of interest. High-quality, real-time ultrasound imaging is therefore

essential and this is usually achieved by means of dynamically focused arrays. Among these, the annular array (mechanically steered) sector scanner and the phased array (electronically steered) sector scanner are two of the most popular configurations for abdominal duplex scanning, although only the latter offers color Doppler (Figure 41–1). In patients in whom a larger acoustic window is available, curvilinear or even linear arrays can be used. In spite of the popularity of such systems that combine abdominal imaging and Doppler in a single probe, the optimum conditions for imaging and Doppler rarely coincide, forcing compromise in scanner and probe design. One example is the choice of transducer frequency. The intensity of the echo scattered by red blood cells moving in a vessel increases with the fourth power of the ultrasound frequency. Thus, doubling the ultrasonic frequency results in an echo from blood that is 16 times stronger. This is responsible for a dramatic difference in performance between Doppler instruments detecting blood flow using different ultrasonic frequencies. Of course, attenuation in soft tissue also rises with frequency and so offsets the advantage of the increased efficiency of scattering at higher frequencies. The optimum ultrasonic frequency with which to perform a Doppler examination is an inevitable compromise based on the strength of the echo from blood and the depth of the structure of interest. This tends to force down the optimum Doppler frequency for an abdominal scan to below that at which the best images are obtained. In general, livers that will be imaged at between 3 and 5 MHz will need Doppler frequencies of between 2 and 3 MHz. Although most modern arrays are capable of operating at a range of frequencies (indeed this is necessary to produce a good image), such a bandwidth is inevitably at the expense of Doppler sensitivity, a key determinant of Doppler performance in deep organs.[4] Many advances have been made in recent years in transducer array design and fabrication, but many consider that the best pulsed Doppler performance is still to be found using single element

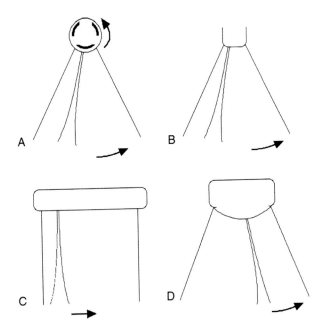

FIGURE 41–1. Four common configurations of duplex color systems for use in the liver. The duplex sample volume and the color region of interest (where applicable) are shown. (A) The mechanical sector scanner. (B) The electronically steered sector scanner. (C) The linear array with electronically steered Doppler beam. (D) The curvilinear (or convex) array.

transducers, which, for the most part, do not produce satisfactory images. The user must therefore be prepared to change transducers between the imaging and Doppler portion of a duplex examination.

Most duplex instruments that employ mechanically moved beams permit selection of the Doppler site only after the real-time image has been frozen and stored on the screen. Electronically steered systems, such as the phased sector, linear or curvilinear arrays, however, employ beams that are sufficiently agile to allow image scan lines to be acquired in rapid alternation with the Doppler data. The result is the simultaneous presentation of the Doppler spectrum and the real-time image. This time-sharing (sometimes called "true duplex" scanning) is the result of some compromise, in which either the frame rate of the real-time image, the pulse-repetition frequency of the Doppler system is reduced, or some interpolation of the Doppler data is implemented during spectral analysis. Though clearly useful in pinpointing a particular vessel in a moving abdomen, the operator should be aware that a price is being paid in performance for the provision of simultaneous Doppler and imaging. The "triplex" mode in which color Doppler and imaging modes are shared with spectral Doppler is usually too slow and noisy for use in the liver.

Color Doppler performance in the abdomen has enjoyed dramatic enhancement in recent years. It should be noted that the color Doppler method is inherently less sensitive to the weaker echoes scattered from low volumes of blood, so that it is possible that small quantities of flowing blood will be detected on duplex scanning but not with color. In addition, the difficulty of rejecting Doppler shifts from moving solid tissue within an image usually forces a higher minimum detectable Doppler shift frequency in a color system. As a result, slow flow—of which there is much in the splanchnic circulation—is detected less easily with a color system than with a duplex scanner. For these reasons, the role of color may be as a real-time tool with which to survey the image for flow, and that of the spectral Doppler to obtain the final Doppler signal for clinical interpretation, including identification of the vessel and its flow characteristics.

Technique

The Doppler examination of deep-lying vessels can be technically demanding. Like all Doppler procedures, satisfactory results rely to a great extent on the coordination of hand, eye, and ear, and the experience of the operator. The nature of Doppler examination in the abdomen involves some considerations that may be new to the peripheral vascular sonographer. The vessels examined are deep and tortuous and often partly hidden by bowel gas, and flow within them is often of low velocity. These characteristics necessitate sensitive instruments, low transducer frequency, and low wall filters and pulse repetition frequency. If duplex scanning is being used to estimate flow velocity, the beam–vessel angle must be less than 60° and it must be measured. Doppler access to abdominal vessels is then confined to those scan planes that contain the vessel axis, a restriction that can cause problems, where, for example, the vessel is tortuous or there is overlying gas. Knowledge of vascular anatomy and flow physiology is essential.

Many of the problems associated with abdominal Doppler examinations have their origin in the relatively poor signal-to-noise ratio of the Doppler signals. The backscattered echo from moving blood is weak, and its detection is confounded by the simultaneous presence of clutter from the moving solid structures of the abdomen. Clutter comprises high-amplitude, low Doppler shift intrusions in the signal that have their origin in moving solid tissue within the sample volume.[5] Such tissue might be the wall of the vessel or surrounding structures experiencing transmitted cardiac or respiratory motion. As the echoes, and hence the Doppler signal, from these structures are many times stronger than those from moving blood, the Doppler detector can be overwhelmed by their presence in the signal. In spectral mode, a low-frequency "thump," heard at the beginning of systole, followed by distortion of the Doppler spectrum, is a common sign of clutter of cardiac origin. As the frequency of the Doppler shifts produced by these motions is quite low, clutter can be eliminated by use of the high-pass filter. However, caution should be exercised when small vessels are being interrogated or when it is necessary to demonstrate or exclude diastolic flow velocities, as these may be obliterated by too high a filter setting. In color mode, a flash from solid tissue obliterates the color associated with vascular flow, forcing the operator to raise the filter, the pulse-repetition frequency, or to engage tissue-motion suppression software that can itself be responsible for additional artifacts.[6]

Shorter ultrasound path lengths to deep organs and vessels mean not only that there is less attenuation, but higher frequencies can be used. This has the simultaneous effect of increasing the backscatter cross section of blood, giving a stronger echo, and increasing the Doppler shift frequencies, so lowering the threshold velocity for the detection of slow flow. The advent of Doppler endosonography has made the largest contribution to the effort to gain closer access to the abdominal and pelvic structures. Although transesophageal, transrectal, transvaginal, endovascular, and endoluminal Doppler are in their infancy, color and duplex systems are already becoming available and it is reasonable to expect that the improved acoustic access they afford to deep structures will continue to be exploited for Doppler studies.

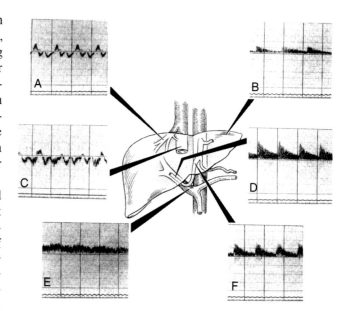

FIGURE 41-2. Time–velocity spectra in (A) right hepatic vein; (B) parenchymal signal; (C) inferior vena cava; (D) proper hepatic artery; (E) portal vein; (f) hepatic artery. (Reproduced with permission from Taylor K, *et al.* Blood flow in deep abdominal and pelvic vessels: Ultrasonic pulsed Doppler analysis. Radiology 1985;154:487–493.)

Interpreting the Doppler Spectrum

Spectral Content

A comparison of normal Doppler signals obtained from the major vessels associated with the liver (Figure 41–2) reveals a variety of waveform and spectral patterns. Each of these features has its origin in the hemodynamic conditions pertaining to that vessel. In interpreting this "flow signature" of a specific vessel's signal it is important to appreciate the major factors that influence its form. Thus, while the waveform shape (that is, the variation of the maximum Doppler shift frequency over the cardiac cycle) can yield information about the vascular impedance distal to the point of measurement, the content of the spectrum reflects aspects of the local flow characteristics, for example, whether the flow is laminar or disturbed, and whether the velocity profile is flat, blunted, or parabolic. Deviations from these appearances are seen to occur with stenosis, as they do in the large peripheral vessels. However, because the normal, laminar flow signal from vessels such as the hepatic artery contains a range of velocities, spectral broadening of itself cannot be taken as a sign of stenosis in smaller, deep-lying vessels. The diagnosis of stenosis in the abdominal arteries therefore relies on the detection of abnormally high velocities, rather than of spectral broadening.

Presence of Flow

Determining whether flow is present is one of the simplest but perhaps most useful applications of Doppler. It may be used to exclude occlusion by thrombosis, or to determine the point of occlusion of a limb vessel during a pressure measurement. It can also be used to differentiate vessels from nonvascular structures that have a similar appearance on the image. An example is the differentiation of suspected biliary tract dilation from an enlarged hepatic artery or from portal venous radicals. The recognition of splenic or hepatic arterial aneurysms and their differentiation from cysts is another application.

Confirming the absence of flow is, by its nature, a little more difficult. It is necessary to be certain that the lack of Doppler signal is a consequence of lack of flow, rather than the acoustic or receiver performance parameters of the system. It is prudent to check that normal flow signals can be detected with the same machine settings from comparable structures at comparable depths before concluding that flow is absent at a particular location.

Direction of Flow

The direction of flow is usually of diagnostic value when an occlusion has produced collateral channels whose flow direction is unusual. This is particularly useful in the investigation of patients with suspected portal venous hypertension. The directional resolution of the Doppler system is best when the beam–vessel angle is relatively small and the signal lies in the middle of the dynamic range of the receiver. If a mirror image of the signal is seen in the reverse-flow sideband of the display, care should be taken with the adjustment of angle and receiver gain so as to obtain a trace showing an unambiguous direction.

Identification of Characteristic Flow

It is apparent that normal flow in various parts of the splanchnic circulation shows distinct characteristics according to location. Those characteristics of waveform shape and spectral distribution are often consequences of hemodynamic factors unique to each vessel. These allow the identification of the origin of a flow signal from the spectral display (and the aural quality of the sound) alone and are particularly useful in circumstances where the image may be ambivalent. Examples are the Doppler "signatures" of the hepatic arterial, portal venous, and hepatic venous structures, which are quite distinct from each other and from that of the biliary tree.

The Role of Doppler in the Study of the Liver

Although angiography is still the gold standard for the investigation of the splanchnic venous system, the roles of computed tomography (CT) and magnetic resonance imaging (MRI) are expanding. The Doppler method coupled with real-time imaging is a relatively new non-invasive method of investigating the liver vasculature and the splanchnic veins. Doppler technology is also evolving rapidly and with it the anatomic and physiologic information that can be gleaned from a vessel and the blood flowing within it. The sensitivity of Doppler machines to the detection of slow flow and flow in vessels far removed from the transducer is improving. Because Doppler sonography is cheaper, faster, and more readily available than CT, MRI, and angiography, it is rapidly becoming the imaging method of choice for screening patients with liver disease or portal hypertension.

Doppler ultrasound is an excellent complement to splanchnic angiography: it can answer queries left by an examination that is necessarily dependent on injection of contrast medium, with or without pharmaceutic manipulation. There sometimes are uncertainties about the direction of flow or about whether a vessel is obstructed or simply inaccessible to the contrast medium (such as in the case of reversed flow in the portal vein). The Doppler findings are a reliable indicator of the direction of flow and assesses the splanchnic system in its physiologic state, without the presence of contrast agent. Hepatic veins are easily identified by ultrasound and their flow pattern and direction by Doppler. They usually are not seen with arterioportography, which outlines the major splanchnic vessels, such as the splenic, mesenteric, and portal veins, but leaves tiny vessels relatively unexplored. This is particularly true of the branches of the left portal vein, which are seldom opacified. Arteriography has therefore added relatively little to our understanding of the intrahepatic portal circulation in health and disease. In contrast, each segmental branch of the portal vein is usually accessible to Doppler interrogation. Regional flow patterns and the result of compression, obstruction, or reversal of flow, or arteriovenous fistulas can be assessed. With angiography, to-and-fro or bidirectional flow in a splanchnic vein is difficult to perceive, whereas the Doppler examination yields clear signals of to-and-fro flow motion both on spectral display (a signal above and then below the baseline) and with color (alternating red and blue regions). If there is any doubt about the details of the examination or if the patient's condition changes, the Doppler examination can be repeated without danger.

These advantages are counterbalanced by certain weaknesses, most of which follow those of real-time sonography. The examination is operator dependent and requires some training, not only in sonography but also in the physics of the Doppler effect and in the normal anatomy and physiology of the liver and splanchnic circulation, both in health and in the presence of pathologic conditions. Doppler sonography is subject to the same physical laws as is real-time ultrasound, and it is wishful thinking to expect a good Doppler examination in a patient in whom a poor real-time sonogram has just been obtained.[7] The alcoholic patient with cirrhosis is often obese, with abundant intestinal gas, ascites, or both. The liver may be enlarged, with increased sound attenuation caused by the cirrhosis. To penetrate all this tissue with a real-time or Doppler beam may be a challenge to present instrumentation.

In comparison with the more superficial peripheral vessels, the splanchnic veins are at present more difficult to examine with color Doppler. Although most portosystemic collateral veins are more readily traced with color Doppler, the crux of the examination of the patient with portal hypertension is still the domain of pulsed Doppler with spectral display. The latter is more sensitive to the low flow velocities in deep veins, especially when these vessels are small. In addition, the influences of cardiac and respiratory motion on flow direction are more easily detected and understood. Most abdominal vessels have a characteristic Doppler flow signature and the experienced examiner can distinguish a splanchnic from a systemic vein and can identify individual abdominal arteries from their spectral display.

The absence of a Doppler signal in a vessel can be a dilemma: is it attributable to technical factors, poor sensitivity of the machine, stagnant flow, or a thrombus? When using a reliable machine with a Doppler beam–vessel angle of less than 60° and low wall filter and pulse repetition frequency, the absence of a Doppler signal implies absence of flow or extremely slow flow. Even so, the possibility always remains that flow is present but remains undetected for technical reasons. The diagnosis of the absence of flow should come, whenever possible, from a positive sign, such as the detection of thrombus or collaterals.

Quantitative analysis of splanchnic blood flow with Doppler instrumentation is a fascinating possibility, as physiologic flow as well as portal hypertension and the response to various drugs could be studied more intensively. However, because the technique depends critically on exact measurements of vessel–beam angle and vessel diameter, the technique is at present fraught with unacceptable inaccuracies.[8,9] Perhaps the arrival of Doppler instrumentation capable of estimating flow volume without measures of vessel–beam angle and vessel diameter will solve these problems.

In the present state of the art, in spite of the above-mentioned weaknesses, the Doppler examination of the splanchnic circulation is valuable. If a noninvasive test can answer questions such as whether the patient has portal hypertension, where the obstruction to blood flow is, and whether there are esophageal varices, it will indeed prove a useful clinical tool.

Clinical Method

The aim of the Doppler examination of a patient with liver disease is to assess the presence and direction of flow in the splanchnic veins, the main portal vein and its segmental intrahepatic branches, the hepatic veins, and the inferior vena cava.[10–12] In addition, the presence of flow in the main hepatic artery and its intrahepatic branches is determined (Figure 41–3). When the clinical or basic Doppler examination raises the suspicion of portal hypertension, a systematic search for portosystemic collateral veins follows. The usual sites for spontaneous portosystemic shunts are outlined in Figure 41–4.[13] The lesser omentum[14] (from the splenomesenteric junction to the esophagus); the renal, splenic, and hepatic hila; as well as the pelvis are screened for the presence of dilated, tortuous veins. Hepatofugal (reversed) flow in a splanchnic vein can be followed to trace the vein to the recipient systemic vessel.

The patient is usually examined after a 6- to 12-h fast. Whenever possible, breathing is stopped during the Doppler examination of a vessel so as to minimize its movement. The usual Doppler frequency is 2 or 3 MHz even though the appropriate real-time frequency for the examination may range from 3 to 7.5 MHz.

Direction of flow in one or several veins comprising the portal venous system may change in portal hypertension, and it is essential to record the flow direction accurately. It is therefore useful to check that orientation of the spectral or color display is not inverted before starting the examination. The Doppler sample volume should be placed in the center of the vessel lumen. The angle between the Doppler beam and the vessel should be kept low whenever possible. If the direction of flow within a vessel is difficult to ascertain, a nearby vessel with known flow direction can be used as a reference, e.g., the splenic or hepatic artery for their adjacent veins. When there is disagreement between the flow direction discerned by the Doppler examination and that seen by angiography, it must be recalled that angiography is not a physiologic examination and may in itself lead to local circulatory changes. During the Doppler recording, a simultaneous electrocardiogram (ECG) tracing may be useful for the comprehension of certain flow fluctuations or pulsations within the system.

The main portal vein and its right hepatic branches are best studied through a right intercostal approach. Sometimes the superior mesenteric vein is also well seen from this position. The left portal vein and three of its four branches (the portal branch to the caudate lobe is rarely seen) and the hepatic veins are best seen through an oblique subcostal approach. The splenic vein is explored through a transverse, and the superior mesenteric vein through a sagittal anterior abdominal approach. The left gastric vein usually ends near the splenoportal junction and is best seen through a medioanterior abdominal infrapancreatic approach. The inferior mesenteric vein may be traced through an anterior, transverse, and longitudinal approach, following the aorta downward from the superior mesenteric artery origin. The inferior mesenteric artery can be seen leaving the anterior surface of the aorta and then lying to the left of the aorta. With a little care, the inferior mesenteric artery can be identified and Doppler flow patterns ascertained in over 90% of persons.

Anatomy

The systematic examination of the liver and the determination of the precise location of a liver lesion presuppose an imaging technique and a good knowledge of liver anatomy.

Before discussing the Doppler examination of the hepatic artery and portal vein and their intrahepatic branches, a brief review of the segmental anatomy of the liver is useful. Sonography has allowed us to explore the liver in many places and trace the intrahepatic vessels and their individual variations with a clarity not possible with

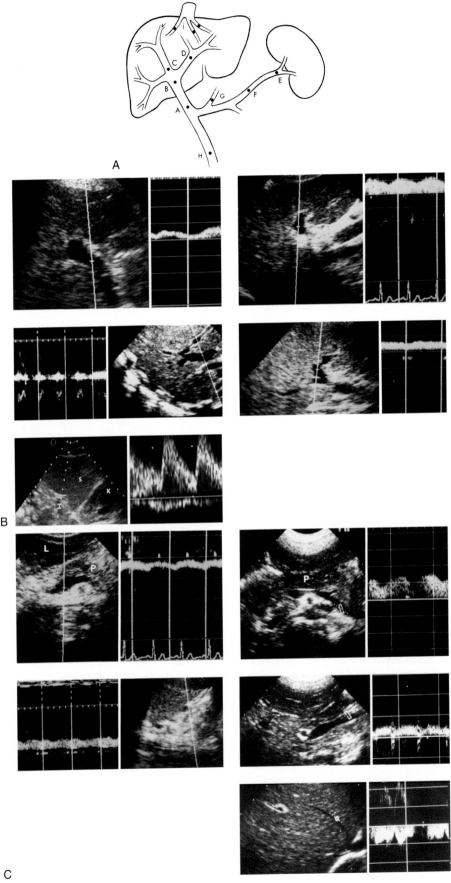

A

B

C

FIGURE 41–3. Diagram of splanchnic veins (A) with corresponding duplex scans (b, c). Lettered points on the diagram correspond to areas examined during a routine Doppler examination. The extrahepatic portal vein (A) is examined through a right anterolateral intercostal approach: blood flows toward the transducer (into the liver). Note the small angle between the vessel axis and Doppler beam. The intrahepatic portal vein signal (B, C) is found through a longitudinal paramedian subcostal approach. Flow fluctuates slightly with the cardiac cycle. The right branch of the portal vein (D) is seen from an oblique subcostal view, with normal flow toward the transducer. The splenic vein can be seen in a transverse view with the Doppler sample volume situated to the left (E) or right (F) of the midline in the vessel's retropancreatic portion. Gently undulating flow is seen toward the liver. A dilated, tortuous left gastric vein (G) is shown in a child with cirrhosis. The vein is seen behind the left lobe of the liver (sagittal left paramedian image). The Doppler sample volume within its lumen shows venous flow directed anteriorly and superiorly toward the esophagus. The superior mesenteric vein (H) is approached from a right paramedian sagittal view. Flow modulation is synchronous with wall pulsations from the adjacent superior mesenteric artery. Flow is directed toward the Doppler sample volume, superiorly into the liver. Tracing from a hepatic vein (I) shows flow modulated by pulsations of the nearby right atrium. (Reproduced with permission from Patriquin H, *et al.* Duplex Doppler examination in portal hypertension: Technique and anatomy. AJR 1987;149;71–76.)

CT or MRI. Despite these possibilities, the anatomy of the liver remains poorly understood by many sonographers; in addition, the nomenclature and definition of segments differ between Europe and North America.

The following simple sonographic approach to the segmental anatomy of the liver is based upon the nomenclature of the French surgeon, Claude Couinaud.[4] It is predicated on the distribution of the portal and hepatic veins. Each segment has a branch (or a group of branches) of the portal vein at its center and a hepatic vein at its periphery. Each lobe of the liver contains four segments. The segments are numbered counterclockwise: 1–4 in the left lobe and 5–8 in the right. Segment 1 is the caudate or Spigel lobe. The right and left lobes are separated by the main hepatic fissure, a line connecting the gallbladder and the left side of the inferior vena cava (IVC) (Figure 41–5).[5] The segmental branches of the portal vein (each one of which leads into a segment) can

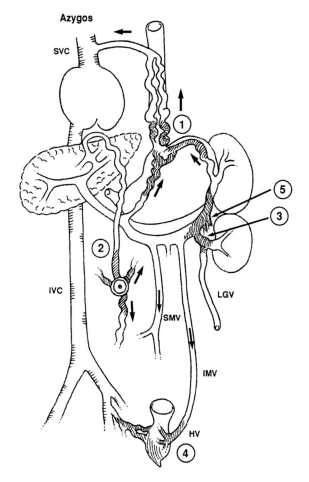

FIGURE 41–4. Diagram of common portosystemic collateral routes in portal hypertension. (Arrows indicate the direction of hepatofugal flow in splanchnic veins and in systemic veins that communicate with them.) Notation of vessels: SVC, superior vena cava; IVC, inferior vena cava; SMV, superior mesenteric vein; IMV, inferior mesenteric vein; HV, hemorrhoidal vein; LGV, left gonadal vein. Notation of routes: 1, esophageal varices: left and short gastric veins communicate with inferior esophageal and azygos veins; 2, caput medusae: paraumbilical veins join veins of the anterior abdominal (or thoracic) wall; 3, splenorenal shunt; 4, IMV: hemorrhoidal vein anastomoses; 5, splenoretroperitoneal shunts: both SMV and IMV may form shunts in the retroperitoneum or pelvis and anastomose with gonadal or retroperitoneal veins.

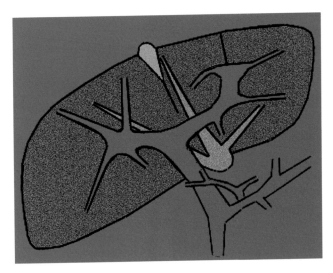

be outlined in the form of two "H"s turned sideways, one for the left lobe (segments 1–4) and one for the right lobe (segments 5–8) (Figure 41–5).

Portal Veins

Left Lobe

The "H" for the left lobe is visualized with an oblique, upwardly tilted subxiphoid view. The "H" is formed by the left portal vein, the branch entering segment 2, the umbilical portion of the left portal vein, and the branches to segments 3 and 4 (Figure 41–5). To this recumbent "H" are attached two ligaments: the ligamentum venosum (also called the lesser omentum or the hepatogastric ligament) and the falciform ligament. The ligamentum venosum separates segment 1 from segment 2. The falciform ligament is seen between the umbilical portion of the left portal vein[4] and the outer surface of the liver; it separates segment 3 from segment 4.

Segment 1 (the caudate lobe) is bordered posteriorly by the IVC, laterally by the ligamentum venosum, and anteriorly by the left portal vein (Figure 41–5). Unlike the other segments of the liver, it may receive branches of the left and right portal veins. The portal veins to segment 1 are usually small and rarely seen sonographically. The caudate lobe has one or more hepatic veins that drain directly into the IVC, separately from the three main hepatic veins.[6,7] This special vascularization is a distinctive characteristic of segment 1. The portal vein leading to segment 2 is a linear continuation of the left portal vein, completing the lower horizontal limb of the "H." Segmental branches to segments 3 and 4 form the other horizontal limb. Segments 2 and 3 are thus located to the left of the umbilical portion of the left portal vein, the ligamentum venosum, and the falciform ligament. Segment

4 (the quadrate lobe) is situated around the right anterior limb of the portal venous "H," to the right of the umbilical portion of the left portal vein and the falciform ligament. Segment 4 is separated from segments 5 and 8 by the middle hepatic vein and by the main fissure (a line between the neck of the gallbladder and the right portal vein).[8] It is separated from segment 1 by the left portal vein.

Right Lobe

The right portal vein and its branches are best seen with a sagittal or oblique midaxillary intercostal approach. In some subjects, a subcostal approach is also useful. The right portal vein follows an oblique or vertical course, directed anteriorly. The branches leading to the segments of the right lobe of the liver are also distributed in the shape of a sideways "H." The right portal vein forms the crossbar of the "H." The branches to segments 5 and 8 form the upper limb of the "H," while the branches to segments 6 and 7 form its lower portion. The branches of segments 6 and 7 are more obliquely oriented, and the transducer should be rotated slightly upward for segment 7 and downward in the direction of the right kidney for segment 6.

The middle hepatic vein separates segments 5 and 8 from segment 4. The right hepatic vein separates the anteriorly situated segments 5 and 8 from the more posteriorly situated segments 6 and 7. Segment 5 is bordered medially by the gallbladder and the middle hepatic vein, and inferiorly by the right hepatic vein. The right portal vein separates segment 5 from segment 8 (Figure 41–5). Segment 8 is separated from segment 7 by the right hepatic vein, from segment 5 by the main right portal vein, and from segment 4 by the middle hepatic vein. Segments 6 and 7 are separated from segments 5 and 8 by the right hepatic vein. Segment 6 is the part of the liver closest to the kidney; its lateral border is the ribcage. Segment 7 is separated from segment 8 by the right hepatic vein and is bordered laterally and cephalad by the rib cage and the dome of the diaphragm.

Hepatic Veins

When seen with an oblique coronal subxiphoid view, the three hepatic veins form a "W," with its base on the IVC. The left and middle hepatic veins join the left anterior part of the IVC (Figure 41–5). The hepatic veins separate the following segments: the left hepatic vein separates segment 2 from segment 3; the middle hepatic vein separates segment 4 from segments 5 and 8; and the right hepatic vein separates segments 5 and 8 from segments 6 and 7. With the oblique coronal subxiphoid view, the right portal vein is seen en face, which helps to separate the superficial segment 5 from the more deeply situated segment 8.

Hepatic Artery

The various possible origins of the hepatic artery are sometimes difficult to recognize; we usually look for the artery at its usual origin from the celiac axis and also as it passes between the portal vein and the main bile duct. When the left hepatic artery arises from the left gastric artery, it passes through the ligamentum venosum. The intrahepatic arterial branches accompany branches of the portal vein and can be detected with a slightly enlarged Doppler sample volume placed over a portal venous branch, even if the arterial branch cannot be seen with real-time ultrasound (Figure 41–3). Flow in the arteries to the right lobe of the liver (especially segments 5, 7, and 8) and to the left portal vein (umbilical portion, coursing toward the round ligament) is usually easily identified in this manner.

Normal Doppler Patterns

Figures 41–2 and 41–3 show normal spectral waveforms from the liver. The portal vein and its intrahepatic branches, the superior mesenteric and splenic veins, have a similar, rather steady flow directed toward the liver (Figure 41–3E).[10] There are small pulsations that mirror the cardiac cycle. After a meal, flow increases. The portal vein and hepatic artery appear to act in consort to nourish the liver. Changes in flow volumes in one affect the other. After a meal, portal venous flow increases in response to intestinal vasodilations and hepatic arterial flow diminishes, probably by vasoconstriction. Diastolic flow is decreased and systolic peaks are lower, when measured at the same sites in the same person.[15–17] Arterial signals within the liver may be difficult to find after a meal. This can be particularly disturbing in the posttransplant period where a false diagnosis of thrombosis may be made. The hepatic veins and IVC usually show three phases of flow: the first two, toward the heart, are reflections of right atrial and ventricular diastole. The third, a short spurt of reversed blood flow, accompanies atrial systole (the p-wave of the ECG) (Figure 41–2a). During expiration, flow velocity in the IVC generally increases. The normal hepatic artery is in a low-resistance system similar to the renal arteries: there is continuous flow throughout diastole (Figure 41–2f). Velocity decreases at the end of systole, but it never reaches zero or flow reversal.

Abnormal Flow Patterns Within the Portal System

Absent Doppler Signal

Proof of the absence of a Doppler signal is much more difficult to establish than its presence. When the examiner fails to obtain a Doppler signal from a given vessel, the usual response is to doubt the sensitivity of the machine and thus to test other nearby vessels. Failure to obtain a Doppler signal from a portal vein examined at an angle of less than 60° with a 3-MHz transducer, full Doppler gain, low pulse repetition frequency, and a 50-Hz wall filter means that blood is flowing at a velocity of less than 2.5 cm/s. This is extremely slow. Thus the absence of a Doppler signal in this situation generally means the absence of flow or a prethrombotic state. A portal venous thrombus, unless very fresh, is usually more echogenic than the blood. When acute, it usually distends the vessel. These sonographic findings are a simple adjunct to the Doppler examination and should be sought using appropriate technical factors to optimize contrast within the vessel.

Arterialized Flow

The normal gently undulating flow within a portal vein is replaced by systolic peaks and high diastolic Doppler shifts in arterialized flow. This pattern may signal the presence of an arterioportal fistula[18] or hyperdynamic flow in certain patients with advanced cirrhosis.

Reversed Flow or To-and-Fro Flow

Reversed flow in a splanchnic or intrahepatic portal vein is the most reliable Doppler sign of portal hypertension. To-and-fro flow, another sign of portal hypertension, is best seen during active breathing. Inspiration draws blood toward the liver (hepatopetal flow), whereas expiration reverses it (hepatofugal flow). Care should be taken that the Doppler sample volume remains in the same part of the portal vein during this maneuver, as to-and-fro flow may be stimulated by the taking of Doppler samples in adjacent loops of the vessel. To-and-fro flow in the portal vein may also be seen in right-sided heart failure. The Doppler spectrum alternates from above the display reference line in inspiration to below the line in expiration or changes color (e.g., blue to red) during a color Doppler examination.

Abnormal Hepatic Arterial Doppler Patterns

Absence of a Doppler signal suggests arterial thrombosis or reduced flow in prethrombotic states.[19] Locally increased systolic Doppler shifts may be the result of stenosis of the hepatic artery, as at any other arterial site. Because the artery and its branches have a variable, often tortuous course and are not always seen with ultrasound imaging, the diagnosis of the localized stenosis is difficult to make. A sudden change in the course of the vessel associated with a much reduced beam–vessel angle will also result in a sudden increase in systolic Doppler shifts. Tumor vessels may likewise show high systolic (and sometimes diastolic) Doppler shifts, ranging from 4 to 10 kHz.[20]

Ease of Detection of Hepatic Arterial Signals Throughout the Liver

Blood flow variations in the portal vein and hepatic artery are intimately related: usually, when portal venous flow is low, such as in the fasting state, arterial flow is high, and vice versa. It is surprisingly easy to detect arterial signals throughout the liver in cirrhotic patients (mainly in alcoholic and biliary cirrhosis). Systolic Doppler shifts are higher and are detected more easily both centrally and peripherally near the portal vein branches than in normal persons. This probably reflects diminishing intrahepatic portal venous flow and a subsequent increase in flow in an enlarged hepatic artery.[21]

Cirrhosis and Portal Hypertension

Morphologic signs that suggest portal hypertension are easily detected sonographically: tortuous collateral vessels, splenomegaly, a thickened lesser omentum in children, changes in liver architecture, and ascites.[13,22–28] The Doppler technique adds another dimension to the standard ultrasound examination—the detection of the presence and direction of blood flow within each of the veins comprising the portal system and its potential portosystemic collaterals. Together, the ultrasound and Doppler examinations achieve a kind of ultrasonographic angiogram that can answer the clinical questions: Is there portal hypertension? What is the direction of flow? Where is the level of obstruction (e.g., portal vein or hepatic vein)?

There are many potential routes for portosystemic derivations of blood flow in portal hypertension. Clinically, the most important route is through the left gastric and paraesophageal veins. The diameter of the left gastric vein is directly related to the size of esophageal varices and probably to the risk of bleeding.[29] In adults, a left gastric venous diameter of greater than 5 mm suggests the presence of portal hypertension. In normal children, this vein is rarely seen; a diameter exceeding 3 mm is suggestive of portal hypertension (Figure 41–3G).[30] The Doppler examination helps to identify the vein as it courses from the esophagus through the lesser omentum to the splenic or portal vein and distinguishes it from a tortuous left gastric artery (Figure 41–6). Flow direction is easily ascertained: hepatofugal flow is proof of portal hypertension. The paraumbilical vein is another common portosystemic route (Figure 41–7),[31] usually with

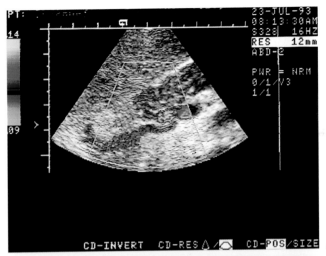

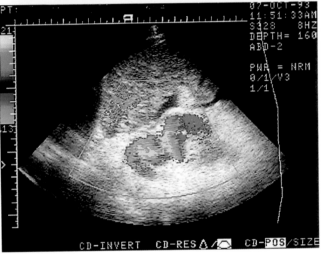

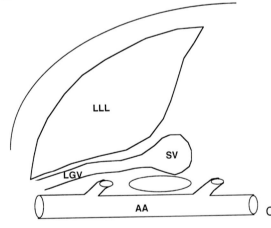

FIGURE 41–6. Coronary (left gastric) vein. Sagittal left paramedian sonograms of the upper abdomen show behind the left lobe of the liver. (A) The color Doppler box shows normal flow toward the splenic vein, which receives the left gastric vein. (B) Flow is reversed away from the splenic vein and toward the esophagus. (C) Schema. LLL, left lobe of liver; SV, splenic vein; LGV, left gastric vein; AA, aorta.

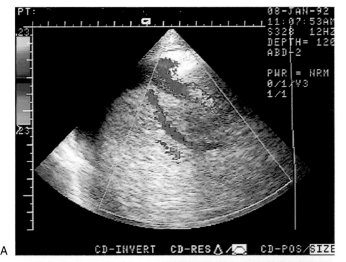

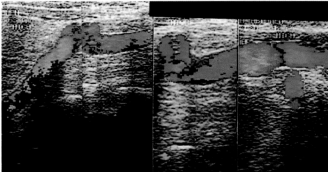

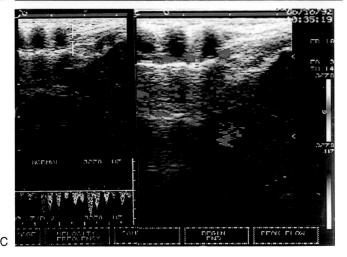

FIGURE 41–7. Recanalized paraumbilical vein in a patient with portal hypertension and ascites. (A) Coronal subcostal view of the left lobe of the liver. Red Doppler signals are seen in two veins. One is the paraumbilical vein and the other is a new vein originating from the portal vein branch of segment 4. (B) Paraumbilical collateral route; composite color Doppler images from the anterior thoracoabdominal wall. Blood flow in a vessel (directed toward the transducer) leaves the liver and flows toward the lower abdomen. Another branch (C) leads beneath the ribs toward the upper thorax.

hepatofugal flow from the left portal vein to the periumbilical venous plexus (Cruveilhier Baumgarten syndrome). Should flow in this vein be toward the liver, thrombosis of the portal vein has probably occurred, and the dilated paraumbilical vein has become a new route of blood flow into the liver.

Whatever the collateral vein discovered during the ultrasound and Doppler examination, the vessel should be traced to its recipient systemic vein (Figure 41–4). The flow pattern of the collateral vein usually changes as it approaches the systemic vein. The latter is usually dilated where it receives blood from the collateral vein. If such a shunt is large, hepatic encephalopathy may ensue.[32,33] The Doppler examination, being "physiologic," at times reveals unusual portosystemic collateral routes difficult to demonstrate with arterioportographic studies: locally inverted flow in intrahepatic portal venous branches, new veins leading from portal veins to the abdominal wall, or hepatofugal flow in the splenic vein.

Portal Vein Thrombosis

With high-resolution grayscale sonography, most thrombi are visible as hyperechoic masses distending the lumen of the vein. Thrombi formed within hours of the examination may be isoechoic with blood.[34-36] The Doppler examination complements the standard sonogram by demonstrating the presence or absence of, or flow around, a clot within the portal vein. Portal venous obstruction may be followed by the formation of a vermiform system of collateral veins at the hepatic hilum, given the descriptive name "cavernoma."[37] Determining the presence and direction of flow in a cavernoma can be difficult. The intrahepatic branches of the portal vein usually become cord-like, without a visible lumen. Tortuous periportal collaterals may develop. A careful Doppler search around the portal branches is nonetheless useful, because flow may be detected even if no vessel lumen is visible (Figure 41–2B).

Budd-Chiari Syndrome

Obstruction of the hepatic veins is often a surgical emergency and difficult to diagnose clinically. Ascites, an enlarged caudate lobe, and hepatic venous thrombi are sonographic signs of the syndrome.[38,39] It should be recalled that Doppler signals should always be distinguishable in patent hepatic veins, even if the vessel lumina are sonographically invisible. We studied eight patients who had Budd-Chiari syndrome and could discern no Doppler signals arising from their hepatic veins. In one patient, a short segment of one hepatic vein gave rise to high Doppler shifts, indicative of stenosis.

Similar high Doppler shifts may arise from hepatic veins compressed by regeneration nodules in cirrhotic patients. The observation that the remainder of the hepatic veins are patent distinguishes cirrhosis from hepatic venous thrombosis. There is an increased incidence of portal vein thrombosis (20%)[40] in patients with Budd-Chiari syndrome. A Doppler examination of the main portal vein and its intrahepatic branches is therefore indicated to assess patency. Treatment consists of portocaval shunting,[41–43] if possible with a transjugular intrahepatic portosystemic shunt (TIPS). A mesenteroatrial shunt may be necessary if the portal vein is thrombosed.

Surgical Portosystemic Shunts

The Doppler examination is most reliable in establishing the patency of surgical portosystemic shunts. Arteriophlebographic studies thus are rarely indicated for diagnostic purposes.

Several types of surgical portosystemic shunts have been devised. Their common aim is to divert high-pressure splanchnic blood flow into the low-pressure systemic venous system to prevent recurrent gastroesophageal hemorrhage in patients with portal hypertension.

The Doppler examination of portosystemic shunts includes study of the shunt site and the splanchnic and hepatic venous system. The site of a shunt may differ according to the surgical technique: if the veins used for a standard shunt are not suitable, the surgeon may use the nearest available vein (e.g., the mesentericocaval shunt). If the shunt is patent, it is often visible sonographically,[44–49] and Doppler signals are usually easily discerned at the site itself (see Figure 41–7). Blood flow often accelerates at and near the site of a patent shunt and there may be some turbulence. Flow direction is hepatofugal (toward the systemic vein). Severe turbulence and sudden high Doppler shifts at the shunt site are signs of stenosis. Should angioplasty be considered, direct imaging of the shunt by phlebography is necessary.[50]

In our experience, a Doppler study of the intrahepatic portal veins is invaluable in the assessment of portocaval shunt patency. In the majority of patent shunts, flow in the intrahepatic portal veins is hepatofugal and easily detected with the Doppler examination. It is easy to understand why this should be so in laterolateral portocaval shunts, where high-pressure intrahepatic venous blood flows through the shunt into the low-pressure vena cava. It is more difficult to explain hepatofugal flow in the intrahepatic portal veins in patients with an end-to-side portocaval shunt, as the hepatic end of the portal vein has been ligated and cut. Blood may leave the liver through a system of collateral veins between intrahepatic branches of the portal vein and low-pressure systemic veins. This phenomenon has been demonstrated angiographically.[51,52]

Signs of shunt obstruction are predictable: the shunt site is difficult or impossible to see sonographically, there are no Doppler flow signals, blood in the splanchnic vein feeding the shunt no longer flows toward the shunt, the direction of intrahepatic portal flow returns to normal, and spontaneous portosystemic shunts (e.g., esophageal varices) and other signs of portal hypertension reappear.

Transjugular Intrahepatic Portosystemic Shunt Surveillance

The TIPS is a new nonsurgical treatment for complications of portal hypertension, variceal bleeding, and refractory ascites.[53–55] In this procedure, a stent is placed between a portal vein (usually the main right portal vein) and a hepatic vein (most often the right, rarely the middle hepatic vein). This creates a direct portosystemic shunt within the liver, whose main function is to decrease portal hypertension. Duplex Doppler ultrasound is ideal for its examination (Figure 41–8).

TIPS is now known to carry its share of complications,[56] primarily recurrent variceal bleeding and ascites. Stenosis and obstruction of the shunt can be depicted by Doppler, hopefully before clinical complications occur.

Doppler signs of TIPS dysfunction are multiple: (1) a localized increase in velocity at the site of a stent stenosis,[57] (2) a decrease of 20% or more of blood flow in the stent, and (3) reversal of flow in intrahepatic portal vein branches or in extrahepatic collaterals in comparison with previous examinations.[58] Our experience showed a frequent occurrence of stent changes over time (27% of patients). A close follow-up examination with Doppler of patients with TIPS should help to discriminate those who need shunt correction.

Doppler Sonography in the Patient Receiving a Liver Transplant

Before transplantation can be considered, the caliber and patency of the main portal vein and IVC must be assessed. This can usually be done with Doppler sonography. If the portal vein diameter is less than 4mm (as it may be in advanced cirrhosis) or if Doppler flow studies are equivocal, MRI or angiography may be performed. Children with biliary atresia sometimes have an associated polysplenia syndrome, which includes intestinal malrotation, bilaterally symmetrical patterns of the major bronchi, abnormal location of the portal vein anterior to the duodenum, and interruption of the IVC. Liver transplantation may be very difficult in these children. It is essential that the surgeon be aware of the anatomic abnormality before transplantation.

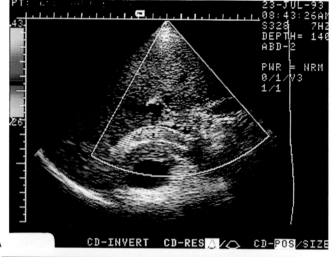

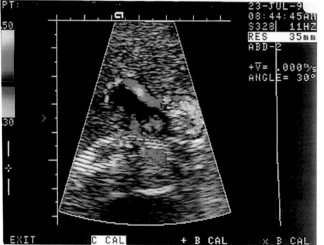

FIGURE 41–8. TIPS (transjugular intrahepatic portosystemic shunt). Color Doppler of a properly functioning shunt. (A) Sagittal right paramedian sonogram shows the right lobe of the liver, the inferior vena cava, and the stent with flow signals directed cranially. Blue is from a nearby portal vein showing flow leaving the liver toward the stent. The mosaic red is from aliased arterial signals. (B) Blue flow from segmental portal veins of the right lobe shows hepatofugal flow (toward the stent). Red mosaic signals originate from nearby arteries.

In addition, portacaval or mesenteric-caval shunts, whether created surgically or occurring naturally, change both the flow pattern and the caliber of the main portal vein and thus alter the surgical approach to transplantation. The anatomic variants of the hepatic artery are not always demonstrated sonographically, but angiography is rarely performed for the purpose of outlining the anatomy of the hepatic artery. (The radiographic examination of the patient before transplantation includes

several organs outside the liver: the kidneys, lungs, heart, and intestinal tract.)[28,31]

Preoperative investigation of the donor (when possible) includes a search for liver masses, stenosis, and possible thrombosis of the portal vein. Most liver transplants are cadaver organs from unrelated donors. The entire liver or segments 2–3 or 5 may be used. Segments 2–3 are used if an adult liver is transplanted into a small child. An adult liver may be divided and used for two recipients.

The common complication in the immediate postoperative period is hepatic artery thrombosis. Although collateral vessels may form in the child and shunt arterial blood into the liver, bile duct necrosis usually occurs, followed by the formation of bile lakes and recurrent infection. Retransplantation is almost invariably necessary.

We usually perform an initial Doppler examination at the patient's bedside soon after the operation and daily for 5 days thereafter to confirm the patency of the anastomosed vessels, before clinical or biochemical liver examinations become abnormal. The hepatic arterial anastomosis is usually difficult to see, and therefore the intrahepatic arterial branches are examined, adjacent to intrahepatic portal veins, where they may be difficult to see with grayscale sonography: however, flow is readily discerned with Doppler techniques. We have found that the following sites are optimal for the detection of hepatic arterial Doppler signals: adjacent to the umbilical branch of the left portal vein and to the branch to segments 3 and 4 (Figure 41–5), and alongside the right portal vein and branches to segments 6 and 7. The presence of arterial signals at these sites usually establishes patency of the hepatic artery.

In patients who are well enough to eat or receive nourishment via a gastric tube, it must be remembered that hepatic arterial Doppler shifts are difficult to detect following a meal. A repeat, fasting examination may show much stronger signals.[17] Failure to detect intrahepatic arterial Doppler shifts signals absent flow in thrombosis or a prethrombotic state. We perform arteriography in doubtful situations. Although hepatic artery interrogation is the most important part of the examination, the Doppler study is also helpful in assessing the patency of the portal and hepatic veins of the graft. Portal venous thrombosis at the anastomosis may occur but is less frequent than arterial occlusion. Turbulence may be expected at the anastomotic site of the portal vein. Stenosis or compression of the portal vein is accompanied by locally increased Doppler shifts. Portal hypertension may follow. Poststenotic dilation of the portal vein may occur without serious sequelae.

Graft rejection does not result in predictable flow alterations of the hepatic artery. Flat, unmodulated Doppler tracings from hepatic veins have been reported as a sign of rejection, but we have not been able to confirm this finding. The Doppler examination is as yet unsatisfactory in assessing the possibility of liver graft rejection.

Malignant Tumors

Malignant tumors depend on a rich, rapidly proliferating network of vessels for their nourishment and growth. These tumor vessels are of two types: large tortuous arteries and veins readily visible angiographically and, more peripherally, microscopic vessels with many arteriovenous fistulas. The microscopic arteriovenous shunts are not visible angiographically,[59] but give rise to very high frequency (up to 10 kHz) systolic Doppler shifts. We have found this tumor Doppler pattern in 5 of 13 hepatomas and in 4 of 5 hepatoblastomas. Because these vessels are not visible sonographically, the Doppler search for them at the periphery of a tumor requires repeated Doppler sampling and is time consuming. Color Doppler may localize these lesions more quickly, because of their high Doppler shift. Spectral analysis can then be performed to recognize the typical Doppler tumor pattern.

Hepatomas typically invade portal veins. The tumor thrombus may be visible sonographically within the venous lumen as an echogenic mass. Residual flow around the clot may be detected with the Doppler examination. The latter may be reversed because of numerous arteriovenous fistulas within the tumor.

Arterioportal Fistula

Arterioportal fistulas are rare lesions that occur within hepatomas or are the result of penetrating trauma (knife wounds, biopsies, liver transplantation). The last three arterioportal fistulas we studied were the result of needle biopsies of the liver performed during portosystemic shunt surgery. Sonographically, large intrahepatic vessels are visible, leading to a network of collateral vessels. At the site of the fistula the Doppler examination shows turbulent, rapid, bidirectional flow.[18] Flow in the recipient portal vein may be "arterialized" (pulsatile flow with systolic peaks and high diastolic Doppler shifts).

Air in the Portal Vein

Usually a grave prognostic sign, air in the portal vein can be difficult to diagnose. Sonographically, air bubbles may be visible in the lumen.[60] The Doppler examination confirms its presence: air mixed with blood produces a high acoustic impedance that results in a mirror-image Doppler tracing with artificial vertical streaks on both sides of the reference line. Air may thus be detected before it is visible on plain radiographs: CT may be used to confirm its presence. Recently, Chezmar et al.[61] have seen portal venous air in transplant recipients. This had no serious prognostic significance.

Monitoring Hepatic Interventional Procedures with Doppler Ultrasound

Prior to needle puncture or drainage of an abdominal "abscess" or fluid-containing structure, it is wise to conduct an examination to determine the presence or absence of blood flow within the lesion. This is especially so at the liver hilum, where aneurysms are particularly frequent. Even if the lesion itself is avascular, knowledge of the anatomy of nearby vessels is essential. These tasks are readily performed with the Doppler examination. During percutaneous interventions, the Doppler mode provides an additional "vascular" perspective to sonographic needle guidance:[62] puncture sites and needle paths can be chosen avoiding major vessels. Examples include cannulating dilated bile ducts and sparing nearby portal venous or arterial branches and locating the ideal injection site during neurolysis of the celiac plexus, again avoiding the hepatic artery. In addition, both the possibility and the success of endovascular interventions can be monitored with the Doppler examination, during or after the procedure. Reduction of flow in an arterioportal fistula or in an artery feeding a hepatoma can be ascertained easily after embolization.

New Methods

Volume Flow Measurement

Noninvasive measurement of volume flow rates in the adult splanchnic system has been the goal of much effort since early invasive measurements. Doppler methods began in 1979 and have since been pursued in a number of directions, to measure arterial inflow as well as portal venous flux.[63] All methods in current clinical use have as a basis measurements of the spatial mean velocity (v) and the cross-sectional area (A) of the vessel. The product of these two quantities is integrated over time to obtain the volume flow rate (Q).

Some of the more commonly used implementations include the following.

Velocity Profile Method

In the velocity profile method the velocity profile is measured at successive intervals throughout the cardiac cycle and integrated to give a volume flow rate. A pulsed Doppler system with a sample volume much smaller than the vessel lumen cross section is required. The sample volume is moved slowly across the vessel lumen and the velocity is calculated using a beam–vessel angle derived from the two-dimensional image. Assuming circular symmetry of the profile, each velocity is multiplied by the corresponding semiannular area, and the resulting flow components are summed. Multigate or "infinite" gate systems that are capable of interrogating an entire vessel at one time have the advantage that they can acquire the necessary data in a single heartbeat and are therefore less prone to problems of beat-to-beat variation. For transcutaneous applications of conventional duplex scanners the method seems to be suitable at present only for large and accessible vessels such as the adult aorta and common carotid arteries. With the newer broad bandwidth color systems (see below) the velocity profile method can be used in vessels of the abdomen with an estimated precision of 10%.[64] At present, clinical validation is awaited.

The Even Insonation Method

The principle of the even insonation method is shown in Figure 41–9. The entire volume of blood whose flow rate is to be assessed is exposed to a uniform ultrasonic beam. The mean Doppler shift corresponding to the mean velocity in the sample volume is then calculated. This velocity is multiplied by the cross-sectional area of the vessels or orifice to give an instantaneous flow value. This product is then integrated into the cardiac cycle yielding the time average rate. For arterial flow the cross-sectional area will change with time, so that ideally the product of the instantaneous mean velocity and the cross-sectional area would be formed at the same moment in time. In practice the goal of simultaneous diameter and flow velocity measurement is not attainable. The optimum ultrasonic approach for the former is perpendicular to the vessel or orifice, whereas for the latter an acute angle of approach to the direction of flow is best. As it is difficult to arrange for two noninterfering beams to be used at the same time, it is usual to measure the mean velocity and mean area separately and take their product after, rather than before, temporal integration. The error thus introduced depends on the rate of change of both the cross-sectional area and the flow velocity over the cardiac cycle. For example, a 4-mm hepatic artery may vary 20% in diameter (that is 40% in cross-sectional area) between systole and diastole.

A common method for the estimation of the cross-sectional area of the vessel orifice is to measure its diameter and assume circular symmetry. Because of the square dependence of area on diameter, the percentage error in diameter measurement will cause an error of approximately double that figure in the flow estimate. For example, a 1 mm uncertainty in the measurement of an 8-mm vessel will produce a 25% variation in the flow circulation. To minimize such errors careful measurement should be made using a consistent technique, preferably with an M-mode beam intersecting the precise location of the Doppler sampler volume. Further errors result if the vessel (for example, the portal vein) is not circular in cross section. Here real-time imaging could be used, but there remains the difficulty of ensuring that the image plane is perpendicular to the flow axis. These considerations alone limit the present usefulness of such measurements in small vessels when when there is no recourse to specially designed equipment.[65]

Assumed Velocity Profile Method

Because of difficulties in achieving insonation of an entire vessel, or of computing the mean Doppler shift frequency, some workers have made measurements at one point in the vessel and assumed a given velocity profile to exist over the vessel lumen.[66] The maximum frequency is then multiplied by a numerical factor that is supposed then gives the mean Doppler shift frequency. Some produce this factor from empirical studies using an animal model: for these studies the factor is really a calibration constant for their particular experiment, and it is necessary to ask whether the physical conditions of the experiment correspond to those of the clinical study. Others dispense with the calculation of the mean frequency and estimate its position from the subjective appearance of the spectral display. This is, however, a rather precarious procedure. The grayscale in a display bears a nonlinear relation (usually square-root or logarithmic) to the spectral power and can therefore mislead the operator. In some cases the assumption may be made that "plug" flow (that is, a perfectly flat velocity profile) exists. This simplifies matters considerably: the spatial mean flow velocity is simply equal to the maximum velocity near the center of the vessel—an easy quantity to measure. The assumptions of this method probably verge on acceptability for the case of the aortic root in the normal adult. Elsewhere its inaccuracies are unacceptable.[9]

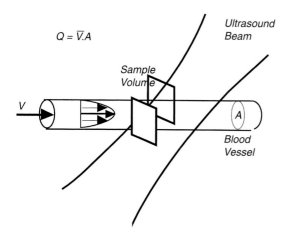

FIGURE 41–9. The principle of the even insonation method for the estimation of volume flow rate Q. The instantaneous mean velocity n is calculated from the mean Doppler shift frequency and multiplied by the cross-sectional area A of the vessel.

Attenuation-Compensated Method

One novel and appealing Doppler method for the measurement of volume flow rate eliminates the need to measure either the beam Doppler angle or the cross-sectional area of the vessel yet makes no severe assumptions about the velocity profile. In the "attenuation-compensated" flowmeter, two ultrasonic beams are used, the first with a uniform sample volume large enough to embrace the entire vessel and the second with a narrower beam along the same path. In principle,[67] volume flow may be measured with knowledge of neither the vessel area nor the angle of insonation. The method was proposed and results of *in vitro* trials were reported in 1979, but further application has had to await practical realization of the required beam geometries. These are beginning to become available, and clinical results (from flow measurements in large vessels such as the adult ascending aorta) are beginning to confirm the validity of the method.

Doppler Instrument Performance

Generally speaking, the sensitivity of color flow imaging instruments to low Doppler signal intensities (associated with the lower number of scatterers in small vessels) and slow Doppler shifts (from the slower moving blood in small vessels) is a major limiting factor in their current use in the abdomen and peripheral circulation. In addition, the spatial resolution of color instruments limits the definition of velocity detail within a large vessel or the ability to localize low-flow structures. At present, color flow imaging sensitivity, especially of flow in deep structures, can be achieved only at the expense of spatial resolution and frame rate, and is generally inferior to that of current duplex scanners. Likewise, color spatial resolution is inferior to that of the grayscale image. Technological developments, however, are likely to narrow these gaps. One of the more promising of these is the use of the so-called time-domain, speckle-tracking methods for the production of color images.[68] These methods do not rely directly on the Doppler shift for the detection of motion; instead they track the movement of structure in the ultrasound image. The principle is quite simple. The echo from blood is the combined result of many small echoes from the individual scatterers, which are the red blood cells themselves. These account for a grainy speckle-like structure within the blood that we would be able to see on the image if the echo from the blood were stronger, much as we see speckle within the parenchyma of the liver, for example. With flow, this pattern moves at the same speed as the blood. By comparing the pattern of the ultrasound echo (usually at the radiofrequency level of the receiver) at a particular location in the beam at one time with that

obtained a moment later at the same location, the distance the speckle has moved can be measured and the blood velocity inferred. Note that this method, like Doppler, yields only the component of velocity along the ultrasound beam, and that to measure true velocity, the beam-flow angle must be known, just as for a Doppler image. This method seems to be particularly suited to the production of high-resolution color images: the cross-correlation method used here works best with the short pulses that give high axial resolution It is possible, however, that the current price for these advantages might be a lower sensitivity to low flow states. Exciting possibilities for the future of the correlation method include two-dimensional Doppler images (albeit with much reduced lateral velocity resolution) and quantitative (volumetric flow)[69] color imaging. Already, promising results have been reported using this method.[64]

In the future, an important role in the detection of low volumes of blood will be played by ultrasound contrast agents, an intravenous injection of a small quantity of which is capable of increasing the echo from deep arterial vessels by a factor of 100 or more.[70] This is one method to raise the received echo intensity of ultrasound scattered from small quantities of blood deep in the body to levels detectable at the skin surface. When this is attained, color flow imaging can be turned to the issue of blood velocity and blood flow imaging itself at the parenchymal level. Success so far in the use of contrast agents has been accompanied by the advent of new imaging techniques such as harmonic and pulse inversion imaging.[71] Quantitative and deep color Doppler is in its infancy at present, with many technical problems remaining to be overcome before specific clinical applications are in sight. However, these and other developments of Doppler technology are likely to ensure that the current proliferation of clinical problems that ultrasonographers have addressed using the Doppler method will be sustained in the foreseeable future.

References

1. Taylor K, Burns P, Woodcock J, Wells P. Blood flow in deep abdominal and pelvic vessels: Ultrasonic pulsed-Doppler analysis. Radiology 1985;154:487–493.
2. Taylor K, Burns P. Duplex Doppler scanning in the pelvis and abdomen. Ultrasound Med Biol 1985;11:643–658.
3. Burns PN. Physical principles of Doppler ultrasound and spectral analysis. Clin Ultrasound 1987;15:567–590.
4. American Institute of Ultrasound in Medicine. *Performance Criteria and Measurements for Doppler Ultrasound Devices.* Rockville, MD: AIUM, 1993.
5. Burns PN. Interpretation and analysis of Doppler signals. In: Taylor KJW, Burns PN, Wells PNT (eds). *Clinical Applicatons of Doppler Ultrasound.* New York: Raven Press, 1988.

6. Mitchell D, Burns PN, Needleman L. Artifactual Doppler noise within anechoic spaces: Differentiation from flow. J Ultrasound Med 1990;9:255–260.

7. Parvey HR, Eisenberg RL, Giyanani V, Krebbs CA. Duplex sonography of the portal venous system: Pitfalls and limitations. AJR 1989;152:765–770.

8. Burns PN, Jaffe CC. Quantitative Doppler flow measurements: Techniques, accuracy and limitations. Radiol Clin North Am 1985;23:641–657.

9. Burns PN, Taylor KJW, Blei AT. Doppler flowmetry and portal hypertension. Gastroenterology 1987;92:824–826.

10. Patriquin H, Lafortune M, Burns PN, Dauzat M. Duplex Doppler examination in portal hypertension: Technique and anatomy. AJR 1987;149:71–76.

11. Patriquin H, Babcock D, Paltiel H. Color Doppler: Applications in children. Ultrasound Q 1989;7:243–269.

12. van Leeuwen MS. Doppler ultrasound in the evaluation of portal hypertension. Clin Diagn Ultrasound 1989;26:53–76.

13. Subramanyam BR, Balthazar EJ, Madamba MR. Sonography of portosystemic venous collaterals in portal hypertension. Radiology 1983;146:161–166.

14. Brunelle F, Alagille D, Pariente D. An ultrasound study of portal hypertension in children. Ann Radiol 1981;24:121–130.

15. Pugliese D, Ohnishi K, Tsunoda T, Sabba C, Albano O. Portal hemodynamics after meal in normal subjects and in patients with chronic liver disease studied by echo-Doppler flowmeter. Am J Gastroenterol 1987;82:1052–1056.

16. Lee SS, Hadengue A, Moreau R, Sayegh R, Hillon P, Lebrec D. Postprandial hemodynamic responses in patients with cirrhosis. Hepatology 1988;8:647–651.

17. Lafortune M, Dauzat M, Pomier-Layrargues G. Hepatic artery: Effect of meal in normal persons and in transplant recipients. Radiology 1993;187:391–394.

18. Lafortune M, Breton G, Charlebois S. Arterioportal fistula demonstrated by pulsed Doppler ultrasonography. J Ultrasound Med 1986;5:105–106.

19. Segel MC, Zajko AB, Bowen A, Bron KM, Skolnick, ML, Penkrot RJ, Starzl TE. Hepatic artery thrombosis after liver transplantation: Radiologic evaluation. AJR 1986;146:137–141.

20. Taylor KJW, Ramos I, Morse SS, Fortune KL, Hammers L, Taylor CR. Focal liver masses: Differential diagnosis with pulsed Doppler US. Radiology 1987;164:643–647.

21. Lautt WW, Greenaway CV. Conceptual review of the hepatic vascular bed. Hepatology 1987;7:952–963.

22. Lafortune M, Constantin A, Bregon G. The recanalized umbilical vein in portal hypertension: A myth. AJR 1985;144:549–553.

23. Kauzlaric D, Petrovic M, Barmeir E. Sonography of cavernous transformation of the portal vein. AJR 1984;142:383–384.

24. Kane RA, Katz SG. The spectrum of sonography findings in portal hypertension: A subject review and new observations. Radiology 1982;142:453–458.

25. Marchal GJF, Holsbeeck MV, Tshibwabwa-Ntumba E. Dilation of the cystic vein in portal hypertension: Sonographic demonstration. Radiology 1985;154:187–189.

26. von Koischwitz D, Paquet KJ, Köster O. Sonographische Beurteiling des portalen Gefassystems bei der portalen Hypertension. Fortschr Rontgenstr 1982;137:509–517.

27. Juttner HV, Jenny JM, Ralls PW. Ultrasound demonstration of portosystemic collaterals in cirrhosis and portal hypertension. Radiology 1982;142:459–463.

28. Waller RM, Oliver TW, McCain AH. Computed tomography and sonography of hepatic cirrhosis and portal hypertension. RadioGraphics 1984;4:677–715.

29. Lebrec D, DeFleury P, Rueff D. Portal hypertension size of oesophageal varices and risk of gastrointestinal bleeding in alcoholic cirrhosis. Gastroenterology 1980;79:1139–1144.

30. Lafortune M, Marleau D, Breton G. Portal venous system measurements in portal hypertension. Radiology 1984;151:27–30.

31. Mostbeck GH, Wittich GR, Herold D. Hemodynamic significance of the paraumbilical vein in portal hypertension: Assessment with duplex US. Radiology 1989;170:339–342.

32. Takayasu K, Moriyama N, Shima Y. Sonographic detection of large spontaneous spleno-renal shunts and its clinical significance. Br J Radiol 1984;57:565–570.

33. Ohnishi K, Saito M, Sata S, Nakayama T, Takashi M, Iida S, Nomura F, Koen H, Okuda K. Direction of splenic venous flow assessed by pulsed Doppler flowmetry in patients with a large splenorenal shunt: Relation to spontaneous hepatic encephalopathy. Gastroenterology 1985;89:180–185.

34. Babcock DS. Ultrasound diagnosis of portal vein thrombosis as a complication of appendicitis. AJR 1979;133:317–319.

35. Miller VE, Berland LL. Pulsed Doppler duplex sonography and CT in portal vein thrombosis. AJR 1985;145:73–76.

36. van Gansbeke D, Avni EF, Delcour C. Sonographic features of portal vein thrombosis. AJR 1985;144:749–752.

37. Weltin G, Taylor K, Carter A, Taylor C. Duplex Doppler: Identification of cavernous transformation of the portal vein. AJR 1985;144:999–1001.

38. Menu Y, Alison D, Lorphelin JM. Budd-Chiari syndrome: US evaluation. Radiology 1985;157:761–764.

39. Baert AL, Fevery J, Marchal, G. Early diagnosis of Budd-Chiari syndrome by computed tomography and ultrasonography: Report of five cases. Gastroenterology 1983;84:587–595.

40. Parker RGF. Occlusion of the hepatic veins in man. Medicine 1959;38:369–402.

41. Orloff MJ. Treatment of Budd-Chiari syndrome by side-to-side portacaval shunt: Experimental and clinical results. Ann Surg 1978;188:494–512.

42. Vons C, Bourstyn E, Bonnet P. Results of portosystemic shunts in Budd-Chiari syndrome. Ann Surg 1986;204:366–370.

43. Prandi D, Rueff B, Benhamou JP. Side-to-side portacaval shunt in the treatment of Budd-Chiari syndrome. Gastroenterology 1975;68:137–141.

44. Foley D, Gleysteen J, Lawson TL. Dynamic computed tomography and pulse Doppler ultrasonography in the

evaluation of splenorenal shunt patency. J Comput Assist Tomogr 1983;7:106–112.

45. Rodgers BM, Kaude JV. Real-time ultrasound in determination of porta-systemic shunt patency in children. J Pediatr Surg 1981;16:968–971.

46. Bolondi L, Mazziotti A, Arienti V. Ultrasonographic study of portal venous shunt system in portal hypertension and after portosystemic shunt operations. Surgery 1984;95:261–269.

47. Ackroyd N, Gill R, Griffiths K. Duplex scanning of the portal vein and portosystemic shunts. Surgery 1986;99:591–597.

48. Forsberg L, Holmin T. Pulsed Doppler and B-mode ultrasound features of interposition meso-caval and porta-caval shunt. Acta Radiol 1983;24:353–357.

49. Lafortune M, Patriquin H, Pomier G, Huet P, Weber A, Lavoie P, Blanchard H, Breton G. Hemodynamic changes in portal circulation after portosystemic shunts: Use of duplex sonography in 43 patients. AJR 1987;149:701–706.

50. Ruff RJ, Chuang VP, Alspaugh JP. Percutaneous vascular intervention after surgical shunting for portal hypertension. Radiology 1987;164:469–474.

51. Nova D, Butzow GH, Becker K. Hepatic occlusion venography with a balloon catheter in patients with end-to-side portacaval shunts. AJR 1976;127:949–953.

52. Reuter SR, Orloff MJ. Wedged hepatic venography in patients with end-to-side portacaval shunts. Radiology 1974;111:563–566.

53. Conn HO. Transjugular intrahepatic portal-systemic shunts: The state of the art. Hepatology 1993;17:148–158.

54. LaBerge JM, Ring EJ, Gordon RL. Creation of transjugular intrahepatic portosystemic shunts with the Wallstent endoprosthesis: Results in 100 patients. Radiology 1993;187:413–420.

55. Richter GM, Noeldge G, Roessle M, Palmaz JC. Evolution and clinical introduction of TIPSS, the transjugular intrahepatic portosystemic stent-shunt. Semin Intervent Radiol 1991;8:331–340.

56. Freedman AM, Sanyal AJ, Tisnado J. Complications of transjugular intrahepatic portosystemic shunt: A comprehensive review. RadioGraphics 1993;13:1185–1210.

57. Ralls PW, Egan RT, Katz MD, Teitelbaum GP. Color Doppler sonography to evaluate transjugular intrahepatic portacaval stent shunt. J Ultrasound Med 1993;12:487–489.

58. Lafortune M, Martinet J-P, Denys A, Dauzat M, Dufresnes M-P, Columbato L, Pomier-Layrargues G. Short and long term hemodynamic effects of TIPS: A Doppler/manometric study. AJR 1995;164:997–1002.

59. Burns PN, Halliwell M, Webb AJ, Wells PNT. Ultrasonic Doppler studies of the breast. Ultrasound Med Biol 1982;8:127–143.

60. Dennis MA, Pretorius D, Manco-Johnson ML. CT detection of portal venous gas associated with suppurative cholangitis and cholecystitis. AJR 1985;145:1017–1018.

61. Chezmar JL, Nelson RC, Bernardino ME. Portal venous gas after hepatic transplantation: Sonographic detection and clinical significance. AJR 1989;53:1203–1205.

62. Ralls RW, Mayekawa DS, Lee KP, Johnson MB, Halls J. The use of color Doppler sonography to distinguish dilated intrahepatic ducts from vascular structures. AJR 1989;152:291–292.

63. Gill RW. Splanchnic blood flow measurement. In: Altobelli SA, Voyles WF, Greene ER (eds). *Cardiovascular Ultrasonic Flowmetry*, pp. 369–389. New York: Elsevier, 1985.

64. Picot PA, Embree PM. Quantitative flow estimation using velocity profiles. IEE Trans Son Ultrason 1994;41:340–345.

65. Gill RW. Measurement of blood flow by ultrasound: Accuracy and sources of error. Ultrasound Med Biol 1985;11:625–641.

66. Ohnishi K, Saito M, Nakayama T, Coen H, Nomura F, Okuda K. Ultrasonic measurements of portal venous flow in chronic liver disease: Effects of posture change and exercise on portal hemodynamics. Radiology 1985;155:757–761.

67. Hottinger C, Meindl J. Blood flow measurement using the attenuation-compensated volume flowmeter. Ultrasonic Imaging 1979;1:1–15.

68. Bonnefous O, Pesqué P. Time domain formulation of pulse-Doppler ultrasound and blood velocity estimation by cross correlation. Ultrasonic Imaging 1986;8:73–85.

69. Embree PM, O'Brien WD. Volumetric blood flow via time-domain correlation: Experimental verification. IEEE Trans Ultrasonic Ferroelec Freq Contr 1990;37:176–189.

70. Burns PN. Ultrasound contrast agents for ultrasound imaging and Doppler. In: Rumack C, Wilson S, Charbonneau W (eds). *Diagnostic Ultrasound*, pp. 57–87. Philadelphia: C.V. Mosby, 1998.

71. Burns PN, Powers JE, Hope Simpson D, Brezina A, Kolin A, Chin CT, Uhlendorf V, Fritzsch T. Harmonic power mode Doppler using microbubble contrast agents: An improved method for small vessel flow imaging. Proc IEEE UFFC 1994;1547–1550.

Recent Readings

1. Zizka J, Elias P, Krajina A, *et al.* Value of Doppler sonography in revealing transjugular intrahepatic portosystemic shunt malformation: a 5-year experience in 216 patients. Am J Roentgenol 2000;175:141–148.

2. Kliewer MA, Hertzberg BS, Heneghan JP, *et al.* Transjugular intrahepatic portosystemic shunts (TIPS): effects of respiratory state and patient position on the measurement of Doppler velocities. Am J Roentgenol 2000;175:149–152.

3. Bodner G, Peer S, Fries D, Dessl A, Jaschke W. Color and pulsed Doppler ultrasound findings in normally functioning transjugular intrahepatic portosystemic shunts. Eur J Ultrasound 2000;12:131–136.

4. Saftoiu A, Ciurea T, Gorunescu F. Hepatic arterial blood flow in large hepatocellular carcinoma with or without portal vein thrombosis: assessment by transcutaneous duplex Doppler sonography. Eur J Gastroenterol Hepatol 2002;14:167–176.

5. Han SH, Rice S, Cohen SM, Reynolds TB, Fong TL. Duplex Doppler ultrasound of the hepatic artery in patients with acute alcoholic hepatitis. J Clin Gastroenterol 2002;34:573–577.

6. Sugimoto H, Kaneko T, Inoue S, Takeda S, Nakao A. Simultaneous Doppler measurement of portal venous peak velocity, hepatic arterial peak velocity, and splenic arterial pulsatility index for assessment of hepatic circulation. Hepatogastroenterology 2002;49:793–797.

7. Tasu JP, Rocher L, Peletier G, et al. Hepatic venous pressure gradients measured by duplex ultrasound. Clin Radiol 2002;57:746–752.

8. Sugimoto H, Kaneko T, Takeda S, Inoue S, Nakao A. The use of quantitative Doppler ultrasonography to predict posthepatectomy complications on the basis of hepatic hemodynamic parameters. Surgery 2002;132:431–440.

9. Ramnarine KV, Leen E, Oppo K. Angerson WJ, McArdle CS. Contrast-enhanced Doppler perfusion index: clinical and experimental evaluation. J Ultrasound Med 2002;21: 1121–1129.

10. Sugimoto H, Kaneko T, Hirota M, Tezel E, Nakao A. Earlier hepatic vein transit-time measured by contrast ultrasonography reflects intrahepatic hemodynamic changes accompanying cirrhosis. J Hepatol 2002;37:578–583.

11. Gorg C, Riera-Knorrenschild J, Dietrich J. Pictorial review: Colour Doppler ultrasound flow patterns in the portal venous system. Br J Radiol 2002;75:919–929.

12. Middleton WD, Teefey SA, Darey MD. Doppler evaluation of transjugular intrahepatic portosystemic shunts. Ultrasound Q 2003;19:56–70.

13. Huang DZ, Le GR, Zhang QP, et al. The value of color Doppler ultrasonography in monitoring normal orthotopic liver transplantation and postoperative complications. Hepatobiliary Pancreat Dis Int 2003;2:54–58.

14. Wachsberg RH. Doppler ultrasound evaluation of transjugular intrahepatic portosystemic shunt function: pitfalls and artifacts. Ultrasound Q 2003;19:139–148.

15. Varsamidis K, Varsamidou E, Mavropoulos G. Doppler ultrasonographic evaluation of hepatic blood flow in clinical sepsis. Ultrasound Med Biol 2003;29:1241–1244.

16. Annet L, Materne R, Danse E, Jamart J, Horsmans Y, Van Beers BE. Hepatic flow parameters measured with MR imaging and Doppler US: correlations with degree of cirrhosis and portal hypertension. Radiology 2003;229: 409–414.

17. Suzuki Y, Fujimoto Y, Hosoki Y, et al. Clinical utility of sequential imaging of hepatocellular carcinoma by contrast-enhanced power Doppler ultrasonography. Eur J Radiol 2003;48:214–219.

18. Kalache K, Romero R, Goncalves LF, et al. Three-dimensional color power imaging of the fetal hepatic circulation. Am J Obstet Gynecol 2003;189:1401–1406.

19. Benito A, Bilbao J, Hernandez T, et al. Doppler ultrasound for TIPS: does it work? Abdom Imaging 2004;29:45–52.

20. Pan Z, Wu XJ, Li JS, Liu FN, Li WS, Han JM. Functional hepatic flow in patients with liver cirrhosis. World J Gastroenterol 2004;10:915–918.

21. Wang Y, Wang WP, Ding H, Huang BJ, Mao F, Xu ZZ. Resistance index in differential diagnosis of liver lesions by color Doppler ultrasonography. World J Gastroenterol 2004;10:965–967.

22. Kruskal JB, Newman PA, Sammons LG, Kane RA. Optimizing Doppler and color flow US: application to hepatic sonography. Radiographics 2004;24:657–675.

23. Kastelan S, Ljubicic N, Kastelan Z, Ostojic R, Uravic M. The role of duplex-Doppler ultrasonography in the diagnosis of renal dysfunction and hepatorenal syndrome in patients with liver cirrhosis. Hepatogastroenterology 2004;51:1408–1412.

24. Yamashita H, Hachisuka Y, Kotegawa H, Fukuhara T, Korayashi N. Effects of posture change on the hemodynamics of the liver. Hepatogastroenterology 2004;51:1797–1800.

25. Kral V, Klein J, Havlik R, Vomacka J, Utikal P, Vrba R. Peripheral portosystemic shunt and its selectivity changes measured on duplex ultrasound. Hepatogastroenterology 2005;52:149–151.

26. Pedersen JF, Dakhil AZ, Jensen DB, Sondergaard B, Bytzer P. Abnormal hepatic vein Doppler waveform in patients without liver disease. Br J Radiol 2005;78:242–244.

27. Sugimoto H, Kaneko T, Hirota M, Inoue S, Takeda S, Nakao A. Physical hemodynamic interaction between portal venous and hepatic arterial blood flow in humans. Liver Int 2005; 25:282–287.

28. Hirota M, Kaneko T, Sugimoto H, Kure S, Inoue S, Takeda S, Nakao A. Intrahepatic circulatory time analysis of an ultrasound contrast agent in liver cirrhosis. Liver Int 2005;25:337–342.

29. Roumen RM, Scheltinga MR, Slooter GD, van der Linden AW. Doppler perfusion index fails to predict the presence of occult hepatic colorectal metastases. Eur J Surg Oncol 2005;31:521–527.

30. Chiu KC, Sheu BS, Chuang CH. Portal venous flow pattern as a useful tool for predicting esophageal varix bleeding in cirrhotic patients. Dig Dis Sci 2005;50:1170–1174.

31. Kaneko T, Sugimoto H, Hirota M, Kure S, Kiuchi T, Nakao A. Intrahepatic venous anastomosis formation of the right liver in living donor liver transplantation: evaluations by Doppler ultrasonography and pulse-inversion ultrasonography with Levovist. Surgery 2005;138:21–27.

42
Duplex Evaluation of the Renal Arteries

Marsha M. Neumyer and John Blebea

Introduction

Hypertension is estimated to affect approximately 50 million people in the United States with 1–6% of them having underlying renal disease as the cause of their elevated blood pressure.[1,2] The true prevalence of renovascular hypertension is unknown and varies with the population studied. In selected patient groups, such as those with severe diastolic hypertension, the prevalence of renal artery stenosis is up to 40% and progression of stenosis occurs in 31–49% of patients depending on the severity of their initial artery stenosis.[3–5] Renal artery stenosis is more likely to be found in adults with abrupt onset or exacerbation of chronic hypertension, angiotensin-converting enzyme inhibitor-induced azotemia, otherwise unexplained renal insufficiency, or pulmonary edema, and in hypertensive children.[6] Although the long-term prognosis for patients with renovascular hypertension is worse than that of patients who do not have identifiable lesions, successful treatment of such lesions is possible and is associated with cure or improvement of the hypertension in the majority of patients.[7] Identification of renal artery stenosis is important because treatment may control or cure renovascular hypertension, prevent loss of renal mass, or stabilize renal function in chronic renal failure.[8]

Since renal artery disease, due to either arterial stenosis or another pathology, is correctable, identification of affected patients is clinically important. Historically, contrast arteriography has been the diagnostic test of choice for renovascular disease. This procedure, however, offers mostly anatomic information without correlative hemodynamic data or causal linkage between identified disease and hypertension or renal dysfunction. In addition, its invasive nature and associated 3–5% complication rates, especially in the setting of associated renal functional impairment, effectively precludes its use as a screening test for renal artery stenosis and, in the majority of cases, even as a confirmatory diagnostic procedure.

For most clinicians, arteriography is performed as a final step in association with planned therapeutic intervention. Other less invasive diagnostic procedures include magnetic resonance angiography (MRA) and computed tomographic angiography (CTA). Both of these modalities, however, are relatively expensive and include the need for intravenous contrast, which, in the case of CTA, can be nephrotoxic. The published sensitivity and specificity of MRA in the diagnosis of renal artery stenosis is greater than 90%, although it has a tendency to overestimate the degree of stenosis and its accuracy in real-life situations is less than that reported from academic centers of excellence.[9] In a similar manner, three-dimensional volume CTA has a reported sensitivity and specificity of 89% and 99%, respectively, in the diagnosis of renal artery stenosis.[10] However, this accuracy is most likely not reflective of community practice results and the procedure requires larger volumes of contrast than used in standard arterial angiography. Because the cost of both MRA and CTA further precludes their use as the initial diagnostic modality, they are most useful as secondary confirmatory studies. Duplex ultrasonography offers the benefits of low cost and absence of ionizing radiation or routine need for intravenous contrast, and is a noninvasive, painless procedure. Technological advances in the past decade with improved low-frequency transducers, Doppler resolution, and digital imaging have made vascular ultrasound the technique of choice in the initial evaluation of the renal arteries. Renal duplex scanning can detect renal artery stenosis, determine its anatomic location, and help define its hemodynamic significance with an overall accuracy of 80–90%.[11]

Etiology of Renal Artery Disease

Atherosclerosis is the cause of 90% of cases of renal artery stenosis.[8,12] It most frequently involves the ostium and proximal third of the renal artery while more distal lesions are seen in 15–20% of patients.[13] Hemodynamically significant lesions may be accompanied by post-stenotic dilation.[3,13] Risk factors for the development of atherosclerotic renal artery stenosis include increasing age, hypertension, tobacco use, coronary artery disease, peripheral vascular disease, hyperlipidemia, and diabetes mellitus. Men are affected twice as frequently as women and bilateral lesions occur in 30% of patients.[14] In contrast, although fibromuscular dysplasia is the second most common cause of renal artery stenosis, it is far less frequent. It usually occurs in females aged 25–50 years old and involves the middle and distal portion of the main renal artery with extension into the first-order branches in 25% of patients. It occurs bilaterally more than 50% of the time although, when involving just one side, the right side is most frequently affected.[15] Angiographically, the renal arteries have a beaded appearance with alternating stenoses and aneurysmal dilations.[16,17] The etiology of fibromuscular dysplasia is unknown. Other less common causes of renal dysfunction include aortic dissections involving the renal vessels, spontaneous or traumatic isolated renal artery dissections or disruptions, renal artery aneurysms, atheroembolization to the renal arteries, progressive atherosclerotic stenosis leading to complete occlusion, arteriovenous fistulas, mid-abdominal aortic coarctation, developmental congenital stenoses, arteritis, and extrinsic compression by tumors or other masses.[13,17]

Renal Duplex Ultrasonography

Greene et al. were the first to use renal duplex ultrasonography to characterize blood flow patterns in the normal and diseased renal artery.[18] Using B-mode imaging and Doppler velocity waveforms, they described renal artery anatomy, blood flow rates, and velocity patterns. Other investigators subsequently developed and validated protocols for the evaluation and classification of normal and pathologic renal artery flow.[11,19–22]

In 1985, Rittgers, Norris, and Barnes created graded renal artery stenoses in a canine model.[23] They demonstrated that disturbances in the Doppler velocity waveform occur before significant reductions in blood flow. Significant stenoses were associated with marked flow disturbance exemplified by blunting of the systolic peak and loss of the systolic spectral window. There was also a decrease in the velocity distal to severe lesions along with associated poststenotic turbulence.

Early studies by Avasthi, Voyles, and Greene proposed criteria for the identification of renal artery lesions in humans: a peak systolic renal artery velocity greater than 100 cm/s, spectral broadening due to turbulence, and loss of the diastolic flow component for hemodynamically significant stenoses while the absence of any detectable flow

identified an occlusion of the renal artery.[24] Subsequent studies found that a peak systolic renal artery velocity of 100 cm/s is too low to yield acceptable sensitivities for detection of flow-reducing stenoses and that the loss of the diastolic flow component will often be reflective of intrinsic parenchymal dysfunction rather than arterial stenosis.[19,20,22] Additionally, flow is commonly detected within the kidney even when the renal artery is occluded because of flow through ureteral and adrenal collateral branches.

The current classification of renal artery stenosis relies on the Doppler-derived systolic velocity, a comparison with the systolic velocity recorded in the proximal abdominal aorta, and flow patterns along the length of the renal artery. Duplex diagnosis of a flow-limiting lesion is dependent on the demonstration of a focal increase in systolic velocity. Hoffman et al. demonstrated a sensitivity of 95% and a specificity of 91% for identification of a significant flow-reducing stenosis, defined as a >60% diameter reduction, using a peak systolic renal artery velocity of >180 cm/s.[25] Absolute velocity measurements may potentially be affected by systemic factors, such as blood pressure and cardiac output, and thus a comparison with aortic peak systolic velocity is routinely used. Kohler et al. have shown that a ratio of the peak systolic velocities of the renal artery to that of the abdominal aorta of >3.5 is predictive of renal artery stenosis of >60% diameter reduction.[19] The usefulness of this ratio has been validated in multiple centers.[11,20–22] Although the velocity in the abdominal aorta, as well as renal artery velocity, decreases with age, flow velocities have fortunately been shown to be independent of body surface area.[18,19]

Examination of the spectral flow patterns within the renal artery is also helpful in diagnosing stenoses. The presence of poststenotic turbulence is confirmatory of a hemodynamically significant lesion. Doppler spectral broadening has not been useful as a diagnostic parameter because the Doppler sample volume size is large in relation to the diameter of the small-caliber renal artery.

Renal artery stenosis is classified into four diagnostic categories based on duplex ultrasound criteria: normal, less than 60% stenosis, greater than 60% stenosis, and occlusion (Table 42–1). Lesions that represent less than 60% diameter-reducing stenosis are distinguished by an elevated systolic velocity but a renal-to-aortic ratio of less than 3.5 and no poststenotic turbulence. Clinically, it is still important to diagnose these lesions in order to identify patients who may benefit from continued monitoring for progression of disease. Confirmation of renal artery occlusion is dependent on the B-mode image of the renal artery to confirm proper location for Doppler insonation and demonstration of absence of flow in the renal artery. False-negative studies may result from insonation of nearby collateral vessels.

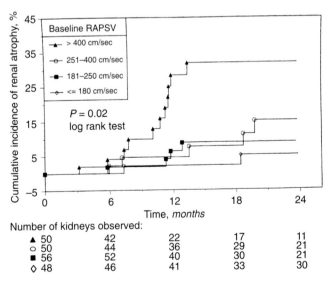

TABLE 42–1. Duplex criteria for classification of renal artery stenosis.[a]

Classification	RAR	PSV	PST
Normal	<3.5	<120 cm/s	Absent
<60% stenosis	<3.5	>180 cm/s	Absent
>60% stenosis	>3.5	>180 cm/s	Present
Occlusion	N/A	N/A	N/A
	Low velocity, low amplitude parenchymal signals		

[a]RAR, renal-aortic velocity ratio; PSV, peak systolic velocity; PST, post-stenotic turbulence; N/A, not applicable.

Renal size, as reflected by the ultrasound-measured length of the kidney, is useful in ascertaining potential intervention for renal artery stenosis. It has been shown that renal length decreases significantly in the presence of severe renal artery stenosis.[26–30] Caps and colleagues reported that kidneys with a renal artery peak systolic velocity greater than 400 cm/s, and cortical end-diastolic velocities less than or equal to 5 cm/s, were at high risk for progression to renal atrophy (Figure 42–1).[31] An atrophic kidney, usually defined as less than 8 cm in length, is unlikely to benefit from revascularization procedures. Although some investigators have been aggressive in such circumstances, the results with either surgical or endovascular revascularization have been disappoint-

ing as reperfusion of the ischemic kidney is not likely to reverse parenchymal changes.[32–34] On the other hand, studies suggest that improved renal function may be expected when intervention is performed prior to progression of the lesion to critical levels of renal impairment[33] or in cases where renal function has acutely deteriorated.[35,36] However, measurement of renal length alone is not a sensitive enough indicator to detect significant renal artery stenosis and progression to arterial occlusion.[31] Therefore, measurement of kidney length is useful to assist in the proper selection of patients for revascularization but inadequate by itself in defining the presence of a hemodynamically significant renal artery stenosis.

Duplex Ultrasound Evaluation of the Renal Arteries

Technique

Patient Preparation and Positioning

Although patients are required to fast for 6–8 h prior to the ultrasound examination to reduce excessive abdominal gas that would make visualization of the renal arteries and veins more difficult, we have not found it necessary to use cathartics. Patients are allowed to take their usual medications with small sips of water. Diabetic patients are permitted to have dry toast and clear liquids in the morning of the study in order to prevent development of hypoglycemia while awaiting their study. Because of this concern, diabetic patients are also the first ones scheduled in the morning. It is recommended that all patients refrain from smoking or chewing gum because these activities increase the amount of swallowed air in the stomach.

Once in the vascular laboratory, the patient is placed on the examination table in the supine position with the head slightly elevated and the feet lower than the heart. This allows the viscera to descend into the lower abdomen and pelvis, increasing the likelihood of finding acceptable acoustic windows. With the patient in this position, the aorta and the mesenteric and proximal-to-mid segments of the renal arteries are visualized. For examination of the distal renal arteries, renal veins, and the kidneys themselves, patients are moved to the right or left lateral decubitus position with the arm raised over their ear and their legs extended to elongate the body. A prone position, using intercostal scan planes, may occasionally be required for a thorough examination of the kidneys and distal renal arteries. In patients with a low rib cage, it may also be helpful to have them raise their arms over their head to elevate the ribs and allow improved access to the proximal renal arteries.

FIGURE 42–1. Cumulative index of renal atrophy stratified according to baseline renal artery peak systolic velocity (RAPSV, in cm/s). Standard error is <10% through 24 months for all plots. (Reproduced with permission from Caps MT, Zierler RE, Polissar NL, et al. The risk of atrophy in kidneys with atherosclerotic renal artery stenosis. Kidney Int 1998;53:735–742).

Equipment

A high-resolution ultrasound system with pulsed Doppler transducers ranging in frequency from 2.25 MHz to 5.0 MHz is required to allow adequate penetration to the depths of the aorta and distal renal arteries. Although color flow and power Doppler imaging are not absolutely required for successful renal vascular examination, these technologies will greatly facilitate visualization of the vessels, identification of regions of flow disturbance, and confirmation of arterial and/or venous occlusion. The sonographer must optimize the B-mode, color, and spectral Doppler information throughout the examination because velocities may vary over focal regions of the renal arterial and venous systems due to tortuosity and short-segment lesions, dissections, or webs.

Examination of the Aorta and Mesenteric and Renal Arteries

The examination is initiated with evaluation of the aorta beginning at the level of the diaphragm and continuing to its bifurcation. B-mode imaging is used to determine the presence of atherosclerotic plaque, aneurysmal dilation, or dissection. The evaluation is complemented with color flow imaging to highlight any regions of disturbed flow. Selective Doppler spectral waveforms are recorded at the level of the celiac and superior mesenteric artery origins. The aortic peak systolic velocity is documented and retained for later utilization in calculation of the renal to aortic velocity ratios.

Branches of the celiac and superior mesenteric arteries may course in close proximity and may be mistaken for accessory or main renal arteries. To help prevent such confusion, Doppler spectral waveforms may be recorded from both the celiac and superior mesenteric arteries with the primary purpose being recognition of the mesenteric flow patterns. A secondary benefit would be detection of unsuspected mesenteric occlusive disease.

The aorta is thereafter imaged in the cross-sectional plane at the level of the superior mesenteric artery. Just inferior to this level, the left renal vein can be identified as it crosses anterior to the aorta (Figure 42–2). Although this vein serves as a useful landmark for locating the renal arteries, it should be recognized that the vein can be completely retroaortic in a small number of patients (1–2%) or may bifurcate with one branch coursing anterior to the aorta and the second following a retroaortic path. The vein diameter and flow patterns should be assessed to rule out thrombosis or extrinsic compression due to overlying small bowel or superior mesenteric artery compression syndrome.

Although the renal arteries usually arise from the mid-lateral or posterolateral wall of the aorta at the level of the second lumbar vertebrae, just posterior to the left

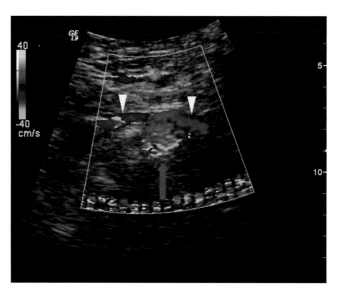

FIGURE 42–2. Cross-sectional color flow image of the left renal vein (white arrowheads) as it crosses over the abdominal aorta (red arrow).

renal vein, there can be much anatomic variability in their location. The location of accessory renal arteries is even more unpredictable and therefore easy to miss. Color flow imaging facilitates the identification of the arteries and makes it easier to follow their course from the origin to the mid-segment of the vessel. When neither color flow nor power Doppler allows satisfactory vessel identification, the use of intravenous ultrasound contrast can be helpful.

To obtain spectral Doppler waveforms, the sample volume is swept slowly from within the lumen of the aorta and through the renal artery ostium to rule out orificial stenotic disease commonly associated with plaque on the aortic wall. In making the transition from the aorta into the renal artery, the high-resistance aortic flow pattern changes to a low-resistance configuration in the renal artery. Using the smallest sample volume, Doppler spectral waveforms are recorded continuously throughout the visualized length of the renal arteries. The highest peak systolic velocity in the vessel is documented being careful to utilize an angle of insonation less than 60° (Figure 42–3). If needed, the patient is moved to the right or left lateral decubitus or prone position for interrogation of the mid-to-distal renal artery and renal parenchymal vessels. Color flow imaging may facilitate appropriate angle correction and identification of vessel tortuosity.

Evaluation of Renal Parenchymal Blood Flow

Blood flow patterns are documented throughout the distal renal artery and the interlobar and arcuate arteries of the renal medulla and cortex. Using a 0° angle of insonation, spectral waveforms are recorded throughout

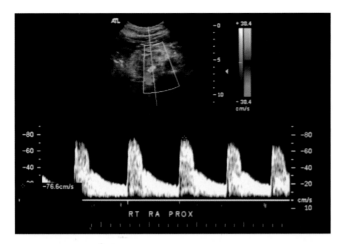

FIGURE 42–3. Color flow image and Doppler spectral waveforms from the proximal right renal artery. A low resistance spectral pattern is evident, which is characteristic of normal renal arterial blood flow.

the kidney, noting regions of increased signal amplitude and disordered or absent flow (Figure 42–4). The signals with the highest peak and end-diastolic velocities are documented from the vessels within the medulla and cortex of the upper, mid, and lower poles of the kidney. The presence of cortical thinning, cysts, masses, renal calculi, hydronephrosis, and/or perinephric fluid collections is noted.

Measurement of Renal Size

Because renal atrophy would be a contraindication to revascularization, the pole-to-pole length of each kidney is documented during each study (Figure 42–5). Normal renal length is between 9 and 13 cm in the greatest longitudinal plane and there is usually less than a 1 cm difference in renal lengths between the two kidneys. The length of the organ is measured during maximum inspi-

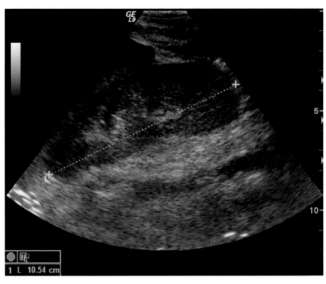

FIGURE 42–5. The pole-to-pole length of the kidney is measured to evaluate suitability for revascularization of stenotic lesions. Normal adult kidney length is greater than 9 cm.

ration using a flank approach to optimize visualization of the renal margins on both poles.

Evaluation for Renal Vein Thrombosis

Although most renal studies are performed for examination of the arterial circulation, renal vein thrombosis can lead to acute renal failure and referral to the vascular laboratory. Confirmation of renal vein thrombosis can be technically challenging. The vein may be dilated with acute thrombus or contracted when it has been chronically thrombosed. Optimization of the grayscale image is needed to demonstrate intraluminal echoes that indicate thrombosis (Figure 42–6). Doppler spectral examination will document the absence of blood flow within the vein and a retrograde, blunted diastolic flow component in the

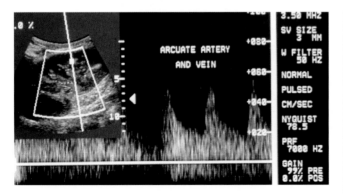

FIGURE 42–4. Color flow image and Doppler spectral waveforms from the arcuate arteries within the renal cortex. Normal renal parenchymal flow is characterized by constant forward diastolic flow.

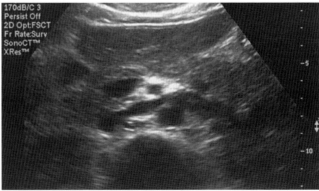

FIGURE 42–6. Transverse abdominal B-mode image of the aorta and left renal vein demonstrates dilation of the vein and intraluminal echoes consistent with thrombus.

renal arterial signals. In the case of renal cell carcinoma, extensive tumor involvement in the renal vein is common with extrusion and propagation into the inferior vena cava. In patients with a thrombosed inferior vena cava, possibly associated with prior placement of a vena caval filter, retrograde thrombosis may extend into the renal veins.

Contrast-Enhanced Imaging

Duplex imaging of renal artery stenosis can be technically challenging and is influenced by both operator expertise and patient factors, such as overlying bowel gas, obesity, and inability to optimally position the patient due to lack of patient cooperation.[11] Contrast enhancement to improve imaging and increase diagnostic accuracy is prevalent in radiologic techniques such as angiography, computed tomography (CT), and magnetic resonance imaging (MRI). Ultrasound contrast agents are stabilized gas microbubbles that enhance ultrasound signals due to the difference between them and the surrounding blood in terms of compressibility and density. They reflect transmitted ultrasound waves strongly, enhancing echogenicity at both fundamental and harmonic frequencies, which provides improved vascular imaging and tissue differentiation.[37,38] Intravenous ultrasound contrast agents have been found to improve ultrasound diagnostic accuracy and are approved for use in the heart with utility also reported in the liver, mesenteric, and peripheral vasculature.[39–41]

More recently, a prospective study examined the use of a perflutren contrast agent (Definity, DuPont) to improve imaging of the renal arteries.[42] This agent is composed of three phospholipids and a perfluoropropane gas that, when mixed together, form lipid- encapsulated gas-filled microbubbles.[40] Because the microbubbles are less than 5μm in diameter, and thus smaller than red blood cells, they pass easily through the pulmonary microcirculation and are rapidly cleared by respiration from the systemic circulation within 5min of their infusion. This particular agent requires mixing for 45s at 4500 oscillations/min in a specific vial shaker. For this study, a volume of 1.3 ml of agitated contrast solution was injected into a 50 ml bag of 0.9% sterile saline solution, which was subsequently infused intravenously at a rate of 2 ml/min via an 18-gauge needle throughout the duration of the duplex examination. The results of the ultrasound examination, with and without contrast enhancement, were compared with intraarterial angiography. Both duplex alone and duplex with contrast demonstrated excellent identification of the renal arteries (Table 42–2). Overall visualization of the renal arteries was 85% for standard duplex and 94% following contrast. Contrast infusion was particularly helpful in identifying additional accessory arteries and visualization of hemodynamically significant stenotic vessels (Figure 42–7). A total of five of seven

TABLE 42–2. Visualization of renal arteries with intravenous contrast.[a]

Renal arteries	Duplex alone	Duplex ± contrast
All renal arteries[48]	41 (85%)	45 (94%)
Main[43]	40 (93%)	42 (98%)
Accessory[5]	1 (20%)	3 (60%)
Normal/minimal disease[32]	30 (94%)	31 (97%)
Stenosis >50%	9 (75%)	12 (100%)
Occlusion[4]	3 (75%)	3 (75%)
Visualized length of artery	3.3 ± 0.3 cm	3.9 ± 0.3 cm

Modified from Blebea et al.[42]

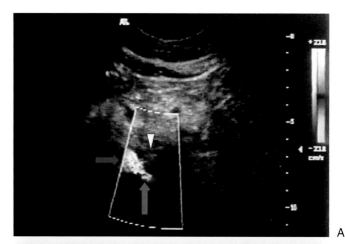

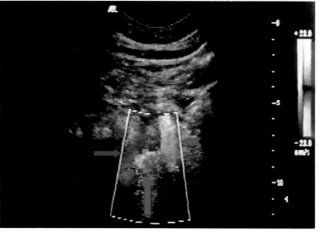

FIGURE 42–7. (A) Transverse abdominal ultrasound image without intravenous contrast barely demonstrates the right renal artery (red arrow) as it travels under the inferior vena cava (blue arrow) at the level of the left renal vein (white arrowhead). (B) With the addition of contrast, the same renal artery shows excellent color filling and its takeoff from the aorta (red arrowhead) is easily visualized and has no turbulent flow to suggest stenosis. (Reproduced with permission from Blebea J, Zickler R, Volteas N, Neumyer M, Assadnia S, Anderson K, Atnip R. Duplex imaging of the renal arteries with contrast enhancement. Vasc Endovasc Surg 2003;37:429–436.)

TABLE 42–3. Doppler velocities following contrast administration.[a]

Renal arteries	Duplex alone	Duplex ± contrast
Normal/minimal disease (cm/s)	112 ± 6	123 ± 7^{b}
Stenosis >50% (cm/s)	173 ± 20^{c}	$194 \pm 18^{b,c}$
All (cm/s)	127 ± 7^{c}	$144 \pm 8^{b,c}$

[a]Modified from Blebea et al.[42]
[b]$p < 0.001$ versus duplex alone.
[c]$p < 0.001$ versus normal.

arteries not visualized by color flow duplex was detected following the infusion of contrast, resulting in an additional 10% (5/48) of vessels visualized. In addition, significantly longer lengths of the renal arteries were visualized in continuity when contrast was infused [3.9 cm as compared to 3.3 cm ($p = 0.001$)].

There were no complications associated with the use of the intravenous contrast. The patients experienced no changes in blood pressure or heart rates during the contrast infusion and no deterioration of renal function as measured by blood urea nitrogen or serum creatinine levels, consistent with the experience of other investigators.[40,43] Insonated Doppler velocities, however, were increased following contrast administration by an average of 10% in normal or minimally diseased vessels and 12% in stenotic vessels (Table 42–3). Although these differences were statistically significant, they did not lead to a change in the category of stenosis. This artifactual increase in measured Doppler velocities has been noted. As contrast agents become more extensively used, separate velocity criteria may need to be established. At the present time, however, the 10–12% increase in peak systolic velocities does not represent a large enough difference to require immediate attention but should be kept in mind for borderline results.

The results from these studies indicate that contrast-enhanced duplex imaging of the renal arteries is safe but not routinely required when an experienced sonographer performs the study. However, it can increase vessel visualization and thus allow more specific placement of the pulsed Doppler sample volume. This may increase the overall accuracy of the study in patients with stenoses and accessory renal arteries or in the approximately 10% of patients whose vessels are not initially successfully visualized. No comparative studies have been done among different contrast agents. Another perflutren-based contrast agent (Optison, Amersham Health) is FDA approved for echocardiography and has the potential benefit of not requiring a specific vial mixer before infusion.

Special Considerations

Accessory and Multiple Renal Arteries

Approximately 20% of the population has multiple renal arteries. These additional vessels usually arise from the lateral aortic wall and are directed toward the upper or lower poles of the kidney rather than the central hilum. For an unknown reason, more accessory renal arteries are seen on the left as compared to the right side. When only a single accessory artery is present, it is usually supplying the lower pole of the kidney. In the presence of an accessory vessel, the main renal artery is usually of normal caliber while the accessory vessels have a smaller diameter. When multiple renal arteries occur, a less commonly seen circumstance, none of the vessels may be dominant and it is quite difficult to be certain that velocity measurements have been acquired from all vessels.

Positive identification of all accessory and multiple renal arteries by B-mode imaging is not generally possible because of the small diameter of these vessels and lack of clinical suspicion for their presence. While color flow imaging may facilitate recognition of accessory renal arteries, it is important to remember that color encodement of Doppler shifted frequencies from blood flow is angle dependent and accessory renal arteries may arise from the aortic wall at angles between 70 and 90° (Figure 42–8). To overcome this problem, power Doppler

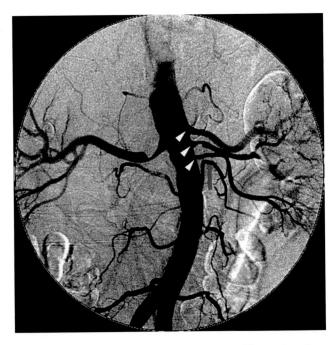

FIGURE 42–8. Digital subtraction angiogram illustrating three renal arteries on the left (white arrowheads) with the midrenal having a 50% stenosis. An adjacent lumbar artery (red arrow) can be misconstrued as an additional accessory artery if it is not followed distally to confirm that it does not lead to the kidney.

imaging, which relies on the amplitude of the returned Doppler signal and is not as angle dependent as color Doppler imaging, may prove beneficial for detection of these small vessels. There can be clues that suggest the presence of multiple renal arteries. It is helpful to increase the size of the Doppler sample volume and scan in the paraaortic region, moving from the level of the main renal artery origin to the aortic bifurcation to detect any additional low-resistance signals that could imply renal arterial flow. Lumbar arteries can be confused with accessory renal arteries but these have a more posterior origin from the aorta. The use of an intravenous contrast agent has improved the detection of accessory renal arteries.[41]

Occlusion of the Main Renal Artery

Diagnosis of an occluded main renal artery can be difficult because the sonographer is appropriately concerned that it has not been possible to adequately visualize flow within the vessel rather than prematurely concluding that the vessel is thrombosed. Excessive overlying abdominal gas that may compromise visualization compounds this hesitation. After optimizing Doppler spectral and color flow parameters for detection of very slow flow, and possibly the use of intravenous contrast, it is possible to look for secondary indications of renal artery occlusion. With chronic occlusion and atrophy, kidney length is less than 8 cm and there can be a significant >3 cm difference in length as compared with the contralateral kidney. Intraparenchymal insonation demonstrates low cortical velocity of <10 cm/s with low amplitude and a delayed systolic upstroke. The presence of cortical blood flow is a result of collateral flow to the kidney through adrenal and ureteral vessels.

Horseshoe Kidney

Horseshoe kidneys are not common, occurring in less than 1% of autopsies. Most often, the organs are fused at the lower pole, with approximately 10% of kidneys joined at the upper pole. This large unified kidney, connected by an isthmus of renal parenchyma of variable size, will lie anterior to the aorta usually at the level of the fourth or fifth lumbar vertebrae. Horseshoe kidneys are usually found in patients who present for investigation of a pulsatile abdominal mass or they may be discovered incidentally during an abdominal ultrasound examination.

Anatomically, the kidney is supplied by multiple renal arteries and drained by multiple renal veins at unpredictable locations. Multiple arteries may arise from the iliac arteries or the distal aorta. Their location, posterior to the body of the kidney, makes it difficult to identify these arteries and even more challenging to diagnose the presence of stenoses. In patients with an underlying abdominal aortic aneurysm, diagnosing renal artery stenosis is best accomplished with contrast angiography.

Renal Aneurysms

Aneurysmal dilation of the renal artery usually involves the main segment of the renal artery or its first order branches. Although aneurysms may also occur intraparenchymally, this location is seen in only approximately 10% of cases. Renal aneurysms are most easily identified with color flow imaging (Figure 42–9). Their large size, compared to the native vessel, makes identification relatively easy. Intervention is generally recommended for aneurysms of 2 cm or greater in diameter. Therefore, it is important to measure the maximal diameter of the aneurysm, either in preparation for surgical repair or as a baseline for monitoring future growth. The specific location is less important, although differentiation between an aneurysm involving the renal artery and an

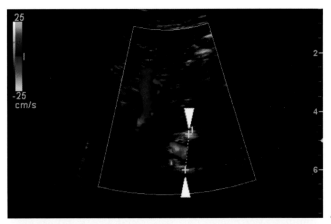

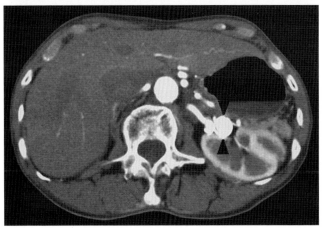

FIGURE 42–9. (A) A left renal artery aneurysm is measured transversely on an ultrasound image. Color flow evaluation is difficult due to circumferential calcification in the wall of the aneurysm. (B) The calcified aneurysm, located just beyond the bifurcation of the renal artery, is seen on CT scan with intravenous contrast.

intraparenchymal position is helpful in selecting proper therapy. Rarely, there is an associated arteriovenous fistula that makes the initial diagnosis more challenging.

Fibromuscular Dysplasia

Fibromuscular dysplasia (FMD) is a term encompassing several histologic forms of arterial wall changes of which medial fibroplasia is the most common. As a group, FMD is the second most common cause of renal artery stenosis and accounts for up to one-third of cases of renovascular hypertension. This nonatherosclerotic disease process is seen almost exclusively in females and presents as a "string of beads" angiographic appearance with weblike stenotic segments alternating with poststenotic dilations. It involves the mid-to-distal segments of the renal artery and will frequently extend into branch vessels with characteristic superimposed high- and low-velocity signals (Figure 42–10). Awareness that this disease affects primarily young women, in the third or fourth decade of life, an age group not usually affected by renal atherosclerosis, may aid in identification of this disorder. The less common variants of FMD, perimedial dysplasia and intimal fibroplasia, are not associated with poststenotic dilations. Intimal fibroplasias in particular produce a smooth concentric stenosis. Differentiation between the types of FMD is neither practical nor necessary during ultrasonographic examination. Because fibromuscular dysplasia is often found bilaterally, it is important to search for similar flow patterns in the contralateral renal artery.

Renal Artery Bypass Grafts

Similar to peripheral bypasses, renal artery bypass procedures are followed postoperatively for the development of stenosis to allow intervention before graft occlusion occurs. When evaluating renal artery bypass grafts, it is helpful to know specific details of the surgical procedure including the origin of the graft, conduit used (prosthetic or autologous saphenous vein), and location and type of distal anastomosis. An operative drawing indicating the donor artery, graft course, and recipient vessel is very useful. Renal artery bypass grafts commonly originate from a prosthetic aortic graft, the native aorta, or the iliac arteries. Other less common inflow sources include the hepatic or gastroduodenal arteries on the right side and the superior mesenteric or splenic arteries on the left side.

As with extremity bypass grafts, the anastomotic regions must be carefully interrogated with spectral and color Doppler because intimal hyperplasia and stenosis most commonly occur at the anastomotic sites. If the conduit is a saphenous vein, attention is given to the possibility of retained valves or stenosis developing at the

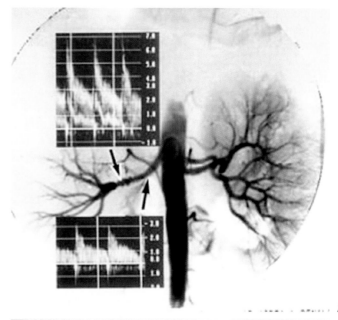

A

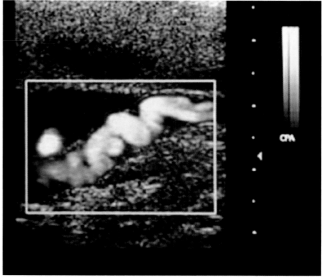

B

FIGURE 42–10. (A) Montage of an arteriogram and Doppler spectral waveforms from a patient with renal medial fibromuscular dysplasia. High-velocity signals are found in the mid-to-distal segment of the renal artery in association with segmental circumferential narrowing of the artery. [Reproduced with permission from Thiele BL, Neumyer MM, Healy DA, Schina MJ. Pitfalls in duplex ultrasonography of the renal arteries. In: Bernstein EF (ed). *Vascular Diagnosis*, 4th ed., p. 664. St. Louis, MO: C.V. Mosby, 1993.) (B) Power Doppler image of fibromuscular dysplasia demonstrating the segmental narrowing and poststenotic dilation associated with this nonatherosclerotic disease process.

site of valve leaflets. The donor and recipient vessels are also examined for progression of atherosclerotic disease. If graft occlusion is suspected, dampening of the velocity spectral waveform is expected within the renal parenchyma.

Renal Artery Stents

The ultrasound evaluation of the renal artery following balloon angioplasty and stenting is identical to that used for evaluation of the native renal artery prior to intervention.[45] In the majority of patients, the metallic stents are well visualized and their location within the renal artery easily determined because the metal stents are brightly echogenic (Figure 42–11). The aortic wall adjacent to the renal artery orifice should be carefully evaluated with high-resolution B-mode, real-time compound or harmonic imaging, to determine how far the stent protrudes into the lumen of the aorta. Similarly, the length of the stented segment should be examined to confirm complete deployment and uniform apposition to the wall of the renal artery without echogenic thrombus or distal dissection.

Using color or power Doppler imaging and Doppler spectral evaluation, the stent is examined throughout its origin, proximal, mid, and distal segments with the study extended into the distal native renal artery and the vessels within the kidney. Marked flow disturbances at the renal artery orifice may indicate that the stent is protruding too far into the aortic lumen. High-velocity signals at this location suggest that aortic flow patterns are severely disrupted and pressure–flow gradients have developed. Minimal flow disturbance is usually noted in the proximal stented segment of the artery. A slight elevation in the systolic velocity may be found due to the rigidity of the stent and consequent decreased vessel wall

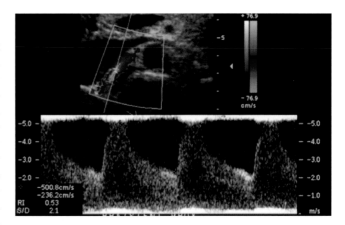

FIGURE 42–12. Color flow image and Doppler spectral waveforms from the distal end of a stent in the right renal artery. The very high velocities noted at peak systole and end diastole suggest flow-reducing stenosis, which would be confirmed by documenting poststenotic turbulence.

compliance. In the absence of flow-limiting stenosis in the proximal stent, the peak systolic velocity range should approximate that seen in normal, unstented renal arteries.

The native renal artery normally tapers as it courses distally. Placement of a renal stent results in slight dilation of the stented segment of the vessel compared to the diameter of the native artery distal to the stent. Given this, a flow gradient may be present at the distal end of the stent because the blood is flowing from a large diameter vessel to a smaller diameter segment. Even though the diameter mismatch across the distal end of the stent is quite small, slightly elevated Doppler velocity signals and disordered color flow patterns may be encountered. Careful attention must be given to the flow patterns at the distal end of the stent to ensure that they are the result of a stent-diameter to vessel-diameter mismatch and not due to flow-reducing stenosis distal to or within the stent. Increased peak and end diastolic velocities with poststenotic turbulence suggest flow-reducing stenosis (Figure 42–12).

Interpretation of Doppler Spectral Waveforms and Images

The Abdominal Aorta

A rapid systolic upstroke and a sharp systolic peak characterize Doppler spectral waveforms recorded from the abdominal aorta proximal to the renal artery origins. Because this segment of the aorta carries flow to the low-resistance vascular beds of the liver, spleen, and kidneys, the flow pattern is most commonly biphasic with a peak

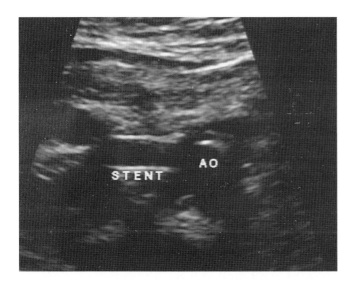

FIGURE 42–11. Cross-sectional abdominal B-mode image of the aorta and the proximal right renal artery demonstrates the echogenic walls of a renal stent. High- resolution imaging confirms uniform apposition of the stent to the walls of the artery and no evidence of intraluminal echoes that might suggest thrombosis of the vessel.

systolic velocity range of 60–100 cm/s. Distal to the renal arteries, the velocity may decrease slightly and the waveform morphology becomes triphasic, consistent with flow to the high-resistance lower extremity peripheral arterial bed.

Flow disturbances may be noted at the renal artery orifices, but high-velocity turbulent signals should not be found in the absence of aortic wall plaque or orificial renal artery lesions. Kohler et al.[19] demonstrated that a ratio of the peak systolic renal artery velocity and the peak systolic aortic velocity that is equal to or less than 3.5 offers excellent sensitivity for confirming the absence of flow-reducing (>60% diameter reduction) renal artery stenosis. Narrowing of the renal artery will result in elevation of velocity while the aortic velocity remains relatively stable. In cases where the aortic velocity exceeds 100 cm/s due to stenotic disease or increased cardiac output, the renal–aortic velocity ratio will be too low and will, therefore, underestimate the severity of renal artery stenosis. For example, if the aortic velocity is 120 cm/s and the renal artery velocity is 240 cm/s, the renal aortic ratio will be 2.0, incorrectly suggesting the absence of any renal artery stenosis. Similarly, in patients with an aortic aneurysm, increased distal impedance due to aortic stenosis or occlusion, or a low cardiac output, lower than normal peak systolic aortic velocities (<40 cm/s) will result in overestimation of the severity of renal disease based on the renal–aortic peak systolic velocity ratio. However, requiring both a renal artery peak systolic velocity >180 cm/s and a poststenotic turbulence will obviate such potential pitfalls in identifying a hemodynamically significant renal artery stenosis (Table 42–1).

Normal Renal Artery

A rapid systolic upstroke and peak systolic velocities ranging from 90 to 120 cm/s characterize the normal renal arterial waveform with the renal–aortic peak systolic velocity ratio being less than or equal to 3.5 (Table 42–1). Systole is followed by rapid deceleration to forward diastolic flow with a velocity at least one-third of the systolic value. Quite often an early systolic, or compliance, peak may be found on the systolic upstroke. This is thought to be a reflection of the expansion and recoil of the artery that occur with each systolic pulse and, indirectly, may reflect the degree of renovascular resistance in the distal parenchymal vessels. The compliance peak may be found either higher or lower than the actual systolic peak. As an indicator of proximal renal artery stenosis, a delay in the systolic acceleration time of more than 100 ms from the onset of systole is abnormal.

Flow patterns throughout the normal renal artery are characterized by constant forward diastolic flow due to the low resistance of the renal arterial system (Figure 42–13). Decreased diastolic flow to zero, or actual flow

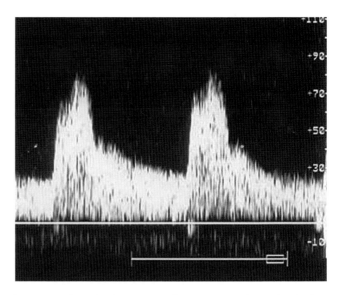

FIGURE 42–13. The flow pattern in normal renal arteries is characterized by rapid systolic upstroke and constant forward diastolic flow.

reversal, should not normally be seen because such findings would be characteristic of impedance to arterial inflow or obstruction to venous outflow from the organ. The ratio of end-diastolic to systolic flow remains fairly constant throughout the normal renal arterial tree although the peak systolic velocity will decrease proportionately from the main renal artery to the level of the renal cortex. Distal renal artery peak systolic velocity is normally 70–90 cm/s. Systolic velocity in the renal medullary arteries averages 30–50 cm/s, assuming a 0° angle of insonation, while more distal cortical velocity averages 10–20 cm/s.

Less than 60% Renal Artery Stenosis

As the severity of renal artery stenosis increases, the peak systolic velocity will increase to meet downstream flow demands. Stenotic lesions that reduce the diameter of the renal artery 30–60% will cause color flow disturbances and the peak systolic renal artery velocity to exceed 180 cm/s. However, the degree of arterial narrowing is not yet severe enough to cause poststenotic turbulence and the renal–aortic peak systolic velocity ratio will remain less than 3.5.

Hemodynamically Significant Renal Artery Stenosis

When reduction of the renal artery diameter exceeds 60%, poststenotic turbulence will become apparent and the peak systolic renal artery velocity will significantly exceed 180 cm/s (Figure 42–14). It is important in cases

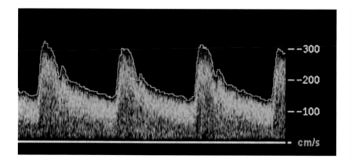

FIGURE 42–14. Flow-reducing renal artery stenosis (>60% diameter reduction) is associated with peak systolic velocities that exceed 180 cm/s and poststenotic turbulence.

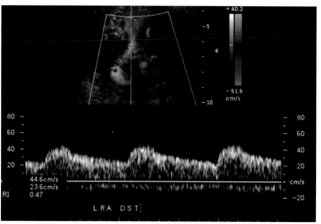

FIGURE 42–15. Distal to critical renal artery lesions (>80% diameter reduction), the systolic upstroke of the Doppler spectral waveform will be delayed, the compliance peak will disappear, and the peak systolic velocity will be decreased.

where the aorta is diseased, thus obviating use of the renal—aortic ratio, to confirm the presence of a post-stenotic signal, as this signifies a pressure-flow gradient and differentiates a hemodynamically significant lesion from a less severe stenosis. Doppler spectral and color flow parameters must be adjusted throughout the interrogation of the lesion to reveal the decrease in velocity that occurs immediately proximal to a stenosis, the high-velocity signals within the lesion, and the decrease in velocity distally that is associated with the poststenotic turbulence that develops downstream. Distal to critical lesions, >80% diameter reduction, systolic upstroke will be delayed, the compliance peak may disappear, and the peak systolic velocity will decrease (Figure 42–15).

Renal Artery Occlusion

Renal artery occlusion is diagnosed by definitively identifying the main renal artery and documenting lack of flow in its lumen. Multiple image planes may be required to ensure the absence of flow in all segments of the renal artery. If the entire length of the renal artery is not well visualized with the patient placed in the supine position, it may be useful to move the patient to the lateral decubitus or prone position. From a near decubitus position, the kidney can be imaged through an intercostal approach using a coronal scan plane from the flank. With the patient lying prone and flexed in the mid-section over a pillow or foam wedge, an intercostal acoustic window

and optimal acute angle of insonation can be obtained for evaluation of the renal hilum and distal renal artery. The lack of arterial flow in a chronically occluded main renal artery produces cortical flow of <10 cm/s with a low-amplitude waveform configuration throughout the renal parenchyma as a result of collateral flow to the kidney (Figure 42–16). After optimizing color, power, and spectral Doppler sensitivity to exclude the very low flow of a preocclusive lesion, it is also useful to compare parenchymal velocity and signals with those in the contralateral kidney.

Renal Parenchymal Dysfunction (Medical Renal Disease)

Doppler spectral waveforms recorded throughout the renal parenchyma help differentiate normal renovascular resistance from patterns associated with intrinsic parenchymal disorders. Normally, the diastolic velocity in the interlobar and arcuate arteries of the renal parenchyma approximates 40–50% of the systolic velocity and resistance remains low even in kidneys with flow-reducing renal artery stenosis. It is thought that the kidney compensates for the reduction in pressure and

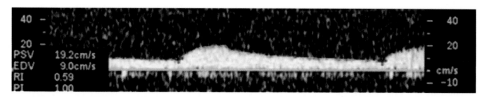

FIGURE 42–16. Blood flow to the kidney may continue via ureteral and adrenal collaterals when the renal artery is chronically occluded. Low-amplitude Doppler spectral waveforms with velocity <10 cm/s may be recorded throughout the parenchyma of the kidney.

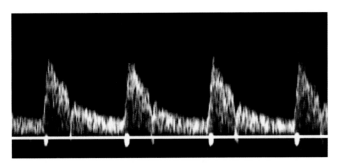

FIGURE 42–17. Doppler spectral waveforms from the interlobar arteries of a kidney with parenchymal dysfunction (medical renal disease). AS renovascular resistance increases and diastolic flow decreases.

flow through vasodilation, which in turn lowers vascular resistance.

When renal function becomes impaired, diastolic flow decreases, suggesting impedance to arterial inflow to the microvasculature of the kidney and increased vascular resistance (Figure 42–17). Although renovascular resistance tends to increase slightly with aging, a marked decrease in diastolic flow can be associated with a wide variety of etiologies including acute tubular necrosis, glomerulonephritis, polycystic disease, diabetic nephropathy, or severe obstructive hydronephrosis. A diastolic-to-systolic velocity ratio less than 0.30 is consistent with parenchymal dysfunction, while ratios less than 0.2 will most often be associated with elevated blood urea nitrogen and serum creatinine levels.

Although it is not uncommon to find low-resistance waveforms in a kidney with a severe proximal renal artery stenosis, the same may not be true for the contralateral nondiseased organ that is unprotected from the hypertensive insult. Therefore, careful sequential monitoring of flow patterns in the contralateral organ is recommended because renovascular resistance will most likely develop.

Renal Hilar Evaluations

With earlier technology, or for those who do not have the experience with direct evaluation of the renal artery and its parenchymal branches, some have advocated a limited examination of the renal arteries within the renal hilum. Such proposed techniques depend on recognizing the distal hemodynamic consequences of more proximal significant stenosis. A limited evaluation offers the attractiveness of lessening the technical challenge and decreasing the length of the examination with possibly a lower incidence of inadequate studies compared with direct evaluation of the entire renal arterial system. Several investigators have reported excellent sensitivities and specificities for detection of significant renal artery stenosis using parameters calculated from the hilar

Doppler spectral waveforms (Figure 42–18).[46–48] An *acceleration index*, defined as the slope of the systolic upstroke (kHz/s) divided by the transmitted frequency, of less than 3.78 (kHz/s/MHz) has been shown by Handa *et al.* to have an accuracy of 95%, sensitivity of 100%, and specificity of 93%.[46] Martin *et al.* calculated the *acceleration time*, defined as the time interval between the onset of systole and the initial compliance peak, to predict flow-reducing proximal renal artery disease.[47] In their study, an acceleration time greater than 0.10s was superior to use of an acceleration index and yielded a sensitivity of 87% and a specificity of 98%. Stavros and his colleagues have additionally used the absence of the compliance peak to suggest significant renal artery stenosis.[48]

The indirect examination of the renal hilar arteries is performed with the patient in a lateral decubitus or prone position using an intercostal scan plane. From a transverse image of the kidney, the distal renal artery is interrogated along its axis using a 0° angle of insonation. It is important to record Doppler velocity waveforms using the highest transducer frequency possible to obtain adequate signals, a large sample volume, and a sweep speed of 100ms.

Although the potential for limited, but accurate, diagnostic evaluations is suggested by these initial investigations, sufficient prospective studies have not been done to validate these criteria. Indeed, in studies from other institutions, acceleration time, acceleration index, and absence of a compliance peak have been shown to be unsatisfactory predictors of 60–79% diameter-reducing renal artery stenosis. Acceptable sensitivity and specificity have been associated only with lesions that exceed 80% diameter reduction by arteriography. Although the limited hilar examination provides complementary information, especially in cases where the entire length of the renal artery cannot be visualized, a complete evaluation of the renal arterial system is much preferred. We do not recommend using hilar evaluations as an alternative to a complete and direct examination of the main renal

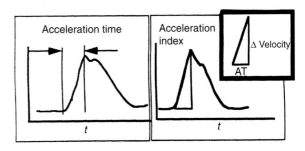

FIGURE 42–18. Diagram illustrating the method of calculation of acceleration time (AT) and acceleration index (AI). AT is the time interval from the onset of flow to the initial (compliance) peak. AI is the slope of the systolic upstroke divided by the transmitted frequency.

artery because it yields no information regarding the anatomic location of a proximal lesion. In addition, a well-collateralized kidney with a proximal renal artery occlusion cannot be differentiated from a high-grade stenosis.[47] In patients with concomitant renal parenchymal disease, the acceleration time and index may be normalized and the acceleration time can be influenced by the peak systolic renal artery velocity.[46–48] The effect of blood flow from multiple renal arteries on hilar Doppler evaluations has also yet to be adequately determined. With present high-quality ultrasound systems, and experienced technologists with certification and adequate training, a complete examination of the renal artery is possible in more than 90% of patients.[41]

Renal Vein Evaluation

When the renal vein is thrombosed or filled with tumor, intraluminal echoes should be demonstrated within the lumen. Care must be taken to optimize the B-mode image because fresh thrombus may have the same acoustic properties as flowing blood. If the patient is thin, the renal vein will be noncompressible and may be dilated if the thrombotic process is acute or contracted with chronic thrombosis. Doppler spectral waveforms should demonstrate an absence of flow in the main trunk of the vein. There will be a lack of phasic flow proximal to the obstructed segment and minimal phasicity in the distal venous segments if the thrombosed segment is recanalized or if venous collaterals have developed. If there is extrinsic compression of the vein, disturbed color flow and high-velocity Doppler signals will be found in the region of venous narrowing.

Evaluation of Renal Artery Stents

A number of factors need to be considered in the interpretation of Doppler velocity waveforms and images in vessels with renal artery stents. The number and the location of renal stents will influence velocity patterns. If stents are placed in sequence in the renal artery, arterial compliance will be decreased along the length of the stented segment and slight elevation of velocities may be noted throughout the vessel. A diameter mismatch between the stented segment and the native renal artery will more likely be noted in stents that are placed in the smaller diameter distal renal artery.

A focal increase in velocity is more likely to be associated with a diameter mismatch while high-velocity flow disturbance that is propagated over a longer distance is commonly found with flow-reducing stenosis. If a significant lesion is suspected it is important to confirm the presence of a poststenotic signal and dampening of the velocity signal downstream. Comparing velocity data to data obtained during previous duplex examinations can yield valuable clues that may help to confirm stenotic disease. Elevated velocities due to vessel diameter mismatch should remain stable while increased velocity due to stenosis may demonstrate a temporal change.

At present, the diagnostic criteria used for the classification of disease in the native renal artery are being applied to interpretation of images and Doppler spectral data from renal arteries with stents. Special consideration must be given, however, to the type, location, and number of stents, reduced arterial compliance in the stented segment, and the possibility of a slight diameter mismatch between the stented segment and the native artery. In the future, it may be necessary to develop stent-specific diagnostic criteria for follow-up monitoring and surveillance.

Prediction of Outcome of Interventions for Renal Artery Stenosis

While success has been attained with both noninvasive and invasive techniques for identification of renal artery stenosis, relatively little success has been achieved with prospective selection of patients whose renal function or blood pressure will improve following correction of the renal stenosis. Multiple factors affect the outcome of surgical or percutaneous intervention including severity of the renal artery stenosis, the procedure used to treat the lesion, nephrotoxicity to the angiographic contrast agents, atheroembolism, and the presence of preexisting intrinsic renal parenchymal disease. Several investigators have evaluated the use of quantitative measurements of Doppler spectral waveform parameters to determine the level of resistance to flow in the segmental arteries of the kidney as predictors of favorable outcome to intervention. Radermacher and his colleagues[49] calculated a resistive index [(1 − end diastolic velocity divided by maximal systolic velocity) × 100] in 138 patients who had either unilateral or bilateral renal artery stenosis of at least 50% diameter reduction and underwent renal angioplasty or surgical bypass. Creatinine clearance and ambulatory blood pressures were documented prior to intervention and at 3, 6, and 12 months and then yearly following the procedure. The mean follow-up was 32 months. Based on this study, they concluded that patients with a renal resistive index value of at least 80 were unlikely to experience significant improvement in blood pressure, renal function, or organ survival following correction of renal artery stenosis. Similarly, Tullis et al. recommended a renal artery end-diastolic ratio from the contralateral kidney in patients with unilateral atherosclerotic renal artery stenosis to predict response to renal revascularization.[50]

Conclusions

Duplex ultrasonography of the renal arteries and kidneys is the diagnostic test of choice in the initial evaluation of renovascular hypertension or suspected renal artery pathology. Beginning with the evaluation of the aorta and the entire length of the main renal artery, color flow ultrasonography is helpful in localizing the vessel, giving a preliminary assessment of disturbed flow and possible underlying stenosis, and allowing accurate placement of sample volume insonation for Doppler velocity measurement and spectral waveform analysis. Peak Doppler systolic velocity measurements in the main renal artery provide the basis for the determination of hemodynamically significant stenoses. In combination with color and/or power Doppler imaging, B-mode visualization is helpful in diagnosing and localizing other arterial and parenchymal pathology, such as fibromuscular dysplasia, aneurysms, dissections, parenchymal masses and cysts, and extrarenal tumors or masses that may induce extrinsic compression. Measurement of kidney length is important in determining the usefulness of therapeutic interventions and sequential monitoring of renal function. Parenchymal assessment, with both Doppler velocity measurements and color and power Doppler flow imaging, provides an indication of intrinsic renal disease and the likelihood of improvement in renal function following revascularization of the kidney. The role of limited, indirect renal hilar scanning is best used as a complement to the complete interrogation of the renal vascular system. Duplex ultrasound is an ideal technology for natural history studies on renal arterial dysfunction and follow-up after endovascular or surgical revascularization. It can be a technically demanding study dependent on the experience and capability of the sonographer. Intravenous contrast agents may be helpful in challenging cases where the vessels are difficult to image.

References

1. Berglund G, Anderson O, Wilhelmensen L. Prevalence of primary and secondary hypertension: Studies in a random population sample. BMJ 1976;II:554–556.
2. Dunnick NR, Sfakianakis GN. Screening for renovascular hypertension. Radiol Clin North Am 1991;29:497–510.
3. Holley KE, Hunt JC, Brown AL, et al. Renal artery stenosis: A clinical-pathologic study in normotensive and hypertensive patients. Am J Med 1964;37:14–18.
4. Eyler WR, Clark MD, Garman JE, et al. Angiography of the renal arteries including a comparative study of renal arterial stenoses in patients with and without hypertension. Radiology 1962;78:879–882.
5. Caps MT, Perissinotto C, Zierler RE, et al. A prospective study of atherosclerotic disease progression in the renal artery. Circulation 1998;98:2866–2872.
6. The Seventh Report of the Joint National Committee on Prevention, Detection, Evaluation, and Treatment of High Blood Pressure. JAMA 2003;289:2560–2572.
7. Martin LG. Renal revascularization using percutaneous balloon angioplasty for fibromuscular dysplasia and atherosclerotic disease. In: Calligaro KD, Dougherty MJ, Dean RH (eds). *Modern Management of Renovascular Hypertension and Renal Salvage*, pp. 125–144. Baltimore: Williams & Wilkins, 1996.
8. Safian RD, Textor SC. Renal artery stenosis. N Engl J Med 2001;344(6):431–442.
9. Hany TF, Leung DA, Pfammatter T, Debatin JF. Contrast-enhanced magnetic resonance angiography of the renal arteries. Invest Radiol 1998;33(9):653–659.
10. Johnson PT, Halpern EJ, Kuszyk BS, Heath DG, et al. Renal artery stenosis: CT angiography: Comparison of real-time volume rendering and maximum intensity projection algorithms. Radiology 1999;211(2):337–343.
11. Hansen KJ, Tribble RW, Reavis SW, et al. Renal duplex sonography: Evaluation of clinical utility. J Vasc Surg 1990;12:227–236.
12. Stanley JC. Natural history of renal artery stenoses and aneurysms. In: Calligaro KD, Dougherty MJ, Dean RH (eds). *Modern Management of Renovascular Hypertension and Renal Salvage*, pp. 15–45. Baltimore: Williams & Wilkins, 1996.
13. Working Group on Renovascular Hypertension. Detection, evaluation, and treatment of renovascular hypertension. Arch Intern Med 1987;147:820–829.
14. Bookstein JJ, Maxwell MH, Abrams HL, et al. Cooperative study of radiologic aspects of renovascular hypertension. JAMA 1977;237:1706–1709.
15. Stanley JC, Gewertz BL, Bove BL, et al. Arterial fibrodysplasia: Histopathologic character and current etiologic concepts. Arch Surg 1975;110:561–566.
16. Harrison EG, McCormack U. Pathological classification of renal artery disease in renovascular hypertension. Mayo Clin Proc 1971;46:161–167.
17. Treadway KK, Slater EE. Renovascular hypertension. Annu Rev Med 1984;35:665–692.
18. Greene ER, et al. Noninvasive characterization of renal artery blood flow. Kidney Int 1981;20:523–529.
19. Kohler TR, Zierler RE, Martin RL, et al. Noninvasive diagnosis of renal artery stenosis by ultrasonic duplex scanning. J Vasc Surg 1986;4:450–456.
20. Taylor DC, Kettler MD, Moneta GL, et al. Duplex ultrasound scanning in the diagnosis of renal artery stenosis: A prospective evaluation. J Vasc Surg 1988;7:363–369.
21. Taylor DC, Moneta GL, Strandness DE Jr. Follow-up renal artery stenosis by duplex ultrasound. J Vasc Surg 1989;9:410–415.
22. Neumyer MM, Wengrovitz M, Ward T, Thiele BL. The differentiation of renal artery stenosis from renal parenchymal disease by duplex ultrasonography. J Vasc Technol 1989;13:205–216.
23. Rittgers SE, Norris CS, Barnes RW. Detection of renal artery stenosis: Experimental and clinical analysis of velocity waveforms. Ultrasound Med Biol 1985;11:523–531.

24. Avasthi PS, Voyles WF, Greene ER. Noninvasive diagnosis of renal artery stenosis by echo-Doppler velocimetry. Kidney Int 1984;25:824–829.

25. Hoffman U, Edwards JM, Carter S, et al. Role of duplex scanning for the detection of atherosclerotic renal artery disease. Kidney Int 1991;39:1232–1239.

26. Moran K, Muihall J, Kelly D, et al. Morphological changes and alterations in regional intrarenal blood flow induced by graded renal ischemia. J Urol 1992;148:1463–1466.

27. Sabbatini M, Sansone G, Uccello F, et al. Functional versus structural changes in the pathophysiology of acute ischemic renal failure in aging rats. Kidney Int 1994;45:1355–1361.

28. Shanley PF. The pathology of chronic renal ischemia. Semin Nephrol 1996;16:21–32.

29. Truong LD, Farhood A, Tasby J, Gillum D. Experimental chronic renal ischemia: Morphologic and immunologic studies. Kidney Int 1992;41:1676–1689.

30. Gob'e GC, Axelsen RA, Searle JW. Cellular events in experimental unilateral ischemic renal atrophy and in regeneration after contralateral nephrectomy. Lab Invest 1990;63:770–779.

31. Caps MT, Zierler RE, Polissar NL, et al. The risk of atrophy in kidneys with atherosclerotic renal artery stenosis. Kidney Int 1998;53:735–742.

32. Hallett JW Jr., Fowl R, O'Brien PC, et al. Renovascular operations in patients with chronic renal insufficiency: Do the benefits justify the risks? J Vasc Surg 1987;5:622–627.

33. Cambria RP, Brewster DC, L'Italien GJ, et al. Renal artery reconstruction for the preservation of renal function. J Vasc Surg 1996;24:371–380.

34. Erdoes LS, Berman SS, Hunter GC, Mills JL. Comparative analysis of percutaneous transluminal angioplasty and operation for renal revascularization. Am J Kidney Dis 1996;27:496–503.

35. Hansen KJ, Thomason RB, Craven TE, et al. Surgical management of dialysis-dependent ischemic nephropathy. J Vasc Surg 1995;21:197–209.

36. Guzman RP, Zierler RE, Isaacson JA, et al. Renal atrophy and renal arterial stenosis: A prospective study with duplex ultrasound. Hypertension 1994;23:346–350.

37. Cotter B, Mahmud E, Kwan OL, DeMaria AN. New ultrasound agents: Expanding upon existing clinical applications. In: Goldberg BB (ed). Ultrasound Contrast Agents, pp. 31–42. St. Louis, MO: Mosby, 1997.

38. Goldberg BB, Liu JB, Forsberg F. Ultrasound contrast agents: A review. Ultrasound Med Biol 1994;20(4):319–333.

39. Robbin ML, Eisenfeld AJ, et al. Perflenapent emulsion: An US contrast agent for diagnostic radiology-multicenter double-blind comparison with a placebo. Radiology 1998; 207:717–722.

40. Kitzman DW, Goldman ME, Gillam LD, Cohen JL, Aurigemma GP, Gottdiener JS. Efficacy and safety of the novel ultrasound contrast agent perflutren (Definity) in patients with suboptimal baseline left ventricular echocardiographic images. Am J Cardiol 2000;86:669–674.

41. Blebea J, Volteas N, Neumyer M, Dawson K, Ingraham J, Assadnia S, et al. Contrast-enhanced duplex ultrasound imaging of the mesenteric arteries. Ann Vasc Surg 2002;16: 77–83.

42. Blebea J, Zickler R, Volteas N, Neumyer M, Assadnia S, Anderson K, Atnip R. Duplex imaging of the renal arteries with contrast enhancement. Vasc Endovasc Surg 2003;37: 429–436.

43. Weissman NJ, Cohen MC, Hack TC, Gillam LD, Cohen JL, Kitzman DW. Infusion versus bolus contrast echocardiography: A multicenter, open-label, crossover trial. Am Heart J 2000;139:399–404.

44. Forsberg F, Liu JB, Burns PN, et al. Artifacts in ultrasonic contrast agent studies. J Ultrasound Med 1994;13:357–365.

45. Neumyer MM. Duplex scanning after renal artery stenting. J Vasc Technol 2003;27(3):177–183.

46. Handa N, Fukunaga R, Etani H, et al. Efficacy of echo-Doppler examination for the evaluation of renovascular disease. Ultrasound Med Biol 1988;14:1–5.

47. Martin RL, Nanra RS, Wlodarczyk J. Renal hilar Doppler analysis in the detection of renal artery stenosis. J Vasc Technol 1991;15(4):173–180.

48. Stavros TA, Parker SH, Yakes YF, et al. Segmental stenosis of the renal artery: Pattern recognition of the tardus and parvus abnormalities with duplex sonography. Radiology 1992;184:487–492.

49. Radermacher J, Chavan A, Bleck J, Vitzhum A, Stoess B, et al. Use of Doppler ultrasonography to predict the outcome of therapy for renal-artery stenosis. N Engl J Med 2001;344(6):410–417.

50. Tullis MJ, Zierler RE, Caps MT, Bergelin RO, Cantwell-Gab K, Strandness DE Jr. Clinical evidence of contralateral renal parenchymal injury in patients with unilateral atherosclerotic renal artery stenosis. Ann Vasc Surg 1998;12(2): 122–127.

43
Duplex Ultrasonography of the Mesenteric Circulation

David G. Neschis and William R. Flinn

Arterial occlusive disease of the celiac and superior mesenteric arteries is rare and patients with symptomatic mesenteric ischemia are encountered infrequently. However, the clinical manifestations of mesenteric arterial occlusive lesions remain enigmatic and range from asymptomatic to catastrophic. Acute occlusions of the celiac artery (CA) and the superior mesenteric artery (SMA) due to thrombosis or embolism can produce extensive, irreversible gut ischemia requiring emergency treatment, and the mortality from these events remains among the highest of all vascular emergencies. The true incidence of chronic atherosclerotic occlusive disease of the main mesenteric vessels is not well established, the precise relationship to symptoms is poorly understood, and the rate of disease progression is undocumented. It is well accepted that severe, multivessel disease may initially produce nonspecific symptoms such as pain after eating ("abdominal angina") and weight loss—symptoms that are often mistaken for more common gastrointestinal disorders such as peptic ulcer, gallstone disease, or an occult malignancy. Early diagnosis and treatment of chronic mesenteric ischemia may be of critical importance since progression to thrombosis with gut infarction is fatal in over 50% of the cases when it occurs. However, the nonspecific clinical manifestations of chronic mesenteric ischemia have led to a delay in diagnosis in most patients since arteriography was required in the past for detection of occlusions of the mesenteric vessels. As duplex ultrasound scanning was applied to an increasing number of peripheral and visceral arterial disorders, it was evident that this technique could be adapted to examine the main mesenteric vessels. In this way, mesenteric duplex scanning might serve as an "entry level" noninvasive diagnostic test for the very small number of patients actually suspected of having mesenteric ischemia. In others it might be used to investigate more thoroughly the significance of mesenteric occlusive lesions found by arteriography performed for unrelated reasons. Finally, it could be useful for follow-up of those patients who have undergone visceral revascularization procedures.

Some deep abdominal duplex scanning, including renal and mesenteric arteries,[1,2] the vena cava,[3] and the portal venous system,[4–6] is now performed in most vascular laboratories or ultrasound departments. However, the low prevalence of mesenteric arterial occlusive disease has resulted in fewer patients to examine routinely compared with other disorders such as carotid artery disease or even renovascular disease. Deep abdominal ultrasonography remains one of the most challenging applications of noninvasive testing due to variations in body habitus and fat distribution, the presence of respiratory motion, and the depth and the variable anatomy of the major abdominal vessels. Even normal mesenteric anatomy is complex with the major vessels and their branches running in a spatially unpredictable fashion. The mesenteric arterial anatomy may become even more variable when large collateral vessels have developed in the presence of occlusive lesions. Duplex scan evaluation of visceral vessels may also be obscured by bowel gas found in normal patients or those with gastrointestinal disorders.

Atherosclerotic lesions of the visceral vessels usually occur at or near the origins of the CA and SMA ("ostial lesions") from the abdominal aorta (Figure 43–1), which is the most predictable part of the mesenteric anatomy even when more distal branchings are complex. Most clinically important lesions will be identified by examination of the origins of the CA and SMA, and scanning of the proximal 2–4cm of these vessels. It is generally felt that significant clinical symptoms and/or the risk of gut infarction exist only when there is severe stenosis or occlusion of at least two main mesenteric vessels. Arteriography is still required to determine the need for treatment and the best therapeutic options, but mesenteric duplex scanning may be useful to select those patients who would benefit most from arteriographic study. Thus, one clinical use of mesenteric

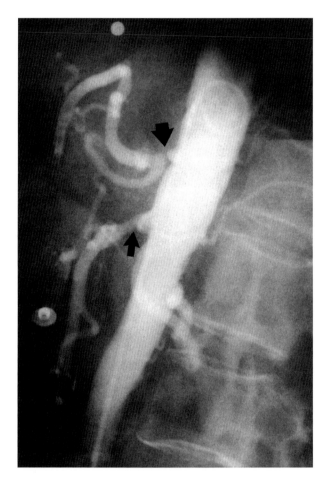

FIGURE 43–1. Lateral view demonstrating the typical ostial location of most atherosclerotic lesions in the main mesenteric vessels. There is a severe stenosis of both the celiac (larger arrow) and superior mesenteric arteries (smaller arrow) near their origins from the aorta.

a problem. In patients with a more acute problem, the ileus produced by any intraabdominal inflammatory processes (e.g., acute mesenteric ischemia, cholecystitis, pancreatitis, diverticulitis) greatly limits the usefulness of mesenteric scanning. When a technically adequate examination can be performed it may be useful in directing further diagnostic evaluation, but in emergent cases where mesenteric ischemia is suspected, arteriography should be performed without delay.

Mesenteric duplex scanning is performed with the patient supine and the head slightly elevated. Low-frequency, dedicated abdominal probes are used for mesenteric, renal, hepatoportal, and vena caval scanning. An anterior–posterior midline approach is used to obtain a sagittal scan of the aorta. The origins of the CA and SMA are usually visualized as they course ventrally from the aorta (Figure 43–2) above the level where the left renal vein crosses the aorta. Most atherosclerotic occlusive lesions in the CA and SMA are at or near the origins of the vessels from the aorta, so insonation of the first few centimeters of each vessel is usually adequate for diagnosis. The inferior mesenteric artery (IMA) originates from the left side of the infrarenal aorta a few centimeters above the aortic bifurcation.

Pulsed Doppler examination is performed using a 1.5–2.0 mm sample volume. Peak systolic velocity (PSV), end-diastolic velocity (EDV), waveform configuration, and direction of flow are recorded. Doppler angles of

duplex scanning would be the identification of normal vessels or those with mild to moderate atherosclerosis where arteriography could be avoided, and another would be to identify accurately severe occlusive disease of the CA and SMA where mesenteric arteriography would determine the subsequent clinical management of the patient.

Mesenteric Duplex Scanning: Technique

As with all deep abdominal duplex scans, intestinal gas will compromise the technical success of a mesenteric examination. An overnight fast is adequate preparation for most elective cases, but simethicone-containing compounds may be useful in cases where bowel gas remains

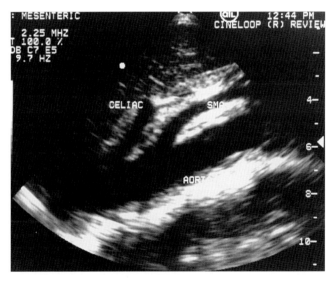

FIGURE 43–2. Sagittal scan of the aorta in a normal patient is similar to the lateral aortogram and demonstrates the origins and proximal portions of the celiac trunk and the superior mesenteric artery. Pulsed Doppler sampling is performed in the proximal portions of these vessels where most occlusive disease occurs. SMA, superior mesenteric artery.

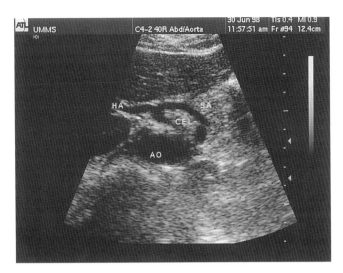

FIGURE 43–3. Doppler spectral analysis in the celiac trunk (CEL) may be challenging due to changes in the angle of insonation produced by its branching into the splenic artery (SA) and the common hepatic artery (HA). These sudden changes in the direction of flow in the celiac branches can produce falsely elevated flow velocities unless the angle of insonation is carefully controlled at 60°. A, aorta.

artery" may originate from the SMA in up to 20% of normal cases. Some patients may even have a common trunk origin of both the CA and SMA. The variable collateral patterns that are present in cases of occlusion of a single main mesenteric artery may be even more confusing. Large gastroduodenal or pancreaticoduodenal branches may serve as collateral communication between the CA and SMA and these may be difficult to interpret by an inexperienced examiner.

The IMA has not been routinely studied but may be identified by scanning down the infrarenal aorta toward the bifurcation where it is generally the only vessel originating from the left side of the aorta. Isolated stenosis or occlusion of the IMA is rare but it may play a major role in the visceral collateral circulation. The presence of a markedly enlarged and thereby easily identifiable IMA may suggest significant occlusive disease of the SMA with the IMA serving as the collateral (Figure 43–4). However, many patients with mesenteric arterial disease have associated aortoiliac occlusions. Here the IMA may be occluded, but large lumbar collaterals may be

insonation of 60° must be employed when sweeping through the vessels. Rizzo et al.[7] observed that pulsed-Doppler arterial flow velocities from the mesenteric vessels should be measured at angles of insonation less than 60° or falsely elevated PSVs will be recorded even in normal vessels. The anatomy of the vessels often produces sudden changes in vessel direction and it is incumbent upon the technologists to be as certain as possible about the location and angle of the sample.

Accurate examination of the celiac trunk may be challenging. The celiac trunk is rarely longer than 1–2 cm and the anatomy of its branches (common hepatic, splenic, and left gastric) may be extremely variable. The left gastric artery is rarely identified by duplex scan and routine examination includes the celiac, hepatic, and splenic arteries. While flow in the origin of the CA roughly parallels that in the SMA ventral from the aorta, the branching of the celiac trunk results in rapid changes in the direction of arterial flow at almost 90° to the right (hepatic) and left (splenic) of the main celiac trunk. These anatomic relationships can be appreciated with a transverse B-mode scan of the CA, which has been termed the "rabbit-ear" or "seagull" appearance (Figure 43–3).

Identification and pulsed Doppler spectral analysis are easier in the SMA than in the celiac trunk. There are generally no major branches of the SMA visualized on routine examination. However, a "replaced right hepatic

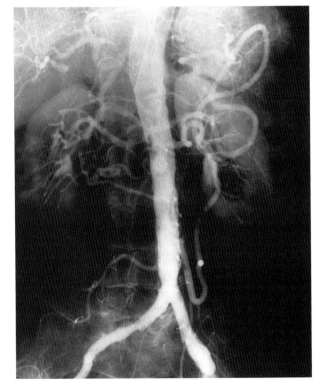

FIGURE 43–4. Aortogram demonstrating a dramatically enlarged inferior mesenteric artery (IMA) originating from the left side of the infrarenal aorta several centimeters above the aortic bifurcation. Retrograde flow through the "meandering mesenteric" collateral is demonstrated in this patient with an SMA occlusion.

mistaken for the IMA on duplex scanning. Another potential source of error in an attempt to scan the IMA is the presence of an accessory lower pole left renal artery that would also originate from the left side of the infrarenal aorta. Overall, in most cases it is sufficient to focus the examination on occlusive lesions at the origins of the CA and SMA, since this is the area of involvement in most clinically relevant disease.

Color Doppler scanning allows more rapid identification of the origins of the CA and SMA from the abdominal aorta and will reduce the time required for an examination. Color-flow scanning may help visually identify focal areas of flow disturbance that require further interrogation, or help in detecting the absence of flow in one or both of the major mesenteric vessels suggesting occlusion. It is important to remember, however, that color assignment is based almost entirely upon direction of flow. The anatomic variations discussed above make it evident that beyond the origins of these vessels, sudden changes in flow direction can produce confusing color-flow patterns even in normal subjects.

Reliable, broadly accepted diagnostic Doppler frequency, or flow velocity parameters have not been developed for the mesenteric circulation as they have been in most other systems (carotid, renal, bypass grafts, etc.). Most reports of visceral arterial duplex scanning emphasize the determination of PSV and EDV, and the presence or absence of early diastolic reversal of flow. Similar to carotid scanning, significant stenoses are most often identified by a focal increase in systolic and diastolic velocities, and occlusions are identified by the absence of flow, or flow reversal. Unlike renal artery duplex scanning, no improvement in diagnostic accuracy has been observed by normalizing visceral arterial velocity measurements to those in the aorta through the calculation of flow velocity ratios.[8,9] Some investigators have reported quantitative blood flow (milliliters/minute) measurements using Doppler-derived velocity information in either the portal venous system,[10,11] or in the mesenteric arterial circulation.[12-15] Although there is considerable research interest in volumetric flow data this estimation is subject to significant error,[16-18] and most diagnostic laboratories do not perform such measurements. The presence of elevated PSV and localized turbulence appears to correlate better with angiographically demonstrated arterial lesions in both the peripheral and the central circulation.

Normal Findings

Mesenteric arterial velocity waveforms have certain specific characteristics. At rest blood flow in a normal SMA has a higher resistance Doppler velocity pattern

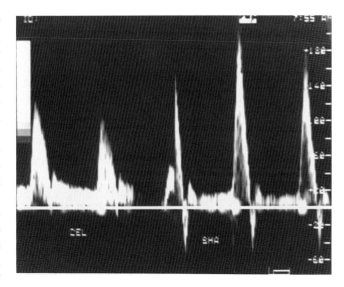

FIGURE 43–5. The normal fasting SMA waveform (right spectra) is recognizably different from celiac artery (CEL, left). The triphasic pattern of the normal SMA is reminiscent of that found in higher resistance peripheral arteries.

with early diastolic flow reversal in most cases, and late diastolic forward flow (triphasic waveform; Figure 43–5). Blood flow in the CA, as in the renal arteries, has a low- resistance Doppler velocity pattern with continuous forward flow during the entire cardiac cycle (Figure 43–6). Spectral waveforms recorded from normal IMA are similar to those from the SMA with a higher resistance pattern with early diastolic flow reversal.

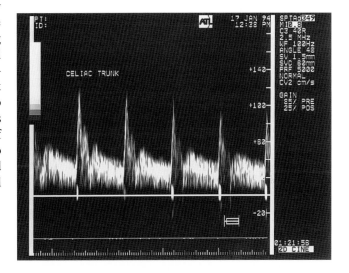

FIGURE 43–6. Velocity spectrum from a normal celiac artery demonstrating continuous forward flow throughout systole and diastole.

Clinical Applications

Physiologic Measurements

Duplex scanning of the mesenteric vessels in normal individuals has been used successfully to characterize the physiologic changes that occur in the visceral circulation after eating. The most reproducible changes occur in the SMA, where significant increases in PSV are seen up to an hour after eating.[19] Also, the SMA flow waveform shifts to a low-resistance pattern characterized by forward flow throughout the cardiac cycle with loss of the early diastolic flow reversal. The composition of the meal, including volume, energy content, and nutritional composition, may influence the observed changes in mesenteric flow velocities after a meal.[1,4,15,20] Fat and carbohydrates appear to be the nutritional components of the meal that produce the most significant postprandial increases in measured PSV.[15]

Duplex scanning has also been used to demonstrate the effects of drugs on intestinal blood flow. Several investigators have demonstrated changes in mesenteric arterial flow following the infusion of splanchnic vasodilators such as glucagon and secretin, and vasoconstrictors such as vasopressin.[19,21] Lilly et al.[19] observed that the changes in superior mesenteric arterial flow following glucagon infusion closely paralleled those observed after a meal.

Visceral Aneurysms

Aneurysms of the mesenteric vessels are extremely rare and the clinical usefulness of duplex scanning for the detection of mesenteric aneurysms remains anecdotal. Ultrasonographic diagnosis of aneurysms of the superior mesenteric,[22–24] hepatic,[25,26] splenic,[27,28] gastroduodenal,[29] middle colic,[30] and pancreaticoduodenal[31] arteries has been reported, but in these cases scanning was often performed due to uncertain gastrointestinal or abdominal complaints. However, duplex scanning may be useful in such cases to select patients for a more thorough, focused vascular examination with computed tomography (CT), magnetic resonance imaging (MRI), or arteriography. Color-flow duplex ultrasonography may be useful for differentiating saccular false aneurysms of the superior mesenteric and splenic artery from other more benign, nonvascular fluid collections in the setting of pancreatitis or other retroperitoneal inflammatory conditions. However, as noted above, an associated ileus with excessive bowel gas may preclude a diagnostic study.

Celiac Artery Compression Syndrome (Median Arcuate Ligament Syndrome)

A focal increase in flow velocities identified at the origin of the celiac artery may be due to extrinsic compression

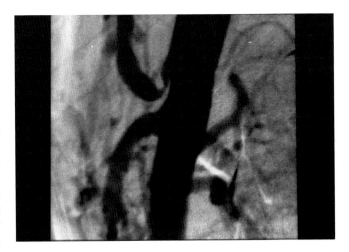

FIGURE 43–7. Characteristic arteriographic appearance of proximal celiac artery stenosis due to compression by the median arcuate ligament of the diaphragm. Note there is no evidence of atherosclerosis in the aorta or the SMA. Deep inspiration in this case produced a normalization of both duplex scan findings and the arteriogram.

of the CA by the median arcuate ligament of the diaphragm, particularly when this finding is detected in a younger individual. Celiac artery compression syndrome has been reported to produce gastrointestinal symptoms in some patients, but most clinicians regard this as a benign condition with little or no risk of intestinal infarction. In fact, duplex scanning of these lesions is more likely to be performed to evaluate the finding of the celiac stenosis on an arteriogram performed for other reasons (Figure 43–7). This "lesion" is usually associated with a normal arterial wall and normal aorta with no evidence of atherosclerotic plaque. Scanning during deep inspiration with breath holding produces a relaxation of the diaphragmatic crus and often results in a return of normal celiac velocities, which confirms the diagnosis.

Visceral Ischemic Syndromes

The use of duplex ultrasonography as a screening test to detect major mesenteric arterial occlusive disease in patients suspected of having chronic intestinal ischemia has attracted interest among clinicians, since the diagnosis of mesenteric occlusive disease in the past required arteriography. Jäger et al.[32] first reported abnormal pulsed Doppler waveforms with increased PSVs and marked spectral broadening in both the CA and SMA of a patient with severe atherosclerotic stenosis in both vessels and symptoms of chronic visceral ischemia. Others[33,34] have used similar criteria of distorted Doppler flow patterns or absence of detectable flow to document high-grade stenosis or occlusion of the intestinal arteries. Moneta et al.[35] reported ultrasound visualization of an enlarged

IMA in several patients with high-grade stenosis or occlusion of the celiac and superior mesenteric vessels where that vessel had become the major collateral supply to the bowel.

Standardized velocity criteria for duplex scan diagnosis of hemodynamically significant lesions of the mesenteric arteries (similar to those used in the diagnosis of extracranial carotid artery disease) have not been thoroughly refined. Considering the low prevalence of mesenteric disease compared to carotid disease and the small number of arteriograms available for comparison, it would appear unlikely that such discrete diagnostic criteria would be forthcoming soon. Nevertheless, several studies can provide general ranges for diagnosis that will be clinically useful for the practitioner. Moneta et al.[9] compared the results of mesenteric duplex scanning to arteriography in 34 patients with known atherosclerosis. This group included patients with suspected visceral ischemia as well as others requiring routine arteriography for lower extremity ischemic symptoms. An analysis of their accumulated data revealed that PSVs above 275 cm/s in the SMA (normal = 125–163 cm/s) could predict a severe SMA stenosis (>70%) with a sensitivity and specificity of 89% and 92%, respectively. A similar diagnostic accuracy was observed by these investigators when PSVs exceeded 200 cm/s in the CA. Total occlusions of the CA and SMA were also accurately diagnosed by duplex scan in this report. This initial retrospective study failed to demonstrate the usefulness of a "mesenteric:aortic" systolic velocity ratio to predict the presence of a severe stenosis in the celiac artery or SMA as has been observed in duplex scanning of the renal arteries. In a subsequent report[36] these investigators prospectively evaluated these diagnostic criteria in 100 patients having arteriograms and demonstrated that mesenteric duplex scanning was indeed sufficiently accurate to be clinically useful as a screening examination in cases with suspected CA or SMA occlusive disease (Figure 43–8).

The usefulness of mesenteric duplex scanning for the diagnosis of significant CA and SMA lesions was confirmed in the report of Bowersox et al.[37] that compared mesenteric duplex scanning with arteriograms in 25 patients, most of whom were suspected of having visceral ischemia. These investigators observed that a >50% stenosis of the SMA could be best predicted by duplex scan measurement of a fasting PSV >300 cm/s or an EDV of >45 cm/s. They were unable to establish reliable duplex scan velocity criteria for CA stenosis. They observed that the anatomy of the CA compromised precise insonation as noted previously in this chapter. Considering the small sample size and the fact that most patients were symptomatic, it is possible that anatomic and collateral variants would account for the observed compromise. Further emphasizing the difficulties encountered in an attempt to

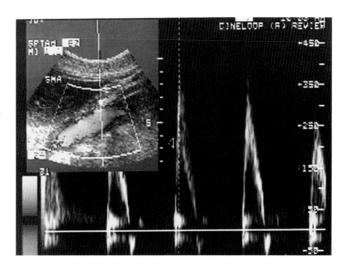

FIGURE 43–8. Duplex scan of the proximal superior mesenteric artery (SMA) reveals a markedly elevated peak systolic velocity >350 cm/s. This suggests the presence of a >70% SMA stenosis.

define precise duplex ultrasound diagnostic criteria for mesenteric occlusive lesions, Healy et al.[38] were unable to identify any definitive velocity criteria for detection of CA or SMA stenoses.

These observations generally serve to reinforce the continued need for prospective studies with arteriographic correlation. However, as noted above, cases available for study are seen infrequently. Nevertheless the general principles of duplex scan detection of a "critical" stenosis or occlusion in any arterial system apply in the mesenteric vessels: (1) a focal marked elevation in PSV, particularly associated with elevated EDV, (2) poststenotic turbulence with reduced flow velocities beyond the stenosis, and (3) absent flow in an anatomically well-defined arterial segment, particularly with flow reversal beyond the lesion (suggestive of occlusion). The key to success in the mesenteric circulation relies not so much upon precise velocity criteria, but in accurate anatomic identification of the vessels and control of the technologic variables for Doppler examination.

Perioperative Applications

Intraoperative Applications

As with all vascular reconstructions, early technical success is essential in the outcome of mesenteric revascularization. Due to the intraabdominal location of the bypass, early graft failure may not be readily apparent. Abdominal pain is an unreliable symptom following laparotomy and if the patient goes on to gut infarction the outcome is almost uniformly fatal. It is clear then that intraoperative assessment of the technical conduct of mesenteric revascularization procedures is an important clinical component of these procedures. The portability of modern ultrasound equipment and increasing surgeon familiarity with these techniques have led to an increase in the use of duplex ultrasound scanning to assess technical success following renal and mesenteric revascularization procedures. Oderich and colleagues evaluated the use of intraoperative duplex scanning in 68 patients undergoing operative visceral revascularization.[39] Patients who were identified as having an abnormal intraoperative mesenteric duplex examination had a higher incidence of early graft thrombosis, reintervention, and higher perioperative mortality. It was concluded that the duplex scan evaluation helped optimize early technical success of mesenteric revascularization procedures.

Postoperative Applications

Revascularization of symptomatic mesenteric arterial occlusions is optimal management, but in the past the patency of these reconstructions, like initial diagnosis, could be determined only by arteriography. Sandager et al.[40] first reported the use of duplex ultrasonography to evaluate the patency of visceral arterial reconstructions. Duplex scanning successfully documented graft function in six of seven visceral bypass grafts and findings were correlated with standard arteriography. McMillan et al.[41] reported successful duplex scan follow-up of mesenteric bypass procedures in 30 cases. Duplex scanning can provide accurate noninvasive documentation of the patency of visceral revascularization procedures without requiring arteriography (Figure 43–9). The role of prospective surveillance of these grafts is unknown at present. However, increased experience with postoperative duplex scanning of mesenteric bypass grafts will allow a more accurate documentation of late patency for these procedures, an aspect that has been incompletely studied in the past due to the requirement for repeated invasive contrast studies.

Endovascular Intervention

Endovascular interventions including balloon angioplasty and stenting have been performed routinely in the renal arteries, and these techniques have also proven to be effective for treatment of mesenteric arterial occlusive lesions (Figure 43–10). Steinmetz and colleagues reported their experience in 19 patients with chronic mesenteric ischemia treated by balloon angioplasty or stenting.[42] The authors reported a 100% technical success rate although in 7 of the 19 cases only one of the two vessels intended for treatment was successfully treated. In seven cases stenting was required due to recoil or residual stenosis. Patients having angioplasty and/or stenting in this series were followed up with duplex ultrasound for a mean of 31 months. The primary patency was 75% and long-term pain relief noted in 85% of patients for whom follow-up was available. Three patients developed symptomatic restenosis and were treated with redo angioplasty with resolution of pain. Two other patients were found to have asymptomatic restenosis and were followed conservatively.[42] AbuRahma and colleagues report on 22 patients with 24 symptomatic mesenteric arterial lesions treated with balloon angioplasty/stenting over a 4.5-year period.[43] In this series the initial technical success as defined, per vessel, as residual stenosis <30%

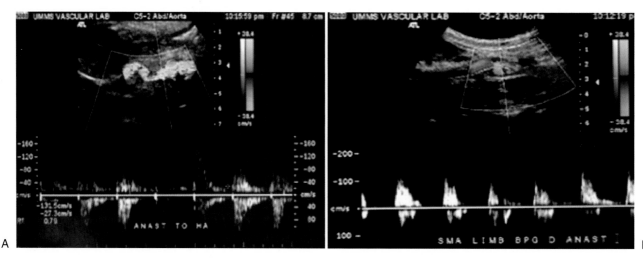

FIGURE 43–9. Duplex scan demonstrating patency of a bifurcated arterial bypass graft with one limb to the hepatic artery (A) and one limb to the SMA (B).

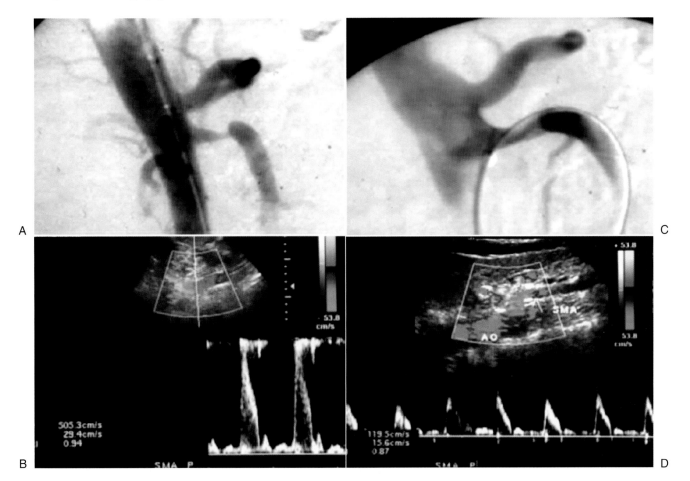

FIGURE 43–10. (A) Aortogram depicting high-grade stenosis in the proximal SMA. (B) Corresponding duplex image demonstrating significantly elevated peak systolic velocities of 505 cm/s at the level of the stenosis. (C) Angiogram post-percutaneous angioplasty and stenting demonstrating resolution of the SMA stenosis. (D) Corresponding duplex image demonstrating a patent stent (arrow) and reduction of peak systolic velocities to normal (120 cm/s).

and pressure gradient <10 mm Hg was 96%. Over a mean follow-up period of 26 months the primary late clinical success rate was 61% with a freedom from restenosis (= 70%), as documented by objective duplex examination, of 30%. Freedom from recurrent symptoms was 67%. Four-year survival rate in these patients was 53%.[43]

Duplex ultrasound has been used to evaluate patency following endovascular revascularization of mesenteric arteries (Figure 43–10). Excellent correlation has been found between a significant decrease in PSV following angioplasty/stenting and a favorable clinical response.[44] PSV following these endovascular treatments may occasionally remain in the abnormal range (>275 cm/s),[44] although the PSV will be significantly lower than pre-procedure levels. Sharafuddin and colleagues suggest scanning the SMA beyond the stent, and performing the study in a strictly fasting state to reduce artifactual increases in PSV observed in the SMA.[44]

Acute Mesenteric Ischemia

Acute mesenteric ischemia is usually produced by mesenteric embolism or mesenteric thrombosis. It would be ideal to provide direct duplex scan identification of discrete mesenteric arterial occlusions in these cases, particularly since the approach to treatment may be different. If patients with acute major mesenteric arterial occlusions were examined very early in the clinical course of these problems, duplex scanning might provide an accurate assessment. However, diagnosis is often delayed in these patients and the associated ileus that rapidly develops renders the scan almost useless. Takahashi et al.[45] reported dramatically reduced portal venous flow by duplex ultrasonography in one patient with acute mesenteric infarction. Reduced portal vein flow is an indirect reflection of severely reduced mesenteric arterial blood flow and its lack of specificity would be of limited clinical usefulness in the majority of cases. Prompt arteriography is the diagnostic examination of choice in such cases since excessive delay in the diagnosis can lead to irreversible intestinal infarction.

Image Enhancement

Unlike vessels in the neck or extremities, the ability to image the mesenteric vessels can often be difficult due to patient body habitus or bowel gas. The low-frequency transducer needed to image at the appropriate depth is hampered by poorer B-mode image resolution. This leads to less accurate placement of the Doppler sample volume. Investigational substances are being developed and studied to assist in enhancing ultrasound imaging of blood vessels. The ideal ultrasound contrast agent would have the appropriate density and acoustic properties to strongly reflect transmitted ultrasound waves. Additionally, the contrast agent would be physiologically inert, small enough to easily pass through capillaries, and persist in the vasculature long enough to complete the study. Perflutren (Definity, Dupont Pharmaceuticals Co.) is one such agent. It can be agitated, injected into a bag of sterile saline solution, and infused intravenously. Blebea et al. studied perflutren in 17 patients to examine its potential usefulness in evaluating the mesenteric arteries.[46] They concluded that the contrast material appeared to be safe, but that it is not routinely required and did not significantly improve the accuracy of standard duplex imaging. However, the use of contrast material may be helpful when visualization is difficult with standard techniques due to patient obesity or excessive abdominal gas.

Population Screening

Although duplex ultrasonography has gained acceptance as a first-line screening test for patients with suspected chronic intestinal ischemia,[47] the incidence of mesenteric arterial stenosis in the general population has not been well studied. Hansen and colleagues studied over 550 elderly volunteers in an effort to estimate the population-based prevalence of mesenteric artery stenosis in elderly Americans.[48] Using criteria of celiac PSV >200cm/s and SMA PSV >270cm/s, or occlusion of either vessel, it was determined that 17.5% of the individuals studied had either a significant celiac or SMA stenosis or occlusion. The majority (10.5%) has isolated celiac stenosis: 1.3% had combined SMA and celiac stenosis, 0.9% had isolated SMA stenosis, and 0.4% had celiac occlusion. When all patients with mesenteric arterial stenosis were considered, there was no association with symptoms of weight loss. It was noted, however, that the combination of celiac occlusion and SMA stenosis was significantly associated with weight loss and concurrent renal artery disease.

Conclusions

Mesenteric duplex scanning can become a routine non-invasive diagnostic testing modality for the evaluation of patients with suspected visceral ischemia since earlier diagnosis and treatment will significantly reduce the risk of catastrophic gut infarction in these patients. Like all deep abdominal duplex scanning, mesenteric scanning is more technologically demanding than scanning vessels of the neck or extremities. However, continued refinement of the duplex instrumentation makes these examinations exciting areas of clinical advancement since there have previously been no other reliable noninvasive techniques for assessment of major intraabdominal vessels. Like other duplex scan applications, mesenteric duplex scanning can be used to ensure the technical efficacy of mesenteric revascularization procedures, whether surgical or endovascular. Mesenteric duplex scanning can then provide a means of late follow-up assessment of these procedures to document their durability or to prevent late procedural failure.

References

1. Flinn WR, Sandager GP, Lilly MP, et al.: Duplex scan of mesenteric and celiac arteries. In: Bergan JJ, Yao JST (eds). *Arterial Surgery: New Diagnostic and Operative Techniques*. Orlando: Grune & Stratton, 1988.
2. Blackburn DR. Color duplex imaging of the mesenteric and renal arteries. J Vasc Technol 1991;15:139.
3. Sandager GP, Zimmer S, Silva MB, Flinn WR. Ultrasonographic characteristics of transvenous vena caval interruption devices. J Vasc Technol 1992;16:17–21.
4. Ackroyd N, Gill R, Griffiths K, et al. Duplex scanning of the portal vein and portasystemic shunts. Surgery 1986;90:591.
5. Ralls PW. Color Doppler sonography of the hepatic artery and portal venous system. AJR 1990;155:517.
6. Grant EG, Tessler FN, Gomes AS, et al. Color Doppler imaging of portosystemic shunts. AJR 1990;154:393.
7. Rizzo RJ, Sandager G, Astleford P, et al. Mesenteric flow velocity variations as a function of angle of insonation. J Vasc Surg 1990;11:688.
8. Healy DA, Neumeyer MM, Atnip RG, Thiele BL. Evaluation of mesenteric vascular disease with duplex ultrasound. Circulation 1990;82(Suppl. III):III-460.
9. Moneta GL, Yeager RA, Dalman R, et al. Duplex ultrasound criteria for diagnosis of splanchnic artery stenosis or occlusion. J Vasc Surg 1991;14:511–520.
10. Moriyasu F, Ban N, Nishida O, et al. Clinical application of an ultrasonic duplex system in the quantitative measurement of portal blood flow. J Clin Ultrasound 1986;14:579.
11. Sato S, Ohnishi K, Sugita S, Okuda K. Splenic artery and superior mesenteric artery blood flow: Nonsurgical

Doppler US measurement in healthy subjects and patients with chronic liver disease. Radiology 1987;164:347.

12. Qamar MI, Read AE, Skidmore R, *et al.* Transcutaneous Doppler ultrasound measurement of coeliac axis blood flow in man. Br J Surg 1985;72:391.

13. Qamar MI, Read AE, Mountford R. Increased superior mesenteric artery blood flow after glucose but not lactulose ingestion. Q J Med 1986;233:893.

14. Jäger K, Bollinger A, Vallie C, Ammann R. Measurement of mesenteric blood flow by duplex scanning. J Vasc Surg 1986;3:462.

15. Moneta GL, Taylor DC, Helton WS, *et al.* Duplex ultrasound measurement of postprandial intestinal blood flow: Effect of meal composition. Gastroenterology 1988; 95:1294.

16. Gill RW. Measurement of blood flow by ultrasound: Accuracy and sources of error. Ultrasound Med Biol 1985; 11:625.

17. Hoskins PR. Measurement of arterial blood flow by Doppler ultrasound. Clin Phys Physiol Meas 1990;11:1.

18. Taylor GA. Blood flow in the superior mesenteric artery: Estimation with Doppler US. Radiology 1990;174:15.

19. Lilly MP, Harward TRS, Flinn WR, *et al.* Duplex ultrasound measurement of changes in mesenteric flow velocity with pharmacologic and physiologic alteration of intestinal blood flow in man. J Vasc Surg 1989;9:18.

20. Flinn WR, Rizzo RJ, Park JS, Sandager GP. Duplex scanning for assessment of mesenteric ischemia. Surg Clin North Am 1990;70:99.

21. Nishida O, Moriyasu F, Nakamura T, *et al.* Relationship between splenic and superior mesenteric venous circulation. Gastroenterology 1990;98:721.

22. Gooding GAW. Ultrasound of a superior mesenteric artery aneurysm secondary to pancreatitis: A plea for real-time ultrasound of sonolucent masses in pancreatitis. J Clin Ultrasound 1981;9:255.

23. Bret PM, Bretagnolle M, Enoch G, *et al.* Ultrasonic features of aneurysms of splanchnic arteries. J Can Assoc Radiol 1985;36:226.

24. Mourad K, Guggiana P, Minasian H. Superior mesenteric artery aneurysm diagnosed by ultrasound. Br J Radiol 1987;60:287.

25. Paolella L, Scola FH, Cronan JJ. Hepatic artery aneurysm: An ultrasound diagnosis. J Clin Ultrasound 1985;13:360.

26. Stokland E, Wihed A, Ceder S, *et al.* Ultrasonic diagnosis of an aneurysm of the common hepatic artery. J Clin Ultrasound 1985;13:369.

27. Bolondi L, Casanova P, Arienti V, *et al.* A case of aneurysm of the splenic artery visualized by dynamic ultrasonography. Br J Radiol 1981;54:1109.

28. Derchi LE, Biggi E, Cicio GR. Aneurysms of the splenic artery: Noninvasive diagnosis by pulsed Doppler sonography. J Ultrasound Med 1984;3:41.

29. Green D, Carroll BA. Aneurysm of the gastroduodenal artery causing biliary obstruction: Real-time ultrasound diagnosis. J Ultrasound Med 1984;3:375.

30. Verma BS, Bose AK, Bhatia HC, Katoch R. Superior mesenteric artery branch aneurysm diagnosed by ultrasound. Br J Radiol 1991;64:169.

31. Grech P, Rowlands P, Crofton M. Aneurysm of the inferior pancreaticoduodenal artery diagnosed by real-time ultrasound and pulsed Doppler. Br J Radiol 1989;62: 753.

32. Jäger KA, Fortner GS, Thiele BL, Strandness DE. Noninvasive diagnosis of intestinal angina. J Clin Ultrasound 1984;12.

33. Nicholls SC, Kohler TR, Martin RL, Strandness ED Jr. Use of hemodynamic parameters in the diagnosis of mesenteric insufficiency. J Vasc Surg 1986;3:507.

34. Hartnell GG, Gibson RN. Doppler ultrasound in the diagnosis of intestinal ischemia. Gastrointest Radiol 1987; 12:285.

35. Moneta GL, Cummings C, Caston J, Porter JM. Duplex ultrasound demonstration of postprandial mesenteric hyperemia in splanchnic circulation collateral vessels. J Vasc Technol 1991;15:37.

36. Moneta GL, Lee RW, Yeager RA, *et al.* Mesenteric duplex scanning: A blinded prospective study. J Vasc Surg 1993;17:79–86.

37. Bowersox JC, Zwolak RM, Walsh DB, *et al.* Duplex ultrasonography in the diagnosis of celiac and mesenteric artery occlusive disease. J Vasc Surg 1991;14:780–788.

38. Healy DA, Neumyer MM, Atnip RG, Thiele, BL. Evaluation of celiac and mesenteric vascular disease with duplex ultrasonography. J Ultrasound Med 1992;11:481–485.

39. Oderich GS, Panneton JM, Macedo TA, *et al.* Intraoperative duplex ultrasound of visceral revascularizations: Optimizing technical success and outcome. J Vasc Surg 2003;38:684–691.

40. Sandager G, Flinn WR, McCarthy WJ, *et al.* Assessment of visceral arterial reconstruction using duplex scan. J Vasc Technol 1987;11:13.

41. McMillan WD, McCarthy WJ, Bresticker MR, *et al.* Mesenteric artery bypass: Objective patency determination. J Vasc Surg 1995;21:729–741.

42. Steinmetz E, Tatou E, Favier-Blavoux C, *et al.* Endovascular treatment as first choice in chronic intestinal ischemia. Ann Vasc Surg 2002;16:693–699.

43. AbuRahma AF, Stone PA, Bates MC, *et al.* Angioplasty/stenting of the superior mesenteric artery and celiac trunk: Early and late outcomes. J Endovasc Ther 2003;10:1046–1053.

44. Sharafuddin MJ, Olson CH, Sun S, *et al.* Endovascular treatment of celiac and mesenteric arteries stenosis: Applications and results. J Vasc Surg 2003;38:692–698.

45. Takahashi H, Takezawa J, Okada T, *et al.* Portal blood flow measured by duplex scanning during mesenteric infarction. Crit Care Med 1986;14:253.

46. Blebea J, Volteas N, Neumyer M, *et al.* Contrast enhanced duplex ultrasound imaging of the mesenteric arteries. Ann Vasc Surg 2002;16:77–83.

47. Moneta GL. Screening for mesenteric vascular insufficiency and follow-up of mesenteric artery bypass procedures. Semin Vasc Surg 2001;14:186–192.

48. Hansen KJ, Wilson DB, Craven TE. Mesenteric disease in the elderly. J Vasc Surg 2004;40:45–52.

44

The Role of Color Duplex Ultrasound in Patients with Abdominal Aortic Aneurysms and Stent Grafts

George H. Meier and Kathleen A. Carter

Although ultrasound is an inexpensive, effective diagnostic tool in abdominal vascular diagnosis in general, its use in abdominal aortic aneurysm (AAA) diagnosis and endograft follow-up has been the subject of controversy and contradictory reports.[1–4] Endograft replacement for abdominal aortic aneurysms has been used for over 10 years in the United States, but controversy still remains as to the role of ultrasound in postimplant surveillance.[5,6] The notable effect of regional variability in the use of ultrasound[7] and the marked differences in expertise from center to center have led to the inconsistent application of ultrasound to both general AAA diagnosis as well as to surveillance after endograft treatment. As a result, many divergent opinions exist as to the ultimate role of color duplex ultrasound in aortic aneurysmal disease.

Clearly ultrasound is a cost-effective tool compared to other modalities used for aortic diagnosis.[8–10] Nonetheless, its perceived subjectivity raises concerns about its reproducibility and reliability. Since ultrasound is generally agreed to be operator dependent, the lack of consistent technical expertise from center to center may mean that results from one institution may not be acceptable at another. This lack of reliability from center to center mandates that each institution maintain a correlation of ultrasound with other vascular imaging modalities to provide an accurate assessment of its local diagnostic value.

When ultrasound is used for vascular diagnosis of the abdominal aorta, the results can be consistent and effective as has been demonstrated in a recent large trial, the UK Small Aneurysm Trial.[11–13] In spite of such trials, computed tomography (CT) scans are the dominant surveillance mode for aneurysmal disease in much of the United States. Such regional variations have led to wide differences in the use of ultrasound in AAA from one region to the next.

History of Aortic Imaging

AAAs for generations have been hidden from diagnosis, with a high rate of sudden death in those individuals possessing such aneurysms. In spite of this, the diagnosis of AAAs has been known for many generations. Until a safe and effective therapy for AAAs was available, diagnosis was not particularly beneficial. With the first successful AAA repair by Dubost in 1951,[14] diagnosis became more important as the natural history of aortic aneurysmal disease was altered for the better.

Physical findings associated with the AAA have also been recognized for generations. In the patient whose CT is seen in Figure 44–1, palpation would be more than adequate due to the size of the aneurysm. Typically, palpation of the abdominal aorta can reproducibly measure AAA diameter with an error of 1–2 cm. The amount of error generated was completely dependent on the patient's body habitus and the depth of the aneurysm from the anterior abdominal wall. Therefore, while reproducible measurements were possible for an individual patient, other patients could not be directly compared based on physical findings alone. In fact, many patients remained undiagnosed until the aneurysm had ruptured, usually resulting in the patient's death. In spite of these limitations, physical examination is claimed to be accurate in up to 88% of the cases.[15]

Initially, X-rays were used to define the aneurysm. Calcification in the wall of the artery could be visualized by plain X-rays and measurements could be performed. By defining the diameter of the aorta in the area of the aneurysm, the natural history of aneurysmal growth and rupture could be defined. Traditionally, a lateral lumbosacral spine film was used to measure the anterior to posterior diameter of the aneurysm. While significant magnification occurs using plain X-ray techniques,

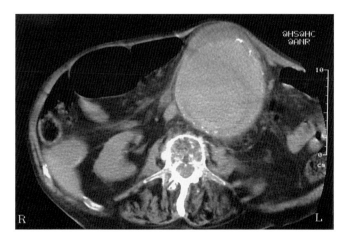

FIGURE 44–1. Large abdominal aortic aneurysm by CT. In this case palpation easily confirms diagnosis and size. CT scan was performed for evaluation for rupture.

correction for this allowed for the first measurements of the rate of aneurysm growth. Based on these techniques, Szylagi *et al.*[16] derived much of the early natural history data available for AAAs. Dr. Szylagi divided aneurysms at the 6 cm anterior to posterior diameter level. Aneurysms smaller than this were not believed to be at risk for impending rupture, while aneurysms larger than this resulting in the patient's death in at least 50% of the cases.

Additional early data had been provided by Estes in the 1950s.[17] Estes divided aneurysms at the 5 cm threshold. The risk of rupture of aneurysms greater than 5 cm was 20% at 5 years, a point at which surgical repair ultimately proved to be of lower risk than observation alone. This threshold has been in use ever since, only to be refined by the UK Small Aneurysm Trial in the 1990s. Again, Estes used plain X-rays to measure the abdominal aortic diameter and derive the natural history data that he published. If calcification was not present in the anterior aneurysm wall, then measurement could be quite difficult if not impossible. Today, plain X-ray imaging of AAAs is of historic interest only. The use of the lateral lumbosacral spine films for aortic diameter measurement has disappeared, although plain films of the abdomen are often the mode of initial diagnosis for many patients with occult aneurysms. Nonetheless, plain X-rays become more important in the follow-up of patients after aortic endografts. The stent portion of the endograft is easily visible on plain X-ray and can be followed for evidence of migration or angulation. Therefore plain X-rays have become a routine adjunct in the assessment of abdominal aortic endografts in follow-up.[18–21]

Ultrasound

The use of ultrasound as a diagnostic technique for AAAs began in the early 1960s and has progressed dramatically since that time. In 1961 Donald and Brown first demonstrated an AAA by ultrasound.[22] While the initial interrogation was with A-mode ultrasound, which provided only one-dimensional data, in the early 1970s B-mode (two-dimensional) ultrasound became the standard and has remained the standard ever since. This ultrasound technique provides two-dimensional data that allow accurate representation of the cross-sectional anatomy of the aorta, providing accurate diameter assessment. Ultrasound has proven to be a reliable technique for assessing aneurysm diameter with measurements reproducible to less than 3%.[23,24] The values are reproducible and consistent, allowing serial surveillance by ultrasound to be used for monitoring AAA size (Figure 44–2). Comparison of abdominal X-rays with ultrasound assessment

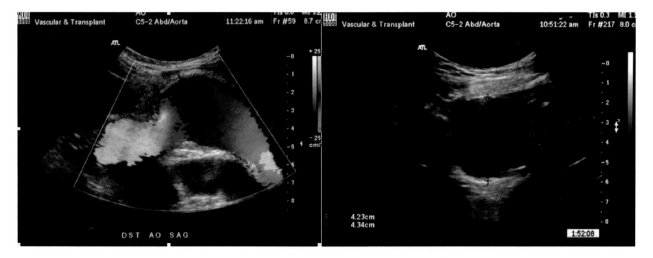

FIGURE 44–2. Ultrasound of native aorta, sagittal and transverse.

demonstrated that there is a high degree of correlation between ultrasound in surgical measurements, much more consistent than that seen with plain X-ray films.[25] Previous studies have demonstrated that ultrasound measurements were identical to operative measurements in 34% of the patients and were within 5mm in 75% of the comparisons.[26] Additionally, the reproducibility of ultrasound measurements has been well established in the surveillance of AAAs by serial studies.[27]

The UK Small Aneurysm Trial reinforced the value of ultrasound for surveillance of AAAs.[11,13,28] In this trial, ultrasound was used as a primary modality for surveillance with an intervention strategy randomized to either early surgery or surveillance until the aneurysm reached 5.5 cm by ultrasound criteria. Using this approach, a benefit to ultrasound surveillance until the aneurysm reached 5.5 cm was seen over that of early surgical intervention in this patient population. Based on this trial, ultrasound surveillance is once again the gold standard for aneurysm monitoring in the abdominal aorta. While CT, as will be discussed below, is an important adjunct in operative aneurysm planning, the routine surveillance of aneurysm size is less expensively achieved by ultrasound alone.

The limitations in ultrasound assessment primarily center on the ability to visualize the aneurysm. While the technique for ultrasound of the abdominal aorta is outlined below, one of the most important adjuncts to quality visualization of the abdominal aorta is performing this examination when the patient is fasting. An empty gastrointestinal (GI) tract and a gasless abdomen are important to provide maximum visualization of the deep abdominal structures such as the abdominal aorta. In spite of these adjuncts, visualization may be complicated in these patients and multiple attempts may be necessary to achieve an optimal examination.

Not to be underestimated in importance relative to abdominal aortic interrogation is the quality of instrumentation employed. Many laboratories rely on older machines without newer technologies that improve imaging of the deeper abdominal structures.[1] To scan the abdominal aorta and its branches, newer transducers and software to improve grayscale imaging are important in achieving successful imaging. While this is more critical in the interrogation of abdominal aortic endografts, visualization of the abdominal aorta can occasionally be problematic and these techniques are beneficial under these circumstances as well.

Technique of Aortic Ultrasound Interrogation of the Native Aorta

Endovascular therapy has dramatically changed the role of the vascular laboratory in many institutions. In addition to being a diagnostic modality, it is often called upon to assist in the determination of the type of therapy used to treat the patient. The vascular laboratory can provide information to direct treatment and assist the physician in determining what type of intervention might best suit individual patient needs. Careful duplex assessment of the aortoiliac artery segments can determine whether the disease is focal or diffuse, determine the exact location of any stenoses, estimate the severity and length of stenoses, and identify aneurysmal disease. Diameter measurements and residual vessel lumen assessment can assist in sizing of endovascular stents and stent grafts. Armed with detailed physiologic and imaging data, physicians may choose to forgo formal angiography in lieu of limited focal angiograms during the interventional procedure, resulting in less contrast to the patient. Many patients today undergo repair of focal arterial disease (aneurysms, arterial stenosis, graft stenosis) based entirely or in part on the duplex findings. The results can also be used as a baseline for postoperative follow-up. This approach to vascular disease management can be cost effective and can save time, but requires high-resolution, high-quality ultrasound systems as well as experienced and qualified examiners and interpreters.

Indications for aortoiliac ultrasound would include hip or buttock claudication that interferes with the patient's occupation or lifestyle, decreased femoral pulses, physiologic studies indicating inflow disease, postoperative angioplasty or poststent evaluation, embolic ischemic digits, and evidence of aneurysmal disease or abdominal bruit. The majority of aneurysms of the abdominal aorta are atherosclerotic and infrarenal. Despite the unique nature of the aneurysmal process, aneurysms can cause the same problems encountered with other arterial diseases such as occlusion, embolism, and hemorrhage. Another abnormality easily recognizable by ultrasound imaging is aortic dissection. Acute dissections are usually readily identified with two channels of flow. More chronic dissections are less easily identified if the false lumen has thrombosed and may be confused with stenosis or atherosclerotic disease.

Contraindications to or limitations on the use of ultrasound in aortoiliac segments are mainly technical in nature. There is a longer learning curve to obtain proficiency in this examination than in peripheral arterial studies and the examiner must be comfortable with abdominal visceral anatomy. Poor patient cooperation or recent abdominal surgery may limit complete assessment as will obesity, extensive bowel gas, and scar tissue. That said, in most instances, these are challenges that can be overcome with good technique and experience.

Patients should be fasted for at least 8 hours prior to the study of aortoiliac segments. Medicines may be taken with water. No gum chewing or smoking is allowed the morning of the examination. Patients should be scheduled in the morning to reduce the amount of air swallowed during the day.

Duplex Ultrasound Protocol

High-resolution real-time ultrasound equipment with color flow capability and spectral Doppler are essential tools for successful aortoiliac ultrasound assessment. Low-frequency transducers ranging from 2 to 5 MHz are generally used but should be appropriate for the girth of the patient. Multiple approaches and transducers may be necessary depending on aortic angulation and bowel gas or obesity. In patients with large abdominal girth, turning the patient onto the left side and using the liver as an acoustic window to image the proximal aorta or turning the patient onto the right side and using the left kidney as an acoustic window may be helpful. Doppler angles ideally should be 45–60° when collecting peak systolic and end-diastolic waveforms. Both B-mode as well as color and spectral Doppler should be used throughout the examination.

The aorta should be evaluated from the diaphragm throughout the iliac arteries to the level of the femoral bifurcation. Anteroposterior and transverse dimensions should be measured and recorded at the site of maximum widening of the vessel. These measurements are taken from outer wall to outer wall, taking care to remain in a true orthogonal 90° angle to the aorta. The examiner should angle the transducer to be perpendicular to the center line of the aorta, not necessarily to the long axis of the body. If thrombus or plaque is present, the diameter of the residual lumen should also be measured. The transverse measurements should include the following:

1. Below the diaphragm including the celiac axis.
2. Inferior to the superior mesenteric artery (SMA).
3. At the level of the renal arteries.
4. Proximal to the iliac bifurcation.
5. The origin of the iliac arteries.

Measurements should be taken of residual diameters of aorta and iliac arteries and anterior-to-posterior wall diameters of iliac (common, external, and internal) and femoral arteries. Doppler waveforms should be documented throughout the aorta and iliac arteries. The entire length of the abdominal aorta in the longitudinal plane should be evaluated by imaging and recording Doppler spectral waveforms including the following:

1. Longitudinal proximal aortic images should include the celiac axis and superior mesenteric artery.
2. Longitudinal mid-aortic assessment taken in the region of the renal arteries and identifying proximity of any aneurysm to the renal arteries.

3. Longitudinal distal aorta (measuring the cranial/caudal extent of any aneurysm).

Scanning Technique

The patient is placed in a supine position with the head slightly elevated (Figure 44–3). Beginning at the level of the celiac axis and extending to the femoral bifurcation, the aorta and iliac arteries should be examined with B-mode in both transverse and sagittal planes. Color flow is especially helpful in assessing the iliac arteries. They are often deep and tortuous as they travel within the pelvis. These arteries are easiest to follow in a sagittal plane sampling with spectral Doppler throughout maintaining an angle of 60° or less. If a hemodynamically significant stenosis is encountered, a transverse view is used to measure percent diameter reduction. The length of the stenosis should also be noted. This can give an approximate length for possible endovascular intervention. Peak systolic velocities are obtained throughout the aorta, common iliac, external iliac, and origins of the internal iliac (or hypogastric) arteries to detect stenosis elevations in velocity. The proximal, mid, and distal common iliac artery, proximal internal iliac artery (hypogastric), and proximal, mid, and distal external iliac artery as well as the common femoral artery, proximal profunda, and proximal superficial femoral artery should be assessed. Denote any areas not well visualized and clearly communicate this to the interpreting physician. Iliac arteries can have focal occlusions with biphasic flow distal to them if collateralization is good. If a stenosis is encountered it is important to document the post-stenotic turbulence.

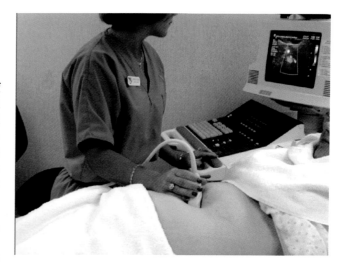

FIGURE 44–3. Positioning for ultrasound scanning of abdominal aorta or aortic endograft.

Computed Tomography Scanning

Body CT scanning became available in the late 1970s as the technology for processing cross-sectional X-ray beams migrated from intracranial evaluation to applications in other areas of the body. While the initial scans done by CT required up to eight rems of radiation exposure to achieve imaging of the abdominal structures, improvements in technology and imaging processing rapidly decreased the radiation exposure. As imaging quality improved so did the techniques used for aortic imaging. While initial scans were performed without intravenous (IV) contrast, determination of aortic diameter required IV contrast to fully visualize the lumen. The combination of IV contrast with more rapid CT techniques allowed for dynamic imaging of the abdominal aorta in ways that were never before possible.

Unfortunately CT scanning requires radiation to define the abdominal anatomy. The dose of radiation is much improved now compared to early CT scans, but the use of radiation is a clear disadvantage when compared to the nontoxic use of ultrasound. Additionally, IV contrast with its associated allergic reactions and nephrotoxicity is another limitation relative to the use of CT scans as routine for aneurysm surveillance. Traditionally, CT scanning has remained more expensive than ultrasound examination, again limiting its usefulness for the routine surveillance of AAAs.

Newer techniques of CT reconstruction allow three-dimensional aortic imaging to be performed based on two-dimensional data sets derived from conventional CT scans. These three-dimensional images allow more accurate assessment of aortic diameter, angulation, and anatomy, particularly relative to abdominal aortic endograft placement (Figure 44–4). Recent studies suggest that the use of three-dimensional CT techniques

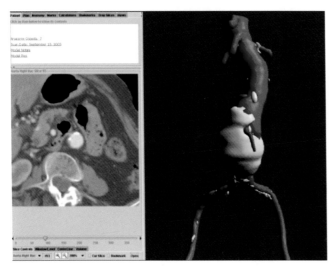

FIGURE 44–4. Three-dimensional reconstruction of CT data.

improves the planning of abdominal aortic endografts for aneurysmal disease, almost eliminating the need for arteriography prior to abdominal aortic surgery.[29–31] While these newer techniques are not universally employed, the benefits of three-dimensional reconstruction appear clear cut relative to endograft placement and surveillance and should be considered in any patient prior to consideration for abdominal aortic endografts.

The Relationship between Computed Tomography-Derived Data and Ultrasound-Derived Data

While both ultrasound and CT have been used for measurement of aortic aneurysm diameter since their development, there has been little correlation until recently between the two modalities. The use of ultrasound for surveillance in the UK Small Aneurysm Trial suggested that ultrasound should be the primary surveillance modality for patients not yet at a size to treat their aneurysms.[32] What about CT scanning? In the United States, most centers relied on CT rather than ultrasound for the routine follow-up of aneurysms. Were the values derived from CT comparable to those derived from color duplex ultrasound? While equivalence had always been assumed between the two modalities, no studies were available to define the areas of correlation or difference.

In 2001 our group attempted to define this relationship.[33] Using the core laboratory data from the Guidant Ancure endograft trial, we evaluated paired ultrasound and CT data reviewed by the core laboratory as part of the trial. In all cases the measurements were made by the core laboratory and were therefore free from observer bias at the institution implanting the endograft. Ultimately paired measurements were available for comparison in 334 patients at the initial follow-up after endograft implantation. In this group, 95% of the CT measurements were larger that those obtained with ultrasound (Figure 44–5) by an average difference of 9.5 mm ($p < 0.01$). Thus, for the first time the differences between CT diameter and ultrasound diameter were demonstrated to be significant. It remained to be defined why this difference occurred.

What are the causes of such a discrepancy in the measurement of aortic diameter? While maximum minor axis diameter measurements have been proposed as a more accurate diameter assessment by CT, these measurements did not completely provide the answer as the measurements were still discrepant using these values. There were several possible causes for the differences. First, it is possible that ultrasound fundamentally measures a different layer of the aortic wall, such as the inner wall, so that measurements were less by ultrasound. Second, ultrasound is operator dependent, raising the question as to whether the operator was manipulating the

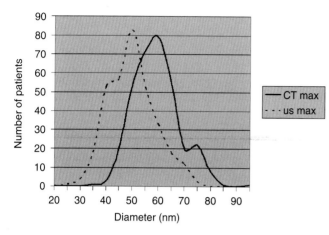

FIGURE 44–5. CT diameter (black line) versus ultrasound diameter (white line) in the same patients. (Adapted from Sprouse LR 2nd, Meier GH 3rd, Lesar CJ, Demasi RJ, Sood J, Parent FN, *et al.* Comparison of abdominal aortic aneurysm diameter measurements obtained with ultrasound and computed tomography: Is there a difference? J Vasc Surg 2003;466–71, with permission.)

image acquired by ultrasound in such a way as to minimize diameter, such as compressing the aorta while imaging. Finally, since the larger diameter aneurysms consistently had larger discrepancies, was there some factor seen with increasing diameter that may account for the differences?

We undertook a review with our sonographers of their technique of aortic aneurysm interrogation. One of the striking features of the ultrasonographers' technique of

aortic imaging was the routine effort to obtain a round cross section for diameter measurements (Figure 44–2). If the aortic image was oblique, then an oval cross section was seen; when the image was corrected for aortic angulation the cross section became rounded. It was immediately apparent that the ultrasonographer was correcting for aortic angulation on cross-sectional duplex imaging of the aorta.

From this we undertook a new study to evaluate aortic angulation and its effect on the differences seen between ultrasound and CT-derived data.[29] To do this, we needed three-dimensional data providing aortic angulation as well as CT-derived diameters perpendicular to the center line of aortic flow. Fortunately, Metrix Media Systems (MMS, Lebanon, NH) had developed an aortic CT reformatting methodology that allowed us to derive these values and compare axial CT data at the same time. We therefore undertook a study in our own patients comparing axial CT diameters, CT diameters perpendicular to flow, ultrasound diameters, and the effect of aortic angulation on all of these measurements. In a group of 38 patients these parameters were assessed and compared prospectively. Since many of these patients were not yet operative candidates, the mean diameter was somewhat smaller than in the previous study, but axial CT diameter was still 4.1 mm larger than ultrasound diameter ($p < 0.05$). When compared to maximum CT diameter perpendicular to the axis of flow, this difference decreased to 0.9 mm, a nonsignificant difference. We then reviewed the effect of aortic angulation on these differences (Figure 44–6). When aortic angulation was less than

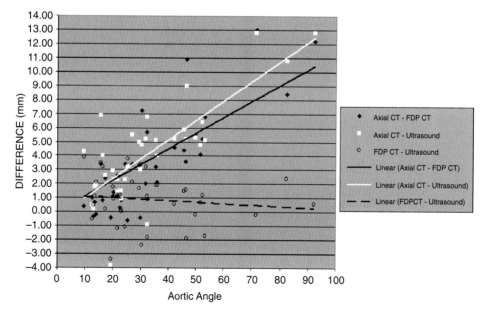

FIGURE 44–6. The effect of aortic angulation on differences between axial CT, flow-directed perpendicular (FDP) CT, and ultrasound. [Reproduced from Sprouse LR 2nd, Meier GH 3rd, Paren FN, DeMasi RJ, Glickman MH, Barber GA. Is ultrasound more accurate than axial computed tomography for determination of maximal abdominal aortic aneurysm diameter? Eur J Vasc Endovasc Surg 2004;28(1):28–35, with permission.]

25° from vertical, there was no significant difference between the two CT-derived diameters and the ultrasound diameter; when the angulation was greater than 25°, the difference between maximum axial CT diameter and the other two diameters became statistically significant.

Other investigators have evaluated the same questions with mixed results.[1,2,34,35] Nonetheless, the tacit acceptance of equivalence between CT and ultrasound-derived data has to be abandoned and differences are the expected result when comparing CT AAA diameter to ultrasound AAA diameter. The larger question centers on the effect of this discrepancy on natural history data relative to the growth and rupture risk of aneurysms. Clearly the UK Small Aneurysm Trial has changed the approach in Europe as to when these patients receive treatment. Whether the more widespread use of CT in the United States for aneurysm surveillance alters the threshold for intervention compared to those who use ultrasound surveillance remains to be seen.

Post-Intervention Surveillance

Once an aneurysm is treated, either by conventional surgery or endograft implantation, surveillance becomes an issue. While the benefits of surveillance after open repair are controversial, the routine use of surveillance after endografting is an accepted routine, with many surgeons refusing endografts in patients unwilling or unable to return for routine postimplantation surveillance. Nonetheless, the theoretical basis for surveillance in these two clinical scenarios is quite different and the goals of the surveillance protocol are dissimilar. In both clinical situations the use of ultrasound is valuable, as long as certain standards can be guaranteed.

Ultrasound Surveillance After Open Aneurysm Repair

Once an aortic graft is surgically implanted, the long-term success of the intervention is quite high, exceeding 90% at 10 years.[36] In spite of these long-term successes, many advocate surveillance at regular intervals even after conventional surgical repair.[37–39] The issues for surveillance are different with open repair, focusing primarily on surveillance for new aneurysm formation, expansion of residual aneurysm segments, or the development of stenoses or occlusions. While these issues may be present early after surgery, in most cases surveillance is warranted only after a period of time—usually 2 years or more after surgical intervention. While advocates of routine surveillance after open repair suggest definite benefits

in discovering pathologic features that warrant intervention, others believe that the routine use of surveillance after open aneurysm surgery is unfounded and unnecessary.[40,41]

With surgical repair, most abnormal pathology is treated with graft replacement and exclusion. Nonetheless, aneurysmal disease is a field defect disease, and with time other arterial segments are at risk for aneurysmal degeneration. Therefore, the focus of postsurgical surveillance is on monitoring for aneurysmal degeneration in arterial segments adjacent to the grafted segments as well as in remote segments at risk for aneurysm. These segments include the proximal aortic segment, the iliac arteries, and other vessels as appropriate. The more segments with aneurysmal degeneration, the greater the risk for further aneurysm formation.

Other areas for surveillance relate to the complications of surgical intervention. The development of stenoses in the reconstruction may represent areas for intervention to prevent occlusive complications. Ultrasound can effectively diagnose and follow areas of stenoses for possible intervention. Conventional arterial velocity and grayscale criteria for stenosis are appropriate for this form of surveillance.

Ultrasound Surveillance After Endovascular Aneurysm Repair

While the best method and interval of follow-up after endovascular aneurysm repair remain controversial, there is generally consensus that some form of surveillance after endograft repair is crucial to the success of this therapy. As a result, many centers have developed independently programs of surveillance that include both CT and ultrasound. As with many imaging techniques the best protocol is likely related to what is available at a given institution. Both CT and ultrasound provide independent information that is valuable in follow-up for the physician implanting endografts for abdominal aortic aneurysms.

CT scans provide standardized information that is reproducible and objective. Ultrasound data are often influenced by the ability of the technologist as well as the quality of the equipment available. Therefore the results obtained with ultrasound are much harder to reproduce from center to center, while CT can be easily standardized using a reproducible protocol for obtaining the scan. Unfortunately, interrogation of aortic endografts by either methodology can be challenging, with many subtleties to the images obtained. As a result, the best methodology for surveillance may not be one or the other, but a combination of the two. The unique ability of ultrasound to look at flow allows interrogation of the residual aneurysm sac around the endograft in ways that are likely not possible using conventional CT scans.

Typically, CT scans are performed using a spiral technique with image acquisition at a 2 mm slice thickness. Baseline scans through the aneurysm and endograft are performed without contrast to better evaluate endograft structure and the presence of structural features within the abdominal aortic aneurysm. IV contrast is administered as a bolus via a peripheral vein, timed to provide maximum enhancement of flow within the aneurysm sac. Importantly, delayed imaging of the aneurysm sac must be performed to allow for late filling of endoleaks within the aneurysm sac. With these techniques endoleaks can be detected in many patients.

Ultrasound, on the other hand, is not nearly as simple. The subjective nature of the images obtained requires that a standardized approach be undertaken to maximize objectivity. The elements of this protocol are described below, but it should be remembered that this is only a guideline. As newer technology becomes available changes in the protocol may be necessary to improve our ability to define endoleak. A good example of this is the use of harmonic imaging and ultrasound contrast (Figure 44–7). These adjuncts will be discussed further in a later section in this chapter.

Endoleak Ultrasound Surveillance Protocol

The purpose of duplex ultrasound evaluation of endovascular aortic stent grafts following device placement is to identify the presence of possible perigraft leaks, enlarging aneurysmal size, or other complications associated with the procedure such as iatrogenic injury. In addition, it is an ideal way of identifying hemodynamic or anatomic abnormalities that may impair graft function. In experienced hands and with adequate protocols, color duplex ultrasound (CDU) can be used to reliably determine the presence of endoleaks, hemodynamic impairment, and changes in aneurysm size.

All patients with endografts potentially can be followed with ultrasound, however, while there are no real contraindications, there are certain limitations. Excessive bowel gas, obesity, or recent abdominal surgery may limit the examination (abdominal tenderness may limit the technologist's ability to obtain an adequate scan). In patients with obesity, if the aorta is located at a depth of more than 15 cm, this will limit good visualization of the device, attachment or fixation sites, and the ability to readily identify endoleak.

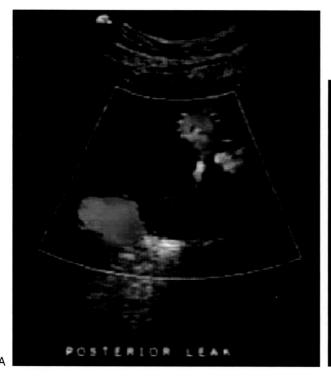
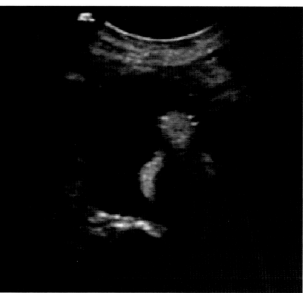

FIGURE 44–7. Color flow duplex showing endoleak (A) and corresponding endoleak demonstrated with intravenous ultrasound contrast (B).

Equipment and Supplies

To adequately assess patients with aortic endografts, a high-resolution duplex ultrasound system with good pulsed Doppler and color flow capability is essential. Low-frequency pulsed Doppler transducers with 2.25–5 MHz frequency are generally used. It may require multiple transducers in the course of the study including curved array, phased array, or mechanical sector transducers. Many of the currently available manufacturers' features to enhance resolution, decrease artifact, and improve color and spectral Doppler deep in the abdomen will help with accuracy and speed of this complex and challenging ultrasound study.

Patient Preparation

Patients should fast overnight to minimize the amount of bowel gas present at the time of the study. Water is usually allowed as it is usually better if the patient is well hydrated. A bowel prep is not usually needed. No smoking or gum chewing is allowed the morning of the examination since this may increase swallowing of air and limit visibility. Occasionally it is helpful to have the patient take a Simethecone-containing over-the-counter medicine if they are known to have excessive abdominal gas.

Patients should be prepared for the procedure to take up to 1.5 hours to perform. The examination is performed with the patient supine in a comfortable position and the head elevated for both comfort and to drop the abdominal contents. In patients with extreme abdominal girth, positioning in a right or left lateral decubitus position may be useful.

Test Protocol

The technologist must know the details of the endovascular aortic repair prior to beginning assessment of the aortic endograft with ultrasound. This is a much more complex evaluation than standard aortic ultrasound and requires more technical expertise. In addition, different complications can arise with different graft configurations. Some stent grafts are totally supported, some are unsupported, some are modular in design, and some are single body construction.

The examiner should be aware of any additional ancillary procedures that may have been performed. Patients may have multiple modular segments placed to accommodate their anatomy and aneurysmal disease. Often a patient with small iliac vessels may have additional procedures to allow introduction of the device including transluminal angioplasty, endarterectomy, placement of a "chimney" graft, or other endovascular procedures. Some patients will require precoiling or ligation of the hypogas-

tric arteries. It is much easier to identify any complications if the details of the procedure are known prior to the ultrasound.

There are different types of aortic stent grafts and most are currently placed infrarenally. Configurations of the devices come in tube, bifurcated, or occasionally aortouniiliac grafts that involve exclusion or occlusion of the contralateral iliac artery to prevent retrograde flow from entering the aneurysmal sac and a femoral-to-femoral bypass to restore flow to the limb. Most aortic endografts placed are bifurcated. Transrenal and thoracic aortic stent graft devices are under investigation and may be encountered.

Begin by identifying the region of the maximum size of the aneurysm in both transverse (transaxial) and sagittal/longitudinal planes. Transverse measurements are made of the maximum diameter of the aneurysm sac. It is important to be perpendicular to the aorta, not necessarily to the long axis of the body. Many patients have tortuous aortoiliac anatomy. The transducer should be angled to accommodate for the tortuosity for the most accurate transverse diameter measurements.

Using B-mode imaging without color, identify superior (proximal) and inferior (distal) attachment sites (also called fixation sites); annotate and record the location. Look for small linear reflective metal struts. In some devices you may see the anchoring hooks that anchor the device to the aortic wall. Other devices are externally or internally supported and should be fairly easily visualized. The superior attachment (fixation) should be located distally inferior to the renal arteries. Also identify and record a systematic assessment of the entire aortic graft and residual aneurysm sac. If the stent graft is a bifurcated graft or aortoiliac graft, identify the inferior iliac attachment site(s) and the native iliac inferior to the attachment site. In unsupported grafts, marked wall motion is likely an indicator of endoleak. The B-mode assessment will also identify hypoechoic areas within the residual endograft, which should be carefully investigated for endoleak (Figure 44–8). In addition, a "spongy" texture to the thrombus within the residual sac is sometimes associated with very subtle, slow flow endoleak, particularly in the accompanying presence of increasing aneurysmal size (Figure 44–9). Endoleak influences aneurysm sac morphology. Asymmetry of the sac is frequently associated with endoleak. Systemic pressures from endoleaks found within the aneurysm sac often appear to be localized to the area of endoleak, indicating that forces applied within the aneurysm sac are not uniform.[42] Aneurysm volume expansion is also more likely to occur in the presence of endoleak.

Continue to scan slowly from above the superior attachment to the inferior attachment in both transverse and sagittal views in both B-mode and with color flow. Optimize B-mode and color settings so that color

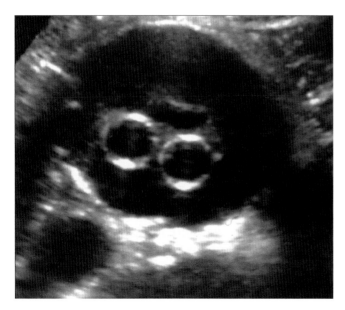

FIGURE 44–8. Grayscale hypoechoic defect within the residual aneurysm suggestive of endoleak.

completely fills the graft lumen without excessive artifact in the color box, and so that the residual aneurysmal sac can be clearly seen. The color box should be large enough to encompass the sac but not too large to encourage artifact. Power Doppler may sometimes be helpful in detecting perigraft flow. Three-dimensional imaging software may make posterior vessels such as lumbars easier to locate. Look for potential sites of perigraft leak at the superior attachment/fixation and inferior attachment/fixation (Type I). Type II endoleaks are those originating from native vessels that arise from the aorta and potentially may flow retrograde into the residual aneurysmal

sac outside of the endograft. These Type II endoleaks include the inferior mesenteric artery (IMA) located anterior to the graft in the mid-portion of the residual aneurysmal sac (usually found near the umbilicus) as well as lumbar arteries usually located posterior to the graft potentially over the entire length of the AAA sac. These are most often found in the transverse approach. Type III endoleaks are those associated with modular disconnection of segments of the endograft. For this reason, it is important to know the configuration of the endograft and which limb is the docking limb and where any additional modular segments are attached. Type IV endoleaks are generally transgraft endoleaks associated with flow through the interstices of the fabric of the graft. Note that more than one type of leak can occur at the same time, for instance, an attachment leak (Type I) exiting through a lumbar or IMA (Type II). Attempt to identify the IMA origin, anterior and near the mid to distal aorta and usually found more toward the patient's left. Try to identify direction of flow in the IMA. The IMA may be occluded at its origin but patent through collaterals, so attempt to determine patency/occlusion at the origin.

It is important to confirm all suspected leaks with spectral Doppler. Record any flow entering or exiting the residual aneurysm sac and attempt to identify the source location and direction. True endoleaks will have reproducible arterial waveforms with spectral characteristics *different* from that of the graft flow. Artifactual pulsatile color may be present if the color sensitivity settings are low enough so that the equipment will prioritize movement as color verses gray when in fact it is only movement secondary to the pulsatility of the adjacent graft structure. Other color artifacts can occur from abdominal gas. The spectral Doppler waveform will differentiate true perigraft leak from color artifact (Figure 44–10).

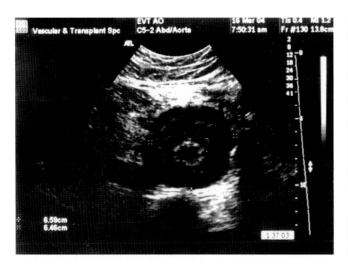

FIGURE 44–9. Heterogeneous thrombus on grayscale image raises concerns of occult endoleak.

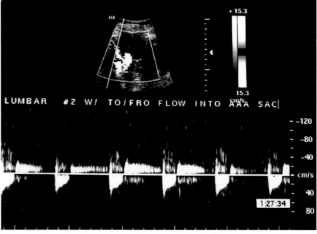

FIGURE 44–10. Example of spectral Doppler confirmation of endoleak to differentiate true flow from color artifact.

Make note of the Doppler characteristics of the waveform (biphasic, monophasic, bidirectional). Differing spectral waveform types can usually be associated with different types of endoleak. Once confirmed by spectral Doppler, try to determine the extent of the leak by color Doppler, i.e., whether the leak extends through the entire length of the residual sac or is confined only to the immediate area of the suspected origin of the leak. If possible, determine direction of flow in the source of the leak and into and/or out of the sac. Even if no leak is suspected, the entire residual sac should be sampled throughout using spectral Doppler both anteriorly and posteriorly to ensure the absence of endoleak. Focus should be directed to potential leak sites (IMA and lumbars as well as attachment sites). Careful assessment in the area between the posterior wall of the aorta and the spine may reveal patent retrograde lumbar arteries.

Assess the graft for any deformity in the graft material such as folding and incomplete deployment, and in bifurcated and aortoiliac stent grafts, assess the limb(s) for twisting, kinking, or any other deformity that may lead to stenosis or potential thrombosis of the limb. Record flow velocity through the body of the graft and limb(s) if a bifurcated or aortoiliac graft is present. Record the peak systolic velocity at the attachment sites. This is important in defining any limb dysfunction that may lead to limb thrombosis. Unsupported endografts are at greater risk for limb dysfunction but it can be seen in any limb. CDU surveillance effectively identifies problems that may threaten the graft patency. Continue down the remainder of the native outflow arterial tree to the femoral arteries, noting any flow abnormalities that could be associated with iatrogenic injury involving the use of the large introducers used in the placement of these devices. Such injuries, while uncommon, can include intimal flaps, dissection, hematoma, pseudoaneurysm, and arteriovenous fistula. In addition, remodeling of the aneurysm residual sac over time can result in redundancy of the graft and cause additional complications.

The advantages of duplex ultrasound in the follow-up of patients with aortic endografts include the ability to collect accurate residual aortic sac diameter measurements serially over time. It is a very sensitive method for endoleak detection with adequate time and when protocol is used. Ultrasound can often identify the source for endoleak classification and can readily evaluate for limb dysfunction or any other hemodynamic impairment. It is inexpensive and reproducible and requires no contrast and there may be an additive effect of CT with ultrasound in the follow-up of patients with these devices placed. The disadvantages of using duplex ultrasound may be the time commitment involved in a busy vascular laboratory. Additionally, there is a need for high-resolution equipment for the adequate performance of this examination. It is a technically challenging, subjective study that is highly dependent on the examiner and interpreter but it can be a valuable tool in the assessment of patients with aortic endografts.

Results of Ultrasound for Endograft Surveillance

The use of ultrasound for endograft surveillance has been advocated by many as an alternative to or an adjunct to routine CT scan surveillance.[5,43–45] Those who support the use of ultrasound believe that it offers information not available from routine CT scans, improving endoleak detection and providing information on limb dysfunction that is not necessarily available by CT imaging. While there is not yet a consensus on the role of ultrasound in endograft surveillance, there are many areas where good data exist supporting the use of ultrasound.

Endoleak Detection

One of the most important aspects of endograft surveillance is the reliable detection of endoleak. While numerous studies have documented the frequency of endoleak, it is still widely recognized that endoleak detection is variable from institution to institution due to differences in imaging technique and frequency. Ultrasound is an ideal agent for measuring flow. While ultrasound is optimized for the detection of arterial and venous flow velocities, the lower velocity seen with endoleaks can still be assessed. The addition of color flow to conventional ultrasound techniques provides a visual assessment of endoleak. In spite of these theoretical advantages, some centers have been unable to reliably detect endoleak with ultrasound.[1]

While the first reports of ultrasound surveillance after endograft aneurysm repair were from Europe in about 1997,[46] many other centers have subsequently reported their experience with ultrasound surveillance.[1,5,6,8,34,35,38,44–54] The relative efficacy of ultrasound for endoleak detection clearly varies from institution to institution, but the experience in many centers suggests that endoleak detection by ultrasound may be superior to that seen with contrast CT alone.[5,19,34,44–48,51,53,54] At this time, a consensus for the use of ultrasound after abdominal aortic endograft implantation is lacking. For the moment, CT scan interrogation of the residual aneurysm sac remains a standard with or without supplementary CDU.

The second issue relative to endoleak relates to the classification of endoleak type (Table 44–1). Type I, or attachment site endoleak, is a greater concern after endograft implantation. Its detection is usually straightforward by either CT or ultrasound as these leaks tend to have high flows associated with their presence. Type II

TABLE 44–1. Classification of endoleak.[61]

Type	Cause of perigraft flow
I	Inadequate seal at proximal end of endograft
	Inadequate seal at distal end of endograft
	Inadequate seal at iliac occluder plug
II	Flow from visceral vessel (lumbar, IMA,[a] accessory renal, hypogastric) without attachment site connection
III	Flow from module disconnection
	Flow from fabric disruption
	Minor (<2 mm)
	Major (≥2 mm)
IV	Flow from porous fabric (<30 days after graft placement)
Endoleak of undefined origin	Flow visualized but source unidentified

[a]IMA, inferior mesenteric artery.

endoleak (branch vessel) can be much more subtle since the rate of flow can be quite low. Typically these endoleaks communicate between lumbar vessels and other branches, primarily the IMA. Occasionally, a to-and-fro pattern can be seen similar to that seen in a femoral pseudoaneurysm after catheterization. This pattern is less worrisome and in most cases does not persist. Type III endoleak occurs at the connections between segments of the endograft. These may occur in isolation or may be combined with branch vessels. Generally these endoleaks are high flow as well, making detection relatively easy. Finally, Type IV endoleak occurs through the fabric of the graft and can be quite subtle. In these situations detection is difficult, but many of these leaks will seal spontaneously.

Definition of endoleak type rests on tracking the endoleak within the aneurysm sac from its origin to its endpoint. Turbulence can make tracking the endoleak quite challenging and in many cases the channels themselves may be poorly developed or irregular. As a result there is no standard for endoleak mapping and many centers find that endoleak classification is poorly defined and inconsistent. Many endoleaks end up being reclassified over time as additional information becomes available from interventions or additional studies. Therefore endoleak classification is more of a goal than a reality at this point.

Limb Dysfunction

After endograft implantation changes in the sac pressurization may result in conformational changes in the endograft limbs. These changes may cause decreased flow in the limbs, a condition referred to as limb dysfunction. This is similar to the forces resulting in modular disconnects in modular aortic endografts, as the leveraging of the attachment sites versus the body of the endograft can create either narrowing of the endograft limb or sufficient force to dislocate the interconnect of the graft modules. Ultrasound is uniquely suited for detecting changes in flow within the limbs and can effectively detect narrowing as an increase in velocity relative to adjacent segments.[55]

Similarly, ultrasound is useful for interrogating the outflow arteries from the endograft limb to detect areas of flow restriction or aneurysmal degeneration that may lead to limb thrombosis. While these changes may be detected with other modalities such as CT, flow changes are the strength of ultrasound evaluation due to the ability to measure Doppler velocities. As flow changes over time, ultrasound can follow these changes to suggest the need for intervention as changes progress. The ability to reliably detect flow changes over time is the strength of ultrasound evaluation of endograft limbs, providing unique information that may not otherwise be apparent.

Aneurysm Growth

As discussed earlier in this chapter, ultrasound provides accurate imaging of aortic diameters, independent of aortic angulation. Therefore, routine surveillance of maximum aneurysm size can be easily performed by ultrasound. The difficulties in ultrasound reside in the relative position of one measurement to the next. While CT scans can measure diameters at given locations relative to fixed branch origins such as the SMA, ultrasound cannot reliably follow the measurements at a given point with accuracy. For the assessment of diameters at a given reference point, CT seems more consistent.

It has been suggested that aneurysm volumes may prove more sensitive than diameter in the assessment of aneurysm behavior.[47,56,57] In spite of this suggestion, the routine assessment of aneurysm volumes by either CT or ultrasound is yet to be achieved. The behavior of aortic aneurysms is not well defined with volume measurements at this time.

Device Migration

Since ultrasound has difficulty in repetitive measurements in three-dimensional space, device migration is often detected late when this modality is used alone. Plain X-ray films remain the mainstay in the detection of device migration, although some controversy remains as to whether the changes seen are truly device migration or aortic neck elongation.[58] Whether three-dimensional ultrasound may better define subtle device changes remains to be seen. Currently, plain X-rays and CT scans are the best modalities for detection of endograft migration.

Ultrasound Contrast

Increasing experience with ultrasound contrast suggests that this modality may provide the best definition for endoleak detection (Figure 44–7). Ultrasound contrast is blood pool based, providing accurate imaging of flowing blood within the aneurysm sac. Many centers view this as the current standard for endoleak detection and mapping.[8,43,47,48,59,60] With greater experience, the routine use of contrast-enhanced ultrasound may provide the standard for endograft interrogation.

In this technique, harmonic imaging is used rather than conventional grayscale. Since the ultrasound beam entrains the microbubbles to resonate at a certain frequency, imaging at that harmonic frequency results in dramatic improvements in blood flow imaging. What is sacrificed is grayscale quality; harmonic imaging loses grayscale quality as blood pool imaging is improved. Therefore the ability to evaluate blood flow is improved while the imaging of the endograft and aneurysm sac is degraded. For endoleak, the advantage is a shortened examination with more certainty as to the presence or absence of perigraft blood flow. The combination of conventional CDU with contrast-enhanced imaging when appropriate may ultimately prove to be the new standard in aortic endograft surveillance.[61]

When Should We Use Ultrasound with Aneurysms?

If a center has experience with deep abdominal ultrasound, then routine use of color flow duplex ultrasound for aortic assessment is logical and effective. If adequate expertise is not yet available, then deep abdominal ultrasound imaging is an adjunct that, over time, will improve in quality and overall clinical benefit. Both the follow-up of AAAs and the surveillance of aortic endografts are appropriate uses of duplex ultrasound. With experience and dedication, these modalities become the preferred technique for aortic assessment and follow-up.

References

1. Raman KG, Missig-Carroll N, Richardson T, Muluk SC, Makaroun MS. Color-flow duplex ultrasound scan versus computed tomographic scan in the surveillance of endovascular aneurysm repair. J Vasc Surg 2003;38(4):645–51.

2. Singh K, Jacobsen BK, Solberg S, Kumar S, Arnesen E. The difference between ultrasound and computed tomography (CT) measurements of aortic diameter increases with aortic diameter: Analysis of axial images of abdominal aortic and common iliac artery diameter in normal and aneurysmal aortas. The Tromso Study, 1994–1995. Eur J Vasc Endovasc Surg 2004;28(2):158–67.

3. Tayal VS, Graf CD, Gibbs MA. Prospective study of accuracy and outcome of emergency ultrasound for abdominal aortic aneurysm over two years. Acad Emerg Med 2003; 10(8):867–71.

4. Walker A, Brenchley J, Sloan JP, Lalanda M, Venables H. Ultrasound by emergency physicians to detect abdominal aortic aneurysms: A UK case series. Emerg Med J 2004;21(2):257–9.

5. Parent FN, Meier GH, Godziachvili V, LeSar CJ, Parker FM, Carter KA, et al. The incidence and natural history of type I and II endoleak: A 5-year follow-up assessment with color duplex ultrasound scan. J Vasc Surg 2002;35(3): 474–81.

6. Teodorescu VJ, Morrissey NJ, Olin JW. Duplex ultrasonography and its impact on providing endograft surveillance. Mt Sinai J Med 2003;70(6):364–6.

7. Cronenwett JL. In: Birkmeyer JD (ed). *The Dartmouth Atlas of Vascular Health Care.* Chicago: AHA Press, 2000.

8. Bendick PJ, Zelenock GB, Bove PG, Long,GW, Shanley CJ, Brown OW. Duplex ultrasound imaging with an ultrasound contrast agent: The economic alternative to CT angiography for aortic stent graft surveillance. Vasc Endovasc Surg 2003;37(3):165–70.

9. Multicentre aneurysm screening study (MASS): Cost effectiveness analysis of screening for abdominal aortic aneurysms based on four year results from randomised controlled trial. BMJ 2002;325(7373):1135.

10. Katz DA, Cronenwet JL. The cost-effectiveness of early surgery versus watchful waiting in the management of small abdominal aortic aneurysms. J Vasc Surg 1994;19(6):980–90; discussion 990–1.

11. The U.K. Small Aneurysm Trial: Design, methods and progress. The UK Small Aneurysm Trial participants. Eur J Vasc Endovasc Surg 1995;9(1):42–8.

12. Mortality results for randomised controlled trial of early elective surgery or ultrasonographic surveillance for small abdominal aortic aneurysms. The UK Small Aneurysm Trial Participants. Lancet 1998;352(9141):1649–55.

13. Brown LC, Powell JT. Risk factors for aneurysm rupture in patients kept under ultrasound surveillance. UK Small Aneurysm Trial Participants. Ann Surg 1999;230(3):289–96; discussion 296–7.

14. Dubost C, Allary M, Oeconomos N. Resection of an aneurysm of the abdominal aorta. Arch Surg 1952;64:405–9.

15. Demos NJ. Severe vascular impairment of the left half of the colon. Surg Gynecol Obstet 1963;117:205–8.

16. Szilagyi DE, Smith RF, DeRusso FJ, Elliott JP, Sherrin FW. Contribution of abdominal aortic aneurysmectomy to the prolongation of life. Ann Surg 1966;164:678–99.

17. Estes JE. Abdominal aortic aneurysm: A study of 102 cases. Circulation 1950;2:258–64.

18. Palombo D, Valenti D, Ferri M, Gaggiano A, Mazzei R, Vola M, et al. Changes in the proximal neck of abdominal aortic

aneurysms early after endovascular treatment. Ann Vasc Surg 2003;17(4):408–10.

19. Thurnher S, Cejna M. Imaging of aortic stent-grafts and endoleaks. Radiol Clin North Am 2002;40(4):799–833.

20. Magennis R, Joekes E, Martin J, White D, McWilliams RG. Complications following endovascular abdominal aortic aneurysm repair. Br J Radiol 2002;75(896):700–7.

21. Whitaker SC. Imaging of abdominal aortic aneurysm before and after endoluminal stent-graft repair. Eur J Radiol 2001;39(1):3–15.

22. Donald L, Brown TG. Demonstration of tissue interfaces within the body by ultrasonic echo sounding. Br J Radiol 1961;34:539.

23. Singh K, Bonaa KH, Solberg S, Sorlie DG, Bjork L. Intra- and interobserver variability in ultrasound measurements of abdominal aortic diameter. The Tromso Study. Eur J Vasc Endovasc Surg 1998;15(6):497–504.

24. Thomas PR, Shaw JC, Ashton HA, Kay DN, Scott RA. Accuracy of ultrasound in a screening programme for abdominal aortic aneurysms. J Med Screen 1994;1(1):3–6.

25. Maloney JD, Pairolero PC, Smith SF Jr, Hattery RR, Brakke DM, Spittell JA Jr. Ultrasound evaluation of abdominal aortic aneurysms. Circulation 1977;56(3 Suppl): II80–5.

26. Hertzer NR, Beven EG. Ultrasound aortic measurement and elective aneurysmectomy. JAMA 1978;240(18):1966–8.

27. Bernstein EF, Dilley RB, Goldberger LE, Gosink BB, Leopold GR. Growth rates of small abdominal aortic aneurysms. Surgery 1976;80(6):765–73.

28. Powell JT, Greenhalgh RM, Ruckley CV, Fowkes FG. The UK Small Aneurysm Trial. Ann NY Acad Sci 1996; 800:249–51.

29. Sprouse LR 2nd, Meier GH 3rd, Paren FN, DeMasi RJ, Glickman MH, Barber GA. Is ultrasound more accurate than axial computed tomography for determination of maximal abdominal aortic aneurysm diameter? Eur J Vasc Endovasc Surg 2004;28(1):28–35.

30. Aziz I, Lee J, Lee JT, Donayre CE, Walot I, Kopchok G, et al. Accuracy of three-dimensional simulation in the sizing of aortic endoluminal devices. Ann Vasc Surg 2003; 17(2):129–36.

31. Sprouse LR 2nd, Meier GH 3rd, Parent FN, DeMasi RJ, Stokes GK, LeSar CJ, et al. Is three-dimensional computed tomography reconstruction justified before endovascular aortic aneurysm repair? J Vasc Surg 2004;40(3):443–7.

32. Long-term outcomes of immediate repair compared with surveillance of small abdominal aortic aneurysms. N Engl J Med 2002;346(19):1445–52.

33. Sprouse LR 2nd, Meier GH 3rd, Lesar CJ, Demasi RJ, Sood J, Parent FN, et al. Comparison of abdominal aortic aneurysm diameter measurements obtained with ultrasound and computed tomography: Is there a difference? J Vasc Surg 2003;466–71; discussion 471–2.

34. Elkouri S, Panneton JM, Andrews JC, Lewis BD, McKusick MA, Noel AA, et al. Computed tomography and ultrasound in follow-up of patients after endovascular repair of abdominal aortic aneurysm. Ann Vasc Surg 2004;18(3):271–9.

35. Wolf YG, Johnson BL, Hill BB, Rubin GD, Fogarty TJ, Zarins CK. Duplex ultrasound scanning versus computed tomographic angiography for postoperative evaluation of

endovascular abdominal aortic aneurysm repair. J Vasc Surg 2000;32(6):1142–8.

36. Plate G, Hollier LA, O'Brien P, Pairolero PC, Cherry KJ, Kazmier FJ. Recurrent aneurysms and late vascular complications following repair of abdominal aortic aneurysms. Arch Surg 1985;120(5):590–4.

37. Mulder EJ, van Bockel JH, Maas J, van den Akker PJ, Hermans J. Morbidity and mortality of reconstructive surgery of noninfected false aneurysms detected long after aortic prosthetic reconstruction. Arch Surg 1998;133(1): 45–9.

38. Raithel D. Surveillance of patients after abdominal aortic aneurysm repair with endovascular grafting or conventional treatment. J Mal Vasc 1998;23(5):390–2.

39. Baker DM, Hinchliffe RJ, Yusuf SW, Whitaker SC, Hopkinson BR. True juxta-anastomotic aneurysms in the residual infra-renal abdominal aorta. Eur J Vasc Endovasc Surg 2003;25(5):412–5.

40. Liapis C, Kakisis J, Kaperonis E, Papavassiliou V, Karousos D, Tzonou A, et al. Changes of the infrarenal aortic segment after conventional abdominal aortic aneurysm repair. Eur J Vasc Endovasc Surg 2000;19(6):643–7.

41. Hallett JW Jr, Marshall DM, Petterson TM, Gray DT, Bower TC, Cherry KJ Jr, et al. Graft-related complications after abdominal aortic aneurysm repair: Reassurance from a 36-year population-based experience. J Vasc Surg 1997;25(2):277–84; discussion 285–6.

42. LeSar CJ, Meier GH. Complications of endovascular abdominal aortic aneurysm exclusion: Evolving concepts. In: Veith FJ, Baum RA (eds). Endoleaks & Endotension: Current Consensus on Their Nature and Significance. New York: Marcel Dekker, 2003.

43. Giannoni MF, Palombo G, Sbarigia E, Speziale F, Zaccaria A, Fiorani P. Contrast-enhanced ultrasound imaging for aortic stent-graft surveillance. J Endovasc Ther 2003;10(2): 208–17.

44. Lie T, Lundbom J, Hatlinghus S, Gronningsaeter A, Ommedal S, Aadahl P, et al. Ultrasound imaging during endovascular abdominal aortic aneurysm repair using the Stentor bifurcated endograft. J Endovasc Surg 1997;4(3): 272–8.

45. Sato DT, Goff CD, Gregory RT, Robinson KD, Carter KA, Herts BR, et al. Endoleak after aortic stent graft repair: Diagnosis by color duplex ultrasound scan versus computed tomography scan. J Vasc Surg 1998;28(4):657–63.

46. Heilberger P, Schunn C, Ritter W, Weber S, Raithel D. Postoperative color flow duplex scanning in aortic endografting. J Endovasc Surg 1997;4(3):262–71.

47. Bargellini I, Napoli V, Petruzzi P, Cioni R, Vignali C, Sardella SG, et al. Type II lumbar endoleaks: Hemodynamic differentiation by contrast-enhanced ultrasound scanning and influence on aneurysm enlargement after endovascular aneurysm repair. J Vasc Surg 2000;41(1):10–8.

48. Bendick PJ, Bove PG, Long GW, Zelenock GB, Brown OW, Shanley CJ. Efficacy of ultrasound scan contrast agents in the noninvasive follow-up of aortic stent grafts. J Vasc Surg 2003;37(2):381–5.

49. McWilliams RG, Martin J, White D, Gould DA, Rowlands PC, Haycox A, et al. Detection of endoleak with enhanced

ultrasound imaging: Comparison with biphasic computed tomography. J Endovasc Ther 2002;9(2):170–9.

50. Pages S, Favre JP, Cerisier A, Pyneeandee S, Boissier C, Veyret C. Comparison of color duplex ultrasound and computed tomography scan for surveillance after aortic endografting. Ann Vasc Surg 2001;15(2):155–62.

51. Johnson BL, Dalman RL. Duplex surveillance of abdominal aortic stent grafts. Semin Vasc Surg 2001;14(3):227–32.

52. Fletcher J, Saker K, Batiste P, Dyer S. Colour Doppler diagnosis of perigraft flow following endovascular repair of abdominal aortic aneurysm. Int Angiol 2000;19(4):326–30.

53. McWilliams RG, Martin J, White D, Gould DA, Harris PL, Fear SC, et al. Use of contrast-enhanced ultrasound in follow-up after endovascular aortic aneurysm repair. J Vasc Intervent Radiol 1999;10(8):1107–14.

54. Fillinger MF. Postoperative imaging after endovascular AAA repair. Semin Vasc Surg 1999;12(4):327–38.

55. Parent FN 3rd, Godziachvili V, Meier GH 3rd, Parker FM, Carter K, Gayle RG, et al. Endograft limb occlusion and stenosis after ANCURE endovascular abdominal aneurysm repair. J Vasc Surg 2002;35(4):686–90.

56. van der Laan MJ, Teutelink A, Meijer R, Wixon CL, Blankensteijn JD. Noninvasive evaluation of the effectiveness of endovascular AAA exclusion. J Endovasc Ther 2003;10(3):458–62.

57. Kaspersen JH, Sjolie E, Wesche J, Asland J, Lundbom J, Odegard A, et al. Three-dimensional ultrasound-based navigation combined with preoperative CT during abdominal interventions: A feasibility study. Cardiovasc Intervent Radiol 2003;26(4):347–56.

58. Lipski DA, Ernst CB. Natural history of the residual infrarenal aorta after infrarenal abdominal aortic aneurysm repair. J Vasc Surg 1998;27(5):805–11; discussion 811–2.

59. Napoli V, Bargellini I, Sardella SG, Petruzzi P, Cioni R, Vignali C, et al. Abdominal aortic aneurysm: Contrast-enhanced US for missed endoleaks after endoluminal repair. Radiology 2004;233(1):217–25.

60. Nelms CR, Carter KA, Meier GH, Gayle RG, Parent FN, Demasi RJ, et al. A technique to improve the confidence of color duplex ultrasound assessment of aortic endografts: The use of contrast agents. J Vasc Technol 2003;27(2):88–92.

61. Chaikof EL, Blankensteijn JD, Harris PL, White GH, Zarins CK, Bernhard VM, et al. Reporting standards for endovascular aortic aneurysm repair. J Vasc Surg 2002;35(5):1048–60.

Section VII
Miscellaneous

45

Transcutaneous Oxygen Tension: Principles and Applications

Jeffrey L. Ballard

Empiric means of assessing foot perfusion are not adequate due to lack of sensitivity and specificity. Fortunately, ongoing research has led to the discovery of a number of different objective tools that can be used to assess the degree of foot ischemia. Among the validated modalities, transcutaneous oxygen ($tcpO_2$) tension has proven to be quite useful in the evaluation of lower extremity ischemia. The unique design of the transcutaneous sensor makes it possible to obtain accurate measurements of oxygen (pO_2) and carbon dioxide (pCO_2) tension on the surface of the skin. This chapter will discuss the physiology of $tcpO_2$ measurements and demonstrate how these measurements can be used for amputation level determination. In addition, $tcpO_2$ measurements will be shown to be essential for the prospective management of diabetic patients with foot ischemia as well as nondiabetic patients with chronic lower extremity ischemia.

Physiology of the Measurement

Modern transcutaneous instrumentation has improved considerably from the viewpoint of maintenance, application, and routine use. A small sensor is applied to the skin with an airtight self-adhesive fixation ring. The heating element of the transcutaneous sensor increases the temperature beneath the sensor to 44°C. Heating the sensor creates local skin hyperemia, a decrease in blood flow resistance, and compensatory arteriolarization of capillary blood. This effectively raises the pO_2 and decreases the pCO_2 values toward arterial levels.[1,2] Contact liquid between the skin and sensor allows the underlying dermal tissue pO_2 to be in equilibrium with the sensor after 15–20 min. In practice, stable $tcpO_2$ readings are generally achieved in 20–30 min.

$TcpO_2$ monitoring is completely noninvasive and atraumatic if sensor placement at one skin site is limited to a maximum of 4 h. The test can be accomplished with the patient comfortably supine at ambient room temperature in an outpatient setting. Oxygen inhalation, change in limb position, and chest wall normalized $tcpO_2$ values are not part of our standard protocol.[3–5] We have experience with the Novametrix 800 monitor (Novametrix Medical Systems, Wallingford, CT), which has three modified Clark electrodes for simultaneous recording of skin oxygen tension at three sites (Figure 45–1). As demonstrated in Figure 45–2, the sensors are usually placed on the dorsal aspect of the forefoot between the great and second toe roughly 5 cm proximal to the second toe tip (forefoot measurement), on the medial aspect of the hindfoot in front of or behind the malleolus (hindfoot measurement), and 10 cm below the patella on the medial aspect of the calf (below-knee measurement). The sensor can also be placed 10 cm above the patella on the medial aspect of the thigh for an above-knee measurement. Inaccurate readings may occur if the sensor is placed over a tendon or exposed bone. For optimal results, the sensor should be placed on skin that is free of edema, ulceration, hyperkeratosis, or cellulitis.

Tissue ischemia or inadequate perfusion to support major wound healing is presumed when the absolute $tcpO_2$ value is less than 30 mm Hg. For practical purposes, a low $tcpO_2$ value can be interpreted as either reduced generalized arterial pO_2, as in the case of patients suffering from cardiopulmonary diseases, or reduced regional blood flow due to impaired arterial pO_2 supply from arteriosclerosis. Many investigators have reported that wound healing can occur in some patients with a low $tcpO_2$ value.[6–16] This can be partially explained by the nonlinear relationship between $tcpO_2$ and cutaneous blood flow. Matsen et al.[12] reported that $tcpO_2$ measurements are mostly dependent on arterial–venous gradients and cutaneous vascular resistance. In essence, there can be nutritive blood flow to the skin even with a $tcpO_2$ level of 0 mm Hg.

One of the techniques used to improve the accuracy of $tcpO_2$ measurements is sensor probe heating (44°C),

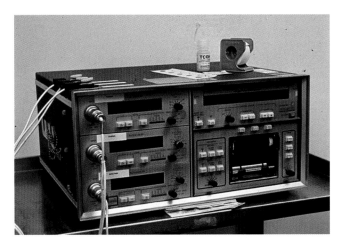

FIGURE 45–1. Novametrix 800 tcpO₂ monitor with three modified Clark electrodes.

quite localized and one value may not represent the overall degree of limb ischemia. Second, as previously mentioned, there may still be some nutritive flow to the skin despite a tcpO₂ level of 0 mm Hg.

Although in theory a tcpO₂ value of 0 mm Hg at a proposed site of amputation does not always indicate ischemia that precludes healing, a tcpO₂ level of 20 mm Hg or less clearly indicates severe limb ischemia. In the Wyss study,[13] a tcpO₂ measurement of 20 mm Hg or less was associated with a rate of failure for amputations distal to the knee that was more than 10 times the 4% rate of failure in patients who had a tcpO₂ level of more than 20 mm Hg.

which minimizes local vascular resistance. This makes tcpO₂ tension more linear with respect to cutaneous blood flow. Additional techniques used to improve tcpO₂ accuracy include measurements performed before and after oxygen inhalation or change in limb position, oxygen isobar extremity mapping, and tcpO₂ recovery half-time.

Wyss et al.[13] evaluated the results of tcpO₂ measurements used as a predictor of successful wound healing following amputation. The study analyzed 162 patients who had 206 lower extremity amputations. It was concluded that tcpO₂ is a reliable indicator of local tissue ischemia and that it can be used to predict failure of amputation healing due to tissue ischemia. However, there are two theoretical inadequacies that must be considered when using tcpO₂ measurements. First, the measurement is

Clinical Applications in Peripheral Vascular Disease

Selecting the Appropriate Amputation Level

There have been numerous reports on the successful use of tcpO₂ measurements to determine the appropriate lower extremity amputation level.[6–16] One of the initial reports on this topic was by Franzeck et al.[7] Mean tcpO₂ levels in patients who experienced primary healing of a lower extremity amputation were compared to those of patients who failed to heal their amputation. The respective values for healing and nonhealing were 36.5 ± 17.5 and less than 30 mm Hg. However, three of nine patients whose tcpO₂ level was less than 10 mm Hg healed primarily.

In a study of below-knee amputations, Burgess et al.[6] noted that all 15 amputations that were associated with a tcpO₂ level greater than 40 mm Hg healed. Primary wound healing was noted in 17 of 19 below-knee amputations with a tcpO₂ measurement between 1 and 40 mm Hg, but none of the three patients with a below-knee level of 0 mm Hg healed the amputation. Katsamouris et al.[9] reported that lower extremity amputations healed in all 17 patients with a tcpO₂ level greater than 38 mm Hg or a pO₂ index (chest wall control site) greater than 0.59. Ratliff et al.[11] reported that below-knee amputations healed in 18 patients with a tcpO₂ measurement greater than 35 mm Hg, whereas healing failed in 10 of 15 patients with a tcpO₂ value less than 35 mm Hg. In a study of 42 lower extremity amputations (28 below-knee and 14 above-knee), Christiansen and Klarke[14] found that 27 of 31 patients with a tcpO₂ level greater than 30 mm Hg healed primarily. Seven patients with values between 20 and 30 mm Hg healed, although four patients had delayed healing. The amputation stumps of all four patients with a value below 20 mm Hg failed to heal because of skin necrosis.

Data from Wyss et al.[13] are comparable to those yielded by a prospective study evaluating multiple tests used for

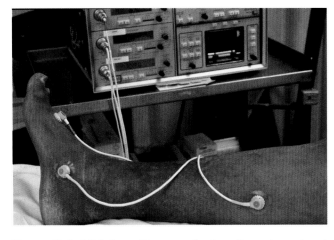

FIGURE 45–2. Right leg with sensors in place. Paper tape, placed over the sensor cup, can assist in keeping the electrode stable and in constant contact with skin.

amputation level selection. In this study, $tcpO_2$ measurements were prospectively compared to transcutaneous carbon dioxide tension, transcutaneous oxygen-to-carbon dioxide tension, foot-to-chest $tcpO_2$ tension, intradermal xenon-133 clearance level, ankle-brachial index (ABI), and the absolute popliteal artery pressure for accuracy in amputation level selection. All metabolic variables exhibited a high degree of statistical accuracy in predicting amputation healing, but none of the other tests showed statistical reliability. All amputations in this study (transmetatarsal, below-knee, and above-knee) healed primarily when the $tcpO_2$ measurement was greater than 20 mm Hg and there were no false-positive or false-negative results.[10] It was also noted that successful prediction of amputation healing for any of the metabolic parameters was not affected by the presence of diabetes mellitus. This finding is similar to the observation of Wyss et al.[13]

In contrast to lower extremity amputations in nondiabetics, which usually result in peripheral vascular disease primarily, most amputations in diabetic patients result from various combinations of contributing causes including neuropathy, ischemia, alterations of white cell function, infection or gangrene, faulty wound healing, cutaneous ulceration, and minor trauma.[15] Malone et al.[10] and Christensen and Klarke[14] concluded that a $tcpO_2$ tension of 20 mm Hg or more accurately predicted amputation site healing and found no difference in the healing rate between diabetics and nondiabetics. Computerized analysis of various transcutaneous metabolic parameters by Malone et al.[10] demonstrated a high association with primary amputation site healing with the following values: $tcpO_2$ tension greater than 20 mm Hg, transcutaneous carbon dioxide value less than 40.5 mm Hg, transcutaneous oxygen-to-transcutaneous carbon dioxide index greater than 0.472, and foot-to-chest $tcpO_2$ index greater than 0.442.

The above data reinforce the fact that elective lower extremity amputation should not be performed without objective testing to ensure selection of the most distal amputation site that will heal primarily yet allow removal of infected, painful, or ischemic tissue.[15,16] A variety of techniques are available to achieve this, depending on available equipment, the amputation level under consideration, and the accuracy of the chosen modality.[16] $TcpO_2$ measurements continue to be a reliable technique; however, they are not suitable for whole limb mapping.

The ultimate role of any method used for amputation level determination is to inform the surgeon of the quantitative risk of nonhealing at the proposed site of surgery. The level of amputation can then be decided on the basis of this objective finding in conjunction with surgeon clinical judgment and patient physical findings. For example, a surgeon might perform an amputation distal to the knee through a site with a very low $tcpO_2$ level in a patient who is well motivated, relatively young, and otherwise healthy. Such an amputation would almost certainly be ruled out in a fragile elderly person who faces a limited prospect for successful rehabilitation.

Prospective Treatment of Diabetic Foot Problems

Successful treatment of the patient with diabetes and limb-threatening ischemia requires an accurate assessment of limb perfusion. Presenting clinical symptoms may be misleading. Physical examination of pedal pulses or ABI may not be accurate due to the noncompressible nature of a diabetic patient's peripheral arteries. Often, the cause of the presenting foot problem is multifactorial and commonly used noninvasive lower extremity hemodynamic studies lack discriminative accuracy. On the other hand, arteriography is ultimately accurate. However, it is invasive, expensive, and carries a small but well-defined set of associated complications.[17,18] In this setting, $tcpO_2$ measurements can be extremely useful as they are noninvasive, inexpensive, and reproducible.[19–24]

In a clinical experience reported by Ballard et al.,[25] $tcpO_2$ measurements were prospectively demonstrated to accurately predict severity of foot ischemia in patients with diabetes. Based on clinical experience and previously published amputation level determination data, an absolute transmetatarsal $tcpO_2$ measurement of 30 mm Hg was used as the threshold value for selection of a treatment option (Table 45–1). If the level was 30 mm Hg or greater, the patient's foot problem was managed conservatively with local wound care, wound debridement, or minor foot amputation. If the level was less than 30 mm Hg, arteriography of the involved limb was performed to plan arterial reconstruction or to perform percutaneous intervention to improve foot perfusion.

Thirty-one of 36 (86%) limbs in the conservatively managed group were treated successfully including 73%

TABLE 45–1. Algorithm for elective management of the diabetic patient with limb-threatening foot ischemia.

A. If forefoot/hindfoot $tcpO_2$ level is ≥30 mm Hg (with or without a palpable pedal pulse):
Outpatient wound care, wound debridement or minor foot amputation.

B. If forefoot/hindfoot $tcpO_2$ level is <30 mm Hg or conservative treatment is unsuccessful after 4–6 weeks:
Arteriography, with revascularization as needed.

C. If forefoot/hindfoot $tcpO_2$ <30 mm Hg and there is pedal edema or cellulitis:
Repeat test after resolution, before proceeding with arteriography.

D. If there is calcaneal gangrene/nonhealing ulcer:
Use higher hindfoot $tcpO_2$ threshold of 40 mm Hg and obtain arteriogram after 2–4 weeks of unsuccessful conservative treatment.

(11/15 feet) of limbs without a palpable pedal pulse. The mean time to wound healing was 6.85 weeks and there were five treatment failures. In the operative/endovascular group, 83.3% of limbs achieved a transmetatarsal (TM) tcpO$_2$ level ≥ 30 mm Hg after treatment. Twenty-two of 26 (85%) limbs in this group had complete resolution of their presenting foot problem. The mean time to wound healing was 9.52 weeks. Treatment failures eventually led to three below-knee amputations (one failed necessitating revision to the above-knee level) and one above-knee amputation.

The pretreatment pedal pulse examination was more accurate than an ABI in predicting forefoot tcpO$_2$ values above or below 30 mm Hg. Further, an abnormal arteriogram was predicted by both a low TM tcpO$_2$ level and the absence of a palpable pedal pulse, but not by an ABI < 0.60. The presence of a pedal pulse was 100% accurate in identifying limbs with a TM tcpO$_2$ ≥ 30 mm Hg, but there were an additional 17 limbs with a measurement ≥ 30 mm Hg and no palpable pedal pulse. Following arterial bypass or angioplasty, a TM tcpO$_2$ level ≥ 30 mm Hg was highly accurate in predicting a successful outcome.[26] Ultimately, an initial or postintervention TM tcpO$_2$ level ≥ 30 mm Hg was more accurate than a palpable pulse in predicting either wound healing or resolution of rest pain. An ABI ≥ 0.60 was also associated with a successful outcome, but due to noncompressible vessels, this was able to be calculated only in 41/62 (66%) limbs.

Certainly diabetic patients without pedal pulses do have arteriosclerotic lesions, some of which can be reconstructed. However, this prospective study demonstrated that such surgical revascularization is not obligatory.[27] In fact, well-performed tcpO$_2$ measurements predicted distal ischemic wound healing in 90% of cases. Furthermore, conservative management was not only cost effective when compared to surgical or endovascular revascularization, but time to wound healing was not statistically significantly different between the two groups (6.84 weeks versus 9.52 weeks, p = 0.169).

As demonstrated in the study just outlined above, an absolute TM tcpO$_2$ level ≥ 30 mm Hg appears to be an accurate cut-off point for the selection of treatment for almost all diabetic foot problems. The conservative management scheme, however, requires diligent patient follow-up. There must be a commitment by the surgeon to perform wound debridements and staged procedures (i.e., minor foot amputations or split-thickness skin grafts). Proper outpatient wound care is essential. Finally, a higher TM tcpO$_2$ threshold (40 mm Hg) should be used to select management of calcaneal gangrene or extensive nonhealing ulcerations. Table 45–1 demonstrates an algorithm for the elective management of diabetic patients with limb-threatening ischemia based on tcpO$_2$ level.

Padberg *et al.*[26] confirmed our previous findings and demonstrated that tcpO$_2$ measurements alone are sufficient to objectively stratify the degree of lower extremity arterial ischemia. They compared tcpO$_2$ measurements to arterial segmental pressures (ASP) and arterial segmental indices (ASI) in 204 ischemic lower extremity sites in patients with either diabetes, chronic renal failure, or neither disease process. Stepwise multiple regression analysis demonstrated that tcpO$_2$ mapping was superior to ASP and ASI for all endpoints. As demonstrated by others, predictive accuracy of tcpO$_2$ measurements was unaffected by the presence of diabetes and ASP and ASI were misleading and inaccurate. Interestingly, because of the reduced accuracy of ASP and ASI, tcpO$_2$ remained the diagnostic modality of choice even for the nondiabetic patient with arterial ischemia of the lower extremity.

Finally, Petrakis and Sciacca[27] used distal limb tcpO$_2$ measurements as a prognostic parameter in the selection of diabetic patients for placement of a permanent spinal cord stimulation device. Sixty diabetic patients had implantation of a spinal cord electrical generator after failed conservative or surgical treatment of severe peripheral vascular disease. The clinical peripheral vascular disease status of each patient was either Fontaine's stage III or IV. Forefoot and hindfoot tcpO$_2$ measurements were compared to toe pressure Doppler measurements before device implantation as well as 2 and 4 weeks postoperatively. Pain relief of over 75% and foot salvage were achieved in 35 patients, while partial success with pain relief greater than 50% and foot salvage for at least 6 months was obtained in 12 other patients. Amputation for persistent gangrene, nonhealing ulceration, or unrelenting rest pain was performed in the remaining 13 patients.

Interestingly, clinical improvement and foot salvage were both associated with a significant increase in the 2-week postoperative tcpO$_2$ measurement while the ABI and toe pressure did not change under spinal cord stimulation. These data suggest that a 2-week testing period before permanent spinal cord stimulation is useful not only for prognosis but also for cost saving. Only patients who experience a significant increase in distal limb tcpO$_2$ in addition to pain relief should be considered for permanent implantation of a spinal cord stimulator.

Prospective Treatment of Nondiabetic Patients with Chronic Lower Extremity Ischemia

Much the same as described above for the treatment of diabetic patients, tcpO$_2$ measurements can be useful for selecting management of ill-defined leg/foot complaints, particularly in elderly patients with multiple medical problems. For instance, an adequate tcpO$_2$ level (≥ 30 mm Hg) at the forefoot and hindfoot may obviate the need for an arteriogram and support nonoperative management. On the other hand, a low tcpO$_2$ level likely indicates a situation that will require a higher level of care. The potential need for arteriography and arterial revascularization can be thoroughly discussed with the patient and family prior to treatment. This ensures reasonable expectations. Finally, a dramatic improvement in tcpO$_2$ measurement following treatment is not only gratifying, but at least 90% of patients will experience a successful outcome.

TcpO$_2$ measurements can also be used to determine whether an invasive intraarterial treatment has been successful at the skin level. Wagner et al.[28] recently demonstrated that percutaneous transluminal angioplasty (PTA) has a positive effect on oxygen supply to the skin in patients with peripheral arterial occlusive disease (PAOD). In this study, 34 patients with PAOD had tcpO$_2$ measurements obtained at the dorsum of the foot 1 day before PTA, during PTA, 1 day after PTA, and 6 weeks after PTA. A significant increase in tcpO$_2$ was noted immediately following PTA as well as 1 day and 6 weeks later.

Arroyo and colleagues[29] used tcpO$_2$ measurements to determine when previously ischemic tissue had adequate perfusion to support major wound healing. Eleven patients with severe chronic limb ischemia defined as a forefoot tcpO$_2 \leq 30\,$mmHg were entered into this prospective study. TcpO$_2$ measurements were recorded prior to lower extremity bypass and on postoperative days 1, 2, and 3. A statistically significant increase in mean tcpO$_2$ pressure was observed between the preoperative and the day 3 postoperative measurements. Despite this finding, some bypass patients still had low tcpO$_2$ values (<30 mmHg) even on postoperative day 3. Nevertheless, this small clinical series suggests that unless urgent, adjunctive minor foot amputation or major debridement should wait until at least 3 days after successful lower extremity bypass. This will ensure that there is now adequate perfusion at the foot level to support major wound healing. This clinical recommendation could also be used to select appropriate timing of minor foot amputations or major debridements that are performed after endovascular procedures.

Finally, tcpO$_2$ measurements are even being used to noninvasively detect lesions in the arterial network supplying blood flow to the hypogastric circulation. A study was recently performed by Abraham et al.[30] in which they selected 43 patients suspected of proximal aortoiliac occlusive disease and 34 without suspected proximal ischemia. TcpO$_2$ measurements were obtained from the buttock region bilaterally in addition to a chest reference value. Arteriography was compared to normalized tcpO$_2$ measurements during and after treadmill exercise in addition to other comparisons. A mean drop in the tcpO$_2$ measurement of at least 15 mmHg in either group was both sensitive (range 79–83%) and specific (range 82–86%) for the diagnosis of a positive arteriogram. The arteriogram was defined as positive when there was at least a 75% stenosis noted on the same side as the tcpO$_2$ drop in one or more of the following arteries: aorta, common iliac, or internal iliac. Thus it appears that an exercise-induced drop in buttock tcpO$_2$ pressure is a sensitive and specific indicator of a hemodynamically significant lesion proximal to or within the hypogastric artery. These measurements could be used to noninvasively and objectively assess the skin level response to endovascular or surgical treatment of infrarenal aortic or proximal iliac artery lesions.

References

1. Baumbach P. Understanding transcutaneous PO$_2$ and PCO$_2$ measurements. Radiometer A/S, Copenhagen 1986;1–54.
2. Steenfos HH, Baumbach P. Transcutaneous PO$_2$ in peripheral vascular disease. Radiometer A/S, Copenhagen 1986;1–18.
3. Moosa HH, Peitzman AB, Makaroun MS, Webster MW, Steed DL. Transcutaneous oxygen measurements in lower extremity ischemia: Effects of position, oxygen inhalation, and arterial reconstruction. Surgery 1988;103(2):193–198.
4. Hauser CJ, Appel P, Shoemaker WC. Pathophysiologic classification of peripheral vascular disease by positional changes in regional transcutaneous oxygen tension. Surgery 1984;95(6):689–693.
5. Larsen JF, Jensen BV, Christensen KS, Egeblad K. Forefoot transcutaneous oxygen tension at different leg positions in patients with peripheral vascular disease. Eur J Vasc Surg 1990;4:185–189.
6. Burgess EM, et al. Segmental transcutaneous measurements of PO$_2$ in patients requiring below the knee amputations for peripheral vascular insufficiency. J Bone Joint Surg (Am) 1982;64:378–392.
7. Franzeck UK, et al. Transcutaneous PO$_2$ measurement in health on peripheral arterial occlusive disease. Surgery 1982;91:156–163.
8. Friedmann LW. The prosthesis—immediate or delayed fitting? Angiology 1972;23:513–524.
9. Katsamouris A, et al. Transcutaneous oxygen tension in selection of amputation level. Am J Surg 1984;147:510–516.
10. Malone JM, et al. Prospective comparison of noninvasive techniques for amputation level selection. Am J Surg 1987;154:179–184.
11. Ratliff DA, et al. Prediction of amputation healing: The role of transcutaneous PO$_2$ assessment. Br J Surg 1984;71:219–222.
12. Matsen FA, et al. The relationship of transcutaneous PO$_2$ and laser Doppler measurements in human model of local arterial insufficiency. Surg Gynecol Obstet 1984;159:418–422.
13. Wyss CR, et al. Transcutaneous oxygen tension as a predictor of success after an amputation. J Bone Joint Surg (Am) 1988;70:203–207.
14. Christensen KS, Klarke M. Transcutaneous oxygen measurement in peripheral occlusive disease: An indicator of wound healing in leg amputation. J Bone Joint Surg (Br) 1986;68:423–426.

(3–8mm thick) than 2D TOF. Very thin (<1mm thick) partitions are reconstructed from these tissue volume slabs, thus increasing spatial resolution. Although 3D MRA can be viewed as a stack of 2D images, better resolution of 3D methods allows for the use of multiplanar reformatting (MPR). MPR creates images from multiple views that optimize the visualization of the tissue. Images are processed using algorithms to display the maximum intensity of the voxels, referred to as *maximum intensity projection* (MIP).[1]

Gadolinium is the most commonly used contrast agent. Gadolinium, a heavy metal analogue chelated with diethylenetriaminepentaacetic acid (DTPA), is excreted by glomerular filtration and is not known to be nephrotoxic. Gadolinium is a potent T_1 relaxing agent and improves image resolution by increasing the contrast between blood and surrounding soft tissue. A dose-timing curve is determined so that proper timing of arterial scanning can be calculated for the particular arterial bed to be examined. Using gadolinium with the 3D TOF technique results in significant imaging time reduction, reduced flow void artifacts, elimination of in-plane flow defects, and improved spatial resolution (Figures 46–1 and 46–2).[4]

The two commonly used methods for imaging the lower extremity peripheral arteries are floating table or bolus chase 3D CE MRA and time-resolved peripheral MRA. Floating table MRA involves a series of 3D acquisitions with chasing of the contrast down the lower extremities. There are usually three stations; the

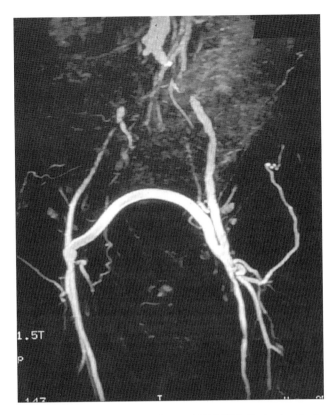

FIGURE 46–2. Gadolinium-enhanced 3D TOF eliminates the in-plane flow defects seen with 2D TOF, allowing visualization of this femoral-to-femoral bypass.

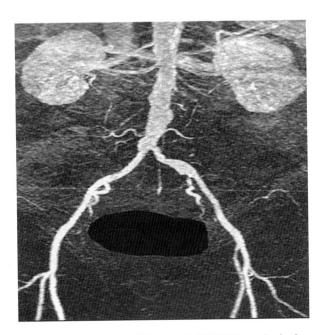

FIGURE 46–1. Using gadolinium with 3D TOF results in fewer flow void artifacts and improved spatial resolution.

aortoiliac segment, thigh segment, and lower leg and foot segment. Unlike 3D CE MRA, time-resolved MRA involves a series of three separate low-dose contrast injections at each station. Image subtraction is used to eliminate signal from the prior injection. These techniques can be used to complement the images obtained from 2D TOF.[5,6]

Phase-contrast MRA (PCA) is another technique better suited for evaluating multiplanar flow through complex vascular beds (intracranial or pelvic vessels). PC angiography takes advantage of the fact that protons undergo a change in the phase of their rotation as they move through a magnetic field.[4] The magnitude of the phase change is proportional to the velocity of the moving protons in the blood. Background suppression is greater for phase contrast than for TOF because only moving protons can generate a signal, thus making PCA even more sensitive to slow flow. In the PCA technique, the sequences are programmed to assign a specific MR signal phase to each velocity of blood flow. Faster moving protons in blood accumulate greater phase shifts relative to slowly flowing blood. Thus, this technique can also be used to measure blood flow velocities.

Use of Magnetic Resonance Arteriography for Lower Extremity Arterial Occlusive Disease

MRA plays an increasingly important role in the diagnosis and management of lower extremity arterial occlusive disease. Because of its noninvasive nature, safety, cost savings, and accuracy, MRA has become the imaging modality of choice at our institution for patients being considered for arterial revascularization procedures. MRA is extremely accurate for localization of disease, detection of hemodynamically significant stenoses, and distinguishing focal from long-segment occlusive disease.

In our practice, we have found that MRA is particularly advantageous for evaluating patients with diabetes mellitus, with complex distal occlusive disease, and for the evaluation of patients with chronic renal insufficiency. In patients with arterial occlusive disease by physical examination and noninvasive studies, MRA is used to confirm the diagnosis and to determine localization of disease and to distinguish focal from long-segment stenosis or occlusion (Figure 46–3). Patients found to have short-segment stenoses can be treated with percutaneous balloon angioplasty and/or stenting (Figure 46–4). The ability of MRA to define the pattern of disease helps in planning arterial access sites (retrograde or antegrade), and makes possible a more focused examination using less ionized con-

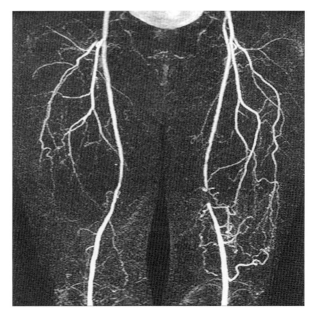

FIGURE 46–3. MRA in this patient with claudication demonstrates a short segment occlusion of the superficial femoral artery. Having this information prior to surgery would influence the decision to proceed with percutaneous revascularization rather than femoral popliteal bypass.

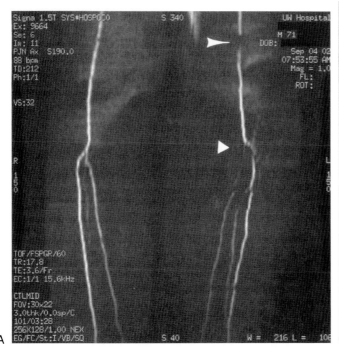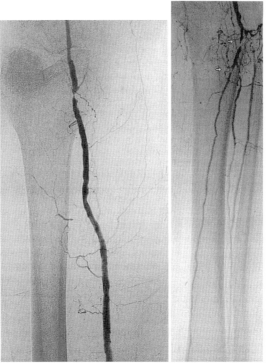

FIGURE 46–4. (A) MRA in a patient with diabetes mellitus who suffered from a nonhealing ulcer demonstrates several areas of focal stenosis. (B) As the patient was at high risk for open surgical revascularization, he was treated with percutaneous angioplasty. This arteriogram performed at the time of PTA confirms the focal lesions seen on MRA.

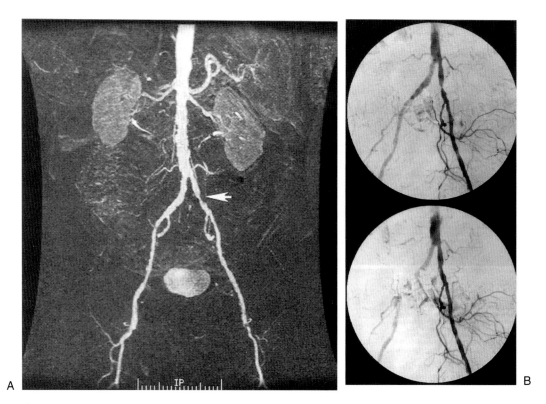

FIGURE 46–5. (A) MRA demonstrates a focal left iliac stenosis (arrow) as well as a left superficial femoral artery occlusion. (B) The lesion was treated intraoperatively at the time of femoral popliteal bypass. The intraoperative arteriogram demonstrates the lesion before (top) and after (bottom) angioplasty of the iliac lesion.

trast. Patients with diffuse disease and limb-threatening ischemia may require hybridized procedures using percutaneous angioplasty and/or stenting for treatment of concomitant focal iliac lesions at the time of distal bypass (Figure 46–5). In patients with previous arteriography and poorly defined distal target vessels, MRA has proven very useful in detecting occult runoff channels that can be used for distal bypass. The additional information obtained from viewing axial images can aid in the identification of soft tissue abnormalities and aneurysmal disease (Figure 46–6).

Several reports have been published demonstrating the utility of MRA in the preoperative planning for lower extremity revascularization. Owen et al. studied 25 extremities with both contrast arteriography and 2D TOF MRA. Discrepancies were found in 18 of the 25 limbs, with superior detection of runoff vessels by MRA. Unlike contrast arteriography, MRA correctly identified all vessels found to be patent at surgery.[7] The use of MRA in these patients avoided the need for blind exploration of runoff vessels and led to limb salvage procedures that had not been previously regarded as possible, based on the preoperative contrast arteriogram. In a study by Hoch et al., 50 ischemic lower limbs in 45 patients were examined with both conventional contrast digital subtraction (DSA) angiography and 2D TOF MRA. Interpretation of MRA and DSA studies correlated exactly in 315 (89.5%) of 352 arterial segments. The MRA and DSA interpretations disagreed in 28 (13.8%) of 203 infrageniculate arteries compared with only 8 (5.6%) disagreements in the suprageniculate arterial segments. MRA predicted the level of arterial reconstruction in all 23 limbs that required arterial bypass and in 18 of 19 (94.7%) limbs treated with percutaneous angioplasty. Importantly, they also noted a 31% ($756) cost savings with MRA compared to DSA.[8]

Using more contemporary 3D CE MRA, Leiner et al. compared DSA to MRA in 23 patients with critical limb ischemia. In their study, MRA detected more patent arteries than DSA in this patient population.[9] Similarly, in a study of 50 patients by Steffens et al., MRA imaging of runoff vessels in the calf in six patients was clearly superior to DSA.[10] Due to problems with timing and low flow states in the distal infrageniculate arteries, DSA may fail to identify a suitable distal target vessel, especially if the injection of contrast is made at the aortic level. Because of its ability to detect low flow states, MRA can be very useful in evaluating these difficult cases (Figure 46–7). In our experience, distal runoff vessels not visualized by MRA are not suitable target vessels for surgical bypass. A meta-analysis by Nelemans et al. clearly demonstrated the superiority of 3D CE MRA to 2D TOF with sensitivities from 92% to 100% and specificities from 91% to 100%.[11]

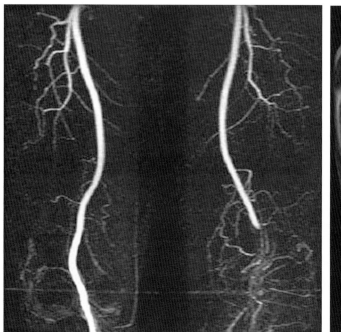

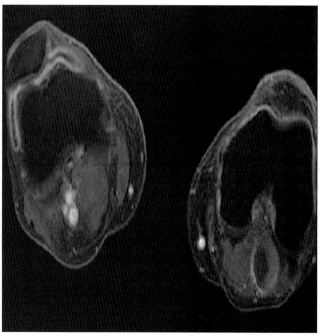

A   B

FIGURE 46–6. (A) MRA demonstrates complete occlusion of the left popliteal artery. (B) Axial images show the thrombosed left popliteal aneurysm.

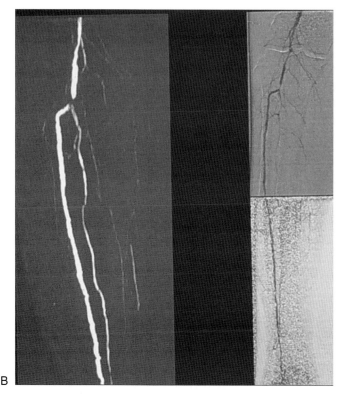

A,B

FIGURE 46–7. (A) Contrast arteriography in this 64-year-old male with a nonhealing ulcer failed to detect adequate runoff vessels. (B) 2D TOF MRA, because of its excellent sensitivity to slow flow, demonstrates a small but patent peroneal artery (arrow).

Use of Magnetic Resonance Arteriography to Detect Restenosis following Lower Extremity Grafting

At our institution, patients undergo routine pulse volume recording and duplex surveillance following lower extremity arterial bypass or percutaneous intervention. When noninvasive tests suggest impending graft failure, MRA is used to identify the location and severity of the occlusive lesions threatening graft function. Stenotic lesions due to intimal hyperplasia at the anastomotic sites or within autogenous grafts can be identified and distinguished from disease progression in host vessels proximal or distal to the graft (Figure 46–8). Surgical revision is usually required for anastomotic or mid autogenous graft stenoses whereas focal stenoses secondary to progressive disease can often be treated with percutaneous angioplasty and/or stenting.

In contrast to the 2D TOF methods, contrast-enhanced MRA does not have the problem with artifacts created by surgical clips. Also, the 3D data set can be viewed in several projections, providing an additional advantage over conventional DSA.[1] In a study by Bendib et al., 3D CE MRA was found to be 91% sensitive and 97% specific for detecting graft stenosis.[12] Meissner et al. studied 26 distal bypass grafts using CE moving table MRA and duplex ultrasound, with DSA as the reference standard. Duplex ultrasound overlooked four high-grade stenoses that were correctly identified by MRA. While duplex

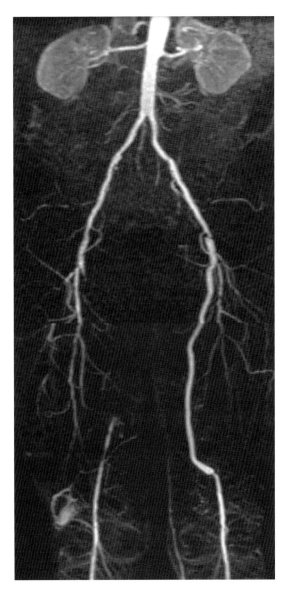

FIGURE 46–8. MRA demonstrating stenosis at both the proximal and distal anastomosis of this femoral popliteal graft.

ultrasound was 90–97% accurate in identifying failing grafts, MRA was 100% accurate. It was suggested that MRA be used routinely for follow-up of patients undergoing infrapopliteal bypass surgery.[13] Similarly, Bertschinger et al. demonstrated 100% accuracy of 3D CE MRA in the surveillance of peripheral artery bypass grafts when compared to DSA.[14]

Limitations of Magnetic Resonance Arteriography

Although 2D and 3D TOF MRA have been shown to be accurate for the assessment of infrainguinal disease, these methods have a few limitations.[2] Disadvantages include sensitivity to flow traveling in the same plane as the magnetic field, creating an imaging void.[15] Motion can severely degrade image quality and spatial resolution resulting in overestimation of disease severity. Areas of turbulent arterial flow within a vessel can also result in signal loss, or a "flow void," because of intervoxel dephasing. Most of these limitations have been overcome by the use of 3D TOF and the addition of gadolinium contrast. Still, because of signal loss at or distal to a stenotic vascular lesion, there is a tendency to overestimate the degree of stenosis. New advances in 3D CE techniques have overcome many of these limitations.

Unfortunately, not all patients are good candidates for MRA. Absolute contraindications to MRA include cardiac pacemakers, automatic cardiac defibrillator devices, cerebral aneurysm clips, and metal within the eyes (such as old shrapnel injuries). Although many patients have problems with claustrophobia, this is usually overcome with mild sedation.[2] With the equipment available at our institution, patients larger than 380 pounds are unable to undergo MRA. MRI is adversely affected by movement during the RF pulse sequences. Problems with swallowing, respiratory motion, and intestinal peristalsis decrease the image quality. When imaging the arterial system of the lower extremities, it is important to have a cooperative patient, as physical movements greatly affect the image quality. Patients with severe respiratory disease may have problems lying flat for the examination. It is important to choose patients who are cooperative and able to follow instructions.[2]

Metallic stents such as the Palmaz stent, vena cava filters, ferromagnetic clips, and prosthetic joints cause significant artifact and severely limit the ability to image the arterial system in that area. Artifacts are caused by the susceptibility effects of the metal, which causes signal dropout in the region of the metal. A metal artifact can be identified due to the signal void that has a characteristic build-up of signal on one side of the void. A simple soft tissue plain film can screen for metallic devices. Artifacts can be minimized, but not completely eliminated, using short TE sequences of 3D contrast MRA.[15] Endovascular surgeons should use nitinol stents when possible, which are totally nonmagnetic.

Future of Magnetic Resonance Arteriography

MR angiography currently provides a noninvasive, accurate, and sensitive method to image the vascular system. Developments in MRA technology, new imaging techniques, and the development of new MR contrast agents have greatly improved the quality and accuracy of MRA. Improved spatial resolution and shortened acquisition time can be achieved by using parallel acquisition imaging. As individual coil sensitivity profiles depend on the position of a voxel, coil sensitivities are used to encode the position of a voxel. These acquisitions are called SMASH or SENSE. The reduction in scan time possible with these spatial encoding techniques depends on the number of coils and how the sensitivities of the coils overlap. SENSE acquisition in the abdominal aorta is combined with manual table translation as part of a three-station single injection peripheral MRA examination. This dramatically reduces the upper station scan time such that high-resolution examinations of the middle and particularly the lower station arteries can be acquired sooner after contrast arrival in the aorta. Using this parallel imaging technology, high-resolution images are obtained in a few minutes (Figure 46–6).[16]

Advances in time-resolved acquisition have also resulted in significantly shortened examination time

and excellent resolution. As images are acquired throughout the passage of the contrast bolus, time-resolved acquisitions have the ability to depict pathologically delayed vessel filling. Using a new TRICKS (time-resolved imaging of contrast kinetics) method of imaging, it is possible to consistently capture an arterial time frame (Figure 46–9). Areas where there is rapid venous return, such as the carotid arteries, can be imaged without venous overlay. In the distal extremities, where bolus chase techniques are sensitive to contrast arrival time and venous overlay, TRICKS is successful in acquiring diagnostic images in patients with severe ischemia (Figure 46–10).[16] In a study of 69 patients being evaluated for surgical intervention, Swan et al. found that compared to DSA, TRICKS had a sensitivity and specificity of 89% and 97%

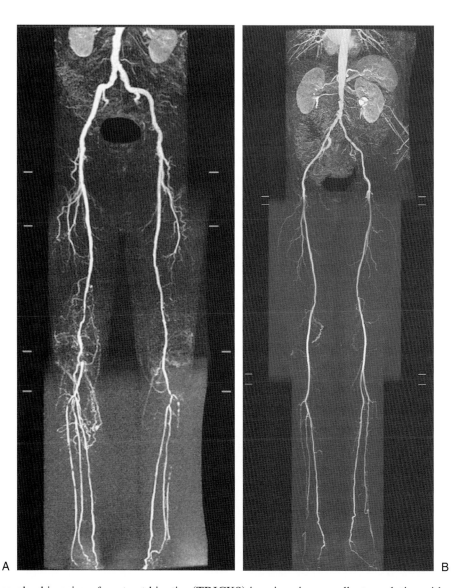

A   B

FIGURE 46–9. Time-resolved imaging of contrast kinetics (TRICKS) imaging gives excellent resolution without venous overlay.

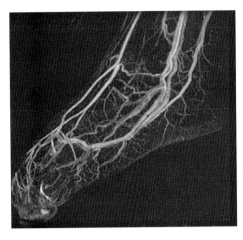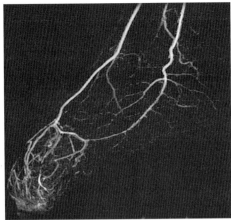

FIGURE 46–10. Time-resolved imaging of contrast kinetics (TRICKS) imaging allows more accurate visualization of pedal vessels, which may be suitable as target vessels for distal bypass.

for occlusion detection and 87% and 90% for detection of significant stenosis.[17]

Many advances in the development of new contrast agents for MRA have been made. Two categories of contrast agents are currently under investigation: extracellular agents and blood pool contrast agents. Extracellular contrast agents are similar to gadolinium and some work to enhance the T_1 relaxivity of the gadolinium chelate. This results in improved signal intensity and better resolution. One of the disadvantages of extracellular contrast agents, including gadolinium, is that leakage of the contrast agent into the extracellular space results in reduced contrast between the intravascular signal and the soft tissues. Blood pool contrast agents are designed to stay within the intravascular space, thus improving the contrast between the vascular phase and the surrounding stationary tissues. Furthermore, the blood pool contrast agents provide a prolonged intravascular signal, allowing the acquisition of high-resolution images. Examples of these new contrast agents include MS-325 and gadomer-17.[16]

Currently, MRA is used for diagnostic "road mapping" and in the planning of therapy for lower extremity vascular occlusive disease. In our practice, patients requiring an endovascular intervention must undergo contrast DSA at the time of the procedure. Research is currently being done to allow MRA-guided endovascular interventions. The application of MR-guided interventions requires the availability of features such as easy patient access within the scanner, high-speed imaging and reconstruction for real-time tracking and imaging, and intuitive interaction with the scanner. Catheters can be imaged by coating the tip with gadolinium contrast or by using tiny

MRI coils on the tip of the catheter. Wacker *et al.* used a new MRA tracking method to follow catheter movements in both phantom and porcine trials. Their system could localize a motionless catheter in the aorta in 100% and a moving catheter in 98% of measured attempts. They were even able to successfully catheterize the renal artery in two pigs.[18]

Conclusions

The development of MRA imaging has greatly improved the vascular surgeon's ability to diagnose and properly treat lower extremity vascular disease. MRA has proven to be a noninvasive, safe, and accurate imaging modality when compared to traditional contrast DSA. Unlike DSA, MRA can provide not only anatomic information, but physiologic information as well. The application of 3D CE MRA can provide enough diagnostic information to plan for surgical or percutaneous intervention in the majority of patients. The limitations of MRA are gradually being overcome by improvements in coil design and software technology and by the addition of new contrast agents. Research in MRA-guided endovascular interventions will eventually make this modality even more useful.

References

1. Sands MJ, Levitin A. Basics of magnetic resonance imaging. Semin Vasc Surg 2004;17(2):66–82.
2. Turnipseed WD, Grist TM. Role of magnetic resonance angiography in peripheral vascular disease. In: Whittemore

AD, Bandyk D, Croenwett J, Hertzer N, White R (eds). *Advances in Vascular Surgery*, pp. 155–169. St. Louis, MO: Mosby Year Book, 1998.

3. Insko EK, Carpenter JP. Magnetic resonance angiography. Semin Vasc Surg 2004;17(2):83–101.

4. Grist TM. MRA of the abdominal aorta and lower extremity. J Magn Reson Imaging 2000;11:32–43.

5. Grist TM. Peripheral MR angiography: Lower extremity. The Experts Guide 2001;9–12.

6. Leiner T, Nejenhuis RJ, Maki JH, Lemaire E, Hoogeveen R, van Engelshoven JM. Use of a three-station phased array coil to improve peripheral contrast-enhanced magnetic resonance angiography. J Magn Reson Imaging 2004;20(3): 417–25.

7. Owen RS, Carpenter JP, Baum RA, Perloff LJ, Cope C. Magnetic resonance imaging of angiographically occult runoff vessels in peripheral arterial occlusive disease. New Engl J Med 1992;11;326(24):1577–81.

8. Hoch JR, Tullis MJ, Kennell TW, McDermott J, Acher CW, Turnipseed WD. Use of magnetic resonance angiography for the preoperative evaluation of patients with infrainguinal arterial occlusive disease. J Vasc Surg 1996;23:792–801.

9. Leiner T, Kessels AG, Schurink GW, Kitslaar PJ, de Hann M, Tordoir JH, van Engelshoven JM. Comparison of contrast-enhanced magnetic resonance angiography and digital subtraction angiography in patients with chronic critical ischemia and tissue loss. Invest Radiol 2004;39:435–44.

10. Steffens JC, Schafer FK, Oberscheid B, Link J, Jahnke T, Heller M, Brossmann J. Bolus-chasing contrast-enhanced 3D MRA of the lower extremities: Comparison with intraarterial DSA. Acta Radiol 2003;44(2):185–92.

11. Nelemans P, Leiner T, de Vet H. Peripheral arterial disease: Meta-analysis of the diagnostic performance of MR angiography. Radiology 2000;217:105–14.

12. Bendib K, Berthezene Y, Croisille P, Villard J, Douek PC. Assessment of complicated arterial bypass grafts: Value of contrast-enhanced subtraction magnetic resonance angiography. J Vasc Surg 1997;26:1036–42.

13. Meissner OA, Verrel F, Tato F, Siebert U, Ramirez, H, Ruppert V, Schoenberg S, Reiser M. Magnetic resonance angiography in the follow-up of distal lower extremity bypass surgery: Comparison with duplex ultrasound and digital subtraction angiography. J Vasc Interv Radiol 2004;15:1269–77.

14. Bertschinger K, Cassina P, Debatin J. Surveillance of peripheral artery bypass grafts with three-dimensional MR angiography: Comparison with digital subtraction angiography. Am J Roentgenol 2001;213:555–60.

15. Turnipseed WD, Sproat IA. A preliminary experience with use of magnetic resonance angiography in assessment of failing lower extremity bypass grafts. Surgery 1992;112:664–9.

16. Carroll TJ, Grist TM. Technical developments in MR angiography. Radiol Clin North Am 2002;40:921–51.

17. Swan JS, Carroll TJ, Kennell TW, Heisey DM, Korosec FR, Frayne R, Mistretta CA, Grist TM. Time-resolved three-dimensional contrast-enhanced MR angiography of the peripheral vessels. Radiology 2002;225(1):43–52.

18. Wacker FK, Elgort D, Hillenbrand CM, Duerk JL, Lewin JS. The catheter-driven MRI scanner: a new approach to intravascular catheter tracking and imaging-parameter adjustment for interventional MRI. Am J Roentgenol 2004;183:391–5.

47
Intravascular Ultrasound Applications

Donald B. Reid, Khalid Irshad, and Edward B. Diethrich

Introduction

Accurate placement of stents and endoluminal grafts in diseased arteries is crucially important in achieving a successful clinical outcome. Intravascular ultrasound (IVUS) is a catheter-based guidance system that facilitates accurate placement during endovascular procedures and while it was originally cardiology led, IVUS is now used in peripheral interventions with great benefit.[1-4] The IVUS probe is passed into the vessel lumen to examine the artery being treated, and because the ultrasound probe is in such close proximity to the artery wall, great detail is possible with significant magnification of the images compared with conventional extracorporeal ultrasound. IVUS provides histologic detail of the vessel wall and also demonstrates blood flow within the lumen.[5,6]

The early IVUS probes rotated mechanically inside a catheter, sweeping an ultrasound signal around 360Å similar to a radar sweeping around a ship at sea. But the disadvantage of such early rotating catheters was that the probe did not configure coaxially with the guidewire. This meant that it did not track smoothly through the artery and could damage it. Furthermore, the images were two-dimensional axial cuts, which being only "black and white" were difficult to interpret. Fortunately many advances have made IVUS much more easily understandable in the operating room environment.[7]

IVUS has two main clinical roles. It provides a diagnostic ability to assess and measure the severity of disease before treatment and also evaluates the completeness of treatment following intervention. In the peripheral arteries IVUS has a complementary role to arteriography, which provides the endovascular surgeon with details of the collateral circulation, vessel contour, quality of flow, and inflow and outflow. IVUS, on the other hand, allows greater appreciation of the vessel wall than the lumen and can distinguish between soft plaque and calcification.

Intimal flaps, thrombus formation, and ulceration are also visible with IVUS and the luminal diameter and cross-sectional areas can also be measured. IVUS can also detect lesions missed on conventional arteriography.[4] IVUS can be used following percutaneous transluminal angioplasty, atherectomy, laser, thrombolysis, and endoluminal grafting.[3,8-10]

This very practical assistance within the operating room environment has become much easier to use with the developments of three-dimensional reconstruction and color-flow IVUS. Its use is described in detail in this chapter together with the latest technical advances of IVUS and its application in many different peripheral arterial situations.

Technical Aspects of Intravascular Ultrasound Applications and Peripheral Interventions

There are two main IVUS systems currently commercially available. The Galaxy system (Boston Scientific, Natick, MA) uses mechanically rotating probes, which provide grayscale IVUS imaging with two- and three-dimensional reconstructions. The second system is the InVision System (Volcano Therapeutics, Rancho Cordova, CA), which uses phased array imaging with probes that are coaxial (with fast exchange versions). The main advantage of the Volcano Therapeutics system is that it also provides colored blood flow imaging. This has significant diagnostic advantages over "grayscale" IVUS.[5]

Probe size varies depending on the situation. In general, high-frequency, low-profile probes are used in the smaller arteries to obtain high-quality resolution, for example, using 20- or even 30-MHz transducers. To achieve a greater penetration of ultrasound distance for larger vessels, 10-MHz catheters are required.[5] We use 2.9F, 20-MHz catheters that configure with 0.014-inch guidewires for the smaller arteries such as the carotid, renal,

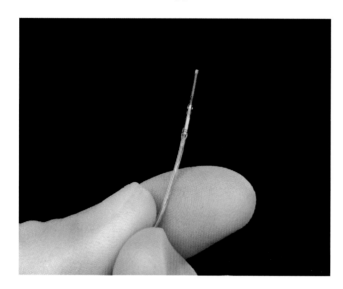

FIGURE 47–1. A 2.9F Eagle Eye IVUS probe compatible with a 0.014-inch guidewire.

powerful computing during a pullback of the ultrasound catheter through the vessel. A computerized edge tracking formula (algorithm) then aligns the consecutive frames.[6] The three-dimensional construction can be viewed as either "longitudinal" or "volume" views. The longitudinal reconstruction is immediately available in the operating room and can be rotated around the longitudinal axis of the catheter to provide oblique and lateral perspectives. The volume view takes 2–3 min longer to create and has some artifact since the raw data are altered. A smooth and steady pullback is necessary to acquire high-quality reconstructions.

Color flow IVUS was developed by EndoSonics (Rancho Cordova, CA, now Volcano Therapeutics). ChromaFlo is the computer software that detects blood flow and colors it red. The software detects the differences between adjacent IVUS frames. As the blood cells move through the artery they move through the IVUS image frames. The software detects differences between adjacent frames and colors the image red. ChromaFlo detects faster flowing blood and colors

superficial femoral, popliteal, and tibial arteries (Figure 47–1). A 3.5F, 135-cm-long, fast-exchange catheter that is coaxial for 30 cm of its length and configures with an 0.018-inch wire has an ultrasound diameter range of 24 mm. We find this suitable for larger arteries such as the iliac. An 8.4F probe with a maximum diameter of 60 mm that is compatible with a 0.035-inch guidewire is used for the great vessels: the abdominal and thoracic aortas. Motorized pullback sled devices are available for peripheral interventions from both Boston Scientific and Volcano Therapeutics (Figure 47–2). However, they are rarely used in peripheral interventions because long-distance pullbacks are necessary compared to coronary artery evaluation and the pullback devices are slow and time consuming. Most have a maximum speed of just 1 mm/s.

The IVUS image created is a circular axial cut with a central disc artifact caused by the catheter. Real-time imaging displays the vessel wall and lumen at 30 frames per second allowing pulsatility of the artery wall to be seen. The ultrasound images display the vessel wall in histologic detail: the thin inner intima reflects the signal brightly while the media is a dark circumferential ring. Outside, the adventitia is also bright and reflective. Calcification typically reflects the ultrasound signal completely causing dark shadowing behind it (Figure 47–3).

Three-dimensional reconstruction of the two-dimensional axial images produces a picture similar in appearance to an angiogram allowing the whole length of the vessel under examination to be viewed at the one time without the need for repeated pullbacks (Figure 47–3). Consecutive axial images are stacked by

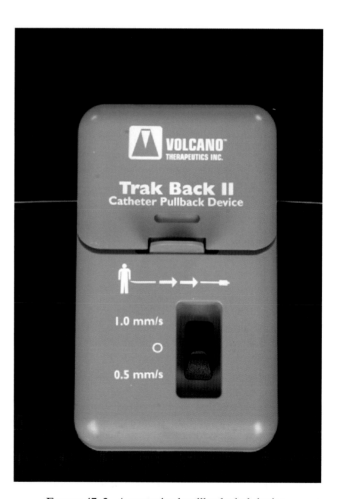

FIGURE 47–2. A motorized pullback sled device.

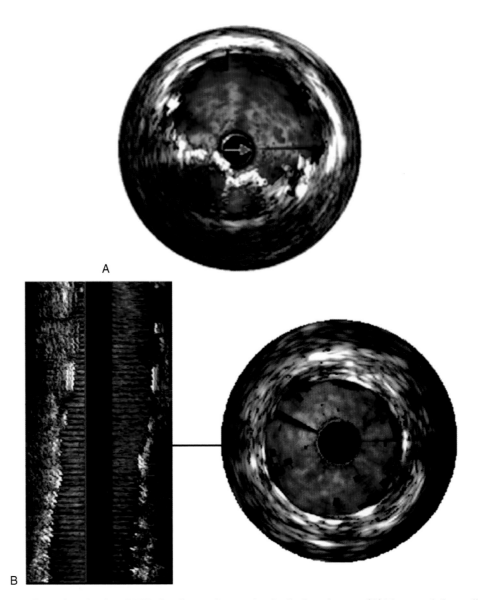

FIGURE 47–3. (A) Two-dimensional color IVUS showing an incompletely deployed stent. (B) Two- and three-dimensional color IVUS showing improved stent deployment following reballooning.

it yellow. However, at present, flow velocities cannot be measured using this technique. ChromaFlo does not utilize the Doppler effect.[5] Color flow IVUS has been a very helpful addition because it shows clearly where the lumen meets the vessel wall. This was not always apparent in "black and white" IVUS, especially if the vessel wall contained dark echolucent plaque or soft thrombus. There are many clinical situations that color IVUS assists in but none more so than arterial dissection. A specific catheter, the Cross Point (Medtronic, MN), has been developed to identify true from false lumen and steer the guidewire (and treatment) accordingly.

Virtual histology IVUS (VH IVUS) is a new advance that is still in development and evaluation.[11–14] Where color IVUS has highlighted the blood flow in the lumen, VH IVUS aims to identify and color code plaque type in the artery wall. Conventional IVUS uses the amplitude of reflected ultrasound from the different components of the vessel and converts it into an image with a grayscale. VH IVUS analyzes the spectrum of reflected radiofrequency (RF) ultrasound signals and then classifies the spectral type into four categories of plaque:

1. Fibrous tissue—densely packed collagen fibers with no evidence of lipid accumulation.

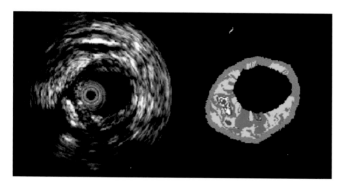

FIGURE 47–4. Color-coded virtual histology IVUS of an arterial plaque containing calcification (white), fibrous plaque (dark green), fibrofatty plaque (light green), and necrotic core plaque (red). (Courtesy of Volcano Therapeutics.)

2. Fibrofatty—loosely packed collagen fibers with regions of fatty deposit resent.
3. Necrotic core—localized areas of loss of matrix containing lipid, typically with microcalcifications.
4. Dense calcium—focal areas of dense calcium.

Each category is color coded (dark green—fibrous, light green—fibrofatty, red—necrotic core, white—calcium) and this is superimposed over the conventional grayscale IVUS image (Figure 47–4). Comparison with histologic examination has produced 80–93% accuracy rates.[11]

The clinical value of VH IVUS is yet to be defined, however, soft lipidic, necrotic core plaques have been implicated in acute ischemic syndromes such as plaque rupture. Detection of such "vulnerable" plaques using VH IVUS could have major treatment implications.[10,15] While to date most work on VH IVUS has been in the coronary arteries, the peripheral arteries merit similar investigation, particularly the carotid arteries, since plaque rupture there has major clinical inplications. Treating such vulnerable plaque by stenting may one day become routine practice despite there being no hemodynamic stenosis. We are participants in a peripheral registry to help define the clinical role of VH IVUS in a worldwide survey of 1500 patients. Long-term follow-up will be necessary.

Performing a Pullback

When the IVUS catheter has been chosen for the artery being treated (based on the size of the artery and the range of ultrasound that the catheter images), the probe is then flushed with heparinized saline and gently introduced over the wire. To obtain color flow a "reference" function needs to be performed on the IVUS machine when the probe is in the arterial lumen. This removes near-field vision artifact, a characteristic of phased array IVUS imaging. This will soon be superseded by new computer software with which we have gained some early clinical experience (NearVu, Volcano Therapeutics, Rancho Cordova, CA). The probe is passed into the artery beyond the disease and a slow and steady pullback is begun through the area in order to interrogate the lesion. Two- and three-dimensional views are then assessed.

Operative and Anatomic Situations

Carotid Angioplasty and Stenting

There are special features to bear in mind when stenting the carotid artery. It is particularly susceptible to incomplete stent deployment since heavy calcification resists complete stent expansion.[16] Furthermore, the internal carotid artery is not always uniform in diameter but is narrower distally and wider near its origin.[17] Stenting can also compromise the origin of the external carotid artery by compression, and recurrent stenosis following carotid endarterectomy may respond differently during stenting compared with a primary atherosclerotic lesion.[18,19] The IVUS operator must appreciate these aspects and avoid dislodging embolic material or causing intimal dissection to the artery through overzealous instrumentation.

IVUS is a powerful tool in carotid stenting; however, the penalties are high if the disease is underestimated or the stent is badly deployed. We use IVUS more frequently now in carotid stenting since the introduction of cerebral protection devices. Immediately after deploying the protection device, IVUS can assess the lesion and take measurements to help stent and balloon sizing. We currently use the Avanar catheter (Volcano Therapeutics, Rancho Cordova, CA), which is a low-profile 2.9F 20-MHz probe that configures with the 0.014-inch wire of most cerebral protection devices (Figure 47–5). The IVUS probe is advanced into the distal internal carotid artery, and the pullback is begun. The distal internal carotid artery has a characteristic appearance on IVUS because it is so thin and usually spared of disease. The histologic layers are elegantly seen. Measurements can be taken just above the lesion to help size balloon and stent diameters, and the degree of stenosis can also be assessed to decide whether predilation is required or whether primary stent deployment can be performed.[20] While currently plaque morphology can be subjectively assessed by IVUS, the new advance of VH IVUS (Volcano Therapeutics, Rancho Cordova, CA) is

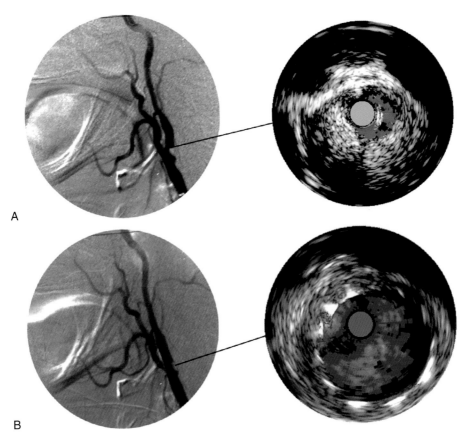

Figure 47–5. (A) Intraoperative carotid angiogram and IVUS showing a stenosis of the internal carotid artery. (B) There is resolution of the stenosis poststenting. IVUS confirms excellent stent deployment.

promising since it will provide classified histologic plaque types.

Following stenting, the IVUS probe is introduced again and a pullback assesses the completeness of stent deployment. IVUS measurements of the minimum stent diameter can be made to decide whether further ballooning is required. Mid-stent waisting is a common finding. In general, a minimum stent diameter of more than 4 mm is recommended in the internal carotid artery to avoid residual hemodynamically significant stenosis.[7] The stent should be uniformly well expanded throughout its length following deployment. It should also appose completely to the artery wall with no space apparent between the stent and the vessel. It is important to make sure that the length of the lesion is covered by the expanded stent such that no proximal or distal disease is left untreated. A careful inspection for intimal dissection is also important.

Despite our enthusiasm for carotid IVUS, passing balloon catheters and the IVUS probes up and down the internal carotid artery is not without hazard even with protection devices. The decision to reballoon or deploy another stent needs to be made cautiously. The advantages must be weighed against the risks of possible complication for the patient. Sometimes it is best to accept a reasonable deployment rather than overpursue it.

Stenting the origin of the common carotid artery from a retrograde carotid approach poses a challenge to all endovascular specialists. The common carotid artery comes off the aortic arch or the innominate artery, and accurate stent location at the origin is difficult using aortography alone because of the natural curvature of the arch[20] (Figure 47–6). Accurate placement is possible using IVUS by passing the IVUS probe down the common carotid artery from above. Fluoroscopy visualizes the radiopaque transducer as it passes down the vessel. Blood flow is displayed in color pulsing red with each cardiac cycle. When the probe passes from the stenosis into the aorta, there is a sudden change in the size of the luminal color. Together with fluoroscopy this technique pinpoints the origin of the vessel exactly for accurate device deployment. The same technique can also be used to stent the origin of all the supraaortic vessels.

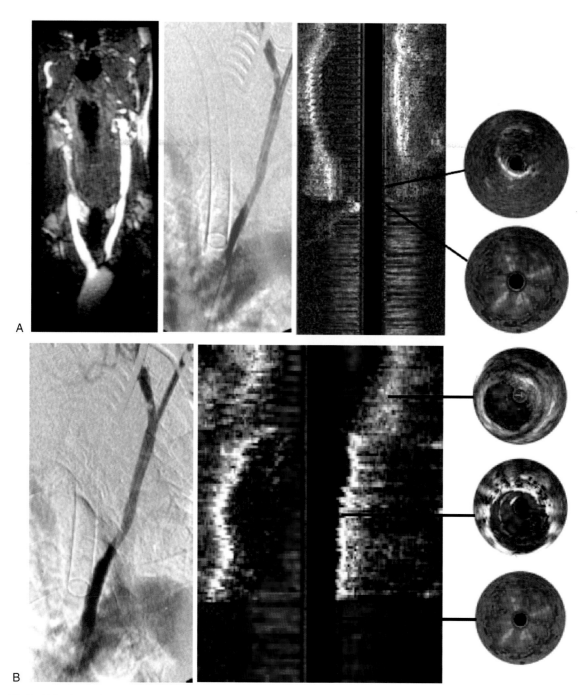

Figure 47–6. (A) Magnetic resonance angiography showing a tight stenosis at the origin of the left common carotid artery. At operation the IVUS probe is passed down from a cervical access assisting road mapping. Two- and three-dimensional color IVUS locates the origin of the carotid artery. (B) Two- and three-dimensional color IVUS showing accurate stenting at the origin of the common carotid artery together with the completion angiogram. [Reprinted from Irshad K, Bain D, Miller PH, *et al.* The role of intravascular ultrasound in carotid angioplasty and stenting. In: Henry M (ed). *Angioplasty and Stenting of the Carotid and Supra-Aortic Trunks*, pp. 127–133. London: Martin Dunitz, 2004. Courtesy of Martin Dunitz, London.]

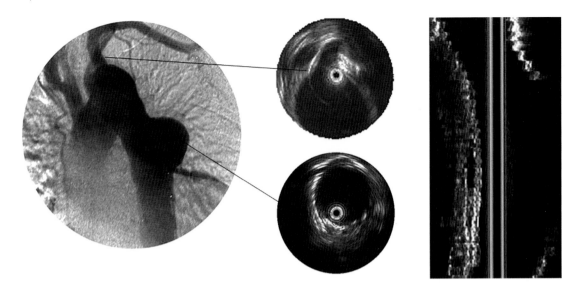

FIGURE 47–7. A thoracic aortic aneurysm. IVUS demonstrates the origin of the left subclavian artery, the neck, and the aneurysm.

Thoracic Aorta

In the thoracic aorta, a larger probe is required (8.4F) with more penetration (10 MHz) and compatibility with a larger guidewire (0.035 inch). IVUS is useful in assessing and measuring the neck of a thoracic aneurysm being treated by endoluminal grafting. The exact origin of the subclavian artery can also be identified (Figure 47–7). IVUS also defines the extent of thoracic dissection and greatly assists treatment of coarctation of the aorta.[21]

Abdominal Aorta

Similarly in endoluminal grafting for abdominal aortic aneurysm, IVUS provides accurate measurements of neck diameters and assessment of the iliac arteries.[3] The IVUS catheter is advanced from the groin to a level just above the renal arteries. The proximal and then the distal necks of the aneurysm are measured together with the luminal length requiring grafting. The amount of calcification and mural thrombus is noted, and assessment of the shape of the proximal and distal necks can indicate how well the endoluminal graft will exclude the aneurysm. IVUS provides a greater understanding of the case than computed tomography (CT) alone (Figure 47–8). Immediately following endoluminal graft deployment it is difficult to obtain good IVUS images because of tiny pockets of air trapped in the endomaterial and because of the metal endoskeleton. These both cause bright reflection

of ultrasound. Further technological advances with IVUS or the endoluminal grafts in this situation are necessary since color IVUS could potentially detect endoleak and its source at the time of device implantation.[4]

In occlusive disease of the aorta, IVUS provides accurate diameters to judge balloon and stent sizing.[1] This is important since ballooning the aorta with too large a balloon to only a few atmospheres can cause aortic rupture.

Iliac Arteries

The iliac arteries are tortuous and deeply placed in the abdomen and pelvis. It is therefore not surprising that IVUS can occasionally detect disease not apparent on arteriography. However, the main use of IVUS in the iliac arteries is to check stent deployment. We use IVUS routinely in this situation together with arteriography and measurements of arterial pressure gradients before and after stenting. This "triple assessment" thoroughly examines the completeness of treatment (Figure 47–9).[4]

Infrainguinal Arteries

We have used IVUS in the infrainguinal arteries, particularly to assist the placement of endoluminal grafts in unfit patients with occlusive disease who might otherwise have undergone distal bypass surgery for critical limb

FIGURE 47–8. (A) CT scan of an aortic aneurysm showing dissection. (B) Two- and three-dimensional IVUS of the abdominal aortic aneurysm demonstrating thrombus with a flapping dissection.

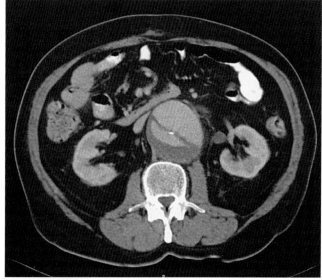

A

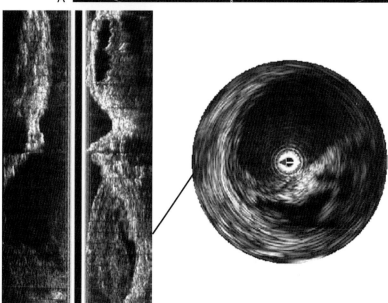

B

ischemia[4] (Figure 47–10). We routinely balloon and stent on 0.018-inch guidewires to avoid time-consuming wire exchanges for IVUS examination.

Unfortunately the combination balloon/IVUS catheters originally developed for coronary angioplasty is no longer commercially available. We found them extremely useful at swiftly checking the results of tibial angioplasty.[4]

Discussion

IVUS is probably more helpful in peripheral interventions than in the coronary situation, assessing the completeness of treatment and providing detailed and accurate luminal measurements. However, it is perceived by many as an expensive guidance system with little support from clinical data and studies. While there are no cost-effectiveness studies of IVUS in the periphery, there are some studies of its clinical value. Arko *et al.* reported in a retrospective study an improved clinical outcome in patients undergoing iliac stenting compared to those who had no IVUS assistance.[22] Another study of 100 consecutive peripheral interventions reported that IVUS detected that 34% of patients had unsatisfactory stent deployment despite a satisfactory completion angiogram. Following retreatment, the cross-sectional area through the stent was increased by 42% (52 of these patients were undergoing carotid stenting).[7]

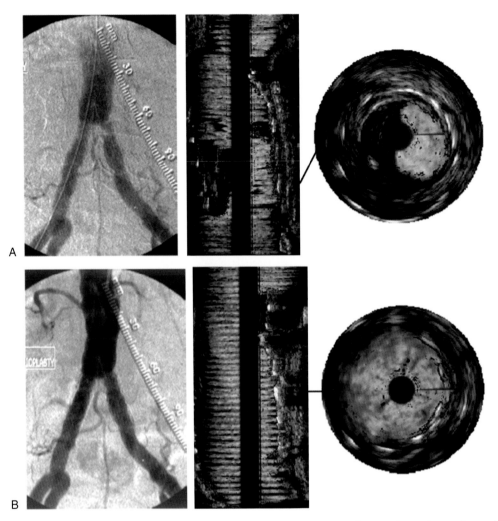

FIGURE 47–9. (A) Angiogram and color IVUS demonstrating restenosis of the left common iliac stent. Neointimal hyperplasia can be seen inside the stent struts. (B) Following reballooning to 16 atmospheres there is angiographic and IVUS resolution together with resolution of the arterial pressure gradient.

In another study, 131 patients underwent renal artery stenting with IVUS evaluation. IVUS detected unsuspected maldeployment of the stent in 23.5% of cases. The IVUS findings included 22 (14.4%) instances of incomplete stent apposition/expansion, 8 (5.2%) dissections, and 6 (3.9%) incompletely covered ostia.[23]

A favorable limb salvage rate in 50 consecutive patients undergoing IVUS-guided treatment for critical limb ischemia also reported the beneficial use of IVUS.[4] IVUS was crucial in 32% of cases, discovering unsuspected disease and inaccurately deployed stents. Limb salvage rate was 79% at 3 years despite the fact that nearly 25% of the patients were diabetic.[4] Such studies lend support to IVUS having clinical outcome benefit, but no randomized controlled peripheral trial has yet been undertaken.

We have become sufficiently familiar with IVUS to use it in patients with renal failure and contrast allergy to treat them without angiography. Together with fluoroscopy the IVUS probe can be used to road map the intervention. This technique of IVUS-guided treatment is very gratifying for the operator and is greatly assisted by the preoperative evaluation of the patient with magnetic resonance angiography.[24]

We have found IVUS especially helpful in complex cases. However, the operating room team needs to frequently use IVUS so that when it is needed (e.g., an emergency case) it is quickly available and used with experience.

Technology has advanced IVUS with great benefit, especially the additions of color flow and three-dimensional reconstruction which make it much more

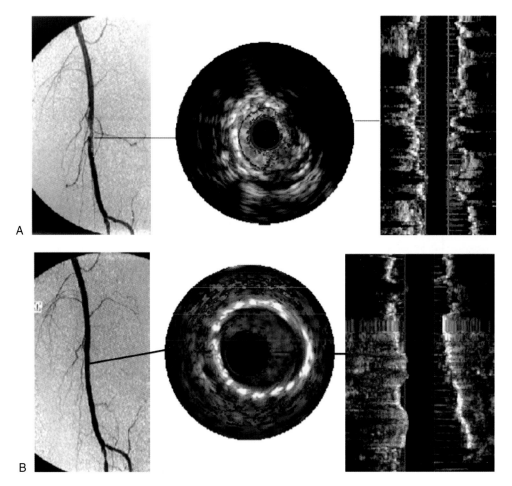

FIGURE 47–10. (A) A critical stenosis of the popliteal artery in a patient with critical limb ischemia. IVUS demonstrates a tight and calcified stenosis. (B) Angiography and IVUS show resolu-tion of the stenosis following deployment of a balloon-mounted endoluminal graft.

user friendly in the operating room. However industry could perhaps do more to manufacture probes specifi-cally for peripheral interventions that have a low profile and are compatible with 0.035-inch guidewires.

Conclusions

Peripheral endovascular procedures have advanced and replaced many vascular surgical operations at an aston-ishing rate in the past decade. There is now an over-whelming variety of devices, and technology being used to treat arterial disease from inside the vessel lumen. The successful use of these new endovascular techniques heavily relies on good imaging. A strong knowledge and understanding of IVUS is important because it is able to guide and assess the completeness of endovascular treat-ment. Its perceived expense has resulted in its underuse in peripheral interventions despite advances of color flow IVUS and three-dimensional reconstruction, which have made it much more readily understandable within the operating room environment.

While IVUS is still driven by interventional cardio-logists, industry has an opportunity to translate much of the technology to the peripheral setting. The latest advance in IVUS is virtual histology, which is potentially promising in improving our understanding of how plaque will behave when treated. If the complexity of endovascular procedures continues to increase and the limitations of conventional imaging continue to be appre-ciated, it is likely that IVUS will increasingly find its role in peripheral inventions.

References

1. Diethrich EB. Endovascular treatment of abdominal occlusive disease; the impact of stents and intravascular ultrasound imaging. Eur J Vasc Surg 1993;7:228–236.

2. Laskey WK, Brady ST, Kussmaul WG, et al. Intravascular ultrasonographic assessment of the results of coronary artery stenting. Am Heart J 1993;125:1576–1583.

3. White RA, Scoccianti M, Back M, et al. Innovations in vascular imaging; arteriography, three-dimensional CT scans, and two- and three-dimensional intravascular ultrasound evaluation of an abdominal aortic aneurysm. Ann Vasc Surg 1994;8:285–289.

4. Irshad K, Rahman N, Bain D, et al. The role of intravascular ultrasound and peripheral endovascular interventions. In: Heuser RR, Henry M (eds). *Textbook of Peripheral Vascular Interventions,* pp. 25–34. London: Martin Dunitz, 2004.

5. Irshad K, Reid DB, Miller PH, et al. Early clinical experience with colour three-dimensional intravascular ultrasound in peripheral interventions. J Endovasc Ther 2001;8:329–338.

6. Reid DB, Douglas M, Diethrich EB. The clinical value of three-dimensional intravascular ultrasound imaging. J Endovasc Surg 1995;2:356–364.

7. Reid DB, Diethrich EB, Marx P, Wrasper R. Clinical application of intravascular ultrasound in peripheral vascular disease. In: Seigel RJ (ed). *Intravascular Ultrasound Imaging in Coronary Artery Disease*, pp. 309–341. New York: Marcel Dekker, 1998.

8. Gussenhoven EJ, van der Lugt A, Pasterkamp G, et al. Intravascular ultrasound predictors of outcome after peripheral balloon angioplasty. Eur J Vasc Endovasc Surg 1995;10:279–288.

9. Cavaye DM, Diethrich EB, Santiago OJM, et al. Intravascular ultrasound imaging: An essential component of angioplasty assessment and vascular stent deployment. Int Angiol 1993;12:212–220.

10. Katzen BT, Benenati JF, Becker GJ, et al. Role of intravascular ultrasound in peripheral atherectomy and stent deployment. Circulation 1991;84:2152. Abstract.

11. Vince DG, Davies SC. Peripheral application of intravascular ultrasound virtual histology. Semin Vasc Surg 2004;17: 119–125.

12. Kuchalakanti P, Rha SW, Cheneau E, et al. Identification of "vulnerable plaque" using virtual histology in angiographically benign looking lesion of proximal left anterior descending artery. Cardiovasc Radiat Med 2003;4:225–227.

13. Nair A, Kuban BD, Obuchowski N, Vince DG. Assessing spectral algorithms to predict atherosclerotic plaque composition with normalized and raw intravascular ultrasound data. Ultrasound Med Biol 2001;27(10):1319–1331.

14. Nair A, Kuban BD, Tuzcu EM, et al. Coronary plaque classification with intravascular ultrasound radiofrequency data analysis. Circulation 2002;106:2200–2206.

15. Schartl M, Bocksch W, Koschyk DH, et al. Use of intravascular ultrasound to compare effects of different strategies of lipid-lowering therapy on plaque volume and composition in patients with coronary artery disease. Circulation 2001;104:387–392.

16. Diethrich EB, Ndiaye M, Reid DB. Stenting in the carotid artery: Initial experience in 110 patients. J Endovasc Surg 1996;3:42–62.

17. Reid DB, Diethrich EB, Marx P, et al. Intravascular ultrasound assessment in carotid interventions. J Endovasc Surg 1996;3:203–210.

18. Diethrich EB, Marx P, Wrasper R, et al. Percutaneous techniques for endoluminal carotid interventions. J Endovasc Surg 1996;3:182–202.

19. Reid DB, Irshad K, Miller S, et al. Endovascular significance of the external carotid artery in the treatment of cerebrovascular insufficiency. J Endovasc Ther 2004;11:727–733.

20. Irshad K, Bain D, Miller PH, et al. The role of intravascular ultrasound in carotid angioplasty and stenting. In: Henry M (ed). *Angioplasty and Stenting of the Carotid and Supra-Aortic Trunks*, pp. 127–133. London: Martin Dunitz, 2004.

21. Irshad K, Miller PH, McKendrick M, et al. The role of IVUS for stentgraft repair in TAA and TAD. In: Amor M, Bergeron P (eds). *Thoracic Aorta Endografting*, pp. 73–77. Marseille: Com & Co, 2004.

22. Arko F, Mattauer M, McCollugh R, et al. Use of intravascular ultrasound improves long-term clinical outcome in the endovascular management of atherosclerotic aorto iliac occlusive disease. J Vasc Surg 1998;27:614–623.

23. Dangas G, Laird JR, Mehran R, et al. Intravascular ultrasound guided renal artery stenting. J Endovasc Ther 2001;8:238–247.

24. Reid AW, Reid DB, Roditi GH. Vascular imaging: An unparalleled decade. J Endovasc Ther 2004;II(Suppl. II): II.163–II.179.

48
Three-Dimensional Vascular Imaging and Three-Dimensional Color Power Angiography Imaging

Ali F. AbuRahma and Phillip J. Bendick

Introduction

From the very early days of bistable ultrasound imaging, it has been the goal of clinicians and engineers to develop techniques for the three-dimensional (3D) imaging of structures and systems within the body. As early as 1956, Howry et al.[1] proposed "stereoscopic" viewing of body structures. Since that time a number of schemes to accomplish 3D imaging have been attempted to realize the potential value of rendering volumetric data,[2–4] but until very recently these have met with limited success in their clinical application.[5–9] Technical limitations of image orientation, low grayscale dynamic range, data storage, and data processing time have affected the usefulness of 3D image reconstruction in direct clinical applications. These early efforts all required extensive off-line, non-realtime processing of image data, often with significant operator interaction, and provided reconstructions with reduced resolution and/or inadequate image registration. Despite these constraints, 3D imaging with off-line processing of grayscale image data has been applied in a wide variety of clinical situations, including fetal imaging, breast ultrasound, urology, ophthalmology, hepatobiliary ultrasound, and echocardiography.[10–17] More recently freehand scanning techniques have been combined with the necessary computational power and high-speed data processing capabilities to produce more timely and accurate 3D images within a more acceptable time frame close to "real time."[18,19] These same limitations for general ultrasound imaging have applied as well to vascular imaging, with the additional constraint that the target organs, in this case the arterial system, are anatomically small structures with increased requirements for high-resolution imaging.[20–22]

For 3D vascular imaging an alternative to visualizing the arterial wall itself is to visualize the flow within the lumen, providing an indirect image of the luminal surface, which is most frequently the area of interest. These efforts have been limited by the requirements for very high resolution to image small anatomic structures and the dependence on some type of volume flow signal that is sensitive enough to detect the very low-flow velocity signals at the vessel wall–blood interface. Technological developments in ultrasound imaging and flow measurement over the past few years have overcome many of these obstacles. Higher frequency ultrasound probes, with center frequencies up to 12 MHz and improved electronic focusing in one or two dimensions, are now widely available to give very high-resolution grayscale data. In addition, intravascular ultrasound probes with the piezoelectric element mounted at the catheter tip are capable of operating at frequencies up to 30 MHz.

A further advantage of vascular imaging is that a fixed probe orientation can be used over short segments of the vascular anatomy, reducing the stringent requirements for an external system for the exact registration of probe location and allowing the use of freehand scanning. Finally, the development of amplitude-dependent Doppler imaging, or so-called power Doppler imaging, has provided a signal related to blood flow volume that is sensitive to very low flow velocities characteristic of those seen near the vessel wall. Rather than display Doppler frequency shift information as is done with conventional color Doppler imaging, power Doppler ultrasound displays an estimate of the entire power contained in that part of the received radiofrequency ultrasound signal for which a phase shift corresponding to motion of the target is detected.[23] The strength of this signal is related to the number of red blood cell scatterers within the sample volume, which in turn is a function of the blood flow dynamics, giving significantly increased sensitivity to low flow velocities and making power Doppler imaging much less angle dependent than conventional color Doppler images.[24] In addition, the power Doppler signal is not subject to aliasing as are conventional pulsed spectral and color Doppler displays.

The extension of two-dimensional (2D) B-mode grayscale imaging of the cardiovascular system to clinical applications has met with limited success thus far. Many of the early problems of image resolution, recognition and registration of probe orientation, and the required data processing time have been at least partially solved.[4,11,22] However, the use of grayscale images obtained using conventional ultrasound scanning remains limited by the large dynamic range of the image data and the artifacts in the image associated with atherosclerotic disease. Even more limiting is the need for off-line processing of the original image data with significant operator dependence to identify tissue interfaces and provide input for arterial edge detection, usually with some type of mechanical tracing device.[9]

Three-Dimensional Intravascular Ultrasound

More recent reports of 3D vascular imaging have used intravascular ultrasound (IVUS) with high-frequency transmit/receive crystals placed at the tip of a catheter, primarily in the coronary arteries.[7,25] Investigators have been able to identify segments of angiographically "silent" atherosclerosis and quantify the degree of narrowing caused by either atherosclerotic lesions or postangioplasty intimal hyperplasia. IVUS has also proved helpful in the placement of coronary stents and investigators have found good correlation between IVUS and conventional angiographic video densitometry in postangioplasty measurements of vessel cross-sectional lumen area.[7,26] The potential exists for increased peripheral vascular utilization of 3D vascular imaging as endovascular stent grafting becomes more widespread, as 3D IVUS has been shown to provide a nearly real-time perspective of the morphologic features of the vascular anatomy and of the stent graft placement during the procedure.[27] Research into the measurement of the mechanical properties of the arterial wall has also been done using 3D IVUS techniques to provide data on wall motion characteristics as a function of intraarterial pressures.[28] However, most of the current work with grayscale 3D vascular imaging remains in the developmental stage using *in vitro* specimens or models; *in vivo* work is primarily experimental in nature and there are very limited data available on its clinical utility.

An alternative to grayscale imaging of the vascular wall and its associated disease is to image the vessel wall–blood interface from the perspective of inside the lumen, using the blood flow signal to separate patent lumen from solid tissue. Power Doppler imaging is ideally suited to this task, for the reasons outlined above, providing very low flow sensitivity, good resolution at the interface, and high-speed processing of the data. Typical applications use a linear array probe with a transmit frequency between 5 and 10 MHz. The vessel(s) of interest are imaged in a cross section and the system gain and filters are set to completely fill the patent lumen with the color-coded flow signal while at the same time minimizing image noise and artifact by adjusting the background signal to the electronic "noise floor" of the system, which is typically color coded in solid blue (Figure 48–1). Once the optimum system settings are obtained, the background can again be displayed as grayscale information (Figure 48–2A) and the vessel(s) slowly scanned at a constant speed in freehand fashion over the region of interest. Figure 48–2 shows an example of scanning in a cephalad direction from just below to just above the carotid artery bifurcation. When the final cross-sectional image is frozen, system memory retains the previous consecutive frames of power Doppler data similar to the cineloop function found on most modern ultrasound scanners. Typically between 32 and 64 frames of data are stored, corresponding to between 3 and 6 s of scanning, depending on the image frame rate during the scanning process. The system then automatically reassembles the stored images, usually in approximately 5–10 s, by stacking successive frames and displaying the resulting image in a 3D format. Figure 48–3A shows the resulting 3D image of the carotid artery bifurcation, outlining the patent lumen that tracks the vessel wall–blood interface. Simple movement of the ultrasound system trac-ball allows rotation of the 3D image to view the luminal contour from any angle

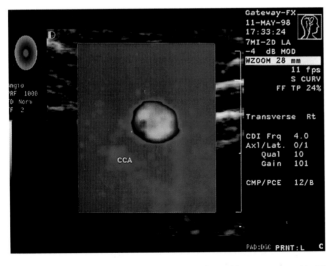

FIGURE 48–1. Cross-sectional view of the mid common carotid artery (CCA) using power Doppler imaging with the background signal color coded in blue representing the electronic "noise floor."

needed to provide a clear view of the vascular anatomy (Figure 48–3B). In addition to the carotid artery bifurcation, other accessible major conduit vessels that are clinically important and appear suitable for 3D power Doppler angiography are the aortoiliac system, including the major visceral branches in the abdomen, the femoropopliteal system, the intracranial vessels comprising the circle of Willis using a transcranial approach, and the portal-hepatic vascular system.

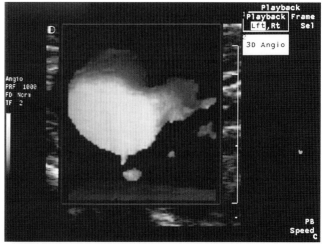

A

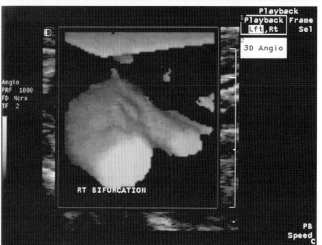

B

FIGURE 48–3. (A) Three-dimensional reconstruction of the images stored in the sequence demonstrated by Figure 48–2. The distal common carotid artery appears nearest, with the internal carotid artery (ICA) (left) and external carotid artery (ECA) (including a small branch artery) extending away from the viewer. (B) Three-dimensional reconstruction of the same image sequence as for (A), with the three-dimensional image rotated approximately 180° so that the ICA (left) and the ECA, with its branch artery, now appear closer to the viewer.

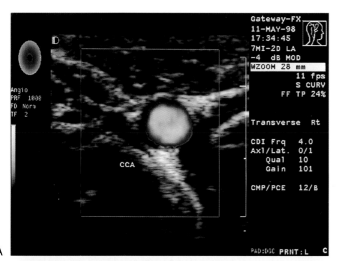

A

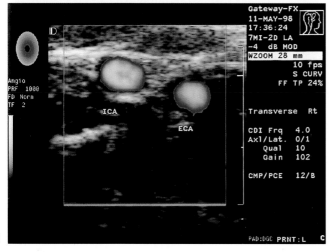

B

FIGURE 48–2. (A) Cross-sectional view of the mid common carotid artery (CCA) using power Doppler imaging with the grayscale image providing the background signal. This represents the initial scanning plane for the collection of images for subsequent three-dimensional reconstruction. (B) Cross-sectional view of the carotid vessels above the bifurcation using power Doppler imaging showing the internal and external carotid arteries (ICA, ECA). This is the final scanning plane and image collected for three-dimensional reconstruction.

Other Clinical Applications

Similar techniques using freehand scanning can be used for 3D imaging of the vascularity of solid organs, such as the kidney. Because of the increased sensitivity of power Doppler to low flow velocities, not only can the major conduit arteries be imaged but the much smaller interlobular and arcuate arteries in the renal cortex can also be displayed, very nearly to the capsule itself. Rubin et al.[24] showed that a 2D power Doppler image of the renal vasculature can be used to estimate the fractional

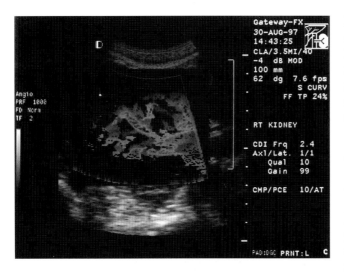

FIGURE 48–4. Three-dimensional reconstruction of the upper lobe of a right kidney demonstrating the major branch arteries and the vascularity of the cortical regions.

moving blood volume within a specific region of the kidney, demonstrating significant changes in this parameter as a function of hydration status as well as the effects of an arteriovenous fistula in a transplant kidney. A cross-sectional scan that sweeps through the kidney will store these consecutive power Doppler image frames to make possible a reconstruction that shows the anatomic extent of perfusion throughout a 3D tissue region of interest (Figure 48–4). Similar displays can be generated for other tissues within the body such as liver, thyroid, breast, and the ophthalmic vasculature.

Three-dimensional power Doppler angiography has been implemented in a number of these vascular beds to investigate specific clinical problems. In a prospective study of 24 patients Carson et al.[29] examined the vascularity of breast masses seen on mammography and correlated their findings with the pathology noted in biopsy specimens. In addition to conventional grayscale image criteria, vascular criteria were identified for grading the 3D angiographic images and a numeric score between 1 (benign extreme) and 5 (malignant extreme) was assigned. These parameters included inner and outside (to 1 cm) vascularity, the presence and number of visible shunt vessels, vessel wrapping around the mass and vessel tortuosity, vessel enlargement, and related (beyond 1 cm) or unusual vascularity indicated by the presence of multiple large vessels with elevated flows.

Most helpful in the discrimination of malignant versus benign lesions were extensive inner vascularity, with a mean score of 3.3 versus 2.2 for malignant versus benign; extensive outside vascularity, 3.7 versus 2.4; the presence of clearly identified, multiple shunt vessels, 2.7 versus 2.1; and significant vessel wrapping around the mass, 3.5 versus 1.9. For a fixed sensitivity of 90%, 3D power

Doppler angiography improved lesion specificity to 85% compared with 79% for 2D conventional color or power Doppler images (which could include the individual frames used to reconstruct the eventual 3D image). Only for the 3D reconstruction data did lesion vascularity display a trend toward statistical significance, which was somewhat limited by the small sample size.

Three-Dimensional Angiography/Carotid Artery

Bendick et al.[30] evaluated the accuracy of 3D angiography in the carotid artery bifurcation compared with digital subtraction contrast angiography and surgical findings at carotid endarterectomy. Thirty-two patients were studied, with 64 vessels available for correlation. Luminal narrowing was categorized as <40%, 40–60%, 60–80%, and >80% diameter reduction, or total occlusion, using direct measurements from the 3D images without knowledge of the angiographic results and applying the methodology of stenosis measurement of the NASCET study (Figure 48–5).

In addition, surface morphology of the 3D images was evaluated to determine the extent of luminal narrowing, defined as focal, moderate (<1 cm), or lengthy (>1 cm), as well as the presence of plaque ulceration. Three carotid bifurcations had atherosclerotic lesions that were too heavily calcified for adequate power Doppler angiogra-

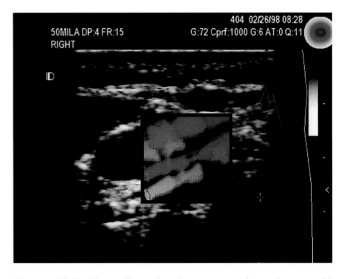

FIGURE 48–5. Three-dimensional reconstruction of a carotid bifurcation region applying the NASCET methodology for stenosis measurement, with ultrasonic calipers on the internal carotid artery showing the minimal lumen diameter (X) and the distal ICA lumen diameter (+). Also note the small ulcerative crater at the distal end of the lesion just beyond the point of maximal narrowing.

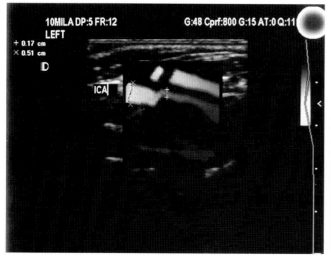

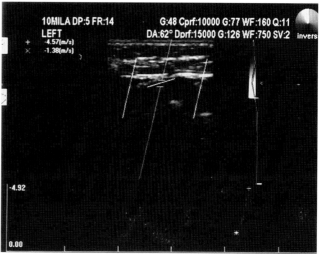

A

B

FIGURE 48–6. (A) Three-dimensional reconstruction of a carotid bifurcation region showing a >60% diameter reduction in the proximal internal carotid artery (ICA); the minimum lumen diameter was 1.7 mm (+) and the distal ICA lumen measured 5.1 mm (X), for a 67% diameter reduction. Angiographic measurements predicted a 50–60% diameter reduction. (B) Spectral Doppler data for the lesion shown in (A) with a peak systolic velocity of 4.57 m/s and an end-diastolic velocity of 1.38 cm/s, corresponding to a >60% diameter reduction.

phy and could not be classified by 3D imaging. Of the remaining 61 bifurcations, 53 were accurately classified as to percent stenosis, giving an overall accuracy of 87%, similar to results obtained when Doppler velocity criteria are used to categorize lesion severity. The sensitivity of 3D imaging to >60% diameter stenoses was 100%, with all such lesions so classified; the positive predictive value for >60% diameter stenosis was 81% (21 of 26 bifurcations). All four total occlusions were correctly identified by 3D imaging. Of the eight lesions that were not accurately classified, all were estimated by 3D imaging to have a higher degree of stenosis than lesions measured by angiography, indicating a possible bias in this technique to slightly underestimate the caliber of the residual lumen at the site of stenosis. Five of these eight lesions were classified as 60–80% diameter stenoses by 3D angiography while subtraction angiography indicated 40–60% diameter reductions; anecdotally in two of these five cases hemodynamic data showed increased flow velocities and poststenotic flow turbulence characteristic of the more severe stenosis, and at endarterectomy the operating surgeon believed that one of the lesions did cause a >60% diameter stenosis (Figure 48–6).

In the evaluation of the extent of lesions, 11 of 13 (85%) were correctly classified as focal, 24 of 29 (83%) as being of moderate extent of <1 cm, and 14 of 14 (100%) as extended lesions of >1 cm. Five lesions were considered to be ulcerated by 3D angiography (Figures 48–5 and 48–7), with four of these ulcerations shown by subtraction angiography. The 3D power Doppler angiography was believed to provide an accurate noninvasive technique comparable to subtraction angiography for the anatomic evaluation of carotid bifurcation atherosclerotic disease, with selectable viewing projections that helped eliminate vessel overlap and other artifacts. The technique complemented the hemodynamic data already available from conventional 2D duplex ultrasound, but at this time could not replace it; instead it allowed a more thorough evaluation of any obstructive disease present without significant additional testing.

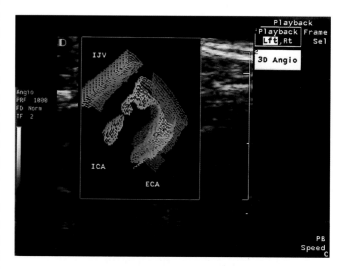

FIGURE 48–7. Three-dimensional reconstruction of a carotid artery bifurcation showing an ulceration in the lesion just past the origin of the internal carotid artery (ICA). IJV, internal jugular vein; ECA, external carotid artery.

Delcker *et al.*[31] investigated 3D power Doppler angiography for transcranial imaging of the major intracranial vessels. Previous studies have shown improved ability for transcranial duplex ultrasound to detect and image the intracranial vessels using power Doppler compared with color Doppler imaging.[32,33] Delcker *et al.* also studied the use of a transpulmonary-stable ultrasound contrast agent. When their 3D studies were compared with diagnostic cerebral angiography, they had imaging success rates of 100% for the ipsilateral anterior cerebral artery, middle cerebral artery (with three or more branches), posterior cerebral artery, and posterior communicating artery, and 90% for the anterior communicating artery. On the side contralateral to the transducer, imaging success rates were 90% for the anterior cerebral artery, 80% for the middle cerebral artery (again with three or more branches), and 100% for the posterior cerebral artery. They concluded that 3D transcranial power Doppler angiography with contrast agent enhancement provided significant improvements in the visualization and evaluation of the major intracranial arteries.

Limitations of Three-Dimensional Imaging and Power Doppler Angiography

Limitations of 3D vascular ultrasound imaging and power Doppler angiography are those that have long been recognized for all applications of ultrasound. Present techniques remain strongly operator dependent, particularly those using freehand scanning to develop the database of image frames for reconstruction. All probe maneuvers must be carefully controlled and done in a smooth, constant speed motion; patient cooperation is also essential during any ultrasound scanning procedure. Specific to vascular imaging and the detection of obstructive disease are the limitations imposed by the lesion itself. Very complex heterogeneous lesions create poor grayscale image quality, degrading the ability to reconstruct image frames and maintain frame-to-frame registration; this is much less a limitation in power Doppler angiography, which is based on a significantly less "noisy" signal for its image. Limiting both techniques, however, is the presence of significant atherosclerotic or vessel wall calcification that prevents the transmission of any ultrasound signals.

Recent Clinical Experience Using Power Doppler Angiography

Few reports have been published on the clinical utility of power Doppler 3D ultrasound in vascular pati-

ents.[30,31,34–39] Following are the results of a study that analyzed our experience concerning the clinical utility of this imaging modality.[40]

Patient Population and Methods

Fifty-three selected patients out of 281 referred to our vascular laboratory during a recent 1-month period underwent conventional color duplex ultrasound and power Doppler imaging for the following indications. All 53 patients had conventional arteriography to verify the results.

Carotid-Vertebral Artery Selection: (1) a question of subtotal versus total carotid occlusion; (2) tortuosity of the artery with limited imaging; (3) the presence of significant disease by Doppler imaging with limited imaging on conventional duplex examination; (4) patients with heavy calcification and limited imaging; and (5) high or deep internal carotid arteries.

Deep Lying Arteries—Renal/Aorta: (1) the arteries are obscured by fat or bowel gas and (2) nonvisualization of the renal orifice.

Peripheral Arteries: (1) a question of subtotal versus total occlusion and (2) a limited view or image on conventional color duplex ultrasound.

The color duplex imaging and the power Doppler examinations were performed by experienced certified vascular technologists in our accredited vascular laboratory using an HDI 5000 Phillips, ATL system (Bothell, WA). Sequential parallel longitudinal views and perpendicular cross-sectional views were obtained on both color duplex and power Doppler imaging. The display quality of both sonographic examinations was classified as satisfactory or unsatisfactory by both the technologist and the interpreting physician, who is also a certified vascular technologist (AFA). A satisfactory image was a well-defined image with clear anatomy and pathology of the examined vessel. The power Doppler imaging portion of the examination was considered to be of positive diagnostic value if the results of that examination were helpful in differentiating subtotal from total occlusion, optimizing image quality, or visualizing deep-lying vessels (e.g., renal artery) that were not seen on conventional duplex examination. If both portions of the examination were inconsistent, the final conclusion was decided based on the results obtained by conventional arteriography.

Results

A positive diagnostic value was achieved using power Doppler imaging in 22 out of 29 (76%) carotid artery examinations. Similarly, 10 out of 14 (71%) peripheral artery examinations had a positive diagnostic value. Four out of five (80%) renal artery examinations had a positive diagnostic value, while three out of five (60%)

TABLE 48–1. Positive diagnostic value of power Doppler imaging.[a]

Arteries	Positive Dx value	No change	Total
Carotid/vertebral	22 (76%)	7 (24%)	29
Peripheral	10 (71%)	4 (29%)	14
Renal	4 (80%)	1 (20%)	5
Aorta/iliacs	3 (60%)	2 (40%)	5
Total	39 (74%)	14 (26%)	53

[a]Overall sensitivity of power Doppler imaging in patients with positive diagnostic value = 95% and positive predictive value = 97%.

TABLE 48–3. Peripheral and renal indications of power Doppler imaging/results.

	Positive Dx value	No change	Total
Peripheral			
Subtotal/total occlusion	6 (75%)	2 (25%)	8
Suboptimal image	4 (67%)	2 (33%)	6
Total	10 (71%)	4 (29%)	14
Renals			
Obscure orifice	3 (100%)	0	3
Suboptimal image	1 (50%)	1 (50%)	2
Total	4 (80%)	1 (20%)	5
Aorta/iliacs			
Suboptimal image	3 (60%)	2 (40%)	5

aortoiliac examinations had a positive diagnostic value. Overall, a positive diagnostic value was achieved by adding power Doppler imaging in 39 out of 53 arteries (74%, Table 48–1). The overall sensitivity of power Doppler imaging in patients with a positive diagnostic value was 95% and the positive predictive value was 97%.

Table 48–2 summarizes the indications of power Doppler imaging and the positive diagnostic value in carotid application. As noted, five out of six patients (83%) who were believed to have total carotid occlusion by conventional color duplex were confirmed to have subtotal occlusion by adding power Doppler imaging. Ten out of 14 (71%) carotid artery patients who were believed to have suboptimal images had a better clearer image on power Doppler imaging (Table 48–2). Table 48–3 summarizes the findings in patients for whom the indications included peripheral arteries, renal arteries, and aortoiliac arteries. As noted in Table 48–3, six out of eight (75%) patients with a questionable subtotal versus total occlusion by conventional duplex examination were confirmed to have subtotal occlusion by power Doppler imaging. Overall, 10 out of 14 (71%) patients with peripheral arterial examinations had a positive diagnostic value. Four out of five (80%) renal examinations resulted in a positive diagnostic value, which included three patients in whom the orifice of the renal arteries was not seen by conventional duplex examina-

tions. Meanwhile, three out of five (60%) aortoiliac examinations resulted in a positive diagnostic value (Table 48–3).

Figures 48–8 through 48–16 illustrate various clinical scenarios where a positive diagnostic value was achieved by adding power Doppler imaging.

In summary, power Doppler imaging is believed to have the following advantages over conventional color Doppler ultrasound: it is sensitive to very low flow velocities, is less angle dependent, is not subject to aliasing, and has a good signal-to-noise ratio.[23,24] Power Doppler imaging is a relatively new sonographic technology that is based on technical principles different from conventional color Doppler imaging for the generation of intravascular color signals.[23,24] The intensity of color signals in this method depends on the reflected echo amplitude from red blood cells, thus reflecting the density of the red blood cells within the examined sample volume. The addition of negative and positive frequency shifts from the moving red blood cells and the use of special filters for blood/tissue discrimination will increase the signal-to-noise ratio, which will result in higher sensitivity to visualizing blood flow and improve the definition of intravascular surfaces. Power Doppler imaging also provides homogeneous color signals, even in tight stenoses, and generates a superior angiographic-like imaging of the vascular lumen surface, as indicated in previous illustrations. This advantage of power Doppler imaging over conventional color duplex imaging minimizes the necessity of conventional arteriography prior to vascular intervention, e.g., prior to carotid endarterectomy. Since power Doppler imaging does not provide information on the direction of the moving blood cells, this modality of imaging must be considered as complementary to conventional color duplex imaging where specific velocity criteria have been determined by many studies for the classification of severity of stenoses.

TABLE 48–2. Carotid indications of power Doppler imaging/results.

	Positive Dx value	No change	Total
Subtotal/total occlusion	5 (83%)	1 (17%)	6
Suboptimal image	10 (71%)	4 (29%)	14
High/deep internal carotids artery	4 (80%)	1 (20%)	5
Tortuous artery	3 (75%)	1 (25%)	4
Total	22	7	29

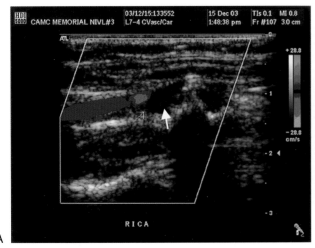

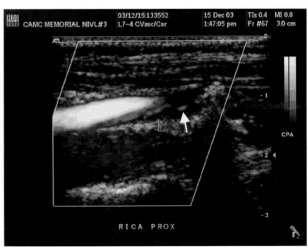

Figure 48–8. (A) Color duplex imaging of a right internal carotid artery suggesting total occlusion. (B) Power Doppler image of the same artery showing string sign (arrow), i.e., subtotal occlusion. (Reproduced with permissions from AbuRhama AF, Jarrett K, Hayes JD. Clinical implications of power Doppler three-dimensional ultrasonography. Vascular 2004;12:293–300, BC Decker, Inc.)

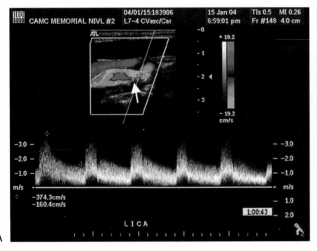

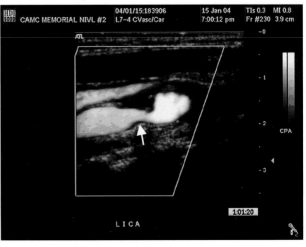

Figure 48–9. (A) Suboptimal image of a left internal carotid artery by conventional duplex ultrasound. (B) A better image is obtained by adding power Doppler ultrasound. (Reproduced with permissions from AbuRhama AF, Jarrett K, Hayes JD. Clinical implications of power Doppler three-dimensional ultrasonography. Vascular 2004;12:293–300, BC Decker, Inc.)

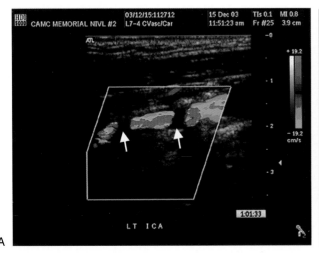

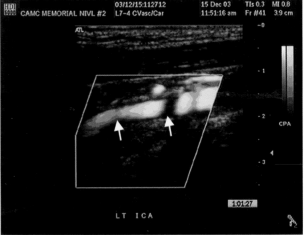

Figure 48–10. (A) Left internal carotid artery with multiple defects of color flow (secondary to shadowing, arrows). (B) Color flow is seen in one area and somewhat seen in the other area (arrows) when power Doppler was added. (Reproduced with permissions from AbuRhama AF, Jarrett K, Hayes JD. Clinical implications of power Doppler three-dimensional ultrasonography. Vascular 2004;12:293–300, BC Decker, Inc.)

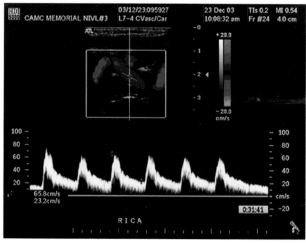

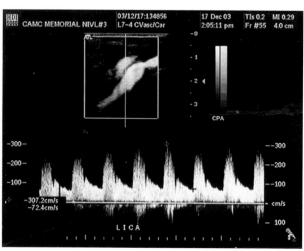

FIGURE 48–11. (A) A deep-lying left internal carotid artery with suboptimal imaging on color duplex ultrasound. (B) A well-defined stenosis using power Doppler ultrasound. (Reproduced with permissions from AbuRhama AF, Jarrett K, Hayes JD. Clinical implications of power Doppler three-dimensional ultrasonography. Vascular 2004;12:293–300, BC Decker, Inc.)

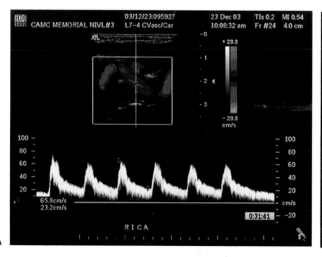

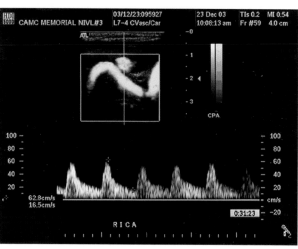

FIGURE 48–12. (A) A tortuous internal carotid artery with poor image of the tortuous segment. (B) Clearly shown tortuosity using power Doppler imaging. (Reproduced with permissions from AbuRhama AF, Jarrett K, Hayes JD. Clinical implications of power Doppler three-dimensional ultrasonography. Vascular 2004;12:293–300, BC Decker, Inc.)

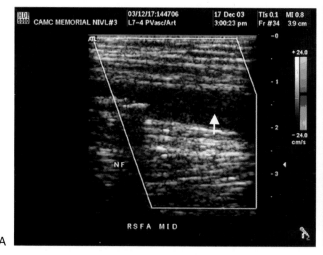

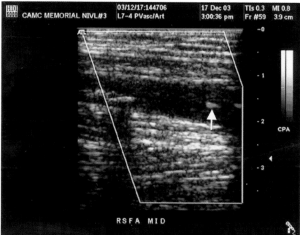

FIGURE 48–13. (A) Color duplex imaging showing a right mid-superficial femoral artery occlusion. (B) A string sign was seen (arrow) when power Doppler imaging was added. (Reproduced with permissions from AbuRhama AF, Jarrett K, Hayes JD. Clinical implications of power Doppler three-dimensional ultrasonography. Vascular 2004;12:293–300, BC Decker, Inc.)

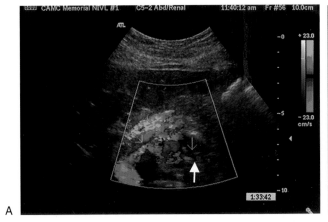
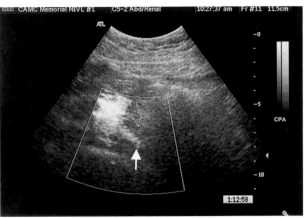

A

B

FIGURE 48–14. (A) A color duplex image of the renal artery that does not clearly show the orifice of the renal artery. (B) The origin of the renal artery (arrow) is well seen using power Doppler imaging. (Reproduced with permissions from AbuRhama AF, Jarrett K, Hayes JD. Clinical implications of power Doppler three-dimensional ultrasonography. Vascular 2004;12:293–300, BC Decker, Inc.)

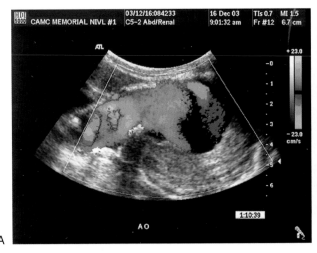
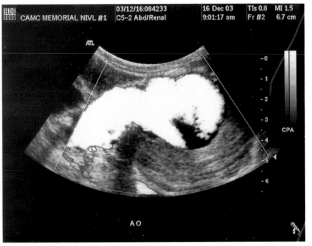

A

B

FIGURE 48–15. (A) A color duplex image of an abdominal aortic aneurysm. (B) A better definition of the color flow and morphology using power Doppler ultrasound. (Reproduced with permissions from AbuRhama AF, Jarrett K, Hayes JD. Clinical implications of power Doppler three-dimensional ultrasonography. Vascular 2004;12:293–300, BC Decker, Inc.)

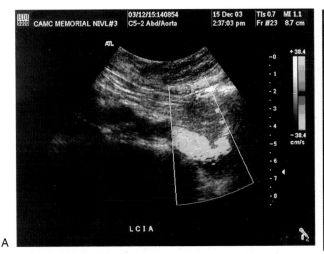
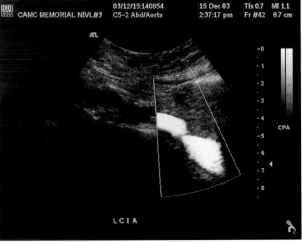

A

B

FIGURE 48–16. (A) A limited color duplex image of a deep-lying left common iliac artery. (B) A clearer image using power Doppler imaging. (Reproduced with permissions from AbuRhama AF, Jarrett K, Hayes JD. Clinical implications of power Doppler three-dimensional ultrasonography. Vascular 2004;12:293–300, BC Decker, Inc.)

Our present study demonstrates that positive diagnostic values were obtained by the addition of power Doppler imaging in 74% of arteries examined. Specifically, this technology was very valuable in differentiating subtotal from total arterial occlusions, which was noted quite clearly in carotid artery examinations in our study (83%). High deep internal carotid arteries (ICAs) were also better seen by adding this technology (80%). This technology was also quite helpful in patients with limited or suboptimal imaging. Three out of three (100%) renal artery orifices that were obscured on conventional color duplex imaging were easily seen by adding power Doppler imaging.

In conclusion, 3D power Doppler imaging, while a more recent technological development, can be more readily applied to clinical practice. This is, in part, because of its ease of use, the ability to use free hand scanning, and a good signal-to-noise ratio, giving a better defined blood–tissue interface, and the speed with which these images can be reconstructed and displayed. Three-dimensional power Doppler imaging has been shown to be capable of defining the severity and extent of atherosclerotic lesions, characterizing the vascularity of other lesions, and extending the use of conventional color power Doppler imaging to further define parameters related to solid organ perfusion, e.g., kidneys.

Future of Three-Dimensional Imaging and Power Doppler Angiography

The future of 3D imaging for vascular applications appears promising. Three-dimensional imaging of the vessel wall remains primarily a research tool, with a variety of imaging and data processing techniques in development. The best results to date have relied on invasive, intravascular ultrasound using high-frequency transducers for good resolution. Reported results have been good for 3D visualization of atherosclerotic lesions, both in peripheral arteries and in the coronary arteries. These images have provided valuable feedback, for example, in the placement of stents and in the assessment following their deployment. The techniques being developed should provide the capability to extend other current 2D applications, making it possible to investigate preoperatively the extent of any tumor invasion of adjacent vascular structures. In addition, 3D imaging will allow more thorough evaluation of extrinsic vascular compression syndromes, guiding the management of cases of May-Thurner syndrome[41,42] or thoracic outlet compression causing Paget-von Schroetter syndrome.[43]

Three-dimensional power Doppler angiography, while a more recent technological development, has been more readily applied to clinical problems. This is in part because of its ease of use, the ability to use freehand scanning, a good signal-to-noise ratio giving a well-defined blood–tissue interface, and the speed with which these 3D images can be reconstructed and displayed. Three-dimensional power Doppler angiography has been shown to be capable of defining the severity and extent of atherosclerotic obstructive lesions, characterizing the vascularity of other lesions, and extending the use of 2D power Doppler imaging to further define parameters related to solid organ perfusion in, for example, the kidneys. The vascular supply and distribution in other organ systems, such as the orbit of the eye, have not been well studied yet, but the technological capability is present, with adequate resolution, to make such studies possible.

References

1. Howry DH, Posakony G, Cushman R, et al. Three dimensional and stereoscopic observation of body structures by ultrasound. J Appl Physiol. 1956;9:304–306.
2. Moritz WE, Medema DK, Ainsworth M, et al. Three-dimensional reconstruction and volume calculation from a series of nonparallel, real-time, ultrasonic images. Circulation 1980;62(Suppl):111–143.
3. Steen E, Olstad B. Volume rendering of 3D medical ultrasound data using direct feature mapping. IEEE Trans Med Imaging 1994;13:517–525.
4. Detmer PR, Bashein G, Hodges T, et al. 3D ultrasonic image feature location based on magnetic scan head tracking: In vitro calibration and validation. Ultrasound Med Biol 1994;20:923–936.
5. Rankin RN, Fenster A, Downey DB, et al. Three-dimensional sonographic reconstruction: Techniques and diagnostic applications. AJR 1993;161:695–702.
6. Roelandt JR, DiMario C, Pandian NG, et al. Three-dimensional reconstruction of intracoronary ultrasound images: Rationale, approaches, problems and directions. Circulation 1994;90:1044–1055.
7. von Birgelen C, Kutryk MJB, Gil R, et al. Quantification of the minimal luminal cross-sectional area after coronary stenting by two- and three-dimensional intravascular ultrasound versus edge detection and videodensitometry. Am J Cardiol. 1996;78:520–525.
8. Di Mario C, von Birgelen C, Prati F, et al. Three-dimensional reconstruction of two-dimensional intravascular ultrasound: Clinical or research tool? Br Heart J 1995;73(Suppl. 2):26–32.
9. Franceschi D, Bondi JA, Rubin JR. A new approach for three-dimensional reconstruction of arterial ultrasonography. J Vasc Surg 1992;15:800–805.
10. Kelly IM, Gardener JE, Brett AD, et al. Three-dimensional US of the fetus: Work in progress. Radiology 1994;192:253–259.
11. Levine RA, Weyman AE, Handschumacher MD. Three-dimensional echocardiography: Techniques and applications. Am J Cardiol 1992;69:121H–130H.

12. Moskalik A, Carson PL, Meyer CR, et al. Registration of three-dimensional compound ultrasound scans of the breast for refraction and motion corrections. Ultrasound Med Biol 1995;21:769–778.

13. Nelson TR, Pretorius DH, Slansky M, et al. Three-dimensional echocardiographic evaluation of fetal heart anatomy and function. J Ultrasound Med 1996;15:1–9.

14. Lee W, Comstock CH, Kirk JS, et al. Birthweight prediction by three-dimensional ultrasound volumes of the fetal thigh and abdomen. J Ultrasound Med 1997;16:799–805.

15. Cusumano A, Coleman DJ, Silverman RH, et al. Three-dimensional ultrasound imaging: Clinical applications. Ophthalmology 1998;105:300–306.

16. Marks LS, Dorey FJ, Macairan ML, et al. Three-dimensional ultrasound device for rapid determination of bladder volume. Urology 1997;50:341–348.

17. Fine D. Three-dimensional ultrasound imaging of the gallbladder and dilated biliary tree: Reconstruction from real-time B-scans. Br J Radiol 1991;64:1056–1057.

18. Barry CD, Allott CP, John NW, et al. Three-dimensional freehand ultrasound: Image reconstruction and volume analysis. Ultrasound Med Biol 1997;23:1209–1224.

19. von Ramm OT, Smith SW, Carroll BA. Real-time volumetric US imaging. Radiology 1994;193(P):308.

20. Rosenfield K, Kaufman J, Pieczek A, et al. Real-time three dimensional reconstruction of intravascular images of iliac arteries. Am J Cardiol 1992;70:412–415.

21. Riccabona M, Nelson TR, Pretorius DH, et al. Distance and volume measurement using three-dimensional ultrasonography. J Ultrasound Med 1995;14:881–886.

22. King DL, King DL Jr, Shao MY. Evaluation of in vitro measurement accuracy of a three-dimensional ultrasound scanner. J Ultrasound Med 1991;10:77–82.

23. Rubin JM, Bude RO, Carson PL, et al. Power Doppler US: A potentially useful alternative to mean frequency-based color Doppler US. Radiology 1994;190:853–856.

24. Rubin JM, Adler RS, Fowlkes JB, et al. Fractional moving blood volume: Estimation with power Doppler US. Radiology 1995;197:183–190.

25. von Birgelen C, DiMario C, Reimers B, et al. Three-dimensional intracoronary ultrasound imaging: Methodology and clinical relevance for the assessment of coronary arteries and bypass grafts. J Cardiovasc Surg 1996;37:129–139.

26. Goldberg SL, Colombo A, Nakamura S, et al. Benefit of intravascular ultrasound in the deployment of Palmaz–Schatz stents. J Am Coll Cardiol 1994;24:996–1003.

27. White RA, Donayre CE, Walot I, et al. Preliminary clinical outcome and imaging criterion for endovascular prosthesis development in high-risk patients who have aortoiliac and traumatic arterial lesions. J Vasc Surg 1996;24:556–571.

28. Vonesh MJ, Cho C-H, Pinto JV, et al. Regional vascular mechanical properties by 3D intravascular ultrasound with finite-element analysis. Am J Physiol 1997;272:H425–H437.

29. Carson PL, Moskalik AP, Govil A, et al. The 3D and 2D color flow display of breast masses. Ultrasound Med Biol 1997;23:837–849.

30. Bendick PJ, Brown OW, Hernandez D, et al. Three-dimensional vascular imaging using Doppler ultrasound. Am J Surg 1998;176:183–187.

31. Delcker A, Turowski B. Diagnostic value of three-dimensional transcranial contrast duplex sonography. J Neuroimaging 1997;7:139–144.

32. Kenton AR, Martin PJ, Evans DH. Power Doppler: An advance over colour Doppler for transcranial imaging? Ultrasound Med Biol 1996;22:313–317.

33. Postert T, Federlein J, Przuntek H, et al. Insufficient and absent acoustic temporal bone window: Potential and limitations of transcranial contrast-enhanced color-coded sonography and contrast-enhanced power-based sonography. Ultrasound Med Biol 1997;23:857–862.

34. Steinke W, Ries S, Artemis N, Schwartz A, Hennerici M. Power Doppler imaging of carotid artery stenosis. Stroke 1997;28:1981–1987.

35. Griewing B, Morgenstern C, Driesner F, Kallwellis G, Walker ML, Kessler C. Cerebrovascular disease assessed by color-flow and power Doppler ultrasonography: Comparison with digital subtraction angiography in internal carotid artery stenosis. Stroke 1996;27:95–100.

36. Keberle M, Jenett M, Beissert M, Jahns R, Haerten R, Hahn D. Three-dimensional power Doppler sonography in screening for carotid artery disease. J Clin Ultrasound 2000;28:441–451.

37. Keberle M, Jenett M, Wittenberg G, Kessler C, Beissert M, Hahn D. Comparison of 3D power Doppler ultrasound, color Doppler ultrasound, and digital subtraction angiography in carotid stenosis. Rofo Fortschr Geb Rontgenstr Neuen Bildgeb Verfahr 2001;173:133–138.

38. von Herbay A, Haussinger D. Abdominal three-dimensional power Doppler imaging. J Ultrasound Med 2001;20:151–157.

39. Bucek RA, Reiter M, Dirisamer A, Haumer M, Fritz A, Minar E, Lammer J. Three-dimensional color Doppler sonography in carotid artery stenosis. AJNR Am J Neuroradiol 2003;24:1294–1299.

40. AbuRahma AF, Jarrett K, Hayes JD. Clinical implications of power Doppler three-dimensional ultrasonography. Vascular 2004;12:293–300.

41. Akers DL Jr, Creado B, Hewitt RL. Iliac vein compression syndrome: Case report and review of the literature. J Vasc Surg 1996;24:477–481.

42. Kogel H. Regarding iliac vein compression syndrome: Case report and review of the literature. J Vasc Surg 1997;26:721–722.

43. Chengelis DL, Glover JL, Bendick P, et al. The use of intravascular ultrasound in the management of thoracic outlet syndrome. Am Surg 1994;60:592–596.

49
Contrast-Enhanced Ultrasound

Lyssa N. Ochoa, Esteban Henao, Alan Lumsden, and Ruth L. Bush

Introduction

Gramiak and Shah first introduced the technique of using contrast enhanced two-dimensional echocardiography in 1968.[1,2] The first contrast agents used were "free" microbubbles that were limited by their low persistence and efficacy. Since that time, the development of contrast agents has followed several methods.[2,3] Aqueous solutions, colloidal suspensions, and emulsions were studied as possible candidates for contrast agents; however, their safety and efficacy were not compatible with ultrasound. Newer contrast agents are composed of stabilized microbubbles that offer adequate safety profiles and improved efficacy. Their properties approach that of the ideal contrast agent, which is nontoxic, injectable intravenously, able to pass through the capillary pulmonary bed, and stable enough to achieve enhancement for the duration of the examination.

Fundamentals of Ultrasound Contrast Agents

Today's contrast agents are stabilized mircrobubbles made with sugar matrices, albumin, lipids, or polymer shells with or without surfactants. These elastic shells enhance their stability by adding physical support and reducing surface tension at the gas–liquid interface. Simple air-filled microbubbles have evolved to incorportate gases with low diffusion coefficients, such as perfluorocarbons. Their low solubility in blood and increased persistence allow longer examination times.[4,5] Manipulation of the type of gas used and the structure of the encapsulating shell is a currently used technique to prolong contrast enhancement.

The classification of contrast agents is dependent on pharmacokinetics (Table 49–1). They are distinguished mainly based on their ability to cross the pulmonary circulation and their half life. Some contrast agents also have tissue- or organ-specific phases in addition to their vascular phase.[6] For example, Levovist (SHU 508A, Schering, Berlin, Germany) once eliminated from the blood pool localizes to the liver and spleen, approximately 20 min after intravenous injection.[7] The mechanism of this phenomenon is not fully understood at this time, but it is believed that the microbubbles adhere to the sinusoids. Other examples include Sonazoid (Nycomed Amersham, Oslo, Norway) and Sonovist (SHU 563A Schering, Berlin, Germany), which are phagocytosed by hepatic Kupffer cells.[8] It is worth noting that Kupffer cells are not found in metastases or hepatic carcinomas, and therefore these agents accumulate only in normal liver (Figure 49–1).

Contrast agents increase the backscatter of the ultrasound signal intensity, thus improving Doppler analysis as well as enhancing the grayscale echostructure on specific imaging sequences by up to 25 dB (a greater than 300-fold increase).[9] The image quality that contrast agents provide is dependent on the properties of the agent as well as the imaging sequence and signal processing. Each agent behaves uniquely within a certain ultrasound field, which allows for signal processing to be manipulated to optimize microbubble detection.[10] Specific contrast-imaging sequences have been developed by tailoring the acoustic power, the transmit and receive frequencies, the pulse frequency, and the pulse phase and amplitude to each contrast agent for maximal efficacy.

Adverse effects are a possible outcome of administration of any drug or contrast agent including ultrasound contrast agents. Most adverse events with ultrasound contrast agents, though, are rare and of mild intensity.[11] Most commonly, patients experience a temporary alteration in taste, pain at the injection site, a warm facial sensation, or a generalized flush.[12] Other reports of adverse events include dyspnea, chest pain, headache, and nausea.[13–15] Studies have reported that the incidence of adverse events with ultrasound contrast agents is similar to that

TABLE 49–1. Ultrasound contrast agents.

Agent	Company	Gas	Shell	Approval
First generation, nontranspulmonary vascular				
Free microbubbles		Air	None	
Echovist (SHU 454)	Schering	Air	Galactose	Europe
Second-generation, transpulmonary vascular, short half-life (<5 min)				
Albunex	Molecular Biosystems	Air	Albumin	United States
Levovist (SHU 508 A)	Schering	Air	Palmitic acid	Europe, Japan
Third-generation, transpulmonary vascular, longer half-life (>5 min)				
Aerosomes (Definity MRX115, DMP115)	Bristol-Meyers-Squibb	Perfluoropropane	Phospholipid	United States
Echogen (QW3600)	SonoGen	Dodecafluoropentane	Surgactant	a
Optison (FSO 69)	Amersham	Octafluoropropane	Albumin	United States, Europe
Sono Vue (BR1)	Bracco	Sulfur hexafluoride	Phospholipid	Europe
Imaivst (AF0150)	Alliance	Perfluorohexane	Surfactant	United States
Transpulmonary with organ-specific phase				
Levovist (SHU 508A)	Schering	Air	Palmitic acid	Europe, Japan
Sonavist (SHU 563A)	Schering	Air	Cyanoacrylate	b
Sonazoid (NC100100)	Amersham	Perfluorocarbon	Surfactant	a

[a]Currently in clinical trials.
[b]Clinical development stopped.

in a control group.[16] Nevertheless, ultrasound contrast agents have a superb safety profile with no specific renal, liver, or cerebral toxicities.

Mechanics of Ultrasonogaphic Contrast

Microbubble behavior is influenced by the local acoustic power.[17] Local acoustic power depends on the output power of the ultrasound system, the transmit frequency, and the attenuation of the ultrasound beam with depth. The mechanical index (MI) reflects output power, and therefore correlates with the local acoustic power. As

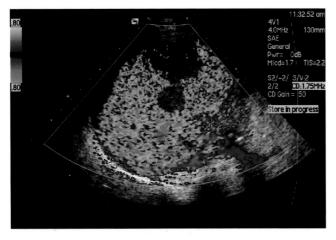

FIGURE 49–1. Imaging 3 min after Levovist injection improves the delineation of tumor metastases. (Image courtesy of Dr. Peter Dawson, University College Hospital, London, UK.)

mentioned above, each contrast agent behaves uniquely at a given MI, and, therefore, each agent will have its own optimal imaging sequence.

Low Acoustic Power (MI < 0.1)

At low MI, microbubbles resonate equally and symmetrically (linear response) with the high and low pressures generated by the incident ultrasound wave with minimal destruction. They act as very efficient signal scatterers, which is attributed to the difference in their compressibility and density compared to the surrounding tissues (Figure 49–2). Scattering efficiency increases as a function of microbubble radius to the sixth power, and therefore larger bubbles display higher backscatter coefficients.[5] As well, increasing shell stiffness or gas density in turn decreases the microbubble response. Under low MI imaging, the intensity of the scattered signal is linearly related to that of the incident ultrasound beam.[9] Low MI is useful in conventional Doppler applications and real-time contrast imaging.

Intermediate Acoustic Power (0.1 < MI < 0.5)

The amplitude of the microbubble oscillations in an ultrasound field increases as the MI is increased. As the amplitude increases, the microbubble oscillations become asynchronous with the ultrasound wave (Figure 49–3). By manipulating the local acoustic power, the microbubbles begin to echo a harmonic response at frequencies that differ from that of the incident wave (fundamental frequency). The highest intensity response is that of the second harmonic response, which is found at twice the

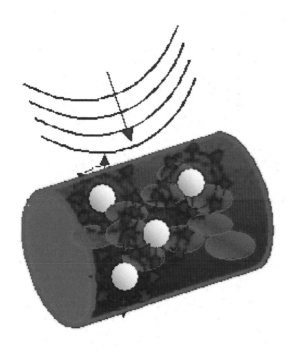

FIGURE 49–2. Resonance of microbubbles. (Image created by Dr. E. Stride, University College London, UK. Reprinted with permission of Dr. Nader Saffari, University College London, UK.)

fundamental frequency. Those responses found at higher frequencies are called higher harmonics. Specific types of harmonics called ultraharmonics can be obtained at specific frequencies such as 1.5 or 3.5 times the fundamental frequency.[5] There two main advantages of intermediate MI imaging. The first is the avoidance of microbubble destruction while eliciting a good harmonic contrast signal. The second is the reduction in the harmonics elicited from the surrounding tissues. Because the advantage of contrast agents is their harmonic echo, any tissue harmonics become the background "noise." Tissue is less

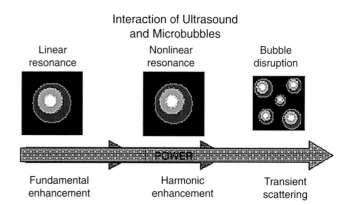

FIGURE 49–4. As acoustic power is increased, microbubbles move from a linear response to a nonlinear, harmonics-producing response. At maximum power, destruction of the microbubbles occurs. (Image courtesy of Dr. David Adams.)

compressible and more dense than the microbubbles, therefore requiring a higher MI for a harmonic response. Intermediate MI scanning allows for a higher contrast-to-tissue ratio compared to a high MI by limiting the tissue harmonic response, and thus eases the removal of the background "noise" from the contrast signal.[17]

High Acoustic Power (MI > 0.5)

The destruction of microbubbles occurs at higher acoustic powers. The encapsulating shell is broken and the gas diffuses into the surrounding fluid. The rupture of the microbubble causes an intense echo, very rich in nonlinear (harmonic) components (Figures 49–4 and 49–5) Although the destruction of contrast agents is often viewed as a limitation, it allows for improved sensitivity in microbubble detection. When color and power Doppler are used, the change in the echo of two consecutive pulses is seen as a particular color pixel. These color signals thus correlate with the distribution of the microbubble with little affect from blood flow characteristics.[5]

FIGURE 49–3. Nonlinear microbubbles return not only the fundamental (transmitted frequency) but also a second harmonic frequency that is at twice the transmitted frequency. (Image courtesy of Dr. David Adams.)

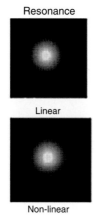

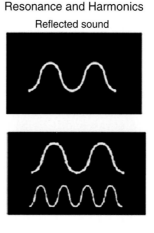

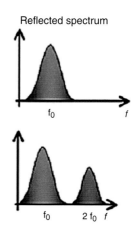

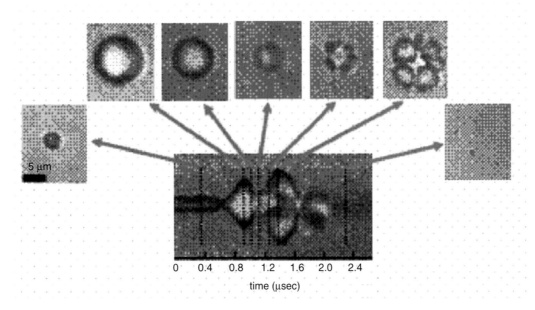

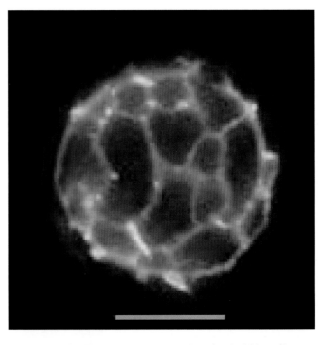

FIGURE 49–5. EM of a microbubble responding to increasing ultrasound MIs.

Microbubble Technology

Newer microbubble engineering techniques have focused on optimizing tissue-specific binding of microbubbles by manipulation of the components of the encapsulating shell. One such strategy exploits the disease-related upregulation of surface receptors in activated leukocytes that bind nonspecifically to either albumin or lipid in the microbubble shell.[18] For example, Linder et al. studied the binding of albumin and lipid shells to activated leukocytes after reperfusion injury and exposure to proinflammatory cytokines. Albumin binds to the β_2-integrin Mac-1 on the activated leukocytes, which in turn binds to intercellular adhesion molecule (ICAM)-1 expressed on endothelial cells in areas of inflammation. Lipids are found to undergo opsonization by complements and bind via a complement receptor to activated leukocytes. By adding phosphatidylserine to the lipid shell, there is a 6-fold increase in the affinity of the microbubble to the activated leukocytes due to increased complement attachment to the lipid shell.[18,19] Inflammation specific binding of microbubbles can augment the visualization of inflammatory atherosclerotic plaques. Since the amount of microbubbles bound correlates with the amount of inflammation, control-enhanced ultrasound (CEUS) will be able to determine the inflammatory phenotype of plaques, thus identifying those plaques with increased vulnerability to thrombose.

Another strategy to enhance the tissue-specific retention of microbubbles is the conjugation of ligands or antibodies that recognize specific antigens or receptors on a specific tissue type (Figure 49–6). One example is the attachment of an oligopeptide to the shell surface that recognizes glycoprotein IIb/IIIa integrin receptor on activated platelets.[20,21] This allows the visualization of thrombus by the binding of microbubbles to platelets, as well as means for clot lysis when the microbubbles are ruptured using an ultrasound beam.[22] A modification of this

FIGURE 49–6. Fluorescent targeted microbubble. (Source: http://ferraralab.bme.ucdavis.edu/index.html?page=http://ferraralab.bme.ucdavis.edu/research.html.)

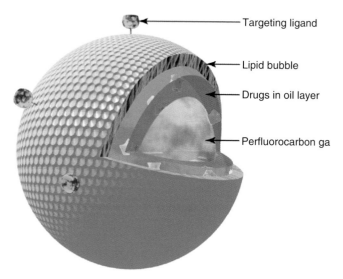

FIGURE 49–7. Schematic of a microbubble with ligands conjugated to its outer shell and encapsulating drugs. (Image courtesy of Drs. Evan Unger and Martin Blomley, ImaRx Therapeutics, Inc., Tucson, AZ.)

strategy by adding the attachment of a chemical spacer, such as polyethylene glycol, allows the ligand to be projected further away from the shell surface, thus increasing its affinity for tissue-specific antigens or receptors.[23]

In addition to tissue-specific binding, new microbubbles are now being used as a vehicle for drug and gene delivery (Figure 49–7). Chemotherapeutic agents, thrombolytics, and plasmid DNA are encapsulated in an oil emulsion within the microbubble. Once the microbubbles have reached their target tissue, an ultrasound beam with a high MI is used to rupture the bubbles and release the agent. This focal destruction of microbubbles decreases the systemic concentration of an agent, thus improving its therapeutic index and limiting systemic toxicities.[24] Encapsulation of genes also protects naked DNA and vectors from plasma endonucleases and hepatic clearance, which limits their stability[24] (Figure 49–8). Engineering microbubbles as target-specific therapeutic delivery vehicles will have a wide range of applications in the diagnosis and therapy of numerous medical conditions.

Ultrasound Imaging Techniques

B-Mode and Color Imaging

Contrast agents can be employed when conventional B-mode imaging and Doppler imaging modalities, including color, power, and spectral imaging. They can be used to opacify fluid-containing cavities such as the bladder, uterus, cardiac chambers (Figure 49–9), and some large venous structures. Echovist (Schering AG, Berlin, Germany) has been used for sonosalpingography[25] and Levovist has been used to detect vesicouteric reflux (Schering).[26] This allows equally sensitive and specific imaging alternatives to conventional radiographs while avoiding ionizing radiation exposure. The limitation of contrast agents with B-mode imaging is that there is no added enhancement in solid structures. Doppler imaging provides excellent detection of microbubbles, but it is limited by color blooming and oversaturation artifacts.[5]

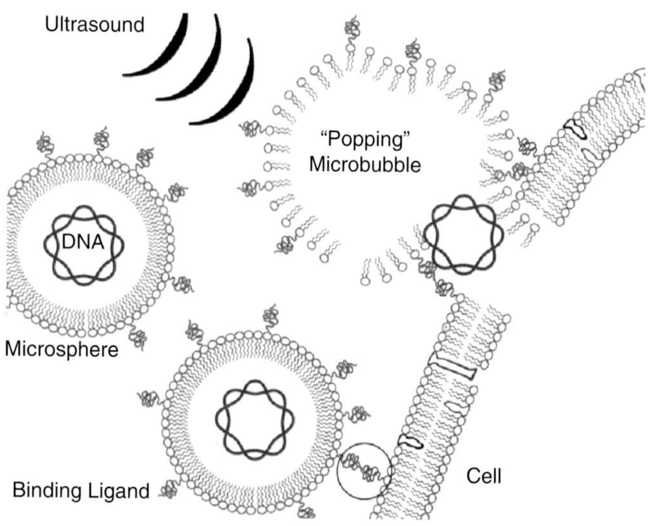

FIGURE 49–8. Schematic of microbubble gene delivery. (Image courtesy of Drs. Evan Unger and Martin Blomley, ImaRx Therapeutics, Inc., Tucson, AZ.)

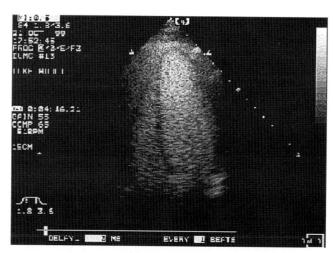

FIGURE 49–9. An apical four-chamber view demonstrating optimal left ventricular opacification with microbubbles. (Image reproduced from McCulloch M, Gresser C, Moos S, et al. Ultrasound contrast physics: A series on contrast echocardiography. J Am Soc Echocardiography 2000;13:962. With permission from Dr. David Adams, Duke University Echo Lab.)

Stimulated Acoustic Emission

This microbubble destructive modality involves an initial wave of ultrasound at a high mechanical index, which ruptures the microbubbles. Signal responses are recorded before and after this destruction, and the loss of correlation between the two signals maps the distribution of the contrast agent.[7] As mentioned above, some organ-specific contrast agents accumulate only in normal liver tissue. This characteristic has been utilized to detect liver metastases using Levovist. Metastases appear as signal defects[27] (Figures 49–10 and 49–11).

Contrast-Enhanced Dynamic Flow

Conventional Doppler imaging can be used with multiple pulse techniques. After the ideal bandwidth is determined, consecutive pulses are emitted. The flow signals are isolated from static tissue signals by amplifying their intercorrelation at different times, and the static tissue signals are removed. This technique, called advanced dynamic flow, allows better spatial delineation of the microvasculature of superficial structures compared to conventional Doppler modes (Figure 49–12). However, its sensitivity is limited by the depth of the structure of interest. The utilization of contrast agents with this technique expands its uses to the visualization of deep structures, hypoperfused structures, and even real-time perfusion imaging using lower MIs to preserve microbubbles.[5]

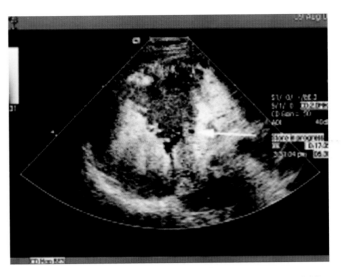

FIGURE 49–11. The presence of liver-specific microbubbles (Levovist) administered 5 min earlier. A defect is clearly seen in the central right lobe of the liver, with several additional defects thought to represent additional satellite foci of hepatocellular carcinoma. (Image courtesy of Drs. Evan Unger and Martin Blomley, ImaRx Therapeutics, Inc., Tucson, AZ.)

Harmonic Imaging

Harmonic imaging is a nonlinear imaging modality that can detect microbubble harmonic responses at a higher sensitivity than the response from the surrounding tissues. The weaker nonharmonic echos from the multiple responses from the body wall (as with obese patients) are filtered from the final image as well, improving the signal-to-noise ratio.[9] Its sensitivity is derived from the fact that the microbubbles produce a unique nonlinear, harmonic response that can be separated from the tissue echos and large vessel blood flow. Currently, there are commercially available transducers that can both emit ultrasound energy and detect the microbubble harmonic response. These transducers are tuned in to detect the resonant frequency of microbubbles, which range in diameter from 1 to 9 μm, in the 1–9 MHz range.[28,29]

Several techniques can be used with harmonic imaging to refine the detection of the nonlinear, harmonic response of the contrast agents including conventional imaging, subtraction techniques using single (coherent imaging mode) or multiple pulses (pulse or phase inversion), and a combination of the latter for multiframe subtraction techniques. Conventional imaging uses a monopulse technique in which a single pulse of ultrasound is emitted and the second harmonic of the microbubble echo is isolated using filters. The microbubble signal returns at 10–15 dB higher than the signal from the surrounding clutter. Harmonic imaging can provide grayscale and Doppler information; however, it

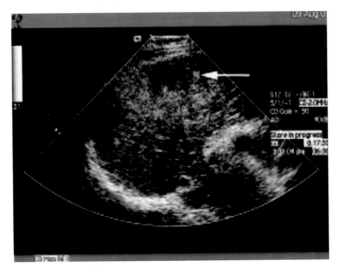

FIGURE 49–10. B-mode imaging shows the liver is heterogeneous with an ill-defined lesion (arrow). (Image courtesy of Drs. Evan Unger and Martin Blomley, ImaRx Therapeutics, Inc., Tucson, AZ.)

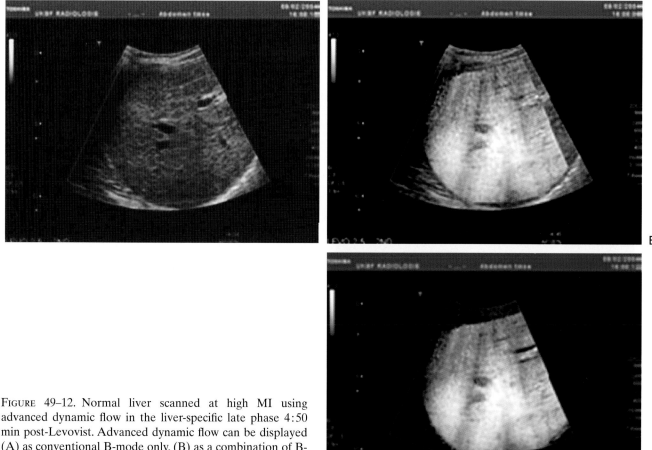

FIGURE 49–12. Normal liver scanned at high MI using advanced dynamic flow in the liver-specific late phase 4:50 min post-Levovist. Advanced dynamic flow can be displayed (A) as conventional B-mode only, (B) as a combination of B-mode and colorized contrast information, or (C) as a contrast only image. (Images courtesy of Dr. Thomas Albrecht, Campus Benjamin Franklin, Berlin, Germany.)

does have its limitations. First, the filtering process to isolate the second harmonic from the fundamental frequency affects the image quality. Also, the increased attenuation of the harmonic frequency compared to the fundamental frequency limits the depth of the imaging capabilities.[5]

Pulse/Phase Inversion

Pulse or phase inversion involves the emission of two consecutive pulses in inverted phases and the detection of the difference of the unique resonance of microbubbles in each phase.[29] Since microbubbles have a unique harmonic response to the consecutive pulses, the difference in the echo signals in the two phases results in an increased sensitivity in the detection of the microbubbles (Figure 49–13). Power pulse inversion utilizes these same principles using a multipulse technique. The multipulse technique adds to the sensitivity of the modality

and improves the differentiation between liquids and solids, as well as limiting motion artifacts.[11]

Intermittent Imaging

Intermittent scanning is employed when using a high MI imaging modality for microbubble destruction.[5] It allows for replenishment of the contrast agent between images. The frame rate is reduced to about one frame per second compared to the conventional 30 frames per second. The frame rate can also be synchronized with the cardiac cycle so that the microbubble can be carried into the area of interest where the microbubbles have been destroyed. Depending on the imaging delay time after the microbubbles have been destroyed, regions with either increased or decreased blood volumes can be determined. Intermittent imaging is, thus, limited by its inability to provide real-time imaging. Another limitation is motion artifact between image acquisitions.

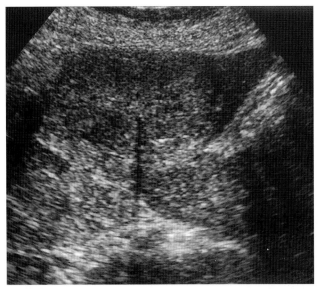

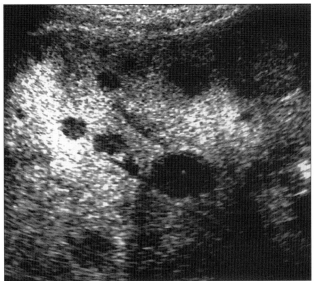

FIGURE 49–13. A 78-year-old man with metastatic liver disease. (A) Native B-mode sonogram shows inhomogeneous parenchyma of the liver, suggestive of focal liver lesions. (B) Contrast-enhanced late-phase pulse-inversion sonogram shows clear demarcation of multiple focal lesions without enhancement surrounded by enhanced liver parenchyma. Liver biopsy revealed metastatic liver disease by adenocarcinoma. Diffuse infiltration of the liver was confirmed on CT. (Source: http://www.ajronline.org/cgi/reprint/179/5/1273. Copyright © American Roentgen Ray Society. Permission requested.)

Flash Echo Imaging

Flash echo imaging is a technique that involves using a low MI between intermittent high MI destructive phases and following the target to be imaged during the entire study. A real-time anatomic image and a contrast-enhanced image during bubble destruction can be viewed simultaneously on the image screen[5] (Toshiba Medical Systems, Tokyo, Japan) (Figure 49–14).

Real-Time Digital Subtraction

Another imaging sequence involves real-time digital subtraction of a bubble-destruction phase image from a consecutively acquired background image taken milliseconds apart. This technique limits motion artifact and improves the visibility of the microbubbles in the resulting image[5] (Figure 49–15).

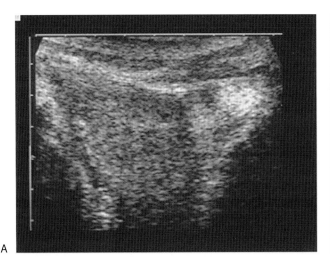

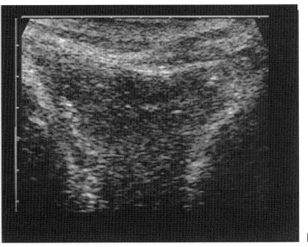

FIGURE 49–14. Contrast echography images obtained using the flash echo imaging system (harmonic imaging): (a, b) first and second frames of intermittent scanning (interval: 4s, multiple-frame scanning: three frames); (c) dual window method (interval: 1s, multiple-frame scanning: two frames); and (d) intermittent scanning (left) with monitoring. (Source: (http://www.sciencedirect.com/science?_ob=MImg&_imagekey =B6TD2–3X23SJT-9-V&_cdi=5186&_user=29261&_orig= search&_coverDate=03%2F31%2F1999&_qd=1&_sk=999749 996&view=c&wchp=dGLbVtb-zSkzS&md5=0d9ee86a23b7c 7afb707e8cfe237ce22&ie=/sdarticle.pdf. Permission requested.)

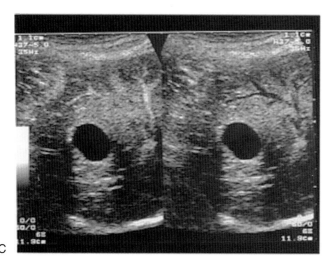

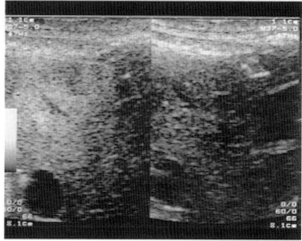

C

D

FIGURE 49–14. *Continued*

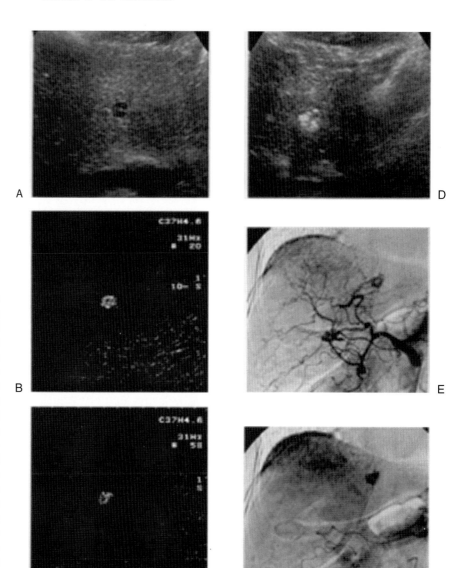

A

B

C

D

E

F

FIGURE 49–15. A 72-year-old woman with a hemangioma (diameter, 12.7mm) on the left liver. (a) Subcostal plain ultrasound (US) scan shows a hypoechoic nodule in the left lobe. (b) Digital subtraction image (DSI) of the same tumor, at 50s after the injection, shows hyperenhancement. (c) DSI of the same tumor, at 5min after the injection, shows hyperenhancement. (d) US angiography of the same tumor, at 5min after the injection, shows hyperenhancement. (e) Hepatic angiogram obtained during the arterial phase shows a hypervascular tumor. (f) Hepatic angiogram obtained during the late phase shows a hypervascular tumor. (Source: Yamamoto K, Shiraki K, Nakanishi S, *et al.* The usefulness of digital subtraction imaging with Levovist in the diagnosis of focal hepatic tumors. Int J Oncol. 2003 Feb;2(2):353–358. Image courtesy of Dr. Shiraki Katsuya.)

Common Application of Ultrasound Contrast Agents

Renovascular Assessment

There are several CEUS applications used for the evaluation of the kidney. Diagnosis of renal artery stenosis, determination of microperfusion and extent of infarcts, as well as delineation of solid or cystic masses are all applications of CEUS that are being studied. It has been shown that using contrast agents with ultrasound evaluation improved the efficacy of the scan by enhancing the operator's ability to visualize the renal arteries and by increasing the number of definitive examinations.

Although angiography has been the gold standard in the evaluation of renal artery stenosis, its invasiveness and exposure to radiation and nephrotoxic contrast agents restrict its use as a screening modality. Conventional Doppler ultrasound is routinely used for renal artery stenosis evaluation; however, studies have shown that there is great variability from center to center in its correlation to angiographic findings. In addition, obtaining technically successful examinations was shown to vary among the studies as well. Avasthi et al. reported good correlation between the studies when evaluating 52 renal arteries with both Doppler ultrasound and angiogram.[30] They reported 89% sensitivity and 73% specificity for Doppler ultrasound in detecting lesions with a greater then 50% lumen reduction. Technically adequate examinations were performed in approximately 84% of the patients. As well, Norris et al. performed successful examinations in 90% of the patients he studied, with Doppler ultrasound having a 73% sensitivity and 97% specificity when compared to angiography.[31] In contrast, Berland et al. obtained adequate examinations in only 58% of their patients, while being unable to identify any of the seven patients who had renal artery stenosis on angiogram. They reported only a 37% specificity, as patients without renal artery stenosis were detected on only 7 out of 19 ultrasound examinations.[32] Desberg et al. reported success in only 51% of ultrasound examinations.[33]

Such variability in the success of Doppler ultrasound in the evaluation of renal artery stenosis is reflective of the technical difficulty of performing an adequate examination in a wide variety of patients. Patient body habitus and variable renal artery anatomy complicate examinations as well. CEUS is proving to be the imaging modality that can overcome these limitations. Claudon et al. reported the results of a randomized crossover study of 198 patients from 14 European centers who were referred for renal arterial angiography because they were suspected of having renal arterial stenosis.[12] They reported a 63.9–83.8% increase in successful examinations when adding contrast to the ultrasound scan, including obese patients and those with renal dysfunction. When comparing Doppler ultrasound to angiography, CEUS results correlated with angiographic results in the diagnosis or exclusion of renal artery stenosis more often than conventional Doppler ultrasound ($p = 0.001$). In addition, Lacourciere et al. reported results from 78 patients involved in a Canadian multicenter controlled pilot study who were undergoing evaluation for renal artery stenosis comparing captopril-enhanced scintography and unenhanced and enhanced ultrasound.[34] Results revealed that CEUS examination yielded a diagnosis in more patients than unenhanced ultrasound or scintography—99%, 82%, and 81%, respectively ($p = 0.002$). The proportion of technically successful ultrasound examinations increased significantly with the addition of contrast.

CEUS has also been used to evaluate the microperfusion of the kidney and to define areas of ischemia or infarct. Renal perfusion has been quantified by using a high MI to destroy microbubbles, then using low MI intermittent harmonic imaging at various pulse intervals to plot pulse interval versus video intensity to derive microbubble velocity and renal blood volume fraction[35] (Figure 49–16). Wei et al. showed that measuring the rate of microbubble replenishment after destruction reflected microbubble velocity (MV). When the tissue is completely replenished with contrast, the signal reflects the tissue blood volume fraction (BVF). The product of MV and BVF correlates with tissue nutrient blood flow (NBF).[36] Total renal blood flow (RBF) is estimated by cortical MV since > 90% of total RBF supplies the renal cortex. Wei et al. showed that CEUS provides an assessment of RBF and tissue nutrient blood flow that correlates with blood flow measurements obtained with a conventional Doppler flow probe.[35] The added assessment of NBF with CEUS allows the evaluation of renal pathologies that affect NBF with little affect on RBF and vice versa. Thus, CEUS provides improved information on the perfusion pattern of the kidneys in conditions such as pyelonephritis, embolism to the kidney, and posttransplant assessment of a transplanted kidney.[37]

In addition to the imaging capabilities of CEUS, recent reports have demonstrated nonvector gene transfer into the kidney using microbubbles and ultrasound as a delivery vehicle. For example, Lan et al. studied the use of ultrasound and microbubbles to transfer a doxycycline-regulated Smad7 gene into the kidney as a potential therapy for renal fibrosis. They found that compared with nonultrasound treatment, the combination of ultrasound–microbubble-mediated delivery largely increased Smad7 transgene expression up to a 1000-fold in all kidney tissues.[38]

CEUS is now becoming both an imaging and therapeutic modality that will hopefully provide a safe, noninvasive, and easily applicable alternative in the management of renal disease.

Baseline   **Stenosis**

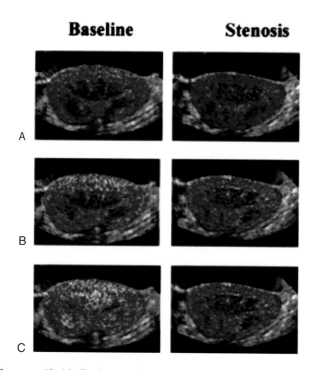

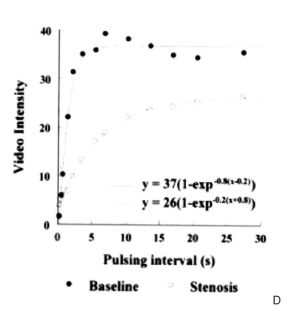

FIGURE 49–16. Background-subtracted color-coded images obtained from an animal at progressively longer pulsing intervals (A–C), at baseline and in the presence of a flow-limiting renal artery stenosis. The pulsing interval versus video intensity curves obtained from the cortex during both stages are shown in (D). The lower rate of rise of video intensity (open versus closed circles) was reflected by a significant decrease in cortical microbubble velocity from 0.8 to 0.2 s^{-1}. (Image courtesy of Dr. Kevin Wei, Oregon Health & Science University, Portland, OR.)

Echocardiography

Left ventricular cavity opacification (LVO) is clinically important in the evaluation of cardiac structure and ventricular function in resting and stress echocardiography. In the United States, contrast agents are FDA approved for ventricular opacification and enhancement of endocardial border definition. CEUS is used in those patients with a technically suboptimal echocardiogram.

Contrast has been shown to increase the diagnostic capability of echocardiograms in numerous studies. In one study with 200 patients, the patient cohort was selected on the basis of suboptimal baseline echocardiograms with nonvisualization of at least two of six segments in the apical four-chamber view. CEUS in these patients converted a nondiagnostic study to a diagnostic echocardiogram in 75% of those patients examined. This added improvement in image quality resulted in a greater ability to answer the primary referral question in as many as 50% of patients.[39] Similar findings have been observed after left ventricular (LV) opacification produced by intravenous injections of investigational contrast agents.[16,40] Administration of an intravenous contrast agent has also been shown to enable more accurate measurement of LV volume and ejection fraction in human beings.[41] It has also been demonstrated clinically that with the use of contrast agents, harmonic imaging produces improvements over fundamental imaging in LVO, endocardial border definition, and reviewer confidence in the assessment of systolic function.[11,12,17,18,30,33,34,42]

The use of contrast agents has been demonstrated in other cardiac pathologies. The diagnosis of complications of myocardial infarction, such as wall rupture and left ventricle pseudoaneurysm formation, has been facilitated by the use of contrast agents. CEUS has also been used to improve the accuracy of transesophageal echocardiography in ascending aortic dissection by discriminating true and false lumina. Intracardiac masses, such as tumors or thrombi, have been easier to identify with the use of ultrasonic contrast.

Other Applications

Plaque Assessment

The significance of inflammation in relation to plaque stability has been well established in animal models of disease. The inflammatory response includes the recruitment of monocyte-derived macrophages and leukocytes to atherosclerotic endothelium leading to plaque propagation, increased susceptibility of rupture, and vascular remodeling.[43] Identifying these inflamed, vulnerable plaques would be valuable in determining which patients would require an immediate intervention to prevent ischemic complications from a ruptured plaque.

Those microbubbles with shells composed of albumin or lipids bind to activated leukocytes in response to ischemic injury or exposure to proinflammatory mediators. The extent of leukocyte binding by these microbubbles correlates with the amount of inflammation, allowing for quantification of the extent of the inflammatory process.[18,44] The albumin and lipid shells of microbubbles bind to these activated leukocytes via different mechanisms, although they both require the upregulated expression of adhesion molecules stimulated by activated leukocytes in response to inflammation. Albumin is bound via the leukocyte β_2-integrin Mac-1 to endothelial ICAM-1, while lipid shells become coated with complement proteins that are recognized by complement receptors on the leukocyte surface.[18,19,24,44] Once the microbubble is bound to the leukocyte, it is phagocytosed

whole by neutrophils and monocytes. Within these cells, the microbubble remains capable of oscillating enough to create an echo response.[19,44]

Another strategy for the targeting of inflamed plaques is the engineering of microbubbles to incorporate ligands to extracellular adhesion molecules (ECAMs) into the encapsulating shell. Targeting of ECAMs allows for tissue-specific binding since they are expressed on the surfaces of plaques, in neovessels of plaques, and in adventitial vessels, and are absent in normal vessels[44,45] (Figure 49–17) ECAMs known to be associated with atherosclerosis include ICAM-1, vascular cell adhesion molecule (VCAM)-1, selectins, and the integrin $\alpha_v\beta_3$.[44,45]

Several investigators have exploited the expression of ECAMs to target regions of inflammation. Villaneueva et al. targeted activated endothelial cells in a flow chamber system by conjugating a monoclonal antibody to ICAM-1 on the surface of a microbubble encapsulated in a lipid shell.[46] Demos et al. employed this same strategy using acoustically active liposomes instead of microbubbles.

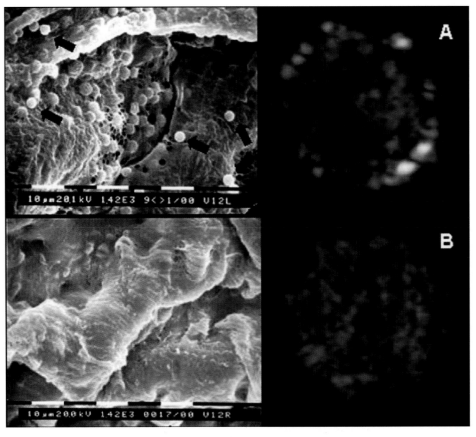

FIGURE 49–17. Ultrasound images with low mechanical index pulse sequence scheme showing the presence of microbubbles binding to the arterial endothelium in a balloon-injured carotid artery (A, right) and the absence of microbubbles in the control noninjured carotid artery (B, right). Scanning electron microscopy revealed sites of injury with endothelial denudation and attachment of microbubbles (black arrows) to the denuded endothelium only in the injured vessel (A) and normal appearing endothelium in the control vessel (B). (Image courtesy of Dr. Thomas R. Porter, The University of Nebraska Medical Center.)

They demonstrated *in vivo* targeting of these antibody-carrying liposomes to inflamed atherosclerotic plaques within the carotid arteries of pigs.[47] Linder *et al.* also used antibodies to P-selectin to target inflamed venules as a means of identifying ischemia-reperfusion injury.[18]

Yet another strategy for identifying inflamed plaques is by targeting the neovessels within their core. Angiogenesis-targeted mircobubbles have been created by attaching antibodies to α_v integrin. Leong-Poi *et al.* demonstrated the adherence of these microbubbles to arterioles, capillaries, and venules in areas of angiogenesis.[48] Currently, the feasibility of creating microbubbles to $\alpha_v\beta_3$ integrin found within the neovessels of the plaque core is being studied as a means of localizing plaque inflammation.

Mesenteric Evaluation

Bowel ischemia is a surgical condition that is often difficult to diagnose. Nonspecific symptoms and laboratory results along with the limitations of diagnostic imaging make the evaluation for bowel ischemia challenging. The gold standard, angiography, is an invasive imaging modality that is not easily performed and provides limited information on the microperfusion of the bowel wall. Its invasiveness limits its use as a screening test for bowel ischemia. Conventional Doppler ultrasound is noninvasive; however, it is limited in its ability to evaluate transmural bowel wall perfusion.

Using CEUS in the evaluation of bowel ischemia is a relatively new application being studied by investigators in Japan[42,49] (Figure 49–18). Early results, which included a study of 51 patients who had evidence of small bowel dilation on plain abdominal radiographs, were reported.

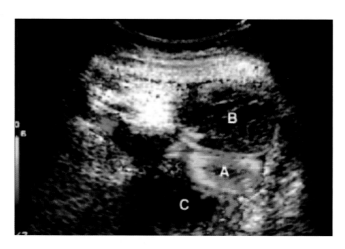

FIGURE 49–18. US scan obtained in a 68-year-old man with bowel strangulation. Bowel segments show normal (A), diminished (B), and absent (C) color signals. (Image courtesy of Dr. Jiro Hata, Department of Clinical Pathology, Kawasaki Medical School, Japan.)

All patients underwent conventional color power Doppler initially to identify the most dilated or nonperistaltic loop of bowel, and then CEUS was performed to evaluate that loop for 2 min at 4 s intervals. Twenty of the 51 patients had bowel ischemia, 5 due to thromboembolism of the superior mesenteric artery and 15 due to strangulation of the small bowel. CEUS signals were classified as normal, diminished, or absent. All 5 patients with thromboembolism were found to have absent signals. Seven of the 15 with strangulation had absent signals, 5 had diminished signals, and 3 had normal signals. All the patients without bowel ischemia had normal CEUS examinations. The sensitivity and specificity of CEUS in identifying bowel ischemia was 85% (95% CI: 62.1%, 96.8%) and 100% (95% CI: 90.8%, 100%), respectively. The positive predictive value was 100% (95% CI: 83.8%, 100%) and negative predictive value was 91.2% (95% CI: 76.3%, 98.1%).[49]

Carotid Assessment

Cerebrovascular accident continues to be a major source of morbidity and mortality in the United States, and duplex ultrasonography is considered the primary modality for screening. However, while it is readily inexpensive and accessible, its ability to discriminate the echogenicity of ulcerations and plaques and the precise degree of stenosis and to differentiate occlusion from "sting sign" stenoses is not optimal. Again, angiography is the gold standard examination, but is limited to outlining the luminal profile in finite angular projections while not truly depicting the plaque or ulceration.[50]

Recently, contrast-enhanced ultrasound was used to evaluate carotid artery disease and was compared with traditional duplex and angiography.[51] Nineteen internal carotid arteries in 10 subjects were evaluated. There was a strong correlation between CEUS and conventional angiography in determining the degree of stenosis ($r = 0.988$). Contrast ultrasound also depicted ulceration in more patients than angiography. A strong correlation was also found between CEUS and *ex vivo* magnetic resonance imaging of the carotid plaque ($r = 0.979$). These results demonstrate the potential utility of ultrasonographic agents in the screening and potential follow-up of carotid disease. Contrast avoids much of the artifact generated by color studies, and does not necessarily suffer from the angular variability found with Doppler evaluations of velocity measurement (Figure 49–19).

Aortic Evaluation

Abdominal aortic aneurysm (AAA) has undergone a paradigm shift in the way it is potentially treated with the advent of endovascular repair. However, while the benefits of the minimally invasive approach are obvious,

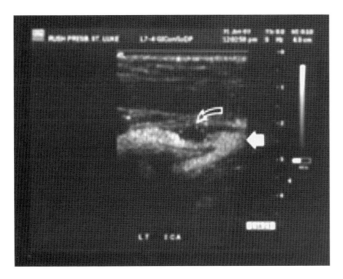

FIGURE 49–19. Contrast-enhanced carotid artery of a patient with a moderate atherosclerotic plaque in the internal carotid artery. (Image courtesy of Dr. Steven B. Feinstein, Rush University Medical Center, Chicago, IL.)

continued surveillance is required in these patients for possible complications, including continued aneurysm growth and rupture. The gold standard is computed tomography (CT), and is associated with increased cost, exposure to nephrotoxic agents, and exposure to ionizing radiation. Several recent reports have shown that contrast-enhanced ultrasound is a possible alternative as a surveillance modality.

Recently, Bendick et al. found eight endoleaks after endovascular repair, two of which were missed on CT. Napoli et al. found one type I, six type II, one type III, and two undefined leaks that were all missed by CT. Bargellini et al. found eight type II endoleaks on CEUS that were missed on CT (Figure 49–20). Our own experience with CEUS after endovascular AAA showed nine endoleaks found with contrast ultrasound, three of which were not demonstrated on CT. Ultrasonographic contrast was shown to be safe and reliable in all of these studies, and is a promising adjunct in the surveillance of AAA after endovascular repair.[52–54]

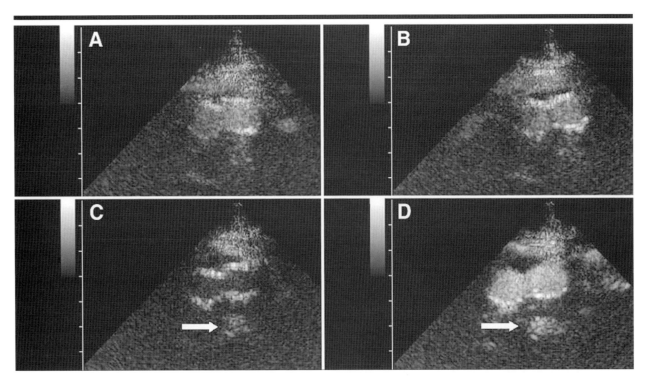

FIGURE 49–20. Transverse contrast-enhanced US scans with an anterior approach of a patient with an enlarging abdominal aortic aneurysm. Endoleak or other complications were not visualized at duplex US and CT angiography. (A–C) Images obtained after administration of an initial bolus of 2.4 ml of second-generation contrast agent show enhancement and slight contrast agent uptake 4 min after contrast agent administration. (A) Image obtained in arterial phase. (B) Image obtained in venous phase. (C) Image shows contrast agent uptake posterior to iliac branches (arrow). (D) Image obtained after administration of a second bolus of 2.4 ml of contrast agent better depicts endoleak (arrow). (Source: Napoli V, Bargellini I, Sardella SG, et al. Abdominal aortic aneurysm: contrast-enhanced US for missed endoleaks after endoluminal repair. Radiology. 2004 Oct;233(1):217–225. Image courtesy of Dr. Irene Bargellini.)

Lower Limb Evaluation

Duplex ultrasonography in the evaluation of infrainguinal arterial disease is important in the evaluation, planning, and follow-up of reconstructive efforts. However, little has been published describing the use of contrast agents as an adjunct. A 2002 European study demonstrated the use of CEUS in 14 patients, and found that all vessels that appeared occluded by the use of contrast-enhanced duplex were also occluded on angiogram. However, the ultrasound study found four cases of patent vessels that were not visualized on conventional angiography. These visualized arteries were thought to be collaterals, rather than the named vessels in question, which was a limitation in the application of CEUS in this study.[55]

Future Directions

Ongoing advances in ultrasound technology and microbubble engineering will expand applications of CEUS as a diagnostic tool as well as a therapeutic modality. As science continues to provide new insight into the body's molecular processes and into disease pathology, these new discoveries will translate into potential targets for microbubbles and improved utility of CEUS. As mentioned above, microbubbles have the ability to target areas of early inflammation. Albumin and lipid-encapsulated microbubbles bind to activated leukocytes in a nonspecific manner. Additional studies have shown the feasibility of targeting-specific imaging via attachment of antibody-coated microbubbles to endothelial adhesion molecules expressed during inflammation as well.[18,44–48]

Recently Weller et al. proposed a means of translating the basic science of target-specific microbubbles and ultrasound to the clinical setting. Their previous studies have shown the importance of microbubble antibody density in the binding of microbubbles to their intended targets.[56] Therefore, in search of a means of improving microbubble adhesion to improve the signal-to-noise ratio of the ultrasound images, Weller et al. attempted to detect inflammation via a multitargeted approach. They compared microbubbles with antibodies to both ICAM-1 and the selectin family of leukocyte adhesion molecules to those with only a single inflammatory target to show that multitargeting inflammation would increase overall microbubble adhesion strength. As well, they proposed that since microbubble binding is linearly related to the degree of inflammation, CEUS with multitargeted microbubbles will allow clinical evaluation of early inflammation before it is evident, as well as a means to monitor the progression of inflammatory plaques or peripheral vascular disease. Microbubbles with equal amounts of anti-ICAM-1 antibody and sialyl Lewis[x] (binds to selectin) were prepared and compared to those with each of them alone.[57] These microbubbles were perfused across endothelial cells activated by interleukin-1β at four different levels, demonstrating four different severities of inflammation, which was assessed by the quantitative determination of ICAM-1 expression. Weller et al. found that ICAM-1-targeted microbubbles had an adhesion strength that was linearly related to the degree of inflammation. As well, microbubble adhesion strength was improved with multitargeted microbubbles when compared to single-targeted microbubbles allowing for improved sensitivity in detecting inflammation. Weller et al. concluded that ultrasound evaluation with multitargeted microbubbles to various ECAMs may be a sensitive, noninvasive means of detecting not only the presence of inflammation, but the severity as well.

Targeting of early, middle, and late inflammatory endothelial surface antigens has the potential of being able to delineate the molecular processes involved in inflammation and determine the "stage" of the inflammatory process.

CEUS has the potential to decrease the requirements for more costly imaging studies, decrease the rate of equivocal, conventional examinations, and increase the diagnostic accuracy and confidence of ultrasound studies in general. More studies are required to fully delineate the indications for its use as a broadly applicable adjunct. Cost analysis studies are needed to justify the potential sweeping changes this modality may bring to its many diagnostic, and potentially, therapeutic applications.

References

1. Gramiak R, Shah P, Kramer DH. Ultrasound cardiography: Contrast studies in anatomy and function. Radiology 1969;92:939.
2. Gramiak R, Shah P. Echocardiography of the aortic root. Invest Radiol 1968;3:356–66.
3. Ophir J, Parker KJ. Contrast agents in diagnostic ultrasound. Ultrasound Med Biol 1989;15(4):319–33.
4. Section 6—mechanical bioeffects in the presence of gas-carrier ultrasound contrast agents. American Institute of Ultrasound in Medicine. J Ultrasound Med 2000;19(2):120–42, 154–68.
5. Correas JM, et al. Ultrasound contrast agents: Properties, principles of action, tolerance, and artifacts. Eur Radiol 2001;11(8):1316–28.
6. Correas JM, et al. Ultrasound contrast agents. Examples of blood pool agents. Acta Radiol Suppl 1997;412:101–12.
7. Blomley MJ, et al. Stimulated acoustic emission to image a late liver and spleen-specific phase of Levovist in normal volunteers and patients with and without liver disease. Ultrasound Med Biol 1999;25(9):1341–52.
8. Marelli C. Preliminary experience with NC100100, a new ultrasound contrast agent for intravenous injection. Eur Radiol 1999;9(Suppl. 3):S343–6.
9. Harvey CJ, et al. Advances in ultrasound. Clin Radiol 2002;57(3):157–77.

10. Burns PN. Harmonic imaging with ultrasound contrast agents. Clin Radiol 1996;51(Suppl. 1):50–5.

11. Tiemann K, et al. Real-time contrast echo assessment of myocardial perfusion at low emission power: First experimental and clinical results using power pulse inversion imaging. Echocardiography 1999;16(8):799–809.

12. Claudon M, et al. Renal arteries in patients at risk of renal arterial stenosis: Multicenter evaluation of the echo-enhancer SH U 508A at color and spectral Doppler US. Levovist Renal Artery Stenosis Study Group. Radiology 2000;214(3):739–46.

13. Cohen JL, et al. Improved left ventricular endocardial border delineation and opacification with OPTISON (FS069), a new echocardiographic contrast agent. Results of a phase III Multicenter Trial. J Am Coll Cardiol 1998;32(3):746–52.

14. Myreng Y, et al. Safety of the transpulmonary ultrasound contrast agent NC100100: A clinical and haemodynamic evaluation in patients with suspected or proved coronary artery disease. Heart 1999;82(3):333–5.

15. Kaps M, et al. Safety and ultrasound-enhancing potentials of a new sulfur hexafluoride-containing agent in the cerebral circulation. J Neuroimaging 1999;(3):150–4.

16. Grayburn PA, et al. Phase III multicenter trial comparing the efficacy of 2% dodecafluoropentane emulsion (EchoGen) and sonicated 5% human albumin (Albunex) as ultrasound contrast agents in patients with suboptimal echocardiograms. J Am Coll Cardiol 1998;32(1):230–6.

17. Averkiou M, et al. Ultrasound contrast imaging research. Ultrasound Q 2003;19(1):27–37.

18. Lindner JR, et al. Microbubble persistence in the microcirculation during ischemia/reperfusion and inflammation is caused by integrin- and complement-mediated adherence to activated leukocytes. Circulation 2000;101(6):668–75.

19. Lindner JR, et al. Noninvasive imaging of inflammation by ultrasound detection of phagocytosed microbubbles. Circulation 2000;102(5):531–8.

20. Unger EC, et al. In vitro studies of a new thrombus-specific ultrasound contrast agent. Am J Cardiol 1998;81(12A):58G–61G.

21. Schumann PA, et al. Targeted-microbubble binding selectively to GPIIb IIIa receptors of platelet thrombi. Invest Radiol 2002;37(11):587–93.

22. Tachibana K, Tachibana S. Albumin microbubble echo-contrast material as an enhancer for ultrasound accelerated thrombolysis. Circulation 1995;92(5):1148–50.

23. Klibanov AL. Targeted delivery of gas-filled microspheres, contrast agents for ultrasound imaging. Adv Drug Deliv Rev 1999;37(1–3):139–57.

24. Lindner JR. Evolving applications for contrast ultrasound. Am J Cardiol 2002;90(10A):72J–80J.

25. Ayida G, et al. Hysterosalpingo-contrast sonography (HyCoSy) using Echovist-200 in the outpatient investigation of infertility patients. Br J Radiol 1996;69(826):910–3.

26. Darge K, et al. Reflux in young patients: Comparison of voiding US of the bladder and retrovesical space with echo enhancement versus voiding cystourethrography for diagnosis. Radiology 1999;210(1):201–7.

27. Blomley MJ, et al. Improved imaging of liver metastases with stimulated acoustic emission in the late phase of enhancement with the US contrast agent SH U 508A: Early experience. Radiology 1999;210(2):409–16.

28. Burns PN, Hope Simpson D, Averkiou MA. Nonlinear imaging. Ultrasound Med Biol 2000;26(Suppl. 1):S19–22.

29. Simpson DH, Burns PN, Averkiou MA. Techniques for perfusion imaging with microbubble contrast agents. IEEE Trans Ultrason Ferroelectr Freq Control 2001;48(6):1483–94.

30. Avasthi PS, Voyles WF, Greene ER. Noninvasive diagnosis of renal artery stenosis by echo-Doppler velocimetry. Kidney Int 1984;25(5):824–9.

31. Norris CS, et al. Noninvasive evaluation of renal artery stenosis and renovascular resistance. Experimental and clinical studies. J Vasc Surg 1984;1(1):192–201.

32. Berland LL, et al. Renal artery stenosis: Prospective evaluation of diagnosis with color duplex US compared with angiography. Work in progress. Radiology 1990;174(2):421–3.

33. Desberg AL, et al. Renal artery stenosis: Evaluation with color Doppler flow imaging. Radiology 1990;177(3):749–53.

34. Lacourciere Y, et al. Impact of Levovist ultrasonographic contrast agent on the diagnosis and management of hypertensive patients with suspected renal artery stenosis: A Canadian multicentre pilot study. Can Assoc Radiol J 2002;53(4):219–27.

35. Wei K, et al. Quantification of renal blood flow with contrast-enhanced ultrasound. J Am Coll Cardiol 2001;37(4):1135–40.

36. Wei K, et al. Quantification of myocardial blood flow with ultrasound-induced destruction of microbubbles administered as a constant venous infusion. Circulation 1998;97(5):473–83.

37. Correas JM, et al. [Contrast-enhanced ultrasonography: Renal applications]. J Radiol 2003;84(12 Pt 2):2041–54.

38. Lan HY, et al. Inhibition of renal fibrosis by gene transfer of inducible Smad7 using ultrasound-microbubble system in rat UUO model. J Am Soc Nephrol 2003;14(6):1535–48.

39. Shaw LJ, et al. Use of an intravenous contrast agent (Optison) to enhance echocardiography: Efficacy and cost implications. Optison Multicenter Study Group. Am J Manag Care 1998;4(Spec No):SP169–76.

40. Kitzman DW, et al. Efficacy and safety of the novel ultrasound contrast agent perflutren (definity) in patients with suboptimal baseline left ventricular echocardiographic images. Am J Cardiol 2000;86(6):669–74.

41. Hundley WG, et al. Administration of an intravenous perfluorocarbon contrast agent improves echocardiographic determination of left ventricular volumes and ejection fraction: Comparison with cine magnetic resonance imaging. J Am Coll Cardiol 1998;32(5):1426–32.

42. Yoshida S, et al. Evaluation of flash echo imaging of the canine gastrointestinal tract. J Ultrasound Med 2000;19(11):751–5.

43. Ross R. Atherosclerosis—an inflammatory disease. N Engl J Med 1999;340(2):115–26.

44. Lindner JR. Detection of inflamed plaques with contrast ultrasound. Am J Cardiol 2002;90(10C):32L–35L.

45. Blankenberg S, Barbaux S, Tiret L. Adhesion molecules and atherosclerosis. Atherosclerosis 2003;170(2):191–203.

46. Villanueva FS, *et al*. Microbubbles targeted to intercellular adhesion molecule-1 bind to activated coronary artery endothelial cells. Circulation 1998;98(1):1–5.

47. Demos SM, *et al*. In vivo targeting of acoustically reflective liposomes for intravascular and transvascular ultrasonic enhancement. J Am Coll Cardiol 1999;33(3):867–75.

48. Leong-Poi H, *et al*. Noninvasive assessment of angiogenesis by ultrasound and microbubbles targeted to alpha(v)-integrins. Circulation 2003;107(3):455–60.

49. Hata J, *et al*. Evaluation of bowel ischemia with contrast-enhanced US: Initial experience. Radiology 2005;236(2):712–5.

50. Van Damme H, Vivario M. Pathologic aspects of carotid plaques: Surgical and clinical significance. Int Angiol 1993;12(4):299–311.

51. Kono Y, *et al*. Carotid arteries: Contrast-enhanced US angiography—preliminary clinical experience. Radiology 2004;230(2):561–8.

52. Bendick PJ, *et al*. Efficacy of ultrasound scan contrast agents in the noninvasive follow-up of aortic stent grafts. J Vasc Surg 2003;37(2):381–5.

53. Napoli V, *et al*. Abdominal aortic aneurysm: Contrast-enhanced US for missed endoleaks after endoluminal repair. Radiology 2004;233(1):217–25.

54. Bargellini I, *et al*. Type II lumbar endoleaks: Hemodynamic differentiation by contrast-enhanced ultrasound scanning and influence on aneurysm enlargement after endovascular aneurysm repair. J Vasc Surg 2005;41(1):10–8.

55. Ubbink DT, Legemate DA, Llull JB. Color-flow duplex scanning of the leg arteries by use of a new echo-enhancing agent. J Vasc Surg 2002;35(2):392–6.

56. Weller GE, *et al*. Modulating targeted adhesion of an ultrasound contrast agent to dysfunctional endothelium. Ann Biomed Eng 2002;30(8):1012–9.

57. Weller GE, *et al*. Targeted ultrasound contrast agents: In vitro assessment of endothelial dysfunction and multi-targeting to ICAM-1 and sialyl Lewis(x). Biotechnol Bioeng 2005;92(6):780–8.

Index

Printed in singapore